Red Book®:

2003 REPORT OF THE COMMITTEE ON INFECTIOUS DISEASES

TWENTY-SIXTH EDITION

Author: Committee on Infectious Diseases
American Academy of Pediatrics

Larry K. Pickering, MD, FAAP, Editor

Carol J. Baker, MD, FAAP, Associate Editor
Gary D. Overturf, MD, FAAP, Associate Editor
Charles G. Prober, MD, FAAP, Associate Editor

American Academy of Pediatrics
141 Northwest Point Blvd
Elk Grove Village, IL 60007-1098

Suggested Citation: American Academy of Pediatrics. [chapter title]. In: Pickering LK, ed. *Red Book: 2003 Report of the Committee on Infectious Diseases.* 26th ed. Elk Grove Village, IL: American Academy of Pediatrics; 2003:[page number]

26th Edition
1st Edition–1938
2nd Edition – 1939
3rd Edition – 1940
4th Edition – 1942
5th Edition – 1943
6th Edition – 1944
7th Edition – 1945
8th Edition – 1947
9th Edition – 1951
10th Edition – 1952
11th Edition – 1955
12th Edition – 1957
13th Edition – 1961
14th Edition – 1964
15th Edition – 1966
16th Edition – 1970
16th Edition Revised – 1971
17th Edition – 1974
18th Edition – 1977
19th Edition – 1982
20th Edition – 1986
21st Edition – 1988
22nd Edition – 1991
23rd Edition – 1994
24th Edition – 1997
25th Edition – 2000

ISSN No. 1080-0131
ISBN No. 1-58110-101-5 hardcover
        1-58110-095-7 softcover
MA0228 hardcover
MA0001-03 softcover

Quantity prices on request. Address all inquiries to:
American Academy of Pediatrics
PO Box 927, 141 Northwest Point Blvd
Elk Grove Village, IL 60009-0927

or Phone:
1-888-227-1770 Publications

The recommendations in this publication do not indicate an exclusive course of treatment or serve as a standard of medical care. Variations, taking into account individual circumstances, may be appropriate.

Committee on Infectious Diseases
2001–2003

Collaborators

On behalf of the American Academy of Pediatrics, the committee gratefully acknowledges the invaluable assistance provided by the following individuals who served as contributors and reviewers in the preparation of this edition of the *Red Book*. Their expertise, critical review, and cooperation are essential in the committee's continuing review and revisions of its recommendations for the management, control, and prevention of infectious diseases in children.

Every attempt has been made to recognize all those who contributed to this edition of the *Red Book;* the Academy regrets any omissions that may have occurred.

Mark Abramowicz, MD, *The Medical Letter,* Rochelle, NY
David G. Addiss, MD, MPH, Centers for Disease Control and Prevention, Atlanta, GA
Renata Albrecht, MD, Food and Drug Administration, Rockville, MD
John Alexander, MD, MPH, Food and Drug Administration, Rockville, MD
Lorraine Alexander, RN, MPH, Centers for Disease Control and Prevention, Atlanta, GA
Miriam J. Alter, PhD, Centers for Disease Control and Prevention, Atlanta, GA
Larry J. Anderson, MD, Centers for Disease Control and Prevention, Atlanta, GA
Lennox Archibald, MD, MRCP(UK), DTM&H, Centers for Disease Control and Prevention, Atlanta, GA
David M. Asher, MD, Food and Drug Administration, Rockville, MD
David Ashford, DVM, MPH, DSc, Centers for Disease Control and Prevention, Atlanta, GA
Chintamani D. Atreya, PhD, Food and Drug Administration, Bethesda, MD
William L. Atkinson, MD, MPH, Centers for Disease Control and Prevention, Atlanta, GA
Kassa Ayalew, MD, Food and Drug Administration, Rockville, MD
Leslie K. Ball, MD, Food and Drug Administration, Office of Human Research Protections, Health and Human Services, Rockville, MD
Margaret C. Bash, MD, Food and Drug Administration, Rockville, MD
Melisse Sloas Baylor, MD, Food and Drug Administration, Rockville, MD
Mark E. Beatty, MD, Centers for Disease Control and Prevention, Atlanta, GA
Judy Beeler, MD, Food and Drug Administration, Rockville, MD
Ermias D. Belay, MD, Centers for Disease Control and Prevention, Atlanta, GA
Beth P. Bell, MD, MPH, Centers for Disease Control and Prevention, Atlanta, GA
David Bell, MD, Centers for Disease Control and Prevention, Atlanta, GA
Stuart M. Berman, MD, ScM, Centers for Disease Control and Prevention, Atlanta, GA
Caryn Bern, MD, MPH, Centers for Disease Control and Prevention, Atlanta, GA

David I. Bernstein, MD, Cincinnati Children's Hospital Medical Center, Cincinnati, OH

Richard E. Besser, MD, Centers for Disease Control and Prevention, Atlanta, GA

Kristine M. Bisgard, DVM, MPH, Centers for Disease Control and Prevention, Atlanta, GA

David Blair, PhD, James Cook University, Townsville, Queensland, Australia

Martin Blaser, MD, Cornell University School of Medicine, Ithaca, NY

Robert Bortolussi, MD, FRCPC, Dalhousie University, Halifax, Nova Scotia, Canada

Christopher R. Braden, MD, Centers for Disease Control and Prevention, Atlanta, GA

Mary L. Brandt, MD, Baylor College of Medicine, Houston, TX

Joseph S. Bresee, MD, Centers for Disease Control and Prevention, Atlanta, GA

Marc Bulterys, MD, PhD, Centers for Disease Control and Prevention, Atlanta, GA

Jane L. Burns, MD, University of Washington, Seattle, WA

William Cameron, MD, Ottawa General Hospital, Ottawa, Ontario, Canada

Neil R. Cashman, MD, FRCP(C), University of Toronto, Toronto, Ontario, Canada

Shadi Chamany, MD, Centers for Disease Control and Prevention, Atlanta, GA

Mary E. Chamberland, MD, MPH, Centers for Disease Control and Prevention, Atlanta, GA

Robert T. Chen, MD, MA, Centers for Disease Control and Prevention, Atlanta, GA

P. Joan Chesney, MD, University of Tennessee Health Science Center, Memphis, TN

James E. Childs, ScD, Centers for Disease Control and Prevention, Atlanta, GA

Tom M. Chiller, MD, MPHTM, Centers for Disease Control and Prevention, Atlanta, GA

Ilin Chuang, MD, Centers for Disease Control and Prevention, Atlanta, GA

Thomas A. Clark, MD, Centers for Disease Control and Prevention, Atlanta, GA

Thomas G. Cleary, MD, University of Texas-Houston Health Science Center, Houston, TX

Joanne Cono, MD, Centers for Disease Control and Prevention, Atlanta, GA

Charles K. Cooper, MD, Food and Drug Administration, Rockville, MD

Ralph Cordell, PhD, Centers for Disease Control and Prevention, Atlanta, GA

Armando G. Correa, MD, Baylor College of Medicine, Houston, TX

Margaret Mary Cortese, MD, Centers for Disease Control and Prevention, Atlanta, GA

Edward M. Cox, MD, MPH, Food and Drug Administration, Rockville, MD

Robert B. Craven, MD, Centers for Disease Control and Prevention, Fort Collins, CO

John A. Crump, MB, ChB, Centers for Disease Control and Prevention, Atlanta, GA

Therese Cvetkovich, MD, Food and Drug Administration, Rockville, MD

Inger Damon, MD, PhD, Centers for Disease Control and Prevention, Atlanta, GA

Alma C. Davidson, MD, Food and Drug Administration, Rockville, MD

Jeffrey P. Davis, MD, Wisconsin Division of Public Health, Madison, WI

Dickson D. Despommier, BS, MS, PhD, Columbia University, New York, NY

Bakary S. Drammeh, DrPH, MT(ASCP), Centers for Disease Control and Prevention, Atlanta, GA

Peter Dull, MD, Centers for Disease Control and Prevention, Atlanta, GA

Eileen F. Dunne, MD, MPH, Centers for Disease Control and Prevention, Atlanta, GA

Morven S. Edwards, MD, Baylor College of Medicine, Houston, TX

Lawrence F. Eichenfield, MD, Children's Hospital San Diego-University of California, San Diego, CA

Dean Erdman, DrPH, Centers for Disease Control and Prevention, Atlanta, GA

Joseph J. Esposito, PhD, Centers for Disease Control and Prevention, Atlanta, GA

Geoffrey Evans, MD, Vaccine Injury Compensation Program, Health Resources and Services Administration, Rockville, MD

Karen M. Farizo, MD, Food and Drug Administration, Rockville, MD

Daniel R. Feikin, MD, MSPH, Centers for Disease Control and Prevention, Atlanta, GA

Stephen M. Feinstone, MD, Food and Drug Administration, Bethesda, MD

Anthony E. Fiore, MD, MPH, Centers for Disease Control and Prevention, Atlanta, GA

Patricia M. Flynn, MD, St. Jude Children's Research Hospital, Memphis, TN

Kimberley K. Fox, MD, MPH, Centers for Disease Control and Prevention, Atlanta, GA

Carl Frasch, PhD, Food and Drug Administration, Bethesda, MD

Scott K. Fridkin, MD, Centers for Disease Control and Prevention, Atlanta, GA

Keiji Fukuda, MD, MPH, Centers for Disease Control and Prevention, Atlanta, GA

D. Futterman, MD, Montefiore Medical Center at the Children's Hospital, Bronx, NY

Karin Galil, MD, MPH, Centers for Disease Control and Prevention, Atlanta, GA

William K. Gallo, Jr, Centers for Disease Control and Prevention, Atlanta, GA

Lawrence Gartner, MD, University of Chicago, Chicago, IL

Michael Gerber, MD, Cincinnati Children's Hospital Medical Center, Cincinnati, OH

Francis Gigliotti, MD, University of Rochester-School of Medicine & Dentistry, Rochester, NY

Laurence B. Givner, MD, Wake Forest University School of Medicine, Winston-Salem, NC

Karen L. Goldenthal, MD, Food and Drug Administration, Rockville, MD

Richard Gorman, MD, University of Maryland, Baltimore, MD

Rachel J. Gorwitz, MD, MPH, Centers for Disease Control and Prevention, Atlanta, GA

David P. Greenberg, MD, Children's Hospital of Pittsburgh, Pittsburgh, PA

Carolyn M. Greene, MD, Centers for Disease Control and Prevention, Atlanta, GA

Amita Gupta, MD, Centers for Disease Control and Prevention, Atlanta, GA

Rana A. Hajjeh, MD, Centers for Disease Control and Prevention, Atlanta, GA

Caroline B. Hall, MD, University of Rochester Medical Center, Rochester, NY

Edward B. Hayes, MD, Centers for Disease Control and Prevention, Fort Collins, CO

Rita F. Helfand, MD, Centers for Disease Control and Prevention, Atlanta, GA

Barbara L. Herwaldt, MD, MPH, Centers for Disease Control and Prevention, Atlanta, GA

David R. Hill, MD, University of Connecticut Health Center, Farmington, CT

Margaret K. Hostetter, MD, Yale University School of Medicine, New Haven, CT

Peter J. Hotez, MD, PhD, The George Washington University, Washington, DC

Ekopimo O. Ibia, MD, MPH, MRCP(UK), MR, Food and Drug Administration, Rockville, MD

Joseph P. Icenogle, PhD, Centers for Disease Control and Prevention, Atlanta, GA

John K. Iskander, MD, MPH, Centers for Disease Control and Prevention, Atlanta, GA

Richard F. Jacobs, MD, University of Arkansas for Medical Sciences, Little Rock, AR

William R. Jarvis, MD, Centers for Disease Control and Prevention, Atlanta, GA

John Jereb, MD, Centers for Disease Control and Prevention, Atlanta, GA

Rosemary Johann-Liang, MD, Food and Drug Administration, Rockville, MD

Robert E. Johnson, MD, MPH, Centers for Disease Control and Prevention, Atlanta, GA

M. Suzanne Johnson-DeLeon, MPH, Centers for Disease Control and Prevention, Atlanta, GA

Jeffrey L. Jones, MD, MPH, Centers for Disease Control and Prevention, Atlanta, GA

Joshua D. Jones, MD, Centers for Disease Control and Prevention, Atlanta, GA

Dennis D. Juranek, DVM, MSc, Centers for Disease Control and Prevention, Atlanta, GA

Pavani Kalluri, MD, Centers for Disease Control and Prevention, Atlanta, GA

Harry Keyserling, MD, Emory University School of Medicine, Atlanta, GA

Nino Khetsuriani, MD, PhD, Centers for Disease Control and Prevention, Atlanta, GA

Martin B. Kleiman, MD, Indiana University School of Medicine, Indianapolis, IN

Dennis J. Kopecko, PhD, Food and Drug Administration, Bethesda, MD

Emilia H. A. Koumans, MD, MPH, Centers for Disease Control and Prevention, Atlanta, GA

Philip R. Krause, MD, Food and Drug Administration, Bethesda, MD

Steven Krug, MD, Northwestern University School of Medicine, Chicago, IL

T. G. Ksiazek, DVM, PhD, Centers for Disease Control and Prevention, Atlanta, GA

Matthew J. Kuehnert, MD, Centers for Disease Control and Prevention, Atlanta, GA

Michael F. Lademarco, Centers for Disease Control and Prevention, Atlanta, GA

Nicole Le Saux, MD, FRCPC, Children's Hospital of Eastern Ontario-University of Ottawa, Ottawa, Ontario, Canada

Lucia Lee, MD, Food and Drug Administration, Bethesda, MD

Linda L. Lewis, MD, Food and Drug Administration, Bethesda, MD

Jay M. Lieberman, MD, Miller Children's Hospital, Long Beach, CA

Jairam R. Lingappa, MD, PhD, Centers for Disease Control and Prevention, Atlanta, GA

Robert W. Linkins, MPH, PhD, Centers for Disease Control and Prevention, Atlanta, GA

Mark N. Lobato, MD, Centers for Disease Control and Prevention, Atlanta, GA

Stephen P. Luby, MD, Centers for Disease Control and Prevention, Atlanta, GA
Ronald E. Lundquist, PhD, Food and Drug Administration, Rockville, MD
James H. Maguire, MD, MPH, Centers for Disease Control and Prevention,
    Atlanta, GA
Susan A. Maloney, MD, MHSc, Centers for Disease Control and Prevention,
    Atlanta, GA
Tahir H. Malik, PhD, Food and Drug Administration, Bethesda, MD
Harold S. Margolis, MD, Centers for Disease Control and Prevention, Atlanta, GA
Lewis Markoff, MD, Food and Drug Administration, Bethesda, MD
Norman Marks, Food and Drug Administration, Rockville, MD
Michael T. Martin, MD, MSc, MPH, Centers for Disease Control and Prevention,
    Atlanta, GA
Eric E. Mast, MD, MPH, Centers for Disease Control and Prevention, Atlanta, GA
Lisa L. Mathis, MD, Food and Drug Administration, Rockville, MD
Leonard W. Mayer, PhD, Centers for Disease Control and Prevention, Atlanta, GA
Anne E. McCarthy, MD, FRCPC, DTM&H, Ottawa Hospital, Ottawa,
    Ontario, Canada
Michael M. McNeil, MD, MPH, Centers for Disease Control and Prevention,
    Atlanta, GA
Jennifer H. McQuiston, DVM, MS, Centers for Disease Control and Prevention,
    Atlanta, GA
Paul Mead, MD, MPH, Centers for Disease Control and Prevention, Atlanta, GA
Michael Merchlinsky, PhD, Food and Drug Administration, Rockville, MD
Richard F. Meyer, PhD, Centers for Disease Control and Prevention, Atlanta, GA
James N. Mills, PhD, Centers for Disease Control and Prevention, Atlanta, GA
ChrisAnna Marie Mink, MD, Food and Drug Administration, Rockville, MD
Douglas K. Mitchell, MD, Eastern Virginia Medical School, Norfolk, VA
John F. Modlin, MD, Dartmouth Medical School, Lebanon, NH
Nasim Moledina, MD, Food and Drug Administration, Rockville, MD
Anne C. Moore, MD, PhD, Centers for Disease Control and Prevention,
    Atlanta, GA
Matthew R. Moore, MD, MPH, Centers for Disease Control and Prevention,
    Atlanta, GA
Gina T. Mootrey, DO, MPH, Centers for Disease Control and Prevention,
    Atlanta, GA
Juliette Morgan, MD, Centers for Disease Control and Prevention, Atlanta, GA
Jean M. Mulinde, MD, Food and Drug Administration, Rockville, MD
Trudy V. Murphy, MD, Centers for Disease Control and Prevention, Atlanta, GA
Dennis Murray, MD, Medical College of Georgia, Augusta, GA
Tippavan Nagachinta, MD, DrPH, Centers for Disease Control and Prevention,
    Atlanta, GA
Sumathi Nambiar, MD, MPH, Food and Drug Administration, Rockville, MD
James P. Nataro, MD, PhD, University of Maryland School of Medicine,
    Baltimore, MD
Stuart T. Nichol, PhD, Centers for Disease Control and Prevention, Atlanta, GA
Glen J. Nowak, PhD, Centers for Disease Control and Prevention, Atlanta, GA

Thomas B. Nutman, MD, National Institutes for Health, Bethesda, MD
Michael O'Reilly, MD, Centers for Disease Control and Prevention, Atlanta, GA
Michael Osterholm, PhD, MPH, Centers for Disease Control and Prevention,
    Atlanta, GA
Christopher D. Paddock, MD, Centers for Disease Control and Prevention,
    Atlanta, GA
Anil A. Panackal, MD, Centers for Disease Control and Prevention, Atlanta, GA
Adelisa L. Panlilio, MD, MPH, Centers for Disease Control and Prevention,
    Atlanta, GA
Mark Papania, MD, MPH, Centers for Disease Control and Prevention,
    Atlanta, GA
Monica E. Parise, MD, Centers for Disease Control and Prevention, Atlanta, GA
Andrew T. Pavia, MD, University of Utah, Salt Lake City, UT
Bradley Perkins, MD, Centers for Disease Control and Prevention, Atlanta, GA
Joseph F. Perz, DrPH, Centers for Disease Control and Prevention, Atlanta, GA
Georges Peter, MD, Brown Medical School, Providence, RI
Lyle R. Petersen, MD, MPH, Centers for Disease Control and Prevention,
    Atlanta, GA
Joseph Piesman, DSc, Centers for Disease Control and Prevention, Fort Collins, CO
Janice K. Pohlman, MD, Food and Drug Administration, Rockville, MD
Jean Popiak, MHA, Centers for Disease Control and Prevention, Atlanta, GA
Tanja Popovic, MD, PhD, Centers for Disease Control and Prevention, Atlanta, GA
Linda Quick, MD, Centers for Disease Control and Prevention, Atlanta, GA
Rob Quick, MD, MPH, Centers for Disease Control and Prevention, Atlanta, GA
Conrad Quinn, PhD, Centers for Disease Control and Prevention, Atlanta, GA
Pratima L. Raghunathan, PhD, MPH, Centers for Disease Control and Prevention,
    Atlanta, GA
Mobeen H. Rathore, MD, University of Florida Health Science Center,
    Jacksonville, FL
Susan Reef, MD, Centers for Disease Control and Prevention, Atlanta, GA
Megan E. Reller, MDCM, Centers for Disease Control and Prevention, Atlanta, GA
Mary G. Reynolds, PhD, MS, Centers for Disease Control and Prevention,
    Atlanta, GA
Frank O. Richards, Jr, MD, Centers for Disease Control and Prevention,
    Atlanta, GA
Rosemary Roberts, MD, Food and Drug Administration, Rockville, MD
Lance Rodewald, MD, Centers for Disease Control and Prevention, Atlanta, GA
William J. Rodriguez, MD, PhD, Food and Drug Administration, Rockville, MD
Patricia J. Rohan, MD, Food and Drug Administration, Rockville, MD
Pierre Rollin, MD, Centers for Disease Control and Prevention, Atlanta, GA
Martha Roper, MD, MPH, Centers for Disease Control and Prevention, Atlanta, GA
James P. Rosen, MD, University of Connecticut Medical School, West Hartford, CT
Nancy E. Rosenstein, MD, Centers for Disease Control and Prevention, Atlanta, GA
Lawrence A. Ross, MD, University of Southern California, Los Angeles, CA
Lorry Rubin, MD, Schneider Children's Hospital, New Hyde Park, NY
Steven A. Rubin, MS, Food and Drug Administration, Bethesda, MD

Charles E. Rupprecht, VMD, MS, PhD, Centers for Disease Control and
    Prevention, Atlanta, GA
Gary Sanden, BS, MS, PhD, Centers for Disease Control and Prevention,
    Atlanta, GA
Jeanne M. Santoli, MD, MPH, Centers for Disease Control and Prevention,
    Atlanta, GA
Lawrence A. Schachner, MD, University of Miami School of Medicine, Miami, FL
Richard J. Schanler, MD, Baylor College of Medicine, Houston, TX
Peter M. Schantz, VMD, PhD, Centers for Disease Control and Prevention,
    Atlanta, GA
Donald Scott Schmid, PhD, Centers for Disease Control and Prevention,
    Atlanta, GA
Lawrence B. Schonberger, MD, MPH, Centers for Disease Control and Prevention,
    Atlanta, GA
Gordon G. Schutze, MD, University of Arkansas for Medical Sciences,
    Little Rock, AR
Benjamin Schwartz, MD, Centers for Disease Control and Prevention, Atlanta, GA
James Sejvar, MD, Centers for Disease Control and Prevention, Atlanta, GA
Jane F. Seward, MBBS, MPH, Centers for Disease Control and Prevention,
    Atlanta, GA
Andi L. Shane, MD, MPH, Centers for Disease Control and Prevention,
    Atlanta, GA
Eugene D. Shapiro, MD, Yale University School of Medicine, New Haven, CT
Colin W. Shepard, MD, Centers for Disease Control and Prevention, Atlanta, GA
Mary E. Sheperd, MDCM, Centers for Disease Control and Prevention,
    Atlanta, GA
Thomas D. Smith, MD, Food and Drug Administration, Rockville, MD
Robert H. Snyder, MA, Centers for Disease Control and Prevention, Atlanta, GA
Jeremy Sobel, MD, MPH, Centers for Disease Control and Prevention, Atlanta, GA
Padmini Srikantiah, MD, Centers for Disease Control and Prevention, Atlanta, GA
Joseph W. St. Geme III, MD, Washington University School of Medicine,
    St. Louis, MO
Mary Allen Staat, MD, MPH, Children's Hospital Medical Center, Cincinnati, OH
David S. Stephens, MD, Centers for Disease Control and Prevention, Atlanta, GA
John A. Stewart, MD, Centers for Disease Control and Prevention, Atlanta, GA
Paul C. Stillwell, MD, Phoenix Children's Hospital, Phoenix, AZ
Peter M. Strebel, MBChB, MPH, Centers for Disease Control and Prevention,
    Atlanta, GA
Raymond Strikas, MD, Centers for Disease Control and Prevention, Atlanta, GA
Kanta Subbarao, MBBS, MPH, Centers for Disease Control and Prevention,
    Atlanta, GA
Madeline Y. Sutton, MD, MPH, Centers for Disease Control and Prevention,
    Atlanta, GA
Robert V. Tauxe, MD, MPH, Centers for Disease Control and Prevention,
    Atlanta, GA
Susan D. Thompson, MD, Food and Drug Administration, Rockville, MD

Rosemary Tiernan, MD, MPH, Food and Drug Administration, Rockville, MD
James Todd, MD, The Children's Hospital, Denver, CO
Elizabeth R. Unger, PhD, MD, Centers for Disease Control and Prevention, Atlanta, GA
Timothy M. Uyeki, MD, MPH, Centers for Disease Control and Prevention, Atlanta, GA
Chris A. Van Beneden, MD, MPH, Centers for Disease Control and Prevention, Atlanta, GA
Jay Varma, MD, Centers for Disease Control and Prevention, Atlanta, GA
Govinda S. Visvesvara, PhD, Centers for Disease Control and Prevention, Atlanta, GA
Ellen R. Wald, MD, University of Pittsburgh School of Medicine, Pittsburgh, PA
Gregory Wallace, MD, MPH, Centers for Disease Control and Prevention, Atlanta, GA
Richard J. Wallace, MD, University of Texas Health Center, Tyler, TX
E. Wang, MDCM, MSc, FRCP(c), Aventis Pasteur Limited, Toronto, Ontario, Canada
David W. Warnock, PhD, Centers for Disease Control and Prevention, Atlanta, GA
Bruce G. Weniger, MD, Centers for Disease Control and Prevention, Atlanta, GA
Melinda Wharton, MD, Centers for Disease Control and Prevention, Atlanta, GA
A. Clinton White Jr, MD, Baylor College of Medicine, Houston, TX
Cynthia G. Whitney, MD, MPH, Centers for Disease Control and Prevention, Atlanta, GA
Ellen A. S. Whitney, MPH, Centers for Disease Control and Prevention, Atlanta, GA
Robert A. Wood, MD, Johns Hopkins University School of Medicine, Baltimore, MD
Kimberly A. Workowski, MD, Centers for Disease Control and Prevention, Atlanta, GA
Fujie Xu, MD, PhD, Centers for Disease Control and Prevention, Atlanta, GA
Kevin Yeskey, MD, Centers for Disease Control and Prevention, Atlanta, GA
Edward J. Young, MD, Baylor College of Medicine, Houston, TX
Hussain Yusuf, MBBS, MPH, Centers for Disease Control and Prevention, Atlanta, GA
Sherif Zaki, MD, PhD, Centers for Disease Control and Prevention, Atlanta, GA

Committee on Infectious Diseases, 2001–2003

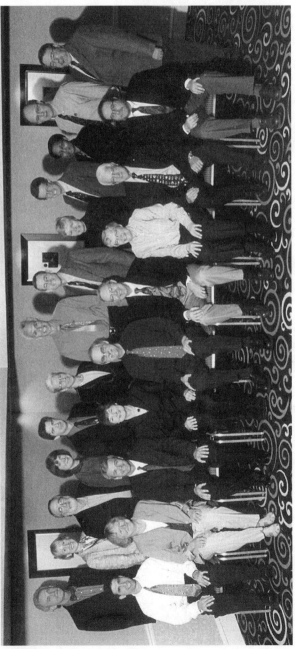

Front row: Marc A. Fischer, Modena E. H. Wilson, Charles G. Prober, Carol J. Baker, Larry K. Pickering, Gary D. Overturf, Margaret C. Fisher, Edgar O. Ledbetter, Robert S. Baltimore

Second row: Keith R. Powell, Trudy V. Murphy, Leonard B. Weiner, Julia A. McMillan, Douglas R. Pratt, Margaret B. Rennels, Jon S. Abramson, H. Cody Meissner, Joanne Embree, Lance Chilton, Mamodikoe Makhene, Jeffrey R. Starke, Thomas N. Saari

Not pictured: Joseph A. Bocchini; Scott F. Dowell, Bruce G. Gellin, Michael Gerber, Sarah S. Long, Martin C. Mahoney, Dennis L. Murray, Martin G. Myers, Katherine L. O'Brien, Walter A. Orenstein, Peter A. Patriarca, Jack Swanson, Richard J. Whitley

Dedication

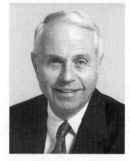

This edition of the *Red Book* is dedicated to Georges Peter, MD, FAAP, who served on the Committee on Infectious Diseases for 21 years and as editor of 5 editions (20th–24th) of the *Red Book* (1986–1997). During his time on the COID, Georges worked with 8 COID chairpersons and many associate editors, providing consistency and institutional memory, not only to the *Red Book* but also to the many issues that are considered by the COID. Georges accomplished this while fulfilling his full-time faculty responsibilities in the Department of Pediatrics at Brown University School of Medicine and Rhode Island Hospital.

The first edition of the *Red Book* that Georges edited in 1986 contained more than 500 pages. This edition was the first in which material was divided into 5 major sections that have constituted the structure of the *Red Book* since then. During the span of Georges' 5 *Red Book* editions, the field of pediatrics as it relates to infectious diseases and immunization underwent many changes, which Georges ensured were included in each edition. Changes during this time consisted of newly recognized diseases or clinical syndromes, rapid methods of diagnosis, recent therapies, and many advances in prevention, particularly in the area of immunization. The structural changes that Georges introduced allowed for easier access to information, and the content changes enabled health care professionals to have access to the most current information.

A major reason that Georges was able to be so successful in his *Red Book* endeavors was Carolyn Peter, his wife of 39 years. Carolyn's continued support, encouragement, and patience formed the underpinning of Georges' success. Carolyn has repeatedly said that Georges is "a man of passionate interests." Second to Carolyn, the *Red Book* was Georges' major passion, a passion that has benefited all of us. Thank you, Georges, we are eternally grateful and are honored to dedicate the 26th edition of the *Red Book* to you.

Preface

The Committee on Infectious Diseases is dedicated to providing practitioners with the most current and accurate information available. Because the practice of pediatric infectious diseases is changing rapidly and because of the emergence of new infectious diseases, the ability to obtain information quickly is paramount. Although the *Red Book* is updated every 3 years, it is important that practitioners who care for children periodically visit the AAP Web site (www.aap.org) and the new Red Book Online Web site (www.aapredbook.org), where interim updates will be provided.

The Committee on Infectious Diseases relies on information and advice from many experts as evidenced by the lengthy list of contributors. We are especially indebted to the many contributors from other AAP committees, the Centers for Disease Control and Prevention, the Food and Drug Administration, the National Institutes of Health, the Canadian Paediatric Society, the World Health Organization, and many other organizations that have made this edition possible. In addition, many suggestions made by individual AAP members to improve the presentation of information on specific issues have been taken into account under the able leadership of Larry K. Pickering, MD, editor, and associate editors Carol J. Baker, MD, Gary D. Overturf, MD, and Charles G. Prober, MD. We also are indebted to Edgar O. Ledbetter, MD, who spent many hours gathering the slide materials that are part of the electronic version of the *Red Book* and provided other invaluable assistance with this edition.

As noted in previous editions of the *Red Book,* some omissions and errors are inevitable in a book of this type. We hope that AAP members will continue to assist the committee actively by suggesting specific ways to improve the quality of future editions.

Jon S. Abramson, MD, FAAP
Chairperson, Committee on Infectious Diseases

Introduction

The Committee on Infectious Diseases (COID) of the American Academy of Pediatrics (AAP) is responsible for developing and revising guidelines of the AAP for control of infectious diseases in children. At intervals of approximately 3 years, the committee issues the *Red Book: Report of the Committee on Infectious Diseases,* which contains a composite summary of current AAP recommendations concerning infectious diseases in and immunizations for infants, children, and adolescents. These recommendations represent a consensus of opinions developed by members of the committee in conjunction with liaison representatives from the Centers for Disease Control and Prevention (CDC), the Food and Drug Administration (FDA), the National Institutes of Health, the National Vaccine Program, the Canadian Paediatric Society, *Red Book* consultants, and numerous collaborators. This edition is based on information available as of January 2003.

Unanswered scientific questions, the complexity of medical practice, the explosion of new information, and inevitable differences of opinion among experts result in inherent limitations of the *Red Book.* In the context of these limitations, the committee endeavors to provide current, relevant, and defensible recommendations for the prevention and management of infectious diseases in infants, children, and adolescents. In some cases, other committees and experts may differ in their interpretation of data and resulting recommendations. In some instances, no single recommendation can be made because several options for management are equally acceptable.

In making recommendations in the *Red Book,* the committee acknowledges these differences in viewpoints by use of the phrases "most experts recommend…" and "some experts recommend…" Both phrases indicate valid recommendations, but the first signifies more support among experts, and the second, less support. Hence "some experts recommend…" indicates a minority view that is based on data and/or experience and is sufficiently valid to warrant consideration.

Inevitably in clinical practice, questions arise that cannot be answered on the basis of currently available data. In such cases, the committee attempts to provide guidelines and information that in conjunction with clinical judgment will facilitate well-reasoned decisions. We appreciate the questions, different perspectives, and alternative recommendations that we have received and encourage any suggestions or correspondence that will improve future editions of the *Red Book.* Through this process, the committee seeks to provide a practical and authoritative guide for physicians and other health care professionals in their care of children.

To aid physicians and other health care professionals in assimilating current changes in the recommendations in the *Red Book,* a list of major changes has been compiled (see Summary of Major Changes, p xxv). However, this listing does not include many changes of lesser importance, and health care professionals should consult individual chapters and sections of the book for further guidelines. In addition, new information inevitably begins to outdate some recommendations in the *Red Book* and necessitates that health care professionals remain informed of new developments and resulting changes in recommendations. Between editions, the AAP publishes new recommendations from the committee in *Pediatrics,* in *AAP News,* and on the AAP Web site (www.aap.org). In this edition, we have provided Web site addresses throughout the text to enable early access to new information.

When using antimicrobial agents, physicians should review the package inserts (product labels) prepared by manufacturers, particularly for information concerning contraindications and adverse events. No attempt has been made in the *Red Book* to provide this information, because it is readily available in the *Physicians' Desk Reference,* online (http://pdrel.thomsonhc.com/pdrel/librarian/action/command. Command), and in package inserts (product labels). As in previous editions, recommended dosage schedules for antimicrobial agents are given (see Section 4, Antimicrobial Agents and Related Therapy). Recommendations in the *Red Book* for drug dosages may differ from those of the manufacturer in the package insert. Physicians also should be familiar with information in the package insert for vaccines and immune globulins as well as recommendations of other committees (see Sources of Vaccine Information, p 2).

This book could not have been prepared without the dedicated professional competence of Edgar O. Ledbetter, MD, who served as the reviewer appointed by the AAP Board of Directors, and Modena E. H. Wilson, MD, MPH, director of the Department of Committees and Sections, who provided valuable suggestions and support. The AAP staff has been outstanding in its committed work and contributions, particularly Martha Cook, manager, who served as the administrative director for the committee and coordinated the preparation of the *Red Book;* Jennifer Pane, senior medical copy editor; Darlene Mattefs, department assistant; Barbara Drelicharz, division assistant; and Peg Mulcahy, graphic designer. Special thanks are given to Tanya Lennon, assistant to the editor, for her work, patience, and support, and to Mimi for her constant encouragement. Marc Fischer, MD, and Douglas Pratt, MD, of the CDC and FDA, respectively, devoted an immense amount of time and effort in providing input from their organizations. I am especially indebted to the associate editors, Carol J. Baker, MD, Gary D. Overturf, MD, and Charles G. Prober, MD, for their expertise, tireless work, and immense contributions in their editorial and committee work. Georges Peter, MD, and Walter A. Orenstein, MD, provided constant support and advice. Members of the committee contributed countless hours and deserve appropriate recognition for their dedication, revisions, and reviews. As a committee, we particularly appreciate the guidance and dedication of our committee Chairperson, Jon Abramson, MD, whose knowledge, dedication, insight, and leadership are reflected in the quality and productivity of the committee's work.

These individuals are only a few of the many contributors whose professional work and commitment have been essential in the committee's preparation of the *Red Book.*

Larry K. Pickering, MD
Editor

Table of Contents

SECTION 2
RECOMMENDATIONS FOR CARE OF CHILDREN
IN SPECIAL CIRCUMSTANCES

SECTION 4
ANTIMICROBIAL AGENTS AND RELATED THERAPY

SECTION 5
ANTIMICROBIAL PROPHYLAXIS

Summary of Major Changes in the 2003 *Red Book*

Several changes in the 2003 *Red Book* affect all sections of this edition. Side bar indicators have been added to facilitate easy access to the specific sections; an expanded number of Web site addresses and references to recommendations of the Committee on Infectious Diseases (COID), Committee on Pediatric AIDS, and other committees of the American Academy of Pediatrics (AAP) as well as the Advisory Committee on Immunization Practices (ACIP) of the Centers for Disease Control and Prevention (CDC) have been included; and for all tables, footnote designators have been changed from symbols to numbers for easier reference. Terms have been updated and standardized throughout the *Red Book,* including changing *hand washing* to *hand hygiene, adverse reactions* to *adverse events,* Mantoux and *PPD (purified protein derivative)* to *tuberculin skin test, nosocomial* to *health care-associated, hepatitis B carrier* to *chronic hepatitis B virus infection;* and *strict isolation precautions* to specific terms (*contact precautions, droplet precautions,* and *airborne precautions*). Several name changes of organisms have been incorporated throughout the book, including:

* *Pneumocystis carinii* to *Pneumocystis jiroveci*
* Tinea versicolor to Pityriasis versicolor
* Norwalk virus to norovirus
* *Ehrlichia phagocytophila* to *Anaplasma phagocytophila*
* *Chlamydia (Chlamydophila) pneumoniae*
* *Chlamydia (Chlamydophila) psittaci*

SECTION 1. ACTIVE AND PASSIVE IMMUNIZATION

1. **Prologue.** Table 1.1 was updated to include the 2001 morbidity and percentage decrease for 9 diseases with vaccines recommended before 1990 for universal use in children in the United States.
2. **Sources of Vaccine Information.** The number of sources is expanded, and Web site addresses are provided for most sources.
3. **Vaccines Produced and/or Licensed in the United States.** Table 1.3 (p 8) lists vaccines produced and/or licensed in the United States and includes a Web site for the US Food and Drug Administration that is updated regularly. Additions since 2000 include hepatitis A-hepatitis B combination vaccine, conjugated pneumococcal vaccine, another diphtheria and tetanus toxoids and acellular pertussis (DTaP) preparation, a DTaP-inactivated poliovirus-hepatitis B combined vaccine, and smallpox vaccine. Several vaccines that no longer are available in the United States have been removed from the table.
4. **Vaccine Handling and Storage.** Information on appropriate handling and storage of all vaccines (Table 1.4, p 11) is updated.

5. **Needle Length.** Recommendations were altered to be consistent with ACIP recommendations and modified for use in preterm infants who have a small muscle mass (pp 18–19).

6. **Immunization Scheduler.** A Web link to an immunization scheduler for parents, physicians, and other health care professionals is provided (p 22).

7. **Scheduling Immunizations.** The 2003 schedule (Figure 1.1, p 24) for recommended childhood and adolescent immunizations is given, and the name of the figure is changed to "Childhood and Adolescent Immunization Schedule." A Web link to the new adult immunization schedule is provided.

8. **Catch-up Immunization Schedules for Children and Adolescents Who Start Late or Who Are >1 Month Behind** have been reformatted for easier use (Table 1.6, p 26).

9. **2003 Standards for Child and Adolescent Immunization Practices** (p 50) has been added (also see Appendix II, p 795).

10. **Internet Resources for Immunization Information.** Twenty-eight resources for information including Web sites have been added (p 52).

11. **Preterm and Low Birth Weight Infants** (p 66) is updated to include recommendations in the AAP statement titled "Immunization of Preterm and Low Birth Weight Infants."

12. **Required or Recommended Travel-Related Immunizations** (p 95). Adverse events associated with yellow fever vaccine have been added (also see Arboviruses, p 199).

13. **New Chapters, Sections, and Tables:**
    - Guidelines for Spacing Live and Inactivated Antigens (Table 1.5, p 23)
    - Minimum Ages and Minimum Intervals Between Vaccine Doses (Table 1.7, p 29)
    - Vaccine Shortages (p 37)
    - Institute of Medicine Immunization Safety Review Committee (p 38)
    - The Brighton Collaboration (p 40)
    - Clinical Immunization Safety Assessment Network (CISA) (p 41)
    - Vaccine Identification Standards Initiative (VISI) (p 43)
    - American Indian/Alaska Native Children (p 84)

SECTION 2. RECOMMENDATIONS FOR CARE OF CHILDREN IN SPECIAL CIRCUMSTANCES

14. **Biological Terrorism.** This chapter has been revised to include only biological agents, with update of the existing 2 tables and addition of Table 2.3 (p 105), which provides emergency contact and educational information.

15. **Blood Safety** (p 106) has been updated to include current information on blood screening measures, potential transfusion-transmitted agents, and improvements in blood safety.

16. **Human Milk** (p 117). This chapter has been revised to include the current recommendations from the AAP statement on breastfeeding and the use of human milk.

17. **Children in Out-of-Home Child Care** (p 123). This chapter has been revised to include the AAP/American Public Health Association National Health and Safety Performance Standards.

18. **Infection Control for Hospitalized Childre**n (p 146) and **Infection Control in Physicians' Offices** (p 155) provide hand hygiene recommendations from the HICPAC/SHEA/APIC/ADSA Hand Hygiene Task Force, including efficacy of alcohol-based hand rubs.

19. **Sexually Transmitted Diseases in Adolescents and Children** (p 157). This chapter has undergone extensive revision to include the 2002 CDC sexually transmitted diseases treatment guidelines. Chapters dealing with specific organisms associated with sexually transmitted diseases also have been updated.

20. **Medical Evaluation of Internationally Adopted Children.** This chapter has been updated to provide guidelines for evaluation of immunization status of internationally adopted children. Table 2.17 (p 175) has been expanded and Table 2.18 (p 179) has been added.

21. **New Section:**
   - Hepatitis and Youth in Corrections Settings (p 167) consolidates old and new recommendations for preventing and controlling infections with hepatitis viruses in corrections settings.

SECTION 3. SUMMARIES OF INFECTIOUS DISEASES

22. **Anthrax** (p 196). This chapter has been updated to include revised treatment and prevention options highlighting the potential use of this organism as a bioterrorist agent.

23. **Arboviruses** (p 199). The chapter has been restructured, and information about West Nile virus has been expanded. Current information about the yellow fever vaccine has been added.

24. **Bacterial Vaginosis** (p 214). Diagnosis and treatment options have been updated to be consistent with the 2002 CDC sexually transmitted diseases treatment guidelines.

25. *Chlamydia trachomatis* (p 238). An update on laboratory diagnostic tests for *C trachomatis* is included.

26. **Cryptosporidiosis** (p 255). Nitazoxanide has been licensed for treatment of children with cryptosporidiosis and giardiasis.

27. **Cytomegalovirus Infections** (p 259). Treatment of cytomegalovirus infection has been updated.

28. **Gonococcal Infections** (p 285). Update on laboratory screening methods to detect *Neisseria gonorrhoeae* is included, and recommendations for treatment are consistent with the 2002 CDC sexually transmitted diseases treatment guidelines.

29. *Helicobacer pylori* **Infections** (p 304). Seven-day therapy including rabeprazole has been added.

30. **Hepatitis A** (p 309). Table 3.15 (p 314) has been updated to include the hepatitis A-hepatitis B combination vaccine.

31. **Hepatitis B** (p 318). Information about new vaccine combinations (hepatitis A-hepatitis B and DTaP-hepatitis B-IPV) is included. Table 3.17 (p 325) has been updated to include all vaccines that contain hepatitis B. Table 3.18 (p 328), which summarizes hepatitis B immunoprophylaxis for preterm and low birth weight infants, has been added.

32. **Hepatitis C** (p 336). Laboratory testing and therapy for hepatitis C virus infection have been updated.

33. **Human Immunodeficiency Virus Infection** (p 360). Recommendations for prevention of opportunistic infections in children with human immunodeficiency virus (HIV) infection and acquired immunodeficiency syndrome have been revised in accordance with the 2002 US Public Health Service/Infectious Diseases Society of America guidelines for prevention of opportunistic infections among HIV-infected persons. Recommendations for using antiretroviral agents among adolescents has been revised according to the 2002 CDC guidelines for using antiretroviral agents among HIV infected adults and adolescents. Web sites where current drugs and treatment recommendations can be found have been added, and the tables in Section 4 showing characteristics of antiretroviral drugs have been updated.

34. **Influenza** (p 382). Updates are provided on the virus, protective immunity, disease burden in children, diagnostic assays, and vaccines. Table 3.29 (p 385) has been added to summarize various aspects of antiviral drugs. Dosages for therapy or prevention of influenza with antiviral drugs has been moved to the Antiviral Drugs for Non-Human Immunodeficiency Virus Infections table in Section 4 (p 729).

35. **Kawasaki syndrome** (p 392). Reference to Kawasaki disease has been changed to Kawasaki syndrome, and a paragraph on incomplete cases has been added.

36. **Malaria** (p 414). Updates on malaria-endemic areas, location of resistant strains, and recommended therapy and prophylaxis are given.

37. **Meningococcal Infections** (p 430). Prophylactic antimicrobial therapy, college requirements for immunization, and air travel as a risk factor have been added. The reimmunization section has been updated.

38. **Human Papillomavirus** (p 448). Section on clinical manifestations attributable to human papillomaviruses has been expanded. Diagnosis and therapy have been updated and are consistent with the 2002 CDC sexually transmitted diseases treatment guidelines.

39. **Parainfluenza Viral Infections** (p 454). The epidemiology and diagnostic tests sections of this chapter have been revised.

40. **Parasitic Diseases** (p 456). Raccoon roundworm *(Baylisascaris procyonis)* has been added to Table 3.38 (p 457).

41. **Parvovirus B19** (p 459). Table 3.39 (p 460), showing clinical manifestations of human parvovirus B19 infection, has been added.

42. **Pediculosis Capitis** (p 463). This chapter includes information contained in the AAP clinical report on head lice.

43. **Pelvic Inflammatory Disease** (p 468). Recommendations for treatment of pelvic inflammatory disease have been updated to be consistent with the 2002 CDC sexually transmitted diseases treatment guidelines.

44. **Pertussis** (p 472). The list of DTaP vaccine products has been updated to include all FDA-licensed preparations (Table 3.42, p 477). The use of DTaP-hepatitis B-IPV combination vaccine is included.

45. **Pneumococcal Infections** (p 490). Information showing susceptibility to penicillin, cefotaxime, and ceftriaxone has been added. Table 3.43 (p 492), showing children at high and moderate risk of invasive pneumococcal disease, and Tables 3.46 (p 497) and 3.47 (p 498), providing recommendations for immunization with PCV7, are included.

46. *Pneumocystis jiroveci* (p 500). The name *Pneumocystis carinii* has been changed to *P jiroveci,* although the term PCP will continue to be used for *Pneumocystis* pneumonia. Recommendations concerning therapy and prevention have been updated and are consistent with the 2002 US Public Health Service/Infectious Diseases Society of America guidelines for prevention of opportunistic infections among HIV-infected persons.

47. Q Fever (p 512). Diagnostic criteria required to confirm a case of Q fever have been added.

48. Respiratory Syncytial Virus (p 523). Recommendations for use of palivizumab in 32- to 35-week-old infants have been clarified, and recommendations for infants and young children with hemodynamically significant congenital heart disease have been added to be consistent with the AAP statement on respiratory syncytial virus infection.

49. Rubella (p 536). The recommended time to wait to become pregnant after rubella immunization has been decreased from 3 months to 28 days.

50. *Salmonella* Infections (p 541). Table 3.52 (p 543), showing the nomenclature for *Salmonella* organisms, is included. The only typhoid vaccine available in the United States for children 6 months to 2 years of age no longer is manufactured (Table 3.53, p 546).

51. Staphylococcal Infections (p 561). Information about vancomycin-resistant *Staphylococcus aureus* has been added. Antimicrobial therapy for bacteremia and other serious *S aureus* infections has been updated (Table 3.55, p 568).

52. Group B Streptococcal Infections (p 584). Recommendations for prevention of perinatal group B streptococcal disease have been updated and are consistent with the 2002 CDC guidelines for prevention of group B streptococcal disease.

53. Non-Group A or B Streptococcal and Enterococcal Infectious (p 591). This chapter has been updated to reflect current nomenclature, clinical manifestations, diagnosis, and therapy.

54. Syphilis (p 595). Table 3.60 (p 604) shows the recommended therapy for syphilis and is consistent with the 2002 CDC sexually transmitted diseases treatment guidelines.

55. Tetanus (p 611). The total number of doses of diphtheria and tetanus toxoids has been changed from "should not exceed 6 before the fourth birthday" to "should not exceed 6 before the seventh birthday."

56. Tuberculosis (p 642). This chapter has been updated to be consistent with the ATS/CDC tuberculosis statement.

57. Diseases Caused by Nontuberculous Mycobacteria (p 661). This chapter has been updated to include current clinical syndromes and their causes, diagnosis, and treatment.

58. New chapters and tables:
- Table 3.4 (p 267) shows human ehrlichiosis by disease, causative agent, vector, and geographic distribution in the United States.
- *Kingella kingae* Infections (p 396)
- Smallpox (p 554)

SECTION 4. ANTIMICROBIAL AGENTS AND RELATED THERAPY

59. The following have been updated:
- Tables of Antibacterial Drug Dosages (Tables 4.1 and 4.2, pp 700–712)
- Sexually Transmitted Diseases (Table 4.3, pp 713–718). This table includes recommendations from the 2002 CDC sexually transmitted diseases treatment guidelines.
- Antifungal Drugs for System Fungal Infections (pp 719–721): caspofungin and voriconazole have been added.
- Antiviral Drugs for Non-Human Immunodeficiency Virus Infections (Table 4.8, pp 729–732).
- Tables 4.13 and 4.14 (pp 744–770), Drugs for Parasitic Infections, reflect the 2002 *Medical Letter on Drugs and Therapeutics* recommendations.

60. Antiretroviral Therapy
- Tables listing nucleoside/nucleotide reverse transcriptase inhibitors (Table 4.9, pp 733–735), nonnucleoside reverse transcriptase inhibitors (Table 4.10, pp 736–737), and protease inhibitors (Table 4.11, pp 738-740) have been updated and simplified.
- The table listing considerations for changing antiretroviral therapy has been deleted.
- Table 4.12 (pp 741–743), showing common class adverse events and drug interactions, has been added.

APPENDICES

61. Appendix I. Directory of Services (p 789) has been updated to include current contact information.

62. Appendix II. Standards for Child and Adolescent Immunization Practices (p 795) has been updated to be consistent with the 2003 Standards.

63. Appendix III. Guide to Contraindications and Precautions to Immunizations, 2003 (p 798) is a separate table that has been updated to include hepatitis A, influenza, and pneumococcal vaccines. Latex allergy as a general precaution is added, immunodeficient household contacts and breastfeeding are added under not a contraindication, and administration guidelines for measles-mumps-rubella vaccine and tuberculin skin testing are clarified.

64. Appendix IV. National Vaccine Injury Act Reporting and Compensation Table (p 802) has been updated.

65. Appendix VII. Prevention of Disease From Potentially Contaminated Food Products (p 814). Information describing food irradiation and shiga-toxin producing *Escherichia coli* infections has been added.

66. Appendix IX. Nationally Notifiable Infectious Diseases in the United States (p 822) now includes Powassan and West Nile virus encephalitis, shiga-toxin producing *E coli*, non-O157:H7 *E coli*, giardiasis, listeriosis, Q fever, *Streptococcus pneumoniae*, invasive diseases in children 5 years of age or younger, and tularemia.

OTHER: SARS

67. Information about severe acute respiratory syndrome (SARS) is not included but may be found at www.cdc.gov/ or www.who.int/en/.

Active and Passive Immunization

••••••••••••••••••••

PROLOGUE

The ultimate goal of immunization is eradication of disease; the immediate goal is prevention of disease in individuals or groups. To accomplish these goals, physicians must make timely immunization, including active and passive immunoprophylaxis, a high priority in the care of infants, children, adolescents, and adults. The global eradication of smallpox in 1977 and elimination of poliomyelitis from the Americas in 1991 serve as models for fulfilling the promise of disease control through immunization. Both of these accomplishments were achieved by combining a comprehensive immunization program providing consistent, high levels of vaccine coverage with intensive surveillance and effective public health disease control measures. Future success in the worldwide elimination of measles, rubella, and hepatitis B is possible through implementation of similar prevention strategies.

High immunization rates have curtailed dramatically or almost eliminated diphtheria, measles, mumps, polio, rubella (congenital and acquired), tetanus, and *Haemophilus influenzae* type b disease (see Table 1.1, p 2) in the United States.

Yet, because organisms that cause these diseases persist in the United States and elsewhere around the world, continued immunization efforts must be maintained and strengthened. Discoveries in immunology, molecular biology, and medical genetics have resulted in burgeoning vaccine research. Licensing of new, improved, and safer vaccines, anticipated arrival of additional combination vaccines, and application of novel vaccine delivery systems promise a new era of preventive medicine. The advent of population-based epidemiologic postlicensure studies of new vaccines provides for detection of rare adverse events temporally associated with immunization that were undetected during prelicensure clinical trials. Studies of the rare occurrence of intussusception after administration of the oral rhesus rotavirus vaccine have confirmed the value of such surveillance systems. Physicians must regularly update their knowledge about specific vaccines, including information about their optimal use, safety, and effectiveness.

Each edition of the *Red Book* provides recommendations for immunization of infants, children, and adolescents based on the knowledge, experience, and premises at the time of publication. The recommendations represent a consensus with which reasonable physicians may at times disagree. No claim is made for infallibility, and the American Academy of Pediatrics Committee on Infectious Diseases acknowledges that individual circumstances may warrant decisions differing from recommendations given herein.

Table 1.1. **Baseline 20th Century Annual Morbidity and 2001 Morbidity From 10 Diseases With Vaccines Recommended Before 1990 for Universal Use in Children: United States[1]**

Disease	Baseline 20th Century Annual Morbidity	2001 Morbidity	% Decrease
Smallpox	48 164[2]	0	100
Diphtheria	175 885[3]	2	>99
Pertussis	147 271[4]	7580	95
Tetanus	1 314[5]	37	97
Poliomyelitis (paralytic)	16 316[6]	0	100
Measles	503 282[7]	116	>99
Mumps	152 209[8]	266	>99
Rubella	47 745[9]	23	>99
Congenital rubella syndrome	823[10]	3	>99
Haemophilus influenzae type b	20 000[11]	181[12]	>99

[1] Adapted from Centers for Disease Control and Prevention. Impact of vaccines universally recommended for children—United States, 1990–1998. *MMWR Morb Mortal Wkly Rep.* 1999;48:243–248; and Centers for Disease Control and Prevention. Notice to readers: final 2001 reports of notifiable diseases. *MMWR Morb Mortal Wkly Rep.* 2002;51:710.

[2] Average annual number of cases during 1900–1904.

[3] Average annual number of reported cases during 1920–1922, 3 years before vaccine development.

[4] Average annual number of reported cases during 1922–1925, 4 years before vaccine development.

[5] Estimated number of cases based on reported number of deaths during 1922–1926, assuming a case-fatality rate of 90%.

[6] Average annual number of reported cases during 1951–1954, 4 years before vaccine licensure.

[7] Average annual number of reported cases during 1958–1962, 5 years before vaccine licensure.

[8] Number of reported cases in 1968, the first year reporting began and the first year after vaccine licensure.

[9] Average annual number of reported cases during 1966–1968, 3 years before vaccine licensure.

[10] Estimated number of cases based on seroprevalence data in the population and on the risk that women infected during a childbearing year would have a fetus with congenital rubella syndrome.

[11] Estimated number of cases from population-based surveillance studies before vaccine licensure in 1985.

[12] Represents invasive disease in children younger than 5 years of age and includes *H influenzae* strains that were not serotyped.

SOURCES OF VACCINE INFORMATION

In addition to the *Red Book,* which is published at intervals of approximately 3 years, physicians should use evidence-based literature and other sources for data to answer specific vaccine questions encountered in practice. Such sources include the following:

• **Pediatrics.** Policy statements developed by the Committee on Infectious Diseases (COID) providing updated recommendations are published in *Pediatrics* between editions of the *Red Book.* Policy statements also may be accessed via the American Academy of Pediatrics (AAP) Web site (www.aap.org).

The updated recommended childhood and adolescent immunization schedule for the United States is published annually in the January issue of *Pediatrics* and elsewhere (see Scheduling Immunizations, p 21).

- **AAP News.** Policy statements (or statement summaries) from the COID often are published initially in *AAP News,* the Academy's monthly newspaper, to inform the AAP membership promptly of new recommendations.
- **Morbidity and Mortality Weekly Report (MMWR).** Published weekly by the Centers for Disease Control and Prevention (CDC), *MMWR* contains current vaccine recommendations, reports of specific disease activity, alerts concerning vaccine availability, changes in formulations and safety, changes in policy statements, and other infectious disease and vaccine information. Recommendations of the Advisory Committee on Immunization Practices (ACIP) of the CDC are published periodically, often as supplements, and are posted on the CDC Web site (www.cdc.gov/mmwr).
- **Manufacturers' package inserts (product labels).** Manufacturers provide product-specific information with each vaccine product. This information also is published in the annual *Physicians' Desk Reference* (Medical Economics, Montvale, NJ). The product label must be in full compliance with US Food and Drug Administration (FDA) regulations pertaining to labeling for prescription drugs, including indications and usage, dosages, routes of administration, clinical pharmacology, contraindications, and adverse events. The package insert lists contents of each vaccine, including preservatives, stabilizers, antimicrobial agents, adjuvants, and suspending fluids, that may cause inflammation or elicit an allergic response. Health care professionals should be familiar with the label for each product they administer. Most manufacturers maintain Web sites with current information concerning new vaccine releases and changes in labeling. Additionally, 24-hour contact telephone numbers for medical questions are available in the *Physicians' Desk Reference* (http://pdrel.thomsonhc.com/pdrel/librarian/action/command.Command).
- **Health Information for International Travel.** This useful monograph is published approximately every 2 years by the CDC as a guide to requirements of various countries for specific immunizations. The monograph also provides information about other vaccines recommended for travel in specific areas and other information for travelers. This document can be purchased from the Superintendent of Documents, US Government Printing Office, Washington, DC 20402-9235. This information also is available on the CDC Web site (www.cdc.gov/travel). For further sources of information on international travel, see International Travel (p 93).
- **CDC materials.** A CDC textbook, *Epidemiology and Prevention of Vaccine-Preventable Diseases* (7th Edition, 2002), provides detailed information on the use and administration of childhood vaccines as well as selected ACIP statements and other vaccine-related information (for copies, contact the Public Health Foundation at 877-252-1200 or visit www.cdc.gov/nip/publications/pink). A CDC publication titled *Manual for Surveillance of Vaccine-Preventable Diseases* provides insight into the principles used to investigate and control outbreaks of disease when immunization levels decrease. The CDC's National Immunization Program (NIP) publishes a series of brochures on immunization topics and produces a CD-ROM that contains a wide range of resources, including vaccine

information statements (VISs) and the complete CDC textbook. To obtain CDC materials, call 1-800-232-2522, fax 1-404-639-8828, or access the NIP Web site (www.cdc.gov/nip).

- **Satellite broadcasts and Web-based training courses.** The NIP, in conjunction with the Public Health Training Network, conducts several immunization-related "train the trainer" courses live via satellite and over the Internet each year. Annual course offerings include the Immunization Update, Vaccines for International Travel, Influenza, and a 4-part introductory course on the Epidemiology and Prevention of Vaccine-Preventable Diseases. The course schedule, slide sets, and written materials can be accessed on the Internet (www.cdc.gov/nip/ed/ newsatellite.htm).

- **Immunization information e-mail-based inquiry system.** The NIP is available to respond to immunization-related questions submitted from health care professionals and members of the public. Individualized responses to inquiries typically are sent within 24 hours. Inquiries should be sent via e-mail (NIPINFO@cdc.gov).

- **National Immunization Hotline.** The hotline is a telephone-based resource for answers to immunization-related questions from health care professionals and members of the public. The English hotline may be reached at 1-800-232-2522, and the Spanish hotline may be reached at 1-800-232-0233.

  Printed information on immunizations also can be obtained from the NIP through the Web site (www.cdc.gov/nip) or by fax at 1-888-CDC-FAXX (1-888-232-3299).

- **Independent sources of reliable immunization information.** Appendix I (p 789) provides a list of reliable immunization information resources that includes facts concerning vaccine efficacy, clinical applications, schedules, and unbiased information about safety. Two organizations are particularly comprehensive in addressing practicing physicians' concerns: the National Network for Immunization Information (www.immunizationinfo.org) and the Immunization Action Coalition (www.immunize.org).

  Other resources include the FDA*; infectious disease experts at university-affiliated hospitals, at medical schools, and in private practice; and state immunization programs and local public health departments. Information can be obtained from state and local health departments about current epidemiology of diseases, immunization recommendations, legal requirements, public health policies, and nursery school, child care, and school health concerns or requirements.

INFORMING PATIENTS AND PARENTS

Parents and patients should be informed about the benefits and risks of disease preventive and therapeutic procedures, including immunization.

The patient, parents, and/or legal guardian should be informed about benefits to be derived from vaccines in preventing disease in individuals and the community in which they live and about the risks of those vaccines. Adequate time should be provided and questions should be encouraged so that the information is understood.

---

* See Appendix I, Directory of Resources, p 789.

The National Childhood Vaccine Injury Act (NCVIA) of 1986 included requirements for notifying *all* patients and parents about vaccine benefits and risks. Whether vaccines are purchased with private or public funds, this legislation mandates that a vaccine information statement (VIS) be provided each time a vaccine covered under the National Vaccine Injury Compensation Program (VICP) is administered (see Table 1.2). For vaccines not yet included in the VICP, VISs are available but are not mandated unless the vaccine is purchased through a contract with the Centers for Disease Control and Prevention (CDC [ie, the Vaccines for Children Program, state immunization grants, or state purchases through the CDC]). Copies of currently available VISs can be obtained from state and local health departments, the CDC, the American Academy of Pediatrics (AAP), and vaccine manufacturers or by calling the National Immunization Hotline (1-800-232-2522 in English and 1-800-232-0233 in Spanish). Copies are available on the NIP Web site (www.cdc.gov/nip/publications/VIS/default.htm) and the Immunization Action Coalition Web site (www.immunize.org) in English and many other languages. Physicians need to ensure that the VIS provided is the current version by noting the date of publication. The latest version can be determined by calling the National Immunization Hotline or by accessing the NIP Web site (www.cdc.gov/nip/publications/VIS/default.htm).

The NCVIA requires physicians administering vaccines covered by the VICP, whether purchased with private or public funds, to record in the patient's medical record information shown in Table 1.2. For vaccines purchased through CDC contract, physicians are required to record the VIS date of publication *and* the date on which the VIS was provided to the patient, parent, and/or legal guardian. Although VIS distribution and vaccine record-keeping requirements do not apply to privately purchased vaccines not covered by the VICP, the AAP recommends using the VISs and following the same record-keeping practices with all vaccines. The AAP also recommends recording the site and route of administration and vaccine expiration date after administering any vaccine.

Table 1.2. **Guidance in Using Vaccine Information Statements (VISs)**

Distribution	Documentation in the Patient's Medical Record
Must be provided each time a VICP-covered vaccine is administered[1]	Vaccine manufacturer, lot number, and date of administration[1]
Given to patient (nonminor), parent, and/or legal guardian[1]	Name and business address of the health care professional administering the vaccine[1]
Must be the current version[2]	VIS version date in addition to date it is provided[2]
Can provide (not substitute) other written materials or audiovisual aids in addition to VISs	Site (eg, deltoid area) and route (eg, intramuscular) of administration and expiration date of the vaccine[3]

VICP indicates Vaccine Injury Compensation Program.
[1] Required under the National Childhood Vaccine Injury Act.
[2] Required by Centers for Disease Control and Prevention (CDC) regulations for vaccines purchased through CDC contract.
[3] Recommended by the American Academy of Pediatrics.

New VISs do not require parents' or patients' signatures to indicate that they have read and understood the material. However, the health care professional has the option to obtain a signature. Whether or not a signature is obtained, the AAP recommends that health care professionals document in the chart that the VIS has been provided and discussed with the patient, parent, and/or legal guardian.

Risk Communication

Health care professionals should anticipate that some parents will question the need for or the safety of immunizations, refuse certain vaccines, or even decide to reject all immunizations for their child. Some parents may have religious or philosophic objections to immunization; others want only to enter into a dialogue with their child's physician about the risks and benefits of one or more vaccines. A nonjudgmental approach to such parents is best. Ideally, health care professionals should determine in general terms what parents understand about vaccines their children will be receiving, the nature of their concerns, their health beliefs, and what information they find credible. Concerns can be reviewed by asking the following questions: (1) Do you have any cultural, religious, or personal beliefs regarding immunizations? (2) Has your child or any child you know had a serious adverse event after an immunization? (3) Do you have any vaccine safety concerns? (4) What vaccine safety information can I provide?

Individuals understand and react to vaccine information on the basis of a variety of factors, including previous experiences, attitudes, health beliefs, personal values, and education. The method in which data are presented about immunizations as well as a person's perceptions of the risks of disease, perceived ability to control those risks, and risk preference also contribute to understanding of immunizations. For some people who use alternative medicine, the risk of immunization may be viewed as disproportionately greater so that immunization is not perceived as beneficial. Others may dwell on sociopolitical issues, such as mandatory immunization, informed consent, and the primacy of individual rights to that of societal benefit.

Parents may be aware through the media or information from nonauthoritative Web sites of controversial issues about vaccines their child is scheduled to receive. Many issues about childhood vaccines communicated by these means are presented incompletely or inaccurately. When a parent initiates discussion about a vaccine controversy, the health care professional should discuss specific concerns and provide factual information, using language appropriate for parents. Through direct dialogue with parents and the use of available resources, health care professionals can help prevent acceptance of inaccurate media reports and information from nonauthoritative sources.

Effective, empathetic vaccine risk communication is essential for responding to misinformation and concerns while recognizing that risk assessment and decision making for some parents may be difficult and confusing. Some vaccines may be acceptable to the resistant parent. Their vaccine safety concerns should be addressed in the context of this information, using the mandated VISs (see p 5) and offering other resource materials (see Parental Misconceptions About Immunizations, p 50). Health care professionals can reinforce important points about each vaccine, including vaccine safety, and emphasize the risks encountered by unimmunized children.

Two helpful information sources that parents can be provided or to which they can be directed, both of which are free, are the National Immunization Program's "Parent's Guide to Childhood Immunization" (visit www.cdc.gov/nip or telephone 1-800-232-2522 for English or 1-800-232-0233 for Spanish) and the National Partnership for Immunizations' "Reference Guide...to Vaccines and Vaccine Safety" (telephone 301-656-0003 or visit www.partnersforimmunization.org). Parents should be advised of state laws pertaining to school or child care entry, which may require that unimmunized children stay home from school during disease outbreaks. Documentation of such discussions in the patient's record may help to decrease any potential liability should a vaccine-preventable disease occur in the unimmunized patient.

....

ACTIVE IMMUNIZATION

Active immunization involves administration of all or part of a microorganism or a modified product of that microorganism (eg, a toxoid, a purified antigen, or an antigen produced by genetic engineering) to evoke an immunologic response mimicking that of natural infection but that usually presents little or no risk to the recipient. Immunization can result in antitoxin, antiadherence, anti-invasive, or neutralizing activity or other types of protective humoral or cellular response in the recipient. Some immunizing agents provide nearly complete lifelong protection against disease, some provide partial protection, and some must be readministered at regular intervals. The effectiveness of a vaccine or toxoid is assessed by evidence of protection against the natural disease. Induction of antibodies commonly is an indirect measure of protection, but for some conditions (eg, pertussis), the magnitude of immunologic response that correlates with protection is poorly understood, and serum antibody concentration does not always predict protection.

Vaccines incorporating an intact infectious agent may be live (attenuated) or killed (inactivated). Vaccines licensed for immunization in the United States are listed in Table 1.3 (p 8). The US Food and Drug Administration (FDA) maintains and updates a Web site listing vaccines licensed for immunization in the United States (www.fda.gov/cber/vaccine/licvacc.htm). Many viral vaccines contain live-attenuated virus. Although active infection (with viral replication) ensues after administration of these vaccines, usually little or no adverse host reaction occurs. The vaccines for some viruses and most bacteria are inactivated (killed), subunit (purified components) preparations or are conjugated chemically to immunobiologically active proteins (eg, tetanus toxoids). Viruses and bacteria in inactivated, subunit, and conjugate vaccine preparations are not capable of replicating in the host; therefore, these vaccines must contain a sufficient antigenic mass to stimulate a desired response. Maintenance of long-lasting immunity with inactivated viral or bacterial vaccines may require periodic administration of booster doses. Inactivated vaccines may not elicit the range of immunologic response provided by live-attenuated agents. For example, an injected inactivated viral vaccine may evoke sufficient serum antibody or cell-mediated immunity but evoke only minimal local antibody in the form of secretory immunoglobulin (Ig) A. Thus, mucosal protection after administration of inactivated vaccines generally is inferior to mucosal immunity

Table 1.3. **Vaccines Produced and/or Licensed in the United States and Their Routes of Administration[1]**

Vaccine	Type	Route
BCG	Live bacteria	ID (preferred) or SC
Diphtheria-tetanus (DT, Td)	Toxoids	IM
DTaP	Toxoids and inactivated bacterial components	IM
DTaP, hepatitis B, and inactivated poliovirus	Toxoids and inactivated bacterial components, recombinant viral antigen, inactivated virus	IM
Hepatitis A	Inactivated viral antigen	IM
Hepatitis B	Recombinant viral antigen	IM
Hepatitis A-hepatitis B	Inactivated and recombinant viral antigens	IM
Hib conjugates[2]	Polysaccharide-protein conjugate	IM
Hib conjugate-DTaP (PRP-T[2] reconstituted with DTaP)	Polysaccharide-protein conjugate with toxoids and inactivated bacterial components	IM
Hib conjugate (PRP-OMP[2])-hepatitis B	Polysaccharide-protein conjugate with recombinant viral antigen	IM
Influenza	Inactivated viral components	IM
Japanese encephalitis	Inactivated virus	SC
Measles	Live-attenuated virus	SC
Meningococcal	Polysaccharide	SC
MMR	Live-attenuated viruses	SC
Mumps	Live-attenuated virus	SC
Pneumococcal	Polysaccharide	IM or SC
Pneumococcal	Polysaccharide-protein conjugate	IM
Poliovirus	Inactivated virus	SC or IM
Rabies	Inactivated virus	IM
Rubella	Live-attenuated virus	SC
Smallpox	Live virus	Scarification only
Tetanus	Toxoid	IM
Typhoid		
Parenteral	Capsular polysaccharide	IM
Oral	Live-attenuated bacteria	Oral
Varicella	Live virus	SC
Yellow fever	Live virus	SC

BCG indicates bacille Calmette-Guérin; ID, intradermal; SC, subcutaneous; IM, intramuscular; DTaP, diphtheria and tetanus toxoids and acellular pertussis, adsorbed; PRP-T, polyribosylribitol phosphate-tetanus toxoid; PRP-OMP, polyribosylribitol phosphate-meningococcal outer membrane protein; Hib, *Haemophilus influenzae* type b; MMR, live measles-mumps-rubella viruses; IPV, inactivated poliovirus; Td, diphtheria and tetanus toxoids (for children 7 years of age or older and adults); DT, diphtheria and tetanus toxoids (for children younger than 7 years of age); OPV, oral poliovirus.

[1] Other vaccines licensed in the United States but not distributed include anthrax vaccine, OPV vaccine, Lyme disease vaccine, and oral tetravalent rotavirus vaccine. The FDA maintains a Web site listing currently licensed vaccines in the United States (www.fda.gov/cber/vaccine/licvacc.htm).

[2] See Table 3.11, p 298.

induced by live vaccines. Although systemic infection is prevented or ameliorated by the presence of serum and cellular factors, local infection or colonization with the agent can occur. However, viruses and bacteria in inactivated vaccines cannot replicate in or be excreted by the vaccine recipient as infectious agents and, thereby, cannot adversely affect immunosuppressed hosts or their contacts.

Recommendations for dose, vaccine storage and handling, route and technique of administration, and immunization schedules should be followed for predictable, effective immunization (see disease-specific chapters in Section 3). Related recommendations are critical to the success of immunization practices.

Immunizing Antigens

Physicians should be familiar with the major constituents of the products they use. The major constituents are listed in the package inserts. If a vaccine is produced by different manufacturers, some differences may exist in the active and inert ingredients and the relative amounts contained in the various products. The major constituents of vaccines include the following:

- **Active immunizing antigens.** Some vaccines consist of a single antigen that is a highly defined constituent (eg, tetanus or diphtheria toxoid). In other vaccines, antigens that provoke protective immune responses vary substantially in chemical composition and number (eg, acellular pertussis components, *Haemophilus influenzae* type b, and pneumococcal and meningococcal products). Vaccines containing live-attenuated (weakened) viruses (measles-mumps-rubella [MMR], varicella, oral poliovirus [OPV]), killed viruses or portions of virus (eg, enhanced inactivated poliovirus [IPV] and inactivated influenza vaccines), and immunologically active viral fragments incorporated into a vaccine through recombinant technology (eg, hepatitis B vaccine) produce both humoral and cellular-mediated responses to ensure long-term protection.

- **Conjugating agents.** Carrier proteins of proven immunologic potential (eg, tetanus toxoid, diphtheria toxoid, meningococcal outer membrane protein), when chemically combined to less immunogenic polysaccharide antigens (eg, *H influenzae* type b, meningococcal and pneumococcal polysaccharides), enhance the type and magnitude of immune responses in patients with immature immune systems, particularly children younger than 2 years of age.

- **Suspending fluid.** The suspending fluid commonly is as simple as sterile water for injection or saline solution, but it may be a complex tissue-culture fluid. This fluid may contain proteins or other constituents derived from the medium and biological system in which the vaccine is produced (eg, egg antigens, gelatin, or tissue culture-derived antigens).

- **Preservatives, stabilizers, and antimicrobial agents.** Trace amounts of chemicals (eg, mercurials, such as thimerosal [see Thimerosal content of some vaccines and immune globulin preparations, p 47]) and certain antimicrobial agents (such as neomycin or streptomycin sulfate) commonly are included to prevent bacterial growth or to stabilize an antigen. Allergic reactions may occur if the recipient is sensitive to one or more of these additives. Whenever feasible, these reactions should be anticipated by identifying known host hypersensitivity to specific vaccine components.

- *Adjuvants.* An aluminum salt commonly is used in varying amounts to increase immunogenicity and to prolong the stimulatory effect, particularly for vaccines containing inactivated microorganisms or their products (eg, hepatitis B and diphtheria and tetanus toxoids).

Vaccine Handling and Storage

Inattention to vaccine storage conditions can contribute to vaccine failure. Certain vaccines, such as measles, varicella, yellow fever, and OPV vaccines, are sensitive to increased temperature. Other vaccines are damaged by freezing; examples include diphtheria and tetanus and pertussis vaccines (diphtheria and tetanus toxoids and acellular pertussis [DTaP]), IPV vaccine, *H influenzae* type b (Hib) vaccine, pneumococcal polysaccharide and conjugate vaccines, hepatitis A and B vaccines, inactivated influenza vaccine, and meningococcal vaccines. Some products may show physical evidence of altered integrity, and others may retain their normal appearance despite a loss of potency. Therefore, all personnel responsible for handling vaccines in an office or clinic setting should be familiar with standard procedures designed to minimize risk of vaccine failure. Recommended storage conditions for commonly used vaccines are listed in Table 1.4 (p 11); new vaccines and new formulations of currently available products may have storage requirements different from those listed. In addition, storage recommendations may be revised by the manufacturer. Revisions require approval by the FDA.

Recommendations for handling and storage of selected biologicals are summarized in the package insert for each product and in a publication, *Vaccine Management,* available from the Centers for Disease Control and Prevention (CDC).* The most current information about recommended vaccine storage conditions and handling instructions can be obtained directly from manufacturers; their telephone numbers are listed in product labels (package inserts) and in the *Physicians' Desk Reference,* which is published yearly. The following guidelines are suggested as part of a quality control system for safe handling and storage of vaccines in an office or clinic setting.

PERSONNEL

- Designate one person as the vaccine coordinator, and assign responsibility for ensuring that vaccines and other biologic agents and products are handled and stored in a careful, safe, recommended, and documentable manner. Assign a backup person to assume these responsibilities during times of illness or vacation.
- Inform all people who will be handling vaccines about specific storage requirements and stability limitations of the products they will encounter (see Table 1.4, p 11). Post the details of proper storage conditions on or near each refrigerator or freezer used for vaccine storage or have them readily available.

---

* Centers for Disease Control and Prevention. *Vaccine Management: Recommendations for Handling and Storage of Selected Biologicals.* Atlanta, GA: US Department of Health and Human Services, Public Health Service; 1999

Table 1.4. Recommended Storage of Commonly Used Vaccines[1]

Vaccine	Recommended Temperature	Duration of Stability	Normal Appearance
Diphtheria and tetanus toxoids and acellular pertussis (DTaP) vaccine, adsorbed	2°C–8°C (35°F–46°F). Do not freeze. As little as 24 hours at <2°C (<35°F) or >25°C (>77°F) may cause antigens to fall from suspension and be difficult to resuspend.	Not more than 18 mo from date of issue from manufacturer's cold storage.	Markedly turbid and whitish suspension. If product contains clumps of material that cannot be resuspended with vigorous shaking, it should NOT be used.
Diphtheria toxoid, adsorbed	2°C–8°C. Do not freeze.	Not more than 2 y from date of issue from manufacturer's cold storage.	Turbid and white, slightly gray, or slightly pink suspension.
DTaP, hepatitis B virus vaccine inactivated (recombinant), and inactivated poliovirus vaccine	2°C–8°C.	See expiration date on vial.	Turbid, white suspension.
Hib conjugate vaccine: HbOC (diphtheria CRM197 protein conjugate)	2°C–8°C. Do not freeze.	Not more than 2 y from date of issue from manufacturer's cold storage.	Clear, colorless liquid.
Hib conjugate vaccine: PRP-OMP (meningococcal protein conjugate)	Lyophilized formulation: 2°C–8°C. Do not freeze.	Not more than 2 y from date of issue from manufacturer's cold storage.	Slightly opaque, white suspension.
Hib conjugate vaccine: PRP-T (tetanus toxoid conjugate)	Lyophilized formulation: 2°C–8°C. Do not freeze formulation.	Not more than 2 y from date of issue from manufacturer's cold storage.	Lyophilized: white, lyophilized cake
	Reconstituted formulation: 2°C–8°C. Do not freeze. Store diluent with product.	Vaccine should be used immediately when reconstituted.	Reconstituted: clear and colorless.
Hepatitis A virus vaccine, inactivated	2°C–8°C. Do not freeze. Do not use if product has been frozen.	3 y, if kept refrigerated.	Opaque, white suspension.
Hepatitis B virus vaccine inactivated (recombinant)	2°C–8°C. Storage outside this temperature range may decrease potency. Freezing substantially decreases potency.	3 y from date of issue from manufacturer's cold storage.	After thorough agitation, a slightly opaque, white suspension.

Table 1.4. Recommended Storage of Commonly Used Vaccines, [1] continued

Vaccine	Recommended Temperature	Duration of Stability	Normal Appearance
Hepatitis A-hepatitis B combination vaccine	2°C–8°C. Do not freeze.	2 y.	Homogeneous white turbid suspension.
Influenza virus vaccine (subvirion)	2°C–8°C. Freezing destroys potency.	Use of vaccine is recommended only during the year for which it is manufactured; antigenic composition differs annually.	Clear, colorless liquid.
Measles-mumps-rubella virus (MMR) vaccine, live	Lyophilized formulation: 2°C–8°C, but may be frozen. Protect from light, which may inactivate virus.	Up to 2 y.	Lyophilized: light yellow compact crystalline plug.
	Diluent: store at room temperature or refrigerate.	Check date on vial.	Diluent: clear, colorless liquid.
	Reconstituted formulation: 2°C–8°C. Protect from light, which may inactivate virus.	Discard reconstituted vial if not used within 8 h (keep refrigerated).	Reconstituted: clear, yellow solution.
Measles virus vaccine, live	See MMR.	See MMR.	See MMR.
Meningococcal vaccine	Lyophilized or reconstituted formulation: 2°C–8°C.	Up to 2 y from date of issue. Discard reconstituted multidose vials after 10 days; use single-dose vial within 30 min.	Lyophilized: white pellet. Reconstituted: clear, colorless.
	Diluent: store with product. Do not freeze.		
Mumps virus vaccine, live	See MMR.	See MMR.	See MMR.
Rubella virus vaccine, live	See MMR.	See MMR.	See MMR.
Pneumococcal polysaccharide vaccine	2°C–8°C. Freezing destroys potency.	See expiration date on vial.	Clear, colorless, or slightly opalescent liquid.

Table 1.4. Recommended Storage of Commonly Used Vaccines,[1] continued

Vaccine	Recommended Temperature	Duration of Stability	Normal Appearance
Pneumococcal conjugate vaccine	2°C–8°C. Do not freeze.	See expiration date on vial.	Homogeneous white suspension after vigorous shaking.
Poliovirus vaccine, inactivated (IPV)	2°C–8°C. Do not freeze.	Up to 18 mo. See expiration date on vial.	Clear, colorless suspension. Vaccine that contains particulate matter, develops turbidity, or changes color should NOT be used.
Poliovirus vaccine, live, oral (OPV)	Must be stored at <0°C (<32°F). Because of sorbitol in the vaccine, it will remain fluid at temperatures above –14°C (7°F). Refreezing the thawed product is acceptable (maximum of 10 thaw-freeze cycles) if the temperature never exceeds 8°C and the cumulative thawing time is <24 h.	Not more than 1 y from date of issue from manufacturer's cold storage.	Clear solution, usually red or pink, from the phenol red (pH indicator) it contains; may be yellow if shipment was packed with dry ice. Color changes that occur during storage or thawing are unimportant, provided the solution remains clear.
Tetanus and diphtheria toxoids, adsorbed (Td)	2°C–8°C. Do not freeze.	Not more than 2 y from date of issue from manufacturer's cold storage.	Markedly turbid and white suspension. If product contains clumps of material that cannot be resuspended with vigorous shaking, it should NOT be used.
Varicella virus vaccine[2]	Lyophilized formulation: keep frozen at –15°C (5°F) or colder. Protect from light. Store in frost-free freezer only.	Lyophilized formulation: 18 mo.	Lyophilized formulation: whitish powder.
	Diluent: store at room temperature or refrigerate.	Check date on vial.	Clear, colorless liquid.

Table 1.4. Recommended Storage of Commonly Used Vaccines, [1] continued

Vaccine	Recommended Temperature	Duration of Stability	Normal Appearance
	For temporary storage, unreconstituted vaccine may be stored at 2°C–8°C for a maximum of 72 h.	Discard unreconstituted vaccine if not used within 72 h (do not refreeze).	
	Reconstituted formulation: use immediately; do not store.	Discard reconstituted vials if not used within 30 min.	Reconstituted formulation: clear, colorless to pale yellow liquid.

Hib indicates *Haemophilus influenzae* type b.

[1] For recently licensed combination vaccines, see package inserts; instructions may be different from those for products listed in the table. Also, any changes in the formulation of currently available immunizing agents may alter their appearance, stability, and storage requirements. Questions about the stability of biologic agents subjected to potentially harmful environmental conditions should be addressed to the manufacturer of the product in question.

[2] For questions about stability, contact the manufacturer by calling 1-800-9-VARIVAX.

EQUIPMENT

- Ensure that refrigerators and freezers in which vaccines are to be stored are working properly and are capable of meeting storage requirements.
- Do not connect refrigerators or freezers to an outlet with a ground-flow circuit interrupter or one activated by a wall switch. Use plug guards to prevent accidental dislodging of the wall plug.
- Equip each refrigerator and freezer compartment with a thermometer located at the center of the storage compartment. This thermometer should be a calibrated, constant recording type with graphed readings or one that indicates upper and lower extremes of temperature during an observation period ("minimum-maximum" thermometer). These thermometers provide a means of determining whether vaccines have been exposed to potentially harmful temperatures. Placement of vaccine cold-chain monitor cards* in refrigerators and freezers can serve to detect potentially harmful increases in temperature.
- Keep a logbook in which temperature readings systematically are recorded daily and in which the date, time, and duration of any mechanical malfunctions or power outages are noted.
- Place all opened vials of vaccine in a refrigerator tray. To avoid mishaps, do not store other pharmaceutical products in the same tray.
- Equip refrigerators with several bottles of chilled water and freezers with several ice trays or ice packs to fill empty space to minimize temperature fluctuations during brief electrical or mechanical failures.

PROCEDURES

- Acceptance of vaccine on receipt of shipment:
  - Ensure that the delivered product is not past the expiration date.
  - Examine the merchandise and its shipping container for any evidence of damage during transport.
  - Consider whether the interval between shipment from the supplier and arrival of the product at its destination is excessive (more than 48 hours) and whether the product has been exposed to excessive heat or cold that might alter its integrity. Review vaccine cold-chain monitor cards if included in the vaccine shipment.
  - Do not accept the shipment if reasonable suspicion exists that the delivered product may have been damaged by environmental insult or improper handling during transport.
  - Contact the vaccine supplier or manufacturer when unusual circumstances raise questions about the stability of a delivered vaccine. Store suspect vaccine under proper conditions until its viability is determined.
- Refrigerator and freezer inspection:
  - Measure the temperature of the central part of the storage compartment daily, and record this temperature in a logbook. If a minimum-maximum thermometer is available, record extremes in temperature fluctuation and reset to baseline. The refrigerator temperature should be maintained between 2°C and 8°C (35°F and 46°F) and the freezer temperature should be at least −15°C (5°F).

---

* Available from 3M Pharmaceuticals, St Paul, Minn.

- Inspect the unit weekly for outdated vaccine and dispose of or return expired products appropriately.
- Routine procedures:
  - Store vaccines according to temperatures recommended in the package insert.
  - Promptly remove expired (outdated) vaccines from the refrigerator or freezer and dispose of them appropriately to avoid accidental use.
  - Keep opened vials of vaccine in a tray so that they are readily identifiable.
  - Indicate on the label of each vaccine vial the date and time it was reconstituted or first opened.
  - Avoid reconstituting multiple doses of vaccine or drawing up multiple doses of vaccine in multiple syringes before immediate use. Predrawing vaccine increases the possibility of mix-ups and uncertainty of vaccine stability.
  - Use prefilled unit-dose syringes to prevent contamination of multidose vials and errors in labeling syringes.
  - Discard reconstituted live-virus and other vaccines if not used within the interval specified in the package insert. Examples include varicella vaccine after 30 minutes, MMR vaccine after 8 hours, and PedvaxHIB (polyribosyl-ribitol phosphate-meningococcal outer membrane protein [PRP-OMP]) after 24 hours (see *Haemophilus influenzae* Infections, p 297), all of which should be refrigerated after reconstitution.
  - Always store vaccines in the refrigerator, including throughout the office day.
  - Do not open more than 1 vial of a specific vaccine at a time.
  - Store vaccine only in the central storage area of the refrigerator, not on the door shelf or in peripheral areas, where temperature fluctuations are greater.
  - Do not keep food or drink in refrigerators where vaccine is stored; this will lead to less frequent opening of the unit and decrease the chance of thermal instability.
  - Do not store radioactive materials in the same refrigerator in which vaccines are stored.
  - Discuss with all clinic or office personnel any violation of handling protocol or any accidental storage problem (eg, electrical failure), and contact vaccine suppliers for information about handling of the affected vaccine.
  - Develop a plan for emergency storage of vaccine in the event of a catastrophic occurrence. Office personnel should have a written procedure that outlines vaccine packing and transport. Vaccines that have been exposed to temperatures outside the recommended storage range may be ineffective. In the event of extended power outages (>4 hours), vaccines should be packed in an appropriate insulated storage box and moved to a location where the appropriate storage temperatures can be maintained. Office personnel need to be aware of alternate storage sites and trained in the correct techniques to store and transport vaccines to avoid warming vaccines that need to be refrigerated or frozen and to avoid freezing vaccines that should be refrigerated (see Table 1.4, page 11).

Vaccine Administration

GENERAL INSTRUCTIONS FOR PEOPLE ADMINISTERING VACCINES

Personnel administering vaccines should take appropriate precautions to minimize the risk of spread of disease to or from patients. Hand hygiene should be used before and after each new patient contact. Gloves are not required when administering vaccines unless the health care professional has open hand lesions or will come into contact with potentially infectious body fluids. Syringes and needles must be sterile and preferably disposable. To prevent accidental needlesticks or reuse, a needle should **not** be recapped after use, and disposable needles and syringes should be discarded promptly in puncture-proof, labeled containers. Changing needles between drawing vaccine into the syringe and injecting it into the child is not necessary. Different vaccines should not be mixed in the same syringe unless specifically licensed and labeled for such use. Needle devices approved by the Occupational Safety and Health Administration are available.

Because of possible hypersensitivity of vaccine recipients to vaccine components, people administering vaccines or other biological products should be prepared to recognize and treat allergic reactions, including anaphylaxis (see Hypersensitivity Reactions to Vaccine Constituents, p 46). Facilities and personnel should be available for treating immediate hypersensitivity reactions. This recommendation does not preclude administration of vaccines in school-based or other nonclinic settings. Whenever possible, patients should be observed for an allergic reaction for 15 to 20 minutes after receiving immunization(s).

Syncope may occur after immunization, particularly in adolescents and young adults. Personnel should be aware of presyncopal manifestations and take appropriate measures to prevent injuries if weakness, dizziness, or loss of consciousness occurs. The relatively rapid onset of syncope in most cases suggests that having vaccine recipients sit or lie down for 15 minutes after immunization could avert many syncopal episodes and secondary injuries. If syncope develops, patients should be observed until they are asymptomatic.

SITE AND ROUTE OF IMMUNIZATION (ACTIVE AND PASSIVE)

Oral vaccines. Breastfeeding does not interfere with successful immunization with oral vaccines (eg, OPV). Vomiting within 10 minutes of receiving an oral dose is an indication for repeating the dose. If the second dose is not retained, neither dose should be counted, and the vaccine should be readministered. In the United States, no oral vaccines currently are recommended for routine immunization.

Parenteral vaccines.* Injectable vaccines should be administered in a site as free as possible from risk of local neural, vascular, or tissue injury. Data do not warrant recommendation of a single preferred site for all injections, and many manufacturers' product recommendations allow flexibility in the site of injection. Preferred sites for

---

* For a review on intramuscular injections, see Centers for Disease Control and Prevention. *Epidemiology and Prevention of Vaccine-Preventable Diseases.* Atlanta, GA: Centers for Disease Control and Prevention; 2002. For copies, contact the Public Health Foundation at 877-252-1200 or visit www.cdc.gov/nip/publications/pink/.

vaccines administered subcutaneously or intramuscularly include the anterolateral aspect of the upper thigh and the deltoid area of the upper arm.

Recommended routes of administration are included in package inserts of vaccines and are listed in Table 1.3 (p 8). The recommended route is based on studies designed to demonstrate maximum safety and efficacy. To minimize untoward local or systemic effects and ensure optimal efficacy of the immunizing procedure, vaccines should be given by the recommended route.

For intramuscular (IM) injections, the choice of site is based on the volume of the injected material and the size of the muscle. In children younger than 1 year of age (ie, infants), the anterolateral aspect of the thigh provides the largest muscle and is the preferred site. In older children, the deltoid muscle is usually large enough for IM injection. Some physicians prefer to use the anterolateral thigh muscles for toddlers. Parents and children, however, often prefer use of the deltoid muscle for immunization at 18 months of age and older because it is associated with less pain in the affected extremity when ambulating.

Ordinarily, the upper, outer aspect of the buttocks should not be used for active immunization, because the gluteal region is covered by a significant layer of subcutaneous fat and because of the possibility of damaging the sciatic nerve. However, clinical information on the use of this area is limited. Because of diminished immunogenicity, hepatitis B and rabies vaccines should not be given in the buttocks at any age. People who were given hepatitis B vaccine in the buttocks should be tested for immunity and reimmunized if antibody concentrations are inadequate (see Hepatitis B, p 318).

When the upper, outer quadrant of the buttocks is used for large-volume passive immunization, such as IM administration of large volumes of Immune Globulin (IG), care must be taken to avoid injury to the sciatic nerve. The site selected should be well into the upper, outer mass of the gluteus maximus, away from the central region of the buttocks, and the needle should be directed anteriorly, that is, if the patient is lying prone, the needle is directed perpendicular to the table's surface, not perpendicular to the skin plane. The ventrogluteal site may be less hazardous for IM injection, because it is free of major nerves and vessels. This site is the center of a triangle for which the boundaries are the anterior superior iliac spine, the tubercle of the iliac crest, and the upper border of the greater trochanter.

Vaccines containing adjuvants (eg, aluminum-adsorbed DTaP, diphtheria and tetanus toxoids for children younger than 7 years of age [DT], diphtheria and tetanus toxoids for children 7 years of age or older and adults [Td], hepatitis B, and hepatitis A) must be injected deep into the muscle mass. These vaccines should not be administered subcutaneously or intracutaneously, because they can cause local irritation, inflammation, granuloma formation, and tissue necrosis. Immune Globulin, Rabies Immune Globulin (RIG), Hepatitis B Immune Globulin, and other similar products for passive immunoprophylaxis also are injected intramuscularly except when RIG is infiltrated around the site of a bite wound.

The needles used for IM injections should be long enough to reach the muscle mass to prevent vaccine from seeping into subcutaneous tissue and, therefore, minimize local reactions and not so long as to involve underlying nerves, blood vessels, or bone. For newborn infants, especially preterm infants, a ⅝-inch long needle usually is adequate. A ⅞- to 1-inch-long needle is recommended to ensure penetration of the thigh muscle of full-term infants 2 to 12 months of age. For injection into the thigh or deltoid muscle in toddlers and older children, a ⅞- to 1¼-inch-long needle is suggested, depending on the size of the muscle. The deltoid is preferred for immunization of adolescents and young adults. The needle length should be 1 to 2 inches, depending on the vaccine recipient's weight (1 inch for females <70 kg; 1.5 inches for females 70–100 kg; 1 to 1.5 inches for males ≤120 kg; and 2 inches for males >120 kg and females >100 kg). A 22- to 25-gauge needle is appropriate for injection of most IM vaccines.

Serious complications resulting from IM injections are rare. Reported adverse events include broken needles, muscle contracture, nerve injury, bacterial (staphylococcal, streptococcal, and clostridial) abscesses, sterile abscesses, skin pigmentation, hemorrhage, cellulitis, tissue necrosis, gangrene, local atrophy, periostitis, cyst or scar formation, and inadvertent injection into a joint space.

Subcutaneous (SC) injections can be administered at a 45° angle into the anterolateral aspect of the thigh or the upper outer triceps area by inserting the needle in a pinched-up fold of skin and SC tissue. A 23- or 25-gauge needle, ⅝ to ¾ inch long is recommended. Immune responses after SC administration of hepatitis B or recombinant rabies vaccine are decreased compared with those after IM administration of either of these vaccines; therefore, these vaccines should not be given subcutaneously. In patients with a bleeding diathesis, the risk of bleeding after IM injection can be minimized by vaccine administration immediately after the patient's receipt of replacement factor, use of a 23-gauge (or smaller) needle, and immediate application of direct pressure to the immunization site for at least 2 minutes. Certain vaccines (eg, Hib vaccines except PRP-OMP [PedvaxHIB]) recommended for IM injection may be given subcutaneously to people at risk of hemorrhage after IM injection, such as people with hemophilia. For these vaccines, immune responses and clinical reactions after IM or SC injection generally have been reported to be similar.

Intradermal (ID) injections usually are given on the volar surface of the forearm. Because of the decreased antigenic mass administered with ID injections, attention to technique is essential to ensure that material is not injected subcutaneously. A 25- or 27-gauge needle is recommended.

A patient should be restrained adequately if indicated before any injection.

When multiple vaccines are administered, separate sites ordinarily should be used if possible, especially if one of the vaccines contains DTaP. When necessary, 2 vaccines can be given in the same limb at a single visit. The anterolateral aspect of the thigh is the preferred site for 2 simultaneous IM injections because of its greater muscle mass. The distance separating the 2 injections is arbitrary but should be at least 1 inch so that local reactions are unlikely to overlap. Multiple vaccines should not be mixed in a single syringe unless specifically licensed and labeled for administration in 1 syringe. A different needle and syringe should be used for each injection.

Although most experts recommend "aspiration" by gently pulling back on the syringe before the injection is given, there are no data to document the necessity for this procedure. If blood appears after negative pressure, the needle should be withdrawn and another site should be selected using a new needle.

A brief period of bleeding at the injection site is common and usually can be controlled by applying gentle pressure.

Managing Injection Pain

Concerns and resulting anxiety about injections are common at any age. Current immunization schedules sometimes require children to receive 4 or more injections during a single visit. Although most children older than 5 years of age usually accept immunization with minimal opposition, some children react vigorously or refuse to receive injections. Effective practical techniques can be used to ameliorate some discomfort of injections.

A planned approach to managing the child before, during, and after immunization is helpful for children of any age. Truthful and empathetic preparation for injections is beneficial. Parents should be advised not to threaten children with injections or use them as a punishment for inappropriate behavior.

If possible, parents should have a role in comforting their child rather than in restraining them. For younger children, parents may soothe, stroke, and calm the child. For older children, parents should be coached to distract the child (see Nonpharmacologic Techniques, p 21).

INJECTION TECHNIQUE AND POSITION

A rapid plunge of the needle through the skin may decrease discomfort associated with skin penetration. The Z-track method of injection also is reported to decrease associated pain; traction is applied to the skin and subcutaneous tissues before insertion of the needle and released after the needle is withdrawn so that the injection track superficial to the muscle is displaced from the track within the muscle to seal vaccine into the muscle. The limb should be positioned to allow relaxation of the muscle to be injected. For the deltoid, some flexion of the arm may be required. For the anterolateral thigh, some degree of internal rotation may be helpful. Infants may exhibit less pain behavior when held on the lap of a parent or other caregiver. Older children may be more comfortable sitting on a parent's lap or examination table edge, hugging their parent chest to chest while an immunization is administered.

If multiple injections are to be given, having different health care professionals administer them simultaneously at multiple sites (eg, right and left anterolateral thighs) may lessen anticipation of the next injection. Allowing older children some choice in selecting the injection site may be helpful by allowing a degree of control.

TOPICAL ANESTHETIC TECHNIQUES

Some physical techniques and topically applied agents reduce the pain of injection. Applying pressure at the site for 10 seconds before injection reduces the pain of injection. Ice provides only 1 to 2 seconds of analgesia at the injection site and, therefore, is not recommended. Local anesthetic agents may be administered by several routes. Eutectic mixture of local anesthetic (EMLA) cream applied topically under an occlusive dressing has been evaluated in placebo-controlled, randomized clinical trials and has been demonstrated to provide pain relief during the injection and for the next 24 hours. Because EMLA requires 1 hour to provide adequate anesthesia, planning is necessary, such as applying the cream before an office visit or immediately on arrival. Lidocaine also may be delivered by iontophoresis to a depth of 8 to 10 mm in approximately 10 minutes, but the electric current causes some discomfort. Vapocoolant spray provides rapid transient analgesia at the injection site and is inexpensive. Studies comparing EMLA and vapocoolant spray at the time of administration demonstrate comparable efficacy.

Additional studies need to be performed on the use of local anesthetic agents to better establish their safety and effectiveness when used to manage injection pain and to ensure that their use does not interfere with the immune response, particularly to SC injections.

NONPHARMACOLOGIC TECHNIQUES

Sucrose placed on the tongue or on a pacifier ameliorates discomfort in newborn infants but has little effect beyond the immediate postnatal period. Stroking or rocking a child after an injection decreases crying and other pain behaviors. For older children, breathing and distraction techniques, such as "blowing the pain away"; use of "party blowers," pinwheels, or soap bubbles; telling children stories; reading books; or use of music, are all effective. Techniques that involve the child in a fantasy or reframe the experience with the use of suggestion ("magic love" or "pain switch") also are effective but may require training.

The younger the child, the greater the reliance on injection techniques and pharmacologic approaches. As the child becomes older, distraction and other psychologic approaches, in addition to pharmacologic and technical approaches to pain reduction, are increasingly effective.

Scheduling Immunizations

A vaccine is intended to be administered to a person who is capable of an appropriate immunologic response and who likely will benefit from the protection given. However, optimal immunologic response for the person must be balanced against the need to achieve effective protection against disease. For example, pertussis-containing vaccines may be less immunogenic in early infancy than in later infancy, but the benefit of conferring protection in young infants dictates that immunization should be given early despite a lessened serum antibody response. For this reason, in some developing countries, OPV vaccine is given at birth, in accordance with recommendations of the World Health Organization.

With parenterally administered live-virus vaccines, the inhibitory effect of residual specific maternal antibody determines the optimal age of administration. For example, live-virus measles vaccine in use in the United States provides suboptimal rates of seroconversion during the first year of life mainly because of interference by transplacentally acquired maternal antibody. If a measles-containing vaccine is administered before 12 months of age, the child should be reimmunized at 12 to 15 months of age with MMR; a third dose is indicated at 4 to 6 years of age.

An additional factor in selecting an immunization schedule is the need to achieve a uniform and regular response. With some products, a response is achieved after 1 dose. For example, live-virus rubella vaccine evokes a predictable response at high rates after a single dose. A single dose of some vaccines confers less-than-optimal response in the recipient. As a result, several doses are needed to complete primary immunization. For example, some people respond only to 1 or 2 types of poliovirus(es) after a single dose of poliovirus vaccine, so multiple doses are given to produce antibody against all 3 types, thereby ensuring complete protection for the person and maximum response rates for the population. For some vaccines, periodic booster doses (eg, with tetanus and diphtheria toxoids) are administered to maintain immunologic protection.

Most vaccines are safe and effective when administered simultaneously, although limited data are available for some products. This information is particularly important for scheduling immunizations for children with lapsed or missed immunizations and for people preparing for international travel (see Simultaneous Administration of Multiple Vaccines, p 33). Inactivated vaccines do not interfere with the immune response to other inactivated vaccines or to live vaccines (Table 1.5, p 23). Limited data indicate possible impaired immune responses when 2 or more live-virus vaccines are given nonsimultaneously but within 28 days of each other; therefore, parenterally administered live-virus vaccines not administered on the same day should be given at least 28 days (4 weeks) apart whenever possible.

The recommended childhood and adolescent immunization schedule in Fig 1.1 (p 24) represents a consensus of the American Academy of Pediatrics (AAP), the Advisory Committee on Immunization Practices (ACIP) of the Centers for Disease Control and Prevention (CDC), and the American Academy of Family Physicians for routine childhood immunizations in the year 2003. This schedule is reviewed regularly, and an updated national schedule is issued annually in January to incorporate new vaccines and revised recommendations. Special attention should be given to footnotes on the schedule, because they summarize major recommendations for routine childhood immunizations. Combination vaccine products may be given whenever any component of the combination is indicated and its other components are not contraindicated, provided they are licensed by the FDA for the child's age.* The use of licensed combination vaccines is preferred over separate injection of their component vaccines. A Web-based childhood immunization scheduler using the current vaccine recommendations is available for parents, caregivers, and health care professionals to make instant immunization schedules for any child 5 years of age or younger (www.cdc.gov/nip). An adult immunization schedule also is available.†

Table 1.6 (p 26) gives the recommended schedule for children who were not immunized appropriately during the first year of life.

For children in whom early or rapid immunization is urgent or for children not immunized on schedule, simultaneous immunization with multiple products allows for more rapid protection. In addition, in some circumstances, immunization can be initiated earlier than at the usually recommended ages and doses can be given at shorter intervals than are recommended routinely (for guidelines, see Table 1.7 [p 29] and the immunization recommendations in the disease-specific chapters in Section 3).

---

* American Academy of Pediatrics, Committee on Infectious Diseases. Combination vaccines for childhood immunization: recommendations of the Advisory Committee on Immunization Practices (ACIP), the American Academy of Pediatrics (AAP), and the American Academy of Family Physicians (AAFP). *Pediatrics.* 1999;103:1064–1077

† Centers for Disease Control and Prevention. Recommended adult immunization schedule— United States, 2002-2003. *MMWR Morb Mortal Wkly Rep.* 2002;51:904–908

Table 1.5. **Guidelines for Spacing of Live and Inactivated Antigens**

Antigen Combination	Recommended Minimum Interval Between Doses
≥2 inactivated	None; can be administered simultaneously or at any interval between doses
Inactivated and live	None; can be administered simultaneously or at any interval between doses
≥2 live parenteral[1]	28-day minimum interval, if not administered simultaneously

[1] Some live oral vaccines (eg, Ty21a typhoid vaccine, oral poliovirus vaccine) can be administered simultaneously or at any interval before or after inactivated or live parenteral vaccines.

The immunization schedule used in the United States may not be appropriate for developing countries because of different disease risks, age-specific immune responses, and vaccine availability. The schedule recommended by the Expanded Programme on Immunization of the World Health Organization should be consulted (www.who.org). Modifications may be made by the ministries of health in individual countries on the basis of local considerations.

Minimum Ages and Minimum Intervals Between Vaccine Doses

Immunizations are recommended for members of the youngest age group at risk of experiencing the disease for whom efficacy, immunogenicity, and safety have been demonstrated. Most vaccines in the childhood and adolescent immunization schedule require 2 or more doses for stimulation of an adequate and persisting antibody response. Studies have demonstrated that the recommended age and interval between doses of the same antigen(s) provide optimal protection and efficacy. Table 1.7 shows the recommended minimum ages and intervals between immunizations for vaccines in the recommended childhood immunization schedule. Administering doses of a multidose vaccine at intervals shorter than those in the recommended childhood and adolescent immunization schedule might be necessary in circumstances in which an infant or child is behind schedule and needs to be brought to date quickly or when international travel is pending. In these cases, an accelerated schedule using minimum age or interval criteria can be used. These accelerated schedules should not be used routinely.

Vaccines should not be administered at intervals less than the recommended minimum or at an earlier age than the recommended minimum (eg, accelerated schedules). Two exceptions to this may occur. The first is for measles vaccine during a measles outbreak, in which case the vaccine may be administered before 12 months of age. However, if a measles-containing vaccine is administered before 12 months of age, the dose is not counted and the child should be reimmunized at 12 to 15 months of age with MMR vaccine (see Measles, p 424). The second consideration involves administering a dose a few days earlier than the minimum interval or age, which is unlikely to have a substantially negative effect on the immune response to that dose. Although immunizations should not be scheduled at an interval or age less than the minimums shown in Table 1.7 (p 29), a child may be in the office early or for an

Figure 1.1. **Childhood and Adolescent Immunization Schedule**

Recommended Childhood and Adolescent Immunization Schedule -- United States, 2003

Legend: range of recommended ages | catch-up vaccination | preadolescent assessment

Vaccine ▶ / Age ▶	Birth	1 mo	2 mos	4 mos	6 mos	12 mos	15 mos	18 mos	24 mos	4-6 yrs	11-12 yrs	13-18 yrs
Hepatitis B[1]	HepB #1 (only if mother HBsAg (-))	HepB #2	HepB #2		HepB #3						HepB series	HepB series
Diphtheria, Tetanus, Pertussis[2]			DTaP	DTaP	DTaP		DTaP	DTaP		DTaP	Td	Td
Haemophilus influenzae Type b[3]			Hib	Hib	Hib	Hib	Hib					
Inactivated Polio			IPV	IPV	IPV	IPV	IPV			IPV		
Measles, Mumps, Rubella[4]						MMR #1	MMR #1			MMR #2	MMR #2	MMR #2
Varicella[5]						Varicella	Varicella	Varicella		Varicella	Varicella	
Pneumococcal[6]			PCV	PCV	PCV	PCV	PCV		PCV	PCV	PPV	PPV
Hepatitis A[7]									Hepatitis A series	Hepatitis A series	Hepatitis A series	Hepatitis A series
Influenza[8]					Influenza (yearly)	Influenza (yearly)	Influenza (yearly)	Influenza (yearly)	Influenza (yearly)	Influenza (yearly)	Influenza (yearly)	Influenza (yearly)

Vaccines below this line are for selected populations

This schedule indicates the recommended ages for routine administration of currently licensed childhood vaccines, as of December 1, 2002, for children through age 18 years. Any dose not given at the recommended age should be given at any subsequent visit when indicated and feasible. ▨ Indicates age groups that warrant special effort to administer those vaccines not previously given. Additional vaccines may be licensed and recommended during the year. Licensed combination vaccines may be used whenever any components of the combination are indicated and the vaccine's other components are not contraindicated. Providers should consult the manufacturers' package inserts for detailed recommendations.

(For necessary footnotes and important information, see next page.)

Figure 1.1. **Childhood and Adolescent Immunization Schedule, continued**

1. Hepatitis B vaccine (HepB). All infants should receive the first dose of hepatitis B vaccine soon after birth and before hospital discharge; the first dose may also be given by age 2 months if the infant's mother is HBsAg-negative. Only monovalent HepB can be used for the birth dose. Monovalent or combination vaccine containing HepB may be used to complete the series. Four doses of vaccine may be administered when a birth dose is given. The second dose should be given at least 4 weeks after the first dose, except for combination vaccines which cannot be administered before age 6 weeks. The third dose should be given at least 16 weeks after the first dose and at least 8 weeks after the second dose. The last dose in the vaccination series (third or fourth dose) should not be administered before age 6 months.

Infants born to HBsAg-positive mothers should receive HepB and 0.5 mL Hepatitis B Immune Globulin (HBIG) within 12 hours of birth at separate sites. The second dose is recommended at age 1-2 months. The last dose in the vaccination series should not be administered before age 6 months. These infants should be tested for HBsAg and anti-HBs at 9-15 months of age.

Infants born to mothers whose HBsAg status is unknown should receive the first dose of the HepB series within 12 hours of birth. Maternal blood should be drawn as soon as possible to determine the mother's HBsAg status; if the HBsAg test is positive, the infant should receive HBIG as soon as possible (no later than age 1 week). The second dose is recommended at age 1-2 months. The last dose in the vaccination series should not be administered before age 6 months.

2. Diphtheria and tetanus toxoids and acellular pertussis

vaccine (DTaP). The fourth dose of DTaP may be administered as early as age 12 months, provided 6 months have elapsed since the third dose and the child is unlikely to return at age 15-18 months. **Tetanus and diphtheria toxoids (Td)** is recommended at age 11-12 years if at least 5 years have elapsed since the last dose of tetanus and diphtheria toxoid-containing vaccine. Subsequent routine Td boosters are recommended every 10 years.

3. *Haemophilus influenzae* type b (Hib) conjugate vaccine. Three Hib conjugate vaccines are licensed for infant use. If PRP-OMP (PedvaxHIB® or ComVax® [Merck]) is administered at ages 2 and 4 months, a dose at age 6 months is not required. DTaP/Hib combination products should not be used for primary immunization in infants at ages 2, 4 or 6 months, but can be used as boosters following any Hib vaccine.

4. Measles, mumps, and rubella vaccine (MMR). The second dose of MMR is recommended routinely at age 4-6 years but may be administered during any visit, provided at least 4 weeks have elapsed since the first dose and that both doses are administered beginning at or after age 12 months. Those who have not previously received the second dose should complete the schedule by the 11-12 year old visit.

5. Varicella vaccine. Varicella vaccine is recommended at any visit at or after age 12 months for susceptible children, i.e. those who lack a reliable history of chickenpox. Susceptible persons aged ≥13 years should receive two doses, given at least 4 weeks apart.

6. Pneumococcal vaccine. The heptavalent **pneumococcal conjugate vaccine (PCV)** is recommended for all children age 2-23 months. It is also recommended for certain children age 24-59 months. **Pneumococcal polysaccharide vaccine (PPV)** is recommended in addition to PCV for certain high-risk groups. See *MMWR* 2000;49(RR-9);1-38.

7. Hepatitis A vaccine. Hepatitis A vaccine is recommended for children and adolescents in selected states and regions, and for certain high-risk groups; consult your local public health authority. Children and adolescents in these states, regions, and high risk groups who have not been immunized against hepatitis A can begin the hepatitis A vaccination series during any visit. The two doses in the series should be administered at least 6 months apart. See *MMWR* 1999;48(RR-12);1-37.

8. Influenza vaccine. Influenza vaccine is recommended annually for children age ≥6 months with certain risk factors (including but not limited to asthma, cardiac disease, sickle cell disease, HIV, diabetes, and household members of persons in groups at high risk; see *MMWR* 2002;51(RR-3);1-31), and can be administered to all others wishing to obtain immunity. In addition, healthy children age 6-23 months are encouraged to receive influenza vaccine if feasible because children in this age group are at substantially increased risk for influenza-related hospitalizations. Children aged ≤12 years should receive vaccine in a dosage appropriate for their age (0.25 mL if age 6-35 months or 0.5 mL if aged ≥3 years). Children aged ≤8 years who are receiving influenza vaccine for the first time should receive two doses separated by at least 4 weeks.

For additional information about vaccines, including precautions and contraindications for immunization and vaccine shortages, please visit the National Immunization Program Website at www.cdc.gov/nip or call the National Immunization Information Hotline at 800-232-2522 (English) or 800-232-0233 (Spanish).

Approved by the Advisory Committee on Immunization Practices (www.cdc.gov/nip/acip), the American Academy of Pediatrics (www.aap.org), and the American Academy of Family Physicians (www.aafp.org).

Table 1.6. **Catch-up Immunization Schedules for Children and Adolescents Who Start Late or Who Are >1 Month Behind***

| Dose 1 (Minimum Age) | Children 4 Months Through 6 Years of Age | | | |
| | Minimum Interval Between Doses | | | |
	Dose 1 to Dose 2	Dose 2 to Dose 3	Dose 3 to Dose 4	Dose 4 to Dose 5
DTaP (6 wk)	4 wk	4 wk	6 mo	6 mo[1]
IPV (6 wk)	4 wk	4 wk	4 wk[2]	
HepB[3] (birth)	4 wk	3 wk (and 16 wk after first dose)		
MMR (12 mo)	4 wk[4]			
Varicella (12 mo)				
Hib[5] (6 wk)	**4 wk:** if first dose given at younger than 12 mo of age / **8 wk (as final dose):** if first dose given at 12 to 14 mo of age / **No further doses needed:** if first dose given at 15 mo of age or older	**4 wk[6]:** if current age younger than 12 mo / **8 wk (as final dose)[6]:** if current age 12 mo or older and second dose given at younger than 15 mo of age / **No further doses needed:** if previous dose given at 15 mo of age or older	**8 wk (as final dose):** this dose only necessary for children 12 mo to 5 y of age who received 3 doses before 12 mo of age	
PCV[7]: (6 wk)	**4 wk:** if first dose given at younger than 12 mo of age and current age younger than 24 mo / **8 wk (as final dose):** if first dose given at 12 mo of age or older or current age 24 to 59 mo / **No further doses needed:** for healthy children if first dose given at 24 mo of age or older	**4 wk:** if current age younger than 12 mo / **8 wk (as final dose):** if current age 12 mo or older / **No further doses needed:** for healthy children if previous dose given at 24 mo of age or older	**8 wk (as final dose):** this dose only necessary for children 12 mo to 5 y of age who received 3 doses before 12 mo of age	

Table 1.6. **Catch-up Immunization Schedules for Children and Adolescents Who Start Late or Who Are >1 Month Behind,** * **continued**

Children 7 Through 18 Years of Age		
Minimum Interval Between Doses		
Dose 1 to Dose 2	Dose 2 to Dose 3	Dose 3 to Booster Dose
Td: **4 wk**	Td: **6 mo**	Td[8]: **6 mo:** if first dose given at younger than 12 mo of age and current age younger than 11 y **5 y:** if first dose given at 12 mo of age or older and third dose given at younger than 7 y of age and current age 11 y or older **10 y:** if third dose given at 7 y of age or older
IPV[9]: **4 wk**	IPV[9]: **4 wk**	IPV[2,9]
HepB: **4 wk**	HepB: **8 wk** (and 16 wk after first dose)	
MMR: **4 wk**		
Varicella[10]: **4 wk**		

* Catch-up schedules and minimum intervals between doses for children who have delayed immunizations. There is no need to restart a vaccine series regardless of the time that has elapsed between doses. Use the chart appropriate for the child's age. For additional information about vaccines, including precautions and contraindications for immunization and vaccine shortages, please visit the National Immunization Program Web site at www.cdc.gov/nip or call the National Immunization Information Hotline at 800-232-2522 (English) or 800-232-0233 (Spanish). Report adverse reactions to vaccines through the federal Vaccine Adverse Event Reporting System. For information on reporting reactions following vaccines, please visit www.vaers.org or call the 24-hour national toll-free information line at 800-822-7967. Report suspected cases of vaccine-preventable diseases to your state or the local health department.

[1] Diphtheria and tetanus toxoids and acellular pertussis (DTaP) vaccine: The fifth dose is not necessary if the fourth dose was given after the fourth birthday.

[2] Inactivated poliovirus (IPV) vaccine: For children who received an all-IPV or all-OPV series, a fourth dose is not necessary if third dose was given at 4 years of age or older. If both OPV and IPV were given as part of a series, a total of 4 doses should be given, regardless of the child's current age.

[3] Hepatitis B (HepB) vaccine: All children and adolescents who have not been immunized against hepatitis B should begin the hepatitis B immunization series during any visit. Providers should make special efforts to immunize children who were born in, or whose parents were born in, areas of the world where hepatitis B virus infection is moderately or highly endemic.

Table 1.6. Catch-up Immunization Schedules for Children and Adolescents Who Start Late or Who Are >1 Month Behind,* continued

[4] Measles-mumps-rubella (MMR) vaccine: The second dose of MMR is recommended routinely at 4 to 6 years of age but may be given earlier if desired.

[5] *Haemophilus influenzae* type b (Hib) vaccine: Vaccine generally is not recommended for children 5 years of age or older.

[6] Hib: If current age younger than 12 months and the first 2 doses were PRP-OMP (PedvaxHIB or ComVax [Merck Vaccine Division, West Point, PA]), the third (and final) dose should be given at 12 to 15 months of age and at least 8 weeks after the second dose.

[7] Pneumococcal conjugate vaccine (PCV): Vaccine generally is not recommended for children 5 years of age or older.

[8] Tetanus and diphtheria toxoids (Td) vaccine: For children 7 to 10 years of age, the interval between the third and booster dose is determined by the age when the first dose was given. For adolescents 11 to 18 years of age, the interval is determined by the age when the third dose was given.

[9] IPV: Vaccine generally is not recommended for people 18 years of age or older.

[10] Varicella: Give 2-dose series to all susceptible adolescents 13 years of age or older.

Table 1.7. Recommended and Minimum Ages and Intervals Between Vaccine Doses[1]

Vaccine and Dose Number	Recommended Age for This Dose	Minimum Age for This Dose	Recommended Interval to Next Dose	Minimum Interval to Next Dose
Hepatitis B1[2]	Birth–2 mo	Birth	1–4 mo	4 wk
Hepatitis B2	1–4 mo	4 wk	2–17 mo	8 wk
Hepatitis B3[3]	6–18 mo	6 mo[4]	—	—
Diphtheria and tetanus toxoids and acellular pertussis (DTaP)1[2]	2 mo	6 wk	2 mo	4 wk
DTaP2	4 mo	10 wk	2 mo	4 wk
DTaP3	6 mo	14 wk	6–12 mo	6 mo[4,5]
DTaP4	15–18 mo	12 mo	3 y	6 mo[4]
DTaP5	4–6 y	4 y	—	—
Haemophilus influenzae type b (Hib)1[2,6]	2 mo	6 wk	2 mo	4 wk
Hib2	4 mo	10 wk	2 mo	4 wk
Hib3[7]	6 mo	14 wk	6–9 mo	8 wk
Hib4	12–15 mo	12 mo	—	—
Inactivated poliovirus (IPV)1[2]	2 mo	6 wk	2 mo	4 wk
IPV2	4 mo	10 wk	2–14 mo	4 wk
IPV3	6–18 mo	14 wk	3.5 y	4 wk
IPV4	4–6 y	18 wk	—	—
Pneumococcal conjugate vaccine (PCV)1[6]	2 mo	6 wk	2 mo	4 wk
PCV2	4 mo	10 wk	2 mo	4 wk

Table 1.7. Recommended and Minimum Ages and Intervals Between Vaccine Doses,[1] continued

Vaccine and Dose Number	Recommended Age for This Dose	Minimum Age for This Dose	Recommended Interval to Next Dose	Minimum Interval to Next Dose
PCV3	6 mo	14 wk	6 mo	8 wk
PCV4	12–15 mo	12 mo	—	—
Measles-mumps-rubella (MMR)1	12–15 mo[8]	12 mo	3–5 y	4 wk
MMR2	4–6 y	13 mo	—	—
Varicella[9]	12–15 mo	12 mo	4 wk[9]	4 wk[9]
Hepatitis A1	≥2 y	2 y	6–18 mo[4]	6 mo[4]
Hepatitis A2	≥30 mo	30 mo	—	—
Influenza[10]	—	6 mo[4]	1 mo	4 wk
Pneumococcal polysaccharide vaccine (PPV)1	—	2 y	5 y[11]	5 y
PPV2	—	7 y[11]	—	—

[1] Combination vaccines are available. Using licensed combination vaccines is preferred over separate injections of their equivalent component vaccines (Source: Centers for Disease Control and Prevention. Combination vaccines for childhood immunization: recommendations of the Advisory Committee on Immunization Practices (ACIP), the American Academy of Pediatrics (AAP), and the American Academy of Family Physicians (AAFP). *MMWR Recomm Rep.* 1999;48(RR-5):1–15). When administering combination vaccines, the minimum age for administration is the oldest age for any of the individual components; the minimum interval between doses is equal to the greatest interval of any of the individual antigens.

[2] A combination hepatitis B-Hib vaccine is available (Comvax, manufactured by Merck Vaccine Division, West Point, PA) and a combination DTaP/hepatitis B/IPV vaccine is available (Pediarix, manufactured by GlaxoSmithKline Biologicals, Rixensart, Belguim). These vaccines should not be administered to infants younger than 6 weeks of age.

[3] Hepatitis B3 should be administered ≥8 weeks after hepatitis B2 and 16 weeks after hepatitis B1, and it should not be administered before 6 months of age.

[4] Calendar months.

Table 1.7. **Recommended and Minimum Ages and Intervals Between Vaccine Doses,** [1] **continued**

5 The minimum interval between DTaP3 and DTaP4 is recommended to be ≥6 months. However, DTaP4 does not need to be repeated if administered ≥4 months after DTaP3.

6 For Hib and PCV, children receiving the first dose of vaccine at 7 months of age or older require fewer doses to complete the series (see Centers for Disease Control and Prevention. Haemophilus b conjugate vaccines for prevention of *Haemophilus influenzae*, type b disease among infants and children two months of age and older: recommendations of the ACIP. *MMWR Recomm Rep.* 1991;40(RR-1):1–7; and Centers for Disease Control and Prevention. Preventing pneumococcal disease among infants and young children: recommendations of the Advisory Committee on Immunization Practices [ACIP]. *MMWR Recomm Rep.* 2000;49(RR-9):1–38).

7 For a regimen of only polyribosylribitol phosphate-meningococcal outer membrane protein (PRP-OMP [PedvaxHIB, manufactured by Merck Vaccine Division, West Point, PA]), a dose administered at 6 months of age is not required.

8 During a measles outbreak, if cases are occurring among infants younger than 12 months of age, measles immunization of infants 6 months of age and older can be undertaken as an outbreak control measure. However, doses administered at younger than 12 months of age should not be counted as part of the series (Source: Centers for Disease Control and Prevention. Measles, mumps, and rubella—vaccine use and strategies for elimination of measles, rubella, and congenital rubella syndrome and control of mumps: recommendations of the Advisory Committee on Immunization Practices [ACIP]. *MMWR Recomm Rep.* 1998;47(RR-8):1–57).

9 Children 12 months to 13 years of age require only 1 dose of varicella vaccine. People 13 years of age and older should receive 2 doses separated by ≥4 weeks.

10 Two doses of inactivated influenza vaccine, separated by 4 weeks, are recommended for children 6 months to 9 years of age who are receiving the vaccine for the first time. Children 6 months to 9 years of age who have previously received influenza vaccine and people 9 years of age and older require only 1 dose per influenza season.

11 Second doses of PPV are recommended for people at highest risk of serious pneumococcal infection and those who are likely to have a rapid decrease in pneumococcal antibody concentration. Reimmunization 3 years after the previous dose can be considered for children at highest risk of severe pneumococcal infection who would be younger than 10 years of age at the time of reimmunization (see Centers for Disease Control and Prevention. Prevention of pneumococcal disease: recommendations of the Advisory Committee on Immunization Practices [ACIP]. *MMWR Recomm Rep.*1997;46(RR-8):1–24).

appointment not specifically for immunization (eg, recheck of otitis media). In this situation, the clinician can consider administering the vaccine before the minimum interval or age. If the child is known to the clinician, rescheduling the child for immunization closer to the recommended interval is preferred. If the parent or child is not known to the clinician or follow-up cannot be ensured (eg, habitually misses appointments), administration of the vaccine at that visit rather than rescheduling the child for a later visit is preferable. Vaccine doses administered 4 days or fewer before the minimum interval or age can be counted as valid. This 4-day recommendation does not apply to rabies vaccine because of the unique schedule for this vaccine. Doses administered 5 days or more before the minimum interval or age should not be counted as valid doses and should be repeated as age appropriate. The repeat dose should be spaced after the invalid dose by a time greater than the recommended minimum interval shown in Table 1.7 (p 29). In certain situations, local or state requirements might mandate that doses of selected vaccines be administered on or after specific ages, precluding these 4-day recommendations.

Interchangeability of Vaccine Products

Similar vaccines made by different manufacturers may differ in the number and amount of their specific antigenic components and formulation of adjuvants and conjugating agents, thereby eliciting different degrees of immune response. However, such vaccines have been considered interchangeable by most experts when administered according to their licensed indications, although data documenting the effects of interchangeability are limited. Licensed vaccines that may be used interchangeably during a vaccine series from different manufacturers according to recommendations from the ACIP or AAP include diphtheria and tetanus toxoids vaccines, live and inactivated poliovirus vaccines, hepatitis A vaccines, hepatitis B vaccines, and rabies vaccines (see Rabies, p 514). An example of similar vaccines used in different schedules that are not recommended as interchangeable are the 2 hepatitis B vaccine options currently available for adolescents 11 through 15 years of age. Adolescent patients begun on a 3-dose hepatitis B regimen are not candidates to complete their series with hepatitis B vaccine used in the 2-dose protocol, and vice versa (see Hepatitis B, p 324).

Licensed Hib conjugate vaccines are considered interchangeable for primary as well as for booster immunization as long as recommendations concerning conversion from a 3-dose regimen (polyribosylribitol-outer membrane complex [PRP-OMC]) to a 4-dose regimen (all other conjugated PRP preparations) are adhered to (see *Haemophilus influenzae* Infections, p 297).

When feasible, the same DTaP vaccine product should be used for the first 3 doses of a pertussis immunization series (see Pertussis, p 476). Minimal data on safety and immunogenicity and no data on efficacy are available for different DTaP vaccines when administered interchangeably in the primary series. However, in circumstances in which the type of DTaP product(s) received previously is not known or the previously administered product(s) is not readily available, any of the DTaP vaccines licensed for use in the primary series may be used. For the fourth and fifth doses of DTaP, any licensed product is acceptable, regardless of previous DTaP or diphtheria and tetanus toxoids and whole-cell pertussis vaccines received. For interchangeability of the DTaP, hepatitis B, and inactivated poliovirus combination vaccine, see Pertussis, p 479. These recommendations may change as additional data become available.

Simultaneous Administration of Multiple Vaccines

Most vaccines can be safely and effectively administered simultaneously. No contraindications to the simultaneous administration of multiple vaccines routinely recommended for infants and children are known. Immune responses to one vaccine generally do not interfere with those to other vaccines. An exception is a decrease in immunogenicity when cholera and yellow fever vaccines are given together or 1 to 3 weeks apart. Simultaneous administration of IPV, MMR, varicella, or DTaP vaccines results in rates of seroconversion and of adverse effects similar to those observed when the vaccines are administered at separate visits. Because simultaneous administration of common vaccines is not known to affect the efficacy or safety of any of the recommended childhood vaccines, simultaneous administration of all vaccines, including DTaP, IPV, MMR, varicella, hepatitis A, hepatitis B, Hib, and pneumococcal conjugate and polysaccharide vaccines that are appropriate for the age and previous immunization status of the recipient, is recommended. When simultaneous vaccines are administered, separate syringes and sites should be used, and injections into the same extremity should be separated by at least 1 inch so that any local reactions can be differentiated. Simultaneous administration of multiple vaccines can increase immunization rates significantly. Individual vaccines should never be mixed in the syringe unless they are specifically licensed and labeled for administration in one syringe. For people preparing for international travel, multiple vaccines generally can be given concurrently.

Lapsed Immunizations

A lapse in the immunization schedule does not require reinstitution of the entire series. If a dose of DTaP, IPV, Hib, pneumococcal conjugate, hepatitis A, or hepatitis B vaccine is missed, subsequent immunizations should be given at the next visit as if the usual interval had elapsed. The medical charts of children in whom immunizations have been missed or postponed should be flagged to remind health care professionals to resume the child's immunization regimen at the next available opportunity. Minimum age and interval criteria should be adhered to for administration of all doses (see Table 1.7, p 29).

Unknown or Uncertain Immunization Status

A physician may encounter children with an uncertain immunization status. Many children, adolescents, and young adults do not have adequate documentation of their immunizations. Parent or guardian recollection of a child's immunization history and the specific vaccines used may not be accurate. In general, when in doubt, these people should be considered disease susceptible, and appropriate immunizations should be initiated without delay on a schedule commensurate with the person's current age. There is no evidence that administration of MMR, varicella,

Hib, hepatitis A, hepatitis B, or poliovirus vaccine to already immune recipients is harmful; Td, rather than DTaP, should be given to those 7 years of age or older (see Pertussis, p 476). Reimmunization with multiple doses of DTaP may result in increased rates of local reactions, including swollen limb reactions; serologic testing for specific antibody to tetanus and diphtheria toxins may be performed before administering additional doses (see Medical Evaluation of Internationally Adopted Children, p 178).

Immunizations Received Outside the United States

People immunized in other countries, including internationally adopted children, refugees, and exchange students, should be immunized according to recommended schedules in the United States for healthy infants, children, and adolescents (see Fig 1.1, p 24, and Table 1.6, p 26). In general, only written documentation should be accepted as evidence of previous immunization. Written records may be considered valid if the vaccines, dates of administration, numbers of doses, intervals between doses, and age of the patient at the time of immunization are comparable with that of the current US schedule. Although some vaccines with inadequate potency have been produced in other countries, most vaccines used worldwide are produced with adequate quality control standards and are reliable. However, immunization records for certain children, especially for those from an orphanage, may not accurately reflect protection because of inaccuracies, lack of vaccine potency, or other problems, such as recording MMR but giving a product that did not contain one of the components (eg, rubella). Therefore, it may be reasonable to ascertain antibody titers for these children. For any child who has received immunizations outside the United States, if any question exists about whether immunizations were administered or were immunogenic, the best course is to repeat the injection of the immunizations in question (see Medical Evaluation of Internationally Adopted Children, p 178).

Vaccine Dose

Reduced or divided doses of DTaP or any other vaccine, including those given to premature or low birth weight infants, should not be administered. The efficacy of this practice in decreasing the frequency of adverse events has not been demonstrated. Also, such a practice may confer less protection against disease than that achieved with recommended doses. A diminished antibody response in both term and premature infants to reduced doses of diphtheria and tetanus and pertussis (DTP) vaccine has been reported. A previous immunization with a dose that was less than the standard dose or one administered by a nonstandard route should not be counted, and the person should be reimmunized as appropriate for age. Exceeding recommended doses also may be hazardous. Excessive local concentrations of injectable inactivated vaccines might result in enhanced tissue or systemic reactions, whereas administering an increased dose of a live vaccine constitutes a theoretic but unproven risk.

Active Immunization of People Who Recently Received Immune Globulin

Live-virus vaccines may have diminished immunogenicity when given shortly before or during the several months after receipt of IG. In particular, IG administration has been demonstrated to inhibit the response to measles vaccine for a prolonged period. Inhibition of immune response to rubella vaccine also has been demonstrated. The appropriate suggested interval between IG administration and measles immunization will vary with the indication for, and dose of, IG and the specific product; suggested intervals are given in Table 3.33 (p 423). If IG must be given within 14 days after administration of measles or measles-containing vaccines, these live-virus vaccines should be administered again after the period specified in Table 3.33 (p 423) unless serologic testing at an appropriate interval after IG administration indicates that adequate serum antibodies were produced.

The effect of administration of IG on antibody response to varicella vaccine is not known. Because of potential inhibition, varicella vaccine administration should be delayed after receipt of an IG preparation or a blood product (except washed Red Blood Cells), as recommended for measles vaccine (see Table 3.33, p 423). In addition, IG preparations ideally should not be administered for 14 days after immunization. If an IG preparation is given in this interval, the vaccine recipient should be reimmunized after the period specified in Table 3.33 (p 423) or tested for varicella immunity at that time and reimmunized if seronegative. Administration of IG preparations does not interfere with antibody responses to yellow fever or OPV vaccines. Hence, OPV and yellow fever vaccines can be administered simultaneously with or at any time before or after IG.

In contrast with live-virus vaccines, administration of IG preparations has not been demonstrated to cause significant inhibition of the immune responses to inactivated vaccines and toxoids. Concurrent administration of recommended doses of Hepatitis B Immune Globulin, Tetanus Immune Globulin, or Rabies Immune Globulin and the corresponding inactivated vaccine or toxoid for postexposure prophylaxis does not impair the efficacy of vaccine and provides immediate and long-term immunity. Standard doses of the corresponding vaccines are recommended. Increases in vaccine dose volume or number of immunizations are not indicated. Vaccines should be administered at different sites from those of intramuscularly administered IG. For further information, see chapters on specific diseases in Section 3.

Administration of hepatitis A vaccine together with IG has been recommended for situations in which immediate *and* prolonged protection against hepatitis A virus infection is desired. Although this combined active-passive immunization has been demonstrated to result in significantly lower serum antibody concentrations than those induced by vaccine administration alone, antibody concentrations still are high enough to be considered protective, and seroconversion rates are not affected.

A possible exception to the lack of inhibition of immune responses to inactivated vaccines may be the effect of Respiratory Syncytial Virus Immune Globulin Intravenous (RSV-IGIV) on antibody responses to some inactivated vaccines. However, data are inconclusive, and supplemental doses of these vaccines for RSV-IGIV recipients are not indicated. Other than deferring MMR and varicella vaccines, RSV-

IGIV recipients should be immunized according to the recommended schedule for routine childhood immunization (see Fig 1.1, p 24). The respiratory syncytial virus monoclonal antibody (palivizumab) does not interfere with response to inactivated or live vaccines.

Tuberculin Testing

Recommendations for tuberculin testing (see Tuberculosis, p 645) are independent of those for immunization. Tuberculin testing at any age is not required before administration of live-virus vaccines, such as MMR, varicella, or yellow fever. A tuberculin skin test can be applied at the same visit during which these vaccines are administered. Because measles vaccine temporarily can suppress tuberculin reactivity, if tuberculin testing is indicated and cannot be done at the same time as measles immunization, tuberculin testing should be postponed for 4 to 6 weeks. The effect of live-virus varicella and yellow fever vaccines on tuberculin skin test reactivity is not known.

Record Keeping and Immunization Registries

PATIENTS' PERSONAL IMMUNIZATION RECORDS

Each state health department has developed an official immunization record. This record should be given to parents of every newborn infant and should be accorded the status of a birth certificate or passport and retained with vital documents for subsequent referral. Physicians should cooperate with this endeavor by recording immunization data in this record and by encouraging patients not only to preserve the record, but also present it at each visit to a health care professional.

The immunization record is especially important for people who move frequently. It facilitates maintaining an accurate patient medical record, enables the physician to evaluate the child's immunization status, and fulfills the need for documentation of immunizations for child care and school attendance and for admission to other institutions and organizations.

Many states are developing state-based computerized immunization registries to record and track immunizations regardless of where in the state the immunization services are provided. In the course of receiving recommended routine immunizations, children encounter an average of 3 different health care professionals. Registry databases can be used to help remind parents and health care professionals when immunizations are due or overdue and to help health care professionals determine the immunization needs of their patients at each visit. Registries also will serve to measure immunization coverage. The AAP urges physicians to cooperate with state and local health officials in providing immunization information for state registry systems. Until such registries are functioning reliably, parents and physicians must rely on the personal immunization record to document each child's immunization status.

PHYSICIANS' IMMUNIZATION RECORDS

Every physician should ensure that the immunization history of each patient is maintained in a permanent confidential record that can be reviewed easily and updated when subsequent immunizations are administered. The medical record maintained by the primary health care professional should document all vaccines received, including those received in another health care setting. The format of the record should facilitate identification and recall of patients in need of immunization.

Records of children whose immunizations have been delayed or missed should be flagged to indicate the need to complete immunizations. For data that are required by the National Childhood Vaccine Injury Act of 1986, as well as data recommended by the AAP to be recorded in each patient's medical record for each immunization, see Informing Patients and Parents (p 4).

Vaccine Shortages

An unprecedented shortage of vaccines in the recommended childhood and adolescent immunization schedule occurred in the United States beginning in 2001 and extending into 2003. These shortages involved 5 vaccines used to prevent 8 of the 11 vaccine-preventable childhood infectious diseases and were more severe in certain regions of the country than others. Because of these shortages, temporary changes in recommendations for immunizing children by the AAP, ACIP, and National Immunization Program at the CDC were necessary, including deferral of certain immunizations in some children, establishment of vaccine priorities for high-risk children, and suspension in some states of school and child care entry immunization requirements. Several national committees and organizations, including the National Vaccine Advisory Committee and the US General Accounting Office, have proposed comprehensive strategies to prevent future shortages and encourage key stakeholders to work together to develop corrective action.

When vaccines are in short supply, physicians and other health care professionals should maintain lists of children and adolescents who do not receive vaccines at the recommended time or age so they can be recalled when the vaccine supply becomes adequate. For additional information about vaccine shortages and resulting recommendations, see the Web sites of the National Immunization Program (www.cdc.gov/nip) or American Academy of Pediatrics (www.aap.org). For recent analyses of vaccine shortages, see the Web sites of the National Vaccine Program Office (www.cdc.gov/od/nvpo) and General Accounting Office (www.gao.gov).

Vaccine Safety and Contraindications

RISKS AND ADVERSE EVENTS

All licensed vaccines in the United States are safe and effective, but no vaccine is completely safe and effective in every person. Some vaccine recipients will have an adverse reaction, and some will not always be fully protected. The goal of vaccine development is to achieve the highest degree of protection with the lowest rate of adverse events.

Risks of immunization may vary from trivial and inconvenient to severe and life threatening. When developing immunization recommendations, vaccine benefits and safety are weighed against the risks of natural disease to the person and the community. Many families lack awareness of the continued threat of certain vaccine-preventable diseases (eg, pertussis and measles) in their community and the risk of tetanus among unimmunized people. Recommendations attempt to maximize protection and minimize risk by providing specific advice on dose, route, and timing of the vaccine and by delineating people who should be immunized and circumstances that warrant precaution or contraindicate immunization.

Common vaccine adverse events usually are mild to moderate in severity (eg, fever or local swelling, redness, and pain at the injection site) and without permanent sequelae. Because such reactions are intrinsic to the immunizing antigen or some other component of the vaccine, they occur frequently and are unavoidable. Examples include local inflammation after administration of DTaP vaccine and fever and rash 1 to 2 weeks after administration of MMR vaccine.

Sterile abscesses have occurred at the site of injection of several inactivated vaccines. These abscesses presumably result from an inflammatory response to the vaccine or its adjuvant; in some instances, they may be caused by inadvertent subcutaneous inoculation of a vaccine intended for intramuscular use. Administration of bacille Calmette-Guérin (BCG) vaccine often is followed by occurrence of local cysts, abscesses, and/or regional lymphadenopathy that will resolve spontaneously (see Tuberculosis, p 659).

Rarely, serious adverse effects of immunization occur, resulting in permanent sequelae or life-threatening illness. The occurrence of an adverse event after immunization does not prove that the vaccine caused the symptoms or signs. Vaccines are administered to infants and children during a period in their lives when certain conditions most commonly become clinically apparent (eg, seizure disorders). Because chance association of an adverse event to the timing of administration of a specific vaccine commonly occurs, a true causal association usually requires that the event occur at a significantly higher rate in vaccine recipients than in unimmunized groups of similar age and residence. Recovery of the vaccine virus from the ill child with compatible symptoms may provide support for a link with the vaccine (eg, vaccine-associated polio with OPV). For most live-virus vaccines, definitive causative association between the vaccine and a subsequent illness requires isolating the vaccine strain from the recipient, although isolation of a vaccine virus still could be a chance association.

Although a specific condition occurring in a single person after immunization does not provide sufficient evidence to establish that the condition was caused by the vaccine, reporting of adverse events after immunization to the Vaccine Adverse Event Reporting System (VAERS, see p 40) is important, because in conjunction with other reports, it may provide clues to an unanticipated adverse reaction. Children and adolescents who develop a vaccine-preventable disease anytime after immunization (vaccine failure) should be reported to the local or state health department and may be reported to the VAERS.

INSTITUTE OF MEDICINE IMMUNIZATION SAFETY REVIEW COMMITTEE

The CDC and the National Institutes of Health commissioned the National Academy of Sciences' Institute of Medicine (IOM) to convene an Immunization Safety Review Committee in 2000. This independent expert committee was charged with examining at least 9 hypotheses about existing and emerging immunization safety concerns through 2003. Through late 2002, the committee had reviewed the following hypotheses:

- That a link exists between MMR vaccine and autism
- That thimerosal-containing vaccines may contribute to neurodevelopmental disorders, such as autism, learning disabilities, and speech delays
- That multiple immunizations may be associated with immune system dysfunction, such as overload of the immune system
- That hepatitis B vaccine may be associated with demyelinating neurologic disorders
- That simian virus (SV)-40 contamination of poliovirus vaccine may be associated with cancer

Information about the IOM, reports of the Immunization Safety Review Committee, and other committee reviews can be found online (www.iom.edu/IOM/IOMHome.nsf/Pages/immunization+safety+review).

MMR vaccine and autism. In 2001, the IOM Immunization Safety Review Committee assessed the scientific plausibility of the hypothesis that MMR vaccine contributes to the onset of autistic spectrum disorder (ASD). The committee concluded that the recent increasing trends in autism diagnoses cannot be attributed to the MMR vaccine. Recognizing that scientific studies can never be absolute in their conclusions, the IOM recommended further research to explore the possibility that exposure to MMR vaccine could be a risk factor for ASD in rare cases. The committee also concluded that the existing recommendations for routine use of MMR at 12 to 15 months of age and 4 to 6 years of age should remain unchanged. The AAP also convened a panel of experts to review this issue before the IOM review, and the panel found that the available evidence does not support the hypothesis that MMR vaccine causes autism, associated disorders, or inflammatory bowel disease.*

Thimerosal and vaccines. The IOM Immunization Safety Review Committee examined the hypothesis that vaccines containing thimerosal could have caused specific neurodevelopmental disorders, including autism, attention-deficit/hyperactivity disorder, and speech or language delay. The committee concluded that the existing evidence was inadequate to accept or reject a causal relationship.

The committee stated, "While the health effects of thimerosal are uncertain, we know for sure that these vaccines protect against real, proven threats to unvaccinated infants, children, and pregnant women." By the end of 2001, all vaccines in the recommended childhood and adolescent immunization schedule contained no thimerosal or only trace amounts of thimerosal.

Multiple immunizations and immune dysfunction. The IOM Immunization Safety Review Committee evaluated the evidence bearing on the hypothesis that multiple immunizations increase the risk of immune dysfunction. Specific considerations were the epidemiologic evidence and potential biologic mechanisms related to infections, type 1 diabetes mellitus, and allergic disorders. The committee found that the epidemiologic evidence favored rejection of a causal relationship between multiple immunizations and increased risk of infections and developing type 1 diabetes mellitus. The epidemiologic evidence regarding risk of developing allergic disease, particularly asthma, was inadequate to accept or reject a causal relationship.

---

* Halsey NA, Hyman SL and the Conference Writing Panel. Measles-mumps-rubella vaccine and autistic spectrum disorder: report from the New Challenges in Immunizations Conference convened in Oak Brook, Illinois, June 12–13, 2000. *Pediatrics.* 2001;107(5). Available at: www.pediatrics.org/cgi/content/full/107/5/e84.

Hepatitis B vaccine and demyelinating neurologic disorders. The IOM
Immunization Safety Review Committee concluded that existing evidence favors
rejection of a causal relationship between hepatitis B vaccine administration to adults
and the incidence and relapse of multiple sclerosis. The committee concluded the
evidence to be inadequate to accept or reject a causal relationship between hepatitis
B vaccine and first episode of a central nervous system demyelinating disorder, acute
disseminated encephalomyelitis, optic neuritis, transverse myelitis, Guillain-Barré
syndrome, and brachial neuritis.

Simian virus-40 contamination of poliovirus vaccine and cancer. The IOM
Safety Review Committee concluded that the evidence was inadequate to determine
whether or not the contaminated poliovirus vaccine from 1955 to 1963 caused
cancer. Poliovirus vaccine used since 1963 has not contained SV-40.

THE BRIGHTON COLLABORATION

The Brighton Collaboration is an international voluntary collaboration formed
to develop globally accepted and standardized case definitions for adverse events
after immunization. These will be known as the Brighton Standardized Case
Definitions. The project began in 2000 with the formation of a steering committee
and the creation of the first 6 working groups. These groups are composed of
international volunteers with expertise in vaccine safety, patient care, pharmaceuticals, regulatory affairs, public health, and vaccine delivery. The guidelines for
interpreting, recording, and presenting safety data developed by the collaboration
will facilitate sharing and comparison of vaccine data among vaccine safety professionals worldwide. Additional information and updates of progress can be found
online (www.brightoncollaboration.org).

REPORTING OF ADVERSE EVENTS

Before administering a dose of any vaccine, parents and patients should be questioned about adverse events and possible reactions after previous doses. No recommendations can anticipate all possible adverse events, particularly with newly
licensed vaccines or a dose being administered as the first in a series. Unexpected
events occurring soon after administration of any vaccine, particularly those severe
enough to require medical attention, should be described in detail in the patient's
medical record, and a VAERS report should be made. There is no time limit for
reporting an adverse event. A possible reaction should be reported when it is recognized. The vaccine injury compensation table provides guidelines for adverse events
and time intervals (see Appendix IV, p 802).

The National Childhood Vaccine Injury Act of 1986 requires physicians and
other health care professionals who administer vaccines covered under the National
Vaccine Injury Compensation Program to maintain permanent immunization
records and to report occurrences of certain adverse events stipulated in the act
(see Appendix IV, p 802) to the VAERS.[*†] The vaccines to which these requirements, as of January 2003, apply are measles, mumps, rubella, varicella, poliovirus,

---

[*] See Appendix I, p 789.
[†] Centers for Disease Control and Prevention. Surveillance for safety after immunization: Vaccine
Adverse Event Reporting System (VAERS)—United States, 1999–2001. *MMWR Surveill Summ.*
2003;52(SS-1):1–24

hepatitis B, pertussis, diphtheria, tetanus, rotavirus, Hib, and pneumococcal conjugate vaccines (see Record Keeping and Immunization Registries, p 36).

Clinically significant adverse events other than those listed in Appendix IV (p 802), those occurring after administration of other vaccines, and vaccine failures (disease in an immunized person) also should be reported to the VAERS. Forms (see Fig 1.2, p 42) can be obtained from the VAERS, or reports can be submitted electronically (www.vaers.org).

All reports of possible adverse events after administration of any vaccine, regardless of the age of the recipient, are accepted. Submission of a report does not necessarily indicate that the vaccine caused the adverse event. All patient-identifying information is kept confidential. Written notification that the report has been received is provided to the person submitting the form. Staff from the VAERS will contact the reporter for follow-up of the patient's condition at 60 days and at 1 year after serious adverse events occur.

CLINICAL IMMUNIZATION SAFETY ASSESSMENT NETWORK

Clinically significant adverse events after immunization rarely occur in clinical trials, and health care professionals see them too infrequently to be able to provide standardized evaluation and management. The Clinical Immunization Safety Assessment (CISA) Network was established in 2001 to evaluate reports of individual patients who believe they have suffered a severe adverse reaction after immunization. The primary goals of this network include developing protocols for the clinical evaluation and management of vaccine adverse events; improving the understanding of adverse events at the individual level, including determining genetic and other risk factors that may predispose individuals to reactions; and serving as a public and health care professional regional referral center for clinical vaccine safety inquiries.

The CISA Network will advise primary care clinicians on evaluation and management of adverse events after immunization. This will be accomplished through telephone consultation, or patients may be referred to a center for further evaluation, generating case series of serious adverse events after immunization. The results of these evaluations will be used to gain a better understanding of how such events might occur and to develop protocols or guidelines for health care professionals that will assist in treating other patients in similar situations. In addition, the CISA Network centers will serve as regional information sources to which clinical vaccine safety questions can be referred. Current information about the CISA Network can be found online (www.partnersforimmunization.org/cisa.pdf).

VACCINE SAFETY DATALINK PROJECT

To supplement the VAERS program, which primarily is a passive surveillance system, the CDC formed partnerships with several large health maintenance organizations to establish the Vaccine Safety Datalink (VSD) project, an active surveillance system designed to continually evaluate vaccine safety. The VSD project includes data on more than 10 million people. Medical records of the study population are monitored for potential adverse events resulting from immunization. The VSD project allows for planned vaccine safety studies as well as for timely investigations of emerging vaccine safety concerns. The VSD concept to evaluate vaccine safety has been proven to be sound; previously known associations between febrile seizures and DTP

Figure 1.2 **VAERS form**

For directions for completing form, see www.fda.gov/cber/vaers/vaers.htm

WEBSITE: www.vaers.org   E-MAIL: info@vaers.org   FAX: 1-877-721-0366

VACCINE ADVERSE EVENT REPORTING SYSTEM
24 Hour Toll-Free Information 1-800-822-7967
P.O. Box 1100, Rockville, MD 20849-1100
PATIENT IDENTITY KEPT CONFIDENTIAL

For CDC/FDA Use Only
VAERS Number _____
Date Received _____

Patient Name:

Last   First   M.I.

Address

City   State   Zip
Telephone no. (____) _____

Vaccine administered by (Name):

Responsible
Physician _____
Facility Name/Address

City   State   Zip
Telephone no. (____) _____

Form completed by (Name):

Relation ☐ Vaccine Provider ☐ Patient/Parent
to Patient ☐ Manufacturer ☐ Other
Address (if different from patient or provider)

City   State   Zip
Telephone no. (____) _____

1. State

2. County where administered

3. Date of birth __/__/__ mm dd yy

4. Patient age

5. Sex ☐ M ☐ F

6. Date form completed __/__/__ mm dd yy

7. Describe adverse events(s) (symptoms, signs, time course) and treatment, if any

8. Check all appropriate:
☐ Patient died (date __/__/__ mm dd yy)
☐ Life threatening illness
☐ Required emergency room/doctor visit
☐ Required hospitalization (_____days)
☐ Resulted in prolongation of hospitalization
☐ Resulted in permanent disability
☐ None of the above

9. Patient recovered ☐ YES ☐ NO ☐ UNKNOWN

10. Date of vaccination __/__/__ mm dd yy   Time _____ AM PM

11. Adverse event onset __/__/__ mm dd yy   Time _____ AM PM

12. Relevant diagnostic tests/laboratory data

13. Enter all vaccines given on date listed in no. 10

	Vaccine (type)	Manufacturer	Lot number	Route/Site	No. Previous Doses
a.					
b.					
c.					
d.					

14. Any other vaccinations within 4 weeks prior to the date listed in no. 10

	Vaccine (type)	Manufacturer	Lot number	Route/Site	No. Previous doses	Date given
a.						
b.						

15. Vaccinated at:
☐ Private doctor's office/hospital ☐ Military clinic/hospital
☐ Public health clinic/hospital ☐ Other/unknown

16. Vaccine purchased with:
☐ Private funds ☐ Military funds
☐ Public funds ☐ Other/unknown

17. Other medications

18. Illness at time of vaccination (specify)

19. Pre-existing physician-diagnosed allergies, birth defects, medical conditions (specify)

20. Have you reported this adverse event previously?
☐ No ☐ To health department
☐ To doctor ☐ To manufacturer

Only for children 5 and under

22. Birth weight _____ lb. _____ oz.

23. No. of brothers and sisters

21. Adverse event following prior vaccination (check all applicable, specify)

	Adverse Event	Onset Age	Type Vaccine	Dose no. in series
☐ In patient				
☐ In brother or sister				

Only for reports submitted by manufacturer/immunization project

24. Mfr./imm. proj. report no.

25. Date received by mfr./imm.proj.

26. 15 day report? ☐ Yes ☐ No

27. Report type ☐ Initial ☐ Follow-Up

Health care providers and manufacturers are required by law (42 USC 300aa-25) to report reactions to vaccines listed in the Table of Reportable Events Following Immunization. Reports for reactions to other vaccines are voluntary except when required as a condition of immunization grant awards.

Form VAERS-1 (FDA)

immunization (day of immunization) and MMR immunization (days 8–14 after immunization) have been replicated in the study. Notable new findings from completed studies include the following: (1) MMR vaccine was not associated with an increased occurrence of chronic arthropathy in women; (2) administration of the Jeryl Lynn-derived strain of mumps virus vaccine in MMR vaccine was not associated with an increased risk of aseptic meningitis; (3) a second dose of MMR vaccine was associated with a greater frequency of adverse events in the 10- to 12-year-old age group than in the 4- to 6-year-old age group; (4) MMR immunization does not increase the risk of inflammatory bowel disease; (5) immunization was not associated with diabetes mellitus; and (6) although febrile seizures were associated rarely with receipt of DTP vaccine and MMR vaccine, these seizures were not associated with any long-term adverse consequences. Additional studies are evaluating the risk of multiple sclerosis after hepatitis B immunization, the risk of rheumatoid arthritis after hepatitis B immunization, and several other vaccine safety issues.

VACCINE IDENTIFICATION STANDARDS INITIATIVE

The Vaccine Identification Standards Initiative (VISI) is a voluntary effort by various partners in the US immunization system to improve the accuracy and convenience of transferring identifying information from vaccine packaging into medical records and onward into immunization registries and other record-keeping systems. Coordinated by the CDC along with liaisons from professional medical and nursing organizations, vaccine manufacturers, state and local immunization program managers, the FDA, health care professional organizations, the bar coding industry, international standards organizations, and other interested parties, the VISI has promulgated guidelines for vaccine packaging and labeling that aim to ease the burden of complying with legal requirements for immunization providers to record the identity and lot number of vaccines administered to patients. Such data enhance passive (see Reporting of Adverse Events, p 40) and active cohort monitoring systems for detecting and studying adverse events after immunization. They also can simplify participation in immunization registries and allow accurate surveys of immunization coverage and calculation of case-control vaccine efficacy rates in the event of disease outbreaks. Components of the VISI include (1) reduced-size bar coding of vaccine identity, lot number, and expiration date on vials and prefilled syringes; (2) peel-off stickers (up to triplicate per dose) on vials and syringes for use by providers still without scanning equipment or computerized practices to capture data into medical records, registry reporting forms, and take-home "immunization passports" (bar-coded stickers also would include equivalent human-readable information); (3) *Vaccine Facts* sidebars on vaccine cartons to group essential information for providers in a standardized format across manufacturers; (4) standardized abbreviations for vaccine types and manufacturers for use on space-constrained stickers; (5) a uniform vaccine administration form to accept such stickers; and (6) a Web-based database to convert the National Drug Code (NDC) found on all vaccine packaging and bar codes into the unique manufacturer, product type, and packaging size it represents and vice-versa. In 2002, the FDA announced proposed rulemaking that would mandate such bar coding on all unit-of-use drug packaging, including vaccines, to help decrease medical errors through the use of scanners at the point of administration in hospitals and other settings. Further information on the VISI is available online (www.cdc.gov/nip/visi), where drafts of the guidelines will be disseminated when ready for public comment and final promulgation.

VACCINE INJURY COMPENSATION

The National Vaccine Injury Compensation Program is a no-fault system in which people may seek compensation if they are thought to have suffered an injury, or a family member is thought to have died, as a result of administration of a covered vaccine. Claims must be filed within 36 months after the first symptom appeared after immunization, and death claims must be filed within 24 months of the death and within 48 months after the onset of the vaccine-related injury from which death occurred. Claims arising from covered vaccines must be adjudicated through the program before civil litigation can be pursued. Developed as an alternative to civil litigation and operational since 1988, the program has decreased the number of lawsuits against health care professionals and vaccine manufacturers and helped to ensure a stable vaccine supply and marketplace while ensuring access to compensation for vaccine-associated injury and death.

The program is based on a Vaccine Injury Table (VIT [see Appendix IV, p 802]) listing the vaccines covered by the program as well as injuries, disabilities, illnesses, and conditions (including death) for which compensation may be awarded. The VIT defines the time during which the first symptoms or significant aggravation of an injury must appear after immunization. If an injury listed in the VIT is proven, claimants receive a "legal presumption of causation," thus avoiding the need to prove causation in an individual case. If the claim pertains to conditions not listed in the VIT, claimants may prevail if they prove causation. Any vaccine that is recommended by the CDC for routine use in children and has an excise tax placed on it by Congress is eligible for coverage by the program.

Additional information about the National Vaccine Injury Compensation Program and the VIT are available from the following:

>National Vaccine Injury Compensation Program
>Division of Vaccine Injury Compensation
>Health Resources and Services Administration

>*Regular mail:*
>Parklawn Building
>5600 Fishers Lane
>Rockville, MD 20857
>Telephone: 800-338-2382
>Web site: www.hrsa.gov/osp/vicp

>*Overnight delivery:*
>East West Towers Building
>4350 East West Highway, 10th Floor
>Bethesda, MD 20814

People wishing to file a claim for a vaccine injury should telephone or write to the following:

>United States Court of Federal Claims
>717 Madison Place, NW
>Washington, DC 20005-1011
>Telephone: 202-219-9657

PRECAUTIONS AND CONTRAINDICATIONS

Precautions and contraindications to immunization are described in specific chapters on vaccine-preventable diseases. A contraindication indicates that a vaccine should not be administered. In contrast, a precaution specifies a situation in which vaccine may be indicated if, after careful assessment, the benefit of immunization to the individual is judged to outweigh the risk of complications. Contraindications and precautions may be generic, applying to all vaccines, or may be specific to one or more vaccines.

Minor illness with or without fever does not contraindicate immunization. Most vaccines are intended for use in healthy people or in people whose diseases or conditions are not affected by immunization. For optimal safety, vaccines should not be used if an adverse reaction to the vaccine may seriously affect or be confused with an underlying illness. Most evidence does not indicate an increased risk of adverse events or a decrease in effectiveness associated with immunization administered during a minor illness with or without fever (body temperature ≥38°C [≥100°F]). Deferring immunization in such situations contributes to missed opportunities and frequently results in unimmunized or inadequately immunized children who may develop or transmit vaccine-preventable disease.

Fever, per se, is not a contraindication to immunization. For the child with an acute febrile illness (body temperature ≥38°C [≥100°F]), guidelines for immunization are based on the physician's assessment of the child's illness and the specific vaccines the child is scheduled to receive. However, if fever or other manifestations suggest a moderate or serious illness, the child should not be immunized until recovered. Specific recommendations are as follows:

- *Live-virus vaccines.* Minor respiratory, gastrointestinal, or other illnesses with or without fever do not contraindicate use of live-virus vaccines, such as MMR or varicella. Children with febrile upper respiratory tract infections have serologic responses similar to those of well children after immunization. The potential benefit of immunization at the recommended age, regardless of the presence of a minor illness, outweighs the possible increased risk of vaccine failure.

- *DTaP vaccine.* Mild illnesses (eg, upper respiratory tract illnesses) do not contraindicate administration of DTaP. However, a moderate or severe illness with or without fever is a reason to delay immunization, in part because evolving signs and symptoms associated with the illness may be difficult to distinguish from a vaccine reaction. Currently available DTaP vaccines have rates of adverse events that are much less than previously licensed DTP vaccines.

- *Child with frequent febrile illnesses.* A child who has moderate or severe febrile illness at the time of scheduled immunizations should be asked to return as soon as the current febrile illness resolves so that immunization can be completed.

- *Immunocompromised children.* Special consideration needs to be given to immunocompromised children, including children with congenital immunodeficiencies, human immunodeficiency virus (HIV) infection, or malignant neoplasm or who are recipients of immunosuppressive therapy (see Immunocompromised Children, p 69).

A concise summary of contraindications to and precautions for immunizations is given in Appendix III (p 798).

HYPERSENSITIVITY REACTIONS TO VACCINE CONSTITUENTS

Hypersensitivity reactions to constituents of vaccines are rare. Facilities and health care professionals should be available for treating immediate hypersensitivity reactions in all settings in which vaccines are administered. This recommendation does not preclude administration of vaccines in school-based or other nonclinic settings.

The 4 types of hypersensitivity reactions considered related to vaccine constituents are (1) allergic reactions to egg-related antigens; (2) mercury sensitivity in some recipients of mercury-containing IG and vaccines (see Thimerosal content of some vaccines and immune globulin preparations, p 47); (3) antimicrobial-induced allergic reactions; and (4) hypersensitivity to other vaccine components, including gelatin, yeast protein, and the infectious agent itself.

Allergic reactions to egg-related antigens. Current measles and mumps vaccines are derived from chicken embryo fibroblast tissue cultures but do not contain significant amounts of egg cross-reacting proteins. Studies indicate that children with egg allergy, even those with severe hypersensitivity, are at low risk of anaphylactic reactions to these vaccines, singly or in combination (eg, MMR) and that skin testing with dilute vaccine is not predictive of an allergic reaction to immunization. Most immediate hypersensitivity reactions after MMR immunization appear to be reactions to other vaccine components, such as gelatin or neomycin. Therefore, children with egg allergy routinely may be given MMR, measles, or mumps vaccine without previous skin testing.

Current yellow fever and inactivated influenza vaccines contain egg proteins and, on rare occasions, may induce immediate allergic reactions, including anaphylaxis. Skin testing with yellow fever vaccines is recommended before administration to people with a history of systemic anaphylactic symptoms (generalized urticaria, hypotension, or manifestations of upper or lower airway obstruction) after egg ingestion. Skin testing also has been used for children with severe anaphylactic reactions to eggs who are to receive inactivated influenza vaccine. However, these children generally should not receive inactivated influenza vaccine because of a risk of adverse reaction, the likely need for yearly immunization, and availability of chemoprophylaxis against influenza infection (see Influenza, p 382). Less severe or local manifestations of allergy to egg or feathers are not contraindications to yellow fever or inactivated influenza vaccine administration and do not warrant vaccine skin testing.

An egg-sensitive person can be tested with vaccine (eg, yellow fever vaccine) before its use as follows:
- *Scratch, prick, or puncture test.* A drop of a 1:10 dilution of vaccine in physiologic saline solution is applied at the site of a superficial scratch, prick, or puncture on the volar surface of the forearm. Positive (histamine) and negative (physiologic saline solution) control tests also should be used. The test is read after 15 to 20 minutes. A positive test result is a wheal 3 mm larger than that of the saline control area, usually with surrounding erythema. The histamine control test result must be positive for valid interpretation. If the result of this test is negative, an ID test is performed.
- *Intradermal test.* A dose of 0.02 mL of a 1:100 dilution of the vaccine in physiologic saline solution is injected intradermally on the volar surface of the forearm; positive- and negative-control skin tests are performed concurrently as described

previously. A wheal 5 mm or larger than the negative control area with surrounding erythema is considered a positive reaction.

If these test results are negative, the vaccine may be given. If the child's test result is positive, the vaccine still may be given using a desensitization procedure if immunization is considered warranted because of a person's risk of complications resulting from the disease. A suggested protocol is SC administration of the following successive doses of vaccine at 15- to 20-minute intervals:

1. 0.05 mL of a 1:10 dilution
2. 0.05 mL of full-strength vaccine
3. 0.10 mL of full-strength vaccine
4. 0.15 mL of full-strength vaccine
5. 0.20 mL of full-strength vaccine

Scratch, prick, or puncture tests with other allergens have resulted in fatalities in highly allergic people. Although such untoward effects have not been reported for vaccine testing, all skin tests and desensitization procedures should be performed by trained personnel experienced in the management of anaphylaxis. Necessary medications and equipment for treatment of anaphylaxis should be readily available (see Treatment of Anaphylactic Reactions, p 63).

Thimerosal content of some vaccines and IG preparations. Thimerosal is a mercury-containing preservative that has been used as an additive to biologic agents and vaccines since the 1930s because of its effectiveness in preventing bacterial and fungal contamination, particularly in open multidose containers. Because of the potential value of decreasing exposures to mercury, vaccine manufacturers, the FDA, other public health service agencies, and the AAP have succeeded in having thimerosal removed from all vaccines currently in the recommended childhood and adolescent immunization schedule. Inactivated poliovirus and live-virus vaccines, such as MMR, OPV, and varicella, never have contained thimerosal. Pneumococcal conjugate vaccine is thimerosal free, and manufacturers of future childhood vaccines will avoid using thimerosal in order to gain licensure and approval. Vaccines available in late 2002 that contain thimerosal as a preservative include DT and Td vaccines, one pneumococcal polysaccharide vaccine, meningococcal vaccines, some inactivated influenza vaccines, and one rabies vaccine (www.fda.gov/cber/vaccine/thimerosal.htm#1).

The only nonvaccine biologic agents that contain thimerosal in active production and US distribution are Vaccinia Immune Globulin and certain antivenins. Immune Globulin Intravenous does not contain thimerosal or other preservatives, and none of the Rh_o (D) Immune Globulin (Human) products contain thimerosal (www.fda.gov/cber/blood/mercplasma.htm).

Antimicrobial-induced allergic reactions. Antimicrobial-induced reactions have been suspected in people with known allergies who received vaccines containing trace amounts of antimicrobial agents (see package insert for each product for specific listing). Proof of a causal relationship is difficult and often impossible to confirm.

The IPV vaccine contains trace amounts of streptomycin, neomycin, and polymyxin B. Live-virus measles, mumps, rubella (singly or in combination as MMR), and varicella vaccines have trace quantities of neomycin. Some people who are allergic to neomycin may experience a delayed-type local reaction 48 to 96 hours after administration of IPV, MMR, or varicella vaccines. The reaction consists of an erythematous, pruritic papule. This minor reaction is of little importance compared with the benefit of immunization and should not be considered a contraindication. However, if a person has a history of anaphylactic reaction to neomycin, neomycin-containing vaccines should not be used. No currently recommended vaccine contains penicillin or its derivatives.

Hypersensitivity to other vaccine components, including the infectious agent. Some live-virus vaccines, such as MMR, varicella, and yellow fever vaccines, contain gelatin as a stabilizer. People with a history of food allergy to gelatin rarely develop anaphylaxis after receipt of gelatin-containing vaccines. Skin testing is a consideration for these people before administration of a gelatin-containing vaccine, but no protocol or reported experience is available. Because gelatin used in the United States as a vaccine stabilizer usually is porcine and food gelatins may be derived solely from bovine sources, a negative food history does not exclude the possibility of an immunization reaction.

Hepatitis B vaccine is manufactured using recombinant technology by harvesting purified hepatitis B surface antigen from genetically engineered yeast cells containing the hepatitis B surface antigen gene. Purification results in a substantial reduction of yeast protein contained in the vaccine, but in rare instances, vaccine recipients with a significant hypersensitivity to yeast products may experience an allergic reaction to hepatitis B vaccine that would contraindicate receiving additional doses.

Reactions occur with DTaP vaccines but are much less common than with DTP vaccines. On occasion, urticarial or anaphylactic reactions have occurred in recipients of DTP, DTaP, DT, Td, or tetanus toxoid vaccine. Tetanus and diphtheria antigen-specific antibodies of the IgE type have been identified in some of these patients. Although attributing a specific sensitivity to vaccine components is difficult, an immediate, severe, or anaphylactic allergic reaction to one of these vaccines is a contraindication to subsequent immunization of the patient with the specific product. A transient urticarial rash, however, is not a contraindication to further doses (see Appendix III, p 798).

People who have high serum concentrations of tetanus IgG antibody, usually as the result of frequent booster immunizations, have an increased incidence and severity of adverse reactions to subsequent vaccine administration (see Tetanus, p 611).

Reactions resembling serum sickness have been reported in approximately 6% of patients after a booster dose of human diploid rabies vaccine, probably resulting from sensitization to human albumin that had been altered chemically by the virus-inactivating agent.

Measles vaccines, including MMR, and rabies vaccines contain Albumin, a derivative of human blood. Because of effective donor screening and product manufacturing processes, the FDA believes the risk of transmission of any viral disease from Albumin in these vaccines is rare.

Japanese encephalitis virus vaccine has been associated with generalized urticaria and angioedema, sometimes with respiratory distress and hypotension, occurring within minutes of immunization to as long as 2 weeks after immunization. The pathogenesis of such reactions is not understood. People with a history of urticaria are at increased risk of this adverse reaction, so vaccine recipients with this history should be observed for 30 minutes after immunization and warned about the possibility of delayed urticaria and potentially life-threatening angioedema.

Significant hypersensitivity reactions occurring as a result of pneumococcal, Hib, hepatitis A, or poliovirus vaccines are rare.

MISCONCEPTIONS ABOUT VACCINE CONTRAINDICATIONS

Contraindications to immunization often are misunderstood by health care professionals and parents. Common conditions or circumstances that are **not** contraindications include:

- Mild acute illness with low-grade fever or mild diarrheal illness in an otherwise well child
- The convalescent phase of illness
- Currently receiving antimicrobial therapy
- Reaction to a previous DTaP or DTP dose that involved only soreness, redness, or swelling in the immediate vicinity of the immunization site or temperature of less than 40.5°C (105°F)
- Prematurity—the appropriate age for initiating most immunizations in the prematurely born infant is the usually recommended chronologic age; vaccine doses should not be reduced for preterm infants (see Preterm Infants, p 66, and Hepatitis B, p 324)
- Pregnancy of mother or other household contact—vaccine viruses in MMR vaccine are not transmitted by vaccine recipients; although varicella vaccine virus has been transmitted by healthy vaccine recipients to contacts, the frequency is rare, only mild or asymptomatic infection has been reported, and use of this vaccine is not contraindicated by pregnancy of the child's mother or other household contacts (see Varicella-Zoster Infections, p 680)
- Recent exposure to an infectious disease
- Breastfeeding—the only vaccine virus that has been isolated from human milk is rubella; no evidence indicates that human milk from women immunized against rubella is harmful to infants
- A history of nonspecific allergies or relatives with allergies
- Allergies to penicillin or any other antimicrobial agent, except anaphylactic reactions to neomycin or streptomycin (see Hypersensitivity Reactions to Vaccine Constituents, p 46)—these reactions occur rarely, if ever; none of the vaccines licensed in the United States contain penicillin
- Allergies to duck meat or duck feathers—no vaccine available in the United States is produced in substrates containing duck antigens
- Family history of seizures in a person considered for pertussis or measles immunization (see Children With a Personal or Family History of Seizures, p 81)
- Family history of sudden infant death syndrome in children considered for DTaP immunization
- Family history of an adverse event, unrelated to immunosuppression, after immunization
- Malnutrition

Reporting of Vaccine-Preventable Diseases

Most vaccine-preventable diseases are reportable throughout the United States. Public health officials depend on health care professionals to report promptly to state or local health departments suspected cases of vaccine-preventable disease. These reports are transmitted weekly to the CDC and are used to detect outbreaks, monitor disease-control strategies, and evaluate national immunization practices and policies. Reporting confirmed and suspected vaccine-preventable diseases is a legal obligation of the physician. Reports provide useful information about vaccine efficacy, changing or current epidemiology of vaccine-preventable diseases, and possible epidemics that could threaten public health.

Standards for Child and Adolescent Immunization Practices (see Appendix II, p 795)

In 2003, national *Standards for Pediatric Immunization Practices* were revised by the National Vaccine Advisory Committee, approved by the US Public Health Service, and endorsed by the AAP and numerous other provider organizations. As part of this revision, the standards were renamed *Standards for Child and Adolescent Immunization Practices.* These standards are recommended for use by all health care professionals providing care in public or private health care settings who are involved in the administration of vaccines or management of immunization services for children. Their use is intended to improve preschool immunization rates, prevent vaccine-preventable disease outbreaks, and achieve national objectives for immunization. The revised standards reflect the increasing role of private practitioners, the importance of adolescent immunization, and recent increases in vaccine safety concerns among the general public.

Parental Misconceptions About Immunizations

Misconceptions about the need for and safety of recommended childhood and adolescent immunizations are potential causes of delayed immunization, underimmunization, or both in the United States. Several common misconceptions of parents have been addressed by the CDC.* In an effort to inform parents further, the AAP has published a brochure titled *Immunizations: What You Should Know,*[†] which addresses common questions about recommended childhood and adolescent immunizations, including the following.

- **"Why should children be immunized when most vaccine-preventable diseases have been eliminated in the United States?"** Although immunizations have decreased dramatically the incidence of a number of childhood diseases in the United States, many of these diseases remain prevalent in other areas of the world and easily could be reintroduced into the United States and, without immunization, could spread quickly. Unimmunized children also will be at risk throughout their lives, including when they travel to countries where vaccine-preventable diseases are endemic.

---

* National Immunization Program. *Six Common Misconceptions About Vaccination and How to Respond to Them.* Atlanta, GA: Centers for Disease Control and Prevention; 1996. Available at: www.cdc.gov/nip/publications/6mishome.htm (to be updated in late 2003)

† For copies, contact the American Academy of Pediatrics at 866-843-2271.

- **"Do immunizations work? Haven't most people who get a vaccine-preventable disease been immunized?"** A few people do not immunologically respond to vaccines, but childhood vaccines are 85% to 98% effective. Most people who get a vaccine-preventable disease have not been fully immunized.
- **"Aren't some vaccine lots more dangerous than others?"** All vaccines are reviewed carefully for safety and efficacy before being licensed by the FDA and recommended for use. No evidence indicates that individual lots of commonly used vaccines differ in safety. The FDA and CDC conduct programs to continue surveillance after licensure for safety and efficacy of all recommended vaccines. Active surveillance for vaccine-associated adverse events after licensure involves numbers of subjects far greater than for many other types of therapeutic agents, reflecting the high standard to which vaccines are held.
- **"Isn't giving children more than one immunization at a time dangerous?"** Numerous studies have shown that multiple recommended childhood and adolescent immunizations can be given safely at the same time. Scientists estimate that the immune system can recognize and respond to hundreds of thousands, if not millions, of antigens. Recommended vaccines use only a small portion of the "memory" of the immune system. The IOM Safety Review Committee found no evidence to support the theory that multiple immunizations increase the risk of immune dysfunction (see p 38).

Health care professionals should obtain and distribute copies of CDC and AAP immunization documents as well as vaccine information statements (VISs) to parents to address their questions and concerns. These resource materials can help parents make informed decisions about immunizing their children. Other sources of objective vaccine information are available (see the list of selected authoritative Web sites, p 52) that can help health care professionals respond to questions and misconceptions about immunizations and vaccine-preventable diseases.

Parents and health care professionals may view scientific data in different ways. Parents often have insufficient education in microbiology, immunology, or epidemiology to judge which vaccine-related studies are well done. Parents often review health issues in a subjective way, relative to how they affect them and their child personally. Health care professionals need to make the risk of disease and benefits of immunization personally relevant.

Alleged adverse events after immunization initially may be published in the mass media. Some parents will want immediate answers to their questions. Health care professionals should refer to the list of Web sites (p 52) to help them address the questions posed by parents. Efforts usually are made by those organizations to address questions raised by the media within 24 to 48 hours. Alternatively, physicians can call the National Immunization Hotline at 1-800-232-2522.

The **National Network for Immunization Information** (NNii), an initiative of the Infectious Diseases Society of America, the Pediatric Infectious Diseases Society, the AAP, and the American Nurses Association, provides education and communication about immunization issues. The NNii also provides additional reliable resources for current immunization information and has published a Resource Kit, "Communicating With Patients About Immunization." Immunization information can be found on the NNii Web site (www.immunizationinfo.org).

INTERNET RESOURCES FOR IMMUNIZATION INFORMATION

Several health professional associations, nonprofit groups, universities, and government organizations provide Internet resources containing immunization information.

Health Professional Associations

American Academy of Family Physicians (AAFP)
    www.familydoctor.org

American Academy of Pediatrics (AAP)
    www.aap.org
    www.cispimmunize.org

American Medical Association (AMA)
    www.ama-assn.org

American Nurses Association (ANA)
    www.nursingworld.org/mods/mod1/cechfull.htm

Association of State and Territorial Health Officials (ASTHO)
    www.astho.org

Association of Teachers of Preventive Medicine (ATPM)
    www.atpm.org/education/education.htm

National Medical Association (NMA)
    www.nmanet.org

Nonprofit Groups and Universities

Albert B. Sabin Vaccine Institute
    www.sabin.org

Allied Vaccine Group (AVG)
    www.vaccine.org

Bill and Melinda Gates Children's Vaccine Program
    www.childrensvaccine.org

Every Child By Two (ECBT)
    www.ecbt.org

Global Alliance for Vaccines and Immunization (GAVI)
    www.vaccinealliance.org

Health on the Net Foundation (HON)
    www.hon.ch

Healthy Mothers, Healthy Babies Coalition (HMHB)
    www.hmhb.org

Immunization Action Coalition (IAC)
    www.immunize.org

Institute for Vaccine Safety (IVS), Johns Hopkins University
    www.vaccinesafety.edu

Institute of Medicine
    www.iom.edu/IOM/IOMHome.nsf/Pages/immunization+safety+review

National Alliance for Hispanic Health
www.hispanichealth.org/immunization.htm

National Network for Immunization Information (NNii)
www.immunizationinfo.org

Parents of Kids with Infectious Diseases (PKIDS)
www.pkids.org

The Vaccine Education Center at the Children's Hospital of Philadelphia
www.vaccine.chop.edu

The Vaccine Page
www.vaccines.com

Government Organizations

Centers for Disease Control and Prevention (CDC)
http://phil.cdc.gov/phil
www.cdc.gov/travel/vaccinat.htm

National Center for Infectious Diseases (NCID)
www.cdc.gov/ncidod

National Immunization Program (NIP)
www.cdc.gov/nip
www.cdc.gov/nip/publications

National Vaccine Program Office (NVPO)
www.cdc.gov/od/nvpo

National Institute of Allergy and Infectious Diseases (NIAID)
www.niaid.nih.gov/dmid/vaccines

World Health Organization
www.who.int/vaccines

....

PASSIVE IMMUNIZATION

Passive immunization entails administration of preformed antibody to a recipient. Passive immunization is indicated in the following general circumstances for prevention or amelioration of infectious diseases:

- When people are deficient in synthesis of antibody as a result of congenital or acquired B-lymphocyte defects, alone or in combination with other immunodeficiencies
- When a person susceptible to a disease is exposed to or has a high likelihood of exposure to that infection, especially when that person has a high risk of complications from the disease (eg, a child with leukemia exposed to a person with varicella or measles) or when time does not permit adequate protection by active immunization alone (eg, some postexposure situations involving measles, rabies, or hepatitis B)
- Therapeutically, when a disease is already present, antibody may ameliorate or aid in suppressing the effects of a toxin (eg, foodborne or wound botulism, diphtheria, or tetanus) or suppress the inflammatory response (eg, Kawasaki syndrome)

Passive immunization has been accomplished with several types of products. The choice is dictated by the types of products available, the type of antibody desired, the route of administration, timing, and other considerations. These products include Immune Globulin (IG) and specific ("hyperimmune") IG preparations given intramuscularly, Immune Globulin Intravenous (IGIV), specific (hyperimmune) IG given by the intravenous (IV) route, human plasma, and antibodies of animal origin.

Indications for administration of IG preparations other than those relevant to infectious diseases are not reviewed in the *Red Book*.

Whole blood and blood components for transfusion (including plasma) from registered blood banks in the United States are tested for the presence of bloodborne pathogens, including syphilis, hepatitis B virus, hepatitis C virus (HCV), human immunodeficiency virus (HIV)-1, HIV-2, and human T-lymphotropic viruses (HTLV)-I and HTLV-II (see Blood Safety, p 106). A similar array of tests is performed by US-licensed establishments that collect plasma used only to manufacture plasma derivatives, such as IGIV, IG, and specific immune globulins. United States-licensed IG and specific immune globulin preparations have not been associated with the transmission of any of these diseases. Hepatitis C virus transmission in 1994 was associated with administration of IGIV produced by a single manufacturer. The US Food and Drug Administration (FDA) now requires that IGIV and other immune globulin preparations for IV or intramuscular (IM) administration undergo additional manufacturing procedures that inactivate or remove viruses.

Immune Globulin

Immune Globulin is derived from the pooled plasma of adults by an alcohol-fractionation procedure. Immune Globulin consists primarily of the immunoglobulin (Ig) fraction (at least 96% IgG and trace amounts of IgA and IgM), is sterile, and is not known to transmit hepatotropic viruses, HIV, or any other infectious disease agent. Immune Globulin is a concentrated protein solution (approximately 16.5% or 165 mg/mL) containing specific antibodies in proportion to the infectious and immunization experience of the population from whose plasma it was prepared. Large numbers of donors (at least 1000 donors per lot of final product) are used to ensure inclusion of a broad spectrum of antibodies.

Immune Globulin is recommended for IM administration. Because some recipients experience local pain and most experience local discomfort, IG should be administered deep into a large muscle mass, usually in the gluteal region or anterior thigh of a child (see Site and Route of Immunization, p 17). No more than 5 mL ordinarily should be administered to one site in an adult or large child; lesser amounts per site (1–3 mL) should be given to small children and infants. Administration of more than 15 mL at any one time is seldom, if ever, warranted. There may be a deferral for blood donation for a person after administration of any IG preparation, depending on the reason for IG administration.

Peak serum concentrations of antibodies usually are achieved 48 to 72 hours after IM administration. The serum half-life generally is 3 to 4 weeks.

Intravenous use of IG is contraindicated. Intradermal use of IG is not recommended.

INDICATIONS FOR THE USE OF IG

Replacement therapy in antibody deficiency disorders. The usual dosage is 100 mg/kg (equivalent to 0.66 mL/kg) per month intramuscularly. Customary practice is to administer twice this dose initially and to adjust the interval between administration of the doses (2–4 weeks) on the basis of trough IgG concentrations and clinical response (absence of or decrease in infections). In most cases, however, IG has been replaced by IGIV. Studies in adolescents and adults with antibody deficiencies indicate that slow subcutaneous administration of IG is safe, less expensive than IGIV, convenient, and suitable for home therapy. Systemic allergic reactions occurred with fewer than 1% of infusions, and local tissue reactions generally were mild.

Hepatitis A prophylaxis. Immune Globulin can prevent hepatitis A in susceptible people for whom immunization is contraindicated when given within 14 days of exposure. Indications include international travel by children younger than 2 years of age and postexposure prophylaxis (see Hepatitis A, p 309).

Measles prophylaxis. Immune Globulin administered to exposed, measles-susceptible people will prevent or modify infection if given within 6 days of exposure (see Measles, p 422).

ADVERSE REACTIONS TO IG

- The most common adverse event encountered with use of IG is discomfort and pain at the site of administration (which is lessened if the preparation is at room temperature at the time of injection). Less common reactions include flushing, headache, chills, and nausea.
- Serious reactions are uncommon; these may involve chest pain or constriction, dyspnea, or anaphylaxis and systemic collapse. An increased risk of systemic reaction results from inadvertent IV administration. People requiring repeated doses of IG have been reported to experience systemic reactions, such as fever, chills, sweating, uncomfortable sensations, and shock.
- Because IG contains trace amounts of IgA, people who are selectively serum IgA deficient rarely can develop anti-IgA antibodies and react to a subsequent dose of IG, whole-blood transfusion, or plasma infusion with systemic symptoms, including chills, fever, and shock-like symptoms. In rare cases in which reactions related to anti-IgA antibodies have occurred, use of IgA-depleted IGIV preparations may decrease the likelihood of further reactions. Because of the rarity of these reactions, routine screening for IgA deficiency is not recommended.
- Healthy people given IG may develop antibodies against heterologous IgG allotypes. Usually, this phenomenon has no clinical significance; however, on rare occasions, a systemic reaction can result.
- Immune Globulin Intravenous, IG, and specific immune globulin preparations (except for Vaccinia Immune Globulin) do not contain thimerosal (see Thimerosal content of some vaccines and immune globulin preparations, p 47).

PRECAUTIONS FOR THE USE OF IG

- Caution should be used when giving IG to a patient with history of adverse reactions to IG.
- Although systemic reactions to IG are rare (see Adverse Reactions to IG, p 55), epinephrine and other means of treating acute reactions should be available immediately.
- Immune Globulin is not licensed by the FDA for use in patients with severe thrombocytopenia or any coagulation disorder that would preclude IM injection. In such cases, use of IGIV is recommended.
- Screening for IgA deficiency is not recommended routinely for potential recipients of IG (see Adverse Reactions to IG, p 55).

Specific Immune Globulins

Specific immune globulins, termed "hyperimmune globulins," differ from other preparations in the selection of donors and may differ in the number of donors whose plasma is included in the pool from which the product is prepared. Donors known to have high titers of the desired antibody, naturally acquired or stimulated by immunization, are selected. Specific immune globulins are prepared by the same procedure as other immune globulin preparations. Specific immune globulin preparations for use in infectious diseases include Hepatitis B Immune Globulin, Rabies Immune Globulin, Tetanus Immune Globulin, Varicella-Zoster Immune Globulin, Vaccinia (smallpox) Immune Globulin, Cytomegalovirus (CMV) Immune Globulin Intravenous, Vaccinia Immune Globulin, and Respiratory Syncytial Virus Immune Globulin Intravenous. An intramuscularly administered monoclonal antibody preparation for prevention of respiratory syncytial virus also is available. Recommendations for use of these globulins are given in the discussion of specific diseases in Section 3. The precautions and adverse reactions for IG and IGIV are applicable to specific immune globulins.

Immune Globulin Intravenous

Immune Globulin Intravenous is derived from pooled plasma of adults by an alcohol-fractionation procedure, which is modified by individual manufacturers to a product suitable for IV use. The donor pool is like that of IG. The FDA specifies that all preparations must have a minimum concentration of measles, diphtheria, poliovirus, and hepatitis B antibodies. Antibody concentrations against common pathogens, such as *Streptococcus pneumoniae,* vary widely among products and even among lots of the same product. Immune Globulin Intravenous consists primarily of the immunoglobulin fraction (more than 95% IgG and trace amounts of IgA and IgM). Protein content varies, depending on the product; liquid and dried products are available. Immune Globulin Intravenous does not contain thimerosal.

INDICATIONS FOR THE USE OF IGIV

Initially, IGIV was developed as an infusion product that allowed patients with primary immunodeficiencies to receive enough IG at monthly intervals to protect them from infection until their next infusion. Subsequently, the FDA and the

National Institutes of Health, through a consensus development conference, have expanded the recommended uses for IGIV (see Table 1.8, p 58). This product also may be useful for other conditions, although demonstrated efficacy from controlled trials is not available in all cases. Since November 1997, periodic shortages of IGIV have existed in the United States because of production impediments related to compliance and product recall based on the theoretic risk of contamination with the Creutzfeldt-Jakob disease (CJD) agent. Other problems causing short supply of IGIV include increased administration for approved and unapproved uses, wastage, and export of IGIV. In August 1998, the US Surgeon General recommended that plasma derivatives including IGIV be withdrawn only if the blood donor developed variant CJD (see Blood Safety, p 106). The FDA is using several methods to improve IGIV distribution to patients. Clinicians should review their IGIV use to ensure consistency with current recommendations. Off-label use of IGIV should be limited until there is adequate scientific evidence of effectiveness.

Licensure by the FDA of specific indications for a manufacturer's IGIV product is based on availability of data from one or more clinical trials. All IGIV products are licensed for primary immunodeficiencies and most are licensed for immune-mediated thrombocytopenia, but not all licensed products are approved for the other indications listed in Table 1.8 (see previous paragraph). In some cases, only a single product has the indication in its product label. Therapeutic differences among IGIV products from different manufacturers are likely to exist but may not have been demonstrated. Recommended indications in children and adolescents for prevention or treatment of infectious diseases include the following:

- **Replacement therapy in antibody deficiency disorders.** The usual dosage of IGIV in immunodeficiency syndromes is 300 to 400 mg/kg administered once a month by IV infusion. Dosage and frequency of infusions, however, should be based on effectiveness in the individual patient. Effective dosages have ranged from 200 to 800 mg/kg monthly. Maintenance of a trough IgG concentration of at least 500 mg/dL (5 g/L) has been demonstrated to correlate with clinical response.
- **Kawasaki syndrome.** Administration of IGIV and aspirin within the first 10 days of onset of fever decreases the frequency of coronary artery abnormalities and shortens the duration of symptoms (see Kawasaki Syndrome, p 392).
- **Pediatric HIV infection.** In children with HIV infection and hypogamma-globulinemia, IGIV is recommended to prevent serious bacterial infection. Immune Globulin Intravenous also should be considered for HIV-infected children who have recurrent serious bacterial infection* (see Human Immunodeficiency Virus Infection, p 360).
- **Hypogammaglobulinemia in chronic B-cell lymphocytic leukemia.** Administration of IGIV to adults with this disease has been demonstrated to decrease the incidence of serious bacterial infections, although its cost-effectiveness has been questioned.

---

* US Public Health Service and Infectious Diseases Society of America. Guidelines for preventing opportunistic infections among HIV-infected persons—2002. *MMWR Recomm Rep.* 2002;51 (RR-8):1–46

Table 1.8. **US Food and Drug Administration and National Institutes of Health (NIH) Recommendations for Use of Immune Globulin Intravenous[1]**

Primary immunodeficiencies

Kawasaki syndrome

Pediatric human immunodeficiency virus infection

Chronic B-cell lymphocytic leukemia

Recent bone marrow transplantation in adults

Immune-mediated thrombocytopenia

Chronic inflammatory demyelinating polyneuropathy[2]

---

[1] From Centers for Disease Control and Prevention. Availability of immune globulin intravenous for treatment of immune deficient patients: United States, 1997–1998. *MMWR Morb Mortal Wkly Rep.* 1999;48:159–162

[2] Approved only by the NIH Consensus Development Conference.

- **Bone marrow transplantation.** Immune Globulin Intravenous may decrease the incidence of infection and death but not acute graft-versus-host disease (GVHD) in pediatric bone marrow transplant recipients. In adult transplant recipients, IGIV decreases the incidence of interstitial pneumonia (presumably caused by CMV), decreases the risk of sepsis and other bacterial infections, decreases the incidence of acute GVHD (but not overall mortality), and in conjunction with ganciclovir, is effective in the treatment of some patients with CMV pneumonia.

  Immune Globulin Intravenous also has been used for many other conditions, some of which are listed below.

- **Low birth weight infants.** Results of most clinical trials have indicated that IGIV does not decrease the incidence or mortality rate of late-onset infections in infants who weigh less than 1500 g at birth. Trials have varied in IGIV dosage, time of administration, and other aspects of study design. At present, IGIV is not recommended for routine use in preterm infants to prevent late-onset infection.

- **Guillain-Barré syndrome.** In Guillain-Barré syndrome and chronic inflammatory demyelinating polyneuropathy, plasmapheresis has been demonstrated to have efficacy equivalent to that of IGIV treatment.

- **Toxic shock syndrome.** Immune Globulin Intravenous has been used in patients with severe staphylococcal or streptococcal toxic shock syndrome. Therapy appears most likely to be beneficial when used early in the course of illness.

- **Other potential uses.** Immune Globulin Intravenous may be useful for anemia caused by parvovirus B19 infection, in patients with stable multiple myeloma who are at high risk of recurrent infection, in CMV-negative recipients of CMV-positive organs, in neonates with hypogammaglobulinemia and a risk factor for infection or morbidity, and for intractable epilepsy, systemic vasculitic syndromes, warm-type autoimmune hemolytic anemia, neonatal alloimmune thrombocytopenia that is unresponsive to other treatments, immune-mediated neutropenia, decompensation in myasthenia gravis, dermatomyositis, polymyositis, and severe thrombocytopenia that is unresponsive to other treatments.

ADVERSE REACTIONS TO IGIV

The reported incidence of adverse events associated with administration of IGIV ranges from 1% to 15%. Adverse events can be decreased by following the package insert for the individual product carefully with regard to the rate of administration. Reactions such as fever, headache, myalgia, chills, nausea, and vomiting often are related to the rate of IGIV infusion and usually are mild to moderate and self-limited. The cause of these reactions may involve formation of IgG aggregates during manufacture or storage. Less common and more severe reactions include hypersensitivity and anaphylactoid reactions marked by flushing, changes in blood pressure, and tachycardia; thromboembolic events; aseptic meningitis; and renal insufficiency and failure. The causes of these reactions are unknown.

Anaphylactic reactions induced by anti-IgA can occur in patients with primary antibody deficiency who have a total absence of circulating IgA and have IgG antibodies to IgA. These reactions are rare in panhypogammaglobulinemic people and potentially more common in patients with selective IgA deficiency and subclass IgG deficiencies. In the rare instances in which reactions related to anti-IgA antibodies have occurred, use of IgA-depleted IGIV preparations may decrease the likelihood of further reactions. Avoidance of anaphylactic reactions, however, may require the use of globulin preparations that are devoid of IgA. Because of the extreme rarity of these reactions, screening for IgA deficiency is not recommended routinely.

An outbreak of HCV infection occurred in the United States in 1994 among recipients of IGIV lots from a single domestic manufacturer. Changes in the preparation of IGIV subsequent to this episode have been instituted to prevent transmission of HCV by IGIV infusion.

PRECAUTIONS FOR THE USE OF IGIV

- Caution should be used when giving IGIV to a patient with a history of adverse reactions to immune globulin.
- Because systemic reactions to IGIV may occur (see Adverse Reactions to IGIV, above), epinephrine and other means of treating acute reactions should be available immediately.
- Adverse reactions often can be alleviated by reducing either the rate or the volume of infusion. For patients with repeated severe reactions unresponsive to these measures, hydrocortisone at a dosage of 1 to 2 mg/kg can be given intravenously 30 minutes before infusion. Using a different IGIV preparation or pretreatment with diphenhydramine, acetaminophen, or aspirin also may be helpful.
- Seriously ill patients with compromised cardiac function who are receiving large volumes of IGIV may be at increased risk of vasomotor or cardiac complications manifested by elevated blood pressure, cardiac failure, or both.
- Screening for IgA deficiency is not recommended routinely for potential recipients of IGIV (see Adverse Reactions to IGIV, above).

Human Plasma

The use of Human Plasma for control of infectious diseases is controversial, and indications are limited. Human Plasma has been administered to patients with burns in an attempt to control *Pseudomonas* infections, but data are insufficient to substantiate this use. Plasma infusions have been useful for treating infants who have protein-losing enteropathy. Plasma infusions also have been substituted for IG for some patients with IgG antibody deficiency when they develop adverse reactions to IG or fail to respond to treatment with IG; however, these immunodeficient patients can be managed with IGIV (or with slow subcutaneous administration of IG).

Antibodies of Animal Origin (Animal Antisera)

Products of animal origin used for prophylaxis of infectious diseases are derived from serum of horses. Experimental products prepared in other species also may be available. These products are derived by concentrating the serum globulin fraction with ammonium sulfate. Some, but not all, products are subjected to an enzyme digestion process to decrease reactions to foreign proteins.

Use of the following products is discussed in the disease-specific chapters in Section 3:

- Botulism Antitoxin (Equine), available from the Centers for Disease Control and Prevention (CDC).
- Diphtheria Antitoxin (Equine), available from the CDC. The sole US manufacturer has stopped producing this product, and current stock supplies will expire in November 2003. Negotiations are underway with another supplier.

INDICATIONS FOR USE OF ANIMAL ANTISERA

Antibody-containing products prepared from animal sera pose a special risk to the recipient, and the use of such products should be limited strictly to certain indications for which specific IG preparations of human origin are not available (eg, diphtheria and botulism).

REACTIONS TO ANIMAL SERA

Before any animal serum is injected, the patient must be questioned about his or her history of asthma, allergic rhinitis, and urticaria after previous exposure to animals or injections of animal sera. Patients with a history of asthma or allergic symptoms, especially from exposure to horses, can be dangerously sensitive to equine sera and should be given these products with the utmost caution. People who previously have received animal sera are at increased risk of developing allergic reactions and serum sickness after administration of sera from the same animal species.

SENSITIVITY TESTS FOR REACTIONS TO ANIMAL SERA

Each patient who is to be given animal serum should be skin tested before administration of the animal serum. Intradermal (ID) skin tests have resulted in fatalities, but the scratch test usually is safe. Therefore, scratch tests always should precede ID tests. Nevertheless, any sensitivity test always should be performed by trained personnel familiar with treatment of acute anaphylaxis; necessary medications and equipment should be readily available (see Treatment of Anaphylactic Reactions, p 63).

Scratch, prick, or puncture test. * Apply 1 drop of a 1:100 dilution of serum in preservative-free isotonic sodium chloride solution to the site of a superficial

---

* Antihistamines may inhibit reactions in the scratch, prick, or puncture test and in the ID test; hence, testing should not be performed for at least 24 hours or, preferably, 48 hours after receipt of these drugs.

scratch, prick, or puncture on the volar aspect of the forearm. Positive (histamine) and negative (physiologic saline solution) control tests for the scratch test also should be applied. A positive test result is a wheal with surrounding erythema at least 3 mm larger than the negative control test area, read at 15 to 20 minutes. The histamine control must be positive for valid interpretation. If the scratch test result is negative, an ID test is performed.

*Intradermal test.** A dose of 0.02 mL of a 1:1000 dilution of preservative-free isotonic saline-diluted serum (enough to raise a small wheal) is administered. Positive and negative control tests as described for the scratch test also should be applied. If the test result is negative, it should be repeated using a 1:100 dilution. For people with negative history for both animal allergy and previous exposure to animal serum, the 1:100 dilution may be used initially if a scratch, prick, or puncture test result with the serum is negative. Interpretation is the same as for the scratch test.

Positive test results not attributable to an irritant reaction indicate sensitivity, but a negative skin test result is not an absolute guarantee of lack of sensitivity. Therefore, animal sera should be administered with caution even to people whose test results are negative. Immediate hypersensitivity testing is performed to identify IgE-mediated disease and does not predict other immune reactions, such as serum sickness.

If the ID test result is positive or if the history of systemic anaphylaxis after previous administration of serum is highly suggestive in a person for whom the need for the serum is unquestioned, desensitization can be undertaken (see Desensitization to Animal Sera, below).

If history and sensitivity test results are negative, the indicated dose of serum can be given intramuscularly. The patient should be observed afterward for at least 30 minutes. Intravenous administration may be indicated if a high concentration of serum antibody is imperative, such as for treatment of diphtheria or botulism. In these instances, serum should be diluted and slowly administered intravenously according to the manufacturer's instructions. The patient should be monitored carefully for signs or symptoms of anaphylaxis.

DESENSITIZATION TO ANIMAL SERA

Tables 1.9 (p 62) and 1.10 (p 63) serve as guides for the desensitization procedures for administration of animal sera. Intravenous (Table 1.9), ID, subcutaneous, or intramuscular (IM) regimens (Table 1.10) may be chosen. The IV route is considered safest, because it offers better control. The desensitization procedure should be performed by trained personnel familiar with treatment of anaphylaxis and with appropriate drugs and available equipment (see Treatment of Anaphylactic Reactions, p 63). Some physicians advocate concurrent use of an oral or parenteral antihistamine (such as diphenhydramine) during the procedure, with or without IV hydrocortisone or methylprednisolone. If signs of anaphylaxis occur, aqueous epinephrine should be administered immediately (see Treatment of Anaphylactic Reactions, p 63). Administration of sera during a desensitization procedure must be continuous, because if administration is interrupted, protection achieved by desensitization will be lost.

---

* Antihistamines may inhibit reactions in the scratch, prick, or puncture test and in the ID test; hence, testing should not be performed for at least 24 hours or, preferably, 48 hours after receipt of these drugs.

Table 1.9. **Desensitization to Serum—Intravenous (IV) Route**

Dose Number[1]	Dilution of Serum in Isotonic Sodium Chloride	Amount of IV Injection, mL
1	1:1000	0.1
2	1:1000	0.3
3	1:1000	0.6
4	1:100	0.1
5	1:100	0.3
6	1:100	0.6
7	1:10	0.1
8	1:10	0.3
9	1:10	0.6
10	Undiluted	0.1
11	Undiluted	0.3
12	Undiluted	0.6
13	Undiluted	1.0

[1] Administer consistently at 15-minute intervals.

TYPES OF REACTIONS TO ANIMAL SERA

The following reactions can occur as the result of administration of animal sera. Of these, only anaphylaxis is mediated by IgE antibodies, and thus, occurrence can be predicted by previous skin testing results.

Acute febrile reactions. These reactions usually are mild and can be treated with antipyretic agents. Severe febrile reactions should be treated with antipyretic agents or other safe available methods to decrease temperature physically.

Serum sickness. Manifestations, which usually begin 7 to 10 days (occasionally as late as 3 weeks) after primary exposure to the foreign protein, consist of fever, urticaria, or a maculopapular rash (90% of cases); arthritis or arthralgia; and lymphadenopathy. Local edema can occur at the serum injection site a few days before systemic signs and symptoms appear. Angioedema, glomerulonephritis, Guillain-Barré syndrome, peripheral neuritis, and myocarditis also can occur. However, serum sickness may be mild and resolve spontaneously within a few days to 2 weeks. People who previously have received serum injections are at an increased risk after readministration; manifestations in these patients usually occur shortly (from hours to 3 days) after administration of serum. Antihistamines can be helpful for management of serum sickness for alleviation of pruritus, edema, and urticaria. Fever, malaise, arthralgia, and arthritis can be controlled in most patients by administration of aspirin or other nonsteroidal anti-inflammatory agents. Corticosteroids may be helpful for controlling serious manifestations that are controlled poorly by other agents; prednisone or prednisolone in therapeutic dosages (1.5–2 mg/kg per day; maximum 60 mg/day) for 5 to 7 days is an appropriate regimen.

Anaphylaxis. The rapidity of onset and overall severity of anaphylaxis may vary considerably. Anaphylaxis usually begins within minutes of exposure to the

Table 1.10. Desensitization to Serum—Intradermal (ID), Subcutaneous (SC), and Intramuscular (IM) Routes

Dose Number[1]	Route of Administration	Dilution of Serum in Isotonic Sodium Chloride	Amount of ID, SC, or IM Injection, mL
1	ID	1:1000	0.1
2	ID	1:1000	0.3
3	SC	1:1000	0.6
4	SC	1:100	0.1
5	SC	1:100	0.3
6	SC	1:100	0.6
7	SC	1:10	0.1
8	SC	1:10	0.3
9	SC	1:10	0.6
10	SC	Undiluted	0.1
11	SC	Undiluted	0.3
12	IM	Undiluted	0.6
13	IM	Undiluted	1.0

[1] Administer consistently at 15-minute intervals.

causative agent, and in general, the more rapid the onset, the more severe the overall course. Major symptomatic manifestations include (1) cutaneous: pruritus, flushing, urticaria, and angioedema; (2) respiratory: hoarse voice and stridor, cough, wheeze, dyspnea, and cyanosis; (3) cardiovascular: rapid weak pulse, hypotension, and arrhythmias; and (4) gastrointestinal: cramps, vomiting, diarrhea, and dry mouth. Anaphylaxis is a medical emergency.

Treatment of Anaphylactic Reactions

Personnel administering biologic products or serum should be prepared to recognize and treat systemic anaphylaxis. The medications, equipment, and competent staff necessary to maintain the patency of the airway and to manage cardiovascular collapse must be available immediately. Appropriate and timely transfer of a patient with anaphylaxis to a pediatric intensive care unit or a hospital emergency department may be necessary.

The emergency treatment of systemic anaphylactic reactions is based on the type of reaction. In all instances, epinephrine is the primary drug. Mild symptoms of pruritus, erythema, urticaria, and angioedema should be treated with epinephrine injected intramuscularly, followed by diphenhydramine, hydroxyzine, or other antihistamine given orally or parenterally (see Tables 1.11, p 64, and 1.12, p 65). Because higher and more rapid concentrations of epinephrine are achieved after IM administration, subcutaneous administration no longer is recommended. If symptoms persist or recur, epinephrine administration may be repeated every 10 to 20 minutes for up to 3 doses. If the patient's condition improves with this management and remains stable, oral antihistamines and possibly oral steroids

Table 1.11. **Epinephrine in the Treatment of Anaphylaxis**[1]

Intramuscular administration

Epinephrine 1:1000 (aqueous): 0.01 mL/kg per dose, up to 0.5 mL, repeated every 10–20 min up to 3 doses.[2]

Intravenous administration

An initial bolus of intravenous epinephrine is given to patients not responding to intramuscular epinephrine using a dilution of 1:10 000 rather than a dilution of 1:1000. This dilution can be made using 1 mL of the 1:1000 dilution in 9 mL of physiologic saline solution. The dose is 1 mg/kg or 0.01 mL/kg of the 1:10 000 dilution. A continuous infusion should be started if repeated doses are required. One milligram (1 mL) of 1:1000 dilution of epinephrine added to 250 mL of 5% dextrose in water, resulting in a concentration of 4 μg/mL, is infused initially at a rate of 0.1 μg/kg per minute and increased gradually to 1.5 μg/kg per minute to maintain blood pressure.

[1] In addition to epinephrine, maintenance of the airway and administration of oxygen are critical.
[2] If agent causing anaphylactic reaction was given by injection, epinephrine can be injected into the same site to slow absorption.

(1.5–2.0 mg/kg per day of prednisone; maximum 60 mg/day) can be given for an additional 24 to 48 hours.

More severe or potentially life-threatening systemic anaphylaxis involving severe bronchospasm, laryngeal edema, other airway compromise, shock, and cardiovascular collapse necessitates additional therapy. Maintenance of the airway and oxygen administration should be instituted promptly. Intravenous epinephrine may be indicated; for this use, it must be diluted from 1:1000 aqueous base to a dilution of 1:10 000 using physiologic saline solution (see Table 1.11, above). A slow continuous infusion is preferable to repeated bolus administration. Nebulized albuterol is indicated for bronchospasm (see Table 1.12, p 65). Rapid IV infusion of physiologic saline solution, lactated Ringer's solution, or other isotonic solution adequate to maintain blood pressure must be instituted to compensate for the loss of circulating intravascular volume.

In some cases, the use of inotropic agents, such as dopamine (see Table 1.12, p 65), may be necessary for blood pressure support. The combination of histamine H_1 and H_2 receptor-blocking agents (see Table 1.12, p 65) can be synergistic in effect and should be used. Corticosteroids should be used in all cases of anaphylaxis except those that are mild and have responded promptly to initial therapy (see Table 1.12, p 65). However, there are no data supporting the usefulness of corticosteroids in treating anaphylaxis, and therefore, they should not be considered primary drugs.

All patients showing signs and symptoms of systemic anaphylaxis, regardless of severity, should be observed for several hours in an appropriate facility. Biphasic and protracted anaphylaxis may be mitigated with early administration of oral corticosteroids; however, usefulness of corticosteroids for these 2 conditions has not been established fully. Therefore, patients should be observed even after remission of immediate symptoms. Although a specific period of observation has not been established, a period of observation of 4 hours would be reasonable for mild episodes and perhaps as long as 24 hours would be reasonable for severe episodes.

Red Book®:

2003 REPORT OF THE COMMITTEE ON INFECTIOUS DISEASES

Erratum

P. 64: Table 1.11: Under the heading "Intravenous administration," in the third sentence, change **1 mg/kg or 0.01 mL/kg** to **0.01 mg/kg or 0.1 mL/kg.**

Table 1.11. Epinephrine in the Treatment of Anaphylaxis[1]

Intramuscular administration

Epinephrine 1:1000 (aqueous): 0.01 mL/kg per dose, up to 0.5 mL, repeated every 10–20 min up to 3 doses.[2]

Intravenous administration

An initial bolus of intravenous epinephrine is given to patients not responding to intramuscular epinephrine using a dilution of 1:10 000 rather than a dilution of 1:1000. This dilution can be made using 1 mL of the 1:1000 dilution in 9 mL of physiologic saline solution. The dose is **0.01 mg/kg or 0.1 mL/kg** of the 1:10 000 dilution. A continuous infusion should be started if repeated doses are required. One milligram (1 mL) of 1:1000 dilution of epinephrine added to 250 mL of 5% dextrose in water, resulting in a concentration of 4 µg/mL, is infused initially at a rate of 0.1 µg/kg per minute and increased gradually to 1.5 µg/kg per minute to maintain blood pressure.

[1] In addition to epinephrine, maintenance of the airway and administration of oxygen are critical.
[2] If agent causing anaphylactic reaction was given by injection, epinephrine can be injected into the same site to slow absorption.

Table 1.12. **Dosages of Commonly Used Secondary Drugs in the Treatment of Anaphylaxis**

Drug	Dose
H$_1$ blocking agents (antihistamines)	
Diphenhydramine	Oral, IM, IV: 1–2 mg/kg, every 4–6 h (100 mg, maximum single dose)
Hydroxyzine	Oral, IM: 0.5–1 mg/kg, every 4–6 h (100 mg, maximum single dose)
H$_2$ blocking agents (also antihistamines)	
Cimetidine	IV: 5 mg/kg, slowly over a 15-min period, every 6–8 h (300 mg, maximum single dose)
Ranitidine	IV: 1 mg/kg, slowly over a 15-min period, every 6–8 h (50 mg, maximum single dose)
Corticosteroids	
Hydrocortisone	IV: 100–200 mg, every 4–6 h
Methylprednisolone	IV: 1.5–2 mg/kg, every 4–6 h (60 mg, maximum single dose)
Prednisone	Oral: 1.5–2 mg/kg, single morning dose (60 mg, maximum single dose); use corticosteroids as long as needed
β$_2$-agonist	
Albuterol	Nebulizer solution: 0.5% (5 mg/mL), 0.05–0.15 mg/kg per dose in 2–3 mL isotonic sodium chloride solution, maximum of 5.0 mg per dose every 20 min over a 1-h to 2-h period or 0.5 mg/kg per hour by continuous nebulization (15 mg/h, maximum dose)
Other	
Dopamine	IV: 5–20 µg/kg per minute. Mixing 150 mg of dopamine with 250 mL of saline or 5% dextrose in water will produce a solution that, if infused at the rate of 1 mL/kg per hour, will deliver 10 µg/kg per min. The solution must be free of bicarbonate, which may inactivate dopamine.

IM indicates intramuscular; IV, intravenous.

Anaphylaxis occurring in people who are already taking β-adrenergic–blocking agents presents a unique situation. In such people, the manifestations are likely to be more profound and significantly less responsive to epinephrine and other β-adrenergic agonist drugs. More aggressive therapy with epinephrine may be adequate to override receptor blockade in some patients. Some experts recommend the use of IV glucagon for cardiovascular manifestations and inhaled atropine for management of bradycardia or bronchospasm.

IMMUNIZATION IN SPECIAL CLINICAL CIRCUMSTANCES

Preterm and Low Birth Weight Infants*

Preterm infants less than 37 weeks' gestation and infants of low birth weight (<2500 g) should, with few exceptions, receive all routinely recommended childhood vaccines at the same chronologic age as should full-term infants. Gestational age and birth weight are not limiting factors when deciding whether a clinically stable premature infant is to be immunized on schedule. Although studies have shown decreased immune responses to some vaccines given to very low birth weight (<1500 g), extremely low birth weight (<1000 g), and very early gestational age (<29 weeks) neonates, most preterm infants produce sufficient vaccine-induced immunity to prevent disease. Vaccine dosages normally given to full-term infants should not be reduced or divided when given to preterm and low birth weight infants.

Preterm and low birth weight infants tolerate most childhood vaccines as well as full-term infants. Apnea, reported to have occurred in some extremely low birth weight infants of fewer than 31 weeks' gestation after use of diphtheria and tetanus toxoids and whole-cell pertussis (DTwP) vaccine, has not been reported after use of acellular pertussis-containing vaccines in small numbers of extremely low birth weight infants. However, preterm infants given heptavalent pneumococcal conjugate vaccine (PCV7) concomitantly with DTwP and *Haemophilus influenzae* type b (Hib) vaccine were reported to experience benign febrile convulsions more frequently than were full-term infants given the same vaccines.

Medically stable preterm infants who remain in the hospital at 2 months of chronologic age should be given all vaccines recommended at that age (see Recommended Childhood and Adolescent Immunization Schedule, Fig 1.1, p 24). A medically stable infant is defined as one who does not require ongoing management for serious infection; metabolic disease; or renal, cardiovascular, or respiratory instability and who demonstrates a clinical course of sustained recovery and pattern of steady growth. All immunizations required at 2 months of age may be administered simultaneously to preterm and low birth weight infants. However, hospitalized preterm infants with limited injection sites may benefit from increasing the intervals between their primary immunizations. The choice of needle lengths used for intra-

---

* American Academy of Pediatrics, Committee on Infectious Diseases. Immunization of preterm and low birth weight infants. *Pediatrics*. In press

muscular vaccine administration is determined by available muscle mass of the premature infant and may be less than the standard ⅞-inch length recommended for full-term infants.

Hepatitis B vaccine given to preterm and low birth weight infants weighing more than 2000 g at birth produces an immune response comparable to that in full-term infants. Therefore, medically stable preterm infants weighing more than 2000 g born to hepatitis B surface antigen (HBsAg)-negative mothers may receive the first dose of hepatitis B vaccine at birth or shortly thereafter. For medically unstable preterm infants weighing >2000 g born to HBsAg-negative mothers, hepatitis B immunization may be deferred until their clinical condition has stabilized. Seroconversion rates and antibody concentrations in very low birth weight and extremely low birth weight infants immunized with hepatitis B vaccine shortly after birth often are lower than those seen in full-term infants immunized at birth and in preterm infants immunized at a later age. Nonetheless, hepatitis B vaccine appears to protect preterm infants born to HBsAg-positive mothers from complications related to perinatal exposure to hepatitis B infection, regardless of birth weight. Several studies confirm that the chronologic age of the medically stable preterm infant at the time of the first dose of hepatitis B vaccine is the best predictor of successful seroconversion regardless of birth weight or gestational age at birth. Consistent weight gain by preterm infants before receipt of the first dose of hepatitis B vaccine also is predictive of immune responsiveness. Medically stable, thriving infants weighing less than 2000 g demonstrate predictable, consistent, and sufficient hepatitis B antibody responses when given hepatitis B vaccine starting at 30 days of age. Preterm infants weighing less than 2000 g who are healthy enough to be released from the hospital before a chronologic age of 30 days may receive hepatitis B vaccine at discharge (see Hepatitis B, p 323). Starting the hepatitis B series at 1 month of age, regardless of the weight of the preterm infant, offers more options for implementing the immunization schedule in the special care nursery setting, lessens the number of simultaneous injections at 2 months of age (when other recommended childhood immunizations are due), provides earlier protection to vulnerable preterm infants more likely to receive multiple blood products and undergo surgical interventions, and decreases the risk of horizontal transmission from occult hepatitis B chronic carriers among family members, hospital visitors, and other caregivers. Studies also have shown that the closer hepatitis B vaccine is given to the infant's birth, the greater the likelihood the complement of childhood vaccines will be completed on time.

All preterm and low birth weight infants born to HBsAg-positive mothers should receive Hepatitis B Immune Globulin (HBIG) within 12 hours of birth and concurrent hepatitis B vaccine at different sites (see Hepatitis B, p 323). If maternal HBsAg status is unknown at birth, preterm or low birth weight infants should receive hepatitis B vaccine in accordance with recommendations for infants born to HBsAg-positive mothers. For hepatitis B immunoprophylaxis schemes for preterm and low birth weight infants born to mothers who are HBsAg negative, HBsAg positive, and HBsAg unknown, see Table 3.18, p 328, and Hepatitis B, Special Considerations, p 327.

Because all preterm infants are considered at increased risk of complications of influenza, 2 doses of inactivated influenza vaccine given 1 month apart should be offered for these infants beginning at 6 months of chronologic age, before the onset of the influenza season (see Influenza, p 386). Preterm infants younger than 6 months of age and infants with chronic complications of prematurity at any age are extremely vulnerable when exposed to influenza virus, making it prudent for household contacts, child care providers, and hospital nursery personnel caring for preterm infants to receive inactivated influenza vaccine yearly (see Influenza, p 386). All preterm infants younger than 32 weeks' gestational age and infants with chronic lung disease and specified cardiovascular conditions up to 2 years of age may benefit from monthly immunoprophylaxis with palivizumab (respiratory syncytial virus monoclonal antibody) during respiratory syncytial virus season. Selected infants of 32 to 35 weeks' gestational age also may benefit from immunoprophylaxis (see Respiratory Syncytial Virus, p 523). Palivizumab use does not interfere with the provision of routine childhood immunizations to preterm or low birth weight infants. Respiratory Syncytial Immune Globulin Intravenous has limited application for use in preterm infants with specific underlying clinical conditions.

Pregnancy

Immunization during pregnancy poses theoretic risks to the developing fetus. Although no evidence indicates that vaccines in use today have detrimental effects on the fetus, pregnant women should receive a vaccine only when the vaccine is unlikely to cause harm, the risk for disease exposure is high, and the infection would pose a significant risk to the mother or fetus. When a vaccine is to be given during pregnancy, delaying administration until the second or third trimester, when possible, is a reasonable precaution to minimize concern about possible teratogenicity.

The only vaccines routinely recommended for administration during pregnancy in the United States, provided they are otherwise indicated (either for primary or booster immunization), are those for tetanus, diphtheria, and influenza. Pregnant women who have not received a diphtheria and tetanus toxoid (Td) booster during the last 10 years should be given a booster dose, and women who are unimmunized or only partially immunized should complete the primary series. In developing countries with a high incidence of neonatal tetanus, Td routinely is administered during pregnancy without evidence of adverse effects and with striking decreases in the occurrence of neonatal tetanus.

Studies indicate that women in the second and third trimesters of pregnancy and early puerperium with absence of other underlying risk factors are at increased risk of complications and hospitalization from influenza. Therefore, the Advisory Committee on Immunization Practices (ACIP) of the Centers for Disease Control and Prevention (CDC) recommends that inactivated influenza vaccine be administered to all women who will be beyond 14 weeks of pregnancy during the influenza season (see Influenza, p 382).

Pneumococcal immunization can be given to a pregnant woman at high risk of serious or complicated illness from infection with *Streptococcus pneumoniae.* Hepatitis A or hepatitis B immunizations, if indicated, should be given to pregnant women. Although data on the safety of these vaccines for the developing fetus are not available, no risk would be expected, because the vaccines contain formalin-inactivated virus (hepatitis A) or noninfectious surface antigen (hepatitis B). In contrast, infection with either agent in a pregnant woman can result in severe disease in the mother and, in the case of hepatitis B, chronic infection in the newborn.

Pregnancy is a contraindication to administration of all live-virus vaccines, except when susceptibility and exposure are highly probable and the disease to be prevented poses a greater threat to the woman or fetus than does the vaccine. Although only a theoretic risk to the fetus of a live-virus vaccine exists, the background rate of anomalies in uncomplicated pregnancies may result in a defect that could be attributed inappropriately to a vaccine. Therefore, live vaccines should be avoided during pregnancy. However, yellow fever vaccine may be given to pregnant women who are at substantial risk of imminent exposure to infection, such as in some circumstances of international travel. Pregnant women who previously received complete or partial immunization against poliovirus may be given IPV vaccine. For unimmunized women, IPV vaccine is recommended for all doses (see Poliovirus Infections, p 505).

Because measles, mumps, rubella, and varicella vaccines are contraindicated for pregnant women, efforts should be made to immunize susceptible women against these illnesses before they become pregnant. Although of theoretic concern, no case of embryopathy caused by rubella vaccine has been reported. Accumulated evidence demonstrates that inadvertent administration of rubella vaccine to susceptible pregnant women rarely, if ever, causes congenital defects. The effect of varicella vaccine on the fetus, if any, is unknown. The manufacturer, in collaboration with the CDC, has established the VARIVAX Pregnancy Registry to monitor the maternal and fetal outcomes of women who inadvertently are given varicella immunization from 3 months before or at any time during pregnancy. From March 1995 to March 2002, 462 women (110 of whom were seronegative) who inadvertently received varicella vaccine before or during pregnancy and whose pregnancy outcomes are known were reported to this registry. No offspring had clinical features of congenital varicella, although 3 have had congenital malformations, which is the rate of congenital anomalies in the general population. Reporting of cases is encouraged and may be done by telephone (1-800-986-8999). A pregnant mother or other household member is not a contraindication for varicella immunization of a child in that household. Transmission of vaccine virus from an immunocompetent vaccine recipient to a susceptible person has been reported only rarely and only in the presence of a vaccine-associated rash (see Varicella-Zoster Infections, p 672).

Immunocompromised Children

PRIMARY AND SECONDARY IMMUNE DEFICIENCIES

The safety and effectiveness of vaccines in people with immune deficiency are determined by the nature and degree of immunosuppression. Immunocompromised people vary in their degree of immunosuppression and susceptibility to infection. Immunocompromised children represent a heterogeneous population with regard to immunization. Immunodeficiency conditions can be grouped into primary and secondary (acquired) disorders. Primary disorders of the immune system generally are inherited and include disorders of B-lymphocyte (humoral) immunity, T-lymphocyte (cell)-mediated immunity, complement, and phagocytic function. Secondary disorders of the immune system are acquired and occur in people with human immunodeficiency virus (HIV) infection, acquired immunodeficiency syndrome, or malignant neoplasms; people who have undergone transplantation; and people receiving immunosuppressive or radiation therapy (see Table 1.13, p 71). Experience with vaccine administration in immunocompromised children is limited. In most situations, theoretic considerations are the only guide to vaccine administration, because experience with specific vaccines in people with a specific disorder is lacking. However, considerable data in HIV-infected infants provide reassurance about the low risk of adverse events in these patients after immunization.

Live vaccines. In general, people who are severely immunocompromised or in whom immune status is uncertain should not receive live vaccines, either viral or bacterial, because of the risk of disease from the vaccine strains. Although precautions, contraindications, and suboptimal efficacy of immunizations in immunocompromised patients are emphasized, some immunocompromised children may benefit from special-use as well as routinely recommended immunizations.

Inactivated vaccines and passive immunization. Inactivated vaccines and Immune Globulin preparations should be used when appropriate, because the risk of complications from these preparations is not increased in immunocompromised people. However, immune responses of immunocompromised children to inactivated vaccines (eg, DTaP, hepatitis B, hepatitis A, inactivated poliovirus, Hib, pneumococcal, and influenza) may vary and may be inadequate. Therefore, a vaccine's immunogenicity in these children may be decreased substantially. In children with secondary immunodeficiency, the ability to develop an adequate immunologic response depends on when immunosuppression occurs. In children in whom immunosuppressive therapy is discontinued, an adequate response occurs usually between 3 months and 1 year after discontinuation. Inactivated influenza vaccine should be given yearly to immunosuppressed children 6 months of age and older before each influenza season. In children with malignant neoplasms, influenza immunization should be given no less than 3 to 4 weeks after chemotherapy is discontinued and when peripheral granulocyte and lymphocyte counts greater than 1000 cells/µL ($1.0 \ 10^9$/L) are achieved.

Primary immunodeficiencies. Measles and varicella vaccines should be considered for children with B-lymphocyte disorders; however, antibody response may not occur because of the underlying disease and because the patient is receiving Immune Globulin Intravenous (IGIV) periodically. All other live vaccines are contraindicated for most patients with B-lymphocyte defects except immunoglobulin (Ig) A deficiency. Live vaccines are contraindicated for all patients with T-lymphocyte–mediated disorders of immune function (see Table 1.13, p 71). Fatal poliomyelitis and measles vaccine virus infections have occurred in children with disorders of T-cell function after administration of live-virus vaccines. Oral poliovirus vaccine no longer is recommended for routine use in the United States.* Inactivated poliovirus vaccine should be administered if available. Children with deficiency in antibody-synthesizing capacity are incapable of developing an antibody response to vaccines and should receive regular doses of Immune Globulin (usually IGIV) to provide passive

---

* American Academy of Pediatrics, Committee on Infectious Diseases. Prevention of poliomyelitis: recommendations for use of only inactivated poliovirus vaccine for routine immunization. *Pediatrics*. 1999;104:1404–1406

Table 1.13. **Immunization of Children and Adolescents With Primary and Secondary Immune Deficiencies**

Category	Specific Immunodeficiency	Vaccine Contraindications	Effectiveness and Comments
Primary			
B-lymphocyte (humoral)	X-linked and common variable agammaglobulinemia	OPV,[1] vaccinia, and live bacterial; consider measles and varicella	Effectiveness of any vaccine dependent on humoral response is doubtful; IGIV interferes with measles and possibly varicella response.
	Selective IgA deficiency and selective subclass IgG deficiency	OPV[1]; other live vaccines seem to be safe, but caution is urged	All vaccines probably effective. Vaccine response may be attenuated.
T-lymphocyte (cell-mediated and humoral)	Severe combined	All live vaccines[2,3]	Effectiveness of any vaccine dependent on humoral or cellular response is doubtful.
Complement	Deficiency of early components (C1, C4, C2, C3)	None	All routine vaccines probably effective. Pneumococcal and meningococcal vaccines recommended.
	Deficiency of late components (C5–C9), properdin, factor B	None	All routine vaccines probably effective. Meningococcal vaccine recommended.
Phagocytic function	Chronic granulomatous disease Leukocyte adhesion defect Myeloperoxidase deficiency	Live bacterial vaccines[3]	All routine vaccines probably effective. Inactivated influenza vaccine should be considered to decrease secondary infection.

Table 1.13. Immunization of Children and Adolescents With Primary and Secondary Immune Deficiencies, continued

Category	Specific Immunodeficiency	Vaccine Contraindications	Effectiveness and Comments
Secondary			
	HIV/AIDS	OPV,[1] vaccinia, BCG; withhold MMR and varicella in severely immunocompromised children	MMR, varicella, and all inactivated vaccines, including influenza, may be effective.[4]
	Malignant neoplasm, transplantation, immunosuppressive or radiation therapy	Live viral and bacterial, depending on immune status[2,3]	Effectiveness of any vaccine depends on degree of immune suppression.

OPV indicates oral poliovirus; IGIV, Immune Globulin Intravenous; Ig, immunoglobulin; HIV, human immunodeficiency virus; AIDS, acquired immunodeficiency syndrome; BCG, bacille Calmette-Guérin; MMR, measles-mumps-rubella.

[1] OPV vaccine no longer is recommended for routine use in the United States.

[2] Live viral vaccines: MMR, OPV, varicella, vaccinia (smallpox). Smallpox vaccine is not recommended for children.

[3] Live bacterial vaccines: BCG and Ty21a *Salmonella typhi* vaccine.

[4] HIV-infected children should receive IG after exposure to measles (see Measles, p 422) and may receive varicella vaccine if CD4+ lymphocyte count = 25% (see Varicella-Zoster Infections, p 684).

protection against many infectious diseases. Specific immune globulins (eg, Varicella-Zoster Immune Globulin [VZIG]) are available for postexposure prophylaxis for some infections (see Specific Immune Globulins, p 56). Children with milder B-lymphocyte and antibody deficiencies have an intermediate degree of vaccine responsiveness and may require monitoring of postimmunization antibody titers to confirm vaccine immunogenicity.

Children with early or late complement deficiencies can receive all immunizations, including live vaccines. Children with phagocytic function disorders, including chronic granulomatous disease and leukocyte adhesion defect, can receive all immunizations except live bacterial vaccines (bacille Calmette-Guérin [BCG] and Ty21a *Salmonella typhi*). Most experts believe that live viral vaccines are safe to administer to children with complement deficiencies and phagocyte disorders.

Secondary (acquired) immunodeficiencies. Several factors should be considered in immunization of children with secondary immunodeficiencies, including the underlying disease, the specific immunosuppressive regimen (dose and schedule), and the infectious disease and immunization history of the person. Live vaccines generally are contraindicated because of an increased risk of serious adverse effects. Exceptions are children with HIV infection who are not severely immunocompromised in whom measles-mumps-rubella (MMR) vaccine is recommended (see Human Immunodeficiency Virus Infections, p 360) and in whom varicella vaccine should be considered if CD4+ lymphocyte counts are 25% or greater (see Varicella-Zoster Infections, p 672). The use of varicella vaccine in children with acute lymphocytic leukemia in remission should be considered, because the risk of natural varicella outweighs the risk from the attenuated vaccine virus (see Varicella-Zoster Infections, p 672).

Live-virus vaccines usually are withheld for an interval of at least 3 months after immunosuppressive cancer chemotherapy has been discontinued. The exception is corticosteroid therapy (see Corticosteroids, p 74), for which the interval is based on the assumption that immune response will have been restored in 3 months and that the underlying disease for which immunosuppressive therapy was given is in remission or under control. However, the interval may vary with the intensity and type of immunosuppressive therapy, radiation therapy, underlying disease, and other factors. Therefore, it often is not possible to make a definitive recommendation for an interval after cessation of immunosuppressive therapy when live-virus vaccines can be administered safely and effectively. In vitro testing of immune function may provide guidelines for safe timing of immunizations in individual patients.

Other considerations. Because patients with congenital or acquired immunodeficiencies may not have an adequate response to an immunizing agent, they may remain susceptible despite having received an appropriate vaccine. Specific serum antibody titers should be determined after immunization to assess immune response and guide further immunization and management of future exposures.

People with certain immune deficiencies may benefit from specific immunizations directed at preventing infections by organisms to which they are particularly susceptible. Examples include administration of pneumococcal and meningococcal vaccines to people with splenic dysfunction, asplenia (see Asplenic Children, p 80), and complement deficiencies who are at increased risk of infection with encapsulated bacteria. Also, annual influenza immunization is indicated for children 6 months of age and older with splenic dysfunction, asplenia, and phagocyte function deficiencies to prevent influenza and decrease the risk of secondary bacterial infections that may occur (see Influenza, p 386).

Household contacts. Immunocompetent siblings and other household contacts of people with an immunologic deficiency should not receive oral poliovirus vaccine, because vaccine virus may be transmitted to immunocompromised people. However, siblings and household contacts should receive MMR vaccine if indicated, because transmission of the vaccine viruses does not occur. Household contacts 6 months of age and older should receive yearly inactivated influenza vaccine to prevent infection and subsequent transmission to the immunocompromised person. Varicella vaccine is recommended for susceptible contacts of immunocompromised children, because transmission of varicella vaccine virus from healthy people is rare, and vaccine-associated illness, if it develops, is mild. No precautions need to be taken after immunization unless the vaccine recipient develops a rash, particularly a vesicular rash. In such instances, the vaccine recipient should avoid direct contact with immunocompromised, susceptible hosts for the duration of the rash. If contact inadvertently occurs, administration of VZIG is not indicated, because risk of transmission is low. Also, when transmission has occurred, the virus has maintained its attenuated characteristics. In most instances, antiviral therapy is not necessary but can be initiated if illness occurs (see Varicella-Zoster Infections, p 674).

CORTICOSTEROIDS

Children who receive corticosteroid therapy can become immunocompromised. The minimal amount of systemic corticosteroids and duration of administration sufficient to cause immunosuppression in an otherwise healthy child are not well defined. The frequency and route of administration of corticosteroids, the underlying disease, and concurrent other therapy are additional factors affecting immunosuppression. Despite these uncertainties, sufficient experience exists to recommend empiric guidelines for administration of live-virus vaccines to previously healthy children receiving corticosteroid therapy for nonimmunocompromising conditions. Many clinicians consider a dosage equivalent to ≥2 mg/kg per day of prednisone or equivalent to a total of ≥20 mg/day for children who weigh more than 10 kg, particularly when given for more than 14 days, sufficient to raise concern about the safety of immunization with live-virus vaccines. Accordingly, guidelines for administration of live-virus vaccines to recipients of corticosteroids are as follows:

- *Topical therapy or local injections of corticosteroids.* Administration of topical corticosteroids on the skin or in the respiratory tract (ie, by aerosol) or eyes and intra-articular, bursal, or tendon injections of corticosteroids usually do not result in immunosuppression that would contraindicate administration of live-virus vaccines. However, live-virus vaccines should not be administered if clinical or laboratory evidence of systemic immunosuppression results from prolonged application until corticosteroid therapy has been discontinued for at least 1 month.
- *Physiologic maintenance doses of corticosteroids.* Children who are receiving only maintenance physiologic doses of corticosteroids can receive live-virus vaccines during corticosteroid treatment.

- *Low or moderate doses of systemic corticosteroids given daily or on alternate days.* Children receiving <2 mg/kg per day of prednisone or its equivalent, or <20 mg/day if they weigh more than 10 kg, can receive live-virus vaccines during corticosteroid treatment.
- *High doses of systemic corticosteroids given daily or on alternate days for fewer than 14 days.* Children receiving ≥2 mg/kg per day of prednisone or its equivalent, or ≥20 mg/day if they weigh more than 10 kg, can receive live-virus vaccines immediately after discontinuation of treatment. Some experts, however, would delay immunization until 2 weeks after corticosteroid therapy has been discontinued, if possible (ie, if the patient's condition allows temporary cessation).
- *High doses of systemic corticosteroids given daily or on alternate days for 14 days or more.* Children receiving ≥2 mg/kg per day of prednisone or its equivalent, or ≥20 mg/day if they weigh more than 10 kg, should not receive live-virus vaccines until corticosteroid therapy has been discontinued for at least 1 month.
- *Children with a disease that, in itself, is considered to suppress the immune response and who are receiving systemic or locally administered corticosteroids.* These children should not be given live-virus vaccines, except in special circumstances.

These guidelines are based on concerns about vaccine safety in recipients of high doses of corticosteroids. In addition, when deciding whether to administer live-virus vaccines, the potential benefits and risks of immunization for an individual patient and in specific circumstances should be considered. For example, some experts recommend immunization of a patient at increased risk of a vaccine-preventable infection (and its complications) if, despite corticosteroid therapy, the patient does not have clinical evidence of immunosuppression.

The guidelines also are based on considerations of safety concerning live-virus vaccines and do not necessarily correlate with those for optimal vaccine immunogenicity. For example, some children receiving moderate doses of prednisone, such as 1.5 mg/kg per day for several weeks or longer, may have a less-than-optimal serum antibody response to some vaccine antigens. Nevertheless, unless immunization can be deferred temporarily until corticosteroids are discontinued without compromising the likelihood of immunization, children should be immunized to enhance the likelihood of protection in the case of exposure to disease. In contrast, some children receiving relatively high doses of corticosteroids (eg, 30 mg/day of prednisone) may respond adequately to immunization.

HODGKIN DISEASE

Patients with Hodgkin disease should be immunized with pneumococcal conjugate and/or polysaccharide vaccine according to age-specific recommendations (see Pneumococcal Infections, p 490); they also should receive Hib vaccine according to age-specific recommendations (see *Haemophilus influenzae* Infections, p 293). These patients are at increased risk of invasive pneumococcal infection; most experts believe they also are at increased risk of invasive Hib infection. Antibody response is likely to be best when patients are immunized at least 10 to 14 days before initiation of therapy for Hodgkin disease. During active chemotherapy and shortly thereafter, antibody responses to the pneumococcal vaccine are impaired. However, the ability of these patients to respond improves rapidly, and immunization as early as 3 months after cessation of chemotherapy is reasonable. Patients who received vaccine during chemotherapy or radiation therapy should be reimmunized 3 months after discontinuation of the therapy.

BONE MARROW TRANSPLANT RECIPIENTS

Many factors can affect immunity to vaccine-preventable diseases for a child recovering from successful bone marrow transplantation (BMT), including the donor's immunity, type of transplantation (ie, autologous or allogeneic, blood or hematopoietic stem cell*), interval since the transplantation, receipt of immunosuppressive medications, and graft-versus-host disease (GVHD). Although many children who are transplant recipients acquire the immunity of the donor, some will lose serologic evidence of immunity. Retention of donor immune memory can be facilitated if recalled by antigenic stimulation soon after transplantation. Clinical studies of bone marrow transplant recipients indicate that pretransplant administration of diphtheria and tetanus toxoids to the bone marrow donor and immediate post-transplant administration to the recipient can facilitate response to these antigens; serum antibody titers did not increase when immunization of the recipient was delayed until 5 weeks after transplantation. In theory, these results could be expected with other inactivated vaccine antigens, including pertussis, Hib, hepatitis B, hepatitis A, IPV, and pneumococcal conjugate and polysaccharide vaccines.

The risk of acquiring diphtheria or tetanus during the year after BMT is low. Some experts elect to reimmunize all children without serologic evaluation, and others base the decision to reimmunize against diphtheria and tetanus on adequacy of serologic titers obtained 1 year after transplantation. Adequate immune responses can be obtained with 3 doses of diphtheria and tetanus toxoids (Td) at 12, 14, and 24 months after transplantation in people 7 years of age or older. In people younger than 7 years of age, DTaP or DT can be used. No data are available on safety and immunogenicity of pertussis immunization for bone marrow transplant recipients. People with tetanus-prone wounds sustained during the first year after transplantation should be given Tetanus Immune Globulin, regardless of their tetanus immunization status.

Data on which to base recommendations for reimmunization against Hib or *S pneumoniae* are limited. Doses of Hib conjugate vaccine appear to provide some protection if given at 12, 14, and 24 months after BMT for recipients of any age. In 1 study, time after transplantation was the most important factor for determining the immune response to pneumococcal polysaccharide vaccine, with the greatest response observed when the vaccine was administered 2 or more years after transplantation. In another study, Hib conjugate and tetanus toxoid vaccines given 12 and 24 months after BMT induced adequate immune responses. Some experts recommend a multiple-dose schedule of pneumococcal conjugate and/or polysaccharide vaccine at 12 and 24 months after transplantation, depending on the age of the patient (see Pneumococcal Infections, p 490). The second dose of pneumo-

---

* Centers for Disease Control and Prevention. Guidelines for preventing opportunistic infections among hematopoietic stem cell transplant recipients. Recommendations of CDC, the Infectious Disease Society of America, and the American Society of Blood and Marrow Transplantation. *MMWR Recomm Rep.* 2000;49(RR-10):1–128

coccal vaccine is not a booster dose but provides a second opportunity for pneumo-coccal immunization for people who fail to respond to the first dose. In patients undergoing autologous BMT, preharvest immunization with Hib-conjugate vaccine resulted in higher anti-Hib antibody concentrations for 2 years after transplantation, compared with patients who were not immunized before harvest. Similar benefit in transplant recipients was noted when allogenic bone marrow donors were immu-nized before harvest.

Two years after BMT, MMR vaccine often is given if the recipient is presumed immunocompetent; data indicate that healthy survivors at that time can receive these live-virus vaccines without untoward effects. A second dose of MMR vaccine should be given 1 month (4 weeks) or more after the first dose unless serologic response to measles is demonstrated after the first dose. The benefit of a second dose in this population has not been evaluated. Patients with chronic GVHD should not receive MMR vaccine because of concern about resulting latent virus infection and its sequelae. Susceptible people who are exposed to measles should receive passive immunoprophylaxis (see Measles, p 419). Varicella vaccine is contraindicated for bone marrow transplant recipients less than 24 months after BMT. Use of varicella vaccine for bone marrow transplant recipients is restricted to research protocols in which the vaccine may be considered 24 months or more after BMT for recipients who are presumed immunocompetent. Passive immunization with VZIG is recom-mended for susceptible people with known exposure to varicella (see Varicella-Zoster Infections, p 672).

Only IPV vaccine should be given to transplant recipients and their household contacts. Bone marrow transplant recipients should be immunized with IPV vaccine at 12, 14, and 24 months after BMT. The effectiveness of giving additional doses is not known; more data are needed on optimal methods and timing of IPV immuni-zation. Recipients can be tested for immunity, but serologic tests for antibody titers against polioviruses are not readily available in commercial or state laboratories.

Inactivated influenza vaccine is not effective when given within the initial 6 months after BMT, but immunization may provide protection when given 1 year after BMT. Because the risk of disease is substantial, inactivated influenza vaccine should be administered annually during early autumn (see Influenza, p 382) to people who underwent BMT more than 6 months previously, even if the interval is fewer than 12 months.

The immunogenicity of hepatitis B vaccine in bone marrow transplant recipients has not been assessed adequately. On the basis of the response of these patients to other protein antigens, initiation of a 3-dose series at 12, 14, and 24 months after transplantation followed by postimmunization serologic testing for antibody to HBsAg is reasonable. Additional doses (maximum of 3) are given to vaccine non-responders. Routine administration of hepatitis A vaccine is not recommended but may be considered 12 months or longer after BMT for people who have chronic liver disease or chronic GVHD, people from hepatitis A-endemic areas, or people in areas experiencing outbreaks. Hepatitis A immunization requires 2 doses (see Hepatitis A, p 309). Household and health care worker contacts of bone marrow and solid organ transplant recipients should have immunity to or be immunized against poliovirus, measles, mumps, rubella, varicella, influenza, and hepatitis A.

SOLID ORGAN TRANSPLANT RECIPIENTS

It is important that children and adolescents being considered for solid organ transplantation receive their recommended immunizations before the transplantation is performed. In general, vaccines will be more immunogenic before transplantation, and live viral vaccines are contraindicated while immunosuppressive therapy is administered. Information about the use of live-virus vaccines in patients after solid organ transplantation is limited. For transplantation candidates who are older than 12 months of age, if previously immunized, serologic antibody titers for measles, mumps, rubella, and varicella should be performed. Children who are susceptible should be given MMR vaccine, varicella vaccine, or both before transplantation. Serum antibody titers to measles, mumps, rubella, and varicella should be measured in all patients 1 year or more after transplantation. Oral poliovirus vaccine is contraindicated for transplant recipients and their household contacts. If protection against polio is indicated, IPV should be used.

Killed and subunit vaccines should not pose a risk to solid organ transplant recipients. After transplantation, DTaP, Hib, hepatitis B, hepatitis A, influenza, and pneumococcal conjugate and polysaccharide vaccines can be administered, if indicated. Safety and immunogenicity data for these vaccines in children after transplantation are limited. Most experts wait at least 6 months after transplantation for resumption of immunization schedules when immune suppression is less intense. However, immunization schedules vary in different transplant centers. Hepatitis A vaccine should be considered for patients undergoing liver transplantation because of an increased mortality rate associated with hepatitis A infection in patients with chronic liver disease. Annual influenza immunization is indicated before and after solid organ transplantation. Solid organ transplant recipients at highest risk of infection with *S pneumoniae* appear to be those who have undergone cardiac transplantation or splenectomy. Pneumococcal conjugate or polysaccharide vaccine should be considered in all transplant recipients (see Pneumococcal Infections, p 490).

The decision to use passive immunization with an Immune Globulin preparation (see Immune Globulin, p 54) should be made on the basis of serologic evidence of susceptibility and exposure to disease. Household and health care worker contacts of bone marrow and solid organ transplant recipients should have immunity to or be immunized against poliovirus, measles, mumps, rubella, varicella, influenza, and hepatitis A.

HUMAN IMMUNODEFICIENCY VIRUS INFECTION (SEE ALSO HUMAN IMMUNODEFICIENCY VIRUS INFECTION, P 360)

Data on the use of currently available live viral and bacterial vaccines in HIV-infected children are limited, but complications have been reported after BCG and measles immunizations, including vaccine-related measles pneumonitis in a severely immunocompromised child 1 year after measles immunization. Because there have been reports of severe measles in symptomatic HIV-infected children, with fatalities in as many as 40% of cases, measles immunization (given as MMR vaccine) is recommended for most HIV-infected children, including children who are symptomatic but are not severely immunocompromised and children who are asymptomatic. Measles-mumps-rubella vaccine should be given at 12 months of age to enhance the likelihood of an appropriate immune response. The second dose after the 12-month immunization may be administered as soon as 1 month (28 days) later in an attempt to induce seroconversion as early as possible. In a measles epidemic, monovalent measles vaccine may be given as young as 6 months of age. Children immunized before their first birthday should be immunized with 2 additional doses of MMR vaccine (see Measles, Immunization During an Outbreak, p 426). Severely immunocompromised patients with HIV infection, as defined by low CD4+ T-lymphocyte counts or low percentage of total circulating lymphocytes, should not receive measles vaccine (see Human Immunodeficiency Virus Infection, p 360, and Table 3.26, p 368).

After the potential risks and benefits are weighed, varicella vaccine should be considered for asymptomatic or mildly symptomatic HIV-infected children with age-specific CD4+ T-lymphocyte percentages of 25% or more (see Varicella-Zoster Infections, p 672).* Children and adolescents with asymptomatic or symptomatic HIV infection also should receive other routinely recommended vaccines, including DTaP, IPV, hepatitis B, Hib, and pneumococcal conjugate vaccines, according to the recommended schedule (see Fig 1.1, p 24). Annual influenza immunization of HIV-infected people is recommended (see Influenza, p 382). Immunization with pneumococcal conjugate and/or polysaccharide vaccine is indicated on the basis of age- and vaccine-specific recommendations (see Pneumococcal Infections, p 490). Data are limited on the effect of routine immunizations on HIV RNA viral load in children. Some studies in adults have demonstrated transient increases of HIV RNA concentrations after immunization with influenza or pneumococcal vaccine, but other studies have shown no increase. No evidence indicates that this transient increase enhances progression of disease. Results of increases in HIV RNA concentrations in children after immunization are variable. Additional studies are needed in infants and children who receive recommended immunizations.

In the United States, BCG vaccine is contraindicated for HIV-infected patients. In areas of the world with a high incidence of tuberculosis, the World Health Organization (WHO) recommends giving BCG vaccine to HIV-infected children who are asymptomatic.

Routine or widespread screening to detect HIV infection in asymptomatic children before routine immunizations is not recommended. Children without clinical manifestations of or known risk factors for HIV infection should be immunized in accordance with the recommended childhood and adolescent immunization schedule.

Because the ability of HIV-infected children to respond to vaccine antigens likely is related to the degree of immunosuppression at the time of immunization and may be inadequate, these children should be considered potentially susceptible to vaccine-preventable diseases, even after appropriate immunization, unless a recent serologic test demonstrates adequate antibody concentrations. Hence, passive immunoprophylaxis or chemoprophylaxis after exposure to these diseases should be considered even if the child previously has received the recommended vaccines.

Vaccine-type varicella-zoster virus rarely has been transmitted from healthy people. Therefore, household contacts of HIV-infected people can be immunized with live-virus varicella vaccine (see Varicella-Zoster Infections, p 672). No precau-

---

* American Academy of Pediatrics, Committee on Infectious Diseases. Varicella vaccine update. *Pediatrics*. 2000;105:136–141

tions are needed after immunization of healthy children who do not develop a rash. Vaccine recipients who develop a rash should avoid direct contact with susceptible immunocompromised hosts for the duration of the rash. If the immunocompromised contact develops varicella, disease will be mild, and use of VZIG to prevent transmission is not indicated.

ASPLENIC CHILDREN

The asplenic state results from the following: (1) surgical removal of the spleen; (2) certain diseases, such as sickle cell disease (functional asplenia); or (3) congenital asplenia. All asplenic infants, children, adolescents, and adults, regardless of the reason for the asplenic state, have an increased risk of fulminant bacteremia, which is associated with a high mortality rate. Susceptibility to fulminant bacteremia is determined largely by the underlying disease. In comparison with immunocompetent children who have not undergone splenectomy, the incidence of and mortality rate from septicemia are increased in children who have had splenectomy after trauma and in children with sickle cell disease by as much as 350-fold, and the rate may be even higher in children who have had splenectomy for thalassemia. The risk of bacteremia is higher in younger children than in older children, and risk may be greater during the years immediately after splenectomy. Fulminant bacteremia, however, has been reported in adults as many as 25 years after splenectomy.

Streptococcus pneumoniae is the most important pathogen in asplenic children. Less common causes of bacteremia include Hib, *Neisseria meningitidis,* other streptococci, *Escherichia coli, Staphylococcus aureus,* and gram-negative bacilli, such as *Salmonella* species, *Klebsiella* species, and *Pseudomonas aeruginosa.* People who are functionally or anatomically asplenic also are at increased risk of fatal malaria and severe babesiosis.

Pneumococcal conjugate and/or polysaccharide vaccine is indicated for all asplenic children at the appropriate age (see Pneumococcal Infections, p 490). Reimmunization of recipients of the conjugate and/or polysaccharide vaccine at or before 24 months of age is recommended (see Pneumococcal Infections, p 490). Immunization against Hib infections should be initiated at 2 months of age, as recommended for otherwise healthy young children (see Fig 1.1, p 24), and for all previously unimmunized children with asplenia. Quadrivalent meningococcal polysaccharide vaccine also should be administered to asplenic children 2 years of age and older (see Meningococcal Infections, p 430). The efficacy of meningococcal vaccine in asplenic children is not certain, although this vaccine probably is as effective as pneumococcal polysaccharide vaccine. No known contraindication exists to giving these vaccines at the same time in separate syringes at different sites. In the United States, the currently licensed meningococcal vaccine is an unconjugated polysaccharide vaccine, which is not as effective for preventing disease in children younger than 5 years of age as it is in older people.

Daily antimicrobial prophylaxis against pneumococcal infections is recommended for many asplenic children, regardless of immunization status. For infants with sickle cell anemia, oral penicillin prophylaxis against invasive pneumococcal disease should be initiated as soon as the diagnosis is established and preferably by 2 months of age. Although the efficacy of antimicrobial prophylaxis has been proven only in patients with sickle cell anemia, other asplenic children at particularly high risk, such as children with malignant neoplasms or thalassemia, also should receive daily chemoprophylaxis. Less agreement exists about the need for prophylaxis for children who have had splenectomy after trauma. In general, antimicrobial prophylaxis (in addition to immunization) should be considered strongly for all asplenic children younger than 5 years of age and for at least 1 year after splenectomy.

The age at which chemoprophylaxis is discontinued often is an empiric decision. On the basis of a multicenter study, prophylactic penicillin can be discontinued at approximately 5 years of age in children with sickle cell anemia who are receiving regular medical attention and who have not had a severe pneumococcal infection or surgical splenectomy. The appropriate duration of prophylaxis for children with asplenia attributable to other causes is unknown. Some experts continue prophylaxis throughout childhood and into adulthood for particularly high-risk patients with asplenia.

For antimicrobial prophylaxis, oral penicillin V (125 mg, twice a day, for children younger than 5 years of age and 250 mg, twice a day, for children 5 years of age and older) is recommended. Some experts recommend amoxicillin (20 mg/kg per day). In recent years, the proportion of pneumococcal isolates that have intermediate or high-level resistance to penicillin has increased in most areas of the United States. Ongoing surveillance for resistant pneumococci is needed to determine whether changes to the recommended chemoprophylaxis will be required.

When antimicrobial prophylaxis is used, the limitations must be stressed to parents and patients, who should recognize that some bacteria capable of causing fulminant sepsis are not susceptible to the antimicrobial agents given for prophylaxis. Parents should be aware that all febrile illnesses are potentially serious in asplenic children and that immediate medical attention should be sought, because the initial signs and symptoms of fulminant bacteremia can be subtle. When bacteremia is a possibility, the physician should hospitalize the child, obtain specimens for blood and other cultures as indicated, and immediately begin treatment with an antimicrobial regimen effective against *S pneumoniae*, *H influenzae*, and *N meningitidis*. In some clinical situations, other antimicrobial agents, such as aminoglycosides, may be indicated. If an asplenic child travels or resides in an area where medical care is not accessible, an appropriate antimicrobial agent should be readily available, and the child's caregiver should be instructed in appropriate use.

Whenever possible, alternatives to splenectomy should be considered. Management options include postponement of splenectomy for as long as possible in congenital hemolytic anemias, preservation of accessory spleens, performance of partial splenectomy for benign tumors of the spleen, conservative (nonoperative) management of splenic trauma, or when feasible, repair rather than removal and, if possible, avoidance of splenectomy when immunodeficiency is present (eg, Wiskott-Aldrich syndrome).

Children With a Personal or Family History of Seizures

Infants and children with a personal or family history of seizures are at increased risk of having a seizure after receipt of DTP or measles (usually as MMR) vaccines. In most cases, these seizures are brief, self-limited, and generalized and occur in conjunction with fever, indicating that such vaccine-associated seizures usually are febrile seizures. No evidence indicates that these seizures cause permanent brain damage or epilepsy, aggravate neurologic disorders, or affect the prognosis for children with underlying disorders.

In the case of pertussis immunization during infancy, administration of DTaP could coincide with or hasten the recognition of a disorder associated with seizures, such as infantile spasms or epilepsy, and cause confusion about the role of pertussis immunization. Hence, pertussis immunization in infants with a history of recent seizures should be deferred until a progressive neurologic disorder is excluded or the cause of the earlier seizure has been determined. In contrast, measles immunization is given at an age when the cause and nature of any seizures and related neurologic status are more likely to have been established. This difference provides the basis for the recommendation that measles immunization should not be deferred for children with a history of recent seizures.

A family history of a seizure disorder is not a contraindication to pertussis or measles immunization or a reason to defer immunization. Postimmunization seizures in these children usually are febrile in origin, have a benign outcome, and are not likely to be confused with manifestations of a previously unrecognized neurologic disorder. In addition, many children have a family history of seizures and would remain susceptible to pertussis and measles if family history were a contraindication to immunization.

Specific recommendations for pertussis and measles immunization of children with a personal or family history of seizures are given in the respective disease-specific chapters (see Pertussis, p 472, and Measles, p 419); a detailed discussion and recommendations about pertussis immunization of children with neurologic disorders also are given.

Children With Chronic Diseases

Some chronic diseases make children more susceptible to the severe manifestations and complications of common infections. In general, immunizations recommended for healthy children should be given to children with these disorders. However, for children with immunologic disorders, live-virus vaccines usually are contraindicated; the major exception is MMR vaccine for HIV-infected children who are not immunocompromised severely (see Immunocompromised Children, p 69). Children with certain chronic diseases (eg, cardiorespiratory, allergic, hematologic, metabolic, and renal disorders; cystic fibrosis; and diabetes mellitus) are at increased risk of complications of influenza, pneumococcal infection, or both and should receive influenza and/or pneumococcal conjugate and/or polysaccharide vaccine (see Influenza, p 382, and Pneumococcal Infections, p 490). People with chronic liver disease are at risk of severe clinical manifestations of acute infection with hepatitis A virus (HAV). Therefore, these children and adolescents should be immunized with HAV vaccine after 2 years of age (see Hepatitis A, p 309).

Determining the appropriateness of administering a live-virus vaccine to a specific child with a rare disorder (eg, galactosemia or renal tubular acidosis) is problematic, particularly if the disease might impair the immune response to the vaccine. Documented experience with immunization and some of these disorders is minimal or nonexistent, and the physician should seek guidance from a specialist before administering the vaccine(s).

Active Immunization After Exposure to Disease

Because not all susceptible people receive vaccines before exposure, active immunization may be considered for a person who has been exposed to a specific disease. The following situations are the most commonly encountered (see the disease-specific chapters in Section 3 for detailed recommendations).

- **Measles.** Live-virus measles vaccine given within 72 hours of exposure will provide protection against measles in some cases. Determining the time of exposure may be difficult, because infected people can spread measles virus for 3 to 5 days before the appearance of a rash and for 1 to 2 days before the onset of symptoms.

  Immune Globulin (IG), administered intramuscularly in a dose of 0.25 mL/kg (maximum dose 15 mL) within 6 days of exposure, also can prevent or modify measles in a healthy susceptible person. Because the measles morbidity rate is high in children younger than 1 year of age, administration of IG is recommended for infants exposed to measles and for immunocompromised people and pregnant women. Exposed immunocompromised people should receive IG at a rate of 0.5 mL/kg (maximum dose 15 mL). Immunocompromised children who receive IGIV regularly are considered to be protected against measles.

- **Varicella.** Susceptible immunocompetent children and household contacts exposed to a person with varicella disease should be given varicella vaccine within 3 days of the appearance of the rash in the index case (see Varicella-Zoster Infections, p 672). Susceptible immunocompromised children should be given passive protection with VZIG as soon as possible after contact with an infected person (see Varicella-Zoster Infections, p 672).

- **Hepatitis B.** Postexposure immunization is highly effective if combined with administration of antibody. Administration of HBIG does not inhibit active immunization with HBV vaccine. For postexposure prophylaxis in a newborn infant whose mother is an HBsAg carrier, administration of HBIG and hepatitis B immunization is essential. For percutaneous or mucosal exposure to HBV, combined active and passive immunization is recommended for susceptible people (see Hepatitis B, p 318). People with continuing household or sexual contact with an HBsAg carrier also should be immunized.

- **Hepatitis A.** Available data are insufficient to recommend HAV vaccine alone for postexposure prophylaxis. Immune Globulin should be administered to household, sexual, and other contacts of HAV-infected people as soon as possible after exposure. If ongoing exposure to HAV is likely, IG and the first dose of HAV vaccine may be administered simultaneously at different sites.

- **Tetanus.** In wound management, unimmunized or incompletely immunized people should be given tetanus toxoid immediately in addition to TIG, depending on the nature of the wound and the immunization history of the person (see Table 3.61, p 614).

- **Rabies.** Postexposure active and passive immunization are essential aspects of immunoprophylaxis for rabies after proven or suspected exposure to rabid animals (see Rabies, p 514).

- *Mumps and Rubella.* Exposed susceptible people are not necessarily protected by postexposure administration of live-virus vaccine. However, a common practice for people exposed to mumps or rubella is to administer vaccine to presumed susceptible people so that permanent immunity will be afforded by immunization if mumps or rubella does not result from the current exposure. Administration of live-virus vaccine is recommended for exposed adults born in the United States in 1957 or after who previously have not had or been immunized against mumps or rubella.

American Indian/Alaska Native Children

American Indian/Alaska Native children are at greater risk of certain vaccine preventable diseases, such as hepatitis A, hepatitis B, and diseases caused by Hib and *S pneumoniae,* than are children of other ethnic groups. For this reason, physicians caring for American Indian/Alaska Native children should consider the following special immunization recommendations, which have been incorporated into current immunization schedules. Although increased risk of these diseases generally is found among American Indian/Alaska Native children who live on reservations or in traditional rural villages as well as in urban settings, there may be some differences in disease risk depending on where the child lives. However, because of the difficulty in ascertaining these risks and the high degree of mobility of the American Indian/Alaska Native population among reservations, rural villages, and urban settings, all American Indian/Alaska Native children should receive the benefit of these special immunization recommendations.

Hepatitis A. American Indian/Alaska Native children living in rural villages, reservations, and urban settings have been shown to have high endemic rates of HAV infection. Routine hepatitis A immunization of all American Indian/Alaska Native children at 2 years of age is recommended. In addition, older children (up to 18 years of age) living on American Indian reservations and in Alaska Native villages as well as in urban settings should be immunized. Most of these children reside in states or communities with previously high rates of hepatitis A and where universal childhood hepatitis A immunization currently is recommended (see Hepatitis A, p 309). For American Indian/Alaska Native children not living in such areas, universal hepatitis A immunization is recommended.

Hepatitis B. Alaska Native children had a high prevalence of chronic HBV infection before implementation of universal infant hepatitis B immunization. Although a high prevalence of chronic HBV infection has not been found among American Indian children, a high incidence of HBV infection has been observed among older adolescents and young adults and is associated with high-risk behaviors, such as injection drug use. All American Indian/Alaska Native children should be given the hepatitis B immunization series as infants, preferably starting in the newborn period. In addition, special efforts should be made to ensure catch-up hepatitis B immunization of previously unimmunized adolescents, including those in correctional settings or substance abuse treatment programs.

As with all pregnant women, Alaska Native women not living in Alaska and all American Indian women should be tested for HBsAg status during pregnancy, and women at high risk of HBV infection during pregnancy (eg, those with sexually transmitted disease[s] or those who use injection drugs) should be retested late in pregnancy. For pregnant Alaska Native women living in Alaska, routine HBsAg testing is no longer recommended, because all infants are immunized beginning at birth, which provides active postexposure prophylaxis against perinatal HBV infection; and the documented prevalence of chronic HBV infection among women of childbearing age has been decreased to low levels through routine hepatitis B immunization programs, which began in 1983. Infants of women who are HBsAg positive should be given postexposure prophylaxis with both HBV vaccine and HBIG within the first 12 hours of life; the vaccine series should be completed by 6 months of age, and postimmunization serologic testing should be performed at 12 to 15 months of age (see Hepatitis B, p 318).

Haemophilus influenzae *type b.* Invasive Hib disease occurred at a high incidence and at young ages in many American Indian/Alaska Native populations before the availability of immunization with conjugated Hib vaccines. Because of the high risk of invasive Hib disease within the first 6 months of life in American Indian/Alaska Native infants, recommendations are that the first dose of Hib conjugate vaccine contain polyribosylribitol phosphate-meningococcal outer membrane protein (PRP-OMP) as a single-antigen vaccine or in a combination vaccine with other antigens. This leads to more rapid seroconversion to protective concentrations of antibody within the first 6 months of life, and not using PRP-OMP vaccine in this population has been shown to result in the occurrence of invasive Hib disease. The same or any of the other Hib conjugate vaccines can be used for subsequent doses with apparently equal efficacy (see *Haemophilus influenzae* Infections, p 293).

Streptococcus pneumoniae. The incidence of invasive pneumococcal disease was 5 to 24 times higher among certain American Indian/Alaska Native children than among other US children before the use of the conjugated pneumococcal vaccine. Now, as with other US children, all American Indian/Alaska Native children should receive conjugated pneumococcal vaccine according to the recommended schedule (see Pneumococcal Infections, p 490). Studies of pneumococcal vaccine in American Indian/Alaska Native infants have shown that the vaccine successfully decreased the incidence of invasive disease in those populations.

Because older American Indian/Alaska Native children also are at higher risk of pneumococcal disease than are other US children, immunization of American Indian/Alaska Native children 2 to 5 years of age with conjugated pneumococcal vaccine or with the 23-valent pneumococcal polysaccharide vaccine should be considered.

Children in Residential Institutions

Children housed in institutions pose special problems for control of certain infectious diseases. Ensuring appropriate immunization is important because of the risk of transmission within the facility and because conditions that led to institutionalization may increase the risk of complications from the disease. All children entering a residential institution should have received recommended immunizations for their age (see Fig 1.1, p 24, and Table 1.6, p 26). If they have not been immunized appropriately, arrangements should be made to administer these immunizations as soon as possible. Staff members should be familiar with standard precautions and procedures for handling contaminated blood and body fluids and for trauma with bleeding. Staff members should be aware of children infected with HBV to ensure prompt and appropriate management in these circumstances. Specific diseases of concern include the following (see the disease-specific chapters in Section 3 for detailed recommendations).

- **Measles.** Epidemics can occur among susceptible children in institutional settings. Recommendations for managing children in an institutional setting when a case of measles is recognized are as follows: (1) within 72 hours of exposure, administer live measles virus vaccine (as MMR vaccine) to all susceptible children 1 year of age or older for whom immunization is not contraindicated; and (2) administer IG in a dose of 0.25 mL/kg, or 0.5 mL/kg to immunocompromised children (maximum dose 15 mL), as soon as possible and within 6 days of exposure to all exposed susceptible children younger than 1 year of age. These IG recipients still will require live-virus vaccine (as MMR vaccine) at 12 months of age or thereafter, depending on the age and dose of IG administration (see Table 3.33, p 423, for the appropriate interval between IG administration and MMR immunization).

- **Mumps.** Epidemics may occur among susceptible unimmunized children in institutions. Major hazards are disruption of activities, the need for acute nursing care in difficult settings, and occasional serious complications (eg, in susceptible adult staff).

    If mumps is introduced into a setting where susceptible people reside, prophylaxis is not available to limit the spread or to modify the disease in a susceptible person. Immune Globulin is not effective, and Mumps Immune Globulin is not available. Although mumps virus vaccine may not be effective after exposure, the vaccine should be administered to susceptible people to protect against infection from future exposures.

- **Influenza.** Influenza can be devastating in a residential or custodial institutional setting. Rapid spread, intensive exposure, and underlying disease can result in a high risk of severe illness that may affect many residents simultaneously or in close sequence. Current measures for control of influenza in institutions include: (1) a program of annual influenza immunization of residents and staff and (2) appropriate use of chemoprophylaxis during influenza epidemics (see Influenza, p 382). When considering the use of chemoprophylaxis, health care professionals can obtain information on which strains of influenza are prevalent in the community from local and state health department personnel.

- **Pertussis.** Because progressive developmental delay may have resulted in a deferral of pertussis immunization, many children in an institutional setting may not be immunized fully or may be immunized incompletely against pertussis. Because pertussis vaccine does not cause progressive neurologic disease and because pertussis disease poses a greater risk than does pertussis immunization to a specific child, children who are not immunized fully and are younger than 7 years of age should be immunized against pertussis. If pertussis is recognized, infected patients and their close contacts should receive chemoprophylaxis.

- *Hepatitis A.* Outbreaks of hepatitis A affecting residents and staff can occur in institutions for custodial care by fecal-oral transmission. Infection usually is mild or asymptomatic in young children but can be severe in adults. Although an effective HAV vaccine is available for children 2 years of age and older, the role of this vaccine in helping to control or prevent outbreaks in these settings has not been determined. If an outbreak occurs, susceptible residents and staff members in close personal contact with patients should receive IG (0.02 mL/kg, intramuscularly).

- *Hepatitis B.* Children living in residential institutions for developmentally disabled children and their caregivers are assumed to be at increased risk of acquiring HBV infection. The high prevalence of HBV markers among children living in these facilities indicates that HBV infections have the propensity for spread in an institutional setting, presumably by exposure to blood and body fluids containing HBV. Factors associated with high prevalence of HBV markers include crowding, high resident-staff ratios, and lack of in-service educational programs for staff. In the presence of such factors, the prevalence of HBV increases with the duration of time spent at the institution. Thus, residents and staff entering or already residing in institutions for the developmentally disabled should be immunized against HBV; preimmunization serologic screening for HBV markers probably is not cost-effective.

    After parenteral exposure or sexual exposure to an institutionalized patient recognized to be an HBsAg carrier, patients or staff who are unimmunized and susceptible should receive active and passive immunoprophylaxis.

- *Pneumococcal Infections.* Children with severe physical or mental disabilities, particularly children who are bedridden, who suffer from a compromised respiratory status, or who are capable of only limited physical activity, may benefit from pneumococcal conjugate and/or polysaccharide vaccine (see Pneumococcal Infections, p 490).

- *Varicella.* Varicella is very contagious and can occur in a high proportion of susceptible children in an institutional setting. All healthy children 1 year of age or older who lack a reliable history of varicella should be immunized. Prophylaxis with VZIG (see Table 3.77, p 679) during outbreaks currently is recommended only for immunocompromised, susceptible children at risk of serious complications or death from varicella.

- *Other Infections.* Other organisms causing diseases that spread in institutions and for which no immunizations are available include *Shigella, E coli* O157:H7, other enteric pathogens, *Streptococcus pyogenes, Staphylococcus aureus,* respiratory tract viruses, cytomegalovirus, scabies, and lice.

Children in Military Populations

In general, children of active-duty military personnel require the same immunizations as their civilian counterparts. If delay in pertussis immunization is recommended for any reason, parents should be warned that the risk of contracting the disease in countries where pertussis immunization is not administered routinely is significantly higher than that in countries where effective vaccine is used. For military dependents traveling internationally, the risk of exposure to HAV, HBV, measles, pertussis, diphtheria, poliovirus, yellow fever, Japanese encephalitis, and other infections may be increased and may necessitate additional immunizations (see International Travel, p 93). In these instances, the choice of immunizations will be dictated by the country of proposed residence, expected travel, and the age and health of the child. For information on the risk of specific diseases in different countries and preventive measures, see International Travel (p 93) or consult the CDC Web site (www.cdc.gov/travel).

Adolescent* and College Populations

Adolescents and young adults may not be protected against all vaccine-preventable diseases. This age group may include people who escaped natural infection and who (1) were not immunized with all recommended vaccines; (2) received appropriate vaccines but at too young an age (eg, measles vaccine before 12 months of age); (3) received incomplete immunization regimens (eg, only 1 or 2 doses of HBV vaccine); or (4) failed to respond to vaccines administered at appropriate ages.

To ensure age-appropriate immunization, all children should have a routine preadolescent appointment at 11 to 12 years of age for the following purposes: (1) to immunize people who previously have not received 2 doses of MMR; (2) to give varicella and/or hepatitis B vaccines as indicated; (3) to provide a booster dose of diphtheria and tetanus (Td) toxoids; and (4) to provide other immunization and preventive services that are indicated. Additional vaccines that may be indicated at this preadolescent visit include influenza, pneumococcal, and hepatitis A vaccines. Specific indications for each of these vaccines are given in the respective disease-specific chapter in Section 3.

Appointments for needed doses of vaccines that are not administered during the aforementioned visit should be scheduled. During all subsequent adolescent visits, the person's immunization status should be reviewed and deficiencies should be corrected, including completion of the 3-dose HBV vaccine series.

School immunization laws encourage "catch-up" programs for older adolescents. Accordingly, school and college health services should establish a system to ensure that all students are protected against vaccine-preventable diseases. Many colleges are implementing the American College Health Association (ACHA) recommendations for prematriculation immunization requirements, mandating protection from measles, mumps, rubella, tetanus, diphtheria, polio, varicella, and HBV (www.acha.org). In addition, *N meningitidis* vaccine is recommended by some colleges and universities and required by law for college students in many states.

- *Measles.* Since 1990, many colleges and universities have experienced measles outbreaks, delaying efforts to eliminate this disease from the United States. To prevent measles outbreaks and ensure high levels of immunity among young adults on college and university campuses, the ACHA has recommended that colleges and universities require 2 doses of measles vaccine as a condition for matriculation. The first dose must have been given on or after the first birthday; the interval between the first and second dose must have been at least 1 month.

* Centers for Disease Control and Prevention. Vaccine-preventable diseases: improving vaccination coverage in children, adolescents, and adults. A report on recommendations from the Task Force on Community Preventive Services. *MMWR Recomm Rep.* 1999;48(RR-8):1–15

Similarly, in postsecondary school educational settings, the American Academy of Pediatrics (AAP) recommends a 2-dose measles immunization schedule, given as MMR vaccine, for people born in 1957 or after.

- **Rubella.** Adolescents and adults should be considered susceptible to rubella if documentation of immunity is lacking. Immunizing adolescents and adults in college decreases the chance of outbreaks and helps to prevent congenital rubella syndrome.

- **Varicella.** Varicella immunity is desirable in adolescents and adults, especially adults in colleges and universities and nonpregnant women of childbearing age.* Adults, adolescents, and children with a reliable history of varicella disease can be assumed to be immune, and immunization is not necessary. Because approximately 70% to 90% of people 18 years of age or older without a reliable history of varicella disease also will be immune, serologic testing of people 13 years of age or older and immunization of people who are seronegative may be cost-effective. If serologic testing is performed, a tracking system for seronegative people should be developed to ensure that susceptible people are immunized. However, serologic testing is not required, because varicella vaccine is well tolerated in those who are immune from immunization or previous disease. In some situations, universal immunization may be easier to implement than may serologic testing and tracking.

- **Hepatitis B.** Hepatitis B virus vaccine is recommended for administration to all adolescents, especially those who have one or more risk factors for HBV infection. Risk factors include multiple sexual partners (defined as more than 1 partner within the previous 6 months), a sexually transmitted disease, sexually active homosexual or bisexual behavior, injection drug use, and occupation or training involving contact with blood or body fluids.

- **Diphtheria, Tetanus, and Pertussis.** Adult-type diphtheria and tetanus toxoids (Td) vaccine should be given at 11 to 12 years of age and no later than 16 years of age. Thereafter, booster immunization with Td is given every 10 years. Studies are underway to address the need for and safety of pertussis immunization in adolescents and adults.

- **Influenza.** Epidemic influenza can affect any closed population. Physicians responsible for health care in schools and colleges should consider annual influenza immunization of students, particularly students residing in dormitories or students who are members of athletic teams, to decrease morbidity and minimize disruption of routine activities during epidemics.

- **Neisseria meningitidis.** Immunization of college students is recommended by the ACHA and required by state law for college students in many states. Pediatricians should inform and educate students and parents about the risk of meningococcal disease and the existence of a safe and effective vaccine and immunize students at their request or if educational institutions or state laws require its use for admission.

- **Other recommendations.** Because adolescents and young adults commonly travel internationally, their immunization status and travel plans should be reviewed 2 or more months before departure to allow time to administer any needed vaccines (see International Travel, p 93).

---

* American Academy of Pediatrics, Committee on Infectious Diseases. Varicella vaccine update. *Pediatrics.* 2000;105:136–141

Some physicians are unaware of the risks of vaccine-preventable diseases to adolescents and young adults and do not give priority to immunization. Pediatricians should assist in providing information on immunization and vaccine-preventable disease to others who care for adolescents in their communities and should work to heighten awareness of the importance of immunizing adolescents and young adults.

The possible occurrence of diseases such as measles, mumps, rubella, hepatitis A, hepatitis B, pertussis, influenza, and *N meningitidis* infections in a school or college should be reported promptly to local health officials.

Health Care Personnel*

Adults whose occupations place them in contact with patients with contagious diseases are at increased risk of contracting vaccine-preventable diseases and, if infected, for transmitting them to their patients. Staff at residential institutions and health care personnel, including physicians, nurses, students, and ancillary personnel, should protect themselves and susceptible patients by receiving appropriate immunizations. Physicians, hospitals, and schools for health care professionals should have a major role in implementing these policies. Vaccine-preventable infections of special concern to those involved in the health care of children are as follows (see the disease-specific chapters in Section 3 for further recommendations).

- **Rubella.** Outbreaks of rubella among health care personnel have been reported. Although the disease is mild in adults, the risk to a fetus necessitates documentation of rubella immunity in hospital personnel of both sexes. People who are at risk of transmitting rubella infection include hospital personnel in pediatrics, physicians and nurses working in pediatric and obstetric ambulatory care (including emergency departments), and all people working in health care areas in which pregnant women are encountered. People should be considered immune only on the basis of serologic tests or documented proof of rubella immunization at or after 12 months of age. A history of rubella disease is unreliable and should not be used in determining immune status. All susceptible people should be immunized with MMR vaccine (or monocomponent rubella vaccine if immunity to measles and mumps has been documented) before initial or continuing contact with pregnant patients.

    Although birth before 1957 generally is considered acceptable evidence of rubella immunity, health care facilities should consider recommending a dose of MMR vaccine to unimmunized workers born before 1957 who lack laboratory evidence of rubella immunity.

- **Measles.** Because measles in health care personnel has contributed to spread of this disease during outbreaks, evidence of immunity to measles should be required for health care personnel born in 1957 or after who will have direct patient contact. Proof of immunity is established by physician-documented measles, a positive serologic test for measles antibody, or documented receipt of 2 doses of live-virus

* Centers for Disease Control and Prevention. Immunization of health-care workers: recommendations of the Advisory Committee on Immunization Practices and the Hospital Infection Control Practices Advisory Committee (HICPAC). *MMWR Recomm Rep.* 1997;46(RR-18):1–42

measles vaccine, the first of which is given on or after the first birthday. Health care personnel born before 1957 generally have been considered immune to measles. However, because measles cases have occurred in health care personnel in this age group, health care facilities should consider offering at least 1 dose of measles-containing vaccine to workers who lack proof of immunity to measles, particularly in communities with documented measles outbreaks.

- *Mumps.* Transmission of mumps in health care facilities can be disruptive and costly. Adults born before 1957 generally have been considered immune to mumps; those born in 1957 or after are considered immune if they have documentation of a single dose of mumps vaccine received on or after their first birthday or laboratory evidence of immunity.

- *Hepatitis B.* Vaccine is recommended for all health care personnel who are likely to be exposed to blood or blood-containing body fluids. The Occupational Safety and Health Administration of the US Department of Labor has issued a regulation requiring employers of workers at risk of occupational exposure to HBV to offer HBV immunization to employees at the employer's expense. Employees who refuse recommended immunizations should sign a refusal document.

- *Influenza.* Certain groups of patients, such as people with chronic cardiovascular or pulmonary disease, are at high risk of serious or complicated influenza infection. Because health care personnel can transmit influenza to their patients and nosocomial outbreaks can occur, influenza immunization programs for hospital personnel and other health care professionals should be recommended each autumn.

- *Varicella.* Proof of varicella immunity is recommended for all susceptible health care personnel. In health care institutions, serologic screening of personnel who have a negative or uncertain history of varicella before immunization is likely to be cost-effective but need not be done. Varicella immunization is recommended for all susceptible people.

- On occasion, susceptible health care personnel immunized adequately with measles, mumps, rubella, varicella, or HBV vaccines fail to develop serologic evidence of immunity against one or more of these antigens. In those instances, an additional 1 to 3 doses of HBV vaccine can be given, followed by serologic testing (see Hepatitis B, p 318). People who fail to develop immunity thereafter are unlikely to benefit from further immunization.

- *Tuberculosis.** Early detection and treatment of patients (or visitors) with communicable tuberculosis is recommended to prevent tuberculosis infection in health care personnel. The risk of transmission of tuberculosis in hospitals varies greatly; the likelihood that a specific institution is a site of transmission of *Mycobacteria tuberculosis* can be determined only by local epidemiologic data. Policies for tuberculin skin testing for health care personnel should reflect local incidence rates. Immunization with BCG vaccine is not recommended for personnel in most circumstances. According to current CDC recommendations, BCG immunization should be considered on an individual basis in settings with a high prevalence of multidrug-resistant *M tuberculosis* infection, in situations

---

* Centers for Disease Control and Prevention. Targeted tuberculin testing and treatment of latent tuberculosis infection. *MMWR Recomm Rep.* 2000;49(RR-6):1–54

in which transmission of resistant organisms is likely, and in facilities where comprehensive infection control precautions against *M tuberculosis* transmission have been implemented and have failed.*

Refugees and Immigrants

Prevention of infectious diseases in refugee and immigrant children presents special problems because of the diseases to which these children have been exposed and the immunization practices unique to their native countries. In 1996, a new subsection was added to the Immigration and Nationality Act (INA) requiring for the first time that people seeking an immigrant visa for permanent residency show proof of having received the recommended vaccines, as established by the ACIP. Although these regulations apply to most immigrant children entering the United States, internationally adopted children who are younger than 10 years of age have been exempted from the international immunization requirements. Adoptive parents are required to sign a waiver indicating their intention to comply with the ACIP immunization requirements after arrival in the United States. Refugees are not required to meet the Immigration and Nationality Act immunization requirements at the time of initial entry into the United States but must show proof of immunization at the time they apply for permanent residency, typically within 3 years of arrival.

Refugee children who have resided in processing camps for a few months often have received medical evaluation and treatment, which may have included certain immunizations. However, they may be underimmunized or without immunization records. For refugee children whose immunizations are not up-to-date, as documented by a written immunization record (see Immunizations Received Outside the United States, p 34), recommended vaccines as indicated for their age should be administered (see Fig 1.1 p 24, and Table 1.6, p 26). For children without documentation of immunizations, a new vaccine schedule may be initiated. Alternatively, measurement of antibody concentrations to diphtheria, tetanus, measles, mumps, rubella, varicella, poliovirus (each serotype), and hepatitis B surface antibody may be considered to determine whether the child needs additional immunizations or whether the vaccine schedule appropriate for that child's age should be initiated (see Table 2.18, Approaches to the Evaluation and Immunization of Internationally Adopted Children, p 179). Although many children will have received DTP, poliovirus, measles, and hepatitis B vaccines, most will not have received Hib, pneumococcal, hepatitis A, MMR, and varicella vaccines. Although measles antibody may be measured to determine whether the child is immune, many children may need a dose of mumps and rubella vaccine, because these vaccines may not have been given in developing countries. Varicella vaccine is not administered in most countries, and history of varicella infection may be unavailable or unreliable in these populations; therefore, children should be immunized for varicella or have antibody testing performed.

Tuberculosis is an important public health problem for refugees and immigrants. Refugees and immigrants have accounted for a substantial and increasing proportion

---

* Centers for Disease Control and Prevention. The role of BCG vaccine in the prevention and control of tuberculosis in the United States: a joint statement by the Advisory Council for the Elimination of Tuberculosis and the Advisory Committee on Immunization Practices. *MMWR Recomm Rep.* 1996;45(RR-4):1–18

of new cases of tuberculosis in the United States during the past decade. For recommendations about diagnosis and treatment, see Tuberculosis, p 642, and International Travel, below.

All refugees and immigrants from hepatitis B-endemic areas, particularly Asia and Africa, should be screened for hepatitis B by performing serologic tests for HBsAg, hepatitis B surface antibody, and hepatitis B core antibody. If the child has HBsAg, the child is infectious and may be defined as a chronic carrier if the surface antigen persists for longer than 6 months. Most children who are HBsAg carriers are asymptomatic and, therefore, screening is important so transmission of disease can be limited. Transmission risks should be minimal among children because of universal infant HBV immunization programs in the United States. However, adult caregivers may be unimmunized and should be given HBV vaccine if they are susceptible and HBIG if they have had a significant exposure to the blood of a carrier (see Hepatitis B, p 318). Serologic screening of all pregnant refugees and immigrants for HBsAg is imperative to identify women whose infants need passive as well as active immunoprophylaxis.

International Travel

Children and adolescents should be up-to-date on routinely recommended immunizations before international travel. In addition, travel requires consideration of additional vaccines to prevent hepatitis A, yellow fever, meningococcal disease, typhoid fever, rabies, and Japanese encephalitis. Vaccines may be required or recommended depending on the destination and type of international travel (see Table 1.14, p 94). Travelers to tropical and subtropical areas often risk exposure to malaria, dengue fever, leptospirosis, diarrhea, and other diseases for which vaccines are not available. For travelers at risk, malaria chemoprophylaxis, insect precautions, and care in hygiene associated with food and liquids are other important preventive behaviors (see Malaria, p 414).

An excellent source of information is *Health Information for International Travel* (the "Yellow Book") published every 2 years by the CDC as a reference for people who advise international travelers of health risks. Every other week, the CDC also publishes a *Summary of Health Information* (the "Blue Sheet"), which lists areas experiencing yellow fever and cholera and provides any changes in recommendations reported by the CDC and WHO for entry into certain countries. Travel information and recommendations can be obtained from the CDC by fax (888-232-3299) or telephone recording (877-394-8747, or 877-FYI-TRIP) or online at (www.cdc.gov/travel). The Yellow Book and Blue Sheet also can be located on the CDC Web site. Local and state health departments and travel clinics also can provide updated information.

RECOMMENDED IMMUNIZATIONS

Infants and children embarking on international travel should be up-to-date on receipt of recommended immunizations appropriate for their age. These include DTaP, IPV, Hib, MMR, varicella, pneumococcal, and HBV vaccines (see Fig 1.1, p 24). For travel to many countries and some areas of the United States with high endemic rates of hepatitis A infection, HAV immunization also may be recom-

Table 1.14. **Recommended Immunizations for Travelers to Developing Countries[1]**

| | Length of Travel | | |
| | Brief, <2 wk | Intermediate, 2 wk to 3 mo | Long-term Residential, >3 mo |
Immunizations			
Review and complete age-appropriate childhood schedule (see text for details)	+	+	+
• DTaP, poliovirus, and *Haemophilus influenzae* type b vaccines may be given at 4-wk intervals if necessary to complete the recommended schedule before departure			
• Measles: 2 additional doses given if younger than 12 mo of age at first dose			
• Varicella			
• Hepatitis B[2]			
Yellow fever[3]	+	+	+
Hepatitis A[4]	+	+	+
Typhoid fever[4]	±	+	+
Meningococcal disease[5]	±	±	±
Rabies[6]	±	+	+
Japanese encephalitis[7]	±	±	+

DTaP indicates diphtheria and tetanus toxoids and acellular pertussis; +, recommended; ±, consider.
[1] See disease-specific chapters in Section 3 for details. For further sources of information, see text.
[2] If insufficient time to complete 6-month primary series, accelerated series can be given (see text for details).
[3] For endemic regions (see *Health Information for International Travel,* p 3).
[4] Indicated for travelers who will consume food and liquids in areas of poor sanitation.
[5] Recommended for endemic regions of Africa, during local epidemics, and required for travel to Saudi Arabia for the Hajj.
[6] Indicated for people with high risk of animal exposure (especially to dogs) and for travelers to endemic countries.
[7] For endemic regions (see *Health Information for International Travel,* p 3). For high-risk activities in areas experiencing outbreaks, vaccine is recommended even for brief travel.

mended (see Hepatitis A, p 309). To ensure immunity before departure, vaccines may need to be given on an accelerated schedule (see Table 1.14, above).

Worldwide poliovirus eradication efforts have decreased the number of countries where travelers are at risk of poliovirus infection. The Western Hemisphere was declared free of wild-type poliovirus in 1994, and the Western Pacific Region was declared free in 2000. However, poliovirus outbreaks still occur; in July 2000, an outbreak of vaccine-derived poliovirus type 1 was reported in the Dominican Republic and Haiti. To ensure protection, pediatric travelers should be fully immunized against poliovirus. Three doses of IPV vaccine should be administered before departure. If necessary, the doses may be given at 4-week intervals, although 6- to 8-week intervals are preferred. Children should receive a supplemental fourth dose at 4 to 6 years of age (see Poliovirus Infections, p 505).

Importation of measles remains an important source for measles cases in the United States. Therefore, people traveling abroad should be immune to measles to provide personal protection and minimize importation of measles. People should be considered susceptible to measles unless they have documentation of appropriate immunization, physician-diagnosed measles, or laboratory evidence of immunity to measles or were born in the United States before 1957. For people born in the United States in 1957 or after, 2 doses of measles vaccine, the first administered at or after 12 months of age, are required to ensure immunity (see Measles, p 419). The age of initiation of measles immunization can be lowered for children traveling to areas with a high rate of measles transmission. Infants 6 to 11 months of age should receive 1 dose of a measles-containing vaccine. These children should be given 2 additional doses of a measles-containing vaccine separated by at least 1 month starting at 12 to 15 months of age.

Hepatitis B vaccine now is recommended for all children but particularly should be considered for travelers of all ages visiting areas where hepatitis B is highly endemic, such as countries in Asia and Africa and some countries in South America (see Hepatitis B, p 318). Risk factors for hepatitis B include close contact with the local population for a prolonged period (>6 months), contact with blood or blood-containing body fluids, or sexual contact with residents of these areas. An accelerated dosing schedule is licensed for one hepatitis B vaccine (Engerix-B, GlaxoSmithKline Biologicals, Rixensart, Belgium), during which the first 3 doses are given at 0, 1, and 2 months. This schedule may benefit travelers who have insufficient time (ie, <6 months) to complete a standard 3-dose schedule before departure. If the accelerated schedule is used, a fourth dose should be given 12 months after the third dose (see Hepatitis B, p 318).

REQUIRED OR RECOMMENDED TRAVEL-RELATED IMMUNIZATIONS

Depending on the destination, planned activity, and length of stay, other immunizations may be required or recommended (see Table 1.14, p 94, and disease-specific chapters in Section 3).

Immunoprophylaxis against hepatitis A is indicated for susceptible people traveling internationally to areas with intermediate or high rates of HAV infection. These include all areas of the world except Australia, Canada, Japan, New Zealand, and Western Europe. Inactivated vaccines and intramuscular Immune Globulin (IG) are effective for immunoprophylaxis; however, only inactivated vaccines will provide long-term protection. For people 2 years of age and older, vaccine is preferred. To ensure immediate protection for people whose departure is imminent, IG and vaccine may be given concurrently at different sites (see Hepatitis A, p 309). For children younger than 2 years of age, IG is indicated, because hepatitis A vaccine is not licensed in the United States for use in this age group. Immune Globulin may interfere with the immune response to varicella, measles, mumps, and rubella vaccines.

Yellow fever vaccine, an attenuated live-virus vaccine, is required by some countries as a condition of entry, including for travelers arriving from endemic regions.* The vaccine is available in the United States only in centers designated by

---

* Centers for Disease Control and Prevention. Yellow fever vaccine. Recommendations of the Advisory Committee on Immunization Practices, 2002. *MMWR Recomm Rep.* 2002;51(RR-17):1–10

state health departments. Current requirements and recommendations for yellow fever immunization based on travel destination can be obtained from the CDC Travelers' Health Web site (www.cdc.gov/travel) or from the CDC Yellow Book, *Health Information for International Travel.* Yellow fever occurs year-round in predominantly rural areas of sub-Saharan Africa and South America; in recent years, outbreaks have been increasing including in some urban areas. Although rare, yellow fever continues to be reported among travelers, particularly unimmunized travelers, and usually is fatal. Prevention measures against yellow fever should include immunization and protection against mosquitoes. Yellow fever vaccine generally is considered to be a safe and effective vaccine. However, the vaccine rarely has been found to be associated with a risk of viscerotropic disease (multiple organ system failure) and neurotropic disease (postvaccinal encephalitis). The vaccine should not be used in children younger than 4 months of age and should be used with caution in children 4 to 8 months of age and only after consultation with a travel medicine expert and/or the CDC to weigh risks and benefits (ie, consider immunization if travel to an area of ongoing yellow fever transmission cannot be avoided and a high level of protection against mosquito bites is not possible). Whenever possible, immunization should be delayed until 9 months of age to minimize the risk of vaccine-associated encephalitis. Medical waivers can be given to children who are too young for immunization and to those who have other contraindications to immunization, such as immunodeficiency. The CDC has stated that, given the risk of serious illness and death attributable to yellow fever, evidence of increasing transmission of the disease, and the known effectiveness of the vaccine, clinicians should continue to use yellow fever vaccine to protect travelers. However, the CDC recommends that health care professionals review carefully travel itineraries so that only people traveling to yellow fever-endemic areas or areas where there is reported yellow fever activity receive yellow fever vaccine.

The whole-cell inactivated cholera vaccine no longer is produced in the United States. According to WHO regulations, no country may require cholera immunization as a condition for entry. However, despite WHO recommendations, some local authorities may require documentation of immunization. In such cases, a notation of vaccine contraindication should be sufficient to satisfy local requirements.

Typhoid vaccine is recommended for travelers who may be exposed to contaminated food or water. In particular, people with anticipated long-term travel or residence in areas with poor sanitation and those who visit remote areas are at greatest risk. Two typhoid vaccines are available for civilian use in the United States: an oral vaccine containing live-attenuated *S typhi* (Ty21a strain), and a parenteral Vi capsular polysaccharide (ViCPS) vaccine (see *Salmonella* Infections, p 541). Whole-cell inactivated vaccine no longer is produced in the United States. For specific recommendations, see *Salmonella* Infections (p 541). Because antimicrobial agents and the antimalarial drug mefloquine (but not chloroquine) can inhibit the growth of the vaccine strain of *S typhi,* the orally administered vaccine should be given at least 24 hours before or after administration of any of these agents. The oral vaccine capsules need to be refrigerated. Because the vaccine is not completely efficacious, typhoid immunization is not a substitute for careful selection of food and drink.

Meningococcal polysaccharide vaccine (quadrivalent groups A, C, Y, and W-135) should be offered for travelers to areas where epidemics occur frequently, such as sub-Saharan Africa, and to countries with current meningococcal epidemics. Saudi Arabia requires a certificate of immunization for pilgrims to Mecca or Medina, where outbreaks with serogroups A and W-135 have been reported in travelers participating in the Hajj. The travel section of the CDC Web site (www.cdc.gov/travel) should be consulted. As in the United States, meningococcal vaccine also should be considered for first-year college students traveling to foreign countries for university training or those living in US in dormitory settings (see Meningococcal Infections, p 430).

Rabies immunization should be considered for children who will be traveling to areas where they may encounter rabid animals (particularly dogs in developing countries) or if they will engage in activities involving increased risk of rabies transmission (eg, spelunking). This is particularly important if they will not have immediate access to appropriate medical care and rabies biological agents. The 3-dose preexposure series is given by intramuscular injection (see Rabies, p 514). In the event of a bite by a potentially rabid animal, all travelers (whether or not they have received preexposure rabies vaccine) should be counseled to thoroughly clean the wound with soap and water and then promptly receive postexposure treatment, including booster doses of rabies vaccine.

Japanese encephalitis virus, which is spread by dusk-to-dawn-biting *Culex* species mosquitoes, is a potential risk in Southeast Asia, China, Eastern Russia, and the Indian subcontinent. Vaccine should be offered to travelers with prolonged residence in endemic or epidemic areas (particularly rural farming areas) during transmission season and to travelers who will engage in high-risk activities with extensive outdoor exposure, such as camping, bicycling, and field work regardless of the duration of travel. Geographic and seasonal risks are discussed in the CDC Yellow Book. Because potentially severe immediate and delayed allergic reactions to Japanese encephalitis vaccine occur in approximately 0.5% of vaccine recipients, potential benefits and risks of vaccine use should be considered carefully. Data are not available on vaccine safety and efficacy in infants younger than 1 year of age. Immunization requires 3 doses administered subcutaneously on days 0, 7, and 30 and should be completed at least 10 days before travel to an endemic area so the patient may be observed for potential delayed allergic reactions. If time constraints necessitate an abbreviated schedule, vaccine can be given at 0, 7, and 14 days (see Arboviruses, p 199).

Influenza immunization may be warranted for international travelers, depending on the destination, duration of travel, risk of acquisition of disease (in part on the basis of the season of the year), and the traveler's underlying health status. The influenza season is different in the northern and southern hemispheres. Because epidemic strains may differ, the antigenic composition of inactivated influenza vaccines used in North America may be different from those used in the Southern Hemisphere (see Influenza, p 382).

The risk of acquiring latent tuberculosis infection (LTBI) during international travel depends on the activities of the traveler and the epidemiology of tuberculosis in the areas in which travel occurs. In general, the risk of acquiring LTBI during usual tourism activities appears to be low, and no pre- or post-travel testing is recommended routinely. When travelers live or work among the general population of a high-prevalence country, the risk may be appreciably higher. In most high prevalence countries, contact investigation of tuberculosis cases is not performed, and treatment of LTBI is not available. Two approaches are acceptable for US children who are going to live temporarily in a high-prevalence country. The first approach is to perform a tuberculin skin test 8 to 12 weeks after return. This approach particularly is recommended for children who spend ≤6 months in a high-prevalence country. The second approach is for the child to receive a pretravel BCG immunization. Although one form of BCG vaccine is available in the United States, few individuals have experience in its administration. Many experts suggest that the child receive BCG immunization immediately after arrival in a high-prevalence country. This approach may be best for infants in whom LTBI can progress rapidly to tuberculosis disease. Some countries may require a BCG vaccine for issuance of work and residency permits for expatriate workers and their families. Children returning to the United States who have signs or symptoms compatible with tuberculosis should be evaluated appropriately for active tuberculosis.

Other considerations. In addition to vaccine-preventable diseases, international travelers to the tropics will be exposed to other diseases, such as malaria, which can be life threatening. Prevention strategies for malaria are twofold: prevention of mosquito bites and antimalarial chemoprophylaxis. For recommendations on appropriate use of chemoprophylaxis, including recommendations for pregnant women, infants, and breastfeeding mothers, see Malaria (p 414).

Prevention of mosquito bites will decrease the risk of malaria, dengue fever, and other mosquito-transmitted diseases. Appropriate personal protective measures, particularly during the malaria mosquito-biting period from dusk to dawn, can be highly effective. These preventive measures include wearing long-sleeved cotton shirts and long trousers; application of insect repellent, such as diethyltoluamide (DEET), to exposed skin; and use of window screens and bed nets. The DEET concentration in repellents should not exceed 20% to 30%; and repellents containing DEET should be used sparingly, applied only to exposed areas of skin avoiding irritated skin and mucous membranes, and washed off when the child comes indoors. Insect sprays and soaks containing the residual insecticide permethrin may be applied to clothing and bed nets.

Traveler's diarrhea is a significant problem that may be mitigated by attention to foods and beverages ingested and appropriately treating suspected water sources, because enteric bacteria, viruses, and parasites are transmitted in contaminated water and food supplies. Chemoprophylaxis generally is not recommended, but educating families about self-treatment, particularly oral rehydration, is important. During international travel, families may want to carry an antimotility agent and an antimicrobial agent for treatment of an older child or adolescent (see *Escherichia coli* Diarrhea, p 275).

Recommendations for Care of Children in Special Circumstances

··

BIOLOGICAL TERRORISM

Some infectious agents have the potential to be used in acts of bioterrorism. The Centers for Disease Control and Prevention (CDC) has designated 3 categories of biological agents according to their potential as weapons of terrorism.* The highest priority agents are designated category A, because they can be easily disseminated or transmitted person-to-person, cause high rates of mortality with potential for major public health effects, could cause public panic and social disruption, and require special action for public health preparedness. Category A agents include organisms that cause anthrax, smallpox, plague, tularemia, botulism, and viral hemorrhagic fevers, including Ebola, Marburg, Lassa, and others. Category B agents are moderately easy to disseminate, cause moderate morbidity and low mortality rates, and require enhanced diagnostic capacity and disease surveillance. These agents include *Coxiella burnetti* (Q fever), *Brucella* species (brucellosis), *Burkholderia mallei* (glanders), alphaviruses (Venezuelan, eastern, and western equine encephalomyelitis), ricin toxin from *Ricinus communis* (castor beans), epsilon toxin of *Clostridium perfringens*, and *Staphylococcus* enterotoxin B. Additional category B agents that are food- or water-borne include, but are not limited to, *Salmonella* species, *Shigella dysenteriae*, *Escherichia coli* O157:H7, *Vibrio cholerae*, and *Cryptosporidium parvum*. Category C agents include emerging pathogens that could be engineered for mass dissemination in the future because of availability, ease of production and dissemination, and potential for high morbidity and mortality rates and major health effects. These include Nipah virus, hantavirus, tickborne hemorrhagic fever viruses, tickborne encephalitis viruses, yellow fever virus, and multidrug-resistant *Mycobacterium tuberculosis*. A classification for deaths and injuries associated with terrorism has been developed.[†]

Children may be particularly vulnerable to a bioterrorist attack, because they have a more rapid respiratory rate, increased skin permeability, higher ratio of skin surface area to mass, and less fluid reserve compared with adults. Accurate and rapid diagnosis may be more difficult in children because of their inability to describe symptoms. In addition, the adults on whom children depend for their health and safety may become ill or require quarantine during a bioterrorist event.

---

* Centers for Disease Control and Prevention. Biological and chemical terrorism: strategic plan for preparedness and response. Recommendations of the CDC Strategic Planning Workgroup. *MMWR Recomm Rep.* 2000;49(RR-4):1–14

[†] Centers for Disease Control and Prevention. Notice to readers: new classification for deaths and injuries involving terrorism. *MMWR Morb Mortal Wkly Rep.* 2002;51(Special Issue):18–19; or www.cdc.gov/nchs/about/otheract/icd9/appendix1.htm

Table 2.1. Prominent Early Clinical Manifestations After Exposure to Bioterrorist Agents[1]

Clinical Manifestations[2]	Agents/Disease
Respiratory	
Influenza-like illness +/– atypical pneumonia	Tularemia, brucellosis, Q fever, alphaviruses (Venezuelan, eastern, and western equine encephalomyelitis)
Influenza-like illness with cough and respiratory distress	Inhalational anthrax, pneumonic plague, inhalational tularemia, ricin, aerosol exposure to *Staphylococcal* enterotoxin B, hantavirus
Exudative pharyngitis and cervical lymphadenopathy	Oropharyngeal tularemia
Dermatologic	
Vesicular rash[3] associated with fever, headache, malaise	Smallpox
Painless ulceration progressing to black eschar	Cutaneous anthrax
Ulcer plus painful regional lymphadenopathy and influenza-like illness	Ulceroglandular tularemia
Petechiae[3] with fever, myalgia, prostration	Viral hemorrhagic fever
Cardiovascular	
Shock after respiratory distress	Inhalational anthrax, ricin, viral hemorrhagic fever
Hematologic	
Thrombocytopenia	Brucellosis, viral hemorrhagic fever, hantavirus
Neutropenia	Viral hemorrhagic fever, alphaviruses (Venezuelan, eastern, and western equine encephalomyelitis)
Hemorrhage	Viral hemorrhagic fever
Disseminated intravascular coagulation	Viral hemorrhagic fever
Neurologic	
Flaccid paralysis	Botulism
Encephalitis	Alphaviruses (Venezuelan, eastern, and western equine encephalomyelitis)
Meningitis	Inhalational anthrax, septicemic and pneumonic plague, alphaviruses (Venezuelan, eastern, and western equine encephalomyelitis)

Table 2.1. Prominent Early Clinical Manifestations After Exposure to Bioterrorist Agents,[1] continued

Clinical Manifestations[2]	Agents/Disease
Gastrointestinal	
Diarrhea	Salmonella species, Shigella dysenteriae, Escherichia coli O157:H7, Vibrio cholerae, Cryptosporidium parvum
Vomiting; abdominal pain, bloody diarrhea, hematemesis	Gastrointestinal anthrax
Renal	
Hemolytic-uremic syndrome, thrombotic thrombocytopenic purpura	Escherichia coli O157:H7 and other shiga toxin-producing E coli; Shigella dysenteriae
Oliguria, renal failure	Viral hemorrhagic fever, hantavirus
Other	
Painful lymphadenopathy	Bubonic plague
Purulent conjunctivitis with preauricular or cervical lymphadenopathy	Oculoglandular tularemia

[1] Only the agents believed by experts in bioterrorism most likely to be used in a bioterrorist attack are included.

[2] The spectrum of clinical manifestations for many of these agents can be protean. The manifestations noted in this table are those that likely would make someone initially seek medical attention and are based on the route of exposure during an attack (eg, the manifestations of anthrax differ for an inhalational versus foodborne exposure). Fever, headache, vomiting, and diarrhea are common early manifestations of many illnesses.

[3] Rashes of diseases that cause petechiae or vesicular skin lesions may start as macular or papular lesions.

Table 2.2. Biological Weapons: Recommended Diagnostic Procedures, Isolation Precautions, and Treatment and Prophylaxis of Children

Agent	Incubation Period	Diagnostic Specimen(s)	Isolation Precautions	Treatment Options	Postexposure Prophylaxis[1]	Comments
Alphaviruses (Venezuelan, eastern, and western equine encephalomyelitis)	2–10 days	CSF for viral isolation, antibody detection in CSF and acute and convalescent serum	Standard; respiratory precautions for western equine encephalitis virus	Supportive	Protection from mosquito vectors	
Anthrax	1–60 days	Gram stain of buffy coat, CSF, pleural fluid, swab of skin lesion; culture of blood, CSF, pleural fluid, skin biopsy	Standard; contact for skin lesions	Ciprofloxacin[2] or doxycycline[3]; combine with 1 or 2 additional antimicrobial agents for inhalational, gastrointestinal, or oropharyngeal disease[4]	Ciprofloxacin[2] or doxycycline[3] or amoxicillin[5]; anthrax vaccine	Additional antimicrobial agents to be used for inhalational, gastrointestinal, or oropharyngeal disease include rifampin, vancomycin, penicillin, ampicillin, chloramphenicol, imipenem, clindamycin, and clarithromycin
Botulism	Foodborne: 2 h– 8 days; inhalational: 24–72 h	Toxin detection from serum, stool, enema fluid, gastric fluid, vomitus, or suspected food samples; culture of stool or gastric secretions; nerve conduction testing	Standard	Supportive care; mechanical ventilation and parenteral nutrition may be required. Equine botulism antitoxin given as soon as possible (CDC)[6]		Type-specific antitoxin should be administered when possible; antitoxin prevents additional nerve damage but does not reverse existing paralysis

Table 2.2. **Biological Weapons: Recommended Diagnostic Procedures, Isolation Precautions, and Treatment and Prophylaxis of Children, continued**

Agent	Incubation Period	Diagnostic Specimen(s)	Isolation Precautions	Treatment Options	Postexposure Prophylaxis[1]	Comments
Brucellosis	5–60 days	Culture of blood or bone marrow; acute and convalescent serum for antibody testing	Standard; contact for draining skin lesions	Doxycycline[3] and rifampin; if younger than 8 years of age, use trimethoprim-sulfamethoxazole (TMP-SMX)	Doxycycline[3] and rifampin	TMP-SMX may substitute for rifampin with doxycycline
Plague	2–4 days	Culture or fluorescent antibody staining of blood, sputum, lymph node aspirate	Droplet	Streptomycin sulfate or gentamicin sulfate; doxycycline[3] or tetracycline[3]	Doxycycline[3]; tetracycline[3]	TMP-SMX is an alternative; chloramphenicol for meningitis
Q fever	10–40 days	Acute and convalescent serum samples	Standard	Doxycycline[3] or tetracycline[3]	Doxycycline[3] or tetracycline[3]	Chloramphenicol is an alternative for treatment or prophylaxis
Smallpox	7–19 days	Culture of pharyngeal swab or skin lesions	Airborne, contact	Supportive care	Vaccine if administered within 4 days	
Staphylococcal enterotoxin B	3–12 h	Serum, urine, and respiratory secretions for toxin; acute and convalescent serum for antibodies	Standard	Supportive care	None available	

Table 2.2. Biological Weapons: Recommended Diagnostic Procedures, Isolation Precautions, and Treatment and Prophylaxis of Children, continued

Agent	Incubation Period	Diagnostic Specimen(s)	Isolation Precautions	Treatment Options	Postexposure Prophylaxis[1]	Comments
Ricin	4–8 h	Serum and/or respiratory secretions for EIA	Standard	Supportive care; gastric lavage and cathartics if toxin is ingested	Protective mask	
Viral hemorrhagic fevers	6–17 days	Culture and/or antigen detection of blood and other body tissues[7]; serum for acute and convalescent antibody detection	Standard, droplet, and contact precautions[8]	IV ribavirin for Lassa fever; plasma from convalescent patients for Argentine hemorrhagic fever; supportive care		

CSF indicates cerebrospinal fluid; CDC, Centers for Disease Control and Prevention; EIA, enzyme immunoassay; IV, intravenous.

[1] Prophylaxis should be administered only after consultation with public health officials and only in situations in which exposure is highly likely. The duration of prophylaxis has not been determined for most agents.

[2] If susceptibility is unknown or indicates resistance to other agents. Ciprofloxacin is not licensed by the US Food and Drug Administration (FDA) for use in people younger than 18 years of age but is indicated for potentially serious or life-threatening infections.

[3] Tetracyclines, including doxycycline, are not licensed by the FDA and usually are contraindicated for children younger than 8 years of age, but treatment is warranted for selected serious infections.

[4] Treatment should be administered parenterally initially but may be changed to oral therapy for cutaneous infection without dissemination.

[5] Amoxicillin may used as prophylaxis only if the organism is known to be susceptible.

[6] Botulism antitoxin must be obtained from the CDC Drug Service, 404-639-3670 (weekdays, 8:00 am–4:30 pm) or 404-639-2888 (weekends, nights, holidays).

[7] Isolation should be attempted only under biosafety level-4 conditions.

[8] Because of the risk of nosocomial transmission, the state health department and the CDC should be contacted for specific advice about management and diagnosis of suspected cases.

Table 2.3. **Emergency Contacts and Educational Resources**

Health Department Information

- State Health Department Web sites, **www.cdc.gov/other.htm#states**
- Phone numbers for state health departments, **www.asmusa.org/pasrc/StateLabContacts.pdf**

Emergency Contacts

- CDC 24-Hour Notification Line, **770-488-7100**
- USAMRIID Emergency Response Line, **888-872-7443**
- National Response Center, **800-424-8802** or **202-267-2675**
- Domestic Preparedness Help Line, **800-368-6498**
- US Public Health Service Emergency Preparedness Office, **800-USA-NDMS** or **www.ndms.dhhs.gov**

Selected Web Information Resources

- American Academy of Pediatrics bioterrorism information, **www.aap.org/terrorism**
- CDC bioterrorism information Web site, **www.bt.cdc.gov/**
- Infectious Diseases Society of America Web site, **www.idsociety.org/BT/ToC.htm**
- American Society for Microbiology Web site, **www.asmusa.org/pcsrc/biodetection.htm**
- Johns Hopkins Center for Civilian Biodefense Studies, **www.hopkins-biodefense.org/**
- US Army Medical Research Institute of Infectious Disease (USAMRIID), **www.usamriid.army.mil/**

Many preventive and therapeutic agents recommended for adults exposed or potentially exposed to agents of bioterrorism have not been studied in infants and children, and pediatric doses have not been established.*

Fever, malaise, headache, vomiting, and diarrhea are common early manifestations of many infectious diseases. Table 2.1 (p 100) describes some of the early signs and symptoms that might be helpful in distinguishing some of the biological agents included in the CDC's category A and category B lists. More extensive discussion of the clinical illnesses associated with these agents can be found in the disease-specific chapters in Section 3. Table 2.2 (p 102) lists incubation periods, diagnostic tests, isolation, and recommended treatment and prophylaxis for selected category A and B agents. Table 2.3 (above) lists resources, including telephone numbers and Internet sites, that provide updated information concerning clinical recognition, prevention, diagnosis, and treatment of illness caused by potential agents of bioterrorism.

---

* American Academy of Pediatrics, Committee on Environmental Health and Committee on Infectious Diseases. Chemical-biological terrorism and its impact on children: a subject review. *Pediatrics* 2000;105:662–670

BLOOD SAFETY: REDUCING THE RISK OF TRANSFUSION-TRANSMITTED INFECTIONS

In the United States, the risk of transmission of infectious agents through transfusion of blood components (Red Blood Cells, Platelets, and Plasma) and plasma derivatives (clotting factor concentrates, immune globulins, and protein-containing plasma volume expanders) is extremely low. Nevertheless, continued vigilance, including improved surveillance and reporting, is crucial as the blood supply remains vulnerable to organisms associated with newly identified or emerging infections. This chapter will review blood and plasma collection procedures in the United States, some factors that have contributed to enhancing the safety of the blood supply, some of the known and emerging infectious agents and related blood safety concerns; and approaches to decreasing the risk of transfusion-transmitted infections.

Blood Components and Plasma Derivatives

Blood collection, preparation, and testing are regulated carefully by the US Food and Drug Administration (FDA). In the United States, whole blood is collected from volunteer donors and separated into **components**, including Red Blood Cells, Platelets, Plasma, Gamma Globulin, and White Blood Cells. Platelets also can be obtained through apheresis, in which blood passes through a machine that separates the platelets and returns other components to the donor. Plasma for transfusion or further manufacturing into plasma derivatives can be prepared from Whole Blood or collected by apheresis. Most Plasma in the United States is obtained from paid donors at specialized collection centers. **Plasma derivatives** are prepared by pooling plasma from many donors and subjecting the plasma to a fractionation process that separates the desired proteins.

From an infection standpoint, plasma derivatives differ from blood components in several ways. For economic and therapeutic reasons, plasma from thousands of donors is pooled, and therefore, recipients of plasma derivatives have vastly greater donor exposure than do blood component recipients. However, plasma derivatives are able to withstand vigorous viral inactivation processes that would destroy Red Blood Cells and Platelets. Development and evaluation of various blood component inactivation strategies are ongoing.

Current Blood Safety Measures

The safety of the blood supply relies on multiple steps, including donor interview and selection, donor screening by serologic tests and other markers of infection, and viral inactivation procedures for plasma-derived products (see Table 2.4, p 107). Blood donors are interviewed to exclude people with a history of exposures or behaviors that increase their risk of an infectious agent. All blood donations are tested routinely for syphilis, hepatitis B virus (HBV), hepatitis C virus (HCV), human T-lymphotropic virus (HTLV) types I and II, and human immunodeficiency virus (HIV) types 1 and 2; selected donations are tested for cytomegalovirus (CMV). In 1997, approximately 226 000 units of Whole Blood were disqualified in the

Table 2.4. **Blood Donor Screening Measures**[1]

Measure	Targeted Infectious Agents
General interview and screening	
• Previous safety of donor (ie, no deferral in effect)	Bloodborne phase of multiple agents
• General health, current illness, temperature at time of donation	Bloodborne phase of multiple agents
• Donor confidential unit exclusion option	Bloodborne phase of multiple agents
• Reminder to notify blood collector of illness (eg, fever, diarrhea) after donation or of any other pertinent information recalled	Bloodborne phase of multiple agents
Specific risk factor history	
• High-risk sexual behaviors or injection drug use in donor or donor's partner(s)	HIV, HCV, HBV, HTLV
• Geographic risks (travel and residence)	Malaria, vCJD
• History of specific infections	HIV, HBV, HCV, other hepatitis agents, parasites (those causing malaria, Chagas disease, babesiosis)
• Previous parenteral exposure to blood via transfusion or occupational exposure; not lifetime deferral	HIV, HCV, HBV
Laboratory screening	HIV-1 and HIV-2 (HIV antibody and HIV-1 [p24] antigen), HCV (antibody), HIV and HCV nucleic acid testing; HBV (HBsAg and anti-HBc) (ALT generally is performed but not recommended by the FDA), HTLV-I/II (antibodies), syphilis

HIV indicates human immunodeficiency virus; HCV, hepatitis C virus; HBV, hepatitis B virus; HTLV, human T-lymphotropic virus; vCJD, variant Creutzfeldt-Jakob disease; HBsAg, hepatitis B surface antigen; anti-HBc, antibody to hepatitis B core antigen; ALT, alanine transaminase; FDA, US Food and Drug Administration.

[1] Screening of Plasma (paid) donors is similar but not identical. For example, because HTLV-I and HTLV-II are cell-borne agents, Plasma donations are not tested for anti-HTLV-I/II. Donors are tested for syphilis at least every 4 months.

United States because of positive results on screening tests for one of these organisms. This represents 1.7% of units collected.

Look-Back Programs

If a person who has donated in the past reveals a new or previously undisclosed risk factor on questioning or is found to be infected with certain agents, product retrieval and notification of the party to whom the product was shipped (hospital, transfusion service, or physician) are conducted by blood establishments according to FDA guidance and recommendations. Records are reviewed to determine whether any previous donations pose a threat to recipients. For example, an earlier donation may have been made during the "window period" of a viral infection, a time when the donor was viremic but serologic test results were not yet positive. As part of look-back, any remaining components that may contain the infectious agent are located and removed from distribution, and potentially exposed recipients are notified, counseled, and tested.

In 1999 in the United States, a major effort was initiated to notify hundreds of thousands of people who may have acquired HCV infection from blood transfusions before the introduction of effective blood donation screening. Two approaches were used to identify these transfusion recipients: (1) a targeted (or directed) approach to identify previous transfusion recipients of donors who tested positive for antibody to HCV after screening tests were implemented (1990 and later); and (2) a general approach to identify all people who had received transfusions before July 1992 (when the more sensitive and specific multiantigen HCV test was implemented). The general notification and education campaign was aimed at health care professionals and the public. People who received a transfusion of blood or blood components before July 1992 should seek counseling and testing for HCV infection. Health care professionals routinely should ascertain their patients' transfusion history and risk factors for previous transfusion, such as hematologic disorders, major surgery, trauma, and premature birth.

Transfusion-Transmitted Agents: Known Threats and Potential Pathogens

Any infectious agent that has a blood phase potentially may be transmitted by blood transfusion. Factors that influence the risk of transfusion-transmission of an infectious agent and the development of clinical disease in the recipient include prevalence and incidence of the agent in donors, duration of hematogenous phase, tolerance of the agent to processing and storage, infectivity and pathogenicity of the agent, and recipient's health status. Table 2.5 (p 109) lists major known transfusion-transmitted infections and some of the emerging agents under investigation.

VIRUSES

Human Immunodeficiency Virus (p 360), HCV (p 336), HBV (p 318). The probability of infection in recipients who are exposed to these viruses is approximately 90% for HIV and HCV and 70% for HBV. Although blood donations are screened for these viruses, there is a small residual risk of infection resulting almost exclusively from donations collected during the "window period" of infection, the period soon after infection during which a blood donor is infectious but screening test results are negative.

To decrease the time period when viral infection can go undetected, nucleic acid testing (NAT) of blood and plasma donations for HIV and HCV was implemented beginning in 1999. Testing is being performed under investigational new drug applications. Although not mandatory at this time, NAT is performed on essentially all blood and plasma donations in the United States. Various estimates suggest that pooled NAT can decrease the preantibody seroconversion "window period" from 22 days to 13 to 15 days for HIV and from 70 days to 10 to 29 days

Table 2.5. **Selected Known and Potential Transfusion-Transmitted Agents[1]**

Agents and Products	Transfusion-Transmitted	Pathogenic	Estimated per Unit Risk of Contamination (US Studies, Except as Noted)
Viruses for which all blood donors tested			
HIV	Yes	Yes	1 in 725 000–835 000
HCV	Yes	Yes	1 in 250 000–500 000
HBV	Yes	Yes	1 in 63 000–500 000
HTLV types I and II	Yes	Yes	1 in 641 000
Other viruses			
CMV	Yes	Yes	Most donors harbor virus
Parvovirus B19	Yes	Yes	1 in 10 000
HAV	Yes	Yes	<1 in 1 million
HGV	Yes	Unknown	1–2 in 100
TTV	Yes	Unknown	1 in 10 (Japan), 1 in 50 (Scotland)
SEN virus	Yes	Yes	Unknown
HHV-8	Unknown	Yes	Unknown
Bacteria			
Red Blood Cells	Yes	Yes	Vary widely depending on study
Platelets			
Random donor	Yes	Yes	Vary widely depending on study
Apheresis	Yes	Yes	Vary widely depending on study
Parasites[2]			
Malaria	Yes	Yes	Vary widely depending on study
Chagas disease (*Trypanosoma cruzi*)	Yes	Yes	Unknown
Prion diseases			
CJD/vCJD	Unknown	Yes	Unknown
Tickborne			
Babesia species	Yes	Yes	Unknown
Rickettsia rickettsii	Yes	Yes	Unknown
Colorado tick fever virus	Yes	Yes	Unknown
Borrelia burgdorferi	Unknown	Yes	Unknown
Ehrlichia species	Unknown	Yes	Unknown

HIV indicates human immunodeficiency virus; HCV, hepatitis C virus; HBV, hepatitis B virus; HTLV, human T-lymphotropic virus; CMV, cytomegalovirus; HAV, hepatitis A virus; HGV, hepatitis G virus; TTV, transfusion-transmitted virus; HHV, human herpesvirus; CJD, Creutzfeldt-Jakob disease; and vCJD, variant CJD.

[1] For additional information, see Goodnough LT, Brecher ME, Kanter MH, AuBuchon JP. Transfusion medicine: first of two parts: blood transfusion. *N Engl J Med.* 1999;340:438-447; and Goodnough LT, Brecher ME, Kanter MH, AuBuchon JP. Transfusion medicine: second of two parts: blood conservation. *N Engl J Med.* 1999;340:525-533.

[2] Other transfusion-transmitted agents include *Toxoplasma gondii* and leishmanial species.

for HCV. Mathematic models have been developed to estimate the current very low risks of transfusion transmission of HIV, HCV, and HBV (Table 2.5).

Human T-Lymphotropic Virus Types I and II. Infections with HTLV are relatively common in certain geographic areas and in specific populations, such as HTLV-I in Japan, the Caribbean, and southern United States and HTLV- II in indigenous people of North, Central, and South America and injection drug users in the United States and Europe. Human T-lymphotropic virus types I and II are transmitted by transfusion of cellular components of blood but not by plasma or plasma derivatives. The risk of HTLV transmission from screened blood donated during the "window period" has been estimated at 1 per 641 000 units screened. However, transmission of HTLV is less likely to lead to infection than is transmission of HIV, HBV, or HCV, with an approximate 27% seroconversion rate in people in the United States who receive cellular blood components from infected donors.

Cytomegalovirus (p 259). Immunocompromised people, including premature infants, bone marrow and solid organ transplant recipients, and others, are at risk of severe, life-threatening illness from transfusion-transmitted CMV. Consequently, in many centers, only blood from donors who lack CMV antibodies is given to these people. Leukoreduction decreases the risk of CMV transmission, because CMV resides in a latent phase within white blood cells.

Parvovirus B19 (p 459). Blood donations are not screened for parvovirus B19, because infection with this virus is relatively ubiquitous in humans. Seroprevalence rates in adult blood donors range from 29% to 79%. Estimates of parvovirus B19 viremia in blood donors have ranged from 0 to 2.6 per 10 000. Parvovirus, like CMV, usually does not cause severe disease in immunocompetent hosts but may be a threat to certain people (eg, nonimmune pregnant women; people with hemoglobinopathies, such as sickle cell disease and thalassemia; and immunocompromised patients). Transmission of parvovirus B19 from single-donor components is thought to occur rarely. However, pooled plasma derivatives commonly are positive for parvovirus B19 DNA, because parvovirus B19 lacks a lipid envelope, making it resistant to solvent and detergent treatment. People with hemophilia have increased rates of seropositivity to parvovirus B19 compared with age-matched control subjects; however, the clinical significance of parvovirus B19 among people with hemophilia is uncertain. To increase safety, some manufacturers of plasma derivatives test plasma mini-pools for parvovirus DNA.

Hepatitis A Virus (p 309). Infection with hepatitis A virus (HAV) leads to a relatively short period of viremia, and a chronic carrier state does not occur. Cases of post-transfusion HAV infection have been reported but are rare. Clusters of HAV infections transmitted from clotting factor concentrates occurred among people with hemophilia in Europe during the early 1990s, in South Africa, and more recently, in the United States. Like parvovirus, HAV lacks a lipid envelope and may survive solvent and detergent treatment.

Non-A Through -E Hepatitis Viruses. A small proportion of people with post-transfusion hepatitis as well as community-acquired hepatitis test negative for all known hepatitis agents. In recent years, several newly discovered viruses have been evaluated as possible etiologic agents. Although 2 of these viruses, hepatitis G virus/GB virus type C (strain variants of a member of the *Flaviviridae* family) and TT virus (TTV) (named for the patient from whom it was first isolated in Japan), can be found in blood donors and can be transmitted by transfusion, neither agent has been found to be associated with development of post-transfusion hepatitis and, hence, are not "hepatitis" viruses.

The SEN virus also is being evaluated as an agent of non-A through -E hepatitis. In one study, tests of stored sera from blood donors and cardiac surgery patients revealed that approximately 2% of donors tested positive for SEN virus DNA, and the proportion of cardiac surgery patients with evidence of new infection with SEN virus was 10 times higher among those who had received transfusions, compared with those who had not. Of 12 recipients with non-A through -E hepatitis, 11 (92%) became SENV positive after transfusion. Extending this early work will be essential to prove that SENV replicates inside hepatocytes. There are no data to date showing that SENV is a cause of fulminant liver failure, and its roles in chronic crytogenic hepatitis and cirrhosis are uncertain.

There are no approved tests for screening donors for any of these viruses, and there are no data to suggest that such tests would be beneficial.

Human Herpesvirus 8. Human herpesvirus 8 (HHV-8) has been associated with Kaposi sarcoma in people with HIV infection, non-HIV Kaposi sarcoma, and certain rare malignant neoplasms. The predominant modes of transmission are male-to-male sexual contact in the United States and close, nonsexual contact in Africa. Because HHV-8 DNA has been detected in peripheral blood mononuclear cells and serum specimens, there has been concern that HHV-8 could be transmitted by blood and blood products. Also, recent studies have found an association between serologic evidence of HHV-8 and injection drug use. Although theoretically possible, HHV-8 transmission has not been detected in studies of small numbers of recipients of blood from known HHV-8–seropositive donors. Also, HHV-8 seroprevalence among people with exposure to blood and blood products (eg, people with hemophilia) generally is comparable to seroprevalence among healthy, HIV-seronegative individuals. Larger populations of recipients of blood or blood products from HHV-8–positive individuals need to be studied to more completely evaluate this possibility.

West Nile Virus. West Nile virus has been shown to be transmitted through blood transfusions. Cases of West Nile virus disease in patients who have received blood transfusions within 4 weeks before onset of illness should be reported to the Centers for Disease Control and Prevention (CDC) through state and local public health authorities. Serum and tissue samples should be retained for later studies. Also, cases of West Nile virus infection diagnosed in people who have donated blood within 2 weeks of onset of illness should be reported.

BACTERIA

Although major advances in blood safety have been made, bacterial contamination of blood products remains an important cause of transfusion reaction. Bacterial contamination can occur during collection, processing, and transfusion of blood components.

Platelets are stored at room temperature, which can facilitate growth of contaminating bacteria. However, suspicion of bacterial contamination often is low, and appropriate testing is not performed regularly for detection. For these reasons, bacterial contamination of blood products may be underestimated and underrecognized. The predominant bacterium that contaminates platelets is *Staphylococcus epidermidis.*

Bacillus species; more virulent organisms, such as *Staphylococcus aureus;* and various gram-negative bacteria also have been reported. Transfusion reactions attributable to contaminated platelets likely are underrecognized, because episodes of bacteremia with skin organisms are common in patients requiring platelets, and the link to the transfusion may not be suspected.

Red Blood Cell units are much less likely than are Platelets to contain bacteria at the time of transfusion, because refrigeration kills or inhibits growth of many bacteria. However, certain bacteria, most notably *Yersinia enterocolitica,* may contaminate Red Blood Cells, because this organism survives cold storage. Cases of septic shock and death attributable to transfusion-transmitted *Y enterocolitica* have been documented.

Reported rates of transfusion-associated bacterial sepsis have varied widely depending on study methodology and microbial detection methods used. A prospective, multisite study (the Assessment of the Frequency of Blood Component Bacterial Contamination Associated with Transfusion Reaction [BaCon] Study), estimated the rate of transfusion-transmitted bacteremia to be 1 in 100 000 units for single-donor and pooled Platelets and 1 in 5 million units for Red Blood Cells. Other studies that did not require matching bacterial cultures and/or molecular typing of both the component and the recipient's blood as in the BaCon Study have found higher rates of infection. For example, one hospital-based surveillance study found that approximately 1 in 13 500 transfusions of single-donor Platelets resulted in clinical septic reactions; this rate increased to approximately 1 in 2500 for pools of platelet concentrates.

PARASITES

Several parasitic agents have been reported to cause transfusion-transmitted infections, including malaria, Chagas disease, babesiosis, toxoplasmosis, and leishmaniasis. Decreasing transfusion transmission of parasites is crucial in endemic regions, but increasing travel to and immigration from endemic areas has led to a need for increased vigilance in the United States.

Malaria (see p 414). The incidence of transfusion-associated malaria has decreased over the last 30 years in the United States. During the last decade, the rate has ranged from 0 to 0.18 cases per million units transfused, that is, no more than 1 to 2 cases per year. Most cases currently are attributed to infectious donors who have immigrated to the United States rather than people born in the United States who traveled to endemic areas. *Plasmodium falciparum* now is the species most commonly transmitted. Prevention of transfusion-transmitted malaria relies on interviewing donors for risk factors related to travel or previous treatment for malaria. There is no approved laboratory test to screen donated blood for malaria.

Chagas Disease (see American Trypanosomiasis, p 640). The immigration of millions of people from *Trypanosoma cruzi*-endemic areas (parts of Central and South America and Mexico) and increased international travel have raised concern about the potential for transfusion-transmitted Chagas disease. To date, 5 cases of transfusion-transmitted Chagas disease have been reported in North America. Studies of blood donors likely to have been born in or to have traveled to endemic areas have found antibodies to *T cruzi* in as many as 0.5% of people tested. Although transfusion transmission of *T cruzi* in the United States appears to be rare, the lack of adequately sensitive and specific donor history questions and/or licensed tests has limited efforts to identify donors who may be at increased risk of infection.

Babesiosis (see p 211). The most commonly reported transfusion-associated tickborne infection in the United States is babesiosis. More than 30 cases of transfusion-induced babesiosis have been documented; most were attributed to *Babesia microti*, but the WA1-type *Babesia* parasite also has been implicated. *Babesia* organisms are intracellular parasites that infect red blood cells. However, at least 4 cases have been associated with receipt of Platelets, which often contain a small number of red blood cells. Although most infections are asymptomatic, *Babesia* infection can cause severe, life-threatening disease, particularly in elderly or splenectomized patients. Severe infection can result in hemolytic anemia, thrombocytopenia, and renal failure. Surveys using indirect immunofluorescence antibody (IFA) assays in highly endemic areas of Connecticut and New York have revealed seropositivity rates for *B microti* in 1.2% and 4.3%, respectively. In a study of blood donors in Connecticut, 19 (56%) of 34 seropositive donors had positive results for nucleic acid, as determined by polymerase chain reaction (PCR) assay. Blood from 3 (20%) of 15 donors with positive PCR assay results was infectious when inoculated into hamsters, and infection was transmitted to recipients of blood from approximately 1 in 4 donors with positive PCR assay results.

No licensed test currently is available to screen donors for *Babesia* organisms. Donors with a history of babesiosis are deferred indefinitely from future donation. Although people with acute illness or fever are not eligible to donate, infected individuals commonly are asymptomatic or experience only mild and nonspecific clinical symptoms. In addition, *Babesia* species can cause chronic, asymptomatic infection for years in otherwise healthy people. Questioning donors about recent tick bites has been shown to be ineffective, because donors who are seropositive for antibody to tickborne agents are no more likely than seronegative donors to recall tick bites.

TRANSMISSIBLE SPONGIFORM ENCEPHALOPATHIES: PRION DISEASE

Creutzfeldt-Jakob Disease and Variant Creutzfeldt-Jakob Disease (p 510).

Creutzfeldt-Jakob disease (CJD) and variant CJD (vCJD) are fatal neurologic illnesses believed to be caused by unique agents known as prions (see Transmissible Spongiform Encephalopathies, p 510).

Sporadic CJD. The risk of CJD transmission through blood is considered theoretic. No cases of CJD resulting from receipt of blood transfusion have been documented, and case-control studies have not found an association between receipt of blood and development of CJD. No cases of CJD in people with hematologic conditions that require frequent transfusion, such as sickle cell disease and thalassemia, have been reported. Studies of recipients of blood from donors who subsequently developed CJD and surveillance for CJD among people with hemophilia also have not detected evidence of transfusion-transmitted CJD. Collectively, these epidemiologic data suggest that the risk of CJD, if any, from transfusion must be extremely rare.

Nevertheless, because of concerns about the theoretic risk of CJD transmission by blood transfusion, people diagnosed with or at increased risk of CJD (eg, receipt of pituitary-derived growth hormone or dura mater transplant or family history of CJD) are deferred from donation. In addition, all available Whole Blood, cellular blood components, and unpooled Plasma from previous donations are discarded. However, withdrawal of plasma derivatives is not required, because epidemiologic and laboratory data suggest that plasma derivatives are unlikely to transmit the CJD agent, and plasma pools undergo extensive fractionation and processing.

Variant CJD. In 1996, a new variant form of CJD (vCJD) was first recognized in the United Kingdom. The agent that causes this new human transmissible spongiform encephalopathy is believed to be the same agent responsible for an outbreak of bovine spongiform encephalopathy (BSE) among cattle in the United Kingdom, which was diagnosed initially in 1986. Clinical features of vCJD are distinct from those of sporadic CJD. As of January 2003, 139 cases of vCJD had been reported, 129 from the United Kingdom, 6 from France, and one each from Canada, Ireland, Italy, and the United States. The Canadian and US patients resided in the United Kingdom during key exposure periods of the population to the BSE agent. Most patients with vCJD were younger than 30 years of age, and several were adolescents.

Transmission of vCJD by blood and blood products has not been observed to date. However, vCJD differs from sporadic CJD in ways that have raised concern about its potential transmissibly by blood and plasma. The prion protein has been detected in white blood-cell rich organs, such as human spleens and tonsils, from people with vCJD but not sporadic CJD. Limited, early evidence suggests that blood from experimentally infected animals may be infectious. In one study, intravenous administration of blood from an asymptomatic donor sheep (at the halfway point in its incubation period after being fed BSE-infected cattle brain) resulted in transmission of BSE to a single recipient sheep. Also, intravenous administration of BSE-infected tissue has been shown to transmit infection in macaque monkeys.

The following categories of potential donors are deferred indefinitely: people who have received a blood or blood component transfusion in the United Kingdom after January 1, 1980; people who have lived in the United Kingdom for 6 months or more between 1980 and 1996; people who have spent 5 years or more in any European country after January 1, 1980; people who have been injected with bovine insulin since January 1, 1980, unless it can be confirmed that the insulin was not manufactured from United Kingdom cattle; and former or current US military personnel, civilian military personnel, or their dependents who resided at US military bases in Northern Europe for 6 months or more between January 1, 1980 and December 31, 1990 or at US military bases elsewhere in Europe for 6 months or more between January 1, 1980 and December 31, 1996.

TICKBORNE INFECTIONS (SEE PREVENTION OF TICKBORNE INFECTIONS, P 186)

Several emerging tickborne agents are of concern in North America (see Prevention of Tickborne Infections, p 186). Babesiosis is the most commonly reported transfusion-transmitted tickborne infection. Other reports of transfusion-transmitted tickborne agents have been limited to 1 case each of Rocky Mountain spotted fever and Colorado tick fever and 1 possible case of human granulocytic ehrlichiosis. *Borrelia burgdorferi* has yet to be reported as being transmitted by blood transfusion, despite Lyme disease being the most commonly reported tickborne disease in the United States. Individuals who become infected with these agents through the bites of infected ticks often are asymptomatic or experience only mild and nonspecific clinical symptoms (eg, fever, headache, myalgia). Hence, blood donors may feel well and healthy but may have circulating organisms that can be transmitted by transfusion. Strategies to prevent transfusion-transmitted tickborne infections are limited at present to deferral of people with acute illness or fever. No licensed test is available to screen donors for any of these agents. Questioning donors about recent tick bites is too nonspecific to be effective.

Improving Blood Safety

A number of strategies have been proposed or implemented to further decrease the risk of transmission of infectious agents through blood and blood products. Various safety strategies are as follows.

ELIMINATION OF INFECTIOUS AGENTS

Agent Inactivation. Virtually all plasma derivatives, including Immune Globulin Intravenous (IGIV) and clotting factors, are treated to eliminate infectious agents that may be present, despite screening measures. Methods used for this include wet and dry heat and treatment with a solvent and a detergent. Solvent- and detergent-treated pooled Plasma for transfusion is available in the United States, and methods of treating single-donor Plasma are under study. Solvent and detergent treatment dissolves the lipid envelope of HIV, HBV, and HCV but is not effective against nonlipid-enveloped viruses, such as HAV and parvovirus B19.

Because of their fragility, pathogen inactivation of Red Blood Cells and Platelets is more difficult. However, several methods have been developed, such as addition of psoralens followed by exposure to ultraviolet A, which binds the nucleic acids and blocks replication of bacteria and viruses. Clinical trials of these treated components are underway.

Agent Removal. Another proposed strategy under FDA review is leukoreduction, whereby filters are used to remove donor white blood cells. The concentration of intracellular or cell-associated agents would be decreased (eg, viruses such as CMV, Epstein-Barr virus, HHV-8, and HTLV). Several countries have adopted this practice. In addition, some experts believe that the theoretic risk of transmission of vCJD through blood may be decreased by white blood cell removal. Additional benefits of this process include decreasing febrile transfusion reactions related to white blood cells and their products and decreasing the immune modulation associated with transfusion.

DECREASING EXPOSURE TO BLOOD PRODUCTS

Alternatives to Human Blood Products. Many alternatives to human blood products have been developed. Established alternatives include recombinant clotting factors for patients with hemophilia and factors such as erythropoietin used to stimulate red blood cell production. Other agents include several red blood cell substitutes currently in clinical trials, such as human hemoglobin extracted from red blood cells, recombinant human hemoglobin, animal hemoglobin, and various oxygen-carrying chemicals.

Autologous Transfusion. Another means of decreasing recipient exposure is autologous transfusion. Blood may be donated by the patient several weeks before a surgical procedure (preoperative autologous donation) or, alternatively, donated immediately before surgery and replaced with a volume expander (acute normovolemic hemodilution). In either case, the patient's blood can be reinfused if needed. Autologous blood is not completely risk free, because bacterial contamination may occur.

Blood recycling techniques (autotransfusion) also are in this category. During surgery, blood lost by the patient may be collected, processed, and reinfused to the patient.

SHORTAGES OF PLASMA DERIVATIVES

Periodically, shortages of plasma derivatives occur. Factors that contribute to these shortages have included: (1) production impediments related to compliance; (2) increase in off-label use of some products (eg, IGIV); (3) waste; and (4) hoarding of product because of concerns about scarcity. For recommendations for use of IGIV, see Indications for the Use of IGIV, p 56.

STRATEGIES TO PREVENT HARM TO THOSE EXPOSED TO CONTAMINATED BLOOD

Preexposure Strategies. Receipt of HBV vaccine is recommended for patients with bleeding disorders who receive clotting factor concentrates (see Hepatitis B, p 318); HAV vaccine also should be given to people in this group (see Hepatitis A, p 309).

STRATEGIES TO IMPROVE SURVEILLANCE

National programs for surveillance include pathogen- and disease-specific systems (eg, HIV, viral hepatitis) and programs that focus on donors and recipients of blood and plasma products. In addition, large-scale repositories of specimens from donors and recipients have been used to study the infectious complications of transfusions.

Transfusion-transmitted infection surveillance is crucial and must be coupled with the capacity to rapidly investigate reported cases and to implement measures needed to prevent additional infections. Serious adverse reactions and product problems should be reported to the manufacturer (or, alternatively, to the supplier for transmission to the manufacturer). Health care professionals also may report such information directly to the FDA through MEDWATCH. This can be done by telephone (1-800-FDA-1088), fax (1-800-FDA-0178), Internet (www.fda.gov/medwatch/report/hcp.htm), or mail (see MEDWATCH, p 771). This voluntary reporting is considered vital for monitoring product safety.

HUMAN MILK

Breastfeeding provides numerous health benefits to infants, including protection against morbidity and mortality from infectious diseases of bacterial, viral, and parasitic origin. In addition to providing an ideal source of infant nutrition, largely uncontaminated by environmental pathogens, human milk contains protective factors, including cells, specific secretory antibodies, innate factors such as glyco-conjugates, and anti-inflammatory components. Breastfed infants have high concentrations of protective bifidobacteria and lactobacillus in their gastrointestinal tracts, which increase resistance to pathogenic organisms. Evidence also indicates that human milk may modulate development of infants' immune systems. Protection by human milk is established most clearly for pathogens causing gastrointestinal tract infection. In addition, human milk seems to provide protection against otitis media, invasive *Haemophilus influenzae* type b infection, respiratory syncytial virus infection, and other causes of upper and lower respiratory tract infections.

The American Academy of Pediatrics (AAP) issues statements and publishes a manual on infant feeding that provides further information about the benefits of breastfeeding and recommended feeding practices.* In the *Pediatric Nutrition Handbook* and in the AAP policy statement on human milk,[†] issues regarding immunization of lactating mothers and breastfeeding infants, transmission of infectious agents via human milk, and potential effects on breastfeeding infants of antimicrobial agents administered to lactating mothers also are addressed.

Immunization of Mothers and Infants

EFFECT OF MATERNAL IMMUNIZATION

Women who have not received recommended immunizations before or during pregnancy may be immunized during the postpartum period regardless of lactation status. No evidence exists to validate concern about the potential presence of live viruses from vaccines in maternal milk if the mother is immunized during lactation. Lactating women may be immunized as recommended for other adults to protect against measles, mumps, rubella, tetanus, diphtheria, influenza, *Streptococcus pneumoniae* infection, hepatitis A, hepatitis B, and varicella. If previously unimmunized or if traveling to a highly endemic area, a lactating mother may be given inactivated poliovirus vaccine. Rubella seronegative mothers who could not be immunized during pregnancy should be immunized during the postpartum period.

EFFICACY OF IMMUNIZATION IN BREASTFED INFANTS

Infants should be immunized according to the recommended schedule regardless of the mode of infant feeding. The immunogenicity of some currently recommended vaccines is enhanced by breastfeeding, but data are lacking as to whether the efficacy of these vaccines is enhanced. Although high concentrations of antipoliovirus anti-

---

* American Academy of Pediatrics, Committee on Nutrition. *Pediatric Nutrition Handbook*. 5th ed. Elk Grove Village, IL: American Academy of Pediatrics. In press
† American Academy of Pediatrics, Section on Breastfeeding. Breastfeeding and the use of human milk. *Pediatrics*. In press

body in milk of some mothers theoretically could interfere with the immunogenicity of oral polio vaccine, no such association has been demonstrated. This is not a concern with inactivated poliovirus vaccine.

Transmission of Infectious Agents via Human Milk

BACTERIA

Mastitis and breast abscesses have been associated with the presence of bacterial pathogens in human milk. In general, infectious mastitis resolves with continued lactation during antimicrobial therapy and does not pose a significant risk for the healthy term infant. Breast abscesses occur rarely and have the potential to rupture into the ductal system, releasing large numbers of organisms, such as *Staphylococcus aureus,* into milk. In general, feeding an infant using a breast affected by an abscess is not recommended. However, some experts recommend that infant feeding using the affected breast may resume once the mother is treated adequately with an appropriate antimicrobial agent and the abscess is drained surgically. Even when breastfeeding is interrupted on the affected breast, breastfeeding may continue on the opposite (unaffected) breast.

Women with tuberculosis who have been treated appropriately for 2 or more weeks and who are not considered contagious may breastfeed. Women with active tuberculosis suspected of being contagious should refrain from breastfeeding or any other close contact with the infant because of potential transmission through respiratory tract droplets (see Tuberculosis, p 642). *Mycobacterium tuberculosis* rarely causes mastitis or a breast abscess, but if a breast abscess caused by *M tuberculosis* is present, breastfeeding should be discontinued until the mother is no longer contagious.

Expressed human milk can become contaminated with a variety of bacterial pathogens, including *Staphylococcus* species and gram-negative enteric bacilli. Outbreaks of gram-negative bacterial infections in neonatal intensive care units occasionally have been attributed to contaminated human milk specimens that have been collected or stored improperly. Human milk fed to infants from women other than the biologic mother should be treated according to the guidelines of the Human Milk Banking Association of North America. Routine culturing or heat treatment of a mother's milk fed to her infant has not been demonstrated to be necessary or cost-effective (see Human Milk Banks, p 121).

VIRUSES

Cytomegalovirus. Cytomegalovirus (CMV) may be shed intermittently in human milk. Although transmission of CMV through human milk has occurred, disease in neonates is uncommon, presumably because of passively transferred maternal antibody. Preterm infants, however, are at greater potential risk of symptomatic disease and sequelae than are term infants. Infants born to CMV-seronegative women who seroconvert during lactation and premature infants with low concentrations of transplacentally acquired maternal antibodies to CMV can develop symptomatic disease with sequelae from acquiring CMV through breastfeeding. Decisions about breastfeeding of premature infants by mothers known to be CMV seropositive should include consideration of the potential benefits of human milk and the risk of CMV transmission. Pasteurization of milk seems to inactivate CMV; freezing milk at −20°C (−4°F) will decrease viral titers but does not reliably eliminate CMV.

Hepatitis B Virus. Hepatitis B surface antigen (HBsAg) has been detected in milk from HBsAg-positive women. However, studies from Taiwan and England have indicated that breastfeeding by HBsAg-positive women does not increase significantly the risk of infection among their infants. In the United States, infants born to known HBsAg-positive women should receive Hepatitis B Immune Globulin and the recommended series of 3 doses of hepatitis B virus vaccine, effectively eliminating any theoretic risk of transmission through breastfeeding. There is no need to delay initiation of breastfeeding until after the infant is immunized. Immunoprophylaxis of infants with hepatitis B vaccine alone also provides protection, but optimal therapy of infants born to HBsAg-positive mothers includes the 3-dose series of hepatitis B virus vaccine and Hepatitis B Immune Globulin (see Hepatitis B, p 318).

Hepatitis C Virus. Hepatitis C virus (HCV) RNA and antibody to HCV have been detected in milk from mothers infected with HCV. Transmission of HCV via breastfeeding has not been documented in anti-HCV–positive, anti-human immunodeficiency virus (HIV)-negative mothers. Mothers infected with HCV should be counseled that transmission of HCV by breastfeeding theoretically is possible but has not been documented. According to current guidelines of the US Public Health Service, maternal HCV infection is not a contraindication to breastfeeding. The decision to breastfeed should be based on informed discussion between a mother and her health care professional.

Human Immunodeficiency Virus. Human immunodeficiency virus has been isolated from human milk and can be transmitted through breastfeeding. The risk of transmission is higher for women who acquire HIV infection during lactation (ie, postpartum) than for women with preexisting infection. In populations such as the United States, in which the risk of mortality from infectious diseases and malnutrition is low and in which safe and effective alternative sources of feeding are available readily, HIV-infected women should be counseled not to breastfeed their infants or donate milk. All pregnant women in the United States should be counseled and encouraged to be tested for HIV infection. Data are not available about the safety of breastfeeding by mothers on highly active antiretroviral therapy. In areas where infectious diseases and malnutrition are important causes of mortality early in life, the feeding decision may be more complex. The World Health Organization states that if a mother is infected with HIV, replacement of human milk to decrease the risk of HIV transmission may be preferable to breastfeeding provided that the risk of replacement feeding is less than the potential risk of HIV transmission. Implementation of this suggestion has many obstacles. The World Health Organization policy stresses the need for continued support for breastfeeding by mothers who are HIV negative or of unknown HIV status, improved access to HIV counseling and testing, and government efforts to ensure uninterrupted access to nutritionally adequate human milk substitutes (see Human Immunodeficiency Virus Infection, p 360).

Human T-Lymphotropic Virus Type I. This retrovirus, which is endemic in Japan, the Caribbean, and parts of South America, is associated with development of malignant neoplasms and neurologic disorders among adults. Epidemiologic and laboratory studies suggest that mother-to-infant transmission of human T-cell lymphotropic virus (HTLV) type I occurs primarily through breastfeeding. Women in the United States who are HTLV-I seropositive should be advised not to breastfeed.

Human T-Lymphotropic Virus Type II. Human T-lymphotropic virus type II, also a retrovirus, has been detected among American and European injection drug users and some American Indian/Alaska Native groups. Although apparent maternal-infant transmission has been reported, the rate and timing of transmission have not been established. Until additional data about possible transmission through breastfeeding become available, women in the United States who are seropositive should be advised not to breastfeed.

Herpes Simplex Virus Type 1. The virus has been isolated from human milk in the absence of vesicular lesions on or drainage from the breast or concurrent positive cultures from the maternal cervix, vagina, or throat. Cases of transmission of herpes simplex virus (HSV) type 1 after breastfeeding in the presence of maternal breast lesions have been reported. Because development of extragenital lesions seems to occur more often with primary than with recurrent HSV infection, some experts recommend that women with primary mucocutaneous disease not breastfeed their infants until all lesions have resolved. Women with herpetic lesions on their breasts should refrain from breastfeeding; active lesions elsewhere should be covered during breastfeeding, and careful hand hygiene should be used.

Rubella. Wild and vaccine strains of rubella virus have been isolated from human milk. However, the presence of rubella virus in human milk has not been associated with significant disease in infants, and transmission is more likely to occur via other routes. Women with rubella or women who have just been immunized with live-attenuated rubella virus vaccine need not refrain from breastfeeding.

Varicella. Whether varicella vaccine virus is secreted in human milk or whether the virus would infect a breastfeeding infant is unknown. Varicella vaccine may be considered for a susceptible breastfeeding mother if the risk of exposure to natural varicella-zoster virus is high. Recommendations on the use of Varicella-Zoster Immune Globulin and varicella vaccine for breastfeeding mothers who have had contact with people in whom varicella has developed or for contacts of a breastfeeding mother in whom varicella has developed are available (see Varicella-Zoster Infections, p 672).

West Nile Virus. West Nile virus RNA has been detected in human milk collected from a woman with disease attributable to West Nile virus; her breastfed infant developed West Nile virus immunoglobulin M antibodies but remained asymptomatic. Animal experiments have shown that West Nile virus can be transmitted in animal milk, and other related flaviviruses can be transmitted to humans via unpasteurized milk from ruminants. The degree to which West Nile virus is transmitted in human milk and the extent to which breastfeeding infants become infected are unknown. Most infants and young children infected with West Nile virus are asymptomatic or develop mild disease; serious neurologic disease is uncommon.

HUMAN MILK BANKS

Some circumstances, such as premature delivery, may preclude breastfeeding. In these instances, infants may be fed milk collected from their own mothers or from individual donors. The potential for transmission of infectious agents through human milk requires appropriate selection and screening of donors and careful collection, processing, and storage of milk. Currently, US donor milk banks that belong to the Human Milk Banking Association of North America voluntarily follow guidelines drafted in consultation with the US Food and Drug Administration and the Centers for Disease Control and Prevention. These guidelines include screening of all donors for antibodies to HIV-1, HIV-2, HTLV-I, HTLV-II, HBsAg, hepatitis C, and syphilis. Donor milk is dispensed only by prescription after it is heat-treated at ≥56°C (≥133°F) for 30 minutes and bacterial cultures reveal no growth. Milk from the birth mother of a premature infant does not require processing if fed to her infant, but proper collection and storage need to be ensured.

Heat treatment at ≥56°C (≥133°F) for 30 minutes reliably eliminates bacteria, inactivates HIV, and decreases titers of other viruses but in 1 study did not completely eliminate CMV. Holder pasteurization (62.5°C [144.5°F] for 30 minutes) reliably inactivates HIV and CMV and eliminates or significantly decreases titers of most other viruses.

Freezing at −20°C (−4°F) eliminates HTLV-I and decreases the concentration of CMV but does not destroy most other viruses or bacteria. Microbiologic quality standards for fresh, unpasteurized, expressed milk are not available. The presence of gram-negative bacteria, S aureus, or α- or β-hemolytic streptococci may preclude use of the milk.

Antimicrobial Agents in Human Milk

Antimicrobial agents taken by a lactating mother often appear in her milk. As a general guideline, an antimicrobial agent is safe to administer to a lactating woman if it is safe to administer to an infant. The American Academy of Pediatrics (AAP) Committee on Drugs has reviewed the risks to infants of specific antimicrobial agents taken by lactating mothers.* Recommendations are included in Table 2.6 (p 122). Although important exceptions exist, most antimicrobial agents that might be taken by lactating mothers are compatible with breastfeeding. When treatment with metronidazole is indicated for a lactating mother, the infant's exposure can be minimized by alteration of the dosing schedule and temporary interruption of breastfeeding. For example, for treatment of *Trichomonas vaginalis* infection, a single 2-g dose of metronidazole may be taken by the lactating mother. She then should pump and discard her milk for 12 to 24 hours to allow excretion of the antimicrobial agent and its metabolites and then resume breastfeeding. The alternative is a 10-day course of metronidazole with cessation of breastfeeding during that time. Women receiving chloramphenicol should not breastfeed because of the theoretic risk of idiosyncratic or dose-related bone marrow suppression in the breastfeeding infant.

---

* American Academy of Pediatrics, Committee on Drugs. The transfer of drugs and other chemicals into human milk. *Pediatrics.* 2001;108:776–789

Table 2.6. Antimicrobial Agents Taken by Mothers That May Be Cause for Concern During Breastfeeding

Maternal Antimicrobial Agent	Reported Sign or Symptom in Infant or Possible Cause for Concern	AAP Committee on Drugs Evaluation
Chloramphenicol	Possible idiosyncratic bone marrow suppression	Unknown effect on breastfeeding infant but may be of concern
Metronidazole	In vitro mutagen	Unknown effect on breastfeeding infant but may be of concern; may discontinue breastfeeding for 12–24 h to allow excretion of dose when single-dose therapy is given to mother
Fluoroquinolones	None for ciprofloxacin or ofloxacin	Data not available for other fluoroquinolones
Isoniazid	None; acetyl metabolite secreted, but no hepato-toxicity reported in infants	Usually compatible with breastfeeding; some experts would give infant pyridoxine hydrochloride
Nalidixic acid	Hemolysis in infant with G6PD deficiency	Usually compatible with breastfeeding
Nitrofurantoin	Hemolysis in infant with G6PD deficiency	Usually compatible with breastfeeding
Sulfonamides	Caution in infant with jaundice or G6PD deficiency and in ill, stressed, or premature infant	Usually compatible with breastfeeding
Tinidazole	See metronidazole	Not licensed by FDA in the United States

AAP indicates American Academy of Pediatrics; G6PD, glucose-6-phosphate dehydrogenase; FDA, Food and Drug Administration.

The AAP Committee on Drugs considers maternal use of isoniazid to be compatible with breastfeeding. Although potential hepatotoxic effects in breastfeeding infants are a concern, no adverse effects have been documented. Some experts recommend that the infant receive pyridoxine hydrochloride (see Tuberculosis, p 642). The use of ciprofloxacin and ofloxacin by the lactating mother is reported by the Committee on Drugs to be safe for her breastfeeding infant. Data are not available on other fluoroquinolones.

Maternal use of doxycycline or other tetracyclines may be compatible with breastfeeding, because absorption of the drugs by the breastfeeding infant is negligible. Some experts recommend that use of tetracycline or doxycycline by a lactating mother be avoided, if possible, because of the potential for staining of the infant's unerupted teeth.

The amount of drug an infant receives from a lactating mother depends on a number of factors, including maternal dose, frequency and duration of administration, absorption, and distribution characteristics of the drug. When a lactating woman receives appropriate doses of an antimicrobial agent, the concentration of the compound in her milk usually is less than the equivalent of a therapeutic dose for the infant. A breastfed infant who requires antimicrobial therapy should receive the recommended doses, even if the same agent is administered to the mother.

Characteristics of the breastfeeding infant should be considered when assessing the potential effect of specific antimicrobial agents taken by the mother. The infant's maturity at birth, postpartum age, and clinical status and the pattern of breastfeeding will alter the possible risks to the infant. If an infant has glucose-6-phosphate dehydrogenase deficiency, maternal use of nalidixic acid, nitrofurantoin, or sulfonamides should be avoided (see Table 2.6, p 122). With premature, jaundiced, stressed, or ill infants, maternal use of sulfonamide compounds should be avoided. In addition, pharmacokinetic properties of the antimicrobial agent may be helpful for determining the safety of a new agent for which appearance in milk is unknown. If the drug is not bioavailable orally (ie, it must be given parenterally), it will not be absorbed from milk by the infant.

Another consideration is the potential for interaction between drugs the mother is receiving and drugs her infant is receiving. Hence, physicians caring for infants who are breastfeeding should be aware of the medications the mother is taking and their potential for adverse interaction with drugs being administered to the infant. When making the decision about use of antimicrobial agents for a lactating woman, the physician should weigh benefits of breastfeeding against the potential risk to the breastfeeding infant of exposure to a drug. In most cases, the benefits exceed the risks. The circumstance would be rare in which the only effective medication for treatment of maternal infection would be contraindicated because of risks to the infant.

CHILDREN IN OUT-OF-HOME CHILD CARE*

Infants and young children who are cared for in group settings have an increased rate of certain infectious diseases and an increased risk of acquiring antimicrobial-resistant organisms. Prevention and control of infection in out-of-home child care settings is influenced by several factors, including the following: (1) caregivers' practice of personal hygiene and immunization status; (2) environmental sanitation; (3) food handling procedures; (4) ages and immunization statuses of children; (5) the ratio of children to caregivers; (6) the physical space and quality of the facilities; and (7) frequency of use of antimicrobial agents in children in child care. Adequately addressing problems of infection control in child care settings requires

* This chapter is modified from American Academy of Pediatrics, American Public Health Association, and Maternal and Child Health Bureau. *Caring for Our Children. National Health and Safety Performance Standards: Guidelines for Out-of-Home Child Care Programs.* 2nd ed. Elk Grove Village, IL: American Academy of Pediatrics; 2002.

collaborative efforts of public health officials, licensing agencies, child care providers, physicians, nurses, parents, employers, and other members of the community.

Child care programs should require that all children and staff members receive age-appropriate immunizations and routine health care. In addition, these programs have the opportunity to provide young, inexperienced parents with day-to-day instruction in child development, hygiene, appropriate nutrition, and management of minor illnesses.

Classification of Care Service

Child care services commonly are classified by the type of setting, number of children in care, and ages and health statuses of the children. **Small family child care homes** provide care and education for up to 6 children at a time, including any preschool children of the care provider, in a residence that usually is the home of the care provider. **Large family child care homes** provide care and education for between 7 and 12 children at a time, including any preschool children of the care provider, in a residence that is usually the home of one of the care providers. A **child care center** is a facility that provides care and education to any number of children in a nonresidential setting, or 13 or more children in any setting if the facility is open on a regular basis. A **facility for ill children** provides care for 1 or more children who temporarily are excluded from their regular child care setting. All 50 states license out-of-home child care; however, licensing is directed toward center-based child care; few states or municipalities license small or large family child care homes.

Grouping of children by age varies, but in child care centers, common groups consist of **infants** (birth–12 months of age), **toddlers** (13–35 months of age), **preschoolers** (36–59 months of age), and **school-aged children** (5–12 years of age).

Infants and toddlers require diapering or assistance in using a toilet, explore the environment with their mouths, have poor control over their secretions and excretions, have immunity to fewer common pathogens, and require hands-on contact with care providers. In addition, toddlers have frequent direct contact with other toddlers. Therefore, child care programs that provide infant and toddler care need to give special attention to infection control measures.

Management and Prevention of Illness

The modes of transmission of bacteria, viruses, parasites, and fungi within child care settings are listed in Table 2.7 (p 125). In most instances, the risk of introducing an infectious agent into a child care group is related directly to prevalence of the agent in the population and to the number of susceptible children in that group. Transmission of an agent within the group depends on the following: (1) characteristics of the organism, such as mode of spread, infective dose, and survival in the environment; (2) frequency of asymptomatic infection or carrier state; and (3) immunity to the respective pathogen. Transmission also can be affected by behaviors of the child care providers, particularly hygienic aspects of child handling; by environmental sanitation practices; and by ages and immunization statuses of the children enrolled. Appropriate hand hygiene is the most important factor for decreasing transmission of disease in child care settings. Children infected in a child

Table 2.7. Modes of Transmission of Organisms in Child Care Settings

Usual Route of Transmission[1]	Bacteria	Viruses	Other[2]
Fecal-oral	Campylobacter organisms, Clostridium difficile, Escherichia coli O157:H7, Salmonella organisms, Shigella organisms	Astrovirus, calicivirus, enteric adenovirus, enteroviruses, hepatitis A virus, rotaviruses	Cryptosporidium parvum, Enterobius vermicularis, Giardia lamblia
Respiratory	Bordetella pertussis, Haemophilus influenzae type b, Mycobacterium tuberculosis, Neisseria meningitidis, Streptococcus pneumoniae, group A streptococcus	Adenovirus, influenza virus, measles virus, mumps virus, parainfluenza virus, parvovirus B19, respiratory syncytial virus, rhinovirus, rubella virus, varicella-zoster virus	…
Person-to-person contact	Group A streptococcus, Staphylococcus aureus	Herpes simplex virus, varicella-zoster virus	Agents causing pediculosis, scabies, and ringworm
Contact with blood, urine, and/or saliva	…	Cytomegalovirus, herpes simplex virus	…
Bloodborne	…	Hepatitis B virus	…

[1] The potential for transmission of microorganisms in the child care setting by food and animals also exists (see Appendix VI, Clinical Syndromes Associated With Foodborne Diseases, p 810, and Appendix VIII, Diseases Transmitted by Animals, p 817).

[2] Parasites, fungi, mites, and lice.

care group subsequently can transmit organisms not only within the group but also within their households and the community.

Major options for management of ill or infected children in child care and for controlling spread of infection include the following: (1) antimicrobial treatment or prophylaxis; (2) immunization when appropriate; (3) exclusion of ill or infected children from the facility; (4) provision of alternative care at a separate site; (5) cohorting to provide care (eg, segregation of infected children in a group with separate staff and facilities); (6) limiting new admissions; and (7) closing the facility (a rarely exercised option). Recommendations for controlling the spread of specific infectious agents differ according to the epidemiology of the pathogen (see disease-specific chapters in Section 3) and nature of the setting.

Certain general and disease-specific infection control procedures in child care programs decrease acquisition and transmission of communicable diseases within and outside the programs. Among these procedures are the following: (1) periodic review of center-maintained child and employee illness records, including current immunization status; (2) hygienic and sanitary procedures for toilet use and toilet training; (3) review and enforcement of hand-hygiene procedures; (4) environmental sanitation; (5) personal hygiene for children and staff; (6) sanitary preparation and handling of food; (7) communicable disease surveillance and reporting; and (8) management of pets. Specific staff policies that include training procedures for full- and part-time employees and staff illness exclusion policies also aid in control of infectious diseases. Health departments should have plans for responding to reportable and nonreportable communicable diseases in child care programs and should provide training, written information, and technical consultation to child care programs when requested. Evaluation of the health status of each child should be performed by a trained staff member each day as the child enters the site and throughout the day. Parents should be encouraged to share information with child care staff about their child's acute and chronic illnesses and medication use. Parents should be required to report their child's immunization status on an ongoing basis.

Recommendations for Inclusion or Exclusion

Mild illness is common among children. Most children will not need to be excluded from their usual source of care for mild respiratory tract illnesses, because transmission is likely to have occurred before symptoms developed in the child. Disease may occur as a result of contact with children with asymptomatic infection. The risk of illness can be decreased by following common-sense hygienic practices.

Exclusion of sick children and adults from out-of-home child care settings has been recommended when such exclusion could decrease the likelihood of secondary cases. In many situations, the expertise of the program's medical consultant and that of the responsible local and state public health authorities are helpful for determining the benefits and risks of excluding children from their usual care program. Most states have laws about isolation of people with specific communicable diseases. Local or state health departments should be contacted about these laws, and public health authorities in these areas should be notified about cases of reportable communicable diseases and unusual outbreaks of other illnesses involving children or adults in the child care environment (see Appendix IX, Nationally Notifiable Infectious Diseases in the United States, p 822).

Children should be excluded from the child care setting for the following:

- Illness that prevents the child from participating comfortably in program activities.
- Illness that results in a need for care that is greater than the staff can provide without compromising the health and safety of other children.
- Any of the following conditions suggesting possible severe illness: fever, lethargy, irritability, persistent crying, difficult breathing, or other manifestations of possible severe illness.
- Diarrhea or stools that contain blood or mucus.
- Shiga toxin-producing *Escherichia coli,* including *E coli* O157:H7, or *Shigella* infection, until diarrhea resolves and results of 2 stool cultures are negative for these organisms.
- Vomiting 2 or more times during the previous 24 hours, unless the vomiting is determined to be caused by a noncommunicable condition and the child is not in danger of dehydration.
- Mouth sores associated with drooling, unless the child's physician or local health department authority states that the child is noninfectious.
- Rash with fever or behavioral change, until a physician has determined the illness is not a communicable disease.
- Purulent conjunctivitis (defined as pink or red conjunctiva with white or yellow eye discharge, often with matted eyelids after sleep and eye pain or redness of the eyelids or skin surrounding the eye), until examined by a physician and approved for readmission.
- Tuberculosis, until the child's physician or local health department authority states that the child is noninfectious.
- Impetigo, until 24 hours after treatment has been initiated.
- Streptococcal pharyngitis, until 24 hours after treatment has been initiated.
- Head lice (pediculosis), until after the first treatment.
- Scabies, until after treatment has been given.
- Varicella, until all lesions have dried and crusted (usually 6 days after onset of rash; see Varicella-Zoster Infections, p 672).
- Pertussis, until 5 days of appropriate antimicrobial therapy (which is to be given for a total of 14 days) have been completed (see Pertussis, p 472).
- Mumps, until 9 days after onset of parotid gland swelling.
- Measles, until 4 days after onset of rash.
- Hepatitis A virus (HAV) infection, until 1 week after onset of illness or jaundice (if symptoms are mild).

Most minor illnesses do not constitute a reason for excluding a child from child care. Examples of illnesses and conditions that do not necessitate exclusion include the following:

- Nonpurulent conjunctivitis (defined as pink conjunctiva with a clear, watery eye discharge without fever, eye pain, or eyelid redness)
- Rash without fever and without behavioral change
- Parvovirus B19 infection in an immunocompetent host
- Cytomegalovirus (CMV) infection

- Chronic hepatitis B virus (HBV) infection (see p 132 for possible exceptions)
- Human immunodeficiency virus (HIV) infection (see p 133 for possible exceptions).

Asymptomatic children who excrete an enteropathogen usually do not need to be excluded, except when an infection with shiga toxin-producing *E coli* or with a *Shigella* species has occurred in the child care program. Because these infections easily are transmitted and can be severe, exclusion is warranted until results of 2 stool cultures are negative for the organism (see *Escherichia coli* Diarrhea, p 275, and *Shigella* Infections, p 551). Local health ordinances may be more stringent with respect to number and timing of specimens.

During the course of an identified outbreak of any communicable illness in a child care setting, a child determined to be contributing to the transmission of the illness at the program may be excluded. The child may be readmitted when the risk of transmission is determined no longer to be present.

Infectious Diseases—Epidemiology and Control

(See also disease-specific chapters in Section 3.)

ENTERIC DISEASES

The close personal contact and poor hygiene of young children provide ready opportunities for spread of enteric bacteria, viruses, and parasites in child care settings. Enteric pathogens transmitted by the person-to-person route, such as rotaviruses, enteric adenoviruses, astroviruses, caliciviruses, *Shigella, E coli* O157:H7, *Giardia lamblia, Cryptosporidium parvum,* and HAV have been the principal organisms implicated in outbreaks. *Salmonella* species, *Clostridium difficile,* and *Campylobacter* species infrequently have been associated with disease in children in child care. Most reptiles carry *Salmonella* organisms, and small reptiles (like turtles) that could be handled by children can transmit *Salmonella* organisms (or other bacteria) to children.

There is an increased frequency of diarrhea and of HAV infection in young children who are not toilet trained. Fecal contamination of the environment is common in child care programs and is highest in infant and toddler areas. Entero-pathogens are spread by the fecal-oral route, either directly by person-to-person transmission or indirectly via fomites, environmental surfaces, and food. The risk of food contamination can be increased when staff members who care for diapered children also prepare or serve food. Several enteric pathogens, including rotaviruses, HAV, *G lamblia* cysts, and *C parvum* oocysts, survive on environmental surfaces for periods ranging from hours to weeks.

Child care programs can be a major source of HAV spread within the community. Hepatitis A virus differs from most other diseases in child care centers, because symptomatic illness occurs primarily among adult contacts of infected asymptomatic children. To recognize outbreaks and initiate appropriate control measures, health care professionals and child care providers need to be aware of this epidemiologic characteristic (see Hepatitis A, p 309). Vaccine for HAV should be considered for the staff of child care centers with ongoing or recurrent outbreaks and in communities where cases in a child care center are a major source of HAV infection.

The single most important procedure to minimize fecal-oral transmission is frequent hand hygiene measures combined with staff training and monitoring of staff procedures. A child in whom acute diarrhea or jaundice develops should be moved to a separate area, away from contact with other children, until the child can be removed by a parent or guardian. Exclusion criteria are provided under Recommendations for Inclusion or Exclusion (p 126).

RESPIRATORY TRACT DISEASES

Organisms spread by the respiratory route include those causing acute upper respiratory tract infections or those associated with invasive diseases, such as *Haemophilus influenzae* type b (Hib), *Streptococcus pneumoniae, Neisseria meningitidis, Bordetella pertussis,* and *Mycobacterium tuberculosis* infections. Possible modes of spread of respiratory tract viruses include aerosols, respiratory droplets, and direct hand contact with contaminated secretions and fomites. The viral pathogens responsible for respiratory tract disease in child care settings are those that cause disease in the community, including respiratory syncytial virus, parainfluenza virus, influenza virus, adenovirus, and rhinovirus. The incidence of viral infections of the respiratory tract is increased in child care settings.

Hand hygiene measures can decrease the incidence of acute respiratory tract disease among children in child care. However, excluding children with respiratory tract symptoms associated with the common cold, croup, bronchitis, pneumonia, sinusitis, or otitis media from child care might not decrease the spread of infection. Children with such conditions may need to be separated from other children in the program and may need to be excluded from the facility (see Recommendations for Inclusion and Exclusion, p 126).

Transmission of Hib may occur among unimmunized young children in group child care settings, especially children younger than 24 months of age. Transmission can originate from an asymptomatic carrier or a carrier with a respiratory tract infection. Appropriate immunization of children with an Hib conjugate vaccine prevents the occurrence of disease and decreases the rate of carriage, thereby decreasing the risk of transmission to others. In an outbreak of invasive Hib disease in child care, rifampin prophylaxis may be indicated for contacts (see *Haemophilus influenzae* Infections, p 293).

Infections caused by *N meningitidis* occur in all age groups. The highest attack rates are in children younger than 1 year of age. Extended close contact between children and staff exposed to an index case of meningococcal disease predisposes to secondary transmission. Because outbreaks may occur in child care settings, chemoprophylaxis is indicated for exposed child care contacts (see Meningococcal Infections, p 430).

The risk of primary invasive disease attributable to *S pneumoniae* among children in child care settings is increased compared with children not in child care settings. Secondary spread of *S pneumoniae* in child care centers has been reported, but the degree of risk of secondary spread in child care facilities is unknown. Prophylaxis for contacts after the occurrence of one or more cases of invasive *S pneumoniae* disease is not recommended. Use of *S pneumoniae* conjugate vaccine should, like use of Hib conjugate vaccine, decrease the incidence of invasive disease and decrease carriage of serotypes of *S pneumoniae* contained in the vaccine.

Group A streptococcal infection among children in child care has not been a common problem. A child with proven group A streptococcal infection should be excluded from classroom contact until 24 hours after initiation of antimicrobial therapy. Although outbreaks of streptococcal pharyngitis in these settings have occurred, the risk of secondary transmission after a single case of mild or even severe invasive group A streptococcal infection remains low. Chemoprophylaxis for contacts after group A streptococcal infection in child care facilities generally is not recommended (see Group A Streptococcal Infections, p 573).

Infants and young children with tuberculosis are not as contagious as are adults, because children are less likely to have cavitary pulmonary lesions and are unable to forcefully expel large numbers of organisms into the air. If approved by health officials, children with tuberculosis may attend group child care after chemotherapy is begun and they are considered noninfectious to others. Infants and young children who have both HIV and tuberculosis infections may need to be excluded from group child care. Because an adult with tuberculosis poses a hazard to children in group child care, tuberculin screening with a tuberculin skin test of all adults who have contact with children in a child care setting is recommended before contact is initiated. Adults with both HIV and tuberculosis may not have a reaction to a tuberculin skin test (see Tuberculosis, p 642). The need for periodic subsequent tuberculin testing of people without clinically important reactions should be determined on the basis of their risk of acquiring a new infection and local or state health department recommendations. Care providers found to have tuberculosis should be excluded from the center and should not be allowed to care for children until chemotherapy has rendered them noninfectious (see Tuberculosis, p 642).

OTHER CONDITIONS

Parvovirus B19. Isolation or exclusion of immunocompetent people with parvovirus B19 infection in child care settings is unwarranted, because little or no virus is present in respiratory tract secretions at the time of occurrence of the rash of erythema infectiosum. In addition, because fewer than 1% of pregnant teachers during erythema infectiosum outbreaks would be expected to experience an adverse fetal outcome, exclusion of pregnant women from employment in child care or teaching is not recommended (see Parvovirus B19, p 459).

Varicella-Zoster Virus. Children with varicella who have been excluded from child care may return after all lesions have dried and crusted, which usually occurs on the sixth day after onset of rash. All staff members and parents should be notified when a case of varicella occurs; they should be informed about the greater likelihood of serious infection in susceptible adults and adolescents and in susceptible immunocompromised people in addition to the potential for fetal damage if infection occurs during pregnancy. Susceptible adults should be offered varicella vaccine unless contraindicated. Susceptible child care staff members who are pregnant and exposed to children with varicella should be referred promptly to a qualified physician or other professional for counseling and management, including potential use of Varicella-Zoster Immune Globulin. The Centers for Disease Control and Prevention (CDC) and the American Academy of Pediatrics recommend the use of varicella vaccine in nonpregnant immunocompetent susceptible people within 72 hours after exposure to varicella (see Varicella-Zoster, p 672).

The decision to exclude staff members or children with herpes zoster infection (shingles) whose lesions cannot be covered should be made on the basis of criteria similar to those for varicella. Herpes zoster lesions that can be covered pose little risk to susceptible people, because transmission usually occurs as a result of direct contact with fluid from lesions.

Herpes Simplex Virus. Children with herpes simplex virus (HSV) gingivostomatitis who do not have control of oral secretions (drooling) should be excluded from child care when active lesions are present. Although HSV can be transmitted from a mother to her fetus or newborn infant, maternal HSV infections that are a threat to offspring usually are acquired by the infant during birth from genital tract infections of the mother; therefore, exposure of a pregnant woman to HSV in a child care setting carries little risk for her fetus. Care providers should be educated on the importance of hand hygiene and other measures for limiting transfer of infected material from children with varicella-zoster virus or HSV infection (eg, saliva, tissue fluid, or fluid from a skin lesion).

Cytomegalovirus Infection. Spread of CMV from asymptomatic infected children in child care to their mothers or to child care providers is the most important consequence of child care-related CMV infection (see Cytomegalovirus Infection, p 259). Children enrolled in child care programs are more likely to acquire CMV than are children primarily cared for at home. The highest rates (eg, 70%) of viral excretion occur in children between 1 and 3 years of age, and excretion commonly continues for years. Studies of CMV seroconversion among child care providers have found annualized seroconversion rates of 8% to 20%. Exposure to CMV with the increased rate of acquisition that occurs in child care staff most likely leads to an increased rate of gestational CMV infection in seronegative female staff members and an increased risk of congenital CMV infection in their offspring. Women who are seropositive before pregnancy are not at risk from exposure to children, but seropositive women whose CMV infection reactivates during pregnancy have a small (approximately 1 in 500) risk of having an infant with congenital CMV infection; approximately 5% of infants infected during reactivation exposure have sequelae, which are mild and consist mostly of moderate hearing loss.

Cytomegalovirus excretion is so prevalent, attempts at isolation or segregation of children who excrete CMV are impractical and inappropriate. Similarly, testing of children to detect CMV excretion is inappropriate, because excretion often is intermittent and results of testing can be misleading. In view of the risk of CMV infection in child care staff and the potential consequences of gestational CMV infection, child care staff members should be counseled about the risks. This counseling may include testing for serum antibody to CMV to determine the child care provider's immunity against CMV, but routine serologic testing currently is not recommended.

BLOODBORNE VIRUS INFECTIONS

Hepatitis B virus, HIV, and hepatitis C virus (HCV) are bloodborne pathogens. Although the risk of contact with blood containing one of these viruses is low in the child care setting, appropriate infection control practices will prevent transmission of bloodborne pathogens if exposure occurs.

Hepatitis B Virus. Transmission of HBV in the child care setting has been described but occurs rarely. Because of the low risk of transmission, children known to have chronic HBV infection (hepatitis B surface antigen [HBsAg] positive) may attend child care in most circumstances.

Transmission of HBV in a child care setting is most likely to occur through direct exposure to blood after an injury or from bites or scratches that break the skin and introduce blood or body secretions from an HBV carrier into another person. Indirect transmission through environmental contamination with blood or saliva is possible. This occurrence has not been documented in a child care setting in the United States. Because saliva contains much less virus than does blood, the potential infectivity of saliva is low. Infectivity of saliva has been demonstrated only when inoculated through the skin of gibbons and chimpanzees.

On the basis of limited data, the risk of disease transmission from a child or staff member who has chronic HBV infection but who behaves normally and is without injury, generalized dermatitis, or bleeding problems is minimal. This slight risk usually does not justify exclusion of a child who has chronic HBV infection from child care or the necessity of HBV immunization of the child's contacts at the care program, most of whom already should be protected by previous HBV immunization as part of their routine immunization schedule.

Routine screening of children for HBsAg before admission to child care is not justified. The admission of a child previously identified to have chronic HBV infection with one or more risk factors for transmission of bloodborne pathogens (eg, biting, frequent scratching, generalized dermatitis, or bleeding problems) should be determined by the child's physician, child care provider, or program director. The responsible public health authority should be consulted when appropriate. Regular assessment of behavioral risk factors and medical conditions of enrolled children with chronic HBV infection is necessary and requires that the child care director and primary child care providers are informed about enrollment of a child known to have chronic HBV infection.

Children who bite pose an additional concern. Existing data in humans suggest a small risk of HBV transmission from the bite of a child with chronic HBV infection. For susceptible victims of bites by children with chronic HBV infection, prophylaxis with Hepatitis B Immune Globulin (HBIG) and hepatitis B immunization is recommended (see Hepatitis B, p 318).

The risk of HBV acquisition when a susceptible child bites a child who has chronic HBV infection is unknown. A theoretic risk exists if HBsAg-positive blood enters the oral cavity of the biter, but transmission by this route has not been reported. Most experts would initiate the hepatitis B vaccine series but not give HBIG to a susceptible biting child who does not have oral mucosal disease when the amount of blood transferred is small.

In the common circumstance in which the HBsAg status of both the biting child and the victim is unknown, the risk of HBV transmission is extremely low because of the expected low seroprevalence of HBsAg in most groups of preschool-aged children, the low efficiency of disease transmission from bites, and routine HBV immunization of preschool children. Serologic testing generally is not warranted for the biting child or the recipient of the bite, but each situation should be evaluated individually.

Efforts to decrease the risk of disease transmission in child care through hygienic and environmental standards generally should focus primarily on precautions for blood exposures and limiting potential saliva contamination of the environment. Toothbrushes should not be shared among children. Accidents that lead to bleeding or contamination with blood-containing body fluids by any child should be handled as follows: (1) disposable gloves should be used when cleaning or removing any blood or blood-containing body fluid spills; (2) the area should be disinfected with a freshly prepared solution of a 1:10 dilution of household bleach applied for at least 30 seconds and wiped after the minimum contact time; (3) people involved in cleaning contaminated surfaces should avoid exposure of open skin lesions or mucous membranes to blood or blood-containing body fluids and to wound or tissue exudates; (4) hands should be washed thoroughly after exposure to blood or blood-containing body fluids after gloves are removed; (5) disposable towels or tissues should be used and properly discarded and mops should be rinsed in disinfectant; (6) blood-contaminated paper towels, diapers, and other materials should be placed in a plastic bag with a secure tie for disposal; and (7) staff members should be educated about standard precautions for handling blood or blood-containing material.

HIV Infection (see also Human Immunodeficiency Virus Infection, p 360). Children who enter child care should not be required to be HIV tested or to disclose their HIV status. There is no need to restrict placement of HIV-infected children without risk factors for transmission of bloodborne pathogens in child care facilities to protect other children or staff members in these settings. Because HIV-infected children whose status is unknown may attend child care, standard precautions should be adopted for handling spills of blood and blood-containing body fluids and wound exudates of all children, as described in the preceding HBV section.

The decision to admit known HIV-infected children to child care is best made on an individual basis by qualified people, including the child's physician, who are able to evaluate whether the child will receive optimal care in the program and whether an HIV-infected child poses a significant risk to others. Specifically, admission of each HIV-infected child with one or more potential risk factors for transmission of bloodborne pathogens (eg, biting, frequent scratching, generalized dermatitis, or bleeding problems) should be assessed by the child's physician and the program director. A responsible public health authority should be consulted as appropriate. If a bite results in blood exposure to either individual involved, the US Public Health Service recommends postexposure follow-up, including consideration of postexposure prophylaxis. Information about a child who has immunodeficiency, regardless of cause, should be available to caregivers who need to know how to help protect the child against other infections. For example, immunodeficient children exposed to measles or varicella immediately should receive postexposure immunoprophylaxis (see Measles, p 419, and Varicella-Zoster Infections, p 672).

Available data provide no reason to support the contention that HIV-infected adults will transmit HIV to children during the course of their normal duties. Therefore, HIV-infected adults who do not have open and uncoverable skin lesions, other conditions that would allow contact with their body fluids, or a transmissible infectious disease may care for children in child care programs. However, immunosuppressed adults with HIV infection may be at increased risk of acquiring infectious agents from children and should consult their physician about the safety of continuing to work in child care.

Hepatitis C Virus. The transmission risks of HCV infection in child care settings are unknown. The general risk of HCV infection from percutaneous exposure to infected blood is estimated to be 10 times greater than that of HIV but lower than that of HBV. The risk of transmission of HCV via contamination of mucous membranes or broken skin probably is between the risk of transmission of HIV and the risk of transmission of HBV via contaminated blood. Standard precautions (see Hepatitis B, p 318) should be followed to prevent infection with HCV.

IMMUNIZATIONS

Routine immunization at appropriate ages is important for children in child care, because preschool-aged children can have high age-specific incidence rates of measles, rubella, Hib disease, invasive *S pneumoniae* disease attributable to serotypes contained in the vaccine, varicella, and pertussis.

Written documentation of immunizations appropriate for age should be provided by parents or guardians of all children enrolling in child care. Unless contraindications exist or children have received religious or philosophic exemptions, immunization records should demonstrate immunizations as shown in the Recommended Childhood and Adolescent Immunization Schedule (see Fig 1.1, p 24). Immunization mandates by state for children in child care can be found online (www.immunize.org/laws).

Children who have not received recommended age-appropriate immunizations before enrollment should be immunized as soon as possible, and the series should be completed according to Fig 1.1 (p 24) and Table 1.6 (p 26). In the interim, unimmunized or inadequately immunized children should be allowed to attend child care unless a vaccine-preventable disease to which they may be susceptible occurs in the child care program. These diseases include measles, mumps, rubella, polio, varicella, diphtheria, pertussis, and HAV infection. In such a situation, all underimmunized children should be excluded for the duration of possible exposure or until they have completed their immunizations.

Child care providers should have received all immunizations routinely recommended for adults.* All staff members should have completed a primary series for tetanus and diphtheria (Td), should receive a Td booster every 10 years, and should have been immunized against measles, mumps, rubella, and poliomyelitis according to guidelines for adult immunization of the Advisory Committee on Immunization Practices of the CDC and the American College of Physicians. Child care providers should be immunized against influenza annually. Hepatitis B virus immunization also should be considered, especially for providers who may manage blood spills. All providers should receive written information about hepatitis B disease and its complications as well as means of prevention.

Child care providers should be asked about a history of varicella. Child care providers with a negative or uncertain history of varicella should be immunized or undergo serologic testing for susceptibility; those who are not immune should be

---

* Centers for Disease Control and Prevention. Recommended adult immunization schedule—United States, 2002-2003. *MMWR Morb Mortal Wkly Report.* 2002;51:904–908

offered varicella vaccine, unless it is contraindicated medically. All child care providers should receive written information about varicella, particularly disease manifestations in adults, complications, and means of prevention.

Because HAV can cause symptomatic illness in adult contacts and because child care programs have been a source of infection in the community, HAV vaccine in some circumstances may be justified (see Hepatitis A, p 309). However, because the prevalence of HAV infection does not seem significantly increased in staff members of child care centers in comparison with the prevalence in the general population, routine immunization of staff members is not recommended. During HAV outbreaks, immunization should be considered (see Hepatitis A, p 309).

General Practices

The following practices are recommended to decrease transmission of infectious agents in a child care setting:

- Each child care facility should have **written policies** for managing child and employee illness in child care.
- **Toilet areas and toilet training equipment** should be maintained in sanitary condition.
- **Diaper changing surfaces** should be nonporous and sanitized between uses. Alternatively, the diaper changing surface should be covered with disposable paper pads, which are discarded after each use. If the surface becomes wet or soiled, it should be cleaned and sanitized.
- **Diaper changing procedures** should be posted at the changing area. Soiled disposable diapers and soiled disposable wiping cloths should be discarded in a secure, foot-activated, plastic-lined container. Diapers should contain all urine and stool and minimize fecal contamination of children, providers, environmental surfaces, and objects in the child care program. The 2 types of diapers that should be used are modern disposable paper diapers with absorbent gelling material or carboxymethylcellulose and single-unit reusable systems with an inner cotton lining attached to an outer waterproof covering that are changed as a unit. Clothes should be worn over diapers while the child is in the child care facility. Soiled reusable diapers should be bagged and sent home for laundering.
- **Diaper changing areas** never should be located in food preparation areas and never should be used for temporary placement of food, drinks, or eating utensils.
- The use of **child-sized toilets** or access to steps and modified toilet seats that provide for easier maintenance should be encouraged in child care programs. The use of potty chairs should be discouraged, but if used, potty chairs should be emptied into a toilet, cleaned in a utility sink, and disinfected after each use. Staff members should sanitize potty chairs, flush toilets, and diaper changing areas with a freshly prepared solution of a 1:64 dilution of household bleach (one quarter cup of bleach diluted in 1 gallon of water) applied for 2 minutes, rinsed, and dried.

- **Written procedures for hand hygiene** should be established and enforced.* Hand-washing sinks should be adjacent to all diaper changing and toilet areas. These sinks should be washed and disinfected at least daily and, when soiled, should not be used for food preparation. These sinks should not be used for rinsing soiled clothing or for cleaning potty chairs. Children should have access to height-appropriate sinks, soap dispensers, and disposable paper towels.
- Written **personal hygiene policies** for staff and children are necessary.
- Written **environmental sanitation policies and procedures** should include cleaning and disinfecting floors, covering sandboxes, cleaning and sanitizing play tables, and cleaning and disinfecting spills of blood or body fluids and wound or tissue exudates. In general, routine housekeeping procedures using a freshly prepared solution of commercially available cleaner (eg, detergents, disinfectant-detergents, or chemical germicides) compatible with most surfaces are satisfactory for cleaning spills of vomitus, urine, and feces. For spills of blood or blood-containing body fluids and of wound and tissue exudates, the material should be removed using gloves to avoid contamination of hands, and the area then should be disinfected using a freshly prepared solution of a 1:10 dilution of household bleach applied for 30 seconds and wiped with a disposable cloth after the minimum contact time.
- Each item of **sleep equipment** should be used only by a single child and should be cleaned and sanitized before being assigned to another child. Crib mattresses should be cleaned and sanitized when soiled or wet. Sleeping mats should be stored so contact with the sleeping surface of another mat does not occur. Bedding (sheets and blankets) should be assigned to each child and cleaned and sanitized when soiled or wet.
- Optimally, **toys** that are placed in children's mouths or otherwise contaminated by body secretions should be cleaned with water and detergent, disinfected, and rinsed before handling by another child. All frequently touched toys in rooms that house infants and toddlers should be cleaned and disinfected daily. Toys in rooms for older (nondiapered) children should be cleaned at least weekly and when soiled. The use of soft, nonwashable toys in infant and toddler areas of child care programs should be discouraged.
- **Food** should be handled safely and appropriately to prevent growth of bacteria and to prevent contamination by other enteropathogens, insects, or rodents.† Tables and countertops used for food preparation and food service should be cleaned and sanitized between uses and before and after eating. No one who has signs or symptoms of illness, including vomiting, diarrhea, or infectious skin lesions that cannot be covered, or who is infected with potential foodborne pathogens should be responsible for food handling. Hands should be washed using soap and water before handling food. Because of their frequent exposure to feces and children with enteric diseases, staff members who work with diapered children should not prepare food for others. Caregivers who prepare food for

---

* Centers for Disease Control and Prevention. Guideline for hand hygiene in health-care settings. Recommendations of the Healthcare Infection Control Practices Advisory Committee and the HIC-PAC/SHEA/APIC/IDSA Hand Hygiene Task Force. *MMWR Recomm Rep.* 2002;51(RR-16):1–45
† Centers for Disease Control and Prevention. Diagnosis and management of foodborne illnesses: a primer for physicians. *MMWR Recomm Rep.* 2001;50(RR-2):1–69

infants especially should be aware of the importance of careful hand hygiene. No unpasteurized milk or milk products should be served (see Appendix VII, Potentially Contaminated Food Products, p 814).

- The living quarters of **pets** should be enclosed and kept clean of waste to decrease the risk of human contact with the waste. Hands should be washed after handling all animals or animal wastes. Dogs and cats should be in good health and immunized appropriately for age and should be kept away from child play areas and handled only with staff supervision. Such animals should be given flea, tick, and worm control programs. Reptiles should not be handled by children.
- Written policies that comply with local and state regulations for filing and regularly updating each child's **immunization record** should be maintained.
- Each child care program should use the services of a **health consultant** to assist in development and implementation of written policies for the prevention and control of communicable diseases and the provision of related health education to children, staff, and parents.
- The child care provider should, when registering each child, **inform parents of the need to share information about illnesses** that could be communicable in the child or in any member of the immediate household to facilitate prompt reporting of disease and institution of any measures necessary to prevent transmission to others. The child care provider or program director, after consulting with the program's health consultant or the responsible public health official, should follow recommendations of the consultant or public health official for **notification of parents** of children who attend the program about exposure of their child to a communicable disease.
- Local and/or state **public health authorities should be notified** about cases of communicable diseases involving children or care providers in the child care setting.

SCHOOL HEALTH

Although clustering of children together in the school setting provides opportunities for spread of infectious diseases, school attendance is important for children and adolescents, and unnecessary barriers and impediments to attending school should be minimized. Determining the likelihood that infection in one or more children will pose a risk for schoolmates depends on an understanding of several factors, including the following: (1) the mechanism by which the organism causing the infection is spread; (2) the ease with which the organism is spread (contagion); and (3) the likelihood that classmates are immune because of immunization or previous infection. Decisions to intervene to prevent spread of infection within a school should be made through collaboration among school officials, local public health officials, and health care professionals, considering the availability and effectiveness of specific methods of prevention and the risk of serious complications from infection.

Infectious agents are spread through one or more of the following routes of transmission: fecal-oral; respiratory; contact with infected skin; and contact with blood, urine, or body secretions. In the school setting, respiratory tract secretions and skin contact provide the most common means of transmission of microorganisms. In the care of preschool children in out-of-home child care (see Children in Out-of-Home Child Care, p 123) and older children with health problems or developmental disabilities, transmission via the fecal-oral route and through contact with urine also is an important consideration. Specific circumstances, such as care of bleeding injuries or intimate contact between classmates, provide an opportunity for spread via blood and other body fluids.

Generic methods for control and prevention of spread of infection in the school setting include the following:

- For vaccine-preventable diseases, documentation of the immunization status of enrolled children should be reviewed. Schools have a legal responsibility to ensure that students have been immunized against vaccine-preventable diseases at the time of enrollment, in accordance with state requirements (see Appendix V, State Immunization Requirements for School Attendance, p 809). Although specific diseases vary by state, most states require proof of protection against poliomyelitis, tetanus, pertussis, diphtheria, measles, mumps, and rubella. Hepatitis B immunization and immunization against varicella, available since 1995, now is mandatory in many states (www.immunize.org/laws or www.cdc.gov/other.htm#states). Hepatitis A virus (HAV) immunization is required for school entry in some states. The Centers for Disease Control and Prevention recommends that all states require that children entering elementary school have received varicella vaccine or have other evidence of immunity to varicella. Policies established by a state health department about exclusions of unimmunized children and exemptions for children with certain underlying medical conditions and families with religious or philosophic objection to immunization should be followed.
- Infected children should be excluded from school until they no longer are considered contagious (for recommendations on specific diseases, see relevant disease-specific chapters in Section 3).
- In many instances, administration of appropriate antimicrobial therapy will limit further spread of infection (eg, streptococcal pharyngitis and pertussis).
- Antimicrobial prophylaxis given to close contacts of children with infections caused by specific pathogens may be warranted in some circumstances (eg, meningococcal infection).
- Temporary school closing can be used in several circumstances: (1) to prevent spread of infection; (2) when an infection is expected to affect a large number of susceptible students and available control measures are considered inadequate (eg, outbreak of influenza); or (3) when an infection is expected to have a high rate of morbidity or mortality.

Physicians involved with school health should be aware of current public health guidelines to prevent and control infectious diseases. In all circumstances requiring intervention to prevent spread of infection within the school setting, the privacy of children who are infected should be protected.

Diseases Preventable by Routine Childhood Immunization

Students who have received 1 dose of varicella vaccine (2 doses for children immunized past their 13th birthday) and 2 doses of measles-mumps-rubella (MMR) vaccine should be considered immune to these diseases. Students with a history of physician-documented infection or serologic evidence of immunity also are considered immune.

Measles and varicella vaccines have been demonstrated to provide protection in some susceptible people if administered within 72 hours after exposure. Measles or varicella immunization should be recommended immediately for all nonimmune people during a measles or varicella outbreak, respectively, except for people with a contraindication to immunization. Students immunized for measles or varicella for the first time under these circumstances should be allowed to return to school immediately.

Mumps vaccine given after exposure has not been demonstrated to prevent infection among susceptible contacts, but immunization should be administered to unimmunized students to protect them from infection from subsequent exposure.

Although rubella infection usually does not pose a major risk to preadolescent school-aged children, the immunization status of contacts should be reviewed, and documentation of rubella immunization should be required for previously unimmunized students. Pregnant contacts who have serologically confirmed immunity against rubella early in pregnancy can be reassured that they are sufficiently protected. Physician consultation should be recommended for susceptible pregnant women who are exposed to rubella (see Rubella, p 536).

Other Infections Spread by the Respiratory Route

Some pathogens that cause severe lower respiratory tract disease in infants and toddlers, such as respiratory syncytial virus, are of less concern in healthy school-aged children. Respiratory tract viruses, however, are associated with exacerbations of reactive airway disease and an increase in the incidence of otitis media and can cause significant complications for children with chronic respiratory tract disease, such as cystic fibrosis, or for children who are immunocompromised.

Although influenza virus infection is a common cause of febrile respiratory tract disease and school absenteeism, mandatory exclusion of children with suspected influenza infection from school is not warranted. Annual influenza immunizations should be given to targeted high-risk groups (see Influenza Vaccine, p 382). Influenza immunization also may be indicated for students to prevent disruption of academic or athletic activities, especially children residing in dormitories or in other circumstances in which close contact occurs.

Mycoplasma pneumoniae causes upper and lower respiratory tract infection in school-aged children, and outbreaks of *M pneumoniae* infection occur in communities and schools. The nonspecific symptoms and signs of this infection and the lack of a rapid diagnostic test make distinguishing M pneumoniae infection from other causes of respiratory tract illness difficult. Antimicrobial therapy does not eradicate the organism or prevent spread necessarily. Thus, intervention to prevent secondary infection in the school setting is difficult.

Symptomatic contacts of students with pharyngitis attributable to group A streptococcal infection should be evaluated and treated if streptococcal infection is demonstrated. Infected students may return to school 24 hours after initiation of antimicrobial therapy. Students awaiting results of culture or antigen detection tests who are not receiving antimicrobial therapy may attend school during the culture incubation period unless there is an associated fever or the infection involves a young child with poor hygiene and poor control of secretions. Asymptomatic contacts usually require neither evaluation nor therapy.

Bacterial meningitis in school-aged children usually is caused by *Neisseria meningitidis*. Infected people are not considered contagious after 24 hours of appropriate antimicrobial therapy. After discharge from the hospital, they pose no risk to classmates and may return to school. Prophylactic antimicrobial therapy is not recommended for school contacts in most circumstances. Close observation of contacts is recommended, and they should be evaluated promptly if a febrile illness develops. Students who have been exposed to oral secretions of an infected student, such as occurs as a result of kissing or sharing of food and drink, should receive chemoprophylaxis (see Meningococcal Infections, p 430). Immunization of school contacts with meningococcal vaccine, which contains polysaccharide antigens for serogroups A, C, Y, and W-135, should be considered, in consultation with local public health authorities, if evidence suggests an outbreak within a school attributable to one of the meningococcal serogroups contained in the vaccine.

Students and staff with documented pertussis should be excluded until they have received 5 days of erythromycin therapy. In some circumstances, chemoprophylaxis is recommended for their school contacts (see Pertussis, p 472).

Children with tuberculosis generally are not contagious, but students who are in close contact with a child, teacher, or other adult with tuberculosis should be evaluated for infection, including tuberculin skin testing (see Tuberculosis, p 642). An adolescent or adult with tuberculosis almost always is the source of infection for young children. If an adult source outside the school is identified (eg, parent or grandparent of a student), efforts should be made to determine whether other students have been exposed to the same source and whether they warrant evaluation for infection.

Children with erythema infectiosum should be allowed to attend school, because the period of contagion occurs before a rash is evident. Parvovirus B19 infection poses no risk of significant illness for healthy classmates, although aplastic crisis can develop in infected children with sickle cell disease and other hemoglobinopathies. The relatively low risk of fetal damage should be explained to pregnant students and teachers exposed to children in the early stages of parvovirus B19 infection, 5 to 10 days before appearance of the rash. These exposed women should be referred to their physician for counseling and possible serologic testing.

Infections Spread by Direct Contact

Infection and infestation of skin, eyes, and hair can spread through direct contact with the infected area or through contact with contaminated hands or fomites, such as hair brushes, hats, and clothing. *Staphylococcus aureus* and group A streptococcal organisms may colonize the skin or the oropharynx of asymptomatic people. Lesions may develop when these organisms are passed from a person with infected skin to another person. Organisms also can be transmitted to open skin lesions in the same child or to other children. Although most skin infections attributable to *S aureus* and group A streptococcal organisms are minor and require only topical or oral antimicrobial therapy, person-to-person spread should be interrupted by appropriate treatment whenever lesions are recognized. Exclusion of affected children before initiation of therapy is necessary unless the risk of skin contact is low on the basis of location of the lesion and age of the child. Severe and disseminated disease from these pathogens, including toxic shock syndrome and necrotizing fasciitis, occurs rarely.

Herpes simplex virus (HSV) infection of the mouth and skin is common among school-aged children. Infection usually is spread through direct contact with infected lesions. In addition, asymptomatic shedding of virus from oral secretions is common. Infection of the fingers (herpetic whitlow) can occur after direct contact with oral or genital secretions. Cutaneous infection can occur after direct contact with infected lesions or after contact of abraded skin with a contaminated surface, as occurs among wrestlers (herpes gladiatorum) and rugby players (scrum pox). Although asymptomatic shedding of virus from pharyngeal and oral secretions is common, spread of infection requires direct contact with these secretions and, thus, is unlikely to occur during normal school activities. "Cold sore" lesions of herpes labialis identify people with active, and probably recurrent, infection, but no evidence suggests that these students pose any greater risk to their classmates than the unidentified asymptomatic shedders. Herpes simplex virus type 1, the usual cause of oropharyngeal and cutaneous lesions, will infect most people by adulthood. Most of these infections are asymptomatic, and although sometimes painful, even symptomatic infection poses virtually no risk of serious disease to a healthy school-aged child. All children should be advised to avoid direct or indirect (eg, sharing cups and bottles) oral contact with other children and to wash their hands, but excluding symptomatic children with HSV infection from normal school activities is not justified. Exclusion of students with obvious skin or oral lesions from wrestling or rugby and careful cleaning of wrestling mats after use with a freshly prepared solution of a 1:64 dilution of household bleach (one quarter cup of bleach diluted in 1 gallon of water) for a minimum of 30 seconds is reasonable. The bleach solution may be wiped off after the minimum contact time or allowed to air dry.

For immunocompromised children and for children with open skin lesions (eg, severe eczema), HSV infection may pose significant risk. Because of the frequency of symptomatic and asymptomatic shedding of HSV among classmates and staff members, careful hygienic practices are the best means of preventing infection.

Infectious conjunctivitis can be caused by bacterial (eg, nontypeable *Haemophilus influenzae* and *Streptococcus pneumoniae*) or viral (eg, adenoviruses, enteroviruses, HSV) pathogens. Bacterial conjunctivitis is less common in children older than 5 years of age. Infection occurs through direct contact or through contamination of hands followed by autoinoculation. Respiratory tract spread from large droplets also may occur. Topical antimicrobial therapy is indicated for bacterial conjunctivitis, which usually is distinguished by a purulent exudate. Herpes simplex virus conjunctivitis usually is unilateral and may be accompanied by vesicles on adjacent skin. Evaluation of HSV conjunctivitis by an ophthalmologist and administration of specific antiviral therapy are indicated. Conjunctivitis attributable to adenoviruses or enteroviruses is self-limited and requires no specific antiviral therapy. Spread of infection is minimized by careful hand hygiene, and infected people should be presumed contagious until symptoms have resolved. Except when viral or bacterial conjunctivitis is accompanied by systemic signs of illness, infected children should be allowed to remain in school once any indicated therapy is implemented, unless their behavior is such that close contact with other students cannot be avoided.

Fungal infections of the skin and hair are spread by direct person-to-person contact and through contact with contaminated surfaces or objects. *Trichophyton tonsurans,* the predominant cause of tinea capitis, remains viable for long periods on combs, hair brushes, furniture, and fabric. The fungi that cause tinea corporis (ringworm) are transmissible by direct contact. Tinea cruris (jock itch) and tinea pedis (athlete's foot) occur in adolescents and young adults. The fungi that cause these infections have a predilection for moist areas and are spread through direct contact and contact with contaminated surfaces. Students with fungal infections of the skin or scalp should be treated for their benefit and to prevent spread of infection. Spread of infection by students with tinea capitis may be decreased by use of selenium sulfide shampoos, but treatment requires systemic antifungal therapy (see Tinea Capitis, p 617). Students with tinea capitis who receive treatment may attend school and participate in their usual activities. Children who fail to obtain treatment do not need to be excluded unless the nature of their contact with other students could potentiate spread. Students with tinea cruris, tinea corporis, or tinea pedis should not be excluded from school even before initiation of therapy. Students with tinea capitis should be instructed not to share combs, hair brushes, hats, or hair ornaments with classmates until they have been treated. Students with tinea pedis should be excluded from swimming pools and from walking barefoot on locker room and shower floors until treatment has been initiated.

Sarcoptes scabiei (scabies) and *Pediculus capitis* (head lice) are transmitted primarily through person-to-person contact. Combs, hair brushes, hats, and hair ornaments can transmit head lice, but away from the scalp, lice do not remain viable. Shampooing with an appropriate pediculocide and manually removing nits by combing usually are effective in eradicating viable lice. Manual removal of nits after treatment with a pediculicide is not necessary to prevent reinfestation (see Pediculosis Capitis, p 463).

Scabies can be transmitted via clothing and bedding to household contacts, but direct skin contact is the predominant means of transmission in the school setting. The parasite survives on clothing for only 3 to 4 days without skin contact. Caregivers who have prolonged skin-to-skin contact with infested students during the school day because of students' physical or mental disabilities may benefit from prophylactic treatment (see Scabies, p 547).

Children identified as having scabies or head lice should be excluded from school only until treatment has been started. School contacts generally should not be treated prophylactically.

Infections Spread by the Fecal-Oral Route

For developmentally typical school-aged children, pathogens spread via the fecal-oral route constitute a risk only if the infected person fails to maintain good hygiene, including after toilet use, or if contaminated food is shared between or among schoolmates.

Outbreaks attributable to HAV can occur in schools, but these outbreaks usually are associated with community outbreaks. Schoolroom exposure generally does not pose an appreciable risk of infection, and Immune Globulin (IG) administration is not indicated. However, if transmission within a school is documented, IG could be used to limit spread (see Hepatitis A, p 309). Alternatively, HAV vaccine should be considered as a means of prophylaxis and prolonged protection. If an outbreak occurs, consultation with local public health authorities is indicated before initiating interventions.

Enteroviral infections probably are spread via the oral-oral route as well as by the fecal-oral route. The attack rate is so high during summer and fall epidemics that control measures specifically aimed at the school classroom likely would be futile. Person-to-person spread of bacterial, viral, and parasitic enteropathogens within school settings occurs infrequently, but foodborne outbreaks attributable to enteric pathogens can occur. Symptomatic people with gastroenteritis attributable to an enteric pathogen should be excluded until symptoms resolve.

Children in diapers at any age and in any setting constitute a far greater risk for spread of gastrointestinal tract infection attributable to enteric pathogens. Guidelines for control of these infections in child care settings should be applied for developmentally disabled school-aged students in diapers (see Children in Out-of-Home Child Care, p 123).

Infections Spread by Blood and Body Fluids*

Contact with blood and other body fluids of another person requires more intimate exposure than usually occurs in the school setting. The care required for developmentally disabled children, however, may result in exposure of caregivers to urine, saliva, and in some cases, blood. The application of Standard Precautions for prevention of transmission of bloodborne pathogens, as recommended for children in out-of-home child care, prevents spread of infection from these exposures (see Children in Out-of-Home Child Care, p 123). School staff members who routinely provide acute care for children with epistaxis or bleeding from injury should wear disposable gloves and use appropriate hand hygiene measures immediately after glove removal to protect themselves from bloodborne pathogens. Staff members at the scene of an injury or bleeding incident who do not have access to gloves need to use some type of barrier to avoid exposure to blood or blood-containing materials, use appropriate hand hygiene measures, and adhere to proper protocols for handling contaminated material. Routine use of these precautions helps avoid the necessity of identifying children known to be infected with human immunodeficiency virus (HIV), hepatitis

---

* See also American Academy of Pediatrics, Committee on Pediatric AIDS and Committee on Infectious Diseases. Issues related to human immunodeficiency virus transmission in schools, child care, medical settings, the home, and community. *Pediatrics.* 1999;104:318–324

B virus (HBV), or hepatitis C virus (HCV) and acknowledges that unrecognized exposure poses at least as much risk as does exposure from an identified infected child.

During adolescence, the likelihood of infection attributable to HBV, HIV, and other sexually transmitted diseases (STDs) increases in proportion to sexual activity. All children should be immunized against HBV before 13 years of age, and adolescents should be instructed in appropriate methods of prevention of STDs.

Students infected with HIV, HBV, or HCV do not need to be identified to school personnel. Because HIV-, HBV-, and HCV-infected children and adolescents will not be identified, policies and procedures to manage potential exposures to blood or blood-containing materials should be established and implemented. Parents and students should be educated about the types of exposure that present a risk for school contacts. Although a student's right to privacy should be maintained, decisions about activities at school should be made by parents or guardians together with a physician on a case-by-case basis, keeping the health needs of the infected student and the student's classmates in mind.

Prospective studies to aid in determining the risk of transmission of HIV, HBV, or HCV during contact sports among high school students have not been performed, but the available evidence indicates that the risk is low. Guidelines for management of bleeding injuries have been developed for college and professional athletes in recognition of the possibility of unidentified HIV, HBV, or HCV infection in any competitor. Recommendations developed by the American Academy of Pediatrics (AAP) for prevention of transmission of HIV and other bloodborne pathogens in the athletic setting were issued in 1999.*

- Athletes infected with HIV, HBV, or HCV should be allowed to participate in all competitive sports.
- The physician should respect the right of infected athletes to confidentiality. This includes not disclosing the patient's infection status to other participants or the staff of athletic programs.
- Testing for bloodborne pathogens should not be mandatory for athletes or sports participants.
- Pediatricians are encouraged to counsel athletes who are infected with HIV, HBV, or HCV and assure them that they have a low risk of infecting other competitors. Infected athletes can consider choosing a sport in which this risk is relatively low. This may be protective for other participants and for infected athletes themselves, decreasing their possible exposure to bloodborne pathogens other than the one(s) with which they are infected. Wrestling and boxing probably have the greatest potential for contamination of injured skin by blood. The AAP opposes boxing as a sport for youth for other reasons.
- Athletic programs should inform athletes and their parents that the program is operating under the policies of the aforementioned recommendations and that the athletes have a low risk of becoming infected with a bloodborne pathogen.

* American Academy of Pediatrics, Committee on Sports Medicine and Fitness. Human immuno-deficiency virus and other blood-borne viral pathogens in the athletic setting. *Pediatrics.* 1999; 104:1400–1403

- Clinicians and staff of athletic programs aggressively should promote HBV immunization among all athletes and among coaches, athletic trainers, equipment handlers, laundry personnel, and any other people at risk of exposure to athletes' blood as an occupational hazard.
- Each coach and athletic trainer must receive training in first aid and emergency care and in prevention of transmission of bloodborne pathogens in the athletic setting. These staff members then can help implement these recommendations.
- Coaches and members of the health care team should educate athletes about the precautions described in these recommendations. Such education should include the greater risks of transmission of HIV and other bloodborne pathogens through sexual activity and needle sharing during the use of injection drugs, including anabolic steroids. Athletes should be told not to share personal items, such as razors, toothbrushes, and nail clippers, that might be contaminated with blood.
- Depending on law in some states, schools may need to comply with Occupational Safety and Health Administration (OSHA) regulations* for prevention of blood-borne pathogens. The athletic program must determine what rules apply. Compliance with OSHA regulations is a reasonable and recommended precaution even if this is not required specifically by the state.
- The following precautions should be adopted in sports with direct body contact and other sports in which an athlete's blood or other body fluids visibly tinged with blood may contaminate the skin or mucous membranes of other participants or staff members of the athletic program. Even if these precautions are adopted, the risk that a participant or staff member may become infected with a blood-borne pathogen in the athletic setting will not be eliminated entirely.
  - Athletes must cover existing cuts, abrasions, wounds, or other areas of broken skin with an occlusive dressing before and during participation. Caregivers should cover their own damaged skin to prevent transmission of infection to or from an injured athlete.
  - Disposable, water-impervious vinyl or latex gloves should be worn to avoid contact with blood or other body fluids visibly tinged with blood and any objects, such as equipment, bandages, or uniforms, contaminated with these fluids. Hands should be cleaned with soap and water or an alcohol-based antiseptic agent as soon as possible after gloves are removed.
  - Athletes with active bleeding should be removed from competition as soon as possible and bleeding should be stopped. Wounds should be cleaned with soap and water. Skin antiseptic agents may be used if soap and water are not available. Wounds must be covered with an occlusive dressing that will remain intact during further play before athletes return to competition.
  - Athletes should be advised to report injuries and wounds in a timely fashion before or during competition.

---

* American Academy of Pediatrics. *OSHA: Materials to Assist the Pediatric Office in Implementing the Bloodborne Pathogen, Hazard Communication, and Other OSHA Standards.* Elk Grove Village, IL: American Academy of Pediatrics; 1994

- Minor cuts or abrasions that are not bleeding do not require interruption of play but can be cleaned and covered during scheduled breaks. During these breaks, if an athlete's equipment or uniform fabric is wet with blood, the equipment should be cleaned and disinfected (see next bullet), or the uniform should be replaced.
- Equipment and playing areas contaminated with blood must be cleaned until all visible blood is gone and then disinfected with an appropriate germicide, such as a freshly made bleach solution containing 1 part bleach in 10 parts of water. The decontaminated equipment or area should be in contact with the bleach solution for at least 30 seconds. The area then may be wiped with a disposable cloth after the minimum contact time or allowed to air dry.
- Emergency care must not be delayed because gloves or other protective equipment is not available. If the caregiver does not have appropriate protective equipment, a towel may be used to cover the wound until an off-the-field location is reached where gloves can be used during more definitive treatment.
- Breathing bags (eg, Ambu manual resuscitators [Ambu Inc, Linthicum, MD]) and oropharyngeal airways should be available for giving resuscitation. Mouth-to-mouth resuscitation is recommended only if this equipment is not available.
- Equipment handlers, laundry personnel, and janitorial staff must be educated in proper procedures for handling washable or disposable materials contaminated with blood.

INFECTION CONTROL FOR HOSPITALIZED CHILDREN

Isolation Precautions

Health care-associated infections are a major cause of morbidity and mortality in hospitalized children, particularly children in intensive care units. Hand hygiene before and after each patient contact remains the single most important practice in the prevention and control of health care-associated infections. Additional policies and procedures are required to prevent infection in critically ill pediatric patients. A comprehensive set of guidelines for preventing and controlling health care-associated infections, including isolation precautions, personnel health recommendations, and guidelines for the prevention of postoperative and device-related infections, can be found on the Center for Disease Control and Prevention (CDC) Web site (www.cdc.gov/ncidod/hip/guide/guide.htm). Additional guidelines are available from the principal infection control societies in the United States, the Society for Healthcare Epidemiology of America and the Association for Professionals in Infection Control and Epidemiology, and specialty societies and regulatory agencies, such as the Occupational Safety and Health Administration. The Joint Commission on Accreditation of Healthcare Organizations has established infection control standards. Physicians and infection control professionals should be familiar with this increasingly complex array of guidelines, regulations, and standards.

In 1996, the Hospital Infection Control Practices Advisory Committee (HICPAC) issued isolation guidelines for the care of hospitalized patients.* These guidelines recommend strategies to prevent the spread of pathogens among hospitalized patients. These isolation policies, supplemented by hospital policies and procedures for other aspects of infection and environmental control and occupational health, should result in policies that are "possible, practical, and prudent" for each hospital.

Routine and optimal performance of an expanded set of universal practices, designated **Standard Precautions,** is designed for the care of all patients regardless of their diagnosis or presumed infection status. Pathogen- and syndrome-based precautions, designated **Transmission-Based Precautions,** are used when caring for patients who are infected or colonized with pathogens spread by the airborne, droplet, or contact routes. To determine which diseases are reportable, see Appendix IX (Nationally Notifiable Infectious Diseases in the United States, p 822).

STANDARD PRECAUTIONS

These precautions are used for contact with blood; all body fluids, secretions, and excretions except sweat (regardless of whether these fluids, secretions, or excretions contain visible blood); nonintact skin; and mucous membranes. Barrier techniques are designed to decrease exposure of health care personnel to body fluids containing human immunodeficiency virus or other bloodborne pathogens. Precautions are used at all times, because medical history and examination cannot reliably identify all patients infected with these agents. **Standard Precautions** decrease transmission of microorganisms from patients who are not recognized as harboring potential pathogens, such as antimicrobial-resistant bacteria. Standard Precautions include the following techniques:

- **Hand hygiene**[†] is necessary before all patient contacts and after touching blood, body fluids, secretions, excretions, and contaminated items, whether gloves are worn or not. Hand hygiene should be performed with waterless antiseptic agents or soap and water immediately after removing gloves, between patient contacts, and when otherwise indicated to avoid transfer of microorganisms to other patients and to items in the environment, such as phones, computer keyboards, and medical charts.
- **Gloves** (clean, nonsterile) should be worn when touching blood, body fluids, secretions, excretions, and items contaminated with these fluids. Clean gloves should be used before touching mucous membranes and nonintact skin. Gloves should be changed between tasks and procedures on the same patient after contact with material that may contain a high concentration of microorganisms. Gloves should be removed promptly after use and hand hygiene should be performed before touching noncontaminated items and environmental surfaces and before contact with another patient.

---

* Garner JS. Hospital Infection Control Practices Advisory Committee. Guideline for isolation precautions in hospitals. *Infect Control Hosp Epidemiol.* 1996;17:53–80
† Centers for Disease Control and Prevention. Guideline for hand hygiene in health-care settings. Recommendations of the Healthcare Infection Control Practices Advisory Committee and the HICPAC/SHEA/APIC/IDSA Hand Hygiene Task Force. *MMWR Recomm Rep.* 2002;51(RR-16):1–45

- **Masks, eye protection, and face shields** should be worn to protect mucous membranes of the eyes, nose, and mouth during procedures and patient care activities likely to generate splashes or sprays of blood, body fluids, secretions, or excretions.
- **Nonsterile gowns** that are fluid-resistant will protect skin and prevent soiling of clothing during procedures and patient care activities likely to generate splashes or sprays of blood, body fluids, secretions, or excretions. Soiled gowns should be removed promptly.
- **Patient care equipment** that has been used should be handled in a manner that prevents skin or mucous membrane exposures and contamination of clothing.
- **All used linen** is considered to be contaminated and should be handled, transported, and processed in a manner that prevents skin and mucous membrane exposure and contamination of clothing.
- **Bloodborne pathogen** exposure should be avoided by taking precautions to prevent injuries when using, cleaning, and disposing of needles, scalpels, and other sharp instruments and devices.
- **Mouthpieces, resuscitation bags, and other ventilation devices** should be readily available in all patient care areas and used instead of mouth-to-mouth resuscitation.

TRANSMISSION-BASED PRECAUTIONS

Transmission-Based Precautions are designed for patients documented or suspected to have colonization of or infection with pathogens for which additional precautions beyond **Standard Precautions** are recommended to interrupt transmission. The 3 types of transmission on which these precautions are based are airborne, droplet, and contact.

- **Airborne transmission** occurs by dissemination of airborne droplet nuclei (small-particle residue [≤5 µm in size] of evaporated droplets containing microorganisms that remain suspended in the air for long periods) or dust particles containing the infectious agent or spores. Microorganisms spread by the airborne route can be dispersed widely by air currents and may be inhaled by or deposited on a susceptible host within the same room or a long distance from the source patient, depending on environmental factors. Special air handling and ventilation are required to prevent airborne transmission. Examples of microorganisms transmitted by airborne droplet nuclei are *Mycobacterium tuberculosis*, measles virus, and varicella-zoster virus. Specific recommendations for **Airborne Precautions** are as follows:
  - Provide infected or colonized patients with a private room (if unavailable, consider cohorting patients with the same disease and consult with an infection control professional).
  - Use negative air-pressure ventilation (6–12 air changes per hour), with air externally exhausted or high-efficiency particulate air (HEPA) filtered, if recirculated.
  - If infectious pulmonary tuberculosis is suspected or proven, respiratory protective devices (ie, National Institute for Occupational Safety and Health-certified personally "fitted" and "sealing" respirator, such as the N95 respirator) should be worn while inside the patient's room.

* Susceptible health care personnel should not enter rooms of patients with measles or varicella-zoster virus infections. If susceptible people must enter the room of a patient with measles or varicella, a mask should be worn. People with proven immunity to these viruses need not wear a mask.
* **Droplet transmission** occurs when droplets containing microorganisms generated from an infected person, primarily during coughing, sneezing, or talking and during the performance of certain procedures, such as suctioning and bronchoscopy, are propelled a short distance ($\leq$3 feet) and deposited on the conjunctivae, nasal mucosa, and/or mouth. Because these relatively large droplets do not remain suspended in the air, special air handling and ventilation are not required to prevent droplet transmission. Droplet transmission should not be confused with airborne transmission via droplet nuclei, which are much smaller. Specific recommendations for Droplet Precautions are as follows:
  * Provide the patient with a private room. (If unavailable, consider cohorting patients infected with the same organism. If no private rooms are available and there are no patients who can be cohorted, separation of at least 3 feet between other patients and visitors should be maintained.)
  * Use a mask if within 3 feet of the patient

  Specific illnesses and infections requiring **Droplet Precautions** include the following:
  * Adenovirus
  * Diphtheria (pharyngeal)
  * *Haemophilus influenzae* type b (invasive)
  * Influenza
  * Mumps
  * *Mycoplasma pneumoniae*
  * *Neisseria meningitidis* (invasive)
  * Parvovirus B19 (during the phase of illness before onset of rash in immunocompetent patients; see Parvovirus B19, p 459)
  * Pertussis
  * Plague (pneumonic)
  * Rubella
  * Streptococcal pharyngitis, pneumonia, or scarlet fever
* **Contact Transmission** is the most important and most common route of transmission of health care-associated infections. *Direct-contact* transmission involves a direct body surface-to-body contact and physical transfer of microorganisms between a susceptible host and an infected or colonized person, such as occurs when a health care worker turns a patient, gives a patient a bath, or performs other patient care activities that require direct personal contact. Direct-contact transmission also can occur between 2 patients when one serves as the source of the infectious microorganisms and the other serves as a susceptible host. *Indirect-contact* transmission involves contact of a susceptible host with a contaminated intermediate object, usually inanimate, such as contaminated instruments, needles, dressings, toys, or contaminated hands that are not cleansed

or gloves that are not changed between patients. Specific recommendations for **Contact Precautions** are as follows:

- Provide patient with a private room (if unavailable, cohorting patients is permissible).
- Gloves (clean, nonsterile) should be used at all times.
- Practice hand hygiene after glove removal.
- Use gowns, unless the patient is continent and substantial contact of clothing with patient or environmental surfaces is not anticipated. Gowns should be removed before leaving the patient's room or area.

Specific illnesses and infections with organisms requiring **Contact Precautions** include the following:

- Multidrug-resistant bacteria (eg, vancomycin-resistant enterococci; methicillin-resistant *Staphylococcus aureus;* multidrug-resistant, gram-negative bacilli) judged by the infection control program on the basis of current state, regional, or national recommendations to be of special clinical and epidemiologic significance
- *Clostridium difficile*
- Conjunctivitis, viral and hemorrhagic
- Diphtheria (cutaneous)
- Enteroviruses
- *Escherichia coli* O157:H7 and other shiga toxin-producing *E coli*
- Hepatitis A virus
- Herpes simplex virus (neonatal, mucocutaneous, or cutaneous)
- Herpes zoster
- Impetigo
- Major (noncontained) abscess, cellulitis, or decubitus ulcer
- Parainfluenza virus
- Pediculosis (lice)
- Respiratory syncytial virus
- Rotavirus
- Scabies
- *Shigella*
- *Staphylococcus aureus* (cutaneous)
- Viral hemorrhagic fevers (Ebola, Lassa, or Marburg)

Airborne, Droplet, and **Contact Precautions** may be combined for diseases caused by organisms that have multiple routes of transmission. When used alone or in combination, these transmission-based precautions always are to be used in addition to **Standard Precautions,** which are recommended for all patients. The specifications for these categories of isolation precautions are summarized in Table 2.8 (p 151). Table 2.9 (p 152) lists syndromes and conditions that are suggestive of contagious infection and require empiric isolation precautions pending identification of a specific pathogen. When the specific pathogen is known, isolation recommendations and duration of isolation are given in the pathogen- or disease-specific chapters in Section 3.

Table 2.8. **Transmission-Based Precautions for Hospitalized Patients[1]**

Category of Precautions	Single Room	Respiratory Protective Devices	Gowns	Gloves
Airborne	Yes, with negative air pressure ventilation	Yes	No[2]	No[2]
Droplet	Yes[3]	Yes, masks[4] for people close to patient	No[2]	No[2]
Contact	Yes[3]	No	Yes	Yes

[1] These recommendations are in addition to those for **Standard Precautions** for all patients.
[2] Gowns and gloves may be required as a component of **Standard Precautions** (eg, for blood collection or during procedures likely to cause blood splashes).
[3] Preferred but not required. Cohorting of children infected with the same pathogen is acceptable.
[4] See text.

PEDIATRIC CONSIDERATIONS

Unique differences in pediatric care from that for adults necessitate possible modifications of these guidelines, including the following: (1) diaper changing; (2) use of single-room isolation; and (3) use of common areas, such as hospital waiting rooms, play rooms, and schoolrooms.

Because diapering does not soil hands routinely, it is not mandatory to wear gloves except when gloves are required as part of transmission-based precautions.

Private rooms are recommended for all patients for **Transmission-Based Precautions** (ie, **Airborne, Droplet,** and **Contact**). Patients placed in transmission-based isolation may not leave their rooms to use common areas, such as child life playrooms, schoolrooms, or waiting areas. The guidelines for **Standard Precautions** state that patients who cannot control body excretions should be in single rooms. Because most young children are incontinent, this recommendation is inappropriate for routine care of uninfected children.

The CDC isolation guidelines specifically are recommended for the care of hospitalized children. These recommendations should not be extrapolated to schools, out-of-home child care centers, and other settings in which healthy children congregate in shared space.

Occupational Health

Prevention of transmission of infectious agents between patients and health care personnel is important in pediatric care. Pregnant health care personnel who follow recommended precautions should not be at increased risk of infections that have possible adverse effects on the fetus (eg, parvovirus B19, cytomegalovirus, rubella, and varicella). For personnel who are immunocompromised and at increased risk of severe infection (eg, *M tuberculosis,* measles virus, herpes simplex virus, and varicella-zoster virus), advice from their health care professional should be sought.

Table 2.9. Clinical Syndromes or Conditions Warranting Precautions in Addition to *Standard Precautions* to Prevent Transmission of Epidemiologically Important Pathogens Pending Confirmation of Diagnosis[1]

Clinical Syndrome or Condition[2]	Potential Pathogens[3]	Empiric Precautions[4]
Diarrhea		
Acute diarrhea with a likely infectious cause	Enteric pathogens[5]	Contact
Diarrhea in patient with a history of recent antimicrobial use	*Clostridium difficile*	Contact
Meningitis	*Neisseria meningitidis*	Droplet
Rash or exanthems, generalized, cause unknown		
Petechial or ecchymotic with fever	*N meningitidis*	Droplet
Vesicular	Varicella virus	Airborne and contact
Maculopapular with coryza and fever	Measles virus	Airborne
Respiratory tract infections		
Pulmonary cavitary disease	*Mycobacterium tuberculosis*	Airborne
Paroxysmal or severe persistent cough during periods of pertussis activity in the community	*Bordetella pertussis*	Droplet
Viral infections, particularly bronchiolitis and croup, in infants and young children	Respiratory syncytial virus or para-influenza virus	Contact and droplet
Risk of multidrug-resistant microorganisms[6]		
History of infection or colonization with multidrug-resistant organisms	Resistant bacteria	Contact
Skin, wound, or urinary tract infection in a patient with a recent hospital or nursing home stay in a facility in which multidrug-resistant organisms are prevalent	Resistant bacteria	Contact
Skin or wound infection		
Abscess or draining wound that cannot be covered	*Staphylococcus aureus,* group A streptococcus	Contact

[1] Infection control professionals are encouraged to modify or adapt this table according to local conditions. To ensure that appropriate empiric precautions are implemented, hospitals must have systems in place to evaluate patients routinely according to these criteria as part of their preadmission and admission care.

[2] Patients with the syndromes or conditions listed may have atypical signs or symptoms (eg, pertussis in neonates, absence of paroxysmal or severe cough in adults). The clinician's index of suspicion should be guided by the prevalence of specific conditions in the community and clinical judgment.

[3] The organisms listed in this column are not intended to represent the complete or even most likely diagnoses but, rather, possible causative agents that require additional precautions beyond **Standard Precautions** until they can be excluded.

[4] Duration of isolation varies by agent (see Garner JS. Hospital Infection Control Practices Advisory Committee. Guidelines for isolation precautions in hospitals. *Infect Control Hosp Epidemiol.* 1996;17:53–80).

[5] These pathogens include shiga toxin-producing *Escherichia coli* including *E coli* O157:H7, *Shigella* organisms, *Salmonella* organisms, *Campylobacter* organisms, hepatitis A virus, enteric viruses including rotavirus, and *Cryptosporidium* organisms.

[6] Resistant bacteria judged by the infection control program on the basis of current state, regional, or national recommendations to be of special clinical or epidemiologic significance.

The consequences to pediatric patients of acquiring infections from adults are significant. Because children likely lack immunity to many common viruses and bacteria, they are a highly susceptible population. Mild illness in adults, such as viral gastroenteritis, upper respiratory tract viral infection (eg, with respiratory syncytial virus), pertussis, herpes simplex infection, or tuberculosis, can cause life-threatening disease in infants and children. People at greatest risk are premature infants, children who have heart disease or chronic pulmonary disease, and immuno-compromised patients.

The transmission of infectious agents within hospitals is facilitated by the inevitable close contact between patients and health care personnel. In addition, children do not follow good hygienic practices routinely.

To limit the risks of infection to and from children and health care personnel, hospitals should have established personnel health policies and services. It particularly is important to ensure that personnel are protected against measles, rubella, mumps, hepatitis B, varicella, influenza, polio, pertussis, tetanus, and diphtheria by establishing appropriate screening and immunization policies.*

For infections that are not vaccine preventable, personnel should be counseled about exposures and the possible need for leave if they are exposed to, ill with, or a carrier of a specific pathogen, whether the exposure occurs in the home, community, or health care setting.

The frequency and need for screening of health care personnel for tuberculosis should be determined by local epidemiologic data. People with common infections, such as gastroenteritis, dermatitis, herpes simplex lesions on exposed skin, or upper respiratory tract infections, should be evaluated to determine the resulting risk of transmission to patients or to other health care personnel.

Health care personnel, including pregnant women, should be educated about pathogens for which they are (and are not) at increased risk if they follow Standard Precautions.

Health care personnel education is of paramount importance in infection control. Pediatric health care professionals should be knowledgeable about the modes of transmission of infectious agents, proper hand hygiene techniques, and the potential serious risks to children from certain mild infections in adults. Frequent educational sessions will reinforce safe techniques and the importance of infection control policies. Written policies and procedures relating to needlestick or sharp injuries are mandated by OSHA.[†] Employees should be educated regarding hospital policies. Recommendations for postinjury prophylaxis is available (see Human Immunodeficiency Virus Infection, p 360 and Table 3.28, p 375).[‡]

---

* Centers for Disease Control and Prevention. Recommended adult immunization schedule—United States, 2002–2003. *MMWR Morb Mortal Wkly Rep.* 2002;51:904–908

† American Academy of Pediatrics. *OSHA: Materials to Assist the Pediatric Office in Implementing the Bloodborne Pathogen, Hazard Communication, and Other OSHA Standards.* Elk Grove Village, IL: American Academy of Pediatrics; 1994

‡ American Academy of Pediatrics, Committee on Pediatric AIDS. Postexposure prophylaxis in children and adolescents for nonoccupational exposure to human immunodeficiency virus. *Pediatrics.* In press

Sibling Visits

Sibling visits to birthing centers, postpartum rooms, pediatric wards, and intensive care units are encouraged. Newborn intensive care, with its increasing sophistication, often results in long hospital stays for the sick newborn, making family visits important. If guidelines are followed, subsequent infection is not increased in the sick or well newborn whom siblings have visited.

Guidelines for sibling visits should be established to maximize opportunities for visiting and to minimize the risks of spread of pathogens brought into the hospital by these young visitors. Guidelines may need to be modified by local nursing, pediatric, obstetric, and infectious diseases staff members to address specific issues in their hospital settings. Basic guidelines for sibling visits to pediatric patients are as follows:

- Sibling visits should be encouraged for all hospitalized infants and children.
- Before the visit, a trained health care professional should interview the parents at a site outside the unit to assess the health of each sibling visitor. No child with fever or symptoms of an acute illness, including upper respiratory tract infection, gastroenteritis, or dermatitis, should be allowed to visit. Siblings who recently have been exposed to a person with a known communicable disease and are susceptible should not be allowed to visit. These interviews should be documented in the patient's record, and approval for each sibling visit should be noted.
- Asymptomatic siblings who recently have been exposed to varicella but have been immunized previously can be assumed to be immune.
- The visiting sibling should visit only his or her sibling.
- Children should perform hand hygiene carefully before any patient contact.
- Throughout the visit, sibling activity should be supervised by parents or a responsible adult and limited to the mother's or patient's private room or other designated areas.

Guidelines should be established for visits by other relatives and close friends. Anyone with fever or contagious illnesses ideally should not visit. Medical and nursing staff members should be vigilant about potential communicable diseases in parents and other adult visitors (eg, a relative with a cough who may have tuberculosis; a parent with a cold visiting a highly immunosuppressed child).

Pet Visitation

Pet visitation in the hospital setting can be separated into 2 categories, visits by a child's personal pet and pet visitation as a part of child life therapeutic programs. Guidelines for pet visitation should be established to minimize risks of transmission of pathogens from pets to humans or injury from animals. The hospital setting and the level of concern for zoonotic disease will influence the establishment of pet visitation policies. The hospital policy should be developed in consultation with pediatricians, infection control practitioners, nursing staff, the hospital epidemiologist, and veterinarians. Basic principles for hospital pet visitation policies are as follows:

- Personal pets other than cats and dogs should be excluded from the hospital. No reptiles (eg, iguanas, turtles, snakes), amphibians, birds, primates, ferrets, or rodents should be allowed to visit.

- Visiting pets should have a certificate of immunization from a licensed veterinarian and verification that the pet is free from contagious diseases.
- The pet should be bathed and groomed for the visit.
- Pet visitation is inappropriate in the intensive care unit.
- The visit of the pet should be approved by appropriate hospital personnel (for example, the director of the child life therapeutic program), who should observe the pet for temperament and general health at the time of visit. The pet should be free of obvious bacterial skin infections, infections caused by superficial dermatophytes, and ectoparasitic infections (fleas and ticks).
- Pet visitation should be confined to designated areas. Contact should be confined to the petting and holding of animals, as appropriate. All contact should be supervised throughout the visit by appropriate hospital personnel. Supervisors should be familiar with hospital policies for managing animal bites and cleaning pet urine, feces, or vomitus.
- Patients having contact with pets must have approval from a physician or physician representative before animal contact. Documented allergy to dogs or cats should be considered before approving contact. For patients who are immunodeficient or for people receiving immunosuppressive therapy, the risks of exposure to the microflora of pets may outweigh the benefits of contact. Contact of children with pets should be approved on a case-by-case basis.
- Care should be taken to protect indwelling catheter sites. These sites should have dressings that provide an effective barrier to pet contact, including licking. Concern for contamination of other body sites should be considered on a case-by-case basis.
- Children should perform appropriate hand hygiene after contact with pets.
- The pet policy should not apply to professionally trained guide animals, such as "seeing eye" dogs. These animals are not pets, and separate policies should govern their uses and presence in the hospital.

INFECTION CONTROL IN PHYSICIANS' OFFICES

Infection control is an integral part of pediatric practice in outpatient settings as well as in hospitals. All health care personnel should be aware of the routes of transmission and techniques used to prevent transmission of infectious agents. Policies for infection control and prevention should be written, readily available, and enforced. Standard precautions, as outlined for the hospitalized child (see Infection Control for Hospitalized Children, p 146), with modifications by the American Academy of Pediatrics,* are appropriate for most patient encounters. Key principles of infection control in an outpatient setting are as follows:

---

* American Academy of Pediatrics, Committee on Infectious Diseases and Committee on Practice and Ambulatory Medicine. Infection control in physicians' offices. *Pediatrics.* 2000;105:1361–1369

- All health care personnel should use hand hygiene before and after patient contact. Parents and children should be taught the importance of hand hygiene.*
- Standard precautions should be used when caring for all patients.
- Contact between contagious children and uninfected children should be minimized. Policies for children who are suspected of having infections, such as varicella or measles, should be implemented. Prompt triage of immunocompromised children should be performed routinely.
- Alcohol is preferred for skin preparation before immunization or routine venipuncture. Skin preparation for incision, suture, or collection of blood for culture requires 10% povidone-iodine, 70% alcohol, alcohol tinctures of iodine, or 2% chlorhexidine.
- Physicians should be familiar with aseptic technique, particularly regarding entry or manipulation of intravascular catheters.[†]
- Needles and sharps should be handled with great care. Needle disposal units that are impermeable and puncture proof should be available adjacent to the spaces used for injection or venipuncture. The containers should not be overfilled and should be kept out of the reach of young children. Policies should be established for removal and incineration or sterilization of contents.
- Policies for management of needlestick injuries should be in place.
- Standard guidelines for decontamination, disinfection, and sterilization should be followed.
- Appropriate use of antimicrobial agents is essential to limit the emergence and spread of drug-resistant bacteria (see Appropriate Use of Antimicrobial Agents, p 695).
- Outpatient offices and clinics should develop policies and procedures for communication with local and state health authorities about reportable diseases and suspected outbreaks.
- Ongoing educational programs that encompass appropriate aspects of infection control should be implemented, reinforced, and evaluated on a regular basis.
- Physicians should be aware of requirements of government agencies, such as the Occupational Safety and Health Administration (OSHA).[‡]

---

* Centers for Disease Control and Prevention. Guideline for hand hygiene in health-care settings. Recommendations of the Healthcare Infection Control Practices Advisory Committee and the HIC-PAC/SHEA/APIC/IDSA Hand Hygiene Task Force. *MMWR Recomm Rep.* 2002;51(RR-16):1–45

† Garland JS, Hendrickson K, Maki DG. The 2002 Hospital Infection Control Practices Advisory Committee Centers for Disease Control and Prevention guideline for prevention of intravascular device-related infection. *Pediatrics.* 2002;110:1009–1013

‡ American Academy of Pediatrics. *OSHA: Materials to Assist the Pediatric Office in Implementing the Bloodborne Pathogen, Hazard Communication, and Other OSHA Standards.* Elk Grove Village, IL: American Academy of Pediatrics; 1994

SEXUALLY TRANSMITTED DISEASES IN ADOLESCENTS AND CHILDREN

Physicians and other health care professionals perform a critical role in preventing and treating sexually transmitted diseases (STDs) in the pediatric population. Sexually transmitted diseases are a major problem for adolescents; an estimated 25% of adolescents will develop an STD before graduating from high school. For infants and children, detection of an STD is an important warning signal of sexual abuse. Sexual abuse of children has been endemic for generations, but the prevalence and potentially devastating psychologic effects of sexual abuse have been recognized only recently. Whenever sexual abuse is suspected, appropriate social service and law enforcement agencies must be involved to ensure the child's protection and to provide appropriate counseling.

Sexually Transmitted Diseases in Adolescents

EPIDEMIOLOGY

Although the incidence of all reported STDs in the United States has decreased during the past decade, adolescents and young adults continue to have higher rates of STDs than any other age group. Adolescents are at greater risk of STDs, because they frequently have unprotected intercourse, are biologically more susceptible to infection, often are engaged in partnerships of limited duration, and face multiple obstacles to use of health care services. In the United States in 2000, case report rates for gonorrhea were 61 per 100 000 for people between 40 and 44 years of age, 307 per 100 000 for people between 25 and 29 years of age, 623 per 100 000 for people between 20 and 24 years, and 516 per 100 000 for people between 15 and 19 years of age. The highest age-specific incidence rate for acquired immunodeficiency syndrome (AIDS) in 2000 was 34 per 100 000, which occurred among young adults 25 to 39 years of age who presumably acquired human immunodeficiency virus (HIV) infections approximately a decade earlier—commonly during adolescence. In 2000, reports based on AIDS surveillance data indicated a substantial decrease in the number of perinatally acquired AIDS cases, reflecting a decreasing rate of perinatal HIV transmission. In the United States in 2000, the rates of chlamydial infection were 1373 per 100 000 for people between 15 and 19 years of age and 521 per 100 000 for people 25 to 29 years of age. These data underestimate the incidence of STDs among sexually experienced adolescents, because *all* adolescents, including the one third of US 10th, 11th, and 12th grade students who never have had sexual intercourse, are included in the denominators used to calculate age-specific STD rates.

MANAGEMENT

Pediatricians should screen for STD risk by asking all adolescent patients whether they ever have had sexual intercourse or been sexually active. Adolescents at increased risk of STDs are listed in Table 2.10, p 158. Physicians can prepare parents and patients for this sensitive question by informing parents of their policies about con-

Table 2.10. Adolescents Whose History Includes One or More of the Following Features Are Considered at Increased Risk of Contracting a Sexually Transmitted Disease (STD)[1]

- Sexual contact with person(s) with known STD or history of STD
- Symptoms or signs of STD
- Multiple sexual partners
- Street involvement (eg, homelessness)
- Sexual intercourse with new partner during last 2 months
- More than 2 sexual partners during previous 12 months
- No contraception or use of nonbarrier methods
- Injection drug use
- Male homosexual activity
- "Survival sex" (eg, exchanging sex for money, drugs, shelter, or food)
- Time spent in detention facilities
- Having been a patient in an STD clinic

---

[1] Modified from Health Canada. *Canadian STD Guidelines: 1998 Edition.* Ottawa, Ontario: Population and Public Health Branch, Health Canada; 1998. Available at: www.hc-sc.gc.ca/hpb/lcdc/publicat/std98/index.html

fidentiality and by ensuring that the annual checkup of every adolescent includes a private interview. More detailed recommendations for preventive health care for adolescents are contained in the American Academy of Pediatrics *Guidelines for Health Supervision III** and the American Medical Association's *Guidelines for Adolescent Preventive Services.*[†] All 50 states allow minors to give their own consent for confidential STD diagnosis and treatment. Despite the prevalence of STDs among adolescents, health care professionals frequently fail to inquire about sexual behavior, assess STD risks, and counsel about risk reduction.

All adolescent women who have had sexual intercourse should have an annual Papanicolaou smear to screen for cervical dysplasia resulting from human papillomavirus infection. In addition, many experts recommend that all sexually active adolescents be screened for gonorrhea and chlamydia semiannually and receive HIV counseling and syphilis screening annually. All adolescents should receive hepatitis B virus immunization if they were not immunized earlier in childhood (see Recommended Childhood and Adolescent Immunization Schedule, Fig 1.1, p 24).

For treatment recommendations for specific STDs, see the disease-specific chapters in Section 3 and Table 4.3, Guidelines for Treatment of Sexually Transmitted Diseases in Children and Adolescents According to Syndrome, p 713. Patients with gonorrhea, *Chlamydia trachomatis* infection, and trichomoniasis

---

* American Academy of Pediatrics, Committee on Psychosocial Aspects of Child and Family Health. *Guidelines for Health Supervision III.* Elk Grove Village, IL: American Academy of Pediatrics; 1997 (updated 2002)

† Elster AB, Kuznets NJ, eds. *AMA Guidelines for Adolescent Preventive Services (GAPS) Recommendations and Rationale.* Baltimore, MD: Williams & Wilkins; 1994

should be advised to refrain from sexual intercourse for 1 week and until their sexual partners have received appropriate treatment for these infections. Retesting to detect therapeutic failure (tests of cure) for patients who receive recommended treatment regimens for *Neisseria gonorrhoeae* or *C trachomatis* infection no longer is recommended unless therapeutic compliance is in question or symptoms persist. If a multiple-dose regimen is used, noncompliance is possible. Retesting for chlamydia infection fewer than 3 weeks after treatment may be falsely positive as a result of residual nonviable organisms. Some experts recommend repeated testing of adolescents 4 to 6 weeks after STD treatment because of the greater likelihood of reinfection in this age group, compared with adults, from a current sexual partner who did not obtain treatment or from a new sexual partner.

PREVENTION

Pediatricians can contribute to primary prevention of STDs by encouraging adolescent patients to postpone their initiation of sexual intercourse for as long as possible and to be prepared to use barrier methods of contraception beginning with the first intercourse experience. Pediatricians should encourage adolescents who already have had sexual intercourse to practice "secondary" abstinence (to be celibate), to minimize their lifetime number of sexual partners, to use barrier methods of contraception consistently and correctly, and to be aware of the strong association between alcohol or drug use and failure to use barrier contraception. The correct use of male and female condoms and some strategies for encouraging condom use are reviewed in Tables 2.11 (p 160) and 2.12 (p 161).

Diagnosis and Treatment of STDs in Children*

Because of the social and legal implications of the diagnosis, STDs in children must be diagnosed using tests with high specificity, because the low prevalence of STDs in children increases the probability that rapid detection tests for STDs will give false-positive results. Therefore, tests that allow for isolation of the organism and have the highest specificities should be used.

Because of the serious implications of the diagnosis of an STD in a child, antimicrobial therapy for children with suspected STDs may need to be withheld until the final outcome of the diagnostic test is known. Specimens for cultures for *N gonorrhoeae* and *C trachomatis* should be obtained from the vagina in girls and urethra in boys and from the rectal area and, for *N gonorrhoeae*, also from the pharyngeal areas. Endocervical specimens are not recommended for prepubertal girls. Vaginal specimens for culture and wet mount for *Trichomonas vaginalis* and bacterial vaginosis and serum specimens for testing for syphilis, HIV, and hepatitis B surface antigen should be obtained. For more detailed diagnosis and treatment recommendations for specific STDs, see Section 3 and Table 4.3, Guidelines for Treatment of Sexually Transmitted Diseases in Children and Adolescents According to Syndrome, p 713.

---

* Centers for Disease Control and Prevention. Sexually transmitted diseases treatment guidelines— 2002. *MMWR Recomm Rep.* 2002;51(RR-6):1–80

Table 2.11. Recommendations for Proper Use of Condoms to Decrease the Risk of Transmission of Sexually Transmitted Diseases[1]

Male Condoms

- Use a new condom with each act of sexual intercourse.
- Carefully handle the condom to avoid damaging it with fingernails, teeth, or other sharp objects.
- Put condom on after the penis is erect and before genital contact with partner.
- Ensure that no air is trapped in the tip of the condom.
- Ensure that adequate lubrication exists during intercourse, possibly requiring the use of external lubricants.
- Use only water-based lubricants (eg, K-Y Jelly,[2] Astroglide,[3] Aqua-Lube,[4] and glycerin) with latex condoms. Oil-based lubricants (eg, petroleum jelly, shortening, mineral oil, massage oils, body lotions, and cooking oil) can weaken latex.
- Hold the condom firmly against the base of the penis during withdrawal, and withdraw while penis is still erect to prevent slippage.

Female Condoms (eg, Reality[4])

- Lubricated polyurethane sheath with a ring on each end, one of which is inserted into the vagina and rests over the cervix like a diaphragm and the other remains outside the vagina and covers the external genitalia.

- When a male condom cannot be used appropriately, consider use of a female condom. Instructions about insertion may be needed.

---

[1] From Centers for Disease Control and Prevention. Sexually transmitted diseases treatment guidelines—2002. *MMWR Recomm Rep.* 2002;51(RR-6):1–80.
[2] Personal Products Co, Skillman, NJ.
[3] Biofilm, Vista, CA.
[4] Mayer Laboratories Inc, Oakland, CA.

Social Implications of STDs in Children

Children can acquire STDs through vertical transmission, by autoinoculation, or by sexual contact. Each of these mechanisms should be given appropriate consideration in the evaluation of a preadolescent child with an STD. Evaluation based solely on suspicion of an STD should not proceed until the STD diagnosis has been confirmed. Factors to be considered in assessing the likelihood of sexual abuse in a child with an STD include whether the child reports a history of sexual victimization, biologic characteristics of the STD in question, and age of the child (see Table 2.13, p 162).

Anogenital gonorrhea in a prepubertal child indicates sexual abuse in virtually every case. All cases of gonorrhea in prepubertal children beyond the neonatal period should be reported to the local child protective services agency for investigation.

Herpes simplex has a short incubation period but can be transmitted by sexual or nonsexual contact with another person or by autoinoculation. In an infant or toddler in diapers, genital herpes may arise from any of these mechanisms. In a prepubertal child whose toilet use activities are independent, the new occurrence of genital herpes should prompt a careful investigation, including a child protective services investigation, for suspected sexual abuse.

Table 2.12. **Barriers to Condom Use and Ways to Overcome Them**[1]

Perceived Barrier	Intervention Strategy
Decreases sexual pleasure (sensation). Note: often perceived by those who never have used a condom.	Encourage patient to try. Put a drop of water-based lubricant or saliva inside the tip of the condom or on the glans of the penis before putting on the condom. Try a thinner latex condom or different brand or more lubrication.
Decreases spontaneity of sexual activity	Encourage incorporation of condom use during foreplay. Remind patient that peace of mind may enhance pleasure for self and partner.
Embarrassing, juvenile, "unmanly"	Remind patient that it is "manly" to protect self and others.
Poor fit (too small or too big, slips off, uncomfortable)	Smaller and larger condoms are available.
Requires prompt withdrawal after ejaculation	Reinforce the protective nature of prompt withdrawal and suggest substitution of other postcoital sexual activities.
Fear of breakage may lead to less vigorous sexual activity	With prolonged intercourse, lubricant wears off and the condom begins to rub. Have a water-soluble lubricant available to reapply.
Nonpenetrative sexual activity	Condoms have been advocated for use during fellatio; unlubricated condoms may prove best for this purpose because of the taste of the lubricant. Other barriers, such as dental dams or an unlubricated condom cut down the middle to form a barrier, have been advocated for use during certain forms of nonpenetrative sexual activity (eg, cunnilingus and anolingual sex).
Allergy to latex	Polyurethane condoms for women are available commercially. A natural skin condom can be used together with a latex condom to protect the male or female from contact with latex.

[1] From Health Canada. *Canadian STD Guidelines: 1998 Edition.* Population and Public Health Branch, Health Canada; 1998. Available at: www.hc-sc.gc.ca/hpb/lcdc/publicat/std98/index.html

Trichomoniasis is transmitted perinatally or by sexual contact. In a perinatally infected infant, vaginal discharge can persist for several weeks; accordingly, intense social investigation may not be warranted. However, a new diagnosis of trichomoniasis in an older infant or child should prompt a careful investigation, including a child protective services investigation, for suspected sexual abuse.

Table 2.13. Implications of Commonly Encountered Sexually Transmitted Diseases (STDs) for Diagnosis and Reporting of Suspected or Diagnosed Sexual Abuse of Infants and Prepubertal Children[1]

STD Confirmed	Sexual Abuse	Suggested Action[2]
Gonorrhea[3]	Diagnostic[4]	Report
Syphilis[3]	Diagnostic	Report
Human immunodeficiency virus infection[5]	Diagnostic	Report
Chlamydia trachomatis infection[3]	Diagnostic[4]	Report
Trichomonas vaginalis infection	Highly suspicious	Report
Condylomata acuminata infection[3] (anogenital warts)	Suspicious	Report
Herpes (genital location)	Suspicious	Report[6]
Bacterial vaginosis	Inconclusive	Medical follow-up

[1] Adapted from American Academy of Pediatrics, Committee on Child Abuse and Neglect. Guidelines for the evaluation of sexual abuse of children: subject review [published correction appears in Pediatrics. 1999;103:1049]. *Pediatrics.* 1999;103:186–191

[2] Reports should be made to the agency mandated in the community to receive reports of suspected sexual abuse.

[3] If not likely to be acquired perinatally.

[4] Only culture using standard confirmation methods should be used; DNA probes should not be used as a diagnostic method.

[5] If not likely to be acquired perinatally or by transfusion.

[6] Unless there is a clear history of autoinoculation.

Infections that have long incubation periods (eg, papillomavirus infection) and that can be asymptomatic for long periods after vertical transmission (eg, syphilis, HIV infection, *C trachomatis* infection) are more problematic. The possibility of vertical transmission should be considered in these cases, but an evaluation of the patient's circumstances by the local child protective services agency usually is warranted.

Although hepatitis B virus, bacterial vaginosis, scabies, and pediculosis pubis may be transmitted sexually, other modes of transmission can occur. The discovery of any of these conditions in a prepubertal child does not warrant child protective services involvement unless the clinician finds other information that suggests abuse.

Sexual Victimization and STDs

GENERAL CONSIDERATIONS

Child sexual abuse has been defined as the exploitation of a child, either by physical contact or by other interactions, for the sexual stimulation of an adult or a minor who is in a position of power over the child. Sexual victimization of a child younger than 18 years of age by a caregiver is termed *abuse;* physicians are required by law to report abuse to their state child protective services agency. Sexual victimization of a child or adolescent by a person who is not a caregiver is termed *assault;* if the assault did not involve a gun or knife injury, the patient or parent makes the decision whether to report sexual assault to the local law enforcement authority. In some instances, sexual victimization involves physical contact permitting the transfer of sexually transmitted microorganisms. Approximately 5% of sexually abused children acquire an STD as a result of the victimization.

SCREENING ASYMPTOMATIC SEXUALLY VICTIMIZED CHILDREN FOR STDS

Factors that influence the likelihood that a sexually victimized child will acquire an STD include the regional prevalence of STDs in the adult population, the number of assailants, the type and frequency of physical contact between the perpetrator(s) and the child, the infectivity of various microorganisms, the child's susceptibility to infection, and whether the child has received intercurrent antimicrobial agent treatment. The time interval between a child's physical contact with an assailant and the medical evaluation influences the likelihood that an exposed child will demonstrate signs or symptoms of an STD.

The decision to obtain genital or other specimens from a child to conduct an STD evaluation must be made on an individual basis. The following situations involve a high risk of STDs and constitute a strong indication for testing:

- The child has or has had signs or symptoms of an STD or an infection that can be transmitted sexually, even in the absence of suspicion of sexual abuse
- A sibling, another child, or an adult in the household or child's immediate environment has an STD
- A suspected assailant is known to have an STD or to be at high risk of STDs (eg, has had multiple sexual partners or a history of STDs)
- The patient or family requests testing
- The prevalence of STDs in the community is high
- Evidence of genital, oral, or anal penetration or ejaculation is present

See Table 2.14, p 164, if STD testing of a child is to be performed.

Most experts recommend universal screening of postpubertal patients, because the prevalence of preexisting asymptomatic infection in this group is high. When STD screening is performed, it should focus on likely anatomic sites of infection (as determined by the patient's history or by epidemiologic considerations) and should include assessment for HIV infection if the patient, family, or both consent to serologic screening; assessment for bacterial vaginosis for female patients and trichomoniasis; a Papanicolaou smear in female patients; and testing for *N gonorrhoeae* infection, *C trachomatis* infection, and syphilis. To preserve the "chain of custody" for information that may later constitute legal evidence, specimens for laboratory analysis obtained from sexually victimized patients should be labeled carefully, and standard hospital procedures for transferring specimens from site to site should be followed carefully. Only tests with high specificities should be used, and specimens should be obtained by health care professionals with experience in the evaluation of sexually abused and assaulted children. A follow-up visit approximately 2 weeks after the most recent sexual exposure may include a repeat physical examination and collection of additional specimens. Another follow-up visit approximately 12 weeks after the most recent sexual exposure may be necessary to collect convalescent sera.

Table 2.14. **Sexually Transmitted Disease (STD) Testing in a Child[1] When Sexual Abuse Is Suspected**

Organism/Syndrome	Specimens
Neisseria gonorrhoeae	Rectal, throat, urethral (male), and/or vaginal cultures[2]
Chlamydia trachomatis	Rectal, urethral (male), and vaginal cultures[2]
Syphilis	Darkfield examination of chancre fluid, if present; blood for serologic tests at time of abuse and 6, 12, and 24 wk later
Human immuno-deficiency virus	Serologic testing of abuser (if possible); serologic testing of child at time of abuse and 6, 12, and 24 wk later
Hepatitis B virus	Serum hepatitis B surface antigen testing of abuser or hepatitis B surface antibody testing of child
Herpes simplex virus	Culture of lesion
Bacterial vaginosis	Wet mount, pH, and potassium hydroxide testing of vaginal discharge or Gram stain
Human papillomavirus	Biopsy of lesion
Trichomonas vaginalis	Wet mount and culture of vaginal discharge
Pediculus pubis	Identification of eggs, nymphs, and lice with naked eye or using hand lens

[1] See text for indications for testing for STDs (Screening Asymptomatic Sexually Victimized Children for STDs, p 163).
[2] Cervical specimens are not recommended for prepubertal girls.

PROPHYLAXIS AFTER SEXUAL VICTIMIZATION

Most experts do not recommend antimicrobial prophylaxis for abused prepubertal children, because their incidence of STDs is low, the risk of spread to the upper genital tract in a prepubertal girl is low, and follow-up usually can be ensured. If a test for an STD is positive, treatment then can be given. Factors that may increase the likelihood of infection or that constitute an indication for prophylaxis are the same as those listed under Screening Asymptomatic Sexually Victimized Children for STDs (p 163).

Many experts believe that prophylaxis is warranted for postpubertal female patients who seek care within 72 hours after an episode of sexual victimization because of the high prevalence of preexisting asymptomatic infection and the substantial risk of pelvic inflammatory disease in this age group. All patients who receive prophylaxis should be screened for relevant STDs (see Table 2.14, above) before treatment is given. Postmenarcheal patients should be tested for pregnancy before antimicrobial treatment or emergency contraception is given. Regimens for prophylaxis are presented in Tables 2.15, p 165 (children) and 2.16, p 166 (adolescents).

Because of the demonstrated effectiveness of prophylaxis to prevent HIV infection after perinatal and occupational exposures, the question arises about HIV prophylaxis for children and adolescents after sexual assault (see also Human Immunodeficiency Virus Infection, Control Measures, p 374, and Table 3.28,

Table 2.15. **Prophylaxis After Sexual Victimization of Preadolescent Children[1]**

Weight <100 lb (<45 kg)	Weight ≥100 lb (≥45 kg)
For prevention of gonorrhea[2]	
1. Ceftriaxone, 125 mg, IM, in a single dose	1. Ceftriaxone, 125 mg, IM, in a single dose
PLUS **For prevention of** *Chlamydia trachomatis* **infection** **PLUS**	
2A. Azithromycin, 20 mg/kg (maximum 1 g), orally, in a single dose	2A. Azithromycin, 1 g, orally, in a single dose
OR	**OR**
2B. Erythromycin base or ethylsuccinate, 50 mg/kg per day, divided into 4 doses for 10–14 days	2B. Doxycycline, 100 mg, twice daily, for 7 days
PLUS **For prevention of** **hepatitis B virus infection** **PLUS**	
3. Begin or complete hepatitis B virus immunization if not fully immunized	3. Begin or complete hepatitis B virus immunization if not fully immunized
PLUS **For prevention of** **trichomoniasis and bacterial vaginosis** **PLUS**	
4. Consideration should be given to adding prophylaxis for trichomoniasis and bacterial vaginosis (metronidazole, 15 mg/kg per day, orally, in 3 divided doses for 7 days)	4. Consideration should be given to adding prophylaxis against trichomoniasis and bacterial vaginosis (metronidazole, 2 g, orally, in a single dose)

IM indicates intramuscularly.

[1] See text for discussion of prophylaxis for human immunodeficiency virus infection in children after sexual abuse or assault.

[2] Cefixime no longer is manufactured in the United States.

p 375.) Data are insufficient concerning the efficacy and safety of postexposure prophylaxis among children and adults. The risk of HIV transmission from a single sexual assault that involves transfer of secretions and/or blood is low, but not zero. Prophylaxis may be considered for patients who seek care within 24 to 48 hours after an assault if the assault involved the transfer of secretions and particularly if the alleged perpetrator is known or suspected to have HIV infection or to have used injection drugs (see Human Immunodeficiency Virus Infection, p 360). Following are recommendations for postexposure assessment of children within 72 hours of sexual assault:

• Review HIV/AIDS local epidemiology and assess risk of HIV infection in the assailant.

• Evaluate circumstances of assault that may affect risk of HIV transmission.

• Consult with a specialist in treating HIV-infected children if postexposure prophylaxis is considered.

Table 2.16. **Prophylaxis After Sexual Victimization of Adolescents[1]**

Antimicrobial prophylaxis[2] is recommended to include an empiric regimen to prevent *Chlamydia trachomatis* infection, gonorrhea, trichomoniasis, and bacterial vaginosis

For gonorrhea[3]	Ceftriaxone, 125 mg, intramuscularly, in a single dose
	OR
	Ciprofloxacin, 500 mg, orally, in a single dose
	OR
	Ofloxacin, 400 mg, orally, in a single dose
	OR
	Levofloxacin, 250 mg, orally, in a single dose
	PLUS
For *C trachomatis* infection	Azithromycin, 1 g, orally, in a single dose
	OR
	Doxycycline, 100 mg, orally, twice a day for 7 days
	PLUS
For trichomoniasis and bacterial vaginosis	Metronidazole, 2 g, orally, in a single dose
	PLUS
For hepatitis B virus infection	Hepatitis B virus immunization at time of initial examination, if not fully immunized. Follow-up doses of vaccine should be administered 1 to 2 and 4 to 6 mo after the first dose.
	PLUS
For human immunodeficiency virus infection[2]	Consider offering prophylaxis for HIV, depending on circumstances (see Table 3.28, p 375)

Emergency Contraception[4]

Oral contraceptive pills containing 50 μg of ethinyl estradiol: 2 pills orally initially, then 2 pills orally 12 h later

OR

Oral contraceptive pills containing 30 μg of ethinyl estradiol: 4 pills orally initially, then 4 pills orally 12 h later

PLUS

An antiemetic

---

[1] Sources: Hampton HL. Care of the woman who has been raped [published correction appears in *N Engl J Med*. 1997;337:56]. *N Engl J Med*. 1995;332:234–237; and Centers for Disease Control and Prevention. Sexually transmitted diseases treatment guidelines—2002. *MMWR Recomm Rep*. 2002;51(RR-6):1–80

[2] See text for discussion of prophylaxis for human immunodeficiency virus (HIV) infection after sexual abuse or assault.

[3] Cefixime no longer is manufactured in the United States. For people 18 years of age and older, a single dose of a fluoroquinolone can be used in areas of low prevalence of fluoroquinolone-resistant *Neisseria gonorrhoeae*. Because of resistance, fluoroquinolones should not be used if infection is acquired in Asia, Pacific Islands (including Hawaii), and California.

[4] The patient should have a negative pregnancy test result before emergency contraception is given.

- If the child appears to be at risk of HIV transmission from the assault, discuss postexposure prophylaxis with the caregiver(s), including its toxicity and its unknown efficacy.
- If caregivers choose for the child to receive antiretroviral postexposure prophylaxis, provide enough medication until the return visit at 3 to 7 days after initial assessment to reevaluate the child and to assess tolerance of medication; dosages should not exceed those for adults.
- Perform HIV antibody test at original assessment and 6, 12, and 24 weeks later.

HEPATITIS AND YOUTH IN CORRECTIONS SETTINGS*

The number of arrests of juveniles younger than 18 years of age in the United States has stabilized at 2.5 million per year but continues to represent nearly 5% of the pediatric population. More than 300 000 youth are maintained annually in detention facilities awaiting court hearings, and on any given day, 126 000 adolescents are incarcerated in juvenile corrections facilities or adult jails. Incarceration periods of at least 90 days await 60% of juvenile inmates, and 15% can expect to spend a year or more behind bars. Incarcerated youth disproportionately are male and are more likely to be members of ethnic or racial minorities. Female juveniles constitute 15% of the incarcerated juvenile population, and pregnancy often presents additional challenges in the provision of medical services in corrections facilities.

Juvenile offenders commonly lack regular access to preventive health care in their communities and suffer significantly greater health deficiencies, including psychosocial disorders, chronic illness, exposure to illicit drugs, and physical trauma when compared with adolescents who avoid the juvenile justice system.* Detained youth are more likely to have contracted sexually transmitted diseases (STDs) early in adolescence, and delayed or incomplete treatment places them at increased risk of chronic complications of chlamydia, gonorrhea, syphilis, and human papillomavirus infections. Tuberculosis (TB) is more common in corrections populations, and although the current population of juvenile detainees continues to have a low prevalence of human immunodeficiency virus (HIV) infection, their lifestyle choices place them at significant risk.† Hepatitis A, B, and C infections, however, are of particular concern because of the increased frequency of alcohol and injection drug use and increased rate of unprotected sex with multiple partners earlier in life. Juvenile crimes involving drug abuse violations have increased 133% over the past several years, and a history of injection drug use has played a major role in explaining the increased incidence of hepatitis C infections in adolescent offenders. Hepatitis may be a comorbid condition of other diseases including TB and HIV infection, and infected juveniles may place their communities at risk after their release from detention.

* Centers for Disease Control and Prevention. Prevention and control of infections with hepatitis viruses in correctional settings. *MMWR Recomm Rep.* 2003;52(RR-1):1–33

† American Academy of Pediatrics, Committee on Adolescence. Health care for children and adolescents in the juvenile correctional care system. *Pediatrics.* 2001;107:799–803

Up to 15% of all chronic hepatitis B infections and more than 30% of all hepatitis C infections known to exist in the United States can be traced to people released from corrections facilities. High-risk behaviors make adolescents predisposed for incarceration particularly vulnerable to hepatitis A, hepatitis B, and hepatitis C infection well before their first incarceration. Fewer than 3% of new hepatitis virus infections of all types are acquired once incarceration has occurred. Most juvenile offenders ultimately are returned to their community and, without intervention, resume a high-risk lifestyle. High recidivism rates lead many juvenile offenders to adult prisons, in which rates of hepatitis B and hepatitis C infection may be significantly higher than those found in juvenile corrections facilities. An encounter by a youthful offender with the juvenile justice system offers an opportunity to initiate hepatitis assessment, prevention, and behavior modification strategies that, if successful, hold the promise of improved outcomes for a group of adolescents at exceptional risk of complications of chronic liver disease.

Hepatitis A

Hepatitis A infection is common in the United States, and many regions of the country have levels and persistence of transmission considered to be endemic (see Hepatitis A, p 309). Corrections facilities in the United States rarely report cases of hepatitis A, and national prevalence data for incarcerated populations are not available. States that have assessed prevalence in incarcerated populations younger than 20 years of age show a similar ethnic distribution of predominance in American Indian/Alaska Native and Hispanic inmates, as is reflected in at-risk populations as a whole. Some estimates suggest an overall hepatitis seroprevalence between 22% and 39% in the adult prison population, with up to a 43% prevalence found in older prisoners between 40 and 49 years of age. Adolescent hepatitis A risk factors that could contribute to outbreaks include using injection and noninjection street drugs, having multiple sexual partners, and participating in protracted homosexual activity. Hepatitis A virus coinfection increases the severity of liver complications in patients with chronic liver disease caused by hepatitis B or hepatitis C virus infection, a matter of importance to incarcerated youth, who experience higher rates of hepatitis C compared with adolescents who remain outside the justice system. Inmates who reside or are detained in facilities located in states and regions of the United States with high hepatitis A endemicity (see Hepatitis A, p 309) particularly are at risk of dual hepatitis virus infections.

Recommendations for Control of Hepatitis A Virus Infections in Incarcerated Youth. Routine screening of incarcerated youth for hepatitis A markers is not recommended. However, adolescents who have signs or symptoms of hepatitis should be screened not only for hepatitis A virus but also for acute and chronic hepatitis B and hepatitis C virus infection. Hepatitis A vaccine (see Hepatitis A Vaccine, p 311) should be given to all adolescents in corrections facilities located in states where routine hepatitis A immunization is recommended before their release from detention. Given the high proportion of juvenile offenders with risk factors predisposing them to hepatitis A, hepatitis B, and hepatitis C virus infection, corrections facilities should consider strongly routine hepatitis A immunization of all adolescents under their care, regardless of regional endemicity. If this is not possible, consideration should be given to providing hepatitis A vaccine to juveniles with known hepatitis B or hepatitis C infection and juveniles with high-risk profiles, including injection drug users and male adolescents who engage in homosexual activity. Postprophylaxis serologic testing is not recommended. There is no contraindication to giving hepatitis A vaccine to an individual who may be immune as the result of a previous hepatitis A infection or immunization. Incarcerated juveniles found to have hepatitis A disease should be reported to the local health department.

Hepatitis B

The rate of hepatitis B infection in the general population in the United States is influenced by well-recognized risk factors that promote exchange of or exposure to blood, saliva, semen, and vaginal fluid (see Hepatitis B, p 318). At-risk adolescents in corrections facilities include inmates from minority populations (Asian, American Indian/Alaska Native, black, and Hispanic, in descending order of hepatitis B disease prevalence); inmates engaged in injection drug use with needle sharing; inmates who have had early initiation of sexual intercourse, unprotected sexual activity, multiple sexual partners, or history of STDs; and male adolescents who engage in homosexual activity. Studies investigating hepatitis B outbreaks in prison settings also suggest that horizontal transmission may occur when chronic carriers of hepatitis B virus are present. Adolescent female inmates present additional challenges for hepatitis B assessment and management if they are discovered to be pregnant during incarceration, in which case care coordination for mother and infant become paramount.

Although no published national studies have determined hepatitis B prevalence rates for incarcerated juveniles, rates of hepatitis B seroprevalence in homeless and high-risk street youth are higher when compared with peers lacking risk factors. Beginning in 1996, widespread use of hepatitis B vaccine in states with hepatitis B immunization requirements for elementary and middle school (www.immunize.org/laws) has contributed to more than 40% of young inmates incarcerated in those states testing positive for anti-HBs (antibody to hepatitis B surface antigen [HBsAg]) when screened. Without hepatitis B core antibody data available, determining seroprevalence resulting from hepatitis B infection is difficult.

The United States embarked on a campaign in 1982 to eradicate hepatitis B as a national health threat. Phase I was directed at high-risk cohorts that included injection drug users, health care personnel, homosexual men, and HBsAg-positive mothers capable of vertical perinatal exposure to their infants. The failure of this strategy to convince high-risk individuals to be tested and immunized led to phase II (1992), the continued encouragement of prenatal testing of pregnant women for HBsAg begun in 1988 coupled with universal immunization of infants with hepatitis B vaccine. Phase III (1996) focused on immunizing all adolescents with hepatitis B vaccine starting with middle school cohorts as the means to hasten the level of protection for an age group likely to engage in high-risk behaviors. Emphasis on phase I target groups of high risk subsequently has been revived, and government support through the Vaccines For Children program has been directed to STD and family planning clinics, adolescent and teen clinics, and juvenile detention and drug treatment sites. The overall success resulting from full implementation of all 3 phases of hepatitis B prevention strategy has been a decrease in estimated annual cases from more than 300 000 new cases in the 1980s to fewer than 79 000 new cases in 1999. Some states have begun to focus their resources toward immunizing their prison populations not only to decrease the spread of hepatitis B within their institutions but also to protect communities and families when prisoners are released back into society.

Recommendations for Control of Hepatitis B Virus Infections in Incarcerated Youth. Routine screening of juvenile inmates for hepatitis B virus markers generally is not recommended. However, in states where high levels of adolescent hepatitis B immunization have been achieved, initial testing for hepatitis B immunity may save vaccine costs provided the speed of testing does not delay hepatitis B immunization should the patient lack immunity. Corrections facilities may wish periodically to survey juvenile inmates for hepatitis B immunity as they enter the institution to approximate hepatitis B prevalence and determine the desirability of preimmunization testing. Adolescent detainees with signs and symptoms of hepatitis should be tested for hepatitis A, hepatitis B, and hepatitis C virus to determine the presence of chronic infection and coinfection. All pregnant adolescents should be tested for HBsAg. High-risk behaviors by this population preclude reliance on negative preincarceration HBsAg test reports or a history of hepatitis B immunization. The history may be fallacious or vaccine failure may have occurred.

All adolescents receiving medical evaluation in a corrections facility should begin the hepatitis B vaccine series or complete a previously begun series unless they have proof of completion of a previous immunization series. Because there are no time limits or interval restraints on completion of a hepatitis B vaccine series, corrections officials should consider providing hepatitis B vaccine to inmates to complete a previously begun series. Flexibility in the hepatitis B immunization schedule, including use of 2-dose regimens for people 11 to 15 years of age, allows considerable latitude when choosing a regimen that maximizes the probability of completing a vaccine series while the adolescent is incarcerated or shortly thereafter (see Hepatitis B, Control Measures, p 323). However, beginning a hepatitis B vaccine series is critical, because a single dose of vaccine may confer protection from the complications of chronic carriage in a high-risk adolescent who may be lost to follow-up. Routine pre- and postimmunization serologic screening is not recommended. In states where hepatitis B vaccine school entry requirements are in place, corrections facilities may use a combination of immunization history, immunization registry data, and serologic testing to develop institutional policies regarding the need for hepatitis B immunization in specific age groups of adolescents. Corrections facilities should have mechanisms in place for completion of the hepatitis B series in the community after release of the juvenile. Immunization information should be made available to the inmate, the parents or legal guardian, the state immunization registry, and the patient's future medical home in the community.

Postexposure hepatitis B prophylaxis regimens for unimmunized incarcerated adolescents after potential percutaneous or sexual exposures to hepatitis B virus are available (see Hepatitis B, Care of Exposed People, p 331). Should the source of the exposure be found to be HBsAg positive, the unimmunized inmate exposed percutaneously should receive Hepatitis B Immune Globulin (HBIG) within 3 days of exposure. Sexual exposures do not require HBIG intervention, only completion of the hepatitis B immunization series. Exposed juveniles who have not completed their vaccine series should receive the remainder of the series as scheduled.

All pregnant adolescents should be tested for HBsAg at the time a pregnancy is discovered, regardless of hepatitis B immunization history and previous HBsAg and anti-HBs results. Pregnant adolescents who are HBsAg negative should begin the hepatitis B vaccine series as soon as possible during the course of pregnancy. Pregnancy is not a contraindication to receiving hepatitis B vaccine in any trimester. The pregnant adolescent's HBsAg status should be reported to the patient's prenatal care facility, the hospital where she will deliver the infant, and the state health department where case management assistance will occur. Infants born to HBsAg-positive mothers must receive hepatitis B vaccine and HBIG within 12 hours of birth (see Hepatitis B, Care of Exposed People, p 331).

Incarcerated adolescents who are found to have evidence of chronic hepatitis B infection should be evaluated by a specialist to determine the extent of their liver disease and their candidacy for antiviral intervention. Detainees who are HBsAg positive should be reported to the local health department to facilitate long-term follow-up on their release.

Fifteen percent to 35% of adolescents who become chronic carriers of hepatitis B virus can be expected to die from complications (cirrhosis and hepatocellular carcinoma) of their hepatitis B infection. Current treatment options for chronic hepatitis B infection include use of interferon-alfa, lamivudine, and adefovir dipivoxil (currently licensed by the US Food and Drug Administration [FDA] for people 16 years of age and older). All chronic carriers of hepatitis B virus should be immunized with hepatitis A vaccine to prevent fulminant liver disease should coinfection with hepatitis A virus occur. Inmates who are chronic hepatitis B carriers should be counseled strongly against the use and abuse of alcohol and street drugs, both of which can seriously degrade liver function in patients with hepatitis B-induced cirrhosis. Chronic carriers of hepatitis B virus may remain infectious to sexual and household contacts for life and must be counseled in this regard to protect sexual partners and household contacts.

Hepatitis C

Of the nearly 4 million cases of hepatitis C virus infection in the United States, approximately 30% can be traced to individuals who spent time within the nation's corrections institutions. Injection drug use accounts for the highest proportion of infected inmates, and exposure to multiple sexual partners is a distant second. Up to 80% of inmates who use injection street drugs will be infected with hepatitis C virus within 5 years after the onset of their drug use. Tattooing and body piercing is not thought to be a significant source of transmission of hepatitis C virus. In contrast to hepatitis A and hepatitis B virus infections, once an individual becomes infected with hepatitis C virus, chronic infection is the rule, not the exception. Up to 80% of patients with acute disease will remain chronically infected, and 20% of those will have progression to cirrhosis. The number of yearly hepatitis C virus-related deaths is now between 8000 and 10 000 individuals, which surpasses the death toll from hepatitis B virus infection by a factor of 2. Coinfection with HIV increases hepatitis C viral loads and speeds the rate of progression to cirrhosis. Coinfection with hepatitis A or hepatitis B virus increases the risk of fulminant and fatal liver disease. The sustainability of hepatitis C virus in a community is mediated through those who are chronically infected. The circulation of a segment of society in and out of the corrections system provides a steady reservoir of chronic hepatitis C virus carriage that has grown each year.

Prevalence studies of hepatitis C virus infection in incarcerated youth are limited but show an approximate twofold to fourfold increase in the rate when compared with youth who stay outside the juvenile justice system. Injection drug use is the predominant hepatitis C virus infection risk factor for detained juveniles, and remarkably, the rate is consistently higher in adolescent females than in males. Repetitive residence within the corrections system increases hepatitis C virus infection prevalence rates in adult inmates to 10 times the rate reported in the US population as a whole.

Testing inmates for hepatitis C virus infection has created conflicts for administrators of corrections facilities. Many do not view the diagnosis and potential treatment of detainees with hepatitis C virus infection as part of the corrections mission and prefer that public health systems devote their resources to dealing with the problem. Inmates commonly refuse testing, even when at high risk of hepatitis, to avoid persecution from fellow prisoners. The lack of a vaccine for hepatitis C places a substantial burden on prevention counseling to elicit changes in high-risk behaviors and health maintenance counseling to decrease health risks in those already infected. This includes lifestyle alterations and avoidance of street drug and alcohol abuse, which strongly affect chronic hepatitis C morbidity and mortality rates.

Recommendations for Control of Hepatitis C Virus Infections in Incarcerated Youth. Routine screening of incarcerated adolescents for hepatitis C virus infection is not recommended at this time. Focused screening of adult inmates on the basis of risk criteria has proven reliable and cost-effective for corrections facilities that use it consistently. Risk factor assessments of newly admitted juvenile inmates being considered for hepatitis C screening might include (1) self-reported history of injection drug use; (2) history of liver disease; (3) presence of hepatitis B core antibody; (4) increased alanine transaminase concentration; or (5) history of hemodialysis or receipt of clotting factors, blood transfusions, or organ transplants. Thirty percent of new male or female juvenile detainees can be expected to have one or more of these criteria, and hepatitis C antibody screening of this group will detect more than 90% of hepatitis C virus infections in corrections facilities. Some juvenile offenders may withhold reporting risk criteria behaviors and yet express interest in hepatitis C testing when offered as an option. These requests in most instances should be accommodated. Adolescents with signs or symptoms of hepatitis should undergo diagnostic testing for hepatitis A, hepatitis B, and hepatitis C virus to determine the presence of chronic hepatitis B and hepatitis C virus infection and susceptibility to coinfection with hepatitis A virus.

Adolescents who test positive for hepatitis C virus should receive ongoing medical attention to determine the likelihood of chronic hepatitis C virus infection, and cases should be reported to the local health department. The presence of hepatitis C virus antibody and the absence of hepatitis C virus RNA nucleic acid does not preclude the possibility of persistent chronic active disease. Hepatitis C virus antigenemia is variable from day to day and occurs in the presence of circulating hepatitis C antibody. Juveniles found to have chronic hepatitis C infection should receive ongoing medical evaluation to monitor the course of their liver disease and to determine their suitability for therapeutic interventions in the future. Incarcerated adolescents with hepatitis C should be enrolled in a risk reduction program for drug and alcohol avoidance and should receive counseling for safe sex practices for the safety of their sexual partners and the protection of the community at large (www.hepprograms.org). Recent studies evaluating antiviral therapy suggest better outcomes if treatment is initiated in a timely fashion. Treatment protocols incorporating the use of interferon-alfa, ribavirin, and pegylated interferon currently are available to adult patients with chronic hepatitis C virus infection. However, these regimens have not been licensed by the FDA for use in patients younger than 18 years of age. Consultation with a specialist familiar with chronic liver disease may help clarify what new treatment options are possible as they are approved for pediatric use (www.niddk.nih.gov/health/digest/pubs/chrnhepc/chrnhepc.htm). Incarcerated adolescents who are diagnosed with hepatitis C virus infection should be immunized against hepatitis A and hepatitis B virus if not already immune.

The pervasive nature of hepatitis in juvenile corrections populations has been established firmly. Corrections facilities, in partnership with public health departments and other community resources, have the opportunity to assess, contain, control, and prevent liver infection in a highly vulnerable segment of society. Hepatitis C presents the greatest challenge to corrections facilities overall because of the lack of a vaccine to protect prisoners and the public. The extremely high rate of chronic carriage in individuals who already are infected increases the risk to their communities on their release. The controlled nature of the corrections system allows the initiation of many hepatitis prevention and treatment strategies for a pediatric population who otherwise are difficult to reach. Pediatricians should work with state and local public health agencies and corrections administrators to address the health needs of youth in detention and to protect the community as a whole.

······························

MEDICAL EVALUATION OF INTERNATIONALLY ADOPTED CHILDREN FOR INFECTIOUS DISEASES*

Annually, more than 18 000 children from other countries are adopted by families in the United States. More than 90% of international adoptees are from Asian (China, South Korea, Vietnam, India, and Cambodia), Central and South American (Guatemala and Colombia), and Eastern European countries (Russia, Romania, Ukraine, Kazakhstan, and Bulgaria). Africa and the Middle East remain uncommon origins for international adoptees. The diverse origins of these children, their unknown medical histories before adoption, their previous living circumstances (eg, orphanages and/or foster care), and the limited availability of reliable health care in some developing countries, make the medical evaluation of internationally adopted children a challenging but important task.

---

* For additional information, see Canadian Paediatric Society. *Children and Youth New to Canada: Health Care Guide.* Ottawa, Ontario: Canadian Paediatric Society; 1998; and the CDC (www.cdc.gov) and World Health Organization (www.who.int) Web sites.

Internationally adopted children may differ from refugee children in terms of their medical evaluation and treatment before arrival in the United States and in the frequency of certain infectious diseases. Refugee children may have resided in processing camps for months and may have received medical care and treatment, but the history of access to and quality of medical care for international adoptees can be variable. All internationally adopted and refugee children are required to have a medical examination performed by a physician designated by the US State Department in their country of origin before admission to the United States. However, this examination is limited to completing legal requirements for screening for certain communicable diseases and examination for serious physical or mental defects that would prevent the issue of a permanent residency visa. This evaluation is not a comprehensive assessment of the child's health. Accompanying health documents for internationally adopted children commonly are out-of-date and may be inaccurate, and there is no simple method of determining whether the records are reliable. Therefore, medical evaluation and treatment based solely on these records may lead to inadequate screening for infectious diseases and delay initiation or result in omission of preventive health care, such as immunizations.

Infectious diseases are among the most common medical diagnoses identified in international adoptees on initial screening after arrival in the United States. Children may be asymptomatic and, therefore, the diagnoses must be made by screening tests in addition to history and physical examination. Because of the lack of perinatal screening for hepatitis B virus, syphilis, and human immunodeficiency virus (HIV) and the high prevalence of certain intestinal parasites and tuberculosis, all international adoptees should be screened for these infections on arrival in the United States. Suggested screening tests for infectious diseases are listed in Table 2.17, p 175 (see also disease-specific chapters in Section 3). In addition to these infections, other medical and developmental issues, including hearing and vision assessment, evaluation of growth and development, nutritional assessment, determining exposure to lead, complete blood cell count with red blood cell indices, and examination for congenital anomalies, should be part of the evaluation of any internationally adopted child.

Internationally adopted children should be examined within 2 weeks of arrival in the United States or earlier if there are immediate health concerns. Parents generally will have limited information about a child before the adoption. It is helpful to have the parents meet with a physician before the adoption to review available information and to discuss common medical issues regarding adoptive children. Parents who have not met with a physician before adoption should notify their physician when their child arrives so that a timely medical evaluation can be arranged.

Viral Hepatitis

The prevalence of markers for hepatitis B virus (HBV) infection, including hepatitis B surface antigen (HBsAg), in internationally adopted children ranges from 1% to 5%, depending on the country of origin and year studied. Hepatitis B is most prevalent in adoptees from Asia, Africa, and some countries in central and eastern Europe (eg, Romania) and the newly independent states of the former Soviet Union (eg, Russia and Ukraine). However, HBV infection also occurs in adoptees coming

Table 2.17. Screening Tests for Infectious Diseases in International Adoptees

Hepatitis B virus serologic testing:
  Hepatitis B surface antigen (HBsAg)
  Hepatitis B surface antibody (anti-HBs)
  Hepatitis B core antibody (anti-HBc)

Hepatitis C virus serologic testing (see text)

Syphilis serologic testing
  Nontreponemal test (RPR, VDRL, ART)
  Treponemal test (MHA-TP, FTA-ABS)

Human immunodeficiency virus 1 and 2 serologic testing

Complete blood cell count with red blood cell indices

Stool examination for ova and parasites (3 specimens)[1]

Stool examination for *Giardia lamblia* and *Cryptosporidia* antigen (1 specimen)[1]

Tuberculin skin test[1]

RPR indicates rapid plasma reagin; VDRL, Venereal Disease Research Laboratories; ART, automated reagin test; MHA-TP, microhemagglutination test for *Treponema pallidum*; FTA-ABS, fluorescent treponemal antibody absorption.

[1] See text.

---

from other countries. Therefore, all children should undergo serologic testing for hepatitis B infection, including HBsAg, antibody to HBsAg (anti-HBs), and antibody to hepatitis B core antigen (anti-HBc), to identify current or chronic infection, past resolved infection, or evidence of immunization (see Hepatitis B, p 318). Hepatitis B virus tests performed in the country of origin may not be useful, because often only a "hepatitis B" test without specific designation is recorded, and even when recorded, accuracy can vary. Because HBV has a long incubation period, the child may have become infected at or near the time testing was performed. Therefore, consideration should be given to a repeated evaluation 6 months after adoption. Chronic HBV infection is indicated by persistence of HBsAg for more than 6 months. Children with HBsAg-positive test results should be evaluated to verify the presence of chronic HBV infection and to assess for biochemical evidence of chronic liver disease and for severity of disease and possible treatment (see Hepatitis B, p 318).

All family members should be immunized against hepatitis B before arrival of the adoptee, regardless of results of hepatitis B testing of the child. Although institution of universal childhood HBV immunization in the United States should help decrease the risk of hepatitis B infection in school and household contacts of the adopted child, many adults may not be immunized against hepatitis B. All susceptible household contacts of a child found to be HBsAg-positive after arrival in the United States should be immunized against HBV. Adopted children who test negative for hepatitis B should receive immunization for HBV as soon as possible according to the recommended childhood and adolescent immunization schedule (Fig 1.1, p 24). Children who test positive for HBsAg and anti-HBc need not be immunized.

Hepatitis D virus, which occurs only in conjunction with active HBV replication, may be found in adoptees, particularly from Eastern Europe, Africa, South America, and the Middle East. Serologic tests for diagnosis of hepatitis D virus infection are available (see Hepatitis D, p 340), but routine testing is not recommended, because a positive test does not alter clinical management.

Many internationally adopted children have acquired hepatitis A virus (HAV) infection early in life and are, therefore, protected. Routine serologic screening for HAV antibody generally is not indicated to detect susceptible children. However, because routine childhood immunization against HAV is recommended in some areas of the United States beginning at 2 years of age (see Hepatitis A, p 309), antibody testing for HAV may be considered to be cost-effective to determine whether these children have evidence of previous infection. If a child has no evidence of previous infection and lives in a high-risk area, the child should be immunized against HAV.

Serologic screening for hepatitis C virus infection is not indicated routinely because of the low prevalence of infection in most areas. However, children from China, Russia, Eastern Europe, and Southeast Asia should be screened. The decision to screen children from other areas should depend on history (eg, receipt of blood products, maternal drug use) and prevalence of infection in the child's country of origin.

Cytomegalovirus

Routine screening for cytomegalovirus is not recommended.

Intestinal Pathogens

Fecal examinations for ova and parasites by an experienced laboratory will identify a pathogen in 15% to 35% of internationally adopted children. The prevalence of intestinal parasites varies by age of the child and country of origin. The most common pathogens identified are *Giardia lamblia, Hymenolepis species, Ascaris lumbricoides,* and *Trichuris trichiura. Strongyloides stercoralis, Entamoeba histolytica,* and hookworm are recovered less commonly. One stool specimen generally is sufficient for testing for intestinal ova and parasites in asymptomatic children, although some experts recommend that 3 specimens be tested to detect *Ascaris* and tapeworm infections, which may be asymptomatic. If gastrointestinal tract signs or symptoms or malnutrition are present, these symptomatic children should have 3 stool specimens examined for ova and parasites in addition to a single stool specimen screened for antigen for *G lamblia* and *Cryptosporidium parvum.* In addition, children with diarrhea should have stool specimens cultured for *Salmonella* species, *Shigella* species, *Campylobacter* species, and *Escherichia coli* O157:H7. Therapy for intestinal parasites generally will be successful, but complete eradication may not occur always. Therefore, repeat ova and parasite testing after treatment in children who remain symptomatic is important to ensure successful elimination of parasites. In addition, children with gastrointestinal tract symptoms or signs that occur or recur months or even years after arrival in the United States should be reevaluated for intestinal parasites. Some intestinal parasites, such as *Cyclospora* species and *S stercoralis,* may not be detected by standard ova and parasite screening.

Tuberculosis

Tuberculosis commonly is encountered in international adoptees. Reported rates of latent *Mycobacterium tuberculosis* infection range from 0.6% to 19%. Because tuberculosis may be more severe in young children and may reactivate in later years, screening with the tuberculin skin test (TST) particularly is important in this high-risk population (see Tuberculosis, p 642). Routine chest radiography is not indicated in asymptomatic children in whom the TST result is negative. However, because malnutrition is common among international adoptees, there is concern that some international adoptees may be anergic. If malnutrition is suspected, the TST should be repeated once the child is better nourished. Receipt of bacille Calmette-Guérin (BCG) vaccine is not a contraindication to a TST, and a positive TST result should not be attributed to BCG vaccine. In these children, further investigation is necessary to determine whether tuberculosis is present and therapy is needed (see Tuberculosis, p 642). When tuberculosis is suspected in an international adoptee, efforts to isolate and test the organism for drug susceptibilities are imperative because of the high prevalence of drug resistance in many countries.

Syphilis

Congenital syphilis, especially with involvement of the central nervous system, may not have been diagnosed or may have been treated inadequately in adoptees from some developing countries. Each international adoptee should be screened for syphilis by reliable nontreponemal and treponemal serologic tests, regardless of history or a report of treatment (see Syphilis, p 595). Children with positive treponemal serologic test results should be evaluated to determine the extent of infection so appropriate treatment can be administered (see Syphilis, p 595).

Human Immunodeficiency Virus Infection

The risk of HIV infection in internationally adopted children depends on the country of origin and individual risk factors. Because of the rapidly changing epidemiology of HIV infection and because adoptees may come from populations at high risk of infection, screening for HIV should be performed on all internationally adopted children. Although many children will have an HIV result documented in their referral information, test results from the child's country of origin may not be reliable. Transplacentally acquired maternal antibody in the absence of infection can be detected in a child younger than 18 months of age. Hence, positive HIV antibody test results in asymptomatic children of this age require clinical evaluation, follow-up testing, and counseling (see Human Immunodeficiency Virus Infection, p 360).

Other Infectious Diseases

Bacterial and fungal skin infections that commonly occur in international adoptees include ectoparasitic infections, such as scabies and pediculosis. Adoptive families should be instructed to examine their child for signs of scabies and pediculosis so that treatment can be initiated and transmission to family members can be prevented (see Scabies, p 547, and Pediculosis, pp 463–467). Diseases such as typhoid fever, malaria, leprosy, or melioidosis are encountered infrequently in internationally adopted children. Although routine screening for these diseases is not recommended, findings of fever, splenomegaly, respiratory tract infection, anemia, or eosinophilia should prompt an appropriate evaluation on the basis of the epidemiology of infectious diseases that occur in the child's country of origin to identify the etiology of the illness. If the child came from a country where malaria is present, malaria should be considered in the differential diagnosis (see Malaria, p 414).

Clinicians should be aware of potential diseases in internationally adopted children and their clinical manifestations. Some diseases, such as central nervous system cysticercosis, may have long incubation periods and, thus, may not be detected during initial screening. Therefore, on the basis of findings of the initial evaluation, consideration should be given to a repeat evaluation 6 months after adoption. In most cases, the longer the interval from adoption to development of a clinical syndrome, the less likely the syndrome can be attributed to a pathogen acquired in the country of origin.

Immunizations

Some international adoptees will have written documentation of immunizations received in their birth country. Although immunizations such as BCG, diphtheria and tetanus toxoids and pertussis (DTP), poliovirus, measles, and hepatitis B often are documented, other immunizations such as *Haemophilus influenzae* type b, mumps, and rubella vaccines infrequently are given, and *Streptococcus pneumoniae* and varicella vaccines rarely are given. Internationally adopted children and adolescents should receive immunizations according to the recommended schedules in the United States for healthy children and adolescents (see Fig 1.1, p 24, and Table 1.6, p 26) or from the World Health Organization. In general, written documentation of immunizations should not be accepted as unequivocal evidence of adequacy of previous immunization unless the vaccines, dates of administration, number of doses, intervals between doses, and age of the patient at the time of immunization are comparable to current US or World Health Organization schedules (see Immunizations Received Outside the United States, p 34). Although some vaccines with inadequate potency have been produced in other countries, most vaccines used worldwide are produced with adequate quality control standards and are reliable. However, information about storage, handling, site of administration, vaccine potency, and provider generally is not available. Given the limited data available regarding verification of immunization records from other countries, evaluation of concentrations of antibody to the antigens given may be an option to ensure that vaccines were given and were immunogenic. Serologic testing may be performed to determine whether protective antibody concentrations are present. An equally acceptable alternative when doubt exists is to reimmunize the child.

Table 2.18 (p 179) lists the vaccines for which antibody testing can be performed, specifies the types of tests to be ordered, and provides a recommended and alternative approaches. In children older than 6 months of age with or without written documentation of immunization, one could consider antibody testing for diphtheria and tetanus, hepatitis B virus, and poliovirus to determine whether the child has protective concentrations of antibody. If the child has protective concentrations, then the immunization series should be completed as appropriate for that child's age.

Table 2.18. Approaches to the Evaluation and Immunization of Internationally Adopted Children[1]

Vaccine	Recommended Approach	Alternative Approach
Hepatitis B	Serologic testing for hepatitis B surface antigen	—
Diphtheria and tetanus toxoids and acellular pertussis (DTaP)	Immunize with DTaP, with serologic testing for specific IgG antibody to tetanus and diphtheria toxins in the event of a severe local reaction to first dose	Children whose records indicate receipt of ≥3 doses: serologic testing for specific IgG antibody to diphtheria and tetanus toxins before administering additional doses or administer a single booster dose of DTaP, followed by serologic testing after 1 month for specific IgG antibody to diphtheria and tetanus toxins with reimmunization as appropriate (see text)
Haemophilus influenzae type b (Hib)	Age-appropriate immunization	—
Poliovirus	Immunize with inactivated poliovirus vaccine (IPV)	Serologic testing for neutralizing antibody to poliovirus types 1, 2, and 3 (limited availability) or administer single dose of IPV, followed by serologic testing for neutralizing antibody to poliovirus types 1, 2, and 3
Measles-mumps-rubella (MMR)	Immunize with MMR or obtain measles antibody and if positive, give MMR for mumps and rubella protection	Serologic testing for immunoglobulin G (IgG) antibody to vaccine viruses indicated by immunization record
Varicella	Age-appropriate immunization of children who lack reliable history of previous varicella disease or serologic evidence of protection	—
Pneumococcal	Age-appropriate immunization	—

[1] Centers for Disease Control and Prevention. General recommendations on immunization. Recommendations of the Advisory Committee on Immunization Practices and the American Academy of Family Physicians. *MMWR Recomm Rep.* 2002;51(RR-2):1–35. Also see Fig 1.1 (p 24) and Table 1.6 (p 26).

Measles, mumps, and rubella antibody may be measured to determine whether the child is immune. Many children will need a dose of mumps and rubella vaccines, because these vaccines are administered infrequently in developing countries. Testing for measles antibody can be performed, and if positive, one dose of MMR could be administered for mumps and rubella coverage. Antibody testing for measles and varicella should not be performed in children younger than 12 months of age because of the potential presence of maternal antibody. At this time, there is no antibody testing that is reliable or available routinely to assess immunity to pertussis. If serologic testing is not available and receipt of immunogenic vaccines cannot be ensured, the prudent course is to repeat the series.

INJURIES FROM DISCARDED NEEDLES IN THE COMMUNITY

Contact with and injuries from hypodermic needles and syringes presumably discarded in public places by injection drug users are perceived by some people as posing a significant risk for transmission of bloodborne pathogens, especially human immunodeficiency virus (HIV). Although these injuries may pose less of a risk than needlestick injuries that occur in health care settings, the injured person often needs evaluation and counseling. Even if the possibility that the discarded syringe might contain a bloodborne pathogen can be estimated from the prevalence rates of these infections in the local community, the need to test the injured or exposed person usually is not influenced significantly by this assessment.

Management of people with needlestick injuries includes acute wound care, consideration of the need for prophylaxis, and prevention. Standard wound cleansing and care is indicated; such wounds rarely require closure. Tetanus toxoid and Tetanus Immune Globulin should be administered as appropriate for the immunization status of the victim (see Tetanus, p 611).

Consideration of the need for prophylaxis for bloodborne viruses, namely hepatitis B virus (HBV), HIV, and hepatitis C virus (HCV), is the next step in exposure management. Risk of acquisition of various pathogens depends on the nature of the wound, the ability of the pathogens to survive on environmental surfaces, prevalence rates among local injection drug users, and the probability that the syringe and needle came from a local injection drug user. Unlike an occupational blood or body fluid exposure in which the status of the exposure source for HBV, HCV, and HIV often is known, these data usually are not available to help in the decision-making process in a nonoccupational exposure.*

Hepatitis B virus is the hardiest of the major bloodborne pathogens and can survive on environmental surfaces for at least 7 days. Children who have not completed the 3-dose HBV immunization series should receive a dose of vaccine and, if indicated, should be scheduled to receive the remaining doses to complete the schedule. Administration of Hepatitis B Immune Globulin usually is not indicated

---

* Centers for Disease Control and Prevention. Updated US Public Health Service guidelines for the management of occupational exposures to HBV, HCV, and HIV and recommendations for postexposure prophylaxis. *MMWR Recomm Rep.* 2001;50(RR-11):1–52

if the child has received the 3-dose regimen of HBV vaccine (see Table 3.22, p 335). However, experts differ in opinion about the need for Hepatitis B Immune Globulin at the time of an injury of an incompletely immunized child. If the child has received 2 doses of HBV vaccine 4 or more months previously, the immediate administration of the third dose of vaccine alone should be sufficient in most cases.

Infection with HIV usually is the greatest concern of the family and victim. The need for initial baseline serologic tests for preexisting HIV infection is controversial. Negative results from these initial tests support the conclusion that any subsequent positive test result reflects infection acquired from the needlestick. A positive test result in the pediatric patient requires further investigation of the cause, such as perinatal transmission, sexual abuse or activity, or drug use. An alternative option is to obtain and save a baseline serum specimen for later testing for HIV antibody in the unlikely event that a subsequent test result is positive. Counseling is necessary before and after testing (see Human Immunodeficiency Virus Infection, p 360).

The risk of HIV transmission from a needle discarded in public is low. Risk of HIV transmission from a puncture wound attributable to a needle found in the community is lower than the 0.3% risk of HIV transmission to a health care worker from a needlestick injury from a person with known HIV infection. Data are not available on the efficacy of postexposure prophylaxis with antiretroviral drugs in these circumstances for adults or children, and as a result, the US Public Health Service is unable to recommend for or against prophylaxis in this circumstance.*† Furthermore, antiretroviral therapy is not without risk and often is associated with significant adverse effects (see Human Immunodeficiency Virus Infection, p 360). Therefore, postexposure prophylaxis is not recommended routinely in this situation. However, some experts recommend that antiretroviral chemoprophylaxis be considered if the needle and/or syringe are available and found to contain visible blood and the source is an HIV-infected person. Other experts recommend chemoprophylaxis if blood was visible on the syringe or needle, and other experts recommend chemoprophylaxis for any needlestick injury. Testing the syringe for HIV is not practical or reliable and is not recommended. Consultation with a specialist in HIV infection should be obtained before deciding to initiate postexposure chemoprophylaxis. If the decision is to begin prophylaxis, any delay before starting the medications should be minimized (see Human Immunodeficiency Virus Infection, p 360). The suggested medication options are the same as for HIV occupational exposure (see Human Immunodeficiency Virus Infection, p 360).

Follow-up testing of a child for serum HIV antibody should include testing at 6 months and also at 6 and 12 weeks after injury. Testing also is indicated if an illness consistent with acute HIV-related syndrome develops before the 6-week testing (see Human Immunodeficiency Virus Infection, p 360).

The third bloodborne pathogen of concern is HCV. Although transmission by sharing syringes among injection drug users is efficient, the risk of transmission from a discarded syringe is low, because the viability of this virus on environmental

---

* Centers for Disease Control and Prevention. Management of possible sexual, injecting-drug-use, or other nonoccupational exposure to HIV, including considerations related to antiretroviral therapy: Public Health Service statement. *MMWR Recomm Rep.* 1998;47(RR-17):1–14
† American Academy of Pediatrics, Committee on Pediatric AIDS. Postexposure prophylaxis in children and adolescents for nonoccupational exposure to human immunodeficiency virus. *Pediatrics.* In press

surfaces is poor. Immune Globulin preparations and antiviral drugs have not been demonstrated to protect against HCV infection. The need for testing for HCV is uncertain. If performed, testing for antibody to HCV should be performed at the time of injury and 6 months later. Positive test results should be confirmed by supplemental confirmatory laboratory tests (see Hepatitis C, p 336).

Needlestick injuries of children can be minimized by public health programs on safe needle disposal and by programs for exchange of used syringes and needles from injection drug users for sterile ones. Needle and syringe exchanges decrease improper disposal and the spread of bloodborne pathogens without increasing the rate of injection drug use. The American Academy of Pediatrics supports needle-exchange programs in conjunction with drug treatment and within the context of continuing research to document their effectiveness.

....

BITE WOUNDS

As many as 1% of all pediatric visits to emergency departments during summer months are for treatment of human or animal bite wounds. An estimated 4.5 million dog bites, 400 000 cat bites, and 250 000 human bites occur annually in the United States. The rate of infection after cat bites can be more than 50%, and rates of infection after dog or human bites can be 15% to 20%. The bites of humans, wild animals, or exotic pets potentially are sources of serious infection. Parents should be informed to teach children to avoid contact with wild animals and should secure garbage containers so that raccoons and other animals will not be attracted to the home and places where children may play. Concern for transmission of rabies should be increased when a bite is from a wild animal (especially a bat or a carnivore) or from a domestic animal that cannot be observed for 10 days after the bite (see Rabies, p 514). Dead animals should be avoided, because they may harbor rabies virus in their nervous system tissues and saliva and they may be infested with arthropods (fleas or ticks) infected with a variety of bacterial, rickettsial, protozoan, or viral agents.

Recommendations for bite wound management are given in Table 2.19 (p 183). Sufficient, prospective, controlled studies on which to base recommendations about the closure of bite wounds are lacking. In general, recent, apparently noninfected, low-risk lesions may be sutured after thorough wound cleansing, irrigation, and débridement. Use of local anesthesia can facilitate these procedures. Because suturing can enhance the risk of wound infection, some clinicians prefer that small wounds be managed by approximation of the wound edges with adhesive strips or tissue adhesive. Bite wounds on the face, which have important cosmetic considerations, seldom become infected and should be closed whenever possible. Hand and foot wounds have a higher risk of infection and should be managed in consultation with an appropriate surgical specialist. Elevation of injured areas to minimize swelling is important.

Limited data exist to guide antimicrobial therapy for patients with wounds that are not infected overtly. The use of an antimicrobial agent within 8 hours of injury for a 2- to 3-day course of therapy may decrease the rate of infection. Children at high risk of infection (eg, who are immunocompromised or when joint penetration occurs) should receive empiric therapy. Patients with mild injuries in which the skin

Table 2.19. **Prophylactic Management of Human or Animal Bite Wounds to Prevent Infection**

Category of Management	Time From Injury	
	<8 h	≥8 h
Method of cleansing	Sponge away visible dirt. Irrigate with a copious volume of sterile saline solution by high-pressure syringe irrigation.[1] Do not irrigate puncture wounds.	Same as that for wounds of <8 h duration
Wound culture	No, unless signs of infection exist	Yes, except in wounds of >24 h duration and without signs of infection
Débridement	Remove devitalized tissue	Same as that for wounds of <8 h duration
Operative débridement and exploration	Yes, if one of the following: • Extensive wounds (devitalized tissue) • Involvement of the metacarpophalangeal joint (closed fist injury) • Cranial bites by large animal[2]	Same as that for wounds of <8 h duration
Wound closure	Yes, for nonpuncture bite wounds	No
Assess tetanus immunization status[3]	Yes	Yes
Assess risk of rabies from animal bites[4]	Yes	Yes
Assess risk of hepatitis B from human bites[5]	Yes	Yes
Assess risk of human immunodeficiency virus from human bites[6]	Yes	Yes

Table 2.19. Prophylactic Management of Human or Animal Bite Wounds to Prevent Infection, continued

Category of Management	Time From Injury	
	<8 h	≥8 h
Initiate antimicrobial therapy[7]	Yes, for: • Moderate or severe bite wounds, especially if edema or crush injury is present • Puncture wounds, especially if penetration of bone, tendon sheath, or joint has occurred • Facial bites • Hand and foot bites • Genital area bites • Wounds in immunocompromised and asplenic people	Same as that for wounds of <8 h duration and for bite wounds with signs of infection
Follow-up	Inspect wound for signs of infection within 48 h	Same as that for wounds of <8 h duration

1. Use of an 18-gauge needle with a large-volume syringe is effective. Antimicrobial or anti-infective solutions offer no advantage and may increase tissue irritation.
2. Radiographic studies in facial and head injuries are indicated if penetrating central nervous system injury is suspected.
3. See Tetanus, p 611.
4. See Rabies, p 514.
5. See Hepatitis B, p 318.
6. See Human Immunodeficiency Virus Infection, p 360.
7. See Table 2.20 (p 185) for suggested drug choices.

Table 2.20. Antimicrobial Agents for Human or Animal Bite Wounds

Source of Bite	Organism(s) Likely to Cause Infection	Antimicrobial Agent			
		Oral Route	Oral Alternatives for Penicillin-Allergic Patients[1]	Intravenous Route	Intravenous Alternatives for Penicillin-Allergic Patients[1]
Dog/cat	Pasteurella species, Staphylococcus aureus, streptococci, anaerobes, Capnocytophaga species, Moraxella species, Corynebacterium species, Neisseria species	Amoxicillin-clavulanate potassium	Extended-spectrum cephalosporin or trimethoprim-sulfamethoxazole PLUS clindamycin hydrochloride	Ampicillin-sulbactam sodium[2]	Extended-spectrum cephalosporin or trimethoprim-sulfamethoxazole PLUS clindamycin
Reptile	Enteric gram-negative bacteria, anaerobes	Amoxicillin-clavulanate	Extended-spectrum cephalosporin or trimethoprim-sulfamethoxazole PLUS clindamycin	Ampicillin-sulbactam[2] PLUS gentamicin sulfate	Clindamycin PLUS gentamicin
Human	Streptococci, S aureus, Eikenella corrodens, anaerobes	Amoxicillin-clavulanate	Trimethoprim-sulfamethoxazole PLUS clindamycin	Ampicillin-sulbactam[2]	Extended-spectrum cephalosporin or trimethoprim-sulfamethoxazole PLUS clindamycin

1 For patients with history of allergy to penicillin or one of its congeners, alternative drugs are recommended. In some circumstances, a cephalosporin or other β-lactam class drug may be acceptable. However, these drugs should not be used for patients with an immediate hypersensitivity (anaphylaxis) to penicillin, because approximately 5% to 15% of penicillin-allergic patients also will be allergic to cephalosporins.

2 Ticarcillin-clavulanate may be used as an alternative.

only is abraded do not need to be treated with antimicrobial agents. Guidelines for choice of antimicrobial therapy regimen for human and animal bites are given in Table 2.20 (p 185) and reflect the organisms likely to cause infection for each biting species. Empiric therapy may be modified when culture results become available.

Prophylaxis or treatment of the penicillin-allergic child with a human or animal bite wound is problematic. Activity of erythromycin or doxycycline against *Staphylococcus aureus* and anaerobes is unpredictable, and the use of tetracyclines, which have activity against *Pasteurella multocida,* in children younger than 8 years of age must be weighed against the risk of permanent dental staining. Azithromycin dihydrate displays good in vitro activity against organisms that commonly cause bite wound infections, except for some strains of staphylococci, but there are no clinical trials documenting its efficacy. Azithromycin should not be used for treatment of bite wound infections. Oral or parenteral treatment with trimethoprim-sulfamethoxazole, which is effective against *S aureus, P multocida,* and *Eikenella corrodens,* in conjunction with clindamycin hydrochloride, which is active in vitro against anaerobic bacteria, streptococci, and *S aureus,* may be effective for preventing bite wound infections. Cefotaxime sodium or ceftriaxone sodium can be used as alternative parenteral therapy for penicillin-allergic patients who can tolerate cephalosporins; clindamycin is an alternative for patients who also are allergic to cephalosporin.

PREVENTION OF TICKBORNE INFECTIONS

Tickborne infectious diseases in the United States include those caused by bacteria (eg, Lyme disease, tularemia, relapsing fever), rickettsia (eg, Rocky Mountain spotted fever, ehrlichiosis), viruses (eg, Colorado tick fever), and protozoa (eg, babesiosis) (see also disease-specific chapters in Section 3). Physicians should be aware of the epidemiology of tickborne infections in their local areas. Prevention of tickborne diseases is accomplished through avoidance of tick-infested habitats, personal protection against tick bites, decreasing tick populations in the environment, and limiting the length of time ticks remain attached to the human host. Control of tick populations in the field often is not practical. Specific measures for prevention are as follows:
- Physicians, parents, and children should be aware that ticks transmit diseases.
- Tick-infested areas should be avoided whenever possible.
- If a tick-infested area is entered, clothing that covers the arms, legs, and other exposed areas should be worn, pants should be tucked into boots or socks, and long-sleeved shirts should be buttoned at the cuff. In addition, permethrin (a synthetic pyrethroid) can be sprayed onto clothes to decrease tick attachment. Permethrin should not be sprayed onto skin.
- Tick and insect repellents that contain diethyltoluamide (DEET) applied to the skin provide additional protection but require reapplication every 1 to 2 hours for maximum effectiveness. Although there have been rare reports of serious neurologic complications in children resulting from the frequent and excessive application of DEET-containing insect repellents, the risk is low when they are used properly. Products with DEET should be applied sparingly according to label instructions and not applied to a child's face, hands, or any skin that is irritated

or abraded. After the child returns indoors, treated skin should be washed with soap and water.

- People should inspect themselves and their children's bodies and clothing daily after possible tick exposure. Special attention should be given to the exposed hairy regions of the body where ticks often attach, including the head and neck in children. Ticks also may attach at areas of tight clothing (eg, belt line, axillae). Ticks should be removed promptly. For removal, a tick should be grasped with a fine tweezers close to the skin and gently pulled straight out without twisting motions. If fingers are used to remove ticks, they should be protected with tissue and washed after removal of the tick.
- Maintaining tick-free pets also may decrease tick exposure. Daily inspection of pets and removal of ticks are indicated, as is the use of appropriate veterinary products to prevent ticks on pets.

Summaries of Infectious Diseases

Actinomycosis

CLINICAL MANIFESTATIONS: The 3 major anatomic types of disease are cervico-facial, thoracic, and abdominal. Cervicofacial lesions are the most common and often occur after tooth extraction, oral surgery, or facial trauma or are associated with carious teeth. Localized pain and induration progress to "woody hard" nodular lesions that can be complicated by draining sinus tracts that usually are located at the angle of the jaw or in the submandibular region. The infection usually spreads by direct invasion of adjacent tissues. Infection also may contribute to chronic obstructive tonsillitis. Thoracic disease most commonly is secondary to aspiration of oropharyngeal secretions and occurs rarely after esophageal disruption secondary to surgery or nonpenetrating trauma or may be an extension of cervicofacial infection. Disease manifests as pneumonia, which can be complicated by abscesses, empyema, and rarely, pleurodermal sinuses. Focal or multifocal masses may be mistaken for tumors. Abdominal actinomycosis usually is attributable to penetrating trauma or intestinal perforation. The appendix and cecum are the most common sites, and symptoms are similar to those of appendicitis. Slowly developing masses may simulate abdominal or retroperitoneal neoplasms. Intra-abdominal abscesses and peritoneal-dermal draining sinuses eventually occur. Chronic localized disease often forms sinus tracts that drain a purulent discharge. Other sites of actinomycosis include pelvic infection, which has been linked to the use of intrauterine devices, and brain abscesses.

ETIOLOGY: *Actinomyces israelii* is the usual cause. *Actinomyces israelii* and at least 5 other *Actinomyces* species are slow-growing, gram-positive, anaerobic, filamentous, branching bacilli that can be part of the normal oral, gastrointestinal, or vaginal flora.

EPIDEMIOLOGY: *Actinomyces* species are worldwide in distribution. Infection is rare in infants and children. The organisms are components of the endogenous gastrointestinal tract flora. *Actinomyces* species are opportunistic pathogens, and disease results from penetrating (including human bite wounds) and nonpenetrating trauma.

The **incubation period** varies from several days to several years.

DIAGNOSTIC TESTS: A microscopic demonstration of beaded, branched, gram-positive bacilli in purulent material or tissue specimens suggests the diagnosis. Acid-fast staining can be used to distinguish *Actinomyces* species, which are acid-fast negative, from *Nocardia* species, which are variably acid-fast positive. "Sulfur granules" in drainage or loculations of purulent material usually are yellow and may be visualized microscopically or macroscopically and suggest the diagnosis when present. A Gram stain of sulfur granules discloses a dense reticulum of filaments; the ends of individual filaments may project around the periphery of the granule, with or without radially arranged hyaline clubs. Immunofluorescence stains for *Actinomyces* species are available. Specimens must be obtained, transported, and cultured anaerobically on semiselective media.

TREATMENT: Initial therapy should include intravenous penicillin G or ampicillin for 4 to 6 weeks followed by high doses of oral penicillin (up to 2 g/day for adults), amoxicillin, erythromycin, clindamycin, doxycycline, or tetracycline for a total of 6 to 12 months. Tetracyclines are not recommended for children younger than 8 years of age. Surgical drainage may be a necessary adjunct to medical management.

ISOLATION OF THE HOSPITALIZED PATIENT: Standard precautions are recommended. There is no person-to-person spread.

CONTROL MEASURES: Appropriate oral hygiene, regular dental care, and careful cleansing of wounds, including human bite wounds, can prevent infection.

Adenovirus Infections

CLINICAL MANIFESTATIONS: The most common site of adenovirus infection is the upper respiratory tract. Manifestations include symptoms of the common cold, pharyngitis, tonsillitis, otitis media, and pharyngoconjunctival fever. Life-threatening disseminated infection, severe pneumonia, meningitis, and encephalitis occasionally occur, especially among young infants and immunocompromised hosts. Adenoviruses are infrequent causes of acute hemorrhagic conjunctivitis, a pertussis-like syndrome, croup, bronchiolitis, and hemorrhagic cystitis. A few adenovirus serotypes cause gastroenteritis.

ETIOLOGY: Adenoviruses are double-stranded, nonenveloped DNA viruses; at least 51 distinct serotypes divided into 6 species (A to F) cause human infections. Some adenovirus serotypes are more commonly associated with specific syndromes; for example, adenovirus types 3, 4, 7, and 21 are associated with acute respiratory tract disease, particularly in unimmunized new military recruits; types 8, 18, and 37 are associated with epidemic keratoconjunctivitis; and types 40, 41, and to a lesser extent, 31 are associated with gastroenteritis.

EPIDEMIOLOGY: Infection in infants and children may occur at any age. Adenoviruses causing respiratory tract infections usually are transmitted by respiratory tract secretions through person-to-person contact, aerosols, and fomites, the latter because adenoviruses are stable in the environment. Other routes of transmission have not been defined clearly and may vary with age, type of infection, and environmental or other factors. The conjunctiva can provide a portal of entry. Community outbreaks of adenovirus-associated pharyngoconjunctival fever have been attributed to exposure to water from contaminated swimming pools and fomites such as shared towels. Nosocomial transmission of adenoviral respiratory and gastrointestinal tract infections can result from exposure to infected health care professionals and contaminated equipment. Epidemic keratoconjunctivitis often has been associated with nosocomial transmission in ophthalmologists' offices. Enteric strains of adenoviruses are transmitted by the fecal-oral route. The incidence of adenovirus-induced respiratory tract disease is increased slightly during late winter, spring, and early summer. Enteric disease occurs during most of the year and primarily affects children younger than 4 years of age. Adenovirus infections are most communicable during the first few days of an acute illness, but persistent and intermittent shedding for longer periods, even months, is common. Asymptomatic infections are common. Reinfection can occur.

The **incubation period** for respiratory tract infection varies from 2 to 14 days; for gastroenteritis, the incubation period is 3 to 10 days.

DIAGNOSTIC TESTS: The preferred method for diagnosis of adenovirus infection is cell culture or antigen detection. Adenoviruses associated with respiratory tract disease can be isolated from pharyngeal and eye secretions and feces by inoculation of specimens into a variety of cell cultures. A pharyngeal isolate is more suggestive of recent infection than is a fecal isolate, which may indicate prolonged carriage or recent infection. Adenovirus antigens can be detected in body fluids of infected people by immunoassay techniques, which are especially useful for diagnosis of diarrheal disease, because enteric adenovirus types 40 and 41 usually cannot be isolated in standard cell cultures. Enteric adenoviruses also can be identified by electron microscopic examination of stool specimens. Multiple methods to detect group-reactive hexon antigens of the virus in body secretions and tissue have been developed. Also, detection of viral DNA can be accomplished using probe hybridization or gene amplification by polymerase chain reaction. Serodiagnosis is used primarily for epidemiologic studies.

TREATMENT: Supportive.

ISOLATION OF THE HOSPITALIZED PATIENT: In addition to standard precautions for young children with respiratory tract infection, contact and droplet precautions are indicated for the duration of hospitalization. For patients with conjunctivitis and for diapered and incontinent children with adenoviral gastroenteritis, contact precautions in addition to standard precautions are indicated for the duration of the illness.

CONTROL MEASURES: Children who participate in group child care, particularly children from 6 months through 2 years of age, are at increased risk of adenoviral respiratory tract infections and gastroenteritis. Effective measures for preventing spread of adenovirus infection in this setting have not been determined, but frequent hand hygiene is recommended.

Adequate chlorination of swimming pools is recommended to prevent pharyngoconjunctival fever. Epidemic keratoconjunctivitis associated with ophthalmologic practice can be difficult to control and requires use of single-dose medication dispensing and strict attention to hand hygiene and instrument sterilization procedures. Effective disinfection can be accomplished by immersing contaminated equipment in a 1% solution of sodium hypochlorite for 10 minutes or by steam autoclaving.

Health care professionals with known or suspected adenoviral conjunctivitis should avoid direct patient contact for 14 days after the onset of disease in their second eye. Because adenoviruses are particularly difficult to eliminate from skin, fomites, and environmental surfaces, assiduous adherence to hand hygiene and use of disposable gloves when caring for infected patients are recommended.

Amebiasis

CLINICAL MANIFESTATIONS: Clinical syndromes associated with *Entamoeba histolytica* infection include noninvasive intestinal infection, intestinal amebiasis, ameboma, and liver abscess. Disease is more severe in the very young, the elderly, and pregnant women. Patients with noninvasive intestinal infection may be asymptomatic or may have nonspecific intestinal tract complaints. People with intestinal amebiasis (amebic colitis) generally have 1 to 3 weeks of increasingly severe diarrhea progressing to grossly bloody dysenteric stools with lower abdominal pain and tenesmus. Weight loss is common, and fever occurs in one third of patients. Symptoms may be chronic and may mimic inflammatory bowel disease. Progressive involvement of the colon may produce toxic megacolon, fulminant colitis, ulceration of the colon and perianal area and, rarely, perforation. Progression may occur in patients inappropriately treated with corticosteroids or antimotility drugs. An ameboma may occur as an annular lesion of the cecum or ascending colon that may be mistaken for colonic carcinoma or as a tender extrahepatic mass mimicking a pyogenic abscess. Amebomas usually resolve with antiamebic therapy and do not require surgery.

In a small proportion of patients, extraintestinal disease may occur. Although the liver is the most common extraintestinal site, the lungs, pleural space, pericardium, brain, skin, and genitourinary tract also may be involved. Liver abscess may be acute with fever, abdominal pain, tachypnea, liver tenderness, and hepatomegaly or chronic with weight loss, vague abdominal symptoms, and irritability. Rupture of abscesses into the abdomen or chest may lead to death. Evidence of recent intestinal infection usually is absent.

ETIOLOGY: *Entamoeba histolytica* has been reclassified into 2 species that are morphologically identical but genetically distinct protozoa. The pathogenic *E histolytica* and the nonpathogenic *Entamoeba dispar* are excreted as cysts or trophozoites in stools of infected people.

EPIDEMIOLOGY: *Entamoeba histolytica* can be found worldwide but is more prevalent in people of lower socioeconomic status who live in developing countries where the prevalence of amebic infection may be as high as 50%. Groups at increased risk of infection in developed nations include immigrants from endemic areas, long-term visitors to endemic areas, institutionalized people, and men who have sex with men. *Entamoeba histolytica* is transmitted via amebic cysts by the fecal-oral route. Ingested cysts, which are unaffected by gastric acid, undergo excystation in the alkaline small intestine and produce trophozoites that infect the colon. Cysts that subsequently develop are the source of transmission, especially from asymptomatic cyst excreters.

Infected patients excrete cysts intermittently, sometimes for years if untreated. Transmission occasionally has been associated with contaminated food, water, and enema equipment.

The **incubation period** is variable, ranging from a few days to months or years, but commonly is 1 to 4 weeks.

DIAGNOSTIC TESTS: Diagnosis of intestinal infection depends on identifying trophozoites or cysts in stool specimens. Examination of serial specimens may be necessary. Specimens of stool, endoscopy scrapings (not swabs), and biopsies should be examined by wet mount within 30 minutes of collection and fixed in formalin and polyvinyl alcohol (available in kits) for concentration and permanent staining. *Entamoeba histolytica* is not distinguished easily from the noninvasive and more prevalent *E dispar,* although trophozoites containing ingested red blood cells are more likely to be *E histolytica.* Polymerase chain reaction, isoenzyme analysis, and monoclonal antibody-based antigen detection assays can differentiate *E histolytica* and *E dispar.*

Detecting serum antibody using indirect hemagglutination assay (IHA) may be helpful, primarily for diagnosis of amebic colitis (85% positive results) and extra-intestinal amebiasis with liver involvement (99% positive results). In surveys of people in developed countries, 5% have positive IHA results. Up to 30% of the population may have antibodies on IHA in endemic areas. Infection with *E dispar* does not result in a positive IHA.

Ultrasonography and computed tomography can effectively identify liver abscesses and other extraintestinal sites of infection. Aspirates from a liver abscess usually show neither trophozoites nor leukocytes.

TREATMENT*: Treatment involves elimination of the tissue-invading trophozoites as well as organisms in the intestinal lumen. *Entamoeba dispar* infection does not require treatment. Corticosteroids and antimotility drugs administered to people with amebiasis can worsen symptoms and the disease process. The following regimens are recommended:

- **Asymptomatic cyst excreters (intraluminal infections):** treat with a luminal amebicide such as iodoquinol, paromomycin, or diloxanide furoate.
- **Patients with mild to moderate or severe intestinal symptoms or extraintestinal disease (including liver abscess):** treat with metronidazole (or tinidazole), followed by a therapeutic course of a luminal amebicide (iodoquinol or paromomycin).

Dehydroemetine followed by a therapeutic course of a luminal amebicide should be considered for patients for whom treatment of invasive disease has failed or cannot be tolerated. An alternate treatment for liver abscess is chloroquine phosphate concomitantly with metronidazole (or tinidazole) or, if necessary, dehydroemetine, followed by a therapeutic course of a luminal amebicide.

To prevent spontaneous rupture of an abscess, patients with large liver abscesses may benefit from percutaneous or surgical aspiration.

---

* For further information, see also Drugs for Parasitic Infections, p 744.

ISOLATION OF THE HOSPITALIZED PATIENT: In addition to standard precautions, contact precautions are recommended for the duration of illness.

CONTROL MEASURES: Careful hand hygiene after defecation, sanitary disposal of fecal material, and treatment of drinking water will control the spread of infection. Sexual transmission may be controlled by the use of condoms.

Amebic Meningoencephalitis and Keratitis
(*Naegleria fowleri, Acanthamoeba* species, and *Balamuthia mandrillaris*)

CLINICAL MANIFESTATIONS: *Naegleria fowleri* can cause a rapidly progressive, almost always fatal, primary amebic meningoencephalitis. Early symptoms include fever, headache, and sometimes, disturbances of smell and taste. The illness rapidly progresses to signs of meningoencephalitis, including nuchal rigidity, lethargy, confusion, and altered level of consciousness. Seizures are common. Death occurs within a week of onset of symptoms. No distinct clinical features differentiate this disease from fulminant bacterial meningitis.

Granulomatous amebic encephalitis caused by *Acanthamoeba* species and *Balamuthia mandrillaris* has a more insidious onset and progression of manifestations occurring weeks to months after exposure. Signs and symptoms may include personality changes, seizures, headaches, nuchal rigidity, ataxia, cranial nerve palsies, hemiparesis, and other focal deficits. Fever is often low-grade and intermittent. The course may resemble that of a bacterial brain abscess or a brain tumor. Skin lesions (pustules, nodules, ulcers) may be present without central nervous system involvement, particularly in patients with acquired immunodeficiency syndrome.

Amebic keratitis, usually attributable to *Acanthamoeba* species and rarely to other species, occurs primarily in people who wear contact lenses and resembles keratitis caused by herpes simplex, bacteria, or fungi except for a usually more indolent course. Corneal inflammation, pain, photophobia, and secondary uveitis are predominant features.

ETIOLOGY: *Naegleria fowleri, Acanthamoeba* species, and *Balamuthia mandrillaris* are free-living amebae that exist as motile, infective trophozoites and environmentally hardy cysts.

EPIDEMIOLOGY: *Naegleria fowleri* is found in warm fresh water and moist soil. Most infections with *N fowleri* have been associated with swimming in warm, natural bodies of water, but other sources have included tap water, contaminated and poorly chlorinated swimming pools, and baths. Small outbreaks associated with swimming in a warm lake or swimming pool have been reported. A few cases with no history of contact with water have occurred. Disease has been reported worldwide but is uncommon. In the United States, infection occurs primarily in the summer and usually affects children and young adults. The trophozoites of the parasite directly invade the brain from the nose along the olfactory nerves via the cribriform plate.

The **incubation period** for *N fowleri* infection is several days to 1 week.

The causative organisms of granulomatous amebic encephalitis, especially *Acanthamoeba* species, are distributed worldwide and are found in soil, fresh and brackish water, dust, hot tubs, and sewage. *Balamuthia mandrillaris,* however, have not been isolated from the environment. Central nervous system infection occurs primarily in debilitated and immunocompromised people. However, some patients have had no demonstrable underlying disease or defect. Acquisition probably occurs by inhalation or direct contact with contaminated soil or water. The primary focus of infection is most likely the skin or respiratory tract, followed by hematogenous spread to the brain.

Acanthamoeba organisms also cause dendritic keratitis, mimicking herpes keratitis in people who wear contact lenses and use contaminated saline solutions or tap water rinses for lens care or swim while wearing contacts.

The **incubation period** for these infections is unknown.

DIAGNOSTIC TESTS: *Naegleria fowleri* infection can be documented by microscopic demonstration of the motile trophozoites on a wet mount of centrifuged cerebrospinal fluid (CSF). The organism also can be cultured on 1.5% nonnutrient agar layered with enteric bacteria held in Page saline solution. Immunofluorescence tests to determine the species of the organism are available through the Centers for Disease Control and Prevention. The CSF shows polymorphonuclear pleocytosis, an increased protein concentration, a slightly decreased glucose concentration, and no bacteria.

In infection with *Acanthamoeba* species, trophozoites and cysts can be visualized in sections of brain or corneal scrapings. The CSF typically shows a mononuclear pleocytosis and an increased protein concentration but no organisms. *Acanthamoeba* species, but not *Balamuthia* species, can be cultured by the same method as used for *N fowleri.*

TREATMENT: If meningoencephalitis caused by *N fowleri* is suspected because of the presence of organisms in the CSF, therapy should not be withheld while waiting for results of confirmatory diagnostic tests. Amphotericin B is the drug of choice, although treatment often is unsuccessful, with only a few cases of complete recovery being documented. Recovery has occurred after treatment with amphotericin B alone or in combination with other agents, such as miconazole and rifampin. Early diagnosis and institution of high-dose drug therapy is probably important for optimizing outcome.

Effective treatment for central nervous system infections caused by *Acanthamoeba* species and *B mandrillaris* has not been established. Experimental infections can be prevented or cured by sulfadiazine. Although *Acanthamoeba* species usually are susceptible in vitro to a variety of antimicrobial agents (eg, pentamidine, flucytosine, ketoconazole, clotrimazole, and to a lesser degree, amphotericin B), recovery is rare.

Patients with keratitis attributable to *Acanthamoeba* organisms have been treated successfully with prolonged courses of combinations of topical propamidine isethionate plus neomycin-polymyxin B sulfate-gramicidin ophthalmic solution or topical polyhexamethylene biguanide or chlorhexidine gluconate and various azoles (eg, miconazole, clotrimazole, fluconazole, or itraconazole) as well as topical corticosteroids. Early diagnosis is important for a good outcome. Some patients with skin lesions attributable to *Acanthamoeba* species have been treated successfully by first washing lesions with chlorhexidine gluconate and then applying topical ketoconazole cream 3 to 4 times a day. Patients also have been given intravenous pentamidine and oral itraconazole (see Drugs for Parasitic Infections, p 744).

ISOLATION OF THE HOSPITALIZED PATIENT: Standard precautions are recommended.

CONTROL MEASURES: People should avoid swimming in warm, stagnant, polluted fresh water. *Acanthamoeba* organisms are resistant to freezing, drying, and the usual concentrations of chlorine found in drinking water and swimming pools.

Only sterile saline solutions should be used to clean contact lenses.

Anthrax

CLINICAL MANIFESTATIONS: Depending on the route of infection, anthrax disease can occur in 3 forms: cutaneous, inhalational, and gastrointestinal. **Cutaneous** anthrax begins as a pruritic papule or vesicle that enlarges and ulcerates in 1 to 2 days, with subsequent formation of a central black eschar. The lesion usually is painless, with surrounding edema, hyperemia, and regional lymphadenopathy. Patients may have associated fever, malaise, and headache. **Inhalational** anthrax is the most lethal form of disease. A prodrome of fever, chills, nonproductive cough, chest pain, headache, myalgias, and malaise may occur initially, but more distinctive clinical hallmarks occur 2 to 5 days later and include a hemorrhagic mediastinal lymphadenitis, hemorrhagic pleural effusion, bacteremia, and toxemia resulting in severe dyspnea, hypoxia, and septic shock. A widened mediastinum is the classic finding on imaging of the chest but initially may be subtle. **Gastrointestinal tract** disease can present as 2 clinical syndromes, intestinal and oropharyngeal. Patients with the intestinal form have symptoms of nausea, anorexia, vomiting, and fever, progressing to severe abdominal pain, massive ascites, hematemesis, and bloody diarrhea. Oropharyngeal anthrax may include posterior oropharyngeal ulcers that typically are unilateral and associated with marked neck swelling, regional adenopathy, and sepsis. Hemorrhagic meningitis can result from hematogenous spread of the organism after acquiring any form of the disease. The case fatality ratio for patients with appropriately treated cutaneous anthrax usually is <1%, but for inhalational or gastrointestinal disease, mortality can exceed 50%.

ETIOLOGY: *Bacillus anthracis* is an aerobic, gram-positive, encapsulated, spore-forming, nonmotile rod. Spore size is approximately 1×2 μm. *Bacillus anthracis* has 3 major virulence factors: an antiphagocytic capsule and 2 exotoxins, called lethal and edema toxins. The toxins are responsible for the primary clinical manifestations of hemorrhage, edema, and necrosis.

EPIDEMIOLOGY: Anthrax is a zoonotic disease that occurs in many rural regions of the world. *Bacillus anthracis* spores remain viable in the soil for many years, representing a potential source of infection for livestock through ingestion. Natural infection of humans occurs through contact with infected animals or contaminated animal products, including carcasses, hides, hair, wool, meat, and bone meal. Internationally, outbreaks of gastrointestinal anthrax have occurred after ingestion of undercooked or raw meat. In the United States, the incidence of naturally occurring human anthrax decreased from an estimated 130 cases annually in the early 1900s to 1 case each in 2000 and 2001. The vast majority (>95%) of these cases were cutaneous infections among animal handlers or mill workers. The last case of naturally acquired inhalational anthrax in the United States occurred in 1976 in a person who worked with imported yarn.

Bacillus anthracis is one of the most likely biological agents to be used as a weapon, because (1) its spores are highly stabile; (2) spores can infect via the respiratory route; and (3) the resulting inhalational disease has a high mortality rate. In addition to aerosolization, there is a theoretic health risk associated with *B anthracis* spores being introduced into food products or water supplies. In 1979, an accidental release of *B anthracis* spores from a military microbiology facility in the former Soviet Union resulted in 69 deaths. In 2001, 22 cases of anthrax (11 inhalational, 11 cutaneous) were identified in the United States after intentional contamination of the mail; 5 (45%) of the inhalational cases were fatal. Use of *B anthracis* in a biological attack would require immediate response and mobilization of public health resources. Because naturally occurring anthrax is rare in the United States, every suspected case should be reported immediately to the local or state health department (see Biological Terrorism, p 99).

The **incubation period** for all forms of anthrax generally is less than 2 weeks. However, because of spore dormancy and slow clearance from the lungs, the incubation period for inhalational anthrax may be prolonged to as long as several months. Discharges from cutaneous lesions potentially are infectious, but person-to-person transmission rarely has been reported. Both inhalational and cutaneous disease have occurred in laboratory workers.

DIAGNOSTIC TESTS: Depending on the clinical presentation, Gram stain and culture should be performed on specimens of blood, pleural fluid, cerebrospinal fluid, and tissue biopsy or discharge from cutaneous lesions. However, previous treatment with antimicrobial agents significantly decreases the yield of these studies. Definitive identification of suspect *B anthracis* isolates can be performed through the Laboratory Response Network in each state. Additional diagnostic tests for anthrax, including immunohistochemistry, real-time polymerase chain reaction, time-resolved fluorescence, and an enzyme immunoassay that measures immunoglobulin G antibodies against *B anthracis* protective antigen, are performed at the Centers for Disease Control and Prevention and can be accessed through state health departments. The clinical evaluation of patients with suspected inhalational anthrax should include a chest radiograph and/or computed tomography scan to evaluate for widened mediastinum and pleural effusion.

TREATMENT: A high index of clinical suspicion and rapid administration of effective antimicrobial therapy is essential for prompt diagnosis and effective treatment of anthrax. No controlled trials in humans have been performed to validate current treatment recommendations for anthrax, and there is limited clinical experience. Case reports suggest that naturally occurring cutaneous disease can be treated effectively with a variety of antimicrobial agents, including penicillins, macrolides, and tetracyclines, for 7 to 10 days. For bioterrorism-associated cutaneous disease in adults or children, ciprofloxacin (500 mg, orally, 2 times/day or 10–15 mg/kg per day for children, orally, divided 2 times/day for children) or doxycycline (100 mg, orally, 2 times/day or 5 mg/kg per day, orally, divided 2 times/day for children younger than 8 years of age) are recommended for initial treatment until antimicrobial susceptibility data are available. Because of the risk of concomitant inhalational exposure, consideration should be given to continuing an appropriate antimicrobial regimen for postexposure prophylaxis.

On the basis of in vitro data and animal studies, ciprofloxacin (400 mg, intravenously, every 8–12 hours) or doxycycline (200 mg, intravenously, every 8–12 hours) should be used initially as part of a multidrug regimen for treating inhalational anthrax, anthrax meningitis, cutaneous anthrax with systemic signs, and gastrointestinal anthrax until results of antimicrobial susceptibility testing are known.* Other agents with in vitro activity suggested for use in conjunction with ciprofloxacin or doxycycline include rifampin, vancomycin hydrochloride, imipenem, chloramphenicol, penicillin, ampicillin, clindamycin, and clarithromycin. Cephalosporins and trimethoprim-sulfamethoxazole should not be used for therapy. Treatment should continue for at least 60 days. Neither ciprofloxacin nor tetracyclines routinely are used in children or pregnant women because of safety concerns. However, ciprofloxacin or tetracycline should be used for treatment of anthrax in children for life-threatening infections until antimicrobial susceptibility patterns are known.

ISOLATION OF THE HOSPITALIZED PATIENT: Standard precautions are recommended. Contaminated dressings and bedclothes should be incinerated or steam sterilized to destroy spores. Autopsies performed on patients with systemic anthrax require special precautions.

CONTROL MEASURES: BioThrax (formerly known as Anthrax Vaccine Adsorbed [manufactured by BioPort Corp, Lansing, MI]) is the only human vaccine for prevention of anthrax licensed in the United States. This vaccine is prepared from a cell-free culture filtrate. Immunization consists of 6 subcutaneous injections at 0, 2, and 4 weeks and 6, 12, and 18 months followed by annual boosters. The vaccine currently is recommended for people at risk of repeated exposures to *B anthracis* spores, including selected laboratory workers and military personnel.† The vaccine

---

* Centers for Disease Control and Prevention. Update: investigation of bioterrorism-related anthrax and interim guidelines for exposure management and antimicrobial therapy, October 2001. *MMWR Morb Mortal Wkly Rep.* 2001;50:909–919; and Centers for Disease Control and Prevention. Notice to readers: update: interim recommendations for antimicrobial prophylaxis for children and breastfeeding mothers and treatment of children with anthrax. *MMWR Morb Mortal Wkly Rep.* 2001;50:1014–1016

† Centers for Disease Control and Prevention. Notice to readers: use of anthrax vaccine in response to terrorism: supplemental recommendations of the Advisory Committee on Immunization Practices. *MMWR Morb Mortal Wkly Rep.* 2002;51:1024–1026

is effective for preventing the occurrence of cutaneous anthrax in adults. Although protection against inhalational disease has not been evaluated in humans, studies in nonhuman primates have shown the vaccine to be effective. Adverse events mainly are local injection site reactions with rare systemic symptoms, including fever, chills, muscle aches, and hypersensitivity. No data on vaccine effectiveness or safety in children are available, and the vaccine is not licensed for use in children or pregnant women. Anthrax vaccine is not licensed for postexposure use in preventing anthrax.

On the basis of limited available data, the best means for prevention of inhalation anthrax after exposure to *B anthracis* spores is prolonged antimicrobial therapy in conjunction with a 3-dose regimen (at 0, 2, and 4 weeks) of anthrax immunization. However, because BioThrax is not licensed for postexposure prophylaxis or for use as a 3-dose regimen or for use in children, this program can be administered only under an investigational new drug (IND) application as part of an emergency public health intervention. When no information is available about the antimicrobial susceptibility of the implicated strain of *B anthracis*, initial postexposure prophylaxis for adults or children with ciprofloxacin or doxycycline is recommended. Although fluoroquinolones and tetracyclines are not recommended as first-choice drugs in children because of adverse effects, these concerns may be outweighed by the need for early treatment of pregnant women and children exposed to *B anthracis* after a terrorist attack. As soon as susceptibility of the organism to penicillin has been confirmed, prophylactic therapy for children should be changed to oral amoxicillin, 80 mg/kg per day, divided every 8 hours (not to exceed 500 mg, 3 times/day). *Bacillus anthracis* is not susceptible to cephalosporins and trimethoprim-sulfamethoxazole; therefore, these agents should not be used for prophylaxis.

Arboviruses
(Including California Encephalitis [Primarily La Crosse], Eastern and Western Equine Encephalitis, Powassan Encephalitis, St Louis Encephalitis, Venezuelan Equine Encephalitis, West Nile Encephalitis, Colorado Tick Fever, Dengue, Japanese Encephalitis, and Yellow Fever)

CLINICAL MANIFESTATIONS: Arboviruses (arthropodborne viruses) are spread by mosquitoes, ticks, or sandflies and produce 4 principal clinical syndromes: (1) central nervous system (CNS) infection (including encephalitis, aseptic meningitis, or myelitis); (2) an undifferentiated febrile illness, often with rash; (3) acute polyarthropathy; and (4) acute hemorrhagic fever, usually accompanied by hepatitis. Infection with some arboviruses produces perinatal illness.

Selected arboviruses transmitted in the Western hemisphere associated with central nervous system involvement are shown in Table 3.1 (p 200). Eastern equine encephalitis (EEE) virus is the most severe arthropodborne encephalitis in the United States. The other principal arboviruses transmitted in North America mainly produce asymptomatic infections. When present, clinical illness ranges in severity from a self-limited febrile illness with headache and vomiting (especially in children) to a syndrome of aseptic meningitis or acute encephalitis. The La Crosse (LAC) virus produces aseptic meningitis or encephalitis with acute seizures and focal findings in

Table 3.1. Important Arboviral Infections of the Central Nervous System Occurring in the Western Hemisphere[1]

Disease (Causal Agent)[2]	Geographic Distribution of Virus	Incubation Period, days
California encephalitis virus (primarily La Crosse and several other California serogroup viruses)	Widespread in the United States and Canada, including the Yukon and Northwest Territories; most prevalent in upper Midwest	5–15
Eastern equine encephalitis (EEE) virus	Eastern seaboard and Gulf states of the US (isolated inland foci); Canada; South and Central America	3–10
Powassan encephalitis virus	Canada; northeastern, north central, and western US	4–18
St Louis encephalitis (SLE) virus	Widespread: central, southern, northeastern, and western US; Manitoba and southern Ontario; Caribbean area; South America	4–14
Venezuelan equine encephalitis (VEE) virus	Central and South America	1–4
Western equine encephalitis (WEE) virus	Central and western US; Canada; Argentina, Uruguay, Brazil	2–10
West Nile encephalitis virus	Asia; Africa; Europe; US	5–15

[1] Although referred to as encephalitis agents, these arboviral infections may cause encephalitis, aseptic meningitis, myelitis, paralysis, or other neurologic findings or systemic illness.
[2] All are mosquitoborne except Powassan encephalitis virus, which is tickborne.

more than 25% of cases and stupor or coma in 50%, but death occurs in less than 1%. Eastern equine encephalitis typically is a fulminant illness leading to coma and death in one third of cases and serious neurologic sequelae in another one third. The clinical severity of western equine encephalitis (WEE) is intermediate, with a case-fatality rate of 5%; neurologic impairment is common in infants. Powassan encephalitis is associated with long-term morbidity and has a case-fatality rate of 10% to 15%. Characteristics of symptomatic infection caused by St Louis encephalitis (SLE) include confusion, fever, headache, slow disease progression, lack of focal findings, generalized weakness, and tremor; 7% of cases are fatal, and children and the elderly experience more severe illness. In 1999, West Nile virus (WNV) was described for the first time in the United States in New York, and since then, laboratory-confirmed human cases of WNV-associated illness have been reported from more than 40 states in the continental United States. Infection with this virus manifests as a nondescript febrile illness associated with rash, arthritis, myalgias, weakness, lymphadenopathy, and meningoencephalitis. The mortality rate is approximately 5%, and death occurs mainly in older individuals.

Japanese encephalitis (JE) virus can produce a severe encephalitis with a geographic distribution in Asia. Japanese encephalitis is characterized by coma, seizures, paralysis, abnormal movements, and death in one third of cases. Serious sequelae occur in 40% of survivors. Most infections are asymptomatic.

There are several arboviruses in the Western hemisphere associated with acute, febrile diseases and hemorrhagic fevers. These arboviruses are not characterized by encephalitis (Table 3.2, below).

Colorado tick fever (CTF) is an acute, self-limited illness consisting of fever, chills, myalgia, arthralgia, severe headache, and ocular pain. Illness is biphasic in 50% of cases and may be complicated by encephalitis, myocarditis, and rarely, fatal systemic illness with hemorrhage. Transient but significant leukopenia, thrombocytopenia, and anemia attributable to infection of bone marrow elements are hallmarks of disease.

Infection with any of the 4 serotypes of **dengue** virus produces dengue fever, an acute febrile illness with headache, retro-orbital pain, myalgia, arthralgia, rash, nausea, and vomiting. Criteria for dengue hemorrhagic fever (DHF) include fever, any hemorrhage including epistaxis and gum bleeding, thrombocytopenia (platelet count $\leq 100 \times 10^3/\mu L$ [$\leq 100 \times 10^9/L$]), and increased capillary fragility and permeability. Fluid leakage into the interstitial, pleural, and peritoneal spaces leads to hemoconcentration, pleural effusion, and acute shock. Dengue hemorrhagic fever is fatal in one third of untreated cases but is fatal in fewer than 3% of cases managed with aggressive fluid resuscitation. Encephalopathy, hepatitis, myocardiopathy, upper intestinal tract bleeding, and pneumonia are complications. Maternal infection during the third trimester can be followed by acute perinatal illness with hemorrhage.

Yellow fever (YF) evolves through 3 periods from a nonspecific febrile illness with headache, malaise, weakness, nausea, and vomiting through a brief period of remission to a hemorrhagic fever with gastrointestinal tract bleeding and hema-

Table 3.2. Acute, Febrile Diseases and Hemorrhagic Fevers Not Characterized by Encephalitis Caused by Arboviruses in the Western Hemisphere

Disease[1]	Geographic Distribution of Virus	Clinical Syndrome	Incubation Period, days
Colorado tick fever	South Dakota, Rocky Mountain and Pacific states; western Canada; Asia	Febrile illness— may be biphasic	1–14
Dengue fever and dengue hemorrhagic fever	Tropical areas worldwide: Caribbean, Central and South America, Asia, Australia, Oceania, Africa[2]	Febrile illness— may be biphasic with rash; hemorrhagic fever and shock	2–7
Yellow fever	Tropical areas of South America and Africa[2]	Febrile illness, hepatitis, hemorrhagic fever	3–6
Mayaro fever	Central and South America	Febrile illness and polyarthritis	1–12
Oropouche virus fever	Central and South America	Febrile illness	2–6

[1] All are mosquitoborne except Colorado tick fever, which is tickborne, and Oropouche virus fever, which is midgeborne.

[2] Mosquito vectors *Aedes aegypti* (yellow fever, dengue) and *Aedes albopictus* (dengue) now are found in the United States and could transmit introduced virus.

temesis, jaundice, hemorrhage, cardiovascular instability, albuminuria, oliguria, and myocarditis; 50% of cases are fatal.

Mayaro fever and Oropouche virus fever occur in Central and South America. Both cause a febrile, grippe-like syndrome.

ETIOLOGY: More than 550 arboviruses are classified in a variety of taxonomic groups, principally in the families Bunyaviridae, Togaviridae, and Flaviviridae (Table 3.3, p 203), with more than 150 associated with human disease. Viruses in these families principally are arthropodborne or spread as zoonoses. In the United States, arboviral infections are considered principally in the differential diagnosis of acute encephalitis.

EPIDEMIOLOGY: Most arboviruses are maintained in nature through cycles of transmission among birds or small mammals by arthropod vectors. Humans and domestic animals are infected incidentally as "dead-end" hosts. Important exceptions are dengue, YF, Oropouche, and chikungunya viruses because infected vectors spread disease from person to person (anthroponotic transmission). For the other arboviruses, direct person-to-person spread does not occur. Colorado tick fever and WNV have been transmitted through blood transfusion (see Blood Safety, p 106), and WNV has been transmitted through transplanted organs.

In the United States, mosquitoborne arboviral infections usually occur during late summer and early autumn, but in the Deep South, EEE cases occur throughout the year. A range of 1 to 5 WEE and EEE cases are reported nationally each year. During epidemics of SLE, people of all ages may be infected, but cases of clinical illness occur more often at the extremes of age, especially in elderly people. Urban SLE outbreaks have led to hundreds of cases, occurring disproportionately in lower socioeconomic-status neighborhoods and among the homeless. Encephalitis attributable to LAC virus is transmitted in an endemic pattern in wooded environments in the eastern and midwestern United States and California. Almost all of the approximately 100 cases that are reported each year are in children younger than 15 years of age. West Nile virus is transmitted between mosquitoes and birds, with humans and horses becoming infected incidentally. Infection also has occurred through blood transfusions and organ transplantation.

The **incubation periods** and geographic distributions of selected medically important arboviral infections are outlined in Tables 3.1 and 3.2 (p 200 and p 201).

DIAGNOSTIC TESTS: A definitive diagnosis is made by serologic testing of cerebrospinal fluid (CSF) or serum or by viral isolation. Detection of virus-specific immunoglobulin M antibody in CSF is confirmatory, and its presence in a serum specimen is presumptive evidence of recent infection in a patient with acute CNS infection. A greater than fourfold change in serum antibody titer in paired serum specimens obtained 2 to 4 weeks apart confirms a case. A single increased antibody titer defines a case as presumptive. Polymerase chain reaction assays to detect several arboviruses have been developed, but they have not been introduced into routine laboratory diagnosis. Serologic testing for dengue and arboviruses transmitted in the United States is available through several commercial, state, research, and reference laboratories. During the acute phase of dengue, YF, CTF, Venezuelan equine encephalitis (VEE), and certain other arboviral infections, virus can be isolated from

Table 3.3. **Taxonomy of Major Arboviruses**

Family	Genus	Representative Agents and Geographic Locations
Bunyaviridae	Bunyavirus	California serogroup viruses (North and South America, Europe, Asia)
		Oropouche virus (South America)
	Phlebovirus	Sandfly fever virus (Europe, Africa, Asia)
		Rift Valley fever (sub-Saharan Africa, Saudi Arabia, Yemen)
		Toscana virus (Europe)
	Nairovirus	Crimean-Congo hemorrhagic fever virus (Africa, Europe, Asia)
	Hantavirus	Hantaan virus of hemorrhagic fever (Asia)
Togaviridae	Alphavirus	Eastern equine encephalitis virus (North and South America)
		Western equine encephalitis virus (North and South America)
		Venezuelan equine encephalitis virus (Central and South America, Florida)
		Mayaro virus (Central and South America)
		Chikungunya virus (Africa, Asia)
		Ross River virus (Australia, Oceania)
		O'nyong-nyong virus (Africa)
		Sindbis virus (Africa, Scandinavia, northern Europe, Asia, Australia)
Flaviviridae	Flavivirus	St Louis encephalitis virus (North and South America)
		Japanese encephalitis virus (Asia)
		Dengue viruses (types 1–4) (tropics, worldwide)
		Yellow fever virus (South America, Africa)
		Murray Valley encephalitis virus (Australia)
		West Nile virus (Europe, Africa, Asia, North America)
		Tickborne encephalitis complex viruses (Europe and Asia)
		Powassan virus (North America, Asia)
Reoviridae	Coltivirus	Colorado tick fever virus (United States, Canada, Asia)
Rhabdoviridae	Vesiculovirus	Vesicular stomatitis virus (Western hemisphere)

blood and, in VEE, from the throat. In patients with encephalitis, viral isolation should be attempted from a CSF specimen or from biopsy or postmortem brain tissue specimens. Serologic results should be interpreted in the context of any previous immunizations with YF and JE vaccines and locations of previous residence and travel.

TREATMENT: Active clinical monitoring and supportive interventions may be life saving in patients with DHF, YF, and acute encephalitis.

ISOLATION OF THE HOSPITALIZED PATIENT: Because VEE virus has been isolated from the oropharynx of acutely infected patients, respiratory precautions are recommended. Patients with acute dengue and acute YF have these viruses circulating in their blood, so they should be kept away from potential vector mosquitoes that could feed on them and subsequently transmit infection to others from whom they subsequently take a blood meal.

CONTROL MEASURES:

Protection Against Vectors. Public health department-administered mosquito control programs are important for controlling vectors. Personal precautions to avoid mosquito bites include repellents, protective clothing, aerosol insecticides, and staying in screened or air-conditioned locations. Although many vector species are most active during twilight hours, certain vectors of EEE and LAC encephalitis are daytime feeders. *Aedes aegypti,* the vector of dengue and urban YF, is found around houses and indoors, even in well-constructed hotels. Travelers to tropical countries should consider bringing mosquito bed nets and aerosol insecticide sprays.

Active Immunization.

*Yellow Fever Vaccine.** Live-attenuated (17D strain) vaccine is available at state-approved immunization centers. A single dose is accepted by international authorities as providing protection for 10 years and may well confer lifelong immunity.

Immunization is recommended for all people 9 months of age or older living in or traveling to endemic areas and is required every 10 years by international regulations for travel to and from certain countries. Infants younger than 4 months of age should not be immunized, because they have increased susceptibility to vaccine-associated encephalitis. The decision to immunize infants between 4 and 9 months of age must balance the infant's risk of exposure (eg, immunization should be considered for people traveling to an area of ongoing endemic or epidemic activity if a high degree of protection against mosquito exposure is not feasible) with the theoretic risks of vaccine-associated encephalitis. The YF vaccine can be given concurrently with either typhoid vaccine licensed by the US Food and Drug Administration, hepatitis A and B virus vaccines, measles vaccine, poliovirus vaccine, and meningococcal vaccine; chloroquine; and Immune Serum Globulin.

Yellow fever vaccine is prepared in embryonated hen eggs and contains egg protein, which may cause allergic reactions. People who have experienced signs or symptoms of anaphylactic reaction after eating eggs should be excused from immunization and issued a medical waiver letter to fulfill health regulations or should undergo skin testing according to the package insert before immunization (also see Hypersensitivity Reactions to Vaccine Constituents, p 46). The vaccine should be administered to pregnant women only if travel to an endemic area is unavoidable and if an increased risk of exposure exists. Administration of YF vaccine to immunocompromised people poses a theoretic risk. The decision to immunize patients who have immunocompromising conditions must balance the traveler's risk of exposure with his or her clinical status. Family members of immunosuppressed people who themselves have no contraindications can receive YF vaccine. Immunization of breastfeeding mothers should be avoided if possible. Advice regarding immunization of 4- to 9-month-old children, pregnant women, or immunocompromised people

---

* Centers for Disease Control and Prevention. Yellow fever vaccine recommendations of the Advisory Committee on Immunization Practices (ACIP), 2002. *MMWR Recomm Rep.* 2002;51(RR-17):1–10

can be obtained from the Division of Vector-Borne Infectious Diseases of the Centers for Disease Control and Prevention (CDC; telephone 970-221-6400).

*Japanese Encephalitis Vaccine.** The inactivated JE vaccine, derived from infected mouse brain, is not recommended for people who travel routinely to Asia. Vaccine-associated hypersensitivity reactions (angioedema, generalized urticaria) occur in 0.3% of vaccine recipients. Therefore, immunization is recommended only for expatriates living in Asia and for travelers who will be residing in areas where JE virus is endemic or epidemic. Vaccine also is recommended for people who are planning prolonged stays (>30 days) in endemic areas during the transmission season, especially if travel includes rural areas or their activities or itinerary place them at increased risk of exposure (eg, travel into an epidemic area or bicycling, camping, or other unprotected outdoor activity in a rural area). Current information on locations of JE virus transmission and detailed information on vaccine recommendations can be obtained from the CDC (www.cdc.gov/travel).

The recommended primary immunization series for people older than 3 years of age is 3 doses of 1.0 mL each, administered subcutaneously on days 0, 7, and 30. An abbreviated schedule of 0, 7, and 14 days can be used when the longer schedule is precluded by time constraints. The regimen for children 1 to 3 years of age is identical, except that each dose is 0.5 mL. No data are available on vaccine safety and efficacy in infants.

Other Arboviral Vaccines. An inactivated vaccine for tickborne encephalitis is licensed in some countries in Europe where the disease is endemic, but this vaccine is not available in the United States.

Arcanobacterium haemolyticum Infections

CLINICAL MANIFESTATIONS: Acute pharyngitis attributable to *Arcanobacterium haemolyticum* often is indistinguishable from that caused by group A streptococci. Fever, pharyngeal exudate, lymphadenopathy, rash, and pruritus are common, but palatal petechiae and strawberry tongue are absent. In almost half of all reported cases, a maculopapular or scarlatiniform exanthem is present, beginning on the extensor surfaces of the distal extremities, spreading centripetally to the chest and back and sparing the face, palms, and soles. Respiratory infections that mimic diphtheria, including membranous pharyngitis, sinusitis, and pneumonia; and skin and soft tissue infections, including chronic ulceration, cellulitis, paronychia, and wound infection have been attributed to *A haemolyticum*. Invasive infections, including septicemia, peritonsillar abscess, brain abscess, meningitis, endocarditis, osteomyelitis, and pneumonia, have been reported.

ETIOLOGY: *Arcanobacterium haemolyticum* is a gram-positive bacillus formerly classified as *Corynebacterium haemolyticum*.

---

* Centers for Disease Control and Prevention. Inactivated Japanese encephalitis virus vaccine: recommendations of the Advisory Committee on Immunization Practices (ACIP). *MMWR Recomm Rep.* 1993;42(RR01):1–15

EPIDEMIOLOGY: Humans are the primary reservoir of *A haemolyticum,* and spread is person-to-person, presumably via droplet respiratory tract secretions. Pharyngitis occurs primarily in adolescents and young adults. Although long-term pharyngeal carriage with *A haemolyticum* has been described after an episode of acute pharyngitis, isolation of the bacterium from the nasopharynx of asymptomatic people is rare. From 0.5% to 3% of acute pharyngitis is estimated to be attributable to *A haemolyticum.*

The **incubation period** is unknown.

DIAGNOSTIC TESTS: *Arcanobacterium haemolyticum* grows on blood-enriched agar, but colonies are small and have narrow bands of hemolysis and may not be visible for 48 to 72 hours. Detection is enhanced by culture on rabbit or human blood agar rather than on more commonly used sheep blood agar because of larger colony size and wider zones of hemolysis. Growth also is enhanced by addition of 5% carbon dioxide. Nonstandardized serologic tests for antibodies to *A haemolyticum* have been developed but are not available commercially.

TREATMENT: Erythromycin is the drug of choice for treating tonsillopharyngitis, but no prospective therapeutic trials have been performed. *Arcanobacterium haemolyticum* is susceptible in vitro to erythromycin, clindamycin, chloramphenicol, and tetracycline; susceptibility to penicillin is variable, and failures in treatment of pharyngitis have been reported. Resistance to trimethoprim-sulfamethoxazole is common. In rare cases of disseminated infection, susceptibility tests should be performed. In disseminated infection, penicillin plus an aminoglycoside may be used initially as empiric treatment.

ISOLATION OF THE HOSPITALIZED PATIENT: Standard precautions are recommended.

CONTROL MEASURES: None.

Ascaris lumbricoides Infections

CLINICAL MANIFESTATIONS: Most infections are asymptomatic, although moderate to heavy infections may lead to malnutrition, and nonspecific gastrointestinal tract symptoms may occur in some patients. During the larval migratory phase, an acute transient pneumonitis (Löffler syndrome) associated with fever and marked eosinophilia may occur. Acute intestinal obstruction may develop in patients with heavy infections. Children are prone to this complication because of the small diameter of the intestinal lumen and heavy worm burden. Worm migration can cause peritonitis, secondary to intestinal wall penetration, and common bile duct obstruction resulting in biliary colic, cholangitis, or pancreatitis. Adult worms can be stimulated to migrate by stressful conditions (eg, fever, illness, or anesthesia) and by some anthelmintic drugs. *Ascaris lumbricoides* has been found in the appendiceal lumen in patients with acute appendicitis, but a causal relationship is uncertain.

ETIOLOGY: *Ascaris lumbricoides* is the most widespread of all human intestinal roundworms.

EPIDEMIOLOGY: The adult worms live in the lumen of the small intestine. Females produce 200 000 eggs per day, which are excreted in stool and must incubate in soil for 2 to 3 weeks for the embryo to form and to become infectious. Ingestion of infective eggs from contaminated soil results in infection. Larvae hatch in the small intestine, penetrate the mucosa, and are transported passively by portal blood to the liver and subsequently to the lungs. Larvae then ascend through the tracheobronchial tree to the pharynx, are swallowed, and mature into adults in the small intestine. Infection with *A lumbricoides* is widespread but is most common in the tropics, in areas of poor sanitation, and where human feces are used as fertilizer. If the infection is untreated, adult worms can live for 12 to 18 months, resulting in daily excretion of large numbers of ova.

The **incubation period** (interval between ingestion of the egg and the development of egg-laying adults) is approximately 8 weeks.

DIAGNOSTIC TESTS: Ova can be detected by microscopic examination of stool. Occasionally, patients pass adult worms from the rectum, from the nose after migration through the nares, and from the mouth in vomitus.

TREATMENT: Pyrantel pamoate in a single dose, albendazole in a single dose, or mebendazole for 3 days is recommended for treatment of asymptomatic and symptomatic infections (see Drugs for Parasitic Infections, p 744). Although limited data suggest that these drugs are safe in children younger than 2 years of age, the risks and benefits of therapy should be considered before drug administration. Reexamination of stool specimens 3 weeks after therapy to determine whether the worms have been eliminated is helpful for assessing therapy but is not essential.

In cases of partial or complete intestinal obstruction attributable to a heavy worm load, piperazine citrate solution (75 mg/kg per day, not to exceed 3.5 g) may be given through a gastrointestinal tube but is not available in many countries, including the United States. Pyrantel pamoate is not recommended, because it can worsen the obstruction. If piperazine is not available, conservative management (nasogastric suction, intravenous fluids) may result in resolution of obstruction, at which point albendazole or mebendazole may be given. Surgical intervention occasionally is necessary to relieve intestinal or biliary tract obstruction or for volvulus or peritonitis secondary to perforation. If surgery is performed for intestinal obstruction, massaging the bowel to eliminate the obstruction is preferable to incision into the intestine. Endoscopic retrograde cholangiopancreatography has been used successfully for extraction of worms from the biliary tree.

ISOLATION OF THE HOSPITALIZED PATIENT: Only standard precautions are recommended, because there is no direct person-to-person transmission.

CONTROL MEASURES: Sanitary disposal of human feces stops transmission. Children's play areas should be given special attention. Vegetables cultivated in areas where uncomposted human feces are used as fertilizer must be thoroughly cooked or soaked in a diluted iodine solution before eating. Household bleach is ineffective in killing *A lumbricoides*. Despite relatively rapid reinfection, periodic deworming targeted at school-aged children has been used to prevent morbidity (nutritional and cognitive deficits) associated with intestinal helminth infections.

Aspergillosis

CLINICAL MANIFESTATIONS: Aspergillosis manifests as noninvasive and invasive disease of the following types:

- Allergic bronchopulmonary aspergillosis is a hypersensitivity lung disease that manifests as episodic wheezing, expectoration of brown mucus plugs, low-grade fever, eosinophilia, and transient pulmonary infiltrates. This form of aspergillosis occurs most commonly in immunocompetent children with chronic asthma or cystic fibrosis.
- Allergic sinusitis is a far less common allergic response to colonization by *Aspergillus* species than is allergic bronchopulmonary syndrome. Allergic sinusitis occurs in children with nasal polyps or previous episodes of sinusitis or in children who have undergone sinus surgery and is characterized by symptoms of chronic sinusitis with dark plugs of nasal discharge.
- Aspergillomas and otomycosis are 2 syndromes of nonallergic colonization by *Aspergillus* species in immunocompetent children. Aspergillomas ("fungal balls") grow in preexisting cavities or bronchogenic cysts without invading pulmonary tissue; almost all patients have underlying lung disease, typically cystic fibrosis. Patients with otomycosis have chronic otitis media with colonization of the external auditory canal by a fungal mat that produces a dark discharge.
- Invasive aspergillosis occurs almost exclusively in immunocompromised patients with prolonged neutropenia (eg, cytotoxic chemotherapy) or impaired phagocyte function (eg, chronic granulomatous disease, immunosuppressive therapy, corticosteroids). Invasive infection usually involves pulmonary, sinus, cerebral, or cutaneous sites. The hallmark of invasive aspergillosis is angio-invasion with resulting thrombosis, dissemination to other organs, and occasionally, erosion of the blood vessel wall with catastrophic hemorrhage. Rarely, endocarditis, osteomyelitis, meningitis, infection of the eye or orbit, and esophagitis occur.

ETIOLOGY: *Aspergillus* species are ubiquitous molds that grow on decaying vegetation and in soil. *Aspergillus fumigatus* is the usual cause of aspergillosis, with *Aspergillus flavus* being the next most common. Several other species, including *Aspergillus teres* and *Aspergillus niger*, cause invasive human infections.

EPIDEMIOLOGY: The principal route of transmission is inhalation of conidia. Most affected patients have impaired phagocytic function. Nosocomial outbreaks of invasive pulmonary aspergillosis in susceptible hosts have occurred in which the probable source of the fungus was a nearby construction site or faulty ventilation system. Transmission by direct inoculation of skin abrasions or wounds is less likely. Person-to-person spread does not occur.

The **incubation period** is unknown.

DIAGNOSTIC TESTS: Dichotomously branched and septate hyphae, identified by microscopic examination of 10% potassium hydroxide wet preparations or of Gomori methenamine-silver nitrate stain of tissue or bronchoalveolar lavage specimens, are suggestive of the diagnosis. Isolation of *Aspergillus* species in culture is required for definitive diagnosis. The organism usually is not recoverable from blood but is isolated readily from lung, sinus, and skin biopsy specimens when cultured on Sabouraud dextrose agar or brain-heart infusion media (without cycloheximide). *Aspergillus* species may be a laboratory contaminant, but when evaluating results from ill, immunocompromised patients, recovery of this organism usually indicates infection. Biopsy of a lesion usually is required to confirm the diagnosis. Rapid antigen tests and polymerase chain reaction-based techniques may be available in the future for diagnosis of invasive disease. Serologic tests have no established value in the diagnosis of invasive aspergillosis. In allergic aspergillosis, diagnosis is suggested by a typical clinical syndrome and increased concentrations of total and *Aspergillus*-specific serum immunoglobulin E, eosinophilia, and a positive result of a skin test to *Aspergillus* antigens. In people with cystic fibrosis, the diagnosis is more difficult, because wheezing, eosinophilia, and a positive skin test result not associated with allergic bronchopulmonary aspergillosis often are present.

TREATMENT: Amphotericin B in high doses (1.0–1.5 mg/kg per day) is the treatment of choice for invasive aspergillosis (see Drugs for Invasive and Other Serious Fungal Infections, p 725); therapy is continued for 4 to 12 weeks or longer. Some experts recommend concomitant itraconazole or rifampin, but other experts do not believe the additional drugs offer any benefit. Lipid formulations of amphotericin B should be considered for children who are intolerant of or in whom the infection is refractory to conventional amphotericin B therapy. Safety and efficacy of these lipid formulations for children younger than 1 month of age have not been established. Itraconazole alone is an alternative for mild to moderate cases of aspergillosis when an isolate is susceptible to itraconazole. The safety and efficacy of itraconazole for use in children, however, has not been established. Caspofungin acetate has been licensed by the US Food and Drug Administration (FDA) for treatment of invasive aspergillosis in adults; use of this agent in children can be considered, but data regarding dosage and safety are limited. Voriconazole has been licensed by the FDA for treatment of invasive aspergillosis in adults. The safety and efficacy of these products in pediatric patients have not been established. Surgical excision of a localized lesion (eg, sinus debris) often is warranted.

Allergic bronchopulmonary or sinus aspergillosis usually is treated with corticosteroids. Systemic antifungal therapy is not indicated for patients with allergic aspergillosis or for nonallergic colonization.

ISOLATION OF THE HOSPITALIZED PATIENT: Standard precautions are recommended.

CONTROL MEASURES: Outbreaks of invasive aspergillosis have occurred among hospitalized immunosuppressed patients during construction in hospitals or at nearby sites. Environmental measures reported to be effective include erecting suitable barriers between patient care areas and construction sites, cleaning of air handling systems, repair of faulty air flow, and replacement of contaminated air filters.

High-efficiency particulate air filters and laminar flow rooms markedly decrease the risk of conidia in patient care areas. These latter measures, however, may be expensive and difficult for patients to tolerate. Low-dose amphotericin B or itraconazole prophylaxis has been reported for people undergoing bone marrow transplantation, but controlled trials have not been performed in pediatric patients.

Astrovirus Infections

CLINICAL MANIFESTATIONS: Illness is characterized by abdominal pain, diarrhea, vomiting, nausea, fever, and malaise. Illness in the immunocompetent host is self-limited, lasting a median of 5 to 6 days. Asymptomatic infections are common.

ETIOLOGY: Astroviruses are nonenveloped, single-stranded RNA viruses with a characteristic starlike appearance when visualized by electron microscopy. Eight human antigenic types are known.

EPIDEMIOLOGY: Human astroviruses have a worldwide distribution. Multiple antigenic types cocirculate in the same region. Astroviruses have been detected in as many as 10% of sporadic cases of nonbacterial gastroenteritis among young children. Astrovirus infections occur predominately in children younger than 4 years of age and have a seasonal peak during winter. Transmission is usually person to person via the fecal-oral route, although outbreaks associated with contaminated food rarely have been documented. Outbreaks tend to occur in closed populations of the young and the elderly, and attack rates are high among hospitalized children and children in child care centers. Excretion lasts a median of 5 days after the onset of symptoms, but asymptomatic excretion after illness can last for several weeks in healthy children. Persistent excretion may occur in immunocompromised hosts.

The **incubation period** is 1 to 4 days.

DIAGNOSTIC TESTS: Commercial tests for diagnosis are not available in the United States, although enzyme immunoassays are available in many other countries. The following tests are available in some research and reference laboratories: electron microscopy for detection of viral particles in stool, enzyme immunoassay for detection of viral antigen in stool or antibody in serum, and reverse transcriptase-polymerase chain reaction assay for detection of viral RNA in stool. Of these tests, reverse transcriptase-polymerase chain reaction assay is the most sensitive.

TREATMENT: Rehydration with oral or intravenous fluid and electrolyte solutions.

ISOLATION OF THE HOSPITALIZED PATIENT: In addition to standard precautions, contact precautions are recommended for diapered or incontinent children with possible or proven astrovirus infection for the duration of the illness.

CONTROL MEASURES: No specific control measures are available. The spread of infection in child care settings can be decreased by using general measures for control of diarrhea, such as training caregivers about infection control procedures, maintaining cleanliness of surfaces and food preparation areas, exercising adequate hand hygiene, and excluding ill child care providers and food handlers and ill children or placing ill children in cohorts. A vaccine to prevent astrovirus infection is not available.

Babesiosis

CLINICAL MANIFESTATIONS: Most infections are subclinical. In people who are symptomatic, gradual onset of malaise, anorexia, and fatigue typically occur, followed by intermittent fever with temperatures as high as 40°C (104°F) and one or more of the following symptoms: chills, sweats, myalgias, arthralgias, nausea, and vomiting. Less common findings are hyperesthesia, headache, sore throat, abdominal pain, conjunctival injection, photophobia, weight loss, and nonproductive cough. Signs on physical examination generally are minimal, often consisting only of fever, although mild splenomegaly, hepatomegaly, or both are noted occasionally. Many clinical features are similar to those of malaria. The illness can last for a few weeks to several months with a prolonged recovery of as long as 18 months. Severe illness is most likely to occur in people older than 40 years of age, people who are asplenic, and people who are immunocompromised. Some people, especially those who are asplenic, can suffer fulminant illness resulting in death or prolonged convalescence.

ETIOLOGY: *Babesia* species are intraerythrocytic protozoa. *Babesia microti* and several other genetically and antigenetically distinct organisms are responsible for disease in the United States.

EPIDEMIOLOGY: In the United States, the primary reservoir host for *B microti* is the white-footed mouse *(Peromyscus leucopus)*, and the primary vector is the tick, *Ixodes scapularis.* This tick also can transmit *Borrelia burgdorferi,* the causative agent of Lyme disease and of human granulocytic ehrlichiosis. Humans acquire the infection from bites of infected ticks. The white-tailed deer *(Odocoileus virginianus)* is an important host for the tick but is not a reservoir host for *B microti*. An increase in the deer population during the past few decades is thought to be a major factor in the spread of *I scapularis* and in the consequent increase in human cases of babesiosis. Babesiosis can be acquired through blood transfusions. Transplacental or perinatal transmission of babesiosis has been described. Human cases of babesiosis have been reported in the Midwest, Northeast and West Coast of the United States (California, Connecticut, Georgia, Massachusetts, Minnesota, Missouri, New Jersey, New York, Rhode Island, Washington, and Wisconsin). Most human cases of babesiosis occur during summer or autumn. In endemic areas, asymptomatic infections are common.

The **incubation period** ranges from 1 to 9 weeks.

DIAGNOSTIC TESTS: Babesiosis is diagnosed by microscopic identification of the organism on Giemsa- or Wright-stained thick or thin blood smears. Multiple thick and thin blood smears should be examined in suspected cases when a single examination result is negative. Serologic tests for detection of *Babesia* antibodies are available at the Centers for Disease Control and Prevention and at several state reference and research laboratories.

TREATMENT: Because many patients have a mild clinical course and recover without specific antibabesial chemotherapy, therapy is reserved for patients who are moderately or seriously ill. The combinations of clindamycin plus oral quinine for 7 days or atovaquone plus azithromycin for 7 to 10 days are equally efficacious (see Drugs for Parasitic Infections, p 744). The latter combination is associated with fewer adverse effects. Exchange blood transfusions have been used successfully in asplenic patients with life-threatening babesiosis and should be considered for all severely ill people with a high degree of parasitemia.

ISOLATION OF THE HOSPITALIZED PATIENT: Standard precautions are recommended.

CONTROL MEASURES: Specific recommendations concern prevention of tick bites and are similar to those for prevention of Lyme disease and other tickborne infections (see Prevention of Tickborne Infections, p 186).

Bacillus cereus Infections

CLINICAL MANIFESTATIONS: Two clinical syndromes are associated with *Bacillus cereus* food poisoning. The first is the emetic syndrome, which, like staphylococcal food poisoning, develops after a short incubation period, and is characterized by nausea, vomiting, abdominal cramps, and diarrhea in approximately one third of patients. The second is the diarrhea syndrome, which, like *Clostridium perfringens* food poisoning, has a longer incubation period, and is characterized predominantly by moderate to severe abdominal cramps and watery diarrhea, with vomiting in approximately one fourth of patients. Both syndromes are mild, usually are not associated with fever, and abate within 24 hours.

   Bacillus cereus also can cause local skin and wound infections, ocular infections, and invasive disease, including bacteremia, central-line associated infection, endocarditis, osteomyelitis, pneumonia, brain abscess and meningitis. Ocular involvement includes panophthalmitis, endophthalmitis, and keratitis.

ETIOLOGY: *Bacillus cereus* is an aerobic and facultatively anaerobic, spore-forming, gram-positive bacillus. The emetic syndrome is caused by a preformed heat-stable toxin. The diarrhea syndrome is caused by in vivo production of a heat-labile enterotoxin. This enterotoxin is cytoxic and can cause tissue necrosis, including fulminant liver failure.

EPIDEMIOLOGY: *Bacillus cereus* is ubiquitous in the environment. It commonly is present in small numbers in raw, dried, and processed foods but is an uncommon cause of food poisoning in the United States. Spores of *B cereus* are heat-resistant and can survive brief cooking or boiling. Vegetative forms can grow and produce enterotoxins over a wide range of temperatures from 25°C to 42°C (77°F–108°F). The emetic syndrome is acquired by eating food containing preformed toxin, most commonly fried or recooked rice. Disease can result from eating food contaminated with *B cereus* spores, which produce toxin in the gastrointestinal tract. Spore-associated disease most commonly is caused by contaminated meat or vegetables and manifests as a diarrhea syndrome. Foodborne illness caused by *B cereus* is not transmissible from person to person.

Risk factors for invasive disease attributable to *B cereus* include history of injection drug use, presence of indwelling intravascular catheters or implanted devices, and immunosuppression. *Bacillus cereus* endophthalmitis has occurred after penetrating ocular trauma and injection drug use.

The **incubation period** for the emetic syndrome is 1 to 6 hours; for the diarrhea syndrome, it is 6 to 24 hours.

DIAGNOSTIC TESTS: For foodborne illness, isolation of *B cereus* in a concentration of $\geq 10^5$/g of epidemiologically incriminated food establishes the diagnosis. Because the organism can be recovered from stool specimens from some well people, the presence of *B cereus* in feces or vomitus of ill people is not definitive evidence for infection unless isolates from several ill patients are demonstrated to be the same serotype or unless stool cultures from a matched control group test negative. Phage typing, DNA hybridization, plasmid analysis, and enzyme electrophoresis have been used as epidemiologic tools in outbreaks of food poisoning.

In patients with risk factors for invasive disease, isolation of *B cereus* from wounds, blood, or other usually sterile body fluids is significant.

TREATMENT: People with *B cereus* food poisoning require only supportive treatment. Oral rehydration or, occasionally, intravenous fluid and electrolyte replacement for patients with severe dehydration is indicated. Antimicrobial agents are not indicated.

Patients with invasive disease require antimicrobial therapy. Prompt removal of any potentially infected foreign bodies, such as catheters or implants, is essential. *Bacillus cereus* usually is susceptible to vancomycin, clindamycin, ciprofloxacin, imipenem, and meropenem. *Bacillus cereus* uniformly is resistant to β-lactam antimicrobial agents.

ISOLATION OF THE HOSPITALIZED PATIENT: Standard precautions are recommended.

CONTROL MEASURES: Proper cooking and storage of foods, particularly rice cooked for later use, will help prevent foodborne outbreaks. Food should be kept at temperatures higher than 60°C (140°F) or rapidly cooled to less than 10°C (50°F) after cooking.

Hand hygiene and strict aseptic technique in caring for immunocompromised patients or patients with indwelling intravascular catheters are important to minimize invasive disease.

Bacterial Vaginosis

CLINICAL MANIFESTATIONS: Bacterial vaginosis (BV), a syndrome primarily occurring in sexually active adolescent and adult females, is characterized by changes in vaginal flora. Symptoms may include a white, homogenous, adherent vaginal discharge with a fishy odor. Bacterial vaginosis may be asymptomatic and is not associated with abdominal pain, significant pruritus, or dysuria.

Vaginitis and vulvitis in prepubertal girls usually have a nonspecific cause and rarely are manifestations of BV. In prepubertal girls, other predisposing causes for vaginal discharge include foreign bodies or infections attributable to group A streptococci, *Trichomonas vaginalis,* herpes simplex virus, *Neisseria gonorrhoeae, Chlamydia trachomatis,* or *Shigella* species.

ETIOLOGY: The microbiologic cause of BV has not been delineated clearly. Typical microbiologic findings of specimens obtained from the vagina include an increase in concentrations of *Gardnerella vaginalis, Mycoplasma hominis, Ureaplasma* species, and anaerobic bacteria and a marked decrease in the concentration of *Lactobacillus* species.

EPIDEMIOLOGY: Bacterial vaginosis is the most prevalent vaginal infection in sexually active adolescents and adult females. It may occur with other conditions associated with vaginal discharge, such as trichomoniasis or cervicitis. Although the evidence for sexual transmission of BV is inconclusive, the condition is uncommon in sexually inexperienced females. Bacterial vaginosis may be a risk factor for pelvic inflammatory disease (PID). Pregnant women with BV are at increased risk of chorioamnionitis, premature rupture of the membranes, premature delivery, and postpartum endometritis. Preexisting symptomatic or asymptomatic bacterial vaginosis also may be a risk factor for postabortion PID. Bacterial vaginosis and chorioamnionitis may increase the risk of perinatal transmission of human immunodeficiency virus (HIV).

Sexually active adolescent and adult females with BV should be evaluated for the presence of sexually transmitted diseases, including syphilis, gonorrhea, *Chlamydia trachomatis* infection, hepatitis B virus infection, and HIV infection, because coinfection may occur. The occurrence of BV in prepubertal girls should raise suspicion of sexual abuse.

The **incubation period** for BV is unknown.

DIAGNOSTIC TESTS: The clinical diagnosis of bacterial vaginosis requires the presence of 3 of the following symptoms or signs:
- Homogenous, white, noninflammatory vaginal discharge that smoothly coats the vaginal walls
- Vaginal fluid pH greater than 4.5
- A fishy odor of vaginal discharge before or after addition of 10% potassium hydroxide (ie, the whiff test)

- Presence of "clue cells" (squamous vaginal epithelial cells covered with bacteria, which cause a stippled or granular appearance and ragged "moth-eaten" borders) on microscopic examination. In BV, clue cells usually constitute at least 20% of vaginal epithelial cells.

A Gram stain of vaginal secretions is an alternative means of establishing a diagnosis. Numerous mixed bacteria, including small curved bacilli and cocci and few large gram-positive bacilli consistent with lactobacilli, are characteristic. Culture for *G vaginalis* is not recommended, because the organism may be found in females without BV, including females who are not sexually active.

TREATMENT: The principal goal of treatment is to relieve vaginal symptoms and signs of infection and decrease the risk of infectious complications. All nonpregnant patients who are symptomatic require treatment. Nonpregnant patients with symptoms should be treated with metronidazole (1.0 g/day, orally, in 2 divided doses) for 7 days; or metronidazole gel, 0.75%, 5 g (1 applicator), intravaginally, once a day for 5 days; or clindamycin cream, 2%, 1 applicator (5 g), intravaginally, at bedtime for 7 days. Alternative regimens that have a lower efficacy for BV are metronidazole, 2 g, orally, in a single dose; clindamycin, 600 mg/day, orally, in 2 divided doses for 7 days; or clindamycin ovules, 100 g, intravaginally, once at bedtime for 3 days. Clindamycin cream is oil-based and may weaken latex condoms for up to 72 hours after completion of therapy.

Pregnant women with symptoms of BV should be treated, regardless of risk factors for adverse pregnancy outcome. Pregnant women at increased risk of adverse pregnancy outcome in association with BV (eg, previous preterm birth) also should be treated if asymptomatic, according to some experts. Metronidazole, 750 mg/day in 3 divided doses daily for 7 days, is the preferred treatment during pregnancy. An alternative regimen is clindamycin, 600 mg/day, orally, in 2 divided doses for 7 days. Because treatment of BV in high-risk pregnant women who are asymptomatic might prevent adverse pregnancy outcomes, a follow-up evaluation 1 month after completion of treatment should be considered to evaluate whether therapy was successful.

For nonpregnant and low-risk pregnant women, routine follow-up visits on completion of therapy for BV are unnecessary, if symptoms resolve. Recurrences are common and can be treated with the same regimen given initially. The presence of a vaginal foreign body should be excluded. Routine treatment of male sexual partners is not recommended, because treatment has no influence on relapse or recurrence rates.

Treatment of BV in females infected with HIV is the same as for HIV-negative patients and especially is important in women who are pregnant, because BV and chorioamnionitis may increase the risk of perinatal transmission of HIV.

ISOLATION OF THE HOSPITALIZED PATIENT: Standard precautions are recommended.

CONTROL MEASURES: None.

Bacteroides and *Prevotella* Infections

CLINICAL MANIFESTATIONS: *Bacteroides* and *Prevotella* species from the oral cavity can cause chronic sinusitis, chronic otitis media, dental infection, peritonsillar abscess, cervical adenitis, retropharyngeal space infection, aspiration pneumonia, lung abscess, empyema, or necrotizing pneumonia. Species from the gastrointestinal tract are recovered in patients with peritonitis, intra-abdominal abscess, pelvic inflammatory disease, postoperative wound infection, or vulvovaginal and perianal infections. Soft tissue infections include synergistic bacterial gangrene and necrotizing fasciitis. Invasion of the bloodstream from the oral cavity or intestinal tract can lead to brain abscess, meningitis, endocarditis, arthritis, or osteomyelitis. Skin involvement includes omphalitis in newborn infants, cellulitis at the site of fetal monitors, human bite wounds, infection of burns adjacent to the mouth or rectum, and decubitus ulcers. Neonatal infections, such as conjunctivitis, pneumonia, bacteremia, or meningitis, occur rarely. Most *Bacteroides* infections are polymicrobial.

ETIOLOGY: Most *Bacteroides* and *Prevotella* organisms associated with human disease are pleomorphic, nonspore-forming, facultatively anaerobic, gram-negative bacilli. *Bacteroides* and *Prevotella* species produce enzymes that play a role in the pathogenesis of disease.

EPIDEMIOLOGY: *Bacteroides* and *Prevotella* species are part of the normal flora of the mouth, gastrointestinal tract, or female genital tract. Members of the *Bacteroides fragilis* group predominate in the gastrointestinal tract flora; members of the *Prevotella melaninogenica* (formerly *Bacteroides melaninogenicus*) and *Prevotella oralis* (formerly *Bacteroides oralis*) groups are more common in the oral cavity. These species cause infection as opportunists, usually after an alteration of the body's physical barrier, and in conjunction with other endogenous species. Endogenous transmission results from aspiration, spillage from the bowel, or damage to mucosal surfaces from trauma, surgery, or chemotherapy. Mucosal injury or granulocytopenia predispose to infection. Except in infections resulting from human bites, no evidence for person-to-person transmission exists.

The **incubation period** is variable and depends on the inoculum and the site of involvement but usually is 1 to 5 days.

DIAGNOSTIC TESTS: Anaerobic culture media are necessary for recovery of *Bacteroides* or *Prevotella* species. Because infections usually are polymicrobial, aerobic cultures also should be obtained. A putrid odor suggests anaerobic infection. Use of an anaerobic transport tube or a sealed syringe is recommended for collection of clinical specimens.

TREATMENT: Abscesses should be drained when feasible; abscesses involving the brain or liver may resolve with effective antimicrobial therapy. Necrotizing lesions should be débrided surgically.

The choice of antimicrobial agent(s) is based on anticipated or known in vitro susceptibility testing. *Bacteroides* infections of the mouth and respiratory tract generally are susceptible to penicillin G, ampicillin sodium, and broad-spectrum penicillins, such as ticarcillin disodium or piperacillin sodium. Clindamycin is active against virtually all mouth and respiratory tract *Bacteroides* and *Prevotella* isolates and is recommended by some experts as the drug of choice for anaerobic infections of the oral cavity and lungs. Some species of *Bacteroides* and *Prevotella* produce β-lactamase. A β-lactam penicillin active against *Bacteroides* combined with a β-lactamase inhibitor can be useful to treat these infections (ampicillin-sulbactam sodium, amoxicillin-clavulanate potassium, ticarcillin-clavulanate, or piperacillin-tazobactam sodium). *Bacteroides* species of the gastrointestinal tract usually are resistant to penicillin G but are predictably susceptible to metronidazole, chloramphenicol, and usually, clindamycin. More than 80% of isolates are susceptible to cefoxitin sodium, ceftizoxime sodium, and imipenem. Cefuroxime, cefotaxime sodium, and ceftriaxone sodium are not reliably effective.

ISOLATION OF THE HOSPITALIZED PATIENT: Standard precautions are recommended.

CONTROL MEASURES: None.

Balantidium coli Infections
(Balantidiasis)

CLINICAL MANIFESTATIONS: Most human infections are asymptomatic. Acute infection is characterized by the rapid onset of nausea, vomiting, abdominal discomfort or pain, and bloody or watery mucoid diarrhea. Infected patients can develop chronic intermittent episodes of diarrhea. Rarely, organisms spread to mesenteric nodes, pleura, or liver. Inflammation of the gastrointestinal tract and local lymphatic vessels can result in bowel dilation, ulceration, and secondary bacterial invasion. Colitis produced by *Balantidium coli* often is indistinguishable from that produced by *Entamoeba histolytica*. Fulminant disease can occur in malnourished or otherwise debilitated patients.

ETIOLOGY: *Balantidium coli,* a ciliated protozoan, is the largest pathogenic protozoan known to infect humans.

EPIDEMIOLOGY: Pigs are believed to be the primary host reservoir of *B coli.* Cysts excreted in feces can be transmitted directly from hand to mouth or indirectly through fecally contaminated water or food. The excysted trophozoites infect the colon. A person is infectious as long as cysts are excreted. The cysts may remain viable in the environment for months.

The **incubation period** is unknown but may be several days.

DIAGNOSTIC TESTS: Diagnosis of infection is established by scraping lesions via sigmoidoscopy, histologic examination of intestinal biopsy specimens, or ova and parasite examination of stool. The diagnosis usually is established by demonstrating trophozoites in stool or tissue specimens. Stool examination is less sensitive, and repeated stool examination may be necessary to diagnose infection, because shedding of organisms can be intermittent. Microscopic examination of fresh diarrheal stools must be performed promptly, because trophozoites quickly degenerate.

TREATMENT: The drug of choice is tetracycline, which is administered for 10 days in a dose of 40 mg/kg per day, maximum of 2 g/day, divided into 4 doses. Tetracycline should not be given to children younger than 8 years of age unless the benefits of therapy are greater than the risks of dental staining (see Antimicrobial Agents and Related Therapy, p 693). Alternative drugs are iodoquinol and metronidazole (see Drugs for Parasitic Infections, p 744).

ISOLATION OF THE HOSPITALIZED PATIENT: In addition to standard precautions, contact precautions are recommended.

CONTROL MEASURES: Control measures include sanitary disposal of human feces and avoidance of contamination of food and water with porcine feces. Despite chlorination of water, waterborne outbreaks of disease have occurred.

Blastocystis hominis Infections

CLINICAL MANIFESTATIONS: The importance of *Blastocystis hominis* as a cause of gastrointestinal tract disease is controversial. The asymptomatic carrier state is well documented. *Blastocystis hominis* has been associated with symptoms of bloating, flatulence, mild to moderate diarrhea without fecal leukocytes or blood, abdominal pain, and nausea. When *B hominis* is identified in stool from symptomatic patients, other causes of this symptom complex, particularly *Giardia lamblia* and *Cryptosporidium parvum,* should be investigated before assuming that *B hominis* is the cause of the signs and symptoms.

ETIOLOGY: *Blastocystis hominis* is classified as a protozoan and has 3 distinct stages: vacuolar, which is observed most commonly in clinical specimens; granular; and ameboid.

EPIDEMIOLOGY: *Blastocystis hominis* is recovered from 1% to 20% of stool specimens examined for ova and parasites. Because transmission is believed to be via the fecal-oral route, the presence of the organism may be a marker for the presence of other pathogens spread by fecal contamination. Transmission from animals occurs.

The **incubation period** is unknown.

DIAGNOSTIC TESTS: Stool specimens should be preserved in polyvinyl alcohol and stained with trichrome or iron-hematoxylin before microscopic examination. The parasite may be present in varying numbers, and infections may be reported as light to heavy. The presence of 5 or more organisms per high-power (×400 magnification) field indicates a heavy infection, which to some experts suggests causation when other enteropathogens are absent.

TREATMENT: Indications for treatment are not established. Some experts recommend that treatment should be reserved for patients who have persistent symptoms and in whom no other pathogen or process is found to explain the gastrointestinal tract symptoms. Other experts believe that *B hominis* does not cause symptomatic disease and recommend only a careful search for other causes of the symptoms. Metronidazole, trimethoprim-sulfamethoxazole, and iodoquinol have been used with limited success (see Drugs for Parasitic Infections, p 744). Controlled treatment trials are not available.

ISOLATION OF THE HOSPITALIZED PATIENT: In addition to standard precautions, contact precautions are recommended for diapered or incontinent children.

CONTROL MEASURES: None.

Blastomycosis

CLINICAL MANIFESTATIONS: Infection may be asymptomatic or associated with acute, chronic, or fulminant disease. The major clinical manifestations of blastomycosis are pulmonary, cutaneous, and disseminated disease. Children commonly have pulmonary disease that can be associated with a variety of symptoms, and radiographic appearances can be misdiagnosed as bacterial pneumonia, tuberculosis, sarcoidosis, or malignant neoplasm. Skin lesions can be nodular, verrucous, or ulcerative, often with minimal inflammation. Abscesses generally are subcutaneous but may involve any organ. Disseminated blastomycosis usually begins with pulmonary infection and can involve the skin, bones, central nervous system, abdominal viscera, and kidneys. Intrauterine or congenital infections occur rarely.

ETIOLOGY: Blastomycosis is caused by *Blastomyces dermatitidis,* a dimorphic fungus existing in the yeast form at 37°C (98°F) and in infected tissues and in a mycelial form at room temperature and in the soil. Conidia, produced from hyphae of the mycelial form, are infectious for humans.

EPIDEMIOLOGY: Infection is acquired through inhalation of conidia from soil. Person-to-person transmission does not occur. Infection may be epidemic or sporadic and has been reported in the United States, Canada, Africa, and India. Endemic areas in the United States are the southeastern and central states and the midwestern states bordering the Great Lakes. Although blastomycosis can occur in immunocompromised hosts, the disease has been reported rarely in people infected with human immunodeficiency virus.

The **incubation period** is approximately 30 to 45 days.

DIAGNOSTIC TESTS: Thick-walled, figure-of-eight shaped, broad-based, single-budding yeast forms may be seen in sputum, tracheal aspirates, cerebrospinal fluid, urine, or material from lesions processed with 10% potassium hydroxide or a silver stain. Children with pneumonia who are unable to produce sputum may require an invasive procedure (eg, open biopsy or bronchoalveolar lavage) to establish the diagnosis. Organisms can be cultured on brain-heart infusion media and Sabouraud dextrose agar at room temperature. Chemiluminescent DNA probes are available for identification of *B dermatitidis*. Because serologic tests lack adequate sensitivity, every effort should be made to obtain appropriate specimens for culture.

TREATMENT: Amphotericin B is the treatment of choice for severe or life-threatening infection (see Drugs for Invasive and Other Serious Fungal Infections, p 725). Oral itraconazole or fluconazole has been used for mild or moderately severe infections alone or following a short course of amphotericin B. Data regarding the safety and efficacy of itraconazole and fluconazole therapy in children are limited. Itraconazole is highly effective for the treatment of nonmeningeal, nonlife-threatening infections in adults, but it does not achieve effective concentrations in the cerebrospinal fluid.

Oral therapy usually is continued for at least 6 months for pulmonary and extrapulmonary disease. Some experts suggest one year of therapy for patients with osteomyelitis.

ISOLATION OF THE HOSPITALIZED PATIENT: Standard precautions are recommended.

CONTROL MEASURES: None.

Borrelia Infections
(Relapsing Fever)

CLINICAL MANIFESTATIONS: Relapsing fever is characterized by the sudden onset of high fever, shaking chills, sweats, headache, muscle and joint pains, and progressive weakness. A fleeting macular rash of the trunk and petechiae of the skin and mucous membranes sometimes occur. Complications include hepatosplenomegaly, jaundice, epistaxis, iridocyclitis, cough with pleuritic pain, pneumonitis, meningitis, and myocarditis. Untreated, an initial febrile period of 3 to 7 days terminates spontaneously by crisis. The initial febrile episode is followed by an afebrile period of several days to weeks, then by one or more relapses. Relapses typically become progressively shorter and milder as the afebrile periods lengthen. Infection during pregnancy often is severe and can result in abortion, stillbirth, or neonatal infection.

ETIOLOGY: Relapsing fever is caused by certain spirochetes of the genus *Borrelia*. *Borrelia recurrentis* is the only species that causes louseborne (epidemic) relapsing fever, and there is no animal reservoir of *B recurrentis*. Worldwide, at least 15 *Borrelia* species cause tickborne (endemic) relapsing fever, including *Borrelia hermsii* and *Borrelia turicatae* in North America.

EPIDEMIOLOGY: Epidemic transmission is by body lice *(Pediculus humanus)*, and tickborne endemic relapsing fever is transmitted by soft-bodied ticks *(Ornithodoros* species). Louseborne epidemic relapsing fever has been reported in Ethiopia, Eritrea, Somalia, and the Sudan, where it sometimes occurs in epidemics, especially among the homeless and in refugee populations. Body lice become infected only by feeding on spirochetemic humans; the infection is transmitted when infected lice are crushed and their body fluids contaminate a bite wound or skin abraded by scratching.

Endemic tickborne relapsing fever is distributed widely throughout the world and occurs sporadically and in small clusters, often within families. Most tickborne relapsing fever in the United States is caused by *B hermsii*. Infection typically results from tick exposures in rodent-infested cabins in western mountainous areas, including state and national parks. *Borrelia turicatae* infections occur less frequently; most cases have been reported from Texas and often are associated with tick exposures in rodent-infested caves. Soft-bodied ticks inflict painless bites and feed briefly (10–30 minutes), usually at night, so people often are unaware of bites. Ticks become infected by feeding on rodents and transmit infection via their saliva and other fluids when they take subsequent blood meals. Ticks may serve as reservoirs of infection as a result of transovarial and trans-stadial transmission.

Infected body lice and ticks remain contagious throughout their lives. Relapsing fever is not contagious, but perinatal transmission from an infected mother to her infant does occur and can result in stillbirth and neonatal death.

The **incubation period** is 4 to 18 days, with a mean of 7 days.

DIAGNOSTIC TESTS: Spirochetes can be observed by dark-field microscopy and in Wright-, Giemsa-, or acridine orange-stained preparations of thin or dehemoglobinized thick smears of peripheral blood or in stained buffy-coat preparations. Organisms are found in blood most commonly during the febrile stage of the illness. Spirochetes can be cultured from blood in Barbour-Stoenner-Kelly medium or by intraperitoneal inoculation of immature laboratory mice. Serum antibodies to *Borrelia* species can be detected by enzyme immunoassay and Western immunoblot analysis at some reference laboratories; these tests are not standardized and are affected by antigenic variations between and within *Borrelia* species and strains. Serologic cross-reactions occur with other spirochetes, including *Borrelia burgdorferi*, the agent causing Lyme disease. Biologic specimens for laboratory testing can be sent to the Division of Vector-Borne Infectious Diseases, Centers for Disease Control and Prevention, Fort Collins, CO 80522.

TREATMENT: Treatment with penicillin, tetracyclines, doxycycline, erythromycin, or chloramphenicol effectively produces prompt clearance of spirochetes and remission of symptoms. For children younger than 8 years of age and for pregnant women, penicillin and erythromycin are the preferred drugs. A Jarisch-Herxheimer reaction (an acute febrile reaction accompanied by headache, myalgia, and an aggravated clinical picture lasting less than 24 hours) commonly is observed during the first few hours after initiating antimicrobial therapy. Because this reaction sometimes is associated with transient hypotension attributable to decreased effective circulating blood volume (especially in louseborne relapsing fever), patients should be monitored closely during the first 12 hours of treatment. However, the Jarisch-Herxheimer reaction in children typically is mild and usually can be managed with antipyretic agents alone.

Penicillin G procaine or intravenous penicillin G is recommended as initial therapy for people who are unable to take oral therapy. For oral therapy, standard doses of penicillin V, erythromycin, or tetracycline or doxycycline (if 8 years of age or older) are recommended. Single-dose treatment is effective for curing louseborne relapsing fever. Less is known about single-dose treatment of tickborne relapsing fever, but single-dose treatment probably is effective. However, treatment for 5 to

7 days, particularly for tickborne relapsing fever, is recommended to ensure prevention of relapses.

ISOLATION OF THE HOSPITALIZED PATIENT: Standard precautions are recommended. If louse infestation is present, contact precautions also are indicated (see Pediculosis, pp 463–467).

CONTROL MEASURES: Contact with ticks can be limited through use of protective clothing, acaricides, and tick repellents (see Prevention of Tickborne Infections, p 186). Prevention of rodent access to foundations and attics of homes or cabins also decreases the potential for tick exposure. Dwellings infested with soft ticks should be treated professionally with chemical agents and rodent-proofed. When in a louse-infested environment, body lice can be controlled by bathing, washing clothing at frequent intervals, and use of pediculicides (see Pediculosis, pp 463–467). Reporting of suspected cases of relapsing fever to health authorities is important for initiating prompt investigation and institution of control measures.

Brucellosis

CLINICAL MANIFESTATIONS: Brucellosis in children commonly is a mild self-limited disease compared with the more chronic disease in adults. However, in areas where *Brucella melitensis* is the endemic species, disease can be severe. Onset of illness can be acute or insidious. Manifestations are nonspecific and include fever, night sweats, weakness, malaise, anorexia, weight loss, arthralgia, myalgia, abdominal pain, and headache. Physical findings include lymphadenopathy, hepatosplenomegaly, and occasionally, arthritis. Serious complications include meningitis, endocarditis, and osteomyelitis.

ETIOLOGY: *Brucella* species are small, nonmotile, gram-negative coccobacilli. The species that infect humans are *Brucella abortus, B melitensis, Brucella suis,* and rarely, *Brucella canis.*

EPIDEMIOLOGY: Brucellosis is a zoonotic disease of wild and domestic animals. Humans are accidental hosts, contracting the disease by direct contact with infected animals and their carcasses or secretions or by ingesting unpasteurized milk or milk products. People in occupations such as farming, ranching, and veterinary medicine as well as abattoir workers, meat inspectors, and laboratory personnel are at increased risk. Infection is transmitted by inoculation through cuts and abrasions in the skin, by inhalation of contaminated aerosols, by contact with the conjunctival mucosa, or by oral ingestion. Approximately 100 cases of brucellosis occur annually in the United States, with fewer than 10% of reported cases occurring in people younger than 19 years of age. Most cases result from travel outside the United States or from ingestion of unpasteurized milk products. Human-to-human transmission has been documented rarely.

The **incubation period** varies from less than 1 week to several months, but most patients become ill within 3 to 4 weeks of exposure.

DIAGNOSTIC TESTS: A definitive diagnosis is established by recovery of *Brucella* from blood, bone marrow, or other tissues. A variety of media will support the growth of *Brucella* species, but laboratory personnel should incubate cultures for a minimum of 4 weeks. In patients with clinically compatible illness, serologic testing can confirm the diagnosis with a fourfold or greater increase in antibody titers in serum specimens collected at least 2 weeks apart. The serum agglutination test (SAT), the most commonly used test, will detect antibodies against *B abortus, B suis,* and *B melitensis,* but not *B canis,* which requires use of *B canis*-specific antigen. Although a single titer is not diagnostic, most patients with active infection have a titer of 1:160 or greater. Lower titers may be found early in the course of infection. Increased concentrations of immunoglobulin (Ig) G agglutinins are found in acute infection, chronic infection, and relapse. When interpreting SAT results, the possibility of cross-reactions of *Brucella* antibodies with those against other gram-negative bacteria, such as *Yersinia enterocolitica* serotype 09, *Francisella tularensis,* and *Vibrio cholerae,* should be considered. To avoid a prozone phenomenon, serum should be diluted to 1:320 or higher before testing. Enzyme immunoassay is a sensitive method for determining IgG, IgA, and IgM anti-*Brucella* antibodies. Until better standardization is established, enzyme immunoassay should be used only for suspected cases with negative SAT results or for evaluation of patients with suspected relapse or reinfection. The polymerase chain reaction test has been developed but is not available in most clinical laboratories.

TREATMENT: Prolonged antimicrobial therapy is imperative for achieving a cure. Relapses generally are not associated with development of *Brucella* resistance but rather with premature discontinuation of therapy.

Oral doxycycline (2–4 mg/kg per day; maximum 200 mg/day, in 2 divided doses) or oral tetracycline (30–40 mg/kg per day; maximum 2 g/day, in 4 divided doses) should be administered for 4 to 6 weeks. However, tetracycline and doxycycline should be avoided, if possible, for children younger than 8 years of age (see Antimicrobial Agents and Related Therapy, p 693). Oral trimethoprim-sulfamethoxazole (trimethoprim, 10 mg/kg per day; maximum 480 mg/day; and sulfamethoxazole, 50 mg/kg per day; maximum 2.4 g/day) divided in 2 doses for 4 to 6 weeks is appropriate therapy for younger patients.

To decrease the incidence of relapse, many experts recommend combination therapy with a tetracycline (or trimethoprim-sulfamethoxazole if tetracyclines are contraindicated) and rifampin (15–20 mg/kg per day; maximum 600–900 mg/day, in 1 or 2 divided doses). Because of the potential emergence of rifampin resistance, rifampin monotherapy is not recommended.

For treatment of serious infection or complications, including endocarditis, meningitis, and osteomyelitis, streptomycin sulfate or gentamicin sulfate for the first 7 to 14 days of therapy in addition to a tetracycline (or trimethoprim-sulfamethoxazole if tetracyclines are contraindicated) is recommended. In addition, rifampin can be used with this regimen to decrease the rate of relapse. For life-threatening complications of brucellosis, such as meningitis or endocarditis, the duration of therapy often is extended for several months.

The benefit of corticosteroids for people with neurobrucellosis is unproven. Occasionally, a Jarisch-Herxheimer-like reaction (an acute febrile reaction accompanied by headache, myalgia, and an aggravated clinical picture lasting less than 24 hours) occurs shortly after initiation of antimicrobial therapy, but this reaction is rarely severe enough to require corticosteroids.

ISOLATION OF THE HOSPITALIZED PATIENT: In addition to standard precautions, contact precautions are indicated for patients with draining wounds.

CONTROL MEASURES: The control of human brucellosis depends on eradication of *Brucella* species from cattle, goats, swine, and other animals. Pasteurization of milk and milk products for human consumption is especially important to prevent disease in children. The certification of raw milk does not eliminate the risk of transmission of *Brucella* organisms. In endemic areas, enforcement of and education about control measures are crucial.

Burkholderia Infections

CLINICAL MANIFESTATIONS: *Burkholderia cepacia* complex has been associated with severe pulmonary infections in patients with cystic fibrosis, with significant bacteremia in premature infants requiring prolonged hospitalization, and with infection in children with chronic granulomatous disease, hemoglobinopathies, or malignant neoplasms. Nosocomial infections include wound and urinary tract infections and pneumonia. Pulmonary infections in people with cystic fibrosis occur late in the course of disease, usually after infection with *Pseudomonas aeruginosa* has been established. Culture-positive patients may experience no change in the rate of pulmonary decompensation, become chronically infected with a more rapid decline in pulmonary function, or experience an unexpectedly rapid deterioration in clinical status that results in death. In chronic granulomatous disease, pneumonia is the most common infection caused by *B cepacia* complex; lymphadenitis also has been reported. Disease onset is insidious, with low-grade fever early in the course and systemic effects occurring 3 to 4 weeks later. Pleural effusion is common, and lung abscess has been described.

Burkholderia pseudomallei is the cause of melioidosis in the rural population of southeast Asia. Melioidosis can manifest as a localized infection or as fulminant septicemia. Localized infection usually is nonfatal and most commonly manifests as pneumonia, but skin, soft tissue, and skeletal infections also occur. In disseminated infection, hepatic and splenic abscesses may occur, and relapses are common.

ETIOLOGY: *Burkholderia* organisms are nutritionally diverse, catalase-producing, nonlactose-fermenting, gram-negative bacilli. *Burkholderia cepacia* complex comprises at least 7 species, and 4 have received species names (*Burkholderia multivorans, Burkholderia vietnamiensis, Burkholderia stabilis,* and *Burkholderia ambifaria*).

EPIDEMIOLOGY: All *Burkholderia* species are animal or plant pathogens but are nonpathogens in immunocompetent human hosts. *Burkholderia* species are water- and soilborne organisms that can survive for prolonged periods when kept moist. Epidemiologic studies of camps and other social events attended by people with cystic fibrosis from different geographic areas have demonstrated person-to-person spread of *B cepacia*. The source for acquisition of *B cepacia* by patients with chronic granulomatous disease has not been identified. Nosocomial spread of *B cepacia* most often is associated with contamination of disinfectant solutions used to clean reusable patient equipment, such as bronchoscopes and pressure transducers, or to disinfect skin. *Burkholderia gladioli* also has been isolated from sputum from people with cystic fibrosis and may be mistaken for *B cepacia*. The clinical significance of *B gladioli* is not known.

    Burkholderia pseudomallei often is acquired early in life, with the highest seroconversion rates between 6 and 42 months of age. Symptomatic infection can occur as early as 1 year of age. Risk factors for disease include diabetes mellitus and renal insufficiency.

DIAGNOSTIC TESTS: Culture is the appropriate test for diagnosis of *B cepacia* infection. In cystic fibrosis lung infection, culture of sputum on selective agar is recommended to decrease the potential for overgrowth by mucoid *P aeruginosa*. *Burkholderia cepacia* and *B gladioli* can be identified by polymerase chain reaction assay, but this assay is not available routinely. Diagnosis of melioidosis is made by isolation of *B pseudomallei* from blood or other infected sites. The indirect hemagglutination assay is used most often for serologic diagnosis of melioidosis in young children, and a positive test result is more predictive of infection in this age group than in older children and adults. Other rapid assays being developed for diagnosis of melioidosis include the direct fluorescent antibody test for identification of the organism in sputum, an immunoglobulin M enzyme immunoassay, a monoclonal antibody test, and DNA probes.

TREATMENT: Meropenem is the most active agent against *B cepacia*. Most experts recommend synergistic combinations of antimicrobial agents. *Burkholderia cepacia* is intrinsically resistant to aminoglycosides and polymyxin B sulfate. Other agents that are variably active against *B pseudomallei* include ceftazidime, piperacillin sodium, chloramphenicol, doxycycline, and trimethoprim-sulfamethoxazole.

ISOLATION OF THE HOSPITALIZED PATIENT: Contact and droplet precautions are recommended for patients infected with multidrug-resistant strains.

CONTROL MEASURES: Because some strains of *B cepacia* are highly transmissible and virulence is not well understood, many cystic fibrosis centers limit contact between *B cepacia*-infected and uninfected patients with cystic fibrosis. This includes inpatient, outpatient, and social settings. For example, cystic fibrosis patients with *B cepacia* are cared for in single rooms and have unique clinic hours, and specialized camps have been disbanded. Education of patients and families about hand hygiene and appropriate personal hygiene is recommended. There are no specific measures to prevent infection with *B pseudomallei* in endemic regions.

Caliciviruses

CLINICAL MANIFESTATIONS: Diarrhea and vomiting, commonly accompanied by fever, headache, malaise, myalgia, and abdominal cramps, are characteristic of calicivirus infection. Symptoms last from 1 day to 2 weeks.

ETIOLOGY: Caliciviruses are nonenveloped RNA viruses. The 2 recognized genera that cause disease in humans are Norwalk-like (noroviruses) and Sapporo-like caliciviruses.

EPIDEMIOLOGY: Human caliciviruses have a worldwide distribution, with multiple antigenic types circulating simultaneously in the same region. Caliciviruses may be a major cause of sporadic cases of gastroenteritis requiring hospitalization, but sensitive diagnostic tools have been applied only recently to study this problem. Most sporadic calicivirus infections have been detected in children younger than 4 years of age. Transmission is by person-to-person spread via the fecal-oral route or through contaminated food or water, but often a route of transmission cannot be determined. Outbreaks of gastroenteritis have been detected in all age groups. Outbreaks tend to occur in closed populations, such as child care centers and on cruise ships, and there is a high attack rate. Common-source outbreaks have been described after ingestion of ice, shellfish, salads, and cookies, usually contaminated by infected food handlers. Airborne transmission may occur, although compelling evidence of this is lacking. Exposure to contaminated surfaces and vomitus has been implicated in some outbreaks. Excretion lasts 5 to 7 days after the onset of symptoms in half of the infected people, and excretion can be as long as 13 days. Prolonged excretion can occur in immunocompromised hosts.

The **incubation period** is 12 to 72 hours.

DIAGNOSTIC TESTS: Commercial assays for diagnosis are not available. The following tests are available in some research and reference laboratories: electron microscopy for detection of viral particles in stool, enzyme immunoassay for detection of viral antigen in stool or antibody in serum, and reverse transcriptase-polymerase chain reaction (RT-PCR) assay for detection of viral RNA in stool. The most sensitive assays are RT-PCR and serologic testing; electron microscopy is relatively insensitive. Laboratory and epidemiologic support for diagnosis of suspected calicivirus outbreaks is available at the Centers for Disease Control and Prevention, and RT-PCR assays for viral detection in stools increasingly are available at state and local health department laboratories.

TREATMENT: Supportive therapy includes oral rehydration solution to replace fluids and electrolytes.

ISOLATION OF THE HOSPITALIZED PATIENT: In addition to standard precautions, contact precautions are recommended for diapered and incontinent children for the duration of illness.

CONTROL MEASURES: No specific control measures are available. The spread of infection can be decreased by standard measures for control of diarrhea, such as teaching child care providers and all food handlers about infection control, maintaining cleanliness of surfaces and food preparation areas, excluding caregivers or food handlers who are ill, exercising adequate hand hygiene, and excluding or grouping ill children in child care. If a mode of transmission can be identified (eg, contaminated food or water) during an outbreak, then specific interventions to interrupt transmission can be effective. Immunization to prevent calicivirus infection is not available.

Campylobacter Infections

CLINICAL MANIFESTATIONS: Predominant symptoms of *Campylobacter* infections include diarrhea, abdominal pain, malaise, and fever. Stools may contain visible or occult blood. In neonates and young infants, bloody diarrhea without fever may be the only manifestation of infection. Abdominal pain can mimic that produced by appendicitis. Mild infection lasts 1 or 2 days and resembles viral gastroenteritis. Most patients recover in less than one week, but 20% have a relapse or a prolonged or severe illness. Severe or persistent infection can mimic acute inflammatory bowel disease. Bacteremia is uncommon, but neonatal septicemia occurs occasionally. Immunocompromised hosts may have prolonged, relapsing, or extraintestinal infections, especially with *Campylobacter fetus* and other "atypical" species. Immunoreactive complications, such as acute idiopathic polyneuritis (Guillain-Barré syndrome), Miller Fisher syndrome (ophthalmoplegia, areflexia, ataxia), reactive arthritis, Reiter syndrome (arthritis, urethritis, and bilateral conjunctivitis), and erythema nodosum, can occur during convalescence.

ETIOLOGY: *Campylobacter* species are motile, comma-shaped, gram-negative bacilli that cause gastroenteritis. *Campylobacter fetus* predominantly causes systemic illness in neonates and debilitated hosts. *Campylobacter jejuni* and *Campylobacter coli* are the most common species isolated from patients with diarrhea. Other *Campylobacter* species, including *Campylobacter upsaliensis, Campylobacter lari,* and *Campylobacter hyointestinalis,* may cause similar diarrheal or systemic illnesses.

EPIDEMIOLOGY: The gastrointestinal tract of domestic and wild birds and animals is the reservoir of infection. *Campylobacter jejuni* and *C coli* have been isolated from feces of 30% to 100% of chickens, turkeys, and water fowl. Poultry carcasses usually are contaminated. Many farm animals and meat sources can harbor the organism, and pets (especially young animals), including dogs, cats, hamsters, and birds, are potential sources. Transmission of *C jejuni* and *C coli* occurs by ingestion of contaminated food, including unpasteurized milk and untreated water, or by direct contact with fecal material from infected animals or people. Improperly cooked poultry, untreated water, and unpasteurized milk have been the main vehicles of transmission. Outbreaks among school children who drank unpasteurized milk in conjunction with field trips to dairy farms have occurred. Person-to-person spread occurs occasionally, particularly from very young children, and outbreaks of diarrhea in child care centers have been reported infrequently. Person-to-person transmission also has occurred in neonates of infected mothers and has resulted in nosocomial outbreaks in nurseries. In perinatal infection, *C jejuni* and *C coli* usually cause neonatal gastroenteritis, whereas *C fetus* often causes neonatal septicemia or meningitis. Enteritis occurs in people of all ages. Communicability is uncommon but is greatest during the acute phase of illness. Excretion of *Campylobacter* organisms usually is brief, typically 2 to 3 weeks, without treatment. *Campylobacter jejuni* and *C coli* are the major organisms detected by the Foodborne Diseases Active Surveillance Network (FoodNet).*

The **incubation period** usually is 1 to 7 days but can be longer.

DIAGNOSTIC TESTS: Rapid presumptive diagnosis is possible in laboratories experienced in examining stool smears by dark-field microscopic or Gram-stain techniques, although the sensitivity of these techniques is low. *Campylobacter jejuni* and *C coli* can be cultured from feces, and *Campylobacter* species, including *C fetus*, can be cultured from blood. Laboratory identification of *C jejuni* and *C coli* in stool specimens requires selective media, microaerophilic conditions, and an incubation temperature of 42°C. Unless the laboratory uses a filtration method in addition to a growth medium containing antimicrobial agents to suppress colonic flora, many *Campylobacter* species other than *C jejuni* and *C coli* will not be detected. *Campylobacter upsaliensis, C hyointestinalis,* and *C fetus* may not be isolated because of susceptibility to antimicrobial agents in *Campylobacter* selective media. *Campylobacter* species can be detected in stool specimens by enzyme immunoassay or polymerase chain reaction, but these tests are not readily available.

TREATMENT: Erythromycin and azithromycin dihydrate shorten the duration of illness and prevent relapse when given early during gastrointestinal tract infection. Treatment with erythromycin or azithromycin usually eradicates the organism from stool within 2 or 3 days. Doxycycline for children 8 years of age or older is an alternative agent. A fluoroquinolone, such as ciprofloxacin, is effective, but fluoroquinolones are not licensed by the US Food and Drug Administration for people younger than 18 years of age (see Antimicrobial Agents and Related Therapy, p 693). If antimicrobial therapy is given for treatment of gastroenteritis, the recommended duration is 5 to 7 days. Antimicrobial agents for bacteremia should be selected on the basis of antimicrobial susceptibility tests; *Campylobacter* species almost always are susceptible to aminoglycosides, meropenem, and imipenem.

ISOLATION OF THE HOSPITALIZED PATIENT: In addition to standard precautions, contact precautions are recommended for diapered and incontinent children for the duration of illness.

CONTROL MEASURES:
- Exercising hand hygiene after handling raw poultry, washing cutting boards and utensils with soap and water after contact with raw poultry, avoiding contact of fruits and vegetables with the juices of raw poultry, and thorough cooking of poultry are critical.
- Exercising hand hygiene after contact with feces of dogs and cats, particularly stool of puppies and kittens with diarrhea, is important.
- Pasteurization of milk and chlorination of water supplies are important.

---

* www.cdc.gov/foodnet

- Symptomatic people should be excluded from food handling, care of patients in hospitals, and care of people in custodial care and child care centers.
- Infected food handlers and hospital employees who are asymptomatic need not be excluded from work if proper personal hygiene measures, including hand hygiene, are maintained.
- Outbreaks are uncommon in child care centers. General measures for interrupting enteric transmission in child care centers are recommended (see Children in Out-of-Home Child Care, p 123). Infants and children in diapers with symptomatic *C jejuni* infection should be excluded from child care or cared for in a separate area until diarrhea has subsided. Erythromycin or azithromycin treatment may further limit the potential for transmission.
- Stool cultures of asymptomatic exposed children are not recommended.

Candidiasis
(Moniliasis, Thrush)

CLINICAL MANIFESTATIONS: Mucocutaneous infection results in oral (thrush) or vaginal candidiasis; intertriginous lesions of the gluteal folds, neck, groin, and axilla; paronychia; and onychia. Chronic mucocutaneous candidiasis can be associated with endocrinologic diseases or immunodeficiency, particularly T-cell disorders. Oral candidiasis can be the manifesting sign of human immunodeficiency virus (HIV) infection. Esophageal and laryngeal candidiasis can occur in immunocompromised patients. Disseminated or invasive candidiasis occurs in very low birth weight newborn infants and in immunocompromised or debilitated hosts and can involve virtually any organ or anatomic site and can be rapidly fatal. The presence of typical retinal lesions, although uncommon in very low birth weight neonates and other immunocompromised patients, can be useful in diagnosis. Candidemia can occur with or without systemic disease in patients with indwelling vascular catheters or patients receiving prolonged intravenous infusions, especially with parenteral alimentation and lipids. Candiduria can occur in patients with indwelling urinary catheters or disseminated disease.

ETIOLOGY: *Candida albicans* causes most infections (50%–60%). Other species, including *Candida tropicalis, Candida parapsilosis, Candida glabrata, Candida krusei, Candida guilliermondii, Candida lusitaniae,* and *Candida dubliniensis,* also can cause serious infections in compromised hosts. *Candida parapsilosis* is a common cause of systemic candidiasis in very low birth weight neonates.

EPIDEMIOLOGY: *Candida albicans* is ubiquitous. Like other *Candida* species, *C albicans* is present on skin and in the mouth, intestinal tract, and vagina of immunocompetent people. Vulvovaginal candidiasis is associated with pregnancy, and newborn infants can acquire the organism in utero, during passage through the vagina, or postnatally. Mild mucocutaneous infection is common in healthy infants. Person-to-person transmission occurs rarely. Invasive disease occurs almost exclusively in people with impaired immunity, with infection usually arising from endogenous colonization sites. People with HIV infection or who are immunodeficient for other reasons, such as extreme prematurity, neutropenia, diabetes mellitus, or treatment with corticosteroids or cytotoxic chemotherapy, are at high risk of invasive infection. Patients with neutrophil defects, such as chronic granulomatous disease or myeloperoxidase deficiency, also are at increased risk. Patients undergoing intravenous hyperalimentation or receiving broad-spectrum antimicrobial agents have increased susceptibility.

The **incubation period** is unknown.

DIAGNOSTIC TESTS: The presumptive diagnosis of mucocutaneous candidiasis or thrush usually can be made clinically, but other organisms or trauma also can cause clinically consistent lesions. Yeast cells and pseudohyphae can be found in *C albicans*-infected tissue and are identifiable by microscopic examination of scrapings stained with Gram stain or suspended in 10% to 20% potassium hydroxide. Endoscopy is useful for the diagnosis of esophagitis. Ophthalmologic examination is required to determine the presence of typical retinal lesions. Lesions in the brain, kidney, liver, or spleen may be detected by ultrasonography or computed tomography; however, these lesions may not appear by imaging until late in the course.

A definitive diagnosis of invasive candidiasis requires isolation of the organism from a typically sterile body fluid or tissue (eg, blood, cerebrospinal fluid, bone marrow, or biopsy specimen) or demonstration of organisms in a tissue biopsy specimen. Cultures that are negative for *Candida* species, however, do not exclude invasive infection in immunocompromised hosts. Recovery of the organism is expedited using blood culture systems capable of biphasic or lysis-centrifugation. A presumptive species identification of *C albicans* can be made by demonstrating germ tube formation.

TREATMENT:

Mucous Membrane and Skin Infections. Oral candidiasis in immunocompetent hosts is treated with oral nystatin suspension or clotrimazole troches.

Fluconazole or itraconazole may be beneficial for immunocompromised patients with oropharyngeal candidiasis. Although cure rates with fluconazole are greater than with nystatin, relapse rates are comparable. The safety and efficacy of fluconazole for use in infants younger than 6 months of age and of itraconazole for use in children of any age have not been established; both drugs have been used safely in a limited number of patients of these ages.

Mild esophagitis caused by *Candida* species can be treated with high-dose oral nystatin; more severe disease is treated with fluconazole or itraconazole for a minimum of 21 days or for at least 14 days after resolution of clinical findings. Alternatively, low-dose intravenous amphotericin B (0.3 mg/kg per day, maximum 1.5 mg/kg every 24 hours) for at least 5 to 7 days can be used. Duration of treatment depends on severity of illness and patient factors such as age and degree of immunocompromise.

Skin infections are treated with topical nystatin, miconazole nitrate, clotrimazole, naftifine hydrochloride, ketoconazole, econazole nitrate, or ciclopirox olamine (see Topical Drugs for Superficial Fungal Infections, p 726). Nystatin usually is effective and is the least expensive of these drugs.

Vulvovaginal candidiasis is treated effectively with many topical formulations, including clotrimazole, miconazole, butoconazole nitrate, terconazole, and tioconazole. Such topically applied azole drugs are more effective than nystatin. Oral azole agents also are effective and should be considered for recurrent or refractory cases (see Recommended Doses of Parenteral and Oral Antifungal Drugs, p 722).

For chronic mucocutaneous candidiasis, fluconazole and itraconazole are effective drugs. Low-dose amphotericin B (0.3 mg/kg per day, maximum 1.5 mg/kg every 24 hours) given intravenously is effective in severe cases. Relapses are common with any of these agents once therapy is terminated; invasive infection is rare.

Keratomycosis is treated with corneal baths of amphotericin B (1 mg/mL of sterile water). Patients with cystitis attributable to *Candida* organisms can be treated successfully with short courses (3–5 days) of low-dose amphotericin B intravenously (0.3 mg/kg per day, maximum 1.5 mg/kg every 24 hours) or fluconazole or with repeated bladder irrigations with amphotericin B (50 µg/mL of sterile water).

Systemic Infections. Amphotericin B is the drug of choice for treating people with invasive candidiasis (see Drugs for Invasive and Other Serious Fungal Infections, p 725). Duration of therapy will vary with the clinical response and presence or absence of neutropenia. Patients at high risk of morbidity and mortality should be treated for a prolonged period and until all signs and symptoms of infection have resolved. For patients with hepatosplenic candidiasis, resolution of lesions may require weeks or months. Patients without immunocompromising conditions usually can be treated adequately with a 7- to 10-day course of therapy. Short-course therapy also can be used for intravenous catheter-associated infections, provided the catheter is removed promptly and there is no evidence of systemic disease (eg, positive blood cultures after catheter removal). Liposomal preparations of amphotericin B can be used if significant nephrotoxicity or clinical failure is observed with conventional amphotericin B therapy. However, these agents should not be used as first-line drugs.

Flucytosine (100–150 mg/kg per day in 4 divided doses, maximum 150 mg/kg every 24 hours) can be given with amphotericin B for *C albicans* infection involving the central nervous system if oral administration is feasible. In vitro and clinical studies suggest flucytosine and amphotericin B may act synergistically against many strains of *C albicans*. The dose of flucytosine should be decreased for patients with renal insufficiency. Peak plasma concentrations of flucytosine should be maintained between 40 and 60 µg/mL; higher concentrations predispose to toxic effects. Adverse effects of flucytosine, which are more common in azotemic patients, include rash, hepatic and renal dysfunction, diarrhea, gastrointestinal tract bleeding, ulcerative colitis, and dose-related bone marrow suppression.

Amphotericin B remains the drug of choice, but fluconazole has been used successfully to treat disseminated candidiasis. Nonneutropenic adults with candidemia respond equally well to fluconazole or amphotericin B. Published reports in adults and anecdotal reports in premature infants indicate that for at least one preparation of liposomal amphotericin B, decreased nephrotoxicity may be attributable to failure of the drug to penetrate the kidney. Thus, patients with renal or systemic infection have failed treatment with this agent.

Chemoprophylaxis. Chemoprophylaxis of *Candida* infections in immunocompromised patients with oral nystatin and fluconazole has been evaluated with variable results. A recent prospective, randomized, controlled trial in neonates weighing less than 1000 g at birth demonstrated the safety and efficacy of fluconazole given intravenously for 6 weeks in preventing *Candida* colonization and systemic infection. Further study is needed, but some experts recommend this regimen according to the dosage schedule studied. Fluconazole can decrease the risk of mucosal (eg, oropharyngeal and esophageal) candidiasis in patients with advanced HIV disease. However, an increased incidence of fluconazole-resistant *C krusei* infections has been reported in non–HIV-infected patients receiving prophylactic fluconazole. Adults undergoing bone marrow transplantation had significantly fewer *Candida* infections when given fluconazole, but children have not been studied in this regard. Prophylaxis is not recommended routinely for immunocompromised children, including children with HIV infection.

ISOLATION OF THE HOSPITALIZED PATIENT: Standard precautions are recommended.

CONTROL MEASURES: Prolonged broad-spectrum antimicrobial therapy and use of corticosteroids in susceptible patients promote overgrowth of, and predispose to, invasive infection with *Candida* organisms. Meticulous care of intravascular catheter sites is recommended for any patient requiring long-term intravenous alimentation.

Cat-Scratch Disease
(Bartonella henselae)

CLINICAL MANIFESTATIONS: The predominant manifestation of cat-scratch disease (CSD) in an immunocompetent person is regional lymphadenopathy. Fever and mild systemic symptoms occur in approximately 30% of patients. A skin papule often is found at the presumed site of bacterial inoculation and usually precedes development of lymphadenopathy by 1 to 2 weeks. Lymphadenopathy involves nodes that drain the site of inoculation—typically axillary, but cervical, epitrochlear, or inguinal nodes can be affected. The skin overlying affected lymph nodes typically is tender, warm, erythematous, and indurated. In approximately 25% to 30% of people with CSD, the affected nodes suppurate spontaneously. Occasionally, infection can produce Parinaud oculoglandular syndrome, in which inoculation of the conjunctiva results in ipsilateral preauricular or submandibular lymph adenopathy. Less common manifestations of CSD include encephalitis, aseptic meningitis, fever of unknown origin, neuroretinitis, osteolytic lesions, hepatitis, granulomata in the liver and spleen, pneumonia, thrombocytopenic purpura, and erythema nodosum.

ETIOLOGY: *Bartonella henselae,* the causative organism of CSD, is a fastidious, slow-growing, gram-negative bacillus that also has been identified as a causative agent of bacillary angiomatosis and bacillary peliosis hepatitis. The latter 2 manifestations of infection are reported primarily in patients with human immunodeficiency virus infection. *Bartonella henselae* is closely related to Bartonella quintana, the agent of trench fever and also a cause of bacillary angiomatosis.

EPIDEMIOLOGY: Cat-scratch disease is a common infection, although the true incidence is unknown. Most cases occur in people younger than 20 years of age. Cats are the common reservoir for human disease, and bacteremia in cats associated with human CSD cases is common. More than 90% of patients with CSD have a history of recent contact with apparently healthy cats, often kittens. No evidence of person-to-person transmission exists. Infection occurs more often during the autumn and winter. Cat fleas *(Ctenocephalides felis)* transmit *B henselae* between cats.

The **incubation period** from the time of the scratch to the appearance of the primary cutaneous lesion is 7 to 12 days; the period from the appearance of the primary lesion to the appearance of lymphadenopathy is 5 to 50 days (median, 12 days).

DIAGNOSTIC TESTS: The indirect immunofluorescence antibody (IFA) assay for detection of serum antibodies to antigens of *Bartonella* species is useful for the diagnosis of CSD. The IFA test is available through the Centers for Disease Control and Prevention. Results of IFA tests performed in some commercial laboratories are not reliable. Enzyme immunoassays for detection of antibodies to *B henselae* have been developed; however, they have not been demonstrated to be more sensitive or specific than the IFA test. Polymerase chain reaction assays are available in some commercial laboratories. If tissue (eg, lymph node) specimens are available, bacilli occasionally may be visualized using Warthin-Starry silver stain; however, this test is not specific for *B henselae*. Early histologic changes in lymph node specimens consist of lymphocytic infiltration with epithelioid granuloma formation. Later changes consist of polymorphonuclear leukocyte infiltration with granulomas that become necrotic and resemble those from patients with tularemia, brucellosis, and mycobacterial infections. A cat-scratch antigen skin test, prepared from aspirated pus from suppurative lymph nodes of patients with apparent CSD, is not recommended.

TREATMENT: Management is aimed primarily at symptoms, because the disease usually is self-limited, resolving spontaneously in 2 to 4 months. Painful suppurative nodes can be treated with needle aspiration for relief of symptoms; incision and drainage should be avoided, and surgical excision generally is unnecessary.

Antimicrobial therapy may hasten recovery for acutely or severely ill patients with systemic CSD, particularly for people with hepatic or splenic involvement, and is recommended uniformly for immunocompromised people. Reports suggest that several oral antimicrobial agents (trimethoprim-sulfamethoxazole, rifampin, azithromycin dihydrate, and ciprofloxacin) and parenteral gentamicin sulfate are effective in the treatment of CSD; the optimal duration of therapy is not known. Doxycycline and erythromycin or azithromycin are effective for the treatment of bacillary angiomatosis and bacillary peliosis; therapy should be administered for several months to prevent relapse in immunocompromised people.

ISOLATION OF THE HOSPITALIZED PATIENT: Standard precautions are recommended.

CONTROL MEASURES: People should avoid playing roughly with cats and kittens to minimize scratches and bites. Immunocompromised people should avoid contact with cats that scratch or bite and when acquiring a new cat, should avoid those younger than 1 year of age. Sites of cat scratches or bites should be washed immediately. Care of cats should include flea control. Testing of cats for *Bartonella* infection is not recommended.

Chancroid

CLINICAL MANIFESTATIONS: Chancroid is an acute ulcerative disease that involves the genitalia. An ulcer begins as a tender erythematous papule, becomes pustular, and erodes over several days, forming a sharply demarcated, somewhat superficial lesion with a serpiginous border. Its base is friable and may be covered with a gray or yellow, necrotic, and purulent exudate. Single or multiple ulcers may be present. Unlike a syphilitic chancre, which is painless, the chancroidal ulcer is often painful, tender, and nonindurated. The ulcer may be associated with a painful, unilateral inguinal adenitis (bubo) which often is suppurative and fluctuant.

In most males, chancroid manifests as a genital ulcer or inguinal tenderness. Many females are asymptomatic but can, depending on the site of the ulcer, have less obvious symptoms, including dysuria, dyspareunia, vaginal discharge, pain on defecation, or rectal bleeding. Constitutional symptoms are unusual.

ETIOLOGY: Chancroid is caused by *Haemophilus ducreyi,* which is a gram-negative coccobacillus.

EPIDEMIOLOGY: Chancroid is a sexually transmitted disease that is associated with poverty, urban prostitution, and illicit drug use. It is endemic in many areas of the United States and also occurs in discrete outbreaks. Coinfection with syphilis or herpes simplex virus (HSV) occurs in as many as 10% of patients. Chancroid is a well-established cofactor for transmission of human immunodeficiency virus (HIV). Because sexual contact is the only known route of transmission, the diagnosis of chancroid in infants and young children is strong evidence of sexual abuse.

The **incubation period** is 3 to 10 days.

DIAGNOSTIC TESTS: The diagnosis of chancroid usually is made on the basis of clinical findings and the exclusion of other infections associated with genital ulcer disease, such as syphilis, HSV infection, or lymphogranuloma venereum. Direct examination of clinical material using Gram stain may suggest strongly the diagnosis if large numbers of gram-negative coccobacilli are seen. Confirmation can be made by recovery of *H ducreyi* from a genital ulcer or lymph node aspirate. However, special culture media and conditions are required for isolation; if chancroid is suspected, the laboratory should be informed. Purulent material recovered from intact buboes almost always is sterile. Fluorescent monoclonal antibody stains and polymerase chain reaction assays can provide more specific diagnosis but are not available in most laboratories.

TREATMENT: Recommended regimens include azithromycin dihydrate in a single dose, ceftriaxone sodium in a single dose, erythromycin base for 7 days, or ciprofloxacin for 3 days (see Table 4.3, p 713). Ciprofloxacin is not approved for people younger than 18 years of age and should not be administered to pregnant or lactating women (see Antimicrobial Agents and Related Therapy, p 693). Patients with HIV infection may need more prolonged therapy.

Clinical improvement occurs within 7 days of onset of successful therapy, and healing is complete in approximately 2 weeks. Adenitis often is slow to resolve and may require needle aspiration or surgical incision. Patients should be reexamined 3 to 7 days after starting therapy to verify that healing is occurring. If healing has not occurred, the diagnosis may be incorrect, and further testing is required. Relapses may occur; however, retreatment with the original regimen usually is effective.

Patients should be evaluated for other sexually transmitted diseases, including syphilis, hepatitis B virus infection, *Chlamydia trachomatis* infection, gonorrhea, and HIV infection at the time of diagnosis. Because chancroid is a risk factor for HIV infection and an enhancer of HIV transmission, if initial HIV or syphilis test results are negative, they should be repeated 3 months after the diagnosis of chancroid is made. All people having sexual contact with patients with chancroid within 10 days before onset of the patient's symptoms need to be examined and treated, even if they are asymptomatic.

ISOLATION OF THE HOSPITALIZED PATIENT: Standard precautions are recommended.

CONTROL MEASURES: Examination and treatment of sexual partners of patients with chancroid are important control measures. "Partner notification" is used increasingly to identify a reservoir of cases of chancroid during outbreaks, usually occurring among prostitutes. This process can lead to epidemic control. Regular condom use may decrease transmission.

CHLAMYDIAL INFECTIONS

Chlamydia (Chlamydophila) pneumoniae

CLINICAL MANIFESTATIONS: Patients may be asymptomatic or mildly to moderately ill with a variety of respiratory tract diseases, including pneumonia, acute bronchitis, prolonged cough, and less commonly, pharyngitis, laryngitis, otitis media, and sinusitis. In some patients, a sore throat precedes the onset of cough by a week or more. Physical examination may reveal nonexudative pharyngitis, pulmonary rales, and bronchospasm. Chest radiography may reveal an infiltrate. Illness is prolonged, with cough persisting 2 to 6 weeks and can have a biphasic course. In addition to acute respiratory tract disease, some investigators have associated *C pneumoniae* with atherosclerotic cardiovascular disease. Prospective, randomized trials are underway to further explore this association and to determine whether treatment is beneficial.

Investigators also have associated *C pneumoniae* with asthma, Alzheimer disease, hypertension, Kawasaki syndrome, multiple sclerosis, and other conditions, but evidence supporting any of these associations is limited.

ETIOLOGY: *Chlamydia pneumoniae* (proposed new name *Chlamydophila pneumoniae*) is a species of *Chlamydia* that is antigenically, genetically, and morphologically distinct from other *Chlamydia* species. All isolates of *C pneumoniae* appear to be closely related serologically.

EPIDEMIOLOGY: *Chlamydia pneumoniae* infection is assumed to be transmitted from person to person via infected respiratory tract secretions. An animal reservoir is unknown. The disease occurs worldwide, but in tropical and less developed areas disease occurs earlier in life than in developed countries in temperate climates. In the United States, approximately 50% of adults have *C pneumoniae*-specific serum antibody by age 20. Initial infection peaks between 5 and 15 years of age. Recurrent infection is common, especially in adults. Clusters of infection have been reported in groups of children and young adults. There is no evidence of seasonality.

The mean **incubation period** is 21 days.

DIAGNOSTIC TESTS: No reliable diagnostic test is available commercially, and none has been licensed by the US Food and Drug Administration for use in the United States. Serologic testing has been the primary laboratory means of diagnosis of *C pneumoniae* infection. The microimmunofluorescence antibody test is the most sensitive and specific serologic test for acute infection and is the only endorsed approach. A fourfold increase in immunoglobulin (Ig) G titer or an IgM titer of ≥16 is evidence of acute infection. Use of a single IgG titer in the diagnosis of acute infection is discouraged. In primary infection, IgM antibody appears approximately 2 to 3 weeks after the onset of illness, but IgG antibody may not peak until 6 to 8 weeks. In reinfection, IgM may not appear, and IgG increases within 1 to 2 weeks. Early antimicrobial therapy may suppress the antibody response. Past exposure is indicated by an IgG titer of ≥16. *Chlamydia pneumoniae* can be isolated from swab specimens obtained from the nasopharynx or oropharynx or from sputum, bronchoalveolar lavage, or tissue biopsy specimens. Specimens are placed into appropriate transport media and held at 4°C (39°F) until inoculated into cell culture; specimens that cannot be processed within 24 hours should be frozen and held at –70°C (–94°F). A positive culture is confirmed by propagation of the isolate or a positive polymerase chain reaction assay. Nasopharyngeal shedding can occur for months after acute disease. Immunohistochemistry, used to detect *C pneumoniae* in tissue specimens, requires control antibodies and tissues in addition to skill in recognizing staining artifacts to avoid false-positive results.

TREATMENT: Erythromycin or tetracycline is recommended. For adolescents and adults, tetracycline or doxycycline for 14 days also is appropriate. Tetracycline or doxycycline should not be given routinely to children younger than 8 years of age (see Antimicrobial Agents and Related Therapy, p 693). Adolescents and older patients have been treated successfully with erythromycin for 5 to 10 days, but a 14- to 21-day course of therapy may be needed, because prolonged or recurrent symptoms are common. The macrolide drugs azithromycin dihydrate and clarithromycin and some of the fluoroquinolones also are effective. The fluoroquinolones are approved for people 18 years of age and older. In vitro data suggest that *C pneumoniae* is not susceptible to sulfonamides.

ISOLATION OF THE HOSPITALIZED PATIENT: Standard precautions are recommended.

CONTROL MEASURES: Reporting of individual cases of *C pneumoniae* to health authorities is not required. Recommended prevention measures include minimizing crowding and maintaining personal hygiene, with careful disposal of nasal and oral discharge and frequent hand hygiene.

Chlamydia (Chlamydophila) psittaci
(Psittacosis, Ornithosis)

CLINICAL MANIFESTATIONS: Psittacosis (ornithosis) is an acute febrile respiratory tract infection with systemic symptoms and signs that often include fever, nonproductive cough, headache, and malaise. Extensive interstitial pneumonia can occur with radiographic changes characteristically more severe than would be expected from physical examination findings. Pericarditis, myocarditis, endocarditis, superficial thrombophlebitis, hepatitis, and encephalopathy are rare complications.

ETIOLOGY: *Chlamydia psittaci* (proposed new name *Chlamydophila psittaci*) is an obligate intracellular bacterial pathogen that is distinct antigenically and genetically from other *Chlamydia* species.

EPIDEMIOLOGY: Birds are the major reservoir of *C psittaci*. Several mammalian species, such as cattle, goats, sheep, and cats, and avian species may become infected and develop systemic and debilitating disease. In the United States, psittacine birds (such as parakeets, parrots, and macaws, especially those smuggled into the country), pigeons, and turkeys are important sources of human disease. Healthy and sick birds may harbor and transmit the organism, usually via the airborne route in fecal dust or secretions. Excretion of *C psittaci* can be intermittent or continuous for weeks or months. People in the environment of infected birds, such as workers at poultry slaughter plants, poultry farms, and pet shops as well as pet owners, are at risk of infection. Laboratory personnel working with *C psittaci* also are at risk. Psittacosis is worldwide in distribution and tends to occur sporadically in any season. Infections are rare in children. Severe illness and abortion have been reported in pregnant women after exposure to infected sheep.

The **incubation period** usually is 7 to 14 days but may be longer.

DIAGNOSTIC TESTS: The usual method of diagnosis is serologic testing with a fourfold increase in antibody titer determined by complement fixation testing between acute and convalescent specimens obtained 2 to 3 weeks apart. In the presence of a compatible clinical illness, a single titer of 1:32 or greater is considered presumptive evidence of infection. Treatment may suppress the antibody response.

The complement fixation test does not distinguish among infections caused by *C psittaci, Chlamydia pneumoniae, Chlamydia trachomatis,* or *C pecorum.* Micro-immunofluorescence and polymerase chain reaction assays that are more specific for *C psittaci* have been developed but are not widely available. Isolation of the agent from the respiratory tract should be attempted only by experienced personnel in laboratories, in which strict measures to prevent spread of the organism are used during collection and handling of all specimens for culture.

TREATMENT: Tetracyclines are the preferred therapy, except for children younger than 8 years of age. Erythromycin is an alternative drug and is recommended for younger children. The macrolide drugs, azithromycin dihydrate and clarithromycin, as well as chloramphenicol also are effective. Therapy should be administered for at least 10 to 14 days after defervescence.

ISOLATION OF THE HOSPITALIZED PATIENT: Standard precautions are recommended.

CONTROL MEASURES: Reporting cases of human psittacosis to health authorities is mandated in most states. All birds suspected to be the source of human infection should be seen by a veterinarian for evaluation and management. Birds with *C psittaci* infection should be isolated and treated with appropriate antimicrobial agents for at least 45 days.* Birds suspected of having infection that have died or have been euthanatized should be sealed in an impermeable container and transported on dry ice to a veterinary laboratory for testing. All potentially contaminated caging and housing areas should be disinfected thoroughly and aired before reuse, because these areas may contain infectious organisms. *Chlamydia psittaci* is susceptible to most household disinfectants and detergents, including 70% alcohol, 1% Lysol (Reckitt Benckiser, Berkshire, United Kingdom), and a 1:100 dilution of household bleach. People cleaning cages and other bird housing areas should avoid scattering the contents. People exposed to common sources of infection should be observed for development of fever or respiratory tract symptoms; early diagnostic tests should be performed and therapy should be initiated if symptoms appear.

Chlamydia trachomatis

CLINICAL MANIFESTATIONS: *Chlamydia trachomatis* is associated with a range of clinical manifestations, including neonatal conjunctivitis, trachoma, pneumonia in young infants, genital tract infection, and lymphogranuloma venereum (LGV). Neonatal chlamydial conjunctivitis is characterized by ocular congestion, edema, and discharge developing a few days to several weeks after birth and lasting for 1 to 2 weeks and sometimes much longer. In contrast to trachoma, scars and pannus formation are rare.

---

* Centers for Disease Control and Prevention, Committee of the National Association of State Public Health Veterinarians. Compendium of measures to control *Chlamydia psittaci* infection among humans (psittacosis) and pet birds (avian chlamydiosis), 2000. *MMWR Recomm Rep.* 2000; 49(No. RR-8):1–17

Trachoma is a chronic follicular keratoconjunctivitis with neovascularization of the cornea that results from repeated and chronic infection. Blindness secondary to extensive local scarring and inflammation occurs in 1% to 15% of people with trachoma. Trachoma is rare in the United States.

Pneumonia in young infants usually is an afebrile illness occurring between 2 and 19 weeks after birth. A repetitive staccato cough, tachypnea, and rales are characteristic but not always present. Wheezing is uncommon. Hyperinflation usually accompanies the infiltrates seen on chest radiographs. Nasal stuffiness and otitis media may occur. Untreated disease can linger or recur. Severe chlamydial pneumonia has occurred in infants and some immunocompromised adults.

Vaginitis in prepubertal girls; urethritis, cervicitis, endometritis, salpingitis, and perihepatitis in postpubertal females; epididymitis in males; and Reiter syndrome (arthritis, urethritis, and bilateral conjunctivitis) also can occur. Infection can persist for months to years. Reinfection is common. In postpubertal females, chlamydial infection can progress to acute or chronic pelvic inflammatory disease and result in ectopic pregnancy or infertility.

Lymphogranuloma venereum is an invasive lymphatic infection with an initial ulcerative lesion on the genitalia accompanied by tender, suppurative, inguinal and/or femoral lymphadenopathy that is most common unilaterally. Anorectal infection and hemorrhagic proctitis resulting in fistula and strictures also have been described in women and homosexually active men. The disease has a chronic low-grade course.

ETIOLOGY: *Chlamydia trachomatis* is an obligate intracellular bacterial agent with at least 18 serologic variants (serovars) divided between the following biologic variants (biovars): oculogenital (serovars A–K) and LGV (serovars L1, L2, and L3). Trachoma usually is caused by serovars A through C, and genital and perinatal infections are caused by B and D through K.

EPIDEMIOLOGY: *Chlamydia trachomatis* is the most common reportable sexually transmitted infection in the United States, with high rates among sexually active adolescents and young adults. Prevalence of the organism in pregnant women varies between 6% and 12% in most populations but can be as low as 2% or as high as 37% in adolescents. Oculogenital serovars of *C trachomatis* can be transmitted from the genital tract of infected mothers to their newborn infants. Acquisition occurs in approximately 50% of infants born vaginally to infected mothers and in some infants delivered by cesarean section with intact membranes. The risk of conjunctivitis is 25% to 50% and that of pneumonia is 5% to 20% in infants who acquire *C trachomatis*. The nasopharynx is the most commonly infected anatomic site.

Genital infection in adolescents and adults is transmitted sexually. The possibility of sexual abuse should be considered in prepubertal children beyond infancy who have vaginal, urethral, or rectal chlamydial infection, although asymptomatic infection acquired at birth can persist for as long as 3 years. Infection is not known to be communicable among infants and children. The degree of contagiousness of pulmonary disease is unknown but seems to be low.

Lymphogranuloma venereum biovars are worldwide in distribution and particularly are prevalent in tropical and subtropical areas; disease occurs rarely in the

United States. Infection often is asymptomatic in women. Perinatal transmission is rare. Lymphogranuloma venereum is infective during active disease, which may last from weeks to many years.

The **incubation period** of chlamydial illness is variable, depending on the type of infection, but usually is at least 1 week.

DIAGNOSTIC TESTS: Definitive diagnosis can be made by isolating the organism in tissue culture and by nucleic acid amplification in selective circumstances.* Because *Chlamydia* species are obligate intracellular organisms, culture specimens must contain epithelial cells, not just exudate. Nucleic acid amplification tests (NAATs), such as polymerase chain reaction, ligase chain reaction, and others, are more sensitive than cell culture, DNA probe, direct fluorescent antibody (DFA) tests, or enzyme immunoassays (EIAs), although specificity is variable.

Tests for detection of chlamydial antigen (EIA, DFA), DNA probe tests, and NAATs are useful for evaluating urethral swab specimens from males, endocervical swab specimens from females, and conjunctival secretion specimens from infants (although not all of these tests have been licensed by the US Food and Drug Administration for this use). The polymerase chain reaction and ligase chain reaction tests are useful for evaluating urine specimens from either sex. Nonculture tests are not recommended for detection of *C trachomatis* in urethral swab specimens from females and vaginal swabs from postmenarcheal adolescents and adults. In addition, NAATs are not recommended for rectal swabs and pharyngeal swabs.

If a false-positive test result is likely to have adverse medical, social, or psychologic consequences, positive DFA test, EIA, DNA probe test, or NAAT results should be verified by culture, a second nonculture test different from the first, or use of a blocking antibody (eg, Chlamydiazyme, Abbott Laboratories, Abbott Park, IL) or competitive probe. When evaluating a child for possible sexual abuse, culture of the organism may be the only acceptable diagnostic test in certain legal jurisdictions. When culture is not available, some experts support using a NAAT if a positive result can be verified by another NAAT. The EIA and DFA tests should not be used for testing rectal, vaginal, or urethral specimens from infants and children because of low sensitivity and specificity.

Neonatal *C trachomatis* conjunctivitis can be diagnosed by Giemsa staining of conjunctival scrapings. The presence of blue-stained intracytoplasmic inclusions within epithelial cells is diagnostic. The sensitivity of the test varies from 22% to 95% depending on the technique of specimen collection and the examiner's expertise.

Serum antibody concentrations are difficult to determine, and only a few clinical laboratories perform this test. In children with pneumonia, an acute microimmunofluorescence serum titer of *C trachomatis*-specific immunoglobulin (Ig) M of ≥1:32 is diagnostic. A fourfold increase in microimmunofluorescence titer to LGV antigens or a complement fixation titer of ≥1:32 is suggestive of LGV in the presence of compatible clinical findings.

Indirect evidence of chlamydial pneumonia includes hyperinflation and bilateral diffuse infiltrates on radiographs, eosinophilia of 0.3 to 0.4 × 10^9/L (300–400/µL) or

---

* Centers for Disease Control and Prevention. Screening to detect *Chlamydia trachomatis* and *Neisseria gonorrhoeae* infections—2002. *MMWR.* 2002;51(RR-15):1–38

more in peripheral blood counts, and increased total serum IgG ($\geq$5 g/L [500 mg/dL]) and IgM ($\geq$1.1 g/L [110 mg/dL]) concentrations. However, the absence of these findings does not exclude the diagnosis. Direct antigen tests and culture now are available so widely that a diagnosis should be made on the basis of specific laboratory tests.

Diagnosis of chlamydial disease in a child, adolescent, or adult should prompt investigation for other sexually transmitted diseases, including syphilis, gonorrhea, hepatitis B virus infection, and human immunodeficiency virus infection. In the case of an infant, examination of the mother also should be considered.

TREATMENT:

- Young infants with **chlamydial conjunctivitis and pneumonia** are treated with oral erythromycin base or ethylsuccinate (50 mg/kg per day in 4 divided doses) for 14 days. Oral sulfonamides may be used after the immediate neonatal period for infants who do not tolerate erythromycin. Topical treatment of conjunctivitis is ineffective and unnecessary. Because the efficacy of erythromycin therapy is approximately 80%, a second course may be required, and follow-up of infants is recommended.

  An association between orally administered erythromycin and infantile hypertrophic pyloric stenosis (IHPS) has been reported in infants younger than 6 weeks of age. The risk of IHPS after treatment with other macrolides (eg, azithromycin dihydrate and clarithromycin) is unknown. Because confirmation of erythromycin as a contributor to cases of IHPS will require additional investigation and because alternative therapies are not as well studied, the American Academy of Pediatrics continues to recommend use of erythromycin for treatment of diseases caused by *C trachomatis*. Physicians who prescribe erythromycin to newborn infants should inform parents about the signs and potential risks of developing IHPS. Cases of pyloric stenosis after use of oral erythromycin should be reported to MEDWATCH (see MEDWATCH, p 771). The need for treatment of infants can be avoided by screening pregnant women to detect and treat *C trachomatis* infection before delivery. A specific diagnosis of *C trachomatis* infection in an infant should prompt treatment of the mother and her sexual partner(s).

- Infants born to mothers known to have untreated chlamydial infection are at high risk of infection; however, prophylactic antimicrobial treatment is not indicated, because the efficacy of such treatment is unknown. Infants should be monitored to ensure appropriate treatment if infection develops. If adequate follow-up cannot be ensured, some experts recommend that prophylaxis be considered.

- Treatment of **trachoma** is more difficult, and recommendations for therapy differ. The most widely used therapy is topical treatment with erythromycin, tetracycline, or sulfacetamide ointment twice a day for 2 months or twice a day for the first 5 days of the month for 6 consecutive months, or oral erythromycin or doxycycline for 40 days is given if the infection is severe. Azithromycin (20 mg/kg, to a maximum of 1 g once per week) for 3 weeks also is effective.

- For uncomplicated *C trachomatis* **genital tract infection** in adolescents or adults, oral doxycycline (200 mg/day in 2 divided doses) for 7 days or azithromycin in a single 1-g oral dose is recommended. Alternatives include oral erythromycin base (2.0 g/day in 4 divided doses) for 7 days, erythromycin ethylsuccinate (3.2 g/day in 4 divided doses) for 7 days, ofloxacin (600 mg/day in 2 divided doses) for 7 days, or levofloxacin (500 mg, orally) for 7 days. Erythromycin or azithromycin is the recommended therapy for children between 6 months and 12 years of age; for infants younger than 6 months of age, erythromycin is recommended. Erythromycin base (2 g/day in 4 divided doses) or amoxicillin (1.5 g/day in 3 divided doses) for 7 days are recommended regimens for pregnant women, because doxycycline and ofloxacin are contraindicated during pregnancy. Because these regimens for pregnant women may not be highly efficacious, a second course of therapy may be required. If a pregnant woman cannot tolerate erythromycin, half doses daily for 14 days may be given. Azithromycin (1 g orally as a single dose) is an alternative.
- For **LGV,** doxycycline (200 mg/day in 2 divided doses) for 21 days is the preferred treatment for children 8 years of age and older. Erythromycin base (2 g/day in 4 divided doses) for 21 days is an alternative regimen.

Follow-up Testing. Patients do not need to be retested for *Chlamydia* infection after completing treatment with doxycycline or azithromycin unless symptoms persist or reinfection is suspected. Retesting may be considered at 3 or more weeks after completing regimens with erythromycin or amoxicillin. However, recently infected women are a high priority for repeat testing for *C trachomatis*. Clinicians should consider advising all women, especially adolescents, with chlamydial infections to be rescreened 3 to 4 months after treatment.

ISOLATION OF THE HOSPITALIZED PATIENT: Standard precautions are recommended.

CONTROL MEASURES:
Pregnancy. The identification and treatment of women with *C trachomatis* genital tract infection during pregnancy can prevent disease in the infant. Pregnant women at high risk of *C trachomatis* infection, in particular women younger than 25 years of age and women with new or multiple sexual partners, should be targeted for screening. Some experts advocate routine testing of pregnant women at high risk during the first trimester and again during the third trimester.

Neonatal Chlamydial Conjunctivitis. The recommended topical prophylaxis with silver nitrate, erythromycin, or tetracycline for all newborns for prevention of gonococcal ophthalmia will not prevent neonatal chlamydial conjunctivitis or extraocular infection (see Prevention of Neonatal Ophthalmia, p 778).

Trachoma. Although not seen in the United States for more than 2 decades, trachoma is the second leading cause of blindness worldwide. Trachoma is transmitted by transfer of ocular discharge, and predictors of scarring and blindness for trachoma include increasing age and constant, severe trachoma. The prevention methods recommended by the World Health Organization for global elimination of blindness attributable to trachoma by 2020 include *s*urgery, *a*ntibiotics, *f*ace washing, and *e*nvironment improvement (SAFE).

Contacts of Infants With C trachomatis Conjunctivitis or Pneumonia. Mothers (and their sexual partners) of infected infants should be treated for *C trachomatis*.

Gynecologic Examination. Sexually active adolescents should be tested routinely for *Chlamydia* infection during gynecologic examination, even if no symptoms are present. Screening of young adult women 20 to 24 years of age also is desirable, particularly women who do not use barrier contraceptives consistently and who have multiple sexual partners.

Management of Sexual Partners. All sexual contacts of patients with *C trachomatis* infection (whether symptomatic or asymptomatic), nongonococcal urethritis, mucopurulent cervicitis, epididymitis, or pelvic inflammatory disease should be evaluated and treated for *C trachomatis* infection if the last sexual contact occurred during the 60 days preceding onset of symptoms in the index case.

Lymphogranuloma Venereum. Nonspecific preventive measures for LGV are the same as measures for sexually transmitted diseases in general and include education, case reporting, condom use, and avoidance of sexual contact with infected people.

CLOSTRIDIAL INFECTIONS

Botulism and Infant Botulism
(Clostridium botulinum)

CLINICAL MANIFESTATIONS: Botulism is a neuroparalytic disorder that can be classified into the following categories: foodborne, infant, wound, and undetermined. Except for infant botulism, which may have a prolonged course, onset of symptoms occurs abruptly within hours or evolves gradually over several days. Cranial nerve palsies are the most common complication of botulism, followed by symmetric, descending, flaccid paralysis of somatic musculature that may progress rapidly. Patients with rapidly evolving illness initially may have generalized weakness and hypotonia. Signs and symptoms in older children or adults can include diplopia, blurred vision, dry mouth, dysphagia, dysphonia, and dysarthria. Classically, infant botulism, which occurs predominantly in infants younger than 6 months of age, is preceded by constipation and manifests as decreased movement, loss of facial expression, poor feeding, weak cry, diminished gag reflex, subtle ocular palsies, and generalized weakness and hypotonia (eg, "floppy infant"). The spectrum of disease ranges from mild (eg, constipation, slow feeding) to rapidly progressive (eg, apnea, sudden infant death).

ETIOLOGY: Seven antigenic toxin types of *Clostridium botulinum* have been identified. Human botulism usually is caused by neurotoxins A, B, E, and rarely, F. Types C and D are associated primarily with botulism in birds and mammals. Almost all cases of infant botulism are caused by types A and B.

EPIDEMIOLOGY: Foodborne botulism (median number of annual cases, 24) results when a food contaminated with spores of *C botulinum* is preserved or stored improperly under anaerobic conditions that permit germination, multiplication, and toxin production. Outbreaks have occurred with restaurant-prepared foods, such as patty-melts; potato salad; aluminum foil-wrapped baked potatoes; home-canned foods; bottled garlic; and cheese sauce. Illness follows ingestion of preformed botulinum toxin. Immunity to botulinum toxin does not develop in foodborne botulism, even after severe disease. Botulism is not transmitted from person to person.

Infant botulism (median number of annual cases, fewer than 100) results after ingested spores of *C botulinum* or related species germinate, multiply, and produce botulinum toxin in the intestine, probably through a mechanism of transient permissiveness of the intestinal microflora. In most cases of infant botulism, the source of spores is not identified, and these may be airborne from soil or dust. Honey that has not been certified to be free of *C botulinum* spores is an identified and avoidable source. Light and dark corn syrups are manufactured under sterile conditions, but the products are neither packaged under aseptic conditions nor terminally sterilized. The manufacturers cannot ensure that any given product will be free of *C botulinum* spores.

Wound botulism results when *C botulinum* contaminates traumatized tissue, multiplies, and produces toxin. Gross trauma or crush injury may be a predisposing event, but during the last decade, injection of contaminated black tar heroin has been associated with most cases. Botulism of undetermined etiology is rare and occurs in people older than 12 months of age in whom no food or wound source is implicated.

The usual **incubation period** for foodborne botulism is 12 to 48 hours (range, 6 hours–8 days). In infant botulism, the incubation period is estimated at 3 to 30 days from the time of exposure to the spore-containing material. For wound botulism, the incubation period is 4 to 14 days from the time of injury until the onset of symptoms.

DIAGNOSTIC TESTS: A toxin neutralization bioassay in mice* is used to identify botulinum toxin in serum, stool, gastric aspirate, or suspect foods. Enriched and selective media are used to culture *C botulinum* from stool and foods. In infant and wound botulism, the diagnosis is made by demonstrating *C botulinum* organisms or toxin in feces, wound exudate, or tissue specimens. Toxin has been demonstrated in serum in only 1% of infants with botulism. To increase the likelihood of diagnosis, serum and stool specimens should be obtained from all people with suspected botulism. In foodborne cases, serum specimens obtained more than 3 days after ingestion of toxin usually are negative. Stool and gastric aspirates are the best diagnostic specimens for culture. Because obtaining a stool specimen may be difficult because of constipation, an enema of sterile nonbacteriostatic water can be given. Because results of laboratory testing can be delayed by several days, treatment with antitoxin should be initiated promptly on the basis of clinical suspicion. The most prominent electromyographic finding is an incremental increase of evoked muscle potentials at high-frequency nerve stimulation (20–50 Hz). In addition, a characteristic pattern of brief, small-amplitude, overly abundant motor action potentials can be seen. This pattern may not be seen in infants, and its absence does not exclude the diagnosis.

---

* For information, consult your state health department.

TREATMENT:

Meticulous Supportive Care. An important aspect of therapy in all forms of botulism is meticulous supportive care, particularly respiratory and nutritional.

Antitoxin. A 5-year, randomized, double-blind, placebo-controlled treatment trial of human-derived botulinum antitoxin (formally known as Botulism Immune Globulin Intravenous [BIGIV]) in infants with botulism showed a significant decrease in hospital days, mechanical ventilation, tube feedings, and cost associated with BIGIV administration ($70 000 decrease in cost per case). The California Department of Health Services (24-hour telephone number, 510-540-2646) should be contacted to procure BIGIV. Treatment with BIGIV should be initiated as early in the illness as possible. Botulism Immune Globulin Intravenous is available only for treatment of infant botulism. Trivalent equine botulinum antitoxin (types A, B, and E) and bivalent antitoxin (types A and B) are available from the Centers for Disease Control and Prevention (CDC) through state health departments for treatment of foodborne or wound botulism. If contact cannot be made with the state health department, the CDC Drug Service should be contacted (see Appendix I, Directory of Resources, p 789). Patients should be tested for hypersensitivity to equine sera before administration. Approximately 9% of treated people experience some degree of hypersensitivity reaction to equine serum, but severe reactions are rare.

Antimicrobial Agents. In infant botulism, antimicrobial agents should be avoided, because lysis of intraluminal *C botulinum* could increase the amount of toxin available for absorption. Aminoglycosides can potentiate the paralytic effects of the toxin and should be avoided.

ISOLATION OF THE HOSPITALIZED PATIENT: Standard precautions are recommended.

CONTROL MEASURES:

- Prophylactic equine antitoxin for asymptomatic people who have ingested a food known to contain botulinum toxin is not recommended. Because of the danger of hypersensitivity reactions, the decision to administer antitoxin requires careful consideration. Consultation about antitoxin use may be obtained from the state health department or the CDC.
- Elimination of recently ingested toxin may be facilitated by inducing vomiting and by gastric lavage, rapid purgation, and high enemas. These measures should not be used in infant botulism. Enemas should not be administered to people with illness except to obtain a stool specimen for diagnostic purposes. Exposed people should have close medical observation.
- Honey should not be given to children younger than 12 months of age.
- Botulinum toxoid (types A, B, C, D, and E) is available from the CDC for immunization of high-risk laboratory workers.

- Education regarding safe practices in food preparation and home-canning methods should be promoted. Use of a pressure cooker (at 116°C [240.8°F]) is necessary to kill spores of *C botulinum*. Bringing the internal temperature of foods to that of boiling for 10 minutes will destroy the toxin. Time-temperature-pressure requirements vary with the product being heated. In addition, food containers that appear to bulge may contain gas produced by *C botulinum* and should be discarded. Other foods that appear to be spoiled should not be eaten or tasted.
- Cases of suspected botulism should be reported immediately to local and state health departments.

Clostridium difficile

CLINICAL MANIFESTATIONS: Syndromes associated with infections include pseudomembranous colitis and antimicrobial-associated diarrhea. Pseudomembranous colitis generally is characterized by diarrhea, abdominal cramps, fever, systemic toxicity, abdominal tenderness, and passage of stools containing blood and mucus. The colonic mucosa often contains small (2- to 5-mm), raised, yellowish plaques. Characteristically, disease begins while the child is in a hospital receiving antimicrobial therapy, but it can occur weeks after hospital discharge or after cessation of therapy. Rarely, the illness is not associated with antimicrobial therapy or hospitalization. Severe or fatal disease is more likely to occur in severely neutropenic children with leukemia, in infants with Hirschsprung disease, and in patients with inflammatory bowel disease. Infection also may result only in mild diarrhea or asymptomatic carriage. Carriage without symptoms is common in newborn infants and in children younger than 1 year of age.

ETIOLOGY: *Clostridium difficile* is a spore-forming, obligately anaerobic, gram-positive bacillus. Disease is related to the action of toxin(s) produced by these organisms. Two toxins, A and B, have been characterized.

EPIDEMIOLOGY: *Clostridium difficile* can be isolated from soil and commonly is present in the environment. Spores of *C difficile* are acquired from the environment or by fecal-oral transmission from colonized people. Intestinal colonization rates in healthy neonates and young infants can be as high as 50% but usually are less than 5% in children older than 2 years of age and in adults. Hospitals, nursing homes, and child care facilities are major reservoirs for *C difficile*. Risk factors for disease are those that increase exposure to organisms and those that diminish the barrier effect of the normal intestinal flora, allowing *C difficile* to proliferate and elaborate toxin(s) in vivo. Risk factors for acquisition include experiencing prolonged hospitalization, having an infected hospital roommate, and having symptomatically infected patients on the same hospital ward. Risk factors for developing disease include undergoing antimicrobial therapy, repeated enemas, prolonged nasogastric tube insertion, and gastrointestinal tract surgery and having renal insufficiency. Penicillins, clindamycin, and cephalosporins are the antimicrobial drugs most commonly associated with

C difficile colitis, but colitis has been associated with almost every antimicrobial agent. Although *C difficile* toxin rarely is recovered from stool specimens of asymptomatic adults, it may be recovered from stool specimens from neonates and infants who have no gastrointestinal tract illness. This finding confounds the interpretation of positive toxin assays in patients younger than 12 months of age.

The **incubation period** is unknown.

DIAGNOSTIC TESTS: Endoscopic findings of pseudomembranes and hyperemic, friable rectal mucosa suggest pseudomembranous colitis. To diagnose *C difficile* disease, stool should be tested for the presence of *C difficile* toxins. Commercially available enzyme immunoassays detect toxins A and B, or an enzyme immunoassay for toxin A may be used in conjunction with cell culture cytotoxicity assay, the "gold standard" for toxin B detection. Latex agglutination tests should not be used. Symptomatic infants younger than 1 year of age should be investigated for causes of diarrhea other than *C difficile*, because the carriage of *C difficile* is the rule rather than the exception in this age group.

TREATMENT:
- Antimicrobial therapy should be discontinued as soon as possible in patients in whom clinically significant diarrhea or colitis develops.
- Antimicrobial therapy for *C difficile* disease is indicated for patients with severe disease or in whom diarrhea persists after antimicrobial therapy is discontinued.
- Strains of *C difficile* are susceptible to metronidazole and vancomycin hydrochloride, and both are effective. Metronidazole (30 mg/kg per day in 4 divided doses, maximum 2 g/day) is the drug of choice for the initial treatment of most patients with colitis. Oral vancomycin (40 mg/kg per day in 4 divided doses, maximum 500 mg) is an alternative drug, but its use should be discouraged because of the potential for promoting vancomycin-resistant organisms. Vancomycin is indicated for patients who do not respond to metronidazole. Metronidazole is effective when given orally or intravenously; vancomycin is effective only when administered orally. Oral bacitracin zinc is another therapeutic choice, but it is less effective.
- Antimicrobial agents usually are administered for 7 to 10 days.
- As many as 10% to 20% of patients experience a relapse after discontinuing therapy, but the infection usually responds to a second course of the same treatment.
- Cholestyramine resin, which binds toxin, can relieve symptoms. However, its effect has not been evaluated in children with disease caused by *C difficile*. Because cholestyramine also binds vancomycin, the drugs should not be administered concurrently.
- Drugs that decrease intestinal motility should not be administered.
- Follow-up testing for toxin is not recommended if symptoms resolve.

ISOLATION OF THE HOSPITALIZED PATIENT: In addition to standard precautions, contact precautions are recommended for the duration of illness.

CONTROL MEASURES:
- Exercising meticulous hand hygiene, properly handling contaminated waste (including diapers), disinfecting fomites, and limiting use of antimicrobial agents are the best available methods for control of *C difficile* disease.
- Thorough cleaning of hospital rooms and bathrooms of patients with *C difficile* colitis is essential. Germicide resistance as a cause of survival of *C difficile* in the environment has not been demonstrated.
- Children with *C difficile* diarrhea should be in a separate protected area in child care settings or excluded from child care for the duration of diarrhea.

Clostridial Myonecrosis
(Gas Gangrene)

CLINICAL MANIFESTATIONS: Onset is heralded by acute pain at the site of the wound, followed by edema, tenderness, exudate, and progression of pain. Systemic findings initially include tachycardia disproportionate to the degree of fever, pallor, diaphoresis, hypotension, renal failure, and later, alterations in mental status. Crepitus is suggestive but not pathognomonic of *Clostridium* infection and is not always present. Diagnosis is based on clinical manifestations, including the characteristic appearance of necrotic muscle at surgery. Untreated gas gangrene can lead to disseminated myonecrosis, suppurative visceral infection, septicemia, and death within hours.

ETIOLOGY: Gas gangrene is caused by *Clostridium* species, most commonly *Clostridium perfringens,* which are large, gram-positive, anaerobic bacilli with blunt ends. Other *Clostridium* species (eg, *Clostridium sordellii, Clostridium septicum, Clostridium novyi*) also can be associated with myonecrosis. Mixed infection with other gram-positive and gram-negative bacteria is common.

EPIDEMIOLOGY: Gas gangrene usually results from contamination of open wounds involving muscle. The sources of *Clostridium* species are soil, contaminated objects, and human and animal feces. Dirty surgical or traumatic wounds with significant devitalized tissue and foreign bodies predispose to disease. Nontraumatic gas gangrene occurs occasionally from *Clostridium* organisms in a person's gastrointestinal tract.

The **incubation period** is 6 hours to 3 weeks, usually 2 to 4 days.

DIAGNOSTIC TESTS: Anaerobic cultures of wound exudate, involved soft tissue and muscle, and blood should be performed. Because *Clostridium* species are ubiquitous, their recovery from a wound is not diagnostic unless typical clinical manifestations are present. A Gram-stained smear of wound discharge demonstrating characteristic gram-positive bacilli and absent or sparse polymorphonuclear leukocytes suggests clostridial infection. Tissue specimens and aspirates (not swab specimens) are appropriate for anaerobic culture. Because some pathogenic *Clostridium* species are exquisitely oxygen sensitive, care should be taken to optimize anaerobic growth conditions. A radiograph of the affected site may demonstrate gas in the tissue.

TREATMENT:
- Early and complete surgical excision of necrotic tissue and removal of foreign material is essential.
- Management of shock, fluid and electrolyte imbalance, hemolytic anemia, and other complications is crucial.
- High-dose penicillin G (250 000–400 000 U/kg per day) should be administered intravenously. Clindamycin, metronidazole, imipenem-cilastatin or meropenem, and chloramphenicol can be considered as alternative drugs for penicillin-allergic patients or for treatment of polymicrobial infections. The combination of penicillin G and clindamycin may have better efficacy than penicillin alone.
- Hyperbaric oxygen may be beneficial, but adequately controlled data on its efficacy are not available.
- Treatment with antitoxin is of no value.

ISOLATION OF THE HOSPITALIZED PATIENT: Standard precautions are recommended.

CONTROL MEASURES: In wound management, prompt and careful débridement, flushing of contaminated wounds, and removal of foreign material should be performed.

Penicillin G (50 000 U/kg per day) or clindamycin (20–30 mg/kg per day) may be of value for prophylaxis in patients with grossly contaminated wounds.

Clostridium perfringens Food Poisoning

CLINICAL MANIFESTATIONS: Food poisoning is characterized by a sudden onset of watery diarrhea and moderate to severe, crampy, midepigastric pain. Vomiting and fever are uncommon. Symptoms usually resolve within 24 hours. The short incubation, short duration, and absence of fever in most patients differentiates *Clostridium perfringens* foodborne disease from shigellosis and salmonellosis, and the infrequency of vomiting and longer incubation period contrast with the clinical features of foodborne disease associated with heavy metals, *Staphylococcus aureus* enterotoxins, and fish and shellfish toxins. Diarrheal illness caused by *Bacillus cereus* enterotoxin may be indistinguishable from that caused by *C perfringens* (see Appendix VI, Clinical Syndromes Associated With Foodborne Diseases, p 810). Enteritis necroticans (known locally as pigbel) is a cause of severe illness and death attributable to *C perfringens* food poisoning among children in Papua, New Guinea.

ETIOLOGY: Food poisoning is caused by a heat-labile toxin produced in vivo by *C perfringens* type A; type C causes enteritis necroticans.

EPIDEMIOLOGY: *Clostridium perfringens* is ubiquitous in the environment and commonly is present in raw meat and poultry. Spores of *C perfringens* may survive cooking. Spores germinate and multiply during slow cooling and storage at temperatures from 20°C to 60°C (68°F–140°F). Once ingested, an enterotoxin produced by the organisms in the lower intestine is responsible for symptoms. Beef, poultry, gravies, and dried or precooked foods are common sources. Infection usually is acquired at banquets or institutions (eg, schools and camps) or from food provided by caterers or restaurants where food is prepared in large quantities and kept warm for prolonged periods. Illness is not transmissible from person to person.

The **incubation period** is 6 to 24 hours, usually 8 to 12 hours.

DIAGNOSTIC TESTS: Because the fecal flora of healthy people commonly includes *C perfringens*, counts of *C perfringens* spores of 10^6/g of feces obtained within 48 hours of onset of illness are required to support the diagnosis in ill people. The diagnosis also can be suggested by detection of *C perfringens* enterotoxin in stool by commercially available kits. To confirm *C perfringens* as the cause, the concentration of organisms should be at least 10^5/g in the epidemiologically implicated food. Although *C perfringens* is an anaerobe, special transport conditions are unnecessary, because the spores are durable. Stool specimens, rather than rectal swab specimens, should be obtained.

TREATMENT: Usually, no treatment is required. As for other acute gastrointestinal tract infections, oral rehydration or, occasionally, intravenous fluid and electrolyte replacement may be indicated to prevent or treat dehydration. Antimicrobial agents are not indicated.

ISOLATION OF THE HOSPITALIZED PATIENT: Standard precautions are recommended.

CONTROL MEASURES: Preventive measures depend on limiting proliferation of *C perfringens* in foods by cooking foods thoroughly and maintaining food at warmer than 60°C (140°F) or cooler than 7°C (45°F). Meat dishes should be served hot shortly after cooking. Foods never should be held at room temperature to cool; they should be refrigerated after removal from warming devices or serving tables. Foods should be reheated to at least 74°C (165.2°F) before serving. Roasts, stews, and similar dishes should be divided into small quantities for cooking and refrigeration to limit the time such foods are at temperatures at which *C perfringens* replicates.

Coccidioidomycosis

CLINICAL MANIFESTATIONS: The primary infection is acquired by the respiratory route and is asymptomatic or self-limited in 60% of children. Symptomatic disease may resemble influenza, with malaise, fever, cough, myalgia, headache, and chest pain. Diffuse erythematous maculopapular rash, erythema multiforme, erythema nodosum, and/or arthralgias commonly occur and may be the only clinical manifestations in some children. Chronic pulmonary lesions are rare, but up to 5% of infected people may develop asymptomatic pulmonary radiographic residua (eg, cysts, coin lesions).

Extrapulmonary primary infection is rare, usually follows trauma, and includes cutaneous lesions or soft tissue infections with associated regional lymphadenitis.

Disseminated disease occurs in fewer than 1% of infected people. The skin, bones and joints, central nervous system (CNS), and lungs are the affected sites. Limited dissemination to one or more sites is common in infants. Meningitis is a serious manifestation of disseminated disease and is almost invariably fatal if untreated. Congenital infection is rare.

ETIOLOGY: *Coccidioides immitis* is a dimorphic fungus. In soil, it exists in hyphal phase. Infectious arthroconidia (eg, spores) produced in some hyphae become airborne, infecting the host after inhalation or inoculation. In tissues, spores enlarge to form spherules; mature spherules release endospores that develop into new spherules and continue the tissue cycle.

EPIDEMIOLOGY: *Coccidioides immitis* is found extensively in soil and is endemic in the southwestern United States, including California, Arizona, New Mexico, Texas, and northwestern Utah; northern Mexico; and certain areas of Central and South America. People are infected through inhalation of dustborne arthroconidia. In endemic areas, clusters of cases of coccidioidomycosis may follow dust storms, seismic events, archeologic digging, or recreational activities. Infection provides lifelong immunity. Person-to-person transmission of coccidioidomycosis does not occur. Black and Filipino people, pregnant women, neonates, elderly people, and immunocompromised people have an increased risk of dissemination and fatal outcome. A small proportion of new cases are identified in individuals who are not currently residing in endemic regions but may have visited these areas.

The **incubation period** typically is 10 to 16 days; the range is less than 1 week to approximately 1 month.

DIAGNOSTIC TESTS: The diagnosis of coccidioidomycosis is best established using serologic, histopathologic, and culture methods. Serologic tests are useful to confirm diagnoses and provide prognostic information. The immunoglobulin (Ig) M response can be detected by latex agglutination test, enzyme immunoassay (EIA), immunodiffusion, or tube precipitin test. Latex agglutination is a rapid, sensitive test that lacks specificity; hence, positive results should be confirmed by other tests. An IgM response is detectable 1 to 3 weeks after symptoms appear and lasts 3 to 4 months in most cases.

The IgG response can be detected by immunodiffusion, EIA, or complement fixation test. Complement fixation antibodies in serum usually are of low titer and are transient if the disease is asymptomatic or mild. High ($\geq$1:32) persistent titers occur with severe disease and almost always in disseminated infection. Cerebrospinal fluid (CSF) antibodies also are detectable by complement fixation test. Increasing serum and CSF titers indicate progressive disease, and decreasing titers suggest improvement. Low or nondetectable titers in immunocompromised patients should be interpreted with caution.

Spherules as large as 80 μm in diameter may be visualized in infected body fluid specimens and biopsy specimens of skin lesions or organs. Culture of the organisms is possible but is potentially hazardous to laboratory personnel, because spherules can convert to arthroconidia-bearing mycelia on culture plates. Suspect cultures should be sealed and thereafter handled using appropriate safety equipment and procedures. A DNA probe can identify *C immitis* in cultures, thereby decreasing the risk of exposure to infectious fungi.

Skin test may be a useful indicator of exposure and, therefore, is used mostly for epidemiologic studies. A delayed hypersensitivity reaction to a coccidioidin or spherulin skin test is indicative of past or current infection. The spherule skin test is preferred for general use, and conversion of the result from negative to positive in a patient with a clinically compatible syndrome strongly suggests coccidioidomycosis. A positive skin test result can appear from 10 to 45 days after infection, but anergy is common in disseminated disease. These skin tests currently are not available in the United States.

TREATMENT: Antifungal therapy is not indicated for uncomplicated primary infection.

Amphotericin B is the recommended initial therapy for severe, progressive, disseminated infection not involving the central nervous system (CNS) and for immunocompromised patients, including people with human immunodeficiency virus (HIV) infection (see Drugs for Invasive and Other Serious Fungal Infections, Table 4.6, p 725). Fluconazole is recommended for CNS infections. Fluconazole and itraconazole also are useful for treatment of less severe disseminated infections. For CNS infections that are unresponsive to fluconazole, intravenous amphotericin B therapy is augmented by repetitive CSF instillation of this drug. A subcutaneous reservoir can facilitate administration into the cisternal space or lateral ventricle. Orally administered fluconazole and itraconazole have suppressed coccidioidal meningitis in many patients, but lifelong therapy may be necessary. Consultation with a specialist for treatment of patients with meningeal disease is recommended.

In some localized infections with sinuses, fistulae, or abscesses, amphotericin B has been instilled locally or used for irrigation of wounds.

The duration of amphotericin B therapy is variable and depends on the site(s) of involvement, clinical response, and mycologic and immunologic test results. In general, therapy is continued until clinical and laboratory evidence indicates that active infection has subsided. The minimum duration of treatment for disseminated coccidioidomycosis is 1 month. The required duration of treatment with azoles is uncertain, except for patients with CNS infection or underlying HIV infection, for whom suppressive therapy is lifelong.

Surgical débridement or excision of lesions in bone and lung has been advocated for localized, symptomatic, persistent, resistant, or progressive lesions.

ISOLATION OF THE HOSPITALIZED PATIENT: Standard precautions are recommended. Care should be taken in handling, changing, and discarding dressings, casts, and similar materials in which arthroconidial contamination could occur.

CONTROL MEASURES: Measures to control dust are recommended in endemic areas at construction sites, archaeologic project sites, or where other activities cause excessive soil disturbance. Immunocompromised people residing in or traveling to endemic areas should be counseled to avoid exposure to activities that may aerosolize spores in contaminated soil.

Coronaviruses

CLINICAL MANIFESTATIONS: Coronaviruses are a common cause of upper respiratory tract infection in adults and children and occasionally have been implicated in lower respiratory tract disease. Signs and symptoms are consistent with these conditions. Coronavirus-like particles that are not confirmed as coronavirus have been associated with several outbreaks of diarrhea in nurseries and, rarely, with neonatal necrotizing enterocolitis.

ETIOLOGY: Coronaviruses are RNA viruses that are large (80–160 nm in diameter), enveloped with lipid-soluble coats, and pleomorphic (spherical or elliptical). At least 2 distinct antigenic groups of respiratory coronaviruses have been identified.

EPIDEMIOLOGY: Human coronaviruses are transmitted via respiratory tract secretions; transmission is facilitated by close contact. Although several animal coronaviruses have antigens in common with human strains, no evidence implicates animals as reservoirs or vectors for human disease. The distribution of coronaviruses is worldwide. In temperate climates, outbreaks occur in the winter, with young children having the highest infection rate during outbreaks. The period of communicability is unknown but probably persists for the duration of respiratory tract symptoms.

The **incubation period** usually is 2 to 5 days.

DIAGNOSTIC TESTS: Diagnostic tests, including antibody assays, for human coronavirus infection are not available commercially. Most strains cannot be isolated by methods commonly used in diagnostic virology laboratories. Viral particles have been visualized by immune electron microscopy, and viral antigens have been detected by immunoassay.

TREATMENT: Supportive.

ISOLATION OF THE HOSPITALIZED PATIENT: Standard precautions are recommended.

CONTROL MEASURES: None.

Cryptococcus neoformans Infections
(Cryptococcosis)

CLINICAL MANIFESTATIONS: Primary infection is acquired by inhalation of aerosolized fungal elements from contaminated soil and often is asymptomatic or mild. Pulmonary disease, when symptomatic, is characterized by cough, hemoptysis, chest pain, and constitutional symptoms. Chest radiographs may reveal a solitary nodule or focal or diffuse infiltrates. Hematogenous dissemination to the central nervous system, bones and joints, skin, and mucous membranes can occur, but dissemination is rare in children without defects in cell-mediated immunity (eg, people having undergone transplantation; people with malignant neoplasm, collagen-vascular disease, or sarcoidosis; or people receiving long-term corticosteroid therapy). Usually, several sites are infected, but manifestations of involvement of one site predominate. Cryptococcal meningitis, the most common and serious form of cryptococcal disease, often follows an indolent course. Symptoms are characteristic of meningitis, meningoencephalitis, or space-occupying lesions but may manifest as only behavioral changes. Cryptococcal fungemia without apparent organ involvement occurs in patients with human immunodeficiency virus (HIV) infection, but in children it is rare.

ETIOLOGY: *Cryptococcus neoformans*, an encapsulated yeast that grows at 37°C (98°F), is the only species of the genus *Cryptococcus* considered to be a human pathogen.

EPIDEMIOLOGY: *Cryptococcus neoformans* var *neoformans* is isolated primarily from soil contaminated with bird droppings and causes most human infections, especially infections in immunocompromised hosts. *Cryptococcus neoformans* var *gattii* occurs most commonly in tropical and subtropical regions and causes disease primarily in immunocompetent people. Person-to-person transmission does not occur. *Cryptococcus* species infect 5% to 10% of adults with acquired immunodeficiency syndrome, but infection is rare in HIV-infected children.

The **incubation period** is unknown.

DIAGNOSTIC TESTS: Encapsulated yeast cells can be visualized using India ink or other stains of cerebrospinal fluid (CSF) specimens containing 10^3 or more colony-forming units of yeast per mL. Definitive diagnosis requires isolation of the organism from body fluid or tissue specimens. The lysis-centrifugation method is the most sensitive technique for recovery of *C neoformans* from blood cultures. Media containing cycloheximide, which inhibits growth of *C neoformans,* should not be used. Sabouraud glucose agar is optimal for isolation of *Cryptococcus* from sputum, bronchopulmonary lavage, tissue, or CSF specimens. Few organisms may be present in the CSF specimen, and a large quantity of CSF may be needed to recover the organism. The latex agglutination test and enzyme immunoassay for detection of cryptococcal capsular polysaccharide antigen in serum or CSF specimens are excellent rapid diagnostic tests. Antigen is detected in CSF or serum specimens from 90% of patients with cryptococcal meningitis. Cryptococcal antibody testing is useful, but skin testing is of no value.

TREATMENT: Amphotericin B (see Drugs for Invasive and Other Serious Fungal Infections, p 725), in combination with oral flucytosine, is indicated for patients with meningeal and other serious cryptococcal infections. Combination antifungal therapy with flucytosine probably is superior to amphotericin B alone. Flucytosine can induce bone marrow suppression, which often necessitates discontinuation of the medication, especially in HIV-infected patients. Other flucytosine adverse effects are hepatic and renal dysfunction, rash, diarrhea, ulcerative colitis, and gastrointestinal tract bleeding, especially in patients with azotemia. When flucytosine is used, serum concentrations should be monitored and maintained between 40 and 60 mg/mL. Patients with meningitis should receive combination therapy for at least 2 weeks or until CSF culture results are negative; at least 6 weeks of total treatment should be completed with amphotericin B or 10 weeks if fluconazole alone is used for therapy. Lipid formulations of amphotericin B can be substituted for conventional amphotericin B in children with renal impairment. Patients with HIV infection should be treated for longer periods than should non–HIV-infected patients, as should patients who are immunosuppressed as a result of organ transplantation. Patients with less severe disease may be treated with fluconazole or itraconazole, but data on use of these drugs for children with *C neoformans* infection are limited. Another potential treatment option for HIV-infected patients with less severe disease is combination therapy with fluconazole and flucytosine; the toxicity associated with this regimen often limits its usefulness.

Children with HIV infection who have completed initial therapy for cryptococcosis should receive lifelong suppressive therapy with low-dose fluconazole. Data regarding discontinuing this secondary prophylaxis following immune reconstitution as a consequence of highly active antiretroviral therapy are available for adults but not children.

ISOLATION OF THE HOSPITALIZED PATIENT: Standard precautions are recommended.

CONTROL MEASURES: None.

Cryptosporidiosis

CLINICAL MANIFESTATIONS: Frequent, nonbloody, watery diarrhea is the most common manifestation of cryptosporidiosis, although infection can be asymptomatic. Other symptoms include abdominal cramps, fatigue, vomiting, anorexia, and weight loss. Fever and vomiting are relatively common among children and often lead to a misdiagnosis of viral gastroenteritis. In infected immunocompetent people, including children, the diarrheal illness is self-limited, usually lasting 1 to 20 days (mean, 10 days). In immunocompromised people, especially people with human immunodeficiency virus (HIV) infection, chronic severe diarrhea can develop, resulting in malnutrition, dehydration, and death. Pulmonary, biliary tract, or disseminated infection can occur in immunocompromised people, although infection usually is limited to the gastrointestinal tract.

ETIOLOGY: *Cryptosporidium parvum* is a spore-forming coccidian protozoan. Oocysts are excreted in feces and are the infectious form.

EPIDEMIOLOGY: *Cryptosporidium parvum* has been found in a variety of hosts, including mammals, birds, and reptiles. Extensive waterborne outbreaks have been associated with contamination of municipal water and exposure to contaminated swimming pools. In children, the incidence of cryptosporidiosis is greatest during summer and early fall, corresponding to the outdoor swimming season. Transmission to humans can occur from farm livestock, particularly young animals including those found in petting zoos, or pets. Person-to-person transmission occurs and can cause outbreaks in child care centers, with attack rates of 30% to 60% reported. *Cryptosporidium parvum* also causes traveler's diarrhea. Because the oocyst form of the parasite is resistant to chlorine, appropriately functioning water filtration systems are critical for the safety of public water supplies. Most sand filters used for swimming pools are ineffective for removing oocysts from contaminated water.

The median **incubation period** is 7 days, with a range of 2 to 14 days.

Oocysts continue to be detected in stool a mean of 7 days after symptoms resolve. In most people, shedding of *C parvum* stops within 2 weeks, but in a few, shedding continues for up to 2 months.

DIAGNOSTIC TESTS: The detection of oocysts on microscopic examination of stool specimens is diagnostic. Unfortunately, routine laboratory examination of stool for ova and parasites will not detect *C parvum,* so physicians should ask laboratory personnel to test specifically for *C parvum.* The sucrose flotation method or formalin-ethyl acetate method is used to concentrate oocysts in stool before staining with a modified Kinyoun acid-fast stain. Monoclonal antibody-based fluorescein-conjugated stain for oocysts in stool and an enzyme immunoassay (EIA) for detecting antigen in stool are available commercially. With EIA methods, false-positive and false-negative results may occur, and confirmation by microscopy should be considered. Because shedding can be intermittent, at least 3 stool specimens collected on separate days should be examined before considering test results to be negative. Oocysts are small (4–6 μm in diameter) and can be missed in a rapid scan of a slide. Organisms also can be identified in intestinal biopsy tissue or intestinal fluid.

TREATMENT: A 3-day course of nitazoxanide oral suspension has been licensed by the Food and Drug Administration for treatment of children with diarrhea attributable to *C parvum* and *Giardia lamblia.* Paromomycin, alone or with azithromycin dihydrate, is minimally effective. In immunocompromised patients with cryptosporidiosis, oral administration of Human Immune Globulin or bovine colostrum has been beneficial. In HIV-infected patients, antiretroviral therapy-associated improvement in CD4 cell count can improve the course of disease.

ISOLATION OF THE HOSPITALIZED PATIENT: In addition to standard precautions, contact precautions are recommended for diapered or incontinent children.

CONTROL MEASURES: In waterborne outbreaks attributable to contaminated drinking water, advisories to boil water may be issued to prevent cases until proper water treatment is restored. People with diarrhea should not use public recreational water (eg, swimming pools, lakes, ponds), and people with a diagnosis of cryptosporidiosis should not use recreational waters for 2 weeks after symptoms resolve.

Cutaneous Larva Migrans

CLINICAL MANIFESTATIONS: Nematode larvae produce pruritic, reddish papules at the site of skin entry, a condition referred to as creeping eruption. As the larvae migrate through the skin advancing several millimeters to a few centimeters a day, intensely pruritic, serpiginous tracks or bullae are formed. Larval activity can continue for several weeks or months but eventually is self-limiting. An advancing serpiginous tunnel in the skin with an associated intense pruritus is virtually pathognomonic. Rarely, in infections with a large burden of parasites, pneumonitis (Löeffler syndrome), which can be severe, and myositis may follow skin lesions. Occasionally, the larvae reach the intestine and may cause eosinophilic enteritis.

ETIOLOGY: Infective larvae of cat and dog hookworms (ie, *Ancylostoma braziliense* and *Ancylostoma caninum*) are the usual causes. Other skin-penetrating nematodes are occasional causes.

EPIDEMIOLOGY: Cutaneous larva migrans is a disease of children, utility workers, gardeners, sunbathers, and others who come in contact with soil contaminated with cat and dog feces. In the United States, the disease is most prevalent in the Southeast.

DIAGNOSTIC TESTS: Because the diagnosis usually is made clinically, biopsies are not indicated. Biopsy specimens typically demonstrate an eosinophilic inflammatory infiltrate, but the migrating parasite is not visualized. Eosinophilia occurs in some cases. Larvae have been detected in sputum and gastric washings in patients with the rare complication of pneumonitis. Enzyme immunoassay or Western blot analysis using antigens of *A caninum* are available in research laboratories, but use is not warranted routinely.

TREATMENT: The disease usually is self-limited, with spontaneous cure after several weeks or months. Orally administered albendazole or ivermectin or topically administered thiabendazole are the recommended therapy.

ISOLATION OF THE HOSPITALIZED PATIENT: Standard precautions are recommended.

CONTROL MEASURES: Skin contact with moist soil contaminated with animal feces should be avoided. In warm climates, beaches should be kept free of dog and cat feces.

Cyclospora Infections
(Cyclosporiasis)

CLINICAL MANIFESTATIONS: Profuse, nonbloody, watery diarrhea is the most common symptom of cyclosporiasis. Vomiting, fatigue, anorexia, abdominal bloating or cramping, and weight loss also can occur. Diarrhea can alternate with constipation. Fever occurs in approximately 50% of patients. Infection usually is self-limited, but diarrhea and systemic symptoms can persist for weeks. Relapse of symptoms also is common in untreated patients. Prolonged symptoms may persist in immunocompromised patients.

ETIOLOGY: *Cyclospora cayetanensis* is a coccidian parasite. This organism previously was called "cyanobacterium-like body" or "coccidian-like body." Noninfectious, unsporulated oocysts are passed in stools. Sporulation outside the host produces infectious organisms.

EPIDEMIOLOGY: *Cyclospora cayetanensis* has a worldwide distribution but is endemic in some countries, such as Nepal, Peru, and Haiti. Outbreaks have been associated with contaminated food (eg, produce) and water. *Cyclospora cayetanensis* has been reported as a cause of traveler's diarrhea and of isolated community-acquired cases of diarrhea.

Direct person-to-person transmission has not been documented, probably because excreted oocysts take days to weeks under favorable environmental conditions to sporulate and become infectious.

The **incubation period** is approximately 7 days (range, 1–14 days).

DIAGNOSTIC TESTS: Diagnosis is made by identification of oocysts (8–10 μm in diameter) in stool. The organisms can be seen after modified acid-fast staining but also can be detected with a safranin-based stain and heating of fecal smears and by autofluorescence.

TREATMENT: Trimethoprim-sulfamethoxazole for 7 to 10 days is effective therapy. People infected with human immunodeficiency virus may need higher doses and long-term maintenance.

ISOLATION OF THE HOSPITALIZED PATIENT: In addition to standard precautions, contact precautions are recommended for diapered or incontinent children for the duration of illness.

CONTROL MEASURES: Fresh produce should be washed thoroughly before it is eaten. This precaution, however, may not entirely eliminate the risk of transmission.

Cytomegalovirus Infection

CLINICAL MANIFESTATIONS: Manifestations of acquired human cytomegalovirus (CMV) infection vary with the age and immunocompetence of the host. Asymptomatic infections are the most common, particularly in children. An infectious mononucleosis-like syndrome with prolonged fever and mild hepatitis, occurring in the absence of heterophil antibody production, can occur in adolescents and adults. Pneumonia, colitis, and retinitis occur in immunocompromised hosts (particularly people receiving treatment for malignant neoplasms), people infected with human immunodeficiency virus (HIV), and people receiving immunosuppressive therapy for organ transplantation.

Congenital infection has a spectrum of manifestations but is usually asymptomatic. Some congenitally infected infants who are asymptomatic at birth are later found to have hearing loss or learning disability. Approximately 10% of infants with congenital CMV infection have profound involvement, evident at birth, with manifestations including intrauterine growth retardation, jaundice, purpura, hepatosplenomegaly, microcephaly, intracerebral calcifications, and retinitis.

Infection acquired at birth or shortly thereafter from maternal cervical secretions or human milk usually is not associated with clinical illness. Infection resulting from transfusion from CMV-seropositive donors to preterm infants has been associated with systemic symptoms, including lower respiratory tract disease.

ETIOLOGY: Human CMV, a DNA virus, is a member of the herpesvirus group.

EPIDEMIOLOGY: Cytomegalovirus is highly species-specific, and only human strains are known to produce human disease. This virus is ubiquitous and is transmitted horizontally (by direct person-to-person contact with virus-containing secretions), vertically (from mother to infant before, during, or after birth), and via transfusions of blood, platelets, and white blood cells from previously infected people (see Blood Safety, p 106). Infections have no seasonal predilection. Cytomegalovirus persists in latent form after a primary infection, and reactivation can occur years later, particularly under conditions of immunosuppression.

Horizontal transmission probably is the result of salivary contamination, but contact with infected urine also can have a role. Spread of CMV in households and child care centers is well documented. Excretion rates in child care centers can be as high as 70% in children 1 to 3 years of age. Young children can transmit CMV to their parents and other caregivers, such as child care staff (see also Children in Out-of-Home Child Care, p 123). In adolescents and adults, sexual transmission also occurs, as evidenced by virus in seminal and cervical fluids.

Seropositive healthy people have latent CMV in their leukocytes and tissues; hence, blood transfusions and organ transplantation can result in viral transmission. Severe CMV disease is more likely to occur if the recipient is seronegative or is a premature infant. Latent CMV commonly will reactivate in immunosuppressed people and can result in disease if immunosuppression is severe (eg, in patients with acquired immunodeficiency syndrome and solid-organ and bone marrow transplant recipients).

Vertical transmission of CMV to an infant occurs by one of the following methods: (1) in utero by transplacental passage of maternal bloodborne virus; (2) at birth by passage through an infected maternal genital tract; or (3) postnatally by ingestion of CMV-positive human milk. Approximately 1% of all live-born infants are infected in utero and excrete CMV at birth. Although in utero fetal infection can occur after maternal primary infection or after reactivation of infection during pregnancy, sequelae are far more common in infants exposed to maternal primary infection, with 10% to 20% diagnosed with mental retardation or sensorineural deafness in childhood and 10% having manifestations evident at birth.

Maternal cervical infection is common, resulting in exposure of many infants to CMV at birth. Cervical excretion rates are highest among young mothers in lower socioeconomic groups. Although interstitial pneumonia caused by CMV can develop during the early months of life, most infected infants remain asymptomatic. Similarly, although symptomatic disease can occur in seronegative infants fed CMV-infected milk, most infants infected from ingestion of human milk do not develop clinical illness, most likely because of the presence of passively transferred maternal antibody. Of infants who acquire infection from maternal cervical secretions or human milk, premature infants are at greater risk of symptomatic disease and sequelae than are full-term infants.

The **incubation period** for horizontally transmitted CMV infections in households is unknown. Infection usually manifests 3 to 12 weeks after blood transfusions and between 1 and 4 months after tissue transplantation.

DIAGNOSTIC TESTS: The diagnosis of CMV disease is confounded by the ubiquity of the virus, the high rate of asymptomatic excretion, the frequency of reactivated infections, development of serum immunoglobulin (Ig) M CMV-specific antibody in some episodes of reactivation, and concurrent infection with other pathogens.

Virus can be isolated in cell culture from urine, pharynx, peripheral blood leukocytes, human milk, semen, cervical secretions, and other tissues and body fluids. Examination of cells shed in urine for intranuclear inclusions is an insensitive test.

Recovery of virus from a target organ provides strong evidence that the disease is caused by CMV infection. A presumptive diagnosis can be made on the basis of a fourfold antibody titer increase in paired serum specimens or by demonstration of virus excretion. Techniques for detection of viral DNA in tissues and some fluids, especially cerebrospinal fluid, by polymerase chain reaction assay or hybridization are available from specialty laboratories. Detection of pp65 antigen in white blood cells is used to detect infection in immunocompromised hosts.

The complement fixation test is the least sensitive serologic method for detecting CMV antibodies and, therefore, should not be used to establish previous infection. Various immunofluorescence assays, indirect hemagglutination assays, latex agglutination assays, and enzyme immunoassays are preferred for this purpose.

Proof of congenital infection requires a positive viral culture obtained within 3 weeks of birth. Differentiation between intrauterine and perinatal infection is difficult later in infancy unless clinical manifestations of the former, such as chorioretinitis or ventriculitis, are present. A strongly positive result of a test for serum IgM anti-CMV antibody is suggestive during early infancy, but IgM antibody assays vary in accuracy for identification of primary infection.

TREATMENT: Ganciclovir (see Antiviral Drugs for Non-Human Immunodeficiency Virus Infections, p 729) is beneficial for treatment of retinitis caused by acquired or recurrent CMV infection in HIV-infected patients. This drug is licensed in the United States for treatment of severe retinitis in immunocompromised adults. Limited data in children suggest that safety and efficacy are similar to those in adults. The combination of oral ganciclovir and an intraocular ganciclovir implant is efficacious in adults with CMV retinitis, but data in children are not available. Ganciclovir often is useful in other types of CMV organ involvement. Although ganciclovir has been used to treat some congenitally infected infants, it is not recommended routinely because of insufficient efficacy data. One study of ganciclovir therapy of congenitally infected newborns with central nervous system (CNS) disease suggested that treatment decreases the risk of hearing impairment. However, because of the potential toxicity of long-term ganciclovir therapy, additional study is necessary before a recommendation can be made. In bone marrow transplant recipients, the combination of CMV Immune Globulin Intravenous and ganciclovir administered intravenously has been reported to be synergistic in treatment of CMV pneumonia. Foscarnet sodium and valganciclovir hydrochloride also have been licensed for treatment of CMV retinitis in adults and are alternative drugs (see Antiviral Drugs for Non-Human Immunodeficiency Virus Infections, p 729). These drugs are more toxic but may be advantageous for some patients with HIV infection, including people with disease caused by ganciclovir-resistant virus or people who are unable to tolerate ganciclovir. Cidofovir is efficacious for treatment of CMV retinitis in adults, but it has not been studied in children and is nephrotoxic. Fomivirsen sodium is licensed by the Food and Drug Administration for intraocular administration.

Cytomegalovirus disease in HIV-infected patients is not cured by currently available antiviral agents. Lifelong prophylaxis should be administered to patients with a history of CMV disease to prevent recurrence. Treatment with highly active antiretroviral therapy (HAART) has significantly decreased severity. For children with CMV disease, no data are available to guide decisions concerning discontinuing secondary prophylaxis (chronic maintenance therapy) when CD4+ T-lymphocyte count has increased in response to HAART.

ISOLATION OF THE HOSPITALIZED PATIENT: Standard precautions are recommended.

CONTROL MEASURES:

Care of Exposed People. When caring for all children, hand hygiene, particularly after changing diapers, is advised to decrease transmission of CMV. Because asymptomatic excretion of CMV is common in people of all ages, a child with congenital CMV infection should not be treated differently from other children and should not be excluded from school or institutions. Institutional screening programs for CMV-excreting children are not indicated.

Although unrecognized exposure to people who are asymptomatically shedding CMV is likely to be common, concern arises when immunocompromised or pregnant patients or health care professionals are exposed to patients with clinically recognizable CMV infection. Serologic testing can be used to identify nonimmune people. If indicated, follow-up serologic testing of seronegative individuals can establish whether infection has occurred, but routine serologic screening is not recommended.

Prevention of exposure of severely immunocompromised patients to recognized cases of CMV infection is prudent. Because unrecognized exposure may occur, infection control procedures, such as careful hand hygiene, should be used.

Pregnant personnel who may be in contact with CMV-infected patients should be counseled about the potential risks of acquisition and urged to practice universal precautions and good hygiene, particularly hand hygiene. Approximately 1% of newborn infants in most nurseries and a higher percentage of older children excrete CMV without clinical manifestations. Risks to the fetus are greatest during the first half of gestation. Amniocentesis has been used in several small series of patients to establish the presence of intrauterine infection.

Child Care (see also Children in Out-of-Home Child Care, p 123). Educational programs about the epidemiology of CMV, its potential risks, and appropriate hygienic measures to minimize occupationally acquired infection should be provided for female workers in child care centers. Risk seems to be greatest for child care personnel who provide care for children younger than 2 years of age. Routine serologic screening of staff at child care centers for antibody to CMV is not recommended.

Immunoprophylaxis. Cytomegalovirus Immune Globulin Intravenous has been developed for prophylaxis of disease in seronegative transplant recipients. Cytomegalovirus Immune Globulin Intravenous seems to be moderately effective in kidney and liver transplant recipients. Results of studies of its use in prevention of CMV transmission to newborn infants are inconclusive. Evaluation of investigational vaccines in healthy volunteers and renal transplant recipients is in progress.

Prevention of Transmission by Blood Transfusion. Transmission of CMV by blood transfusion to newborn infants or other compromised hosts virtually has been eliminated by the use of CMV antibody-negative donors, by freezing red blood cells in glycerol before administration, by removal of the buffy coat, or by filtration to remove white blood cells.

Prevention of Transmission by Human Milk. Pasteurization or freezing of donated human milk can decrease the likelihood of CMV transmission. If fresh donated milk is needed for infants born to CMV antibody-negative mothers, providing these infants with milk from only CMV antibody-negative women should be considered. For further information on human milk banks, see Human Milk (p 117).

Prevention of Transmission in Transplant Recipients. Cytomegalovirus antibody-negative people who receive tissue from CMV-seropositive donors are at high risk of CMV disease. If such circumstances cannot be avoided, administration of Cytomegalovirus Immune Globulin Intravenous is beneficial for decreasing this risk. Treatment of transplant recipients with acyclovir or ganciclovir at the onset of CMV infection may prevent serious CMV disease.

Diphtheria

CLINICAL MANIFESTATIONS: Diphtheria usually occurs as membranous nasopharyngitis or obstructive laryngotracheitis. Local infections are associated with a low-grade fever and the gradual onset of manifestations over 1 to 2 days. Less commonly, the disease presents as cutaneous, vaginal, conjunctival, or otic infection. Cutaneous diphtheria is more common in tropical areas and among the homeless. Serious complications of diphtheria include upper airway obstruction caused by extensive membrane formation, toxic myocarditis, and peripheral neuropathies.

ETIOLOGY: *Corynebacterium diphtheriae* is an irregularly staining, gram-positive, nonspore-forming, nonmotile, pleomorphic bacillus with 4 colony types (mitis, intermedius, bellanti, and gravis). Strains of *C diphtheriae* may be toxigenic or nontoxigenic. Extracellular toxin consists of an enzymatically active A domain and a binding B domain, which promotes the entry of A into the cell. The toxin gene is carried by a family of related corynebacteria phages. The toxin inactivates elongation factor-2, thereby inhibiting protein synthesis, in myocardial and peripheral nerve cells.

EPIDEMIOLOGY: Humans are the only known reservoir of *C diphtheriae,* which is present in discharges from the nose, throat, and eye and skin lesions for 2 to 6 weeks after infection. Patients treated with an appropriate antimicrobial agent usually are communicable for fewer than 4 days. Transmission results primarily from intimate contact with a patient or carrier; rarely, fomites and foodborne sources serve as vehicles of transmission. Although infection can occur in people who are immunized, partially immunized, or not immunized, disease is most common and most severe in people who are not immunized or inadequately immunized. The incidence of respiratory diphtheria is greatest during autumn and winter, but summer epidemics may occur in warm, moist climates in which skin infections are prevalent. After 1990, epidemic diphtheria occurred throughout the newly independent states of the former Soviet Union, including Russia, the Ukraine, and the central Asian republics. Case-fatality rates ranged from 3% to 23% in these epidemics.

The **incubation period** usually is 2 to 7 days but occasionally is longer.

DIAGNOSTIC TESTS: Specimens for culture should be obtained from the nose or throat or any mucosal or cutaneous lesion. Material should be obtained from beneath the membrane, or a portion of the membrane itself should be submitted for culture. Because special media are required, laboratory personnel should be notified that *C diphtheriae* is suspected. In remote areas, collected culture materials can be placed in silica gel packs or any transport medium or sterile container and sent to a reference laboratory for culture. When *C diphtheriae* is recovered, the strain should be tested for toxigenicity at a laboratory recommended by state and local authorities. All *C diphtheriae* isolates also should be sent through the state health department to the National Center for Infectious Diseases of the Centers for Disease Control and Prevention (CDC).

TREATMENT:

Antitoxin. Because the condition of patients with diphtheria may deteriorate rapidly, a single dose of equine antitoxin should be administered on the basis of clinical diagnosis even before culture results are available. To neutralize toxin as rapidly as possible, the preferred route of administration is intravenous. Before intravenous administration of antitoxin, tests for sensitivity to horse serum should be performed, initially with a scratch test of a 1:1000 dilution of antitoxin in saline solution (see Sensitivity Tests for Reactions to Animal Sera, p 60). If the patient is sensitive to equine antitoxin, desensitization is necessary (see Desensitization to Animal Sera, p 61). Although intravenous immune globulin preparations may contain variable amounts of antibodies to diphtheria toxin, use of Immune Globulin Intravenous for therapy of cutaneous or respiratory diphtheria has not been approved. Antitoxin can be obtained from the National Immunization Program of the CDC (see Directory of Resources, p 789). The site and size of the diphtheria membrane, the degree of toxic effects, and the duration of illness are guides for estimating the dose of antitoxin; the presence of soft, diffuse cervical lymphadenitis suggests moderate to severe toxin absorption. Suggested dose ranges are the following: pharyngeal or laryngeal disease of 48 hours' duration or less, 20 000 to 40 000 U; nasopharyngeal lesions, 40 000 to 60 000 U; extensive disease of 3 or more days' duration or diffuse swelling of the neck, 80 000 to 120 000 U. Antitoxin probably is of no value for cutaneous disease, but some experts recommend 20 000 to 40 000 U of antitoxin, because toxic sequelae have been reported.

    Antimicrobial Therapy. Erythromycin given orally or parenterally for 14 days, penicillin G given intramuscularly or intravenously for 14 days, or penicillin G procaine given intramuscularly for 14 days constitute acceptable therapy. Antimicrobial therapy is required to eradicate the organism and prevent spread. Antimicrobial therapy is not a substitute for antitoxin. Elimination of the organism should be documented by 2 consecutive negative cultures after completion of treatment.

    Cutaneous Diphtheria. Thorough cleansing of the lesion with soap and water and administration of an appropriate antimicrobial agent for 10 days are recommended.

    Carriers. If not immunized, carriers should receive active immunization promptly, and measures should be taken to ensure completion of the immunization schedule. If a carrier has been immunized previously but has not received a booster within 1 year, a booster dose of a preparation containing diphtheria toxoid (DTaP, DT, or Td, depending on age) should be given. Carriers should be given oral erythromycin or penicillin G for 7 days or a single intramuscular dose of penicillin G benzathine (600 000 U for those weighing <30 kg and 1.2 million U for children weighing ≥30 kg and adults). Follow-up cultures should be obtained at least 2 weeks after completion of therapy; if results of cultures are positive, an additional 10-day course of oral erythromycin should be given, and follow-up cultures should be performed. Erythromycin-resistant strains have been identified, but their epidemiologic significance has not been determined. Fluoroquinolones, rifampin, clarithromycin, and azithromycin dihydrate have good in vitro activity and may be better tolerated than erythromycin, but they have not been critically evaluated in clinical infection or in carriers.

ISOLATION OF THE HOSPITALIZED PATIENT: In addition to standard precautions, droplet precautions are recommended for patients and carriers with pharyngeal diphtheria until 2 cultures from both the nose and the throat are negative for *C diphtheriae*. Contact precautions are recommended for patients with cutaneous diphtheria until 2 cultures of skin lesions taken at least 24 hours apart after cessation of antimicrobial therapy are negative.

CONTROL MEASURES:

Care of Exposed People. Whenever the diagnosis of diphtheria is strongly suspected or proven, local public health officials should be notified promptly. Management of exposed people is based on individual circumstances, including immunization status and likelihood of compliance with follow-up and prophylaxis. The following is recommended:

- Identification of close contacts of a person suspected to have diphtheria should be initiated promptly. Contact tracing should begin in the household and usually can be limited to household members and other people with a history of habitual close contact with the person suspected of having the disease.
- For close contacts, *regardless of their immunization status,* the following measures should be taken: (1) surveillance for 7 days for evidence of disease; (2) culture for *C diphtheriae;* and (3) antimicrobial prophylaxis with oral erythromycin (40–50 mg/kg per day for 7 days, maximum 2 g/day) or a single intramuscular injection of penicillin G benzathine (600 000 U for those weighing <30 kg and 1.2 million U for children weighing ≥30 kg and adults). The efficacy of antimicrobial prophylaxis is presumed but not proven. Follow-up pharyngeal cultures should be obtained from contacts proven to be carriers at a minimum of 2 weeks after completion of therapy (see Carriers, p 264). If cultures are positive, an additional 10-day course of erythromycin should be given, and follow-up cultures should be performed.
- Asymptomatic, previously immunized close contacts should receive a booster dose of a preparation containing diphtheria toxoid (DTaP, DT, or Td, depending on age) if they have not received a booster dose of diphtheria toxoid within 5 years. Children in need of their fourth dose should be immunized.
- For asymptomatic close contacts who are not immunized fully (defined as having had fewer than 3 doses of diphtheria toxoid) or whose immunization status is not known, active immunization should be undertaken with DTaP, DT, or Td, depending on age.
- Contacts who cannot be kept under surveillance should receive penicillin G benzathine but not erythromycin, because adherence to an oral regimen is less likely, and a dose of DTaP, DT, or Td, depending on the person's age and immunization history.

The use of equine diphtheria antitoxin in unimmunized close contacts is not recommended, because there is no evidence that antitoxin provides additional benefit for contacts who have received antimicrobial prophylaxis and because of the 5% to 20% risk of allergic reactions to horse serum.

Immunization. Universal immunization with diphtheria toxoid is the only effective control measure. For all indications, diphtheria immunization is administered with tetanus toxoid-containing vaccines. The schedules for immunization against diphtheria are presented in the chapter on tetanus (see Tetanus, p 611). The value of diphtheria toxoid immunization is proven by the rarity of disease in countries in which high rates of immunization with diphtheria toxoid have been achieved. Fewer than 5 cases have been reported annually in the United States in recent years. However, the decreased frequency of exposure to the organism implies decreased maintenance of immunity secondary to community contact. Therefore, ensuring continuing immunity requires regular booster injections of diphtheria toxoid (as Td) every 10 years after completion of the initial immunization series.

Haemophilus influenzae or pneumococcal conjugate vaccines containing diphtheria toxoid (eg, PRP-D) or CRM197 protein, a nontoxic variant of diphtheria toxin (eg, HbOC, pneumococcal conjugate vaccines), are not substitutes for diphtheria toxoid immunization. Vaccine is given intramuscularly.

Immunization for children from 2 months of age to the seventh birthday (see Fig 1.1, p 24, and Table 1.6, p 26) should consist of 5 doses of diphtheria and tetanus toxoid-containing vaccines (see Tetanus, p 611). This typically is accomplished with DTaP. Immunization against diphtheria and tetanus for children younger than 7 years of age in whom pertussis immunization is contraindicated (see Pertussis, p 472) should be accomplished with DT instead of DTaP (see Tetanus, p 611).

Other recommendations for diphtheria immunization, including those for older children, can be found in the chapter on tetanus (see Tetanus, p 611).

- When children and adults require tetanus toxoid for wound management (see Tetanus, p 611), the use of preparations containing diphtheria toxoid (DTaP, DT, or Td as appropriate for age or specific contraindication to pertussis immunization) will help ensure continuing diphtheria immunity.
- Active immunization against diphtheria should be undertaken during convalescence from diphtheria, because disease does not necessarily confer immunity.
- Travelers to countries with endemic or epidemic diphtheria should have their diphtheria immunization status reviewed and updated when necessary.

Precautions and Contraindications. See Pertussis (p 472) and Tetanus (p 611).

Ehrlichia Infections
(Human Ehrlichioses)

CLINICAL MANIFESTATIONS: Human ehrlichioses in the United States are attributable to at least 3 distinct tickborne pathogens: *Ehrlichia chaffeensis* (human monocytic ehrlichiosis [HME]), *Anaplasma* (formerly *Ehrlichia*) *phagocytophila* agent (human granulocytic ehrlichiosis [HGE]), and *Ehrlichia ewingii* (Table 3.4, p 267). These 3 infections have different causes but similar signs, symptoms, and clinical courses. All are acute, systemic, febrile illnesses that are similar clinically to Rocky Mountain spotted fever but often demonstrate leukopenia, anemia, and hepatitis and are associated less commonly with rash. The febrile illness often is accompanied by

Table 3.4. **Human Ehrlichioses in the United States**

Disease	Causal Agent	Vector	Geographic Distribution
Human monocytic ehrlichiosis (HME)	*Ehrlichia chaffeensis*	Lone star tick (*Amblyomma americanum*)	Predominately southeast, south central, and Midwest states
Human granulocytic ehrlichiosis (HGE)	*Anaplasma* (formerly *Ehrlichia*) *phagocytophila*	Black-legged or deer tick (*Ixodes scapularis*)	Northeastern and north central states and northern California
Granulocytic ehrlichiosis	*Ehrlichia ewingii*	Lone star tick (*A americanum*)	Southeast, south central, and Midwest states

one or more systemic manifestations, including headache, chills, malaise, myalgia, arthralgia, nausea, vomiting, anorexia, and acute weight loss. Rash is variable in appearance and location, typically develops approximately 1 week after onset of illness, and occurs only in approximately 60% of children and 25% of adults with reported cases of HME and fewer than 10% of people with HGE. Diarrhea, abdominal pain, cough, or change in mental status occur rarely. More severe manifestations of these diseases include pulmonary infiltrates, bone marrow hypoplasia, respiratory failure, encephalopathy, meningitis, disseminated intravascular coagulation, spontaneous hemorrhage, and renal failure. *Ehrlichia* species do not cause the vasculitis or endothelial damage characteristic of other rickettsial diseases. Anemia, hyponatremia, thrombocytopenia, increased liver transaminase concentrations, and cerebrospinal fluid abnormalities (ie, pleocytosis with a predominance of lymphocytes and increased total protein concentration) are common. Symptoms typically last 1 to 2 weeks, and recovery generally occurs without sequelae; however, reports suggest the occurrence of neurologic complications in some children after severe disease. Fatal infections have been reported. Secondary or opportunistic infections may occur in severe illness, resulting in possible delayed recognition of ehrlichiosis and appropriate antimicrobial treatment. People with underlying immunosuppression are at greater risk of severe disease.

ETIOLOGY: In the United States, human ehrlichioses may be caused by at least 3 distinct species of obligate intracellular bacteria. Human monocytic ehrlichiosis results from infection with *E chaffeensis*. Human granulocytic ehrlichiosis is caused by *A phagocytophila* and *E ewingii*. *Ehrlichia* species are gram-negative cocci that measure 0.5 to 1.5 μm in diameter.

EPIDEMIOLOGY: Most HME infections occur in people from the southeastern and south central United States, but a small number of cases have been described from other areas. Ehrlichial infections caused by *Ehrlichia chaffeensis* and *E ewingii* are associated with the bite of the lone star tick (*Amblyomma americanum*). Cases of HME infection occurring in states beyond the geographic distribution of *A americanum* suggest transmission by additional tick species. Most cases of HGE have been reported in the north central and northeastern United States, particularly Wisconsin, Minnesota, Connecticut, and New York, but cases in many other states, particularly along the West Coast, have been reported. Human granulocytic ehrlichiosis is transmitted by the black-legged or deer tick *(Ixodes scapularis)*, which also is the vector of *Borrelia burgdorferi* (the agent of Lyme disease). Various mammalian reservoirs for the agents of human ehrlichioses have been identified, including white-tailed deer and white-footed mice. In the western United States, *Ixodes pacificus* is the main vector of *Ehrlichia phagocytophila*. Compared with patients with Rocky Mountain spotted fever (see p 532), reported cases of symptomatic ehrlichiosis characteristically are in patients who are older, with age-specific incidences greatest in people older than 40 years of age. However, recent seroprevalence data indicate that infection with *E chaffensis* or a closely related bacterium is common in children. Most human infections occur between April and September, and the peak occurrence is from May through July. The incidence of reported cases seems to be increasing. Coinfections of HGE with other tickborne diseases, including babesiosis and Lyme disease, are recognized.

The **incubation period** of human ehrlichiosis typically is 5 to 10 days after a tick bite or exposure (median, 9 days).

DIAGNOSTIC TESTS: The Centers for Disease Control and Prevention (CDC) defines a confirmed case of ehrlichiosis as isolation of *Ehrlichia* organisms from blood or cerebrospinal fluid, a fourfold or greater change in antibody titer by indirect immunofluorescence antibody (IFA) assay between acute and convalescent serum specimens (ideally collected 3 to 6 weeks apart), polymerase chain reaction assay amplification of ehrlichial DNA from a clinical specimen, or detection of an intraleukocytoplasmic cluster of bacteria (morulae) in conjunction with a single IFA titer of ≥64. A probable case is defined as a single IFA titer of ≥64 or the presence of morulae within infected leukocytes. *Ehrlichia chaffeensis* is used as the antigen for the serologic diagnosis of HME, and *A phagocytophila* is used as the antigen in assays for the diagnosis of HGE. These tests are available in reference laboratories, in some commercial laboratories and state health departments, and at the CDC. Examination of peripheral blood smears to detect morulae in peripheral blood monocytes or granulocytes is insensitive. Use of polymerase chain reaction assay to amplify nucleic acid from acute phase peripheral blood of patients with ehrlichiosis seems sensitive, specific, and promising for early diagnosis.

TREATMENT: Doxycycline is the drug of choice for treatment of human ehrlichioses. The recommended dosage of doxycycline is 4.4 mg/kg per day, every 12 hours intravenously or orally (maximum 100 mg/dose). Ehrlichioses may be severe or fatal in untreated patients, and initiation of therapy early in the course of disease helps minimize complications of illness. Failure to respond to doxycycline within the first 3 days should suggest infection with an agent other than *Ehrlichia* species. Despite concerns regarding dental staining with tetracycline-class antimicrobial agents in young children (see Antimicrobial Agents and Related Therapy, p 693), doxycycline provides superior therapy for this potentially life-threatening disease. Available data suggest that courses of doxycycline ≤14 days do not cause significant discoloration of permanent teeth. Treatment should continue for at least 3 days after defervescence for a minimum total course of 5 to 10 days; unequivocal evidence of clinical improvement generally will be evident by 1 week. Severe or complicated disease may require longer treatment courses.

The clinical manifestations and geographic distributions of ehrlichioses and Rocky Mountain spotted fever overlap. As with other rickettsial diseases, when a presumptive diagnosis of ehrlichiosis is made, doxycycline should be started.

ISOLATION OF THE HOSPITALIZED PATIENT: Standard precautions are recommended.

CONTROL MEASURES: Specific measures focus on limiting exposures to ticks and are similar to those for Rocky Mountain spotted fever and other tickborne diseases (see Prevention of Tickborne Infections, p 186). Prophylactic administration of doxycycline after a tick bite is not indicated because of the low risk of infection.

Enterovirus (Nonpoliovirus) Infections
(Group A and B Coxsackieviruses, Echoviruses, and Enteroviruses)

CLINICAL MANIFESTATIONS: Nonpolio enteroviruses are responsible for significant and frequent illnesses in infants and children and result in protean clinical manifestations. The most common manifestation is nonspecific febrile illness, which, in young infants, may lead to evaluation for bacterial sepsis. Neonates who acquire infection without maternal antibody are at risk of severe disease with a high mortality rate. Manifestations can include the following: (1) respiratory: common cold, pharyngitis, herpangina, stomatitis, pneumonia, and pleurodynia; (2) skin: exanthem; (3) neurologic: aseptic meningitis, encephalitis, and paralysis; (4) gastrointestinal: vomiting, diarrhea, abdominal pain, and hepatitis; (5) eye: acute hemorrhagic conjunctivitis; and (6) heart: myopericarditis. Although each of these findings can be caused by several different enteroviruses, some associations between specific virus and disease particularly are noteworthy. These associations include coxsackievirus A16 and enterovirus 71 with hand-foot-and-mouth syndrome; coxsackievirus A24 variant and enterovirus 70 with acute hemorrhagic conjunctivitis; enterovirus 71 with brainstem encephalitis and polio-like paralysis; echovirus 9 with a petechial exanthem and meningitis; and coxsackieviruses B1 through B5 with pleurodynia and myopericarditis.

Immunocompromised patients with humoral immune deficiencies can have persistent central nervous system infections and/or a dermatomyositis-like syndrome lasting for several months or more.

ETIOLOGY: The nonpolio enteroviruses are RNA viruses, which include 23 group-A coxsackieviruses (types A1–A24, except type A23, which was reclassified as echovirus 9), 6 group-B coxsackieviruses (types B1–B6), 28 echoviruses (types 1–33, except types 8, 10, 22, 23, and 28), and 5 enteroviruses (types 68–71 and 73).

EPIDEMIOLOGY: Enterovirus infections are common and are spread by fecal-oral and respiratory routes and from mother to infant in the peripartum period. Enteroviruses may survive on environmental surfaces for periods long enough to allow transmission from fomites. Infections and clinical attack rates typically are highest in young children, and infections occur more frequently in tropical areas and when hygiene is poor. In temperate climates, enteroviral infections are most common during summer and early fall, but seasonal patterns are less evident in the tropics. Fecal viral shedding can continue for several weeks after onset of infection, but respiratory tract shedding usually is limited to a week or less. Viral shedding can occur without signs of clinical illness.

The usual **incubation period** is 3 to 6 days, except for acute hemorrhagic conjunctivitis, in which the incubation period is 24 to 72 hours.

DIAGNOSTIC TESTS: Specimens providing the highest rate of viral isolation are those obtained from the throat, stool, and rectal swab specimens. Specimens also should be obtained from any other sites of infection, such as cerebrospinal fluid (CSF). Enteroviruses also may be recovered from blood and urine specimens during the acute febrile phase and, rarely, from biopsy specimens. Specimens should be sent to the laboratory at 4°C (39°F). Repeatedly freezing, thawing, and drying specimens is detrimental to viral recovery. In patients with serious illness, viral isolation as a means of diagnosis particularly is important. Virus isolated from any specimen usually can be considered causally related to the patient's illness. Isolation of an enterovirus from stool alone may be less specific than isolation from other sites, because some asymptomatic infected people may shed virus in feces for as long as 6 to 12 weeks. Most viral diagnostic laboratories use cell culture techniques that are capable of recovering echoviruses, group-B coxsackieviruses, and some group-A coxsackieviruses. Suckling mouse inoculation, which is not a routine procedure, is required for recovery of certain group-A coxsackievirus serotypes. Polymerase chain reaction testing for the presence of enterovirus RNA in CSF and other specimens, which is available in a few research laboratories, is more sensitive than viral isolation. Serum specimens for antibody testing can be obtained at the onset of illness and 4 weeks later and stored frozen. The demonstration of an increase in titer of virus-specific neutralizing antibody can be used to confirm infection, particularly when the specific virus has been identified previously during a community outbreak. Serologic screening without a suspected serotype generally is not performed.

TREATMENT: No specific therapy is available, although an antiviral agent, pleconaril, is undergoing clinical evaluation. Pleconaril can be obtained from the manufacturer (ViroPharma Inc, Exton, PA; telephone, 610-458-7300) for compassionate use in children with serious and life-threatening enterovirus infections. Immune Globulin Intravenous (IGIV) containing high antibody titer to the infecting virus may be beneficial for chronic enteroviral meningoencephalitis in immunodeficient patients. Immune Globulin Intravenous also has been used in life-threatening neonatal infections, although there is no evidence of efficacy for this use. Because IGIV preparations vary in the amount of enteroviral antibody, specific manufacturer information should be consulted.

ISOLATION OF THE HOSPITALIZED PATIENT: In addition to standard precautions, contact precautions are indicated for infants and young children for the duration of hospitalization.

CONTROL MEASURES: Particular attention should be given to hand hygiene, especially after diaper changing.

Epstein-Barr Virus Infections
(Infectious Mononucleosis)

CLINICAL MANIFESTATIONS: Infectious mononucleosis manifests typically as fever, exudative pharyngitis, lymphadenopathy, hepatosplenomegaly, and atypical lymphocytosis. The spectrum of diseases is wide, ranging from asymptomatic to fatal infection. Infections commonly are unrecognized in infants and young children. Rash can occur and is more common in patients treated with ampicillin as well as with other penicillins. Central nervous system (CNS) complications include aseptic meningitis, encephalitis, and Guillain-Barré syndrome. Rare complications include splenic rupture, thrombocytopenia, agranulocytosis, hemolytic anemia, hemophagocytic syndrome, orchitis, and myocarditis. Replication of Epstein-Barr virus (EBV) in B lymphocytes and the resulting lymphoproliferation usually is inhibited by natural killer- and T-cell responses. In patients who have congenital or acquired cellular immune deficiencies, fatal disseminated infection or B-cell lymphomas can occur.

Epstein-Barr virus causes several other distinct disorders, including X-linked lymphoproliferative syndrome, post-transplantation lymphoproliferative disorders, Burkitt lymphoma, nasopharyngeal carcinoma, and undifferentiated B-cell lymphomas of the CNS. X-linked lymphoproliferative syndrome occurs in people with an inherited, maternally derived, recessive genetic defect characterized by several phenotypic expressions, including occurrence of infectious mononucleosis early in life among boys, nodular B-cell lymphomas often with CNS involvement, and profound hypogammaglobulinemia.

Epstein-Barr virus-associated lymphoproliferative disorders result in a number of complex syndromes in patients who are immunocompromised, such as transplant recipients or people infected with human immunodeficiency virus (HIV). The highest incidence of these disorders occurs in liver and heart transplant recipients. Other EBV syndromes are of greater importance outside the United States, including Burkitt lymphoma (a B-cell tumor), found primarily in Central Africa, and nasopharyngeal carcinoma, found in Southeast Asia.

Chronic fatigue syndrome is not related specifically to EBV infection. A small group of patients with recurring or persistent symptoms have abnormal serologic test results for EBV, as well as for other viruses.

ETIOLOGY: Epstein-Barr virus, a B-lymphotropic herpesvirus, is the most common cause of infectious mononucleosis.

EPIDEMIOLOGY: Humans are the only source of EBV. Close personal contact usually is required for transmission. The virus is viable in saliva for several hours outside the body, but the role of fomites in transmission is unknown. Epstein-Barr virus also is transmitted occasionally by blood transfusion. Infection commonly is contracted early in life, particularly among members of lower socioeconomic groups, in which intrafamilial spread is common. Endemic infectious mononucleosis is common in group settings of adolescents, such as in educational institutions. No seasonal pattern has been documented. Respiratory tract viral excretion can occur for many months after infection, and asymptomatic carriage is common. Intermittent excretion is lifelong. The period of communicability is indeterminate.

The **incubation period** of infectious mononucleosis is estimated to be 30 to 50 days.

DIAGNOSTIC TESTS: Isolation of EBV from oropharyngeal secretions is possible, but techniques for performing this procedure usually are not available in routine diagnostic laboratories, and viral isolation does not necessarily indicate acute infection. Hence, diagnosis depends on serologic testing. Nonspecific tests for heterophil antibody, including the Paul-Bunnell test and slide agglutination reaction test, are available most commonly. The heterophil antibody principally is immunoglobulin (Ig) M, appears during the first 2 weeks of illness, and gradually disappears over a 6-month period. The results of heterophil antibody tests often are negative in children younger than 4 years of age with EBV infection, but they identify approximately 90% of cases (proven by EBV-specific serologic testing) in older children and adults. An absolute increase in atypical lymphocytes during the second week of illness with infectious mononucleosis is a characteristic but nonspecific finding. However, the finding of >10% atypical lymphocytes together with a positive heterophil antibody test result is considered diagnostic of acute infection.

Multiple specific serologic antibody tests for EBV infection are available in diagnostic virology laboratories (see Table 3.5, p 273). The most commonly performed test is for antibody against the viral capsid antigen (VCA). Because IgG antibody against VCA occurs in high titers early after onset of infection, testing of acute and convalescent serum specimens for anti-VCA may not be useful for establishing the presence of infection. Testing for IgM anti-VCA antibody and for antibodies against early antigen is useful for identifying recent infections. Because serum antibody against EBV nuclear antigen (EBNA) is not present until several weeks to months after onset of infection, a positive anti-EBNA antibody test excludes primary infection.

Serologic tests for EBV particularly are useful for evaluating patients who have heterophil-negative infectious mononucleosis. Testing for other viral agents, especially cytomegalovirus, also may be indicated for these patients. In research -studies, culture of saliva specimens or peripheral blood mononuclear cells for EBV, in situ DNA hybridization, or polymerase chain reaction assay can determine the presence of EBV or EBV DNA and may implicate EBV in a syndrome, such as lymphoproliferation.

TREATMENT: Contact sports should be avoided until the patient is recovered fully from infectious mononucleosis and the spleen no longer is palpable. Patients suspected to have infectious mononucleosis should not be given ampicillin or amoxicillin, which cause nonallergic morbilliform rashes in a high proportion of patients with mononucleosis. Although therapy with short-course corticosteroids may have a beneficial effect on acute symptoms, because of potential adverse effects, their use should be considered only for patients with complications such as marked tonsillar inflammation with impending airway obstruction, massive splenomegaly, myocarditis, hemolytic anemia, or hemophagocytic syndrome. The dosage of prednisone usually is 1 mg/kg per day, orally (maximum 20 mg if >10 kg), for 7 days with subsequent tapering. Although acyclovir has in vitro antiviral activity against EBV, therapy is of no proven value in EBV lymphoproliferative syndromes. Decreasing

Table 3.5 **Serum Epstein-Barr Virus (EBV) Antibodies in EBV Infection**

Infection	VCA IgG	VCA IgM	EA (D)	EBNA
No previous infection	–	–	–	–
Acute infection	+	+	+/–	–
Recent infection	+	+/–	+/–	+/–
Past infection	+	–	–	+

VCA IgG indicates immunoglobulin (Ig) G class antibody to viral capsid antigen; VCA IgM, IgM class antibody to VCA; EA (D), early antigen diffuse staining; and EBNA, EBV nuclear antigen.

immunosuppressive therapy is beneficial for patients with EBV-induced lympho-proliferation, such as the post-transplant lymphoproliferative disorders.

ISOLATION OF THE HOSPITALIZED PATIENT: Standard precautions are recommended.

CONTROL MEASURES: Patients with a recent history of EBV infection or an illness similar to infectious mononucleosis should not donate blood.

Escherichia coli and Other Gram-Negative Bacilli
(Septicemia and Meningitis in Neonates)

CLINICAL MANIFESTATIONS: Neonatal septicemia or meningitis caused by *Escherichia coli* and other gram-negative bacilli cannot be differentiated clinically from serious infections caused by other infectious agents. The first signs of sepsis may be subtle and similar to those observed in noninfectious processes. Clinical signs of septicemia include fever, temperature instability, grunting respirations, apnea, cyanosis, lethargy, irritability, anorexia, vomiting, jaundice, hepatomegaly, abdominal distention, and diarrhea. Meningitis may occur without overt signs suggesting central nervous system involvement. Some gram-negative bacilli, such as *Citrobacter koseri, Enterobacter sakazakii,* and *Serratia marcescens,* are associated with brain abscesses in infants with meningitis caused by these organisms.

ETIOLOGY: *Escherichia coli* strains with the K1 capsular polysaccharide antigen cause approximately 40% of cases of septicemia and 80% of cases of meningitis caused by *E coli.* Other important gram-negative bacilli causing neonatal septicemia include non-K1 strains of *E coli, Klebsiella, Enterobacter, Proteus, Citrobacter, Salmonella, Pseudomonas,* and *Serratia* species. Nonencapsulated strains of *Haemophilus influenzae; Streptococcus pneumoniae;* group A, C, or G streptococci; *Neisseria meningitidis;* and anaerobic gram-negative bacilli are rare causes.

EPIDEMIOLOGY: The source of *E coli* and other gram-negative bacterial pathogens in neonatal infections usually is the maternal genital tract. In addition, nosocomial acquisition of gram-negative organisms through person-to-person transmission among nursery personnel and from nursery environmental sites, such as sinks, multiple-use solutions, and countertops, has been documented, especially in preterm infants who require prolonged intensive care management. Predisposing factors in neonatal gram-negative bacterial infections include maternal intrapartum infections, gestation <37 weeks, low birth weight, prolonged rupture of membranes, and traumatic delivery. Metabolic abnormalities, such as galactosemia, fetal hypoxia, and acidosis also have been implicated as predisposing factors. Neonates with defects in the integrity of skin or mucosa (eg, myelomeningocele) are at increased risk of gram-negative bacterial infections. In intensive care nurseries, sophisticated systems for respiratory and metabolic support, invasive or surgical procedures, indwelling vascular lines, and the frequent use of antimicrobial agents enable selection and proliferation of strains of pathogenic gram-negative bacilli that are resistant to multiple antimicrobial agents.

The **incubation period** is highly variable; time of onset of infection ranges from birth to several weeks after birth or longer in very low birth weight, preterm infants.

DIAGNOSTIC TESTS: The diagnosis is established by growth of *E coli* or other gram-negative bacilli from blood, cerebrospinal fluid, or otherwise sterile sites.

TREATMENT:
- Initial empiric treatment for suspected bacterial septicemia or meningitis in neonates is ampicillin and an aminoglycoside. An alternative regimen of ampicillin and an expanded-spectrum cephalosporin (such as cefotaxime) can be used, but rapid emergence of cephalosporin-resistant strains, especially *Enterobacter cloacae* and *Klebsiella* and *Serratia* species, can occur when use is routine. Hence, routine use of an expanded-spectrum cephalosporin is not recommended unless gram-negative bacterial meningitis is strongly suspected.
- Once the causative agent and its in vitro antimicrobial susceptibility pattern is known, nonmeningeal infections should be treated with ampicillin, an appropriate aminoglycoside, or an expanded-spectrum cephalosporin (such as cefotaxime). Many experts would treat nonmeningeal infections caused by *Enterobacter, Serratia,* or *Pseudomonas* species and some other less commonly occurring gram-negative bacilli with a β-lactam antimicrobial agent and an aminoglycoside. Meningitis usually is treated with ampicillin or an expanded-spectrum cephalosporin in combination with an aminoglycoside. Expert advice from an infectious disease specialist can be helpful for management of meningitis.
- Duration of therapy is based on the patient's clinical and bacteriologic response and the site(s) of infection; the usual duration of therapy for uncomplicated septicemia is 10 to 14 days, and for meningitis, the minimum duration is 21 days.
- A therapeutic role for Immune Globulin or other adjunctive therapies in septicemia or meningitis caused by *E coli* or other gram-negative organisms has not been established.
- All infants with meningitis should undergo careful follow-up examinations, including testing for hearing loss and neurologic abnormalities.

ISOLATION OF THE HOSPITALIZED PATIENT: Standard precautions are recommended. Exceptions include nursery epidemics, infants with *Salmonella* infection, and infants with infection caused by gram-negative bacilli that are resistant to multiple antimicrobial agents; in these situations, contact precautions in addition to standard precautions are indicated.

CONTROL MEASURES: The physician director of the nursery and infection control personnel should be aware of pathogens causing infections in infants and nursery personnel so that clusters of infections are recognized and investigated appropriately. Several cases of infection caused by the same genus and species of bacteria occurring in infants in physical proximity or caused by an unusual pathogen indicate the need for an epidemiologic investigation (see Infection Control for Hospitalized Children, p 146). Periodic review of the in vitro antimicrobial susceptibility patterns of clinically important bacterial isolates from newborn infants, especially infants in the intensive care nursery, can provide useful epidemiologic and therapeutic information.

Escherichia coli Diarrhea
(Including Hemolytic-Uremic Syndrome)

CLINICAL MANIFESTATIONS: At least 5 pathotypes of diarrhea-producing *Escherichia coli* strains have been identified. Clinical features of disease caused by each pathotype are summarized as follows (see also Table 3.6, p 276):

- Shiga toxin-producing *E coli* (STEC), formerly known as enterohemorrhagic *E coli* or verotoxin-producing *E coli,* strains are associated with diarrhea, hemorrhagic colitis, hemolytic-uremic syndrome (HUS), and postdiarrheal thrombotic thrombocytopenic purpura (TTP). Shiga toxin-producing *E coli* O157:H7 is the prototype and the most virulent member of this *E coli* pathotype. Illness caused by STEC often begins as nonbloody diarrhea but usually progresses to diarrhea with visible or occult blood. Severe abdominal pain is typical; fever occurs in fewer than one third of cases. Severe infection may result in hemorrhagic colitis.
- Diarrhea caused by enteropathogenic *E coli* (EPEC) is watery and often is severe enough to result in dehydration. Severe EPEC diarrhea is characteristically persistent and leads to growth retardation. Illness occurs almost exclusively in neonates and children younger than 2 years of age and predominantly (but not exclusively) in resource-limited countries, either sporadically or in epidemics.
- Diarrhea caused by enterotoxigenic *E coli* (ETEC) is a brief (1–5 days) self-limited illness of moderate severity with watery stools and abdominal cramps.
- Diarrhea caused by enteroinvasive *E coli* (EIEC) is similar clinically to infection caused by *Shigella* species. Although dysentery can occur, diarrhea usually is watery without blood or mucus. Patients often are febrile, and stools may contain leukocytes.

Table 3.6. Classification of *Escherichia coli* Associated With Diarrhea

E coli Pathotype	Epidemiology	Type of Diarrhea	Mechanism of Pathogenesis
Shiga toxin-producing (STEC)	Hemorrhagic colitis and hemolytic uremic syndrome in all ages and postdiarrheal thrombotic thrombocytopenic purpura in adults	Bloody or nonbloody	Adherence and effacement, cytotoxin production
Enteropathogenic (EPEC)	Acute and chronic endemic and epidemic diarrhea in infants	Watery	Adherence, effacement
Enterotoxigenic (ETEC)	Infantile diarrhea in resource-limited countries and traveler's diarrhea in all ages	Watery	Adherence, enterotoxin production
Enteroinvasive (EIEC)	Diarrhea with fever in all ages	Bloody or nonbloody; dysentery	Adherence, mucosal invasion and inflammation
Enteroaggregative (EAEC)	Acute and chronic diarrhea in infants	Watery, occasionally bloody	Adherence, mucosal damage

- Enteroaggregative *E coli* (EAEC) causes watery diarrhea, predominantly in infants and young children in resource-limited countries, but all ages can be affected. Enteroaggregative *E coli* has been associated with prolonged diarrhea (>14 days). Asymptomatic infection may be accompanied by a subclinical inflammatory enteritis, which may cause growth disturbances.

Late Sequelae of STEC Infection. Hemolytic-uremic syndrome is a serious sequela of STEC enteric infection, especially with *E coli* O157:H7. Hemolytic-uremic syndrome is defined by the triad of microangiopathic hemolytic anemia, thrombocytopenia, and acute renal dysfunction. In many children with diarrhea caused by *E coli* O157:H7, mild, self-limited, microangiopathic hematologic changes; thrombocytopenia; and/or nephropathy develop during the 2 weeks after onset of diarrhea. Thrombocytopenic purpura occurs in adults, may follow STEC infection, includes central nervous system involvement and fever, may have a more gradual onset than HUS, and is part of a disease spectrum often designated as TTP-HUS. Although most cases of childhood HUS in the United States are caused by *E coli* O157:H7, most cases of TTP in adults are of unknown cause.

ETIOLOGY: Each *E coli* pathotype has specific virulence characteristics, some of which are encoded on pathotype-specific plasmids. Each pathotype has a distinct set of somatic (O) and flagellar (H) antigens. Pathogenetic characteristics are as follows:
- Illness caused by *E coli* O157:H7 occurs in a 2-step process. The intestinal phase is characterized by formation of the so-called attaching and effacing lesion, resulting in secretory diarrhea. This phase is followed by elaboration

of Shiga toxin, a potent cytotoxin also found in *Shigella dysenteriae* 1. The action of Shiga toxin on intestinal cells results in hemorrhagic colitis, and absorption of the toxin in the circulation results in systemic complications including HUS and neurologic sequelae.

- Strains of EPEC adhere to the small bowel mucosa and, like *E coli* O157:H7, produce attaching and effacing lesions. Strains of EPEC historically were defined as members of specific *E coli* serotypes that were incriminated epidemiologically as causes of infantile-diarrhea; now a more precise pathogenic definition includes the capacity to form the attaching and effacing lesions in the absence of Shiga toxin production.
- Strains of ETEC colonize the small intestine without invading and produce heat-labile enterotoxin, heat-stable enterotoxin, or both. Heat-stable enterotoxin-producing strains are responsible for most human illness.
- Enteroinvasive *E coli*, like *Shigella* species, typically are lactose nonfermenting and invade the colonic mucosa, where they spread laterally and induce a local inflammatory response.
- Enteroaggregative *E coli* are defined by their characteristic "stacked brick" adherence pattern in cell culture-based assays. These organisms elaborate one or more enterotoxins and elicit damage to the intestinal mucosa.

EPIDEMIOLOGY: Transmission of most diarrhea-associated *E coli* strains is from infected symptomatic people or carriers or from food or water contaminated with human or animal feces. The only *E coli* pathotype that commonly causes diarrhea in children living in the United States is STEC, including *E coli* O157:H7, which is shed in feces of cattle and, to a lesser extent, of sheep, deer, and other ruminants and is transmitted by undercooked ground beef, unpasteurized milk, and a wide variety of vehicles contaminated with bovine feces. Infections caused by *E coli* O157:H7 are increasingly common in the United States and can occur sporadically or during outbreaks. Outbreaks have been linked to contaminated apple cider, raw vegetables, salami, yogurt, drinking water, and ingestion of water in recreational areas. The infectious dose is low (approximately 100 organisms), and person-to-person transmission is common during outbreaks. The frequency of HUS as a complication of *E coli* O157:H7 infection in children has been estimated to be 5% to 10% but can be higher during outbreaks. Diarrhea and sometimes HUS caused by STEC strains other than O157:H7 are common outside the United States.

Non-STEC pathotypes are associated with disease predominantly in resource-limited countries, where food and water supplies commonly are contaminated and facilities and supplies for hand hygiene are suboptimal. Epidemic EPEC disease in newborn nurseries now is uncommon, but EPEC and *E coli* O157:H7 have caused numerous outbreaks of diarrhea in child care centers. Diarrhea attributable to ETEC occurs in people of all ages but is especially important in infants. Outbreaks have occurred in adults, usually from ingestion of contaminated food or water. Enterotoxigenic *E coli* is the major cause of traveler's diarrhea. Outbreaks of infection attributable to EIEC and EAEC have occurred, usually secondary to contaminated food, among people of all ages in resource-rich countries. The period of communicability is for the duration of excretion of the specific pathogen.

The **incubation period** for most *E coli* strains is 10 hours to 6 days; for *E coli* O157:H7, the incubation period usually is 3 to 4 days but ranges from 1 to 8 days.

DIAGNOSTIC TESTS: Diagnosis of infection caused by diarrhea-associated *E coli* usually is difficult, because most clinical laboratories cannot differentiate diarrhea-associated *E coli* strains from stool flora *E coli* strains. The exceptions are *E coli* O157:H7 and EIEC, which can be identified presumptively or specifically. For definitive identification, isolates suspected to be associated with diarrhea should be sent to reference or research laboratories.

Clinical laboratories can screen for *E coli* O157:H7 by using MacConkey agar base with sorbitol substituted for lactose. Approximately 90% of human intestinal *E coli* strains rapidly ferment sorbitol, whereas *E coli* O157:H7 strains do not. Sorbitol-negative *E coli* then can be serotyped, using commercially available antisera, to determine whether they are O157:H7. If a case or outbreak attributable to diarrhea-associated *E coli* other than O157:H7 is suspected, *E coli* isolates should be sent to the state health laboratory or another reference laboratory for serotyping and identification of pathotypes. Several sensitive, specific, and rapid immunologic assays for detection of Shiga toxin are available commercially.

Strains of STEC should be sought for patients with bloody diarrhea (indicated by history, inspection of stool, or guaiac), HUS, and postdiarrheal TTP as well as contacts of patients with HUS who have any type of diarrhea. People with presumptive diagnoses of intussusception, inflammatory bowel disease, or ischemic colitis sometimes have disease caused by *E coli* O157:H7. Methods of definitive identification of STEC that are used in reference or research laboratories include DNA probes, polymerase chain reaction assay, enzyme immunoassay, and phenotypic testing of strains or stool specimens for Shiga toxin. Serologic diagnosis using enzyme immunoassay to detect serum antibodies to *E coli* O157:H7 lipopolysaccharide is available in reference laboratories.

Hemolytic-Uremic Syndrome. For all patients with HUS, stool specimens should be cultured for *E coli* O157:H7 and, if results are negative, for other STEC serotypes. However, the absence of STEC in feces does not preclude the diagnosis of STEC-associated HUS, because HUS typically is diagnosed a week or more after onset of diarrhea, when the organism no longer may be detectable. When STEC infection is considered, a stool culture should be obtained as early in the illness as possible.

TREATMENT: Dehydration and electrolyte abnormalities should be corrected. Orally administered solutions usually are adequate.* Antimotility agents should not be administered to children with inflammatory or bloody diarrhea. Careful follow-up of patients with hemorrhagic colitis (including complete blood cell count with smear, blood urea nitrogen concentration, and creatinine concentration) is recommended to detect changes suggestive of HUS. If patients have no laboratory evidence of hemolysis, thrombocytopenia, or nephropathy 3 days after resolution of diarrhea, their risk of developing HUS is low.

---

* For further information and detailed recommendations, see American Academy of Pediatrics, Provisional Committee on Quality Improvement, Subcommittee on Gastroenteritis. Practice parameter: the management of acute gastroenteritis in young children. *Pediatrics.* 1996;97:424–435

Antimicrobial Therapy. Although some studies have suggested that children with hemorrhagic colitis caused by STEC have a greater risk of developing HUS if treated with antimicrobial agents when compared with children not treated with antimicrobial agents, a meta-analysis failed to confirm this increased risk or to show a benefit. A randomized trial with adequate power is needed to determine the risks and benefits of antimicrobial therapy for children with *E coli* O157:H7 enteritis. However, until results of such a trial are available, most experts would not treat children with *E coli* O157:H7 enteritis with an antimicrobial agent. If severe watery ETEC diarrhea is suspected in a traveler to a resource-limited country, therapy may be provided. The optimal therapy for ETEC is not established, and resistance to antimicrobial agents is common. Trimethoprim-sulfamethoxazole, azithromycin dihydrate, or ciprofloxacin, which is not licensed for use in people younger than 18 years of age, should be considered if diarrhea is severe or intractable and if the organism is susceptible. If systemic infection is suspected in diarrhea patients, parenteral antimicrobial therapy should be given. For dysentery caused by EIEC strains, antimicrobial agents, such as trimethoprim-sulfamethoxazole, azithromycin, or ciprofloxacin, can be given orally. Whenever possible, antimicrobial selection should be based on susceptibility testing of the isolates.

ISOLATION OF THE HOSPITALIZED PATIENT: In addition to standard precautions, contact precautions are indicated for patients with all types of *E coli* diarrhea for the duration of illness. During outbreaks, contact precautions for infants with diarrhea caused by EPEC strains should be maintained until cultures of stool taken after cessation of antimicrobial therapy are negative for the infecting strain. For patients with HUS or hemorrhagic colitis attributable to STEC, contact precautions should be continued until diarrhea resolves and results of 2 consecutive stool cultures are negative for *E coli* O157:H7.

CONTROL MEASURES:

Escherichia coli O157:H7 Infection. All ground beef should be cooked thoroughly until no pink meat remains and the juices are clear. Raw milk should not be ingested, and only pasteurized apple juice products should be consumed.

Outbreaks in Child Care Centers. If an outbreak of HUS or diarrhea attributable to *E coli* O157:H7 occurs in a child care center, immediate involvement of public health authorities is critical. Infection caused by *E coli* O157:H7 is reportable, and rapid reporting of cases can lead to intervention to prevent further disease. Ill children should not be permitted to reenter the child care center until diarrhea has resolved and results of 2 stool cultures are negative for *E coli* O157:H7. Strict attention to hand hygiene is important but may be insufficient to prevent continued transmission. A child care center should be closed to new admissions, and care should be exercised to prevent transfer of exposed children to other centers.

Nursery and Other Institutional Outbreaks. Strict attention to hand hygiene is essential for limiting spread. Exposed patients should be observed closely, their stools should be cultured for the causative organism, and they should be separated from unexposed infants. In a newborn nursery, EPEC infection is considered a serious hazard, and strict enteric precautions should be maintained.

Traveler's Diarrhea. Traveler's diarrhea has been associated with many entero-pathogens (including ETEC, EAEC, and EIEC), usually is acquired by ingestion of contaminated food or water, and is a significant problem for people traveling in resource-limited countries. Diarrhea attributable to STEC is rare in travelers. Travelers should be advised to drink only bottled or canned beverages and boiled or bottled water; they should avoid ice, salads, and fruit that they have not peeled themselves. Foods should be eaten hot. Antimicrobial agents usually are not recommended for prevention of traveler's diarrhea in children. Although several antimicrobial agents, such as trimethoprim-sulfamethoxazole, doxycycline, and ciprofloxacin, are effective in decreasing the incidence of traveler's diarrhea, the benefit usually is outweighed by the potential risks, including allergic drug reactions, antimicrobial-associated colitis, and the selective pressure of widespread use of antimicrobial agents leading to antimicrobial resistance. If diarrhea occurs, packets of oral rehydration salts can be constituted and ingested to help maintain fluid balance. If diarrhea in a traveler is moderate or severe or is associated with fever or bloody stools, empiric antimicrobial therapy may be indicated until symptoms resolve; empiric therapy should be continued for no more than 3 days.

Fungal Diseases

In addition to the mycoses listed by individual agents in Section 3, infants and children can have infections caused by uncommonly encountered fungi. Infections caused by these additional agents usually occur in children with immunosuppression or other underlying conditions predisposing them to invasive fungal infection. Children who are immunocompetent can acquire infection with these fungi through inhalation via the respiratory tract or direct inoculation after traumatic disruption of cutaneous barriers. A list of these fungal agents and the pertinent underlying host conditions, reservoir or route of entry, clinical manifestations, diagnostic laboratory tests, and treatment for each can be found in Table 3.7 (p 281). Taken as a group, few fungal susceptibility data are available on which to base treatment recommendations for these infections, especially in children. Consultation with a pediatric infectious disease specialist should be considered when caring for a child infected with one of these mycoses.

Table 3.7. Additional Fungal Diseases

Disease and Agent	Underlying Host Condition(s)	Reservoir(s) or Route(s) of Entry	Common Clinical Manifestations	Diagnostic Laboratory Test(s)	Treatment
Hyalohyphomycosis					
Fusarium species	Granulocytopenia; bone marrow transplantation	Respiratory tract; sinuses; skin	Pulmonary infiltrates; cutaneous lesions; sinusitis; disseminated infection	Culture of blood or tissue specimen	High-dose amphotericin B (AmB) deoxycholate (1–1.5 mg/kg per day)[1,2]
Malassezia species	Immunosuppression; prematurity; exposure to parenteral nutrition that includes fat emulsions	Skin	Catheter-associated bloodstream infection; interstitial pneumonitis; urinary tract infection; meningitis	Culture of blood, catheter tip, or tissue specimen	Removal of catheters and temporary cessation of lipid infusions; fluconazole or AmB
Penicilliosis					
Penicillium marneffei	Human immunodeficiency virus infection	Respiratory tract	Pneumonitis; invasive dermatitis; disseminated infection	Culture of blood, bone marrow or tissue; histopathologic examination of tissue	Itraconazole or AmB
Phaeohyphomycosis					
Bipolaris species	None or immunosuppression	Environment	Sinusitis; disseminated infection	Culture and histopathologic examination of tissue	Itraconazole or AmB; surgical excision
Curvularia species	Immunosuppression; altered skin integrity; asthma or nasal polyps; chronic sinusitis	Environment	Allergic fungal sinusitis; invasive dermatitis; disseminated infection	Culture and histopathologic examination of tissue	Allergic fungal sinusitis: surgery and corticosteroids Invasive disease: itraconazole[3] or AmB
Exserohilum species	None or immunosuppression	Environment	Sinusitis; cutaneous lesions; disseminated infection	Culture and histopathologic examination of tissue	Itraconazole[3] or AmB; surgical excision

Table 3.7. Additional Fungal Diseases, continued

Disease and Agent	Underlying Host Condition(s)	Reservoir(s) or Route(s) of Entry	Common Clinical Manifestations	Diagnostic Laboratory Test(s)	Treatment
Phaeohyphomycosis, continued					
Pseudallescheria boydii	None or immunosuppression	Environment	Pneumonia; disseminated infection; mycetoma (immunocompetent patients); endocarditis	Culture and histopathologic examination of tissue	Itraconazole[4]; surgical excision for pulmonary infection, as feasible
Scedosporium species	None or immunosuppression	Environment	Pneumonia; disseminated infection; osteomyelitis or septic arthritis (immunocompetent patients)	Culture and histo pathologic examination of tissue	Itraconazole[3] or AmB
Trichosporonosis					
Trichosporon beigelii	Immunosuppression	Normal flora of gastrointestinal tract	Bloodstream infection; endocarditis; pneumonitis	Blood culture; histopathologic examination of tissue	AmB or fluconazole
Zygomycosis					
Rhizopus; Mucor; Absidia; Rhizomucor species	Immunosuppression; hematologic malignant neoplasm; renal failure; diabetes mellitus; use of nonsterile adhesive dressings	Respiratory tract; skin	Rhinocerebral infection; pulmonary infection; disseminated infection; skin and gastrointestinal tract less commonly	Histopathologic examination of tissue and culture	High dose of AmB (1.5 mg/kg per day)[1] and surgical excision, as feasible

1 Consider use of a lipid formulation of amphotericin B (AmB).

2 Infection may be refractory to AmB; use of investigational antifungal compounds may be required.

3 Itraconazole is the treatment of choice, but data on use in children are limited.

4 Immunocompromised patients may fail to respond. AmB has activity against some strains. Enhanced fungal activity may be observed when AmB is combined with itraconazole or fluconazole.

Giardia lamblia Infections
(Giardiasis)

CLINICAL MANIFESTATIONS: Symptomatic infection causes a broad spectrum of clinical manifestations. Children can have occasional days of acute watery diarrhea with abdominal pain, or they may experience a protracted, intermittent, often debilitating disease, which is characterized by passage of foul-smelling stools associated with flatulence, abdominal distention, and anorexia. Anorexia combined with malabsorption can lead to significant weight loss, failure to thrive, and anemia. Asymptomatic infection is common.

ETIOLOGY: *Giardia lamblia* is a flagellate protozoan that exists in trophozoite and cyst forms; the infective form is the cyst. Infection is limited to the small intestine and biliary tract.

EPIDEMIOLOGY: Giardiasis has a worldwide distribution. Humans are the principal reservoir of infection, but *Giardia* organisms can infect dogs, cats, beavers, and other animals. These animals can contaminate water with feces containing cysts that are infectious for humans. People become infected directly (by hand-to-mouth transfer of cysts from feces of an infected person) or indirectly (by ingestion of fecally contaminated water or food). Many people who become infected with *G lamblia* remain asymptomatic. Most community-wide epidemics have resulted from a contaminated water supply. Epidemics resulting from person-to-person transmission occur in child care centers and in institutions for people with developmental disabilities. Staff and family members in contact with people in these settings occasionally become infected. Humoral immunodeficiencies predispose to chronic symptomatic *G lamblia* infections. Surveys conducted in the United States have demonstrated prevalence rates of *Giardia* organisms in stool specimens that range from 1% to 20%, depending on geographic location and age. Duration of cyst excretion is variable and may be months. The disease is communicable for as long as the infected person excretes cysts.

The **incubation period** usually is 1 to 4 weeks.

DIAGNOSTIC TESTS: Identification of trophozoites or cysts in direct smear examination or immunofluorescence antibody testing of stool specimens or duodenal fluid is diagnostic. Stool usually is collected and preserved in neutral-buffered 10% formalin, but other preservatives can be used, or fresh stool can be examined. A single direct smear examination of stool has a sensitivity of 75% to 95%. Sensitivity is higher for diarrheal stool specimens, because these contain a higher concentration of organisms. Sensitivity is increased by examining 3 or more specimens collected every other day. To enhance detection, microscopic examination of stool specimens or duodenal fluid should be performed soon after collection, or stool should be placed in fixative, concentrated, and examined by wet mount using permanent stain such as trichrome. Commercially available stool collection kits containing a vial of neutral-buffered 10% formalin and a vial of polyvinyl alcohol fixative in childproof containers are convenient for preserving stool specimens collected at home. When giardiasis is suspected clinically, but the organism is not found on repeated stool examination, examination of duodenal contents obtained by direct aspiration or by using a commercially available string test (Enterotest, HDC Corporation, San Jose, CA) may be diagnostic. Rarely, duodenal biopsy is required for diagnosis. Several enzyme immunoassay kits also are available commercially, but because of recurring problems with false-positive and false-negative results, enzyme immunoassay results for *Giardia* species should be interpreted with caution. The direct fluorescent antibody test kit (Meridian Diagnostics, Dallas, TX) has the advantage that the organisms are visualized, providing a greater level of confidence in a positive diagnosis than with enzyme immunoassay.

TREATMENT: Dehydration and electrolyte abnormalities should be corrected. Metronidazole is the drug of choice; a 5- to 7-day course of therapy has a cure rate of 80% to 95%. Tinidazole, a nitroimidazole, has a cure rate of 90% to 100% after a single dose, but limited safety and efficacy data are available in children; this drug is not available in the United States. Furazolidone is 72% to 100% effective when given for 7 to 10 days and is available in a liquid form for pediatric use. Albendazole has been shown to be as effective as metronidazole for treating giardiasis in children, and it has fewer adverse effects. A 3-day course of nitazoxanide oral suspension has been licensed by the Food and Drug Administration for treatment of children with diarrhea attributable to *G lamblia* and *Cryptosporidium parvum*. Paromomycin, a nonabsorbable aminoglycoside that is 50% to 70% effective, is recommended for treatment of symptomatic infection in pregnant women.

If therapy fails, a course can be repeated with the same drug. Relapse is common in immunocompromised patients, who may require prolonged treatment. Some experts recommend combination therapy for giardiasis in immunocompromised patients who are unresponsive to courses of 2 drugs used separately.

Treatment of asymptomatic carriers generally is not recommended. Possible exceptions to prevent transmission are carriers in households of patients with hypogammaglobulinemia or cystic fibrosis and pregnant women with toddlers.

ISOLATION OF THE HOSPITALIZED PATIENT: In addition to standard precautions, contact precautions for the duration of illness are recommended for diapered and incontinent children.

CONTROL MEASURES:
- In child care centers, improved sanitation and personal hygiene should be emphasized (see also Children in Out-of-Home Child Care, p 123). Hand hygiene by staff and children should be emphasized, especially after toilet use or handling of soiled diapers. When an outbreak is suspected, the local health department should be contacted, and an epidemiologic investigation should be undertaken to identify and treat all symptomatic children, child care workers, and family members infected with *G lamblia*. People with diarrhea should be excluded from the child care center until they become asymptomatic. Treatment of asymptomatic carriers is not effective for outbreak control. Exclusion of carriers from child care is not recommended.
- Waterborne outbreaks can be prevented by the combination of adequate filtration of water from surface water sources (eg, lakes, rivers, streams), chlorination, and maintenance of water distribution systems.

- Backpackers, campers, and people likely to be exposed to contaminated water should avoid drinking directly from streams. Boiling of water will kill the infective cysts and other waterborne pathogens.

Gonococcal Infections

CLINICAL MANIFESTATIONS: Gonococcal infections in children occur in 3 distinct age groups.
- Infection in the **newborn infant** usually involves the eyes. Other sites of infection include scalp abscess (which can be associated with fetal monitoring), vaginitis, and disseminated disease with bacteremia, arthritis, or meningitis.
- In children beyond the newborn period, including **prepubertal children,** gonococcal infection may occur in the genital tract and almost always is sexually transmitted. Rarely, nonsexual transmission from household contact can occur. Vaginitis is the most common manifestation; pelvic inflammatory disease (PID) and perihepatitis can occur but are rare. Gonococcal urethritis in the prepubertal male is uncommon. Anorectal and tonsillopharyngeal infection also can occur in prepubertal children.
- In **sexually active adolescents,** as in adults, gonococcal infection of the genital tract in females often is asymptomatic, and common clinical syndromes are urethritis, endocervicitis, and salpingitis. In males, infection usually is symptomatic, and the primary site is the urethra. Infection of the rectum and pharynx can occur alone or with genitourinary tract infection in either sex. Rectal and pharyngeal infections often are asymptomatic. Extension from primary genital mucosal sites can lead to epididymitis, bartholinitis, PID, and perihepatitis (Fitz-Hugh-Curtis syndrome). Even asymptomatic infection can progress to PID, with tubal scarring that can result in ectopic pregnancy or infertility. Infection involving other mucous membranes can produce conjunctivitis, pharyngitis, or proctitis. Hematogenous spread can involve skin and joints (arthritis-dermatitis syndrome) and occurs in up to 3% of untreated people with mucosal gonorrhea. Bacteremia causes a maculopapular rash with necrosis, tenosynovitis, and migratory arthritis. Arthritis may be reactive (sterile) or septic in nature. Meningitis and endocarditis occur rarely. Dissemination is more common in females infected within 1 week of menstruation.

ETIOLOGY: *Neisseria gonorrhoeae* is a gram-negative oxidase-positive diplococcus.

EPIDEMIOLOGY: Gonococcal infections occur only in humans. The source of the organism is exudate and secretions from infected mucosal surfaces; *N gonorrhoeae* is communicable as long as a person harbors the organism. Transmission results from intimate contact, such as sexual acts, parturition, and rarely, household exposure in prepubertal children. Sexual abuse should be considered strongly when genital, rectal, or pharyngeal colonization or infection are diagnosed in children beyond the newborn period and before puberty. An estimated 650 000 new cases of gonococcal infection occur annually in the United States. Adolescents between 15 and

19 years of age have the highest reported incidence of infection, followed by people 20 to 24 years of age. Concurrent infection with *Chlamydia trachomatis* is common.

The **incubation period** is usually 2 to 7 days.

DIAGNOSTIC TESTS: Microscopic examination of Gram-stained smears of exudate from the eyes, endocervix of postpubertal females, vagina of prepubertal girls, male urethra, skin lesions, synovial fluid, and when clinically warranted, cerebrospinal fluid (CSF) is useful in the initial evaluation. Identification of gram-negative intracellular diplococci in these smears can be helpful, particularly if the organism is not recovered in culture. Gram stains of material obtained from the endocervix of postpubertal females are less sensitive than culture for detection of infection, but they can be of help in the differential diagnosis of a patient with acute abdominal pain or when immediate therapy is indicated. However, other *Neisseria* species and gram-negative cocci may be present in the female genital tract, although these organisms seldom are observed within polymorphonuclear leukocytes. Gram-stained smears of anorectal exudate also may be useful, especially when specimens are obtained by direct visualization using an anoscope. Gram-stained smears of pharyngeal secretion specimens are not recommended for the diagnosis of gonorrhea. In prepubertal girls, vaginal secretion specimens are adequate for diagnosis, and endocervical tissue specimens are unnecessary.

Neisseria gonorrhoeae can be cultured from normally sterile sites, such as blood, CSF, or synovial fluid, using nonselective chocolate agar with incubation in 5% to 10% carbon dioxide. Selective media that inhibit normal flora and nonpathogenic *Neisseria* organisms are used for culture from nonsterile sites, such as the cervix, vagina, rectum, urethra, and pharynx. Specimens for *N gonorrhoeae* culture from mucosal sites should be inoculated immediately onto the appropriate agar or placed in transport medium, because *N gonorrhoeae* is extremely sensitive to drying and temperature changes.

Caution should be exercised when interpreting the significance of the isolation of *Neisseria* organisms, because *N gonorrhoeae* can be confused with other *Neisseria* species that colonize the genitourinary tract or pharynx. At least 2 confirmatory bacteriologic tests involving different principles (eg, biochemical, enzyme substrate, or serologic) should be performed. Interpretation of culture results as *N gonorrhoeae* from the pharynx of young children necessitates particular caution because of the high carriage rate of nonpathogenic *Neisseria* species.

During the last few years, nucleic acid amplification tests (NAATs) using polymerase or ligase chain reaction assay have become available clinically.* These tests are highly sensitive and specific when used on urethral (males) and endocervical swab specimens. These tests also are sensitive and specific when used on first-void urine specimens. Use of urine specimens increases compliance with initial testing and follow-up of hard-to-access populations, such as adolescents. These techniques also permit dual testing of urine for *C trachomatis* and *N gonorrhoeae*. These tests are not recommended for vaginal, rectal, or pharyngeal swabs. A limited number of nonculture tests are licensed by the Food and Drug Administration for conjunctival specimens.

---

* Centers for Disease Control and Prevention. Screening to detect *Chlamydia trachomatis* and *Neisseria gonorrhoeae* infections—2002. *MMWR Recomm Rep.* 2002;51(RR-15):1–38

Sexual Abuse. *In all prepubertal children beyond the newborn period and in nonsexually active adolescents who have gonococcal infection, sexual abuse must be considered to have occurred unless proven otherwise. Genital, rectal, and pharyngeal secretion cultures should be performed for all patients before antimicrobial treatment is given. All gonococcal isolates from such patients should be preserved. Nonculture gonococcal tests including Gram stain, DNA probes, enzyme immunoassays, or nucleic acid amplification tests of oropharyngeal, rectal, or genital tract specimens in children cannot be relied on for diagnosis of gonococcal infection for this purpose, because false-positive results can occur. In prepubertal children when culture is not available, some experts support use of nucleic acid amplification tests on vaginal swabs if a positive result can be verified by another nucleic acid amplification test. Appropriate cultures should be obtained from people who have had contact with a child suspected to have been sexually abused. Children in whom sexual abuse is suspected because of detection of gonorrhea should be evaluated for other sexually transmitted diseases, such as *C trachomatis* infection, syphilis, hepatitis B virus infection, and human immunodeficiency virus (HIV) infection.

TREATMENT: Because of the prevalence of penicillin- and tetracycline-resistant *N gonorrhoeae*, an extended-spectrum cephalosporin (eg, ceftriaxone sodium) is recommended as initial therapy for children, and either an extended-spectrum cephalosporin or fluoroquinolone is recommended for adults (see Table 4.3, p 713). Occasional isolates of quinolone-resistant *N gonorrhoeae* have been isolated in many parts of the United States. Because of resistance, fluoroquinolones should not be used if infection is acquired in Asia, the Pacific Islands including Hawaii, and California. Resistance to spectinomycin is uncommon.

Parenteral cephalosporins are recommended for use in young children; ceftriaxone is approved for all gonococcal infections in children, and cefotaxime sodium is approved only for gonococcal ophthalmia. Antimicrobial agents administered orally that have been demonstrated to be effective for treating gonococcal urethritis and cervicitis in adults and older adolescents include ciprofloxacin, ofloxacin, and levofloxacin. Cefixime no longer is manufactured in the United States. Fluoroquinolones generally are not recommended for people younger than 18 years of age (see Antimicrobial Agents and Related Therapy, p 693) and are contraindicated in pregnant or nursing women.

All patients with presumed or proven gonorrhea should be evaluated for concurrent syphilis, hepatitis B virus, HIV, and *C trachomatis* infections. Patients beyond the neonatal period should be treated presumptively for *C trachomatis* infection (see *Chlamydia trachomatis*, p 238).

A test of cure culture need not be performed in adolescents and adults with uncomplicated gonorrhea who are asymptomatic after being treated with one of the recommended antimicrobial regimens. Children treated with ceftriaxone do not require follow-up cultures, but if treated with other regimens, follow-up culture is indicated.

---

* American Academy of Pediatrics, Committee on Child Abuse and Neglect. Guidelines for the evaluation of sexual abuse of children: subject review [published correction appears in *Pediatrics*. 1999;103:1049]. *Pediatrics*. 1999;103:186–191

Specific recommendations for management and antimicrobial therapy are as follows:

Neonatal Disease. Infants with clinical evidence of ophthalmia neonatorum, scalp abscess, or disseminated infections should be hospitalized. Cultures of blood, eye discharge, or other sites of infection, such as CSF, should be performed for infants to confirm the diagnosis and determine antimicrobial susceptibility. Tests for concomitant infection with *C trachomatis,* congenital syphilis, and HIV infection should be performed. Results of the maternal test for HBsAg should be confirmed. The mother and her partner(s) also need appropriate examination and management for *N gonorrhoeae.*

Nondisseminated Infections. Recommended antimicrobial therapy, including that for ophthalmia neonatorum, is ceftriaxone (25–50 mg/kg, intravenously or intramuscularly, not to exceed 125 mg) given once. Infants with gonococcal ophthalmia should receive eye irrigations with saline solution immediately and at frequent intervals until the discharge is eliminated. Topical antimicrobial treatment alone is inadequate and is unnecessary when recommended systemic antimicrobial treatment is given. Infants with gonococcal ophthalmia should be hospitalized and evaluated for disseminated infection (sepsis, arthritis, meningitis).

Disseminated Infections. Recommended therapy for arthritis and septicemia is ceftriaxone or cefotaxime for 7 days. Cefotaxime is recommended for infants with hyperbilirubinemia. If meningitis is documented, treatment should be continued for a total of 10 to 14 days.

Gonococcal Infections in Children Beyond the Neonatal Period and in Adolescents. Recommendations for treatment of gonococcal infections, by age and weight, are given in Tables 3.8 (p 289) and 3.9 (p 290).

Special Problems in Treatment of Children (Beyond the Neonatal Period) and Adolescents. Patients with uncomplicated endocervical infection, urethritis, or proctitis who are allergic to cephalosporins should be treated with spectinomycin (40 mg/kg, maximum 2 g, given intramuscularly as a single dose) if they are not old enough to receive a fluoroquinolone. Doxycycline or azithromycin dihydrate should be used for the concurrent treatment of presumptive *C trachomatis* infection.

Patients with uncomplicated pharyngeal gonococcal infection should be treated with ceftriaxone (125 mg, intramuscularly) in a single dose. Those who cannot tolerate ceftriaxone should be treated with ciprofloxacin (500 mg, orally, in a single dose). Spectinomycin is approximately 50% effective for the treatment of pharyngeal gonorrhea, so it should be used only in people who are unable to take ceftriaxone or ciprofloxacin, and a pharyngeal culture should be obtained 3 to 5 days after treatment to verify eradication.

A single dose of ceftriaxone is not effective treatment for concurrent infection with syphilis (see Syphilis, p 595). Fluoroquinolones and spectinomycin are not active against *Treponema pallidum.*

Children or adolescents with HIV infection should receive the same treatment for gonococcal infection as those without HIV infection.

Acute PID. *Neisseria gonorrhoeae* and *C trachomatis* are implicated in most cases of PID; many cases have a polymicrobial etiology. No reliable clinical criteria distinguish gonococcal from nongonococcal PID. Hence, broad-spectrum treatment regimens are recommended (see Pelvic Inflammatory Disease, p 468).

Table 3.8. Uncomplicated Gonococcal Infection: Treatment of Children Beyond the Newborn Period and Adolescents[1]

Disease[2]	Prepubertal Children Who Weigh <100 lb (<45 kg)	Disease[2]	Patients Who Weigh ≥100 lb (≥45 kg) and Who Are 8 Years or Older
Uncomplicated vulvovaginitis, cervicitis, urethritis, proctitis, or pharyngitis	Ceftriaxone sodium, 125 mg, IM, in a single dose **OR** Spectinomycin,[3] 40 mg/kg (maximum 2 g), IM, in a single dose **PLUS[1]** Azithromycin, 20 mg/kg (maximum 1 g), orally, in a single dose **OR** Erythromycin, 50 mg/kg per day (maximum 2 g/day), orally, in 4 divided doses for 14 days	Uncomplicated endocervicitis, urethritis, epididymitis, proctitis, or pharyngitis[4]	Ceftriaxone, 125 mg, IM, in a single dose **OR** Ciprofloxacin,[5] 500 mg, orally, in a single dose **OR** Ofloxacin,[5] 400 mg, orally, in a single dose **OR** Levofloxacin,[5] 250 mg, orally, in a single dose **PLUS[1]** Azithromycin (1 g, orally, in a single dose) **OR** Doxycycline (100 mg, orally, twice a day for 7 days)

IM indicates intramuscularly.

[1] In addition to the recommended treatment for gonococcal infection, therapy for *Chlamydia trachomatis* is recommended on the presumption that the patient has concomitant infection.

[2] Hospitalization should be considered, especially for people treated as outpatients whose infection has failed to respond and for people who are unlikely to adhere to treatment regimens.

[3] Spectinomycin is not recommended for treatment of pharyngeal infections; in people who cannot take ceftriaxone or ciprofloxacin, spectromycin may be used for pharyngitis, but a follow-up culture is necessary.

[4] Alternative regimens include spectinomycin (2 g, IM, in a single dose), ceftizoxime, cefotaxime, and cefoxitin. Only ceftriaxone and ciprofloxacin are recommended for pharyngitis; in people who cannot take either of these, spectromycin may be used, but a follow-up culture is necessary.

[5] Fluoroquinolones are contraindicated for pregnant women, nursing women, and usually for people younger than 18 years of age (see Antimicrobial Agents and Related Therapy, p 693). Fluoroquinolones should not be used for infections acquired in Asia, the Pacific Islands including Hawaii, or California.

Table 3.9. Complicated Gonococcal Infection: Treatment of Children Beyond the Newborn Period and Adolescents[1]

Disease[2]	Prepubertal Children Who Weigh <100 lb (<45 kg)	Disease[2]	Patients Who Weigh ≥100 lb (≥45 kg) and Who Are 8 Years or Older
Disseminated gonococcal infection (eg, arthritis–dermatitis syndrome)	Ceftriaxone, 50 mg/kg per day (maximum 1 g/day), IV or IM, once a day for 7 days **PLUS[1]** Azithromycin or erythromycin	Disseminated gonococcal infections[3]	Ceftriaxone, 1 g, IV or IM, given once a day for 7 days[4] **OR** Cefotaxime, 1 g, IV, every 8 hours for 7 days[4] **PLUS[1]** Azithromycin, 1 g, orally, in a single dose **OR** Doxycycline, 100 mg, orally, twice a day for 7 days
Meningitis or endocarditis	Ceftriaxone, 50 mg/kg per day (maximum 2 g/day), IV or IM, given every 12 h; for meningitis, duration is 10–14 days; for endocarditis, duration is at least 28 days **PLUS[1]** Azithromycin or erythromycin	Meningitis or endocarditis	Ceftriaxone, 1–2 g, IV, every 12 h; for meningitis, duration is 10–14 days; for endocarditis, duration is at least 28 days
Conjunctivitis[5]	Ceftriaxone, 50 mg/kg (maximum 1g), IM, in a single dose	Conjunctivitis[5]	Ceftriaxone, 1 g, IM, in a single dose
		Pelvic inflammatory disease	See Table 3.41 (p 471)

IV indicates intravenously, and IM, intramuscularly.

[1] In addition to the recommended treatment for gonococcal infection, therapy for *Chlamydia trachomatis* is recommended on the presumption that the patient has concomitant infection.

[2] Hospitalization should be considered, especially for people treated as outpatients whose infection has failed to respond and for people who are unlikely to adhere to treatment regimens.

[3] For people who are allergic to β-lactam drugs: ciprofloxacin (400 mg, IV, every 12 h) *or* ofloxacin (400 mg, IV, every 12 h) *or* levofloxacin (250 mg, IV, daily), or spectinomycin (2 g, IM, every 12 h). Spectinomycin treatment requires a follow-up culture if pharyngeal infection exists. Hospitalization recommended.

[4] Alternatively, parenteral therapy can be discontinued 24 to 48 hours after improvement occurs and a 7-day course is completed with an appropriate oral antimicrobial agent such as ciprofloxacin (500 mg, orally, twice a day), ofloxacin (400 mg, orally twice a day), or levofloxacin (500 mg, orally, once daily). Fluoroquinolones are contraindicated for pregnant women, nursing women, and usually for people younger than 18 years of age (see Antimicrobial Agents and Related Therapy, p 693). Some experts advise a longer course of therapy. Fluoroquinolones should not be used for infections acquired in Asia, the Pacific Islands including Hawaii, or California.

[5] Eyes should be lavaged with saline solution to clear accumulated secretions.

Acute Epididymitis. Sexually transmitted organisms, such as *N gonorrhoeae* or *C trachomatis,* can cause acute epididymitis in sexually active adolescents and young adults but rarely cause acute epididymitis in prepubertal children. The recommended regimen for sexually transmitted epididymitis is ceftriaxone plus erythromycin, azithromycin, or doxycycline, depending on the patient's age (see Table 3.8, p 289).

ISOLATION OF THE HOSPITALIZED PATIENT: Standard precautions are recommended, including for newborns with ophthalmia.

CONTROL MEASURES:

Neonatal Ophthalmia. For routine prophylaxis of infants immediately after birth, a 1% solution of silver nitrate, or 1% tetracycline or 0.5% erythromycin ophthalmic ointment, is instilled into each eye; subsequent irrigation should not be performed (see Prevention of Neonatal Ophthalmia, p 778). Prophylaxis may be delayed for as long as 1 hour after birth to facilitate parent-infant bonding. Topical antimicrobial agents are less likely to cause a chemical irritation than silver nitrate. None of the topical agents are effective against *C trachomatis,* likely because they do not eradicate this organism from the nasopharynx.

Infants Born to Mothers With Gonococcal Infections. When prophylaxis is administered correctly, infants born to mothers with gonococcal infection rarely develop gonococcal ophthalmia. However, because gonococcal ophthalmia or disseminated infection occasionally can occur in this situation, infants born to mothers known to have gonorrhea should receive a single dose of ceftriaxone, 125 mg intravenously or intramuscularly; for premature and low-birth-weight infants, the dose is 25 to 50 mg/kg, to a maximum of 125 mg.

Children and Adolescents With Sexual Exposure to a Patient Known to Have Gonorrhea. Exposed individuals should undergo examination, culture, and the same treatment as people known to have gonorrhea.

Pregnancy. All pregnant women should have an endocervical culture for gonococci at the time of their first prenatal visit. A second culture late in the third trimester is recommended for women at high risk of exposure to gonococcal infection. Recommended therapeutic regimens for patients found to be infected are those previously described for uncomplicated gonorrhea, except that a tetracycline or fluoroquinolone should not be used because of the potential toxic effects on the fetus. Women who are allergic to cephalosporins should be treated with spectinomycin.

Case Reporting and Management of Sexual Partners. All cases of gonorrhea must be reported to public health officials (see Appendix IX, Nationally Notifiable Infectious Diseases in the United States, p 822). Cases in prepubertal children must be investigated to determine the source of infection. Ensuring that sexual contacts are treated and counseled to use condoms is essential for community control, prevention of reinfection, and prevention of complications in the contact.

Granuloma Inguinale
(Donovanosis)

CLINICAL MANIFESTATIONS: Initial lesions are single or multiple subcutaneous nodules that progress to form painless, highly vascular, friable, granulomatous ulcers without regional adenopathy. Lesions usually involve the genitalia, but anal infections occur in 5% to 10% of patients; lesions at distant sites (eg, face, mouth, or liver) are rare. Subcutaneous extension into the inguinal area results in induration that can mimic inguinal adenopathy (ie, the "pseudobubo" of granuloma inguinale). Fibrosis manifests as sinus tracts, adhesions, and lymphedema, resulting in extreme genital deformity.

ETIOLOGY: The disease is caused by *Calymmatobacterium granulomatis,* an intracellular gram-negative bacillus.

EPIDEMIOLOGY: Indigenous granuloma inguinale no longer occurs in the United States and most developed countries. Cases that occur in the United States are imported. Donovanosis is endemic in Papua, New Guinea and parts of India, southern Africa, central Australia, and to a much lesser extent, the Caribbean and parts of South America, most notably Brazil. The highest incidence of disease occurs in tropical and subtropical environments. The incidence of infection seems to correlate strongly with sustained high temperatures and high relative humidity. Infection usually is acquired by sexual intercourse, most commonly with a person with active infection, but possibly also from a person with asymptomatic rectal infection. Granuloma inguinale is mildly contagious, and repeated exposure may be necessary for development of disease. Young children can acquire infection by contact with infected secretions. The period of communicability extends throughout the duration of active lesions or rectal colonization.

The **incubation period** is 8 to 80 days.

DIAGNOSTIC TESTS: The causative organism is difficult to culture, and diagnosis requires microscopic demonstration of dark staining intracytoplasmic Donovan bodies on Wright or Giemsa staining of a crush preparation from subsurface scrapings of a lesion or tissue. The microorganism also can be detected by histologic examination of biopsy specimens. Lesions, however, should be cultured for *Haemophilus ducreyi* to exclude chancroid (pseudogranuloma inguinale). Granuloma inguinale often is misdiagnosed as carcinoma, which can be excluded by histologic examination of tissue or by response of the lesion to antimicrobial agents. Diagnosis by polymerase chain reaction assay and serologic testing is available on a research basis.

TREATMENT: Doxycycline (which ordinarily should not be given to children younger than 8 years of age) and trimethoprim-sulfamethoxazole have been reported to be effective. Ciprofloxacin, which is not recommended for use in pregnant women or children younger than 18 years of age, and gentamicin sulfate are effective but reserved for resistant cases. Erythromycin base has been used in treatment of pregnant patients. Azithromycin dihydrate also is an alternative drug. Antimicrobial therapy is continued for at least 3 weeks or until the lesions have resolved. If antimicrobial therapy is effective, partial healing usually is noted within 7 days. Relapse can occur, especially if the antimicrobial agent is stopped before the primary lesion has healed completely.

Patients should be evaluated for other sexually transmitted diseases, such as gonorrhea, syphilis, and infection with *Chlamydia trachomatis,* hepatitis B virus, and human immunodeficiency virus.

ISOLATION OF THE HOSPITALIZED PATIENT: Standard precautions are recommended.

CONTROL MEASURES: Sexual partners should be examined, counseled to use condoms, and offered antimicrobial therapy. The value of empiric therapy in the absence of signs and symptoms has not been established.

Haemophilus influenzae Infections

CLINICAL MANIFESTATIONS: *Haemophilus influenzae* causes conjunctivitis, otitis media, sinusitis, epiglottitis, pneumonia, empyema, septic arthritis, cellulitis, meningitis, and occult febrile bacteremia. Other *H influenzae* infections include purulent pericarditis, endocarditis, endophthalmitis, osteomyelitis, peritonitis, glossitis, uvulitis, and septic thrombophlebitis. Occasionally, other encapsulated and nonencapsulated strains cause septicemia, otitis media, sinusitis, bronchitis, pneumonia, and meningitis, including infection in neonates.

ETIOLOGY: *Haemophilus influenzae* is a pleomorphic gram-negative coccobacillus. Encapsulated strains express 1 of 6 antigenically distinct capsular polysaccharides (a through f); nonencapsulated strains fail to react with typing antisera against capsular serotypes a through f and are designated nontypeable.

EPIDEMIOLOGY: The natural habitat of the organism is the human upper respiratory tract. The mode of transmission is person-to-person by inhalation of respiratory droplets or by direct contact with respiratory secretions. In neonates, infection is acquired intrapartum by aspiration of amniotic fluid or by contact with genital tract secretions containing the organism. Asymptomatic colonization by *H influenzae* strains is common; nonencapsulated strains are recovered from the nasopharynx of 40% to 80% of children. Colonization by type b organisms is rare, occurring in 2% to 5% of children in the prevaccine era and even fewer individuals currently, because immunization decreases pharyngeal colonization. The exact period of communicability is unknown.

Before introduction of effective *H influenzae* type b (Hib) conjugate vaccines, Hib was the most common cause of bacterial meningitis in children in the United States. The peak incidence of meningitis and most other invasive Hib infections occurred between 6 and 18 months of age, accounting for approximately 45% of cases in children younger than 5 years of age. In contrast, the peak for epiglottitis was 2 to 4 years.

Unimmunized children younger than 4 years of age are at increased risk of invasive Hib disease, especially if they are in prolonged close contact (such as in a household setting) with a child with invasive Hib disease. Other factors that predispose to invasive disease include sickle cell disease, asplenia, human immunodeficiency virus (HIV) infection, certain immunodeficiency syndromes, and malignant neoplasms. Historically, invasive Hib was more common in boys; black, Alaska Native, Apache, and Navajo individuals; child care attendees; children living in crowded conditions; and children who were not breastfed.

Since 1988, when Hib conjugate vaccines were introduced first in toddlers and then 2 years later in infants, the incidence of invasive Hib disease in infants and young children has decreased by 99% to fewer than 1 case per 100 000 children younger than 5 years of age. The incidence of invasive infections caused by all other encapsulated and nontypeable strains combined is similarly low. Currently, invasive Hib disease occurs primarily in underimmunized children and among infants too young to have completed the primary immunization series. *Haemophilus influenzae* type b remains an important pathogen in developing countries where routine vaccines are not available to most of the population.

The **incubation period** is unknown.

DIAGNOSTIC TESTS: Cerebrospinal fluid (CSF), blood, synovial fluid, and pleural fluid specimens and middle ear aspirates should be cultured on a medium such as chocolate agar enriched with factors X and V. Gram stain of an infected body fluid specimen can facilitate presumptive diagnosis. Latex particle agglutination for detection of type b capsular antigen in CSF may be helpful, but a negative test result does not exclude the diagnosis, and false-positive results have been recorded. Antigen testing of serum and urine specimens is not recommended. All *H influenzae* isolates associated with an invasive infection should be serotyped. Serotyping discrepancies have been noted between slide agglutination and polymerase chain reaction capsular typing, with misidentification by slide agglutination of nontypeable strains as encapsulated. If serotyping is not available locally, isolates should be submitted to the state health department or to a reference laboratory for testing.

TREATMENT:
- Initial therapy for children with meningitis possibly caused by Hib is cefotaxime sodium or ceftriaxone sodium or ampicillin in combination with chloramphenicol. Ampicillin alone should not be used because of frequent resistance.
- For antimicrobial treatment of other invasive *H influenzae* infections, including those caused by strains other than type b, recommendations are similar but are based primarily on empiric experience.
- For patients with uncomplicated meningitis who respond rapidly, antimicrobial therapy for 10 days administered intravenously usually is satisfactory. More than 10 days of therapy may be indicated in complicated cases.
- Dexamethasone may be beneficial for treatment of infants and children with Hib meningitis to diminish the risk of neurologic sequelae including hearing loss.

- Epiglottitis is a medical emergency. An airway must be established promptly with an endotracheal tube or by tracheostomy.
- Infected synovial, pleural, or pericardial fluid should be drained.
- For empiric therapy of acute otitis media, most experts recommend oral amoxicillin (see details in Pneumococcal Infections, p 490). Duration of therapy is 5 to 10 days. The 5-day course is considered for children 2 years of age and older. In the United States, 30% to 40% of *H influenzae* isolates produce β-lactamase, necessitating a β-lactamase–resistant agent, such as amoxicillin-clavulanate potassium, an oral cephalosporin, or a newer macrolide. In vitro susceptibility testing of isolates from middle ear fluid specimens may help guide therapy in complicated or persistent cases.

ISOLATION OF THE HOSPITALIZED PATIENT: In patients with invasive Hib disease, droplet precautions are recommended for 24 hours after initiation of antimicrobial therapy.

CONTROL MEASURES (FOR INVASIVE HIB DISEASE):

Care of Exposed People.

Careful observation of exposed unimmunized or incompletely immunized household, child care, or nursery contacts is essential. Exposed children in whom a febrile illness develops should receive prompt medical evaluation. If indicated, antimicrobial therapy appropriate for invasive Hib disease should be initiated.

Chemoprophylaxis. The risk of invasive Hib disease is increased among unimmunized household contacts younger than 4 years of age. Rifampin eradicates Hib from the pharynx in approximately 95% of carriers. Limited data indicate that rifampin prophylaxis also decreases the risk of secondary invasive illness in exposed household contacts. Nursery and child care center contacts also may be at increased risk of secondary disease, but experts disagree about the magnitude of the risk. The risk of secondary disease in children attending child care centers seems to be lower than that observed for age-susceptible household contacts, and secondary disease in child care contacts is rare when all contacts are older than 2 years of age. The efficacy of rifampin in preventing disease in child care groups is not established.

Indications and guidelines for chemoprophylaxis in different circumstances are summarized in Table 3.10 (p 296).

- *Household.* In households with at least 1 contact who is younger than 48 months of age and unimmunized or incompletely immunized against Hib, rifampin prophylaxis is recommended for all household contacts, regardless of age. In households with an immunocompromised child, even if the child is older than 48 months and fully immunized, all members of the household should receive rifampin because of the possibility that immunization may not have been effective. Similarly, in households with a child younger than 12 months of age who has not received the 3-dose primary series of Hib conjugate vaccine, all household members should receive rifampin prophylaxis. Chemoprophylaxis is not recommended for occupants of households that do not have children younger than 48 months of age (other than the index case) or when all household contacts 12 to 48 months of age are immunocompetent and have completed their Hib immunization series (see Table 3.10, p 296).

Table 3.10. Indications and Guidelines for Rifampin Chemoprophylaxis for Contacts of Index Cases of Invasive *Haemophilus influenzae* Type b (Hib) Disease

Chemoprophylaxis Recommended
- For all household contacts[1] in the following circumstances:
  - Household with at least 1 contact younger than 4 years of age who is unimmunized or incompletely immunized[2]
  - Household with a child younger than 12 months of age if the child has not received the primary series.
  - Household with an immunocompromised child, regardless of that child's Hib immunization status
- For nursery school and child care center contacts, regardless of age, when 2 or more cases of Hib invasive disease have occurred within 60 days
- For index case, if younger than 2 years of age or member of a household with a susceptible contact and treated with a regimen other than cefotaxime sodium or ceftriaxone sodium, chemoprophylaxis usually is provided just before discharge from hospital

Chemoprophylaxis Not Recommended
- For occupants of households with no children younger than 4 years of age other than the index patient
- For occupants of households when all household contacts younger than 12 to 48 months of age have completed their Hib immunization series
- For nursery school and child care contacts of 1 index case, especially those older than 2 years of age
- For pregnant women

---

[1] Defined as people residing with the index patient or nonresidents who spent 4 or more hours with the index case for at least 5 of the 7 days preceding the day of hospital admission of the index case.
[2] Complete immunization is defined as having had at least 1 dose of conjugate vaccine at 15 months of age or older; 2 doses between 12 and 14 months of age; or a 2- or 3-dose primary series when younger than 12 months with a booster dose at 12 months of age or older.

Given that most secondary cases in households occur during the first week after hospitalization of the index case, when indicated, prophylaxis should be initiated as soon as possible. Because some secondary cases occur later, initiation of prophylaxis 7 days or more after hospitalization of the index patient may still be of some benefit.
- *Child care and nursery school.* When 2 or more cases of invasive disease have occurred within 60 days and unimmunized or incompletely immunized children attend the child care facility, rifampin prophylaxis for attendees and supervisory personnel should be considered. When a single case has occurred, the advisability of rifampin prophylaxis in exposed child care groups with unimmunized or incompletely immunized children is controversial, but many experts recommend no prophylaxis.

In addition to these recommendations for chemoprophylaxis, unimmunized or incompletely immunized children should receive a dose of vaccine and should be scheduled for completion of the recommended age-specific immunization schedule (see Immunization, below).

- *Index case.* Treatment of Hib disease with cefotaxime sodium or ceftriaxone sodium generally eradicates Hib colonization, eliminating the need for prophylaxis of the index patient. Patients who are treated with ampicillin or chloramphenicol and who are younger than 2 years of age or have a susceptible household contact should receive rifampin prophylaxis.
- *Dosage.* Rifampin should be given orally once a day for 4 days (in a dose of 20 mg/kg; maximum dose 600 mg). The dose for infants younger than 1 month of age is not established; some experts recommend lowering the dose to 10 mg/kg. For adults, each dose is 600 mg.

Immunization.

Three Hib conjugate vaccines currently are available in the United States (see Table 3.11, p 298). The Hib conjugate vaccines consist of the Hib capsular polysaccharide (ie, polyribosylribotol phosphate [PRP] or PRP oligomers) covalently linked to a carrier protein directly or via an intervening spacer molecule. Protective antibodies are directed against PRP. Conjugate vaccines vary in composition and immunogenicity, and as a result, recommendations for their use differ. Given the increased risk of disease in early infancy among American Indian/Alaska Native children, use of PRP-OMP (outer membrane protein complex) for the first dose in a series because of the substantial antibody response after 1 dose is recommended (see American Indian/Alaska Native Children, *Haemophilus influenzae* type b, p 293).

Depending on the vaccine, the recommended primary series consists of 3 doses given at 2, 4, and 6 months of age or 2 doses given at 2 and 4 months of age (see Recommendations for Immunization, p 298, and Table 3.12, p 299). The recommended doses may be given as combination vaccines. The regimens in Table 3.12 are likely to be equivalent in protection after completion of the recommended primary series.

After administration of the primary series, serum antibody concentrations decrease rapidly. An additional booster dose of any conjugate vaccine is recommended at 12 to 15 months of age, regardless of which regimen was used for the primary series. This dose may be given as a combination vaccine.

Vaccine Interchangeability. The available Hib conjugate vaccines are considered interchangeable for primary and booster immunization. If PRP-OMP is administered as only part of a primary series, the recommended number of doses to complete the series is determined by the other Hib conjugate vaccine.

Dosage and Route of Administration. The dose of each Hib conjugate vaccine is 0.5 mL, given intramuscularly.

Children With Immunologic Impairment. Children at increased risk of Hib disease may have impaired anti-PRP antibody responses to conjugate vaccines. Examples include children with HIV infection, immunoglobulin deficiency, anatomic or functional asplenia, and sickle cell disease; recipients of bone marrow transplants; and recipients of chemotherapy for a malignant neoplasm. Some children with immunologic impairment may benefit from more doses of conjugate vaccine than usually indicated (see Recommendations for Immunization, p 298).

Table 3.11. *Haemophilus influenzae* Type b Conjugate Vaccines Licensed for Use in Infants and Children in the United States[1]

Manufacturer	Abbreviation	Trade Name	Carrier Protein
Wyeth-Lederle Vaccines (Philadelphia, PA)	HbOC	HibTITER	CRM$_{197}$ (a nontoxic mutant diphtheria toxin)
Merck & Co, Inc (West Point, PA)	PRP-OMP	PedvaxHIB	OMP (an outer membrane protein complex from *Neisseria meningitidis*)
Aventis Pasteur (Swiftwater, PA)	PRP-T	ActHIB OmniHIB	Tetanus toxoid
Merck & Co, Inc (West Point, PA)[2]	PRP-OMP/Hep B	Comvax	OMP

[1] These vaccines may be given in combination products or as reconstituted products with diphtheria and tetanus toxoids and acellular pertussis (DTaP), provided the combination or reconstituted vaccine is licensed by the US Food and Drug Administration for the child's age and administration of the other vaccine component(s) also is justified. DTaP/Hib combination products should not be used for primary immunization in infants at 2, 4, or 6 months of age but can be used as a booster dose following any Hib vaccine. The license for ProHIBiT (PRP-D) was revoked at the request of the manufacturer in February 2001.

[2] A combination of *H influenzae* (PRP-OMP) and hepatitis B (Recombivax, 5 μg) vaccine is licensed for use at 2, 4, and 12 to 15 months of age (Comvax).

Vaccine Failure. Even in individuals who have been immunized with a conjugate vaccine, Hib disease can occur. Because serum antibody responses do not occur for 1 to 2 weeks after immunization, recipients are not expected to be protected during this immediate postimmunization period. Data from US surveillance indicates that there are approximately 15 cases of Hib invasive disease annually in children younger than 5 years of age who have previously received the primary Hib conjugate vaccine series.

Adverse Reactions. Adverse reactions to the Hib conjugate vaccines are few. Pain, redness, and swelling at the injection site occur in approximately 25% of recipients, but these symptoms typically are mild and last fewer than 24 hours. Systemic reactions are rare. When conjugate vaccines are administered during the same visit that diphtheria and tetanus toxoids and acellular pertussis (DTaP) vaccine is given, the rates of systemic reactions do not differ from those observed when DTaP vaccine is administered alone.

Recommendations for Immunization.

Indications and Schedule

- All children should be immunized with an Hib conjugate vaccine beginning at approximately 2 months of age or as soon as possible thereafter (see Table 3.12, p 299). Other general recommendations are as follows:
  - Immunization can be initiated as early as 6 weeks of age.

Table 3.12. Currently Recommended Regimens for Routine *Haemophilus influenzae* Type b Conjugate Immunization for Children Immunized Beginning at 2 to 6 Months of Age[1]

Vaccine Product at Initiation	Total No. of Doses To Be Administered	Recommended Regimen
HbOC or PRP-T	4	3 doses at 2-mo intervals initially; fourth dose at 12 to 15 mo of age; any conjugate vaccine for dose 4[2]
PRP-OMP	3	2 doses 2 months apart; when feasible, same vaccine for doses 1 and 2[3]; third dose at 12–15 mo of age; any conjugate vaccine for dose 3[†]

[1] See text and Table 3.11 (p 298) for further information about specific vaccines and for explanation of the abbreviations. These vaccines may be given in combination products or as reconstituted products with diphtheria and tetanus toxoids and acellular pertussis (DTaP), provided the combination or reconstituted vaccine is licensed by the US Food and Drug Administration for the child's age and administration of the other vaccine component(s) also is justified.

[2] The safety and efficacy of PRP-OMP, PRP-T, and HbOC are likely to be equivalent for children 12 months of age and older.

[3] If interchanging vaccines in the primary series, 3 doses plus a booster are needed.

- Vaccine may be given during visits when DTaP, pneumococcus, poliovirus, hepatitis A, hepatitis B, measles-mumps-rubella (MMR), and varicella vaccines are administered (see Simultaneous Administration of Multiple Vaccines, p 33). No known contraindications exist to simultaneous administration of Hib conjugate vaccine with meningococcal vaccine when given in separate syringes at different sites.
- For routine immunization of children younger than 7 months of age, the following guidelines are recommended:
  - *Primary series.* A 3-dose regimen of HbOC (diphtheria CRM_{197} protein conjugate) or PRP-T (tetanus toxoid conjugate) or a 2-dose regimen of PRP-OMP should be administered (see Table 3.12, above). Doses are given at approximately 2-month intervals. When sequential doses of different vaccine products are given or uncertainty exists about which products previously were administered, 3 doses of any conjugate vaccine are considered sufficient to complete the primary series, regardless of the regimen used.
  - *Booster immunization at 12 to 15 months of age.* For children who have completed a primary series, an additional dose of conjugate vaccine is recommended at 12 to 15 months of age or as soon as possible thereafter. Any conjugate vaccine or DTaP-Hib combination vaccine is acceptable for this dose.
- Children younger than 5 years of age who did not receive Hib conjugate vaccine during the first 6 months of life should be immunized according to the following recommended schedules (see Table 1.6, p 26). For accelerated immunization, a minimum of a 4-week interval between doses may be used.

- For children in whom immunization is initiated at 7 to 11 months of age, the recommended schedules for HbOC, PRP-OMP, and PRP-T are identical and require 3 doses. The first 2 doses are given 2 months apart. The third (booster) dose should be given at 12 to 15 months of age, preferably 2 months after the second dose.
- For children in whom immunization is initiated at 12 to 14 months of age, the recommended regimens for HbOC, PRP-OMP, and PRP-T are identical and include 2 doses given 2 months apart.
- For children in whom immunization is initiated at 15 to 59 months of age, the recommended regimen is a single dose of any licensed conjugate vaccine.
- If circumstances are such that more rapid catch-up immunization is desirable, the recommended interval between doses is 4 weeks.
- Special circumstances are as follows:
  - *Lapsed immunizations.* Recommendations for children who have had a lapse in the schedule of immunizations are based on limited data. The current recommendations are summarized in Table 1.6 (p 26).
  - *Premature infants.* For infants born prematurely, immunization should be based on chronologic age and should be initiated at 2 months of age according to recommendations in Table 3.12 (p 299). This recommendation is based on available data suggesting that even very low birth weight infants have adequate antibody responses to these vaccines, although the serum concentrations of antibody may be decreased in chronically ill infants in comparison with responses in full-term infants.
  - *Children who may be at increased risk of invasive Hib disease resulting from immunologic or other host defense abnormalities (eg, sickle cell disease and anatomic asplenia).* Children with decreased or absent splenic function who have received a primary series of Hib immunizations and a booster dose at 12 months of age or older need not be immunized further. Children who have received a primary series and a booster dose and are undergoing scheduled splenectomy (eg, for Hodgkin disease, spherocytosis, immune thrombocytopenia, or hypersplenism) may benefit from an additional dose of any licensed conjugate vaccine. This dose should be provided at least 7 to 10 days before the procedure. Patients with HIV infection or immunoglobulin (Ig) G2 subclass deficiency and those receiving chemotherapy for malignant neoplasms also are at increased risk of invasive Hib disease. Whether these children will benefit from additional doses after completion of the primary series of immunizations and the booster dose at 12 months of age or later is unknown. Providers should make every effort to ensure completion of the primary immunization and booster series.

    For children 12 to 59 months of age with an underlying condition predisposing to Hib disease who are not immunized or have received only 1 dose of conjugate vaccine before 12 months of age, 2 doses of any conjugate vaccine, separated by 2 months, are recommended. For children in this age group who received 2 doses before 12 months of age, 1 additional dose of conjugate vaccine is recommended.

- *Unimmunized children with an underlying disease possibly predisposing to Hib disease who are older than 59 months of age.* These children should be immunized with any licensed conjugate vaccine. On the basis of limited data, 2 doses separated by 1 to 2 months are suggested for children with HIV infection or IgG2 deficiency.
- *Haemophilus influenzae* type b invasive infection. Children who develop invasive disease when younger than 24 months of age commonly have low anticapsular antibody concentrations in convalescent serum specimens and may remain at risk of developing a second episode of disease. These patients should be immunized according to the age-appropriate schedule for unimmunized children and as if they had received no previous Hib vaccine doses (see Table 3.12, p 299, and Table 1.6, p 26). Immunization should be initiated 1 month after onset of disease or as soon as possible thereafter. Children who develop disease at 24 months of age or older do not need immunization, because disease almost always induces a protective immune response, making second episodes of disease in this age group rare.

Immunologic evaluation should be performed in children who experience invasive Hib disease despite 2 to 3 doses of vaccine and in children with recurrent invasive disease attributable to type b strains.

Reporting. All cases of *H influenzae* invasive disease, including type b and nontype b, should be reported to the Centers for Disease Control and Prevention through the local or state public health department.

Hantavirus Pulmonary Syndrome

CLINICAL MANIFESTATIONS: Hantaviruses in humans cause hantavirus pulmonary syndrome (HPS), a noncardiogenic pulmonary edema, or hemorrhagic fever with renal syndrome (HFRS) (see Hemorrhagic Fevers and Related Syndromes, p 307). The prodromal illness of HPS is 3 to 7 days and is characterized by fever; chills; headache; myalgias of the shoulders, lower back, and thighs; nausea; vomiting; diarrhea; and dizziness. Respiratory tract symptoms or signs do not occur for the first 3 to 7 days until pulmonary edema and severe hypoxemia appear abruptly and progress over a few hours. In severe cases, persistent hypotension caused by myocardial dysfunction is present.

The extensive bilateral interstitial and alveolar pulmonary edema and pleural effusions are the result of a diffuse pulmonary capillary leak and appear to be immune mediated. Intubation and assisted ventilation usually are required for only 2 to 4 days, with resolution heralded by the onset of diuresis and rapid clinical improvement.

The severe myocardial depression is different from that of septic shock; the cardiac indices and the stroke volume index are low, the pulmonary wedge pressure is normal, and systemic vascular resistance is increased. Poor prognostic indicators include persistent hypotension, marked hemoconcentration, a cardiac index of less than 2, and the abrupt onset of lactic acidosis with a serum lactate concentration of greater than 4 mmol/L (36 mg/dL).

The mortality rate for patients with HPS is 45%. Asymptomatic and mild disease are rare in adults, but limited information suggests they may be more common in children. Serious sequelae are uncommon.

ETIOLOGY: Hantaviruses are RNA viruses of the Bunyaviridae family. Within the hantavirus genus, Sin Nombre virus (SNV) is the major cause of HPS in the 4-corners region of the United States. Bayou virus, Black Creek Canal virus, and New York virus are responsible for sporadic cases in Louisiana, Texas, Florida, and New York. In recent years, new hantavirus serotypes, including Andes virus associated with an HPS syndrome, have been reported in South America.

EPIDEMIOLOGY: Rodents, the natural hosts for the hantaviruses, acquire a lifelong, asymptomatic, chronic infection with prolonged viruria and virus in saliva. Humans acquire infection through direct contact with infected rodents, rodent droppings, nests, or inhalation of aerosolized virus particles from rodent urine, droppings, or saliva. Rarely, infection may be acquired from rodent bites or contamination of broken skin with excreta. Person-to-person transmission of the viruses in the United States has not been demonstrated, but a few cases of person-to-person spread of Andes virus have been reported from Patagonia, South America. At-risk activities include handling or trapping rodents, cleaning or entering closed, rarely used rodent-infested structures, cleaning feed storage or animal shelter areas, hand plowing, and living in a home with an increased density of mice in or around the home. For backpackers or campers, sleeping in a structure also inhabited by rodents has been associated with HPS. Weather conditions resulting in exceptionally heavy rainfall and improved rodent food supplies can result in a large increase in the rodent population. The increased rodent population results in more frequent contact between humans and infected mice and may account for recently recognized outbreaks. Most cases occur during spring and summer, and the geographic location is determined by the habitat of the rodent carrier.

Sin Nombre virus is transmitted by the deer mouse, *Peromyscus maniculatus;* Black Creek Canal virus is transmitted by the cotton rat, *Sigmodon hispidus;* Bayou virus is transmitted by the rice rat, *Oryzomys palustris;* and New York virus is transmitted by the white-footed mouse, *Peromyscus leucopus.*

The **incubation period** may be 1 to 6 weeks after exposure to infected rodents, their saliva, or excreta but has not been established definitely.

DIAGNOSTIC TESTS: Characteristic laboratory findings include neutrophilic leukocytosis with immature granulocytes, more than 10% immunoblasts (basophilic cytoplasm, prominent nucleoli, and an increased nuclear-cytoplasmic ratio), thrombocytopenia, and increased hematocrit. In fatal cases, SNV has been identified by immunohistochemical staining of capillary endothelial cells in almost every organ in the body. Sin Nombre virus RNA has been detected uniformly by the reverse transcriptase-polymerase chain reaction assay of peripheral blood mononuclear cells and other clinical specimens from the first few days of hospitalization up to 10 to 21 days after symptom onset, and the duration of viremia is unknown. Viral RNA is not detected readily in bronchoalveolar lavage fluids.

Hantavirus-specific immunoglobulin (Ig) G and IgM antibodies are present at the onset of clinical disease. A rapid diagnostic test can facilitate immediate appropriate supportive therapy, early transfer to a tertiary care facility, and potential enrollment in antiviral trials. The rapid immunoblot assay is a simple dipstick-like assay that takes 5 hours, requires minimal equipment, and can be performed in rural laboratories. Enzyme immunoassay (available through many state health departments and the Centers for Disease Control and Prevention) and Western blot are assays that use recombinant antigens and have a high degree of specificity for detection of IgG and IgM antibody. Viral culture is not useful for diagnosis and is available only in research laboratories that have specialized facilities to protect laboratory workers.

TREATMENT: Patients with suspected HPS should be transferred immediately to a tertiary care facility. Supportive management of pulmonary edema, severe hypoxemia, and hypotension during the first 24 to 48 hours is critical for recovery. A flow-directed pulmonary catheter for monitoring fluid administration and the use of inotropic support, vasopressors, and careful ventilatory control are important.

Extracorporeal membrane oxygenation (ECMO) may provide particularly important short-term support for the severe capillary leak syndrome in the lungs. Venoarterial ECMO, which also can provide circulatory support, has provided encouraging early results with rapid and dramatic hemodynamic improvement in patients after only 12 hours and a total duration of only 4 to 5 days.

Ribavirin is active in vitro against previously isolated hantaviruses including SNV. A controlled clinical evaluation of ribavirin is being conducted.

ISOLATION OF THE HOSPITALIZED PATIENT: Standard precautions are recommended. Hantavirus pulmonary syndrome has not been associated with nosocomial or person-to-person transmission in the United States.

CONTROL MEASURES:

Care of Exposed People. Serial clinical examinations should be used to monitor individuals assessed to be at high risk of infection after a high-risk exposure (see Epidemiology, p 302).

Environmental Control. Hantavirus infections of humans occur primarily in adults and are associated with domestic, occupational, or leisure activities bringing humans into contact with infected rodents, usually in a rural setting. Eradicating the host reservoir is not feasible. The best currently available approach for disease control and prevention is risk reduction through environmental hygiene practices that discourage rodents from colonizing the home and work environment and that minimize aerosolization and contact with virus in saliva and excreta. Hantaviruses, because of their lipid envelope, are susceptible to most disinfectants, including diluted bleach solutions, detergents, and most general household disinfectants.

Measures to decrease exposure in the home and workplace include eliminating food sources available to rodents in structures used by humans, limiting possible nesting sites, sealing holes and other possible entrances for rodents, and using "snap traps" and rodenticides. Other methods include using a 10% bleach solution to disinfect dead rodents and wearing rubber gloves before handling trapped or dead rodents. Gloves and traps should be disinfected after use. Before entering areas with potential rodent infestations, doors and windows should be opened to ventilate the enclosure. People entering these areas should avoid stirring up or breathing potentially contaminated dust. Dusty or dirty areas or articles should be moistened with a 10% bleach or other disinfectant solution before being cleaned. Brooms and vacuum cleaners should not be used to clean rodent-infested areas.

Efficacious chemoprophylaxis measures or vaccines are not available.

Public Health Reporting. Confirmed cases should be reported immediately to the local and state public health authorities.

Helicobacter pylori Infections

CLINICAL MANIFESTATIONS: Acute infection can manifest as epigastric pain, nausea, vomiting, hematemesis, and guaiac-positive stools. Symptoms usually resolve within a few days despite persistence of the organism for years or life. *Helicobacter pylori* causes chronic active gastritis and increases the risk of duodenal and gastric ulcers; persistence increases the risk of gastric cancer. *Helicobacter pylori* infection is not associated with autoimmune or chemical gastritis.

ETIOLOGY: *Helicobacter pylori* is a gram-negative and spiral, curved, or U-shaped microaerophilic bacillus that has 2 to 6 sheathed flagella at one end.

EPIDEMIOLOGY: *Helicobacter pylori* has been isolated from humans and other primates. An animal reservoir for human transmission has not been demonstrated. The routes by which organisms are transmitted from infected humans are unknown, but fecal-oral transmission may occur. Infection rates are low in children in resource-rich countries, but prevalence increases until 60 years of age. Most carriage is asymptomatic, but almost all infected people have histologic findings of chronic gastritis. Infection is acquired at a younger age in resource-limited countries and by people from lower socioeconomic groups.

The **incubation period** is unknown.

DIAGNOSTIC TESTS: *Helicobacter pylori* infection can be diagnosed by culture of gastric biopsy tissue on nonselective media (eg, chocolate agar) or selective media (eg, Skirrow) at 37°C (98°F) under microaerobic conditions for 2 to 5 days. Organisms usually can be visualized on histologic sections with Warthin-Starry silver, Steiner, Giemsa, or Genta staining. Infection with *H pylori* can be diagnosed but not excluded on the basis of hematoxylin-eosin stains. Because of production of urease by the organisms, urease testing of a gastric specimen can give a rapid and specific microbiologic diagnosis. Each of these tests requires endoscopy and biopsy. Noninvasive, commercially available tests include breath or blood tests, which detect labeled carbon dioxide in expired air or blood after oral administration of isotopically labeled urea, and serologic tests for the presence of immunoglobulin G specific for *H pylori*. Each of these commercially available tests has a sensitivity and specificity of 95% or more. A stool antigen test also has been developed.

TREATMENT: Treatment is recommended only for infected patients who have a history of or active peptic ulcer disease, gastric mucosa-associated lymphoid tissue-type lymphoma, or early gastric cancer. *Helicobacter pylori* is susceptible to a variety of antimicrobial agents, including amoxicillin, tetracycline, metronidazole, clarithro-mycin, and bismuth subsalicylate salts, but none have proven therapeutic effectiveness as single agents. Therapy for *H pylori* infection consists of at least 7 days of treatment, although eradication rates are higher for regimens of 14 days. Effective regimens include 2 antimicrobial agents (eg, amoxicillin, clarithromycin, or metronidazole) plus bismuth subsalicylate or a proton pump inhibitor (lansoprazole, omeprazole, esometrazon, or rabeprazole sodium). These regimens are effective in eliminating the organism, healing the ulcer, and avoiding recurrence. The tolerance and efficacy of regimens in children are unknown, although children have been treated with a proton pump inhibitor plus 2 antimicrobial agents. Such therapies result in eradica-tion rates ranging from 61% to 94% in adults, depending on the regimen used. A 7-day treatment using rabeprazole plus 2 antimicrobial agents (amoxicillin and clarithromycin) has been licensed by the US Food and Drug Administration.

ISOLATION OF THE HOSPITALIZED PATIENT: Standard precautions are recommended.

CONTROL MEASURES: Disinfection of gastroscopes prevents transmission of the organism between patients.

Hemorrhagic Fevers Caused by Arenaviruses

CLINICAL MANIFESTATIONS: The arenaviruses include lymphocytic chori-omeningitis and the agents of 5 hemorrhagic fevers: Bolivian, Argentine, Sabia-virus associated, Venezuelan, and Lassa. These zoonotic diseases range in severity from mild, acute, febrile infections to severe illnesses in which shock is a prominent feature. Fever, headache, myalgia, conjunctival suffusion, and abdominal pain are common early symptoms in all infections. Lymphocytic choriomeningitis causes aseptic meningitis that may be associated with a variety of complications. Axillary petechiae are usual in Argentine hemorrhagic fever (AHF), Bolivian hemorrhagic fever (BHF), and Venezuelan hemorrhagic fever (VHF), and exudative pharyngitis often occurs in Lassa fever. Mucosal bleeding occurs in severe cases as a consequence of vascular damage, thrombocytopenia, and platelet dysfunction. Proteinuria is common, but renal failure is unusual. Increased serum concentrations of aspartate transaminase can indicate an adverse or fatal outcome of Lassa fever. Shock develops 7 to 9 days after onset of the illness in more severely ill patients with these infections. Upper and lower respiratory tract symptoms can develop in people with Lassa fever. Encephalopathic signs with tremor, alterations in consciousness, and seizures can occur in the South American hemorrhagic fevers and in severe cases of Lassa fever.

ETIOLOGY: Arenaviruses are RNA viruses. The major New World arenavirus hemorrhagic fevers occurring in the Western hemisphere, AHF, BHF, and VHF, are caused by Junin, Machupo, and Guanarito viruses, respectively. A fourth are-navirus, sabia virus, caused a single case of naturally occurring hemorrhagic fever in Brazil. The Old World complex of arenaviruses includes Lassa virus, which causes Lassa fever, a disease occurring in West Africa, and lymphocytic choriomeningitis virus (see Lymphocytic Choriomeningitis, p 413), which produces the least severe infection of the arenaviruses.

EPIDEMIOLOGY: Arenaviruses are maintained in nature by association with specific rodent hosts, in which they produce chronic viremia and viruria. Inhalation and mucous membrane and skin contact (eg, through cuts, scratches, or abrasions) with urine and salivary secretions from these persistently infected rodents are the principal routes of infection. All arenaviruses are infectious as aerosols; those causing hemorrhagic fever should be considered highly hazardous to those working with the virus in the laboratory. The geographic distribution and habitats of the specific rodents that serve as reservoir hosts largely determine the endemic areas and populations at risk. Before immunization became available, several hundred cases of AHF occurred yearly in agricultural workers and inhabitants of the Argentine pampas. Epidemics of BHF occurred in small towns from 1962 to 1964; sporadic disease activity in the countryside has continued since then. Venezuelan hemorrhagic fever first was identified in 1989 and occurs in rural north-central Venezuela. Lassa fever is endemic in most of West Africa, where its rodent host lives in proximity with humans, causing thousands of infections annually. Lassa fever has been reported in the United States in travelers from West Africa.

The **incubation periods** are from 6 to 17 days.

DIAGNOSTIC TESTS: Acute infection is diagnosed by demonstrating virus-specific serum immunoglobulin (Ig) M or viral antigen. The IgG antibody response is delayed. Viral nucleic acid also can be detected in acute disease by reverse transcriptase-polymerase chain reaction assay. These viruses may be recovered from the blood of acutely ill patients as well as from various tissues obtained postmortem, but isolation should only be attempted under biosafety level-4 conditions.

TREATMENT: Administration of plasma from convalescent patients has proven effective in decreasing the mortality rate associated with AHF from 15% to 30% in untreated patients to less than 1% in those receiving appropriate quantities (based on neutralizing antibody content) within the first 8 days of illness. Intravenous ribavirin decreases the mortality rate significantly in patients with severe Lassa fever, particularly if they are treated during the first week of illness, and is probably beneficial in treating South American arenavirus infections.

ISOLATION OF THE HOSPITALIZED PATIENT: In addition to standard precautions, contact and droplet precautions, including careful prevention of needlestick injuries, and careful handling of clinical specimens for the duration of illness are recommended for all the hemorrhagic fevers caused by arenaviruses. Respiratory precautions also may be required in certain circumstances.

CONTROL MEASURES:

Care of Exposed People. No specific measures are warranted for exposed people unless direct contamination with blood, excretions, or secretions from an infected patient has occurred. If such contamination has occurred, recording daily temperature for 21 days is recommended, with prompt reporting of fever.

Immunoprophylaxis. An investigational live-attenuated Junin vaccine protects against AHF and probably against BHF. The vaccine is associated with minimal adverse effects in adults; similar findings have been obtained from limited safety studies in children 4 years of age and older.

Environmental. In town-based outbreaks of BHF, rodent control has proven successful. Area rodent control is not practical for control of AHF or VHF. Intensive rodent control efforts modestly have decreased the rate of peridomestic Lassa virus infection, but rodents eventually reinvade human dwellings, and infection still occurs in rural occupational settings.

Public Health Reporting. Because of the risk of nosocomial transmission, the state health department and the Centers for Disease Control and Prevention should be contacted for specific advice about management and diagnosis of suspected cases.

Hemorrhagic Fevers and Related Syndromes, Excluding Hantavirus Pulmonary Syndrome, Caused by Viruses of the Family Bunyaviridae

CLINICAL MANIFESTATIONS: These zoonotic infections are severe febrile diseases in which shock and bleeding can be significant and multisystem involvement can occur. In the United States, one of these infections causes an illness marked by acute respiratory and cardiovascular failure (see Hantavirus Pulmonary Syndrome, p 301).

Hemorrhagic fever with renal syndrome (HFRS) is a complex multiphasic disease characterized by vascular instability and varying degrees of renal insufficiency. Fever, flushing, conjunctival injection, abdominal pain, and lumbar pain are followed by hypotension, oliguria, and subsequently, polyuria. Petechiae and more serious bleeding manifestations are common. Shock and acute renal insufficiency may occur. Nephropathia epidemica, the clinical syndrome of HFRS in Europe, is a milder disease characterized by an influenza-like illness with abdominal pain and proteinuria. Acute renal dysfunction also occurs, but hypotensive shock or a requirement for dialysis are rare.

Hantavirus pulmonary syndrome (HPS) is an acute febrile illness that can progress to acute respiratory failure and shock and is associated with a high case-fatality rate (see Hantavirus Pulmonary Syndrome, p 301).

Crimean-Congo hemorrhagic fever (CCHF) is a multisystem disease characterized by hepatitis and, often, profuse bleeding. Fever, headache, and myalgia are followed by signs of a diffuse capillary leak syndrome with facial suffusion, conjunctivitis, and proteinuria. Petechiae and purpura often appear on the skin and mucous membranes. A hypotensive crisis often occurs after the appearance of frank hemorrhage from the gastrointestinal tract, nose, mouth, or uterus.

Rift Valley fever (RVF), in most cases, is a self-limited febrile illness. Occasionally, hemorrhagic fever with shock and icterus, encephalitis, or retinitis develops.

ETIOLOGY: Bunyaviridae are single-stranded RNA viruses with different geographic distributions depending on their vector. Hemorrhagic fever syndromes are associated with viruses from 3 genera: hantaviruses, nairoviruses (CCHF virus), and phlebo-viruses (RVF and sandfly fever viruses). Old World hantaviruses (Hantaan, Seoul, Dobrava, and Puumula) cause HFRS, and New World hantaviruses (Sin Nombre and related viruses) cause HPS (see Table 3.3, p 203).

EPIDEMIOLOGY: The epidemiology of these diseases mainly is a function of the distribution and behavior of their reservoirs and vectors. All genera except hantaviruses are associated with arthropod vectors, and hantaviruses are associated with exposure to infected rodents.

Classic HFRS occurs throughout much of Asia and Eastern and Western Europe and causes up to 100 000 cases per year. The most severe form of the disease is caused by the prototype Hantaan virus and Dobrava viruses in rural Asia and Europe, respectively; Puumula virus is associated with milder disease (nephropathia epidem-ica) in Europe. Seoul virus is distributed worldwide in association with *Rattus* species and often causes an urban disease of variable severity. Person-to-person transmission never has been reported with HFRS.

Crimean-Congo hemorrhagic fever occurs in much of sub-Saharan Africa, the Middle East, areas in West and Central Asia, and Eastern Europe. The CCHF virus is transmitted by ticks and, occasionally, at the slaughter of domestic animals. Nosocomial transmission of CCHF is a serious hazard.

Rift Valley fever occurs throughout sub-Saharan Africa and has caused epidemics in Egypt in 1977 and 1993–1995 and in Saudi Arabia in 2000. The virus is arthro-podborne and is transmitted from domestic livestock to humans by mosquitoes. It also can be transmitted by aerosol and by direct contact with infected fresh animal carcasses. Person-to-person transmission has not been reported.

The **incubation periods** for CCHF and RVF range from 2 to 10 days; for HFRS, incubation periods usually are longer, ranging from 7 to 42 days.

DIAGNOSTIC TESTS: The CCHF and RVF viruses, but not hantaviruses, can be cultivated readily from blood and tissue specimens of infected patients. Detection of viral antigen is a useful alternative for diagnosis of CCHF and RVF but has been unsuccessful for HFRS. Serum immunoglobulin (Ig) M and IgG virus-specific antibodies typically develop early in convalescence in CCHF and RVF. In HFRS, IgM and IgG antibodies usually are detectable at the time of onset of illness or within 48 hours. Immunoglobulin M antibodies or rising IgG titers in paired serum specimens, as demonstrated by enzyme immunoassay, are diagnostic; neutral-izing antibody tests provide greater virus-strain specificity. Immunofluorescence and complement-fixing antibody tests also are used for serologic diagnosis. Polymerase chain reaction assay can be a useful complement to serodiagnostic assays.

TREATMENT: Ribavirin given intravenously to patients with HFRS within the first 4 days of illness seems effective in decreasing renal dysfunction, vascular instability, and mortality. Supportive therapy for HFRS should include: (1) avoid-ance of transporting patients; (2) treatment of shock; (3) prevention of overhydration (particularly with crystalloid solutions); (4) dialysis for complications of renal failure;

(5) control of hypertension during the oliguric phase; and (6) early recognition of possible myocardial failure with appropriate therapy.

Ribavirin given to patients with CCHF has resulted in clinical responses, although no controlled studies have been performed. Experimental animal data also suggest the potential benefit of ribavirin in treatment of hemorrhagic RVF.

ISOLATION OF THE HOSPITALIZED PATIENT: In addition to standard precautions, contact and droplet precautions, including careful prevention of needlestick injuries and management of clinical specimens, are indicated for patients with CCHF for the duration for their illness. Respiratory precautions also may be required in certain circumstances. Rift Valley fever and HFRS have not been demonstrated to be contagious, but standard precautions should be followed.

CONTROL MEASURES:

Care of Exposed People. People having direct contact with blood or other secretions from patients with CCHF should be observed closely for 14 days with daily monitoring for fever. Immediate therapy with intravenous ribavirin should be considered at the first sign of disease.

Environmental Immunoprophylaxis. Monitoring of laboratory rat colonies and urban rodent control may be effective for ratborne HFRS.

CCHF. Arachnicides for tick control generally have limited benefit but should be used in stockyard settings. Personal protective measures (eg, physical tick removal and protective clothing with permethrin sprays) may be effective.

RVF. Immunization of domestic animals is important for limiting or preventing RVF outbreaks and protecting humans. Mosquito control usually is not effective.

Public Health Reporting. Because of the risk of nosocomial transmission of CCHF and diagnostic confusion with other viral hemorrhagic fevers, the state health department and the Centers for Disease Control and Prevention should be contacted about any suspected diagnosis of viral hemorrhagic fever and the management plan for the patient.

Hepatitis A

CLINICAL MANIFESTATIONS: Hepatitis A virus (HAV) infection characteristically is an acute, self-limited illness associated with fever, malaise, jaundice, anorexia, and nausea. Symptomatic hepatitis A infection occurs in approximately 30% of infected children younger than 6 years of age; few of these children will have jaundice. Among older children and adults, infection usually is symptomatic and typically lasts several weeks, with jaundice occurring in approximately 70%. Prolonged or relapsing disease lasting as long as 6 months can occur. Fulminant hepatitis is rare but is more common in people with underlying liver disease. Chronic infection does not occur.

ETIOLOGY: Hepatitis A virus is an RNA virus classified as a member of the picornavirus group.

EPIDEMIOLOGY: The most common mode of transmission is person-to-person, resulting from fecal contamination and oral ingestion (ie, the fecal-oral route). Age at infection varies with socioeconomic status and associated living conditions. In developing countries, where infection is endemic, most people are infected during the first decade of life. In the United States, hepatitis A is one of the most commonly reported vaccine-preventable diseases; in 2001, approximately 10 600 clinical cases were reported to the Centers for Disease Control and Prevention (CDC). The highest rates occurred among children 5 to 14 years of age, and the lowest rates occurred among adults older than 40 years of age. During the past several decades, reported cases of hepatitis A infection have had an unequal geographic distribution, with the highest rates of disease occurring in a limited number of states and communities. Although yearly rates in these areas may fluctuate, they consistently remain above the US national average. Continued surveillance is needed to determine whether this decrease is sustained and whether it can be attributed to routine immunization of children in areas with consistently higher rates (see Recommendations for Immunoprophylaxis, p 314).

Among cases of hepatitis A infection reported to the CDC, the identified sources of infection include close personal contact with a person infected with hepatitis A virus, household or personal contact with a child care center, international travel, a recognized foodborne or waterborne outbreak, male homosexual activity, and use of injection drugs. Transmission by blood transfusion or from mother to newborn infant (ie, vertical transmission) is rare. Infection has been contracted rarely from nonhuman primates not born in captivity. In approximately 50% of reported cases, the source cannot be determined. Fecal-oral spread from people with asymptomatic infections, particularly young children, likely accounts for many of these cases with an unknown source.

Most HAV infection and illness occurs in the context of community-wide epidemics, in which infection primarily is transmitted in households and extended family settings. Common-source foodborne outbreaks occur; waterborne outbreaks are rare. Nosocomial transmission is unusual, but outbreaks caused by transmission from hospitalized patients to health care professionals have been reported. In addition, outbreaks have occurred in neonatal intensive care units from neonates infected through transfused blood who subsequently transmitted HAV to other neonates and staff.

In child care centers, recognized symptomatic (icteric) illness occurs primarily among adult contacts of children. Most infected children in child care are asymptomatic or have nonspecific manifestations. Hence, spread of HAV infection within and outside a child care center often occurs before recognition of the index case(s). Outbreaks occur most commonly in large child care centers and those that enroll children in diapers.

In most infected people, the highest titers of HAV in stool, when patients are most likely to transmit HAV, occur during the 1 to 2 weeks before the onset of illness. The risk of transmission subsequently diminishes and is minimal by 1 week after the onset of jaundice. However, HAV can be detected in stool for longer periods, especially in neonates and young children.

The **incubation period** is 15 to 50 days, with an average of 25 to 30 days.

DIAGNOSTIC TESTS: Serologic tests for HAV-specific total and immunoglobulin (Ig) M antibody are available commercially. Serum IgM is present at the onset of illness and usually disappears within 4 months but may persist for 6 months or longer. Presence of serum IgM indicates current or recent infection, although false-positive results can occur. Anti-HAV IgG is detectable shortly after the appearance of IgM. The presence of anti-HAV without IgM anti-HAV indicates past infection and immunity.

TREATMENT: Supportive.

ISOLATION OF THE HOSPITALIZED PATIENT: In addition to standard precautions, contact precautions are recommended for diapered and incontinent patients for 1 week after the onset of symptoms.

CONTROL MEASURES:

General Measures. The major methods for prevention of HAV infections are improved sanitation (eg, of water sources and in food preparation) and personal hygiene (eg, hand hygiene after diaper changes in child care settings), hepatitis A immunization, and administration of Immune Globulin (IG).

Schools, Child Care, and Work. Children and adults with acute HAV infection who work as food handlers or attend or work in child care settings should be excluded for 1 week after onset of the illness.

Immune Globulin. Immune Globulin for intramuscular administration, when given within 2 weeks after exposure to HAV, is greater than 85% effective in preventing symptomatic infection. Recommended preexposure and postexposure IG doses and duration of protection are given in Table 3.13 (p 312) and Table 3.14 (p 313).

Hepatitis A Vaccine. Two inactivated hepatitis A vaccines, Havrix (manufactured by GlaxoSmithKline Biologicals, Rixensart, Belgium) and Vaqta (Merck & Co Inc, West Point, PA), are available in the United States. The vaccines are prepared from cell culture-adapted HAV, which is propagated in human fibroblasts, purified from cell lysates, formalin inactivated, and adsorbed to an aluminum hydroxide adjuvant. Havrix is formulated with the preservative 2-phenoxyethanol; Vaqta is formulated without a preservative.

Administration, Dosages, and Schedules (see Table 3.15, p 314). Both hepatitis A vaccines are approved for people 2 years of age and older and have pediatric and adult formulations that are given in a 2-dose schedule. The adult formulations are recommended for people 19 years of age and older. Currently licensed vaccines are given intramuscularly. Recommended doses and schedules for these different products and formulations are given in Table 3.15 (p 314). A combination hepatitis A/hepatitis B vaccine (Twinrix, GlaxoSmithKline Biologicals, Rixensart, Belgium) is approved in the United States for people 18 years of age and older and given in a 3-dose schedule.

Detection of Anti-HAV After Immunization. The concentrations of anti-HAV resulting from hepatitis A immunization are 10- to 100-fold lower than those produced after natural infection and may be below the detection concentration of commercially available assays. The lower concentrations of antibody induced by single dose immunization can be measured by modified immunoassays, expressed as

Table 3.13. **Recommendations for Preexposure Immunoprophylaxis of Hepatitis A for Travelers**

Age, y	Likely Exposure Duration, mo	Recommended Prophylaxis
<2	<3	IG, 0.02 mL/kg[1]
	3–5	IG, 0.06 mL/kg[1]
	Long-term	IG, 0.06 mL/kg at departure and every 5 mo if exposure to HAV continues[1]
≥2	<3[2]	Hepatitis A vaccine[3,4] **OR** IG, 0.02 mL/kg[1]
	3–5[2]	Hepatitis A vaccine[3,4] **OR** IG, 0.06 mL/kg[1]
	Long-term	Hepatitis A vaccine[3,4]

IG indicates Immune Globulin; HAV, hepatitis A virus.

[1] Immune Globulin should be administered deep into a large muscle mass. Ordinarily, no more than 5 mL should be administered in 1 site in an adult or large child; lesser amounts (maximum 3 mL) should be given to small children and infants.

[2] Vaccine is preferable, but IG is an acceptable alternative.

[3] To ensure protection in travelers whose departure is imminent, IG also may be given (see text).

[4] Dose and schedule of hepatitis A vaccine as recommended according to age in Table 3.15, p 314.

mIU/mL. Antibody concentrations after the booster dose usually can be detected by the standard commercial antibody test. The lower limit of antibody needed to confer immunity has not been defined. In most studies conducted with Havrix, concentrations of 20 mIU/mL or greater as measured with a modified enzyme immunoassay were considered to be protective; studies with Vaqta have been based on concentrations of greater than 10 mIU/mL, measured using a modified radioimmunoassay.

Immunoglobulin M Anti-HAV After Immunization. Immunoglobulin M anti-HAV occasionally is detectable by standard assays in adults 2 weeks after receiving hepatitis A vaccine. No data are available for children at 2 weeks after immunization; in 1 study, none had detectable IgM anti-HAV one month after immunization.

Immunogenicity. The different vaccine formulations are similarly immunogenic when given in their respective recommended schedules and doses. One dose of Havrix induced seroconversion by 15 days in 88% to 93% of children, adolescents, and adults and by 1 month in 95% to 99%; 1 month after a second dose, which was administered 6 months after the first dose, 100% had protective serum antibody concentrations with high geometric mean titers. Similar results were achieved with Vaqta. One month after the first dose of vaccine, 95% to 100% of children, adolescents, and adults had protective concentrations of antibody. One month after a second dose, which was administered 6 months after the first dose, 100% had seroconverted.

Limited data on immunogenicity of hepatitis A vaccine in infants indicate high rates of seroconversion, but the geometric mean serum antibody titers are signifi-

Table 3.14. Recommendations for Postexposure Immunoprophylaxis of Hepatitis A

Time Since Exposure, wk	Future Exposure Likely, or Immunization Recommended	Age of Patient, y	Recommended Prophylaxis
≤2	No	All ages	IG, 0.02 mL/kg[1]
	Yes	≥2	IG, 0.02 mL/kg[1] **AND** Hepatitis A vaccine[2]
>2	No	All ages	No prophylaxis
	Yes	≥2	Hepatitis A vaccine[2]

IG indicates Immune Globulin.

1 Immune Globulin should be administered deep into a large muscle mass. Ordinarily, no more than 5 mL should be administered in 1 site in an adult or large child; lesser amounts (maximum 3 mL) should be given to small children and infants.

2 Dosage and schedule of hepatitis A vaccine as recommended according to age in Table 3.15, p 314.

cantly less in infants with passively acquired maternal anti-HAV in comparison with vaccine recipients lacking anti-HAV. Further studies of the immunogenicity of hepatitis A vaccine in infants are in progress.

Efficacy. In double-blind, controlled, randomized trials, the protective efficacy in preventing clinical hepatitis A infection was 94% to 100%.

Duration of Protection. The need for booster doses cannot be determined, because long-term efficacy of hepatitis A vaccines has not been established. Detectable antibody, however, persists after a 2-dose series for at least 8 years in adults and 5 years in children. Kinetic models suggest that protective antibody concentrations will persist for at least 20 years.

Vaccine in Immunocompromised Patients. The immune response in immunocompromised people, including people with human immunodeficiency virus, may be suboptimal.

Effect of IG on Vaccine Immunogenicity. Seroconversion rates are not impaired by simultaneous administration of IG with the first vaccine dose, but lower serum antibody concentrations may be achieved. This decreased immunogenicity is not likely to be clinically important. If rapid protection is needed (ie, in <2 weeks) after the first dose of vaccine, concomitant administration of IG is indicated.

Vaccine Interchangeability. Vaqta and Havrix, when given as recommended, seem to be similarly effective. Studies among adults have found no difference in the immunogenicity of a vaccine series that mixed the 2 currently available vaccines, compared with using the same vaccine throughout the licensed schedule. Therefore, although completion of the immunization regimen with the same product is preferable, immunization with either product is acceptable.

Administration With Other Vaccines. Limited data from studies among adults indicate that hepatitis A vaccine may be administered simultaneously with other vaccines. Vaccines should be given in a separate syringe and at a separate site (see Simultaneous Administration of Multiple Vaccines, p 33).

Table 3.15. **Recommended Doses and Schedules for Inactivated Hepatitis A Vaccines**[1]

Age, y	Vaccine	Hepatitis A Antigen Dose	Volume per Dose, mL	No. of Doses	Schedule
2–18	Havrix	720 ELU	0.5	2	Initial and 6–12 mo later
2–18	Vaqta	25 U[2]	0.5	2	Initial and 6–18 mo later
≥19	Havrix	1440 ELU	1.0	2	Initial and 6–12 mo later
≥19	Vaqta	50 U[2]	1.0	2	Initial and 6–12 mo later
≥18	Twinrix[3]	720 ELU	1.0	3	Initial and 1 and 6 mo later

ELU indicates enzyme-linked immunoassay units.

[1] Havrix and Twinrix are manufactured by GlaxoSmithKline Biologicals, Rixenart, Belgium; Vaqta is manufactured and distributed by Merck & Co Inc, West Point, PA.

[2] Antigen units (each unit is equivalent to approximately 1 µg of viral protein).

[3] A combination of hepatitis B (Engerix-B, 20 µg) and hepatitis A (Havrix, 720 ELU) vaccine (Twinrix) is licensed for use in people 18 years of age and older in a 3-dose schedule.

Adverse Events. Adverse reactions are mild and include local pain and, less commonly, induration at the injection site. No serious adverse events attributed definitively to hepatitis A vaccine have been reported.

Precautions and Contraindications. The vaccine should not be administered to people with hypersensitivity to any of the vaccine components. Safety data in pregnant women are not available, but the risk is considered to be low or nonexistent, because the vaccine contains inactivated, purified, viral proteins.

Preimmunization Serologic Testing. Preimmunization testing for anti-HAV generally is not recommended for children. Testing may be cost-effective for people who have a high likelihood of immunity from previous infection, including people whose early childhood was spent in an area of high endemicity, people with a history of jaundice potentially caused by HAV, and people older than 40 years of age.

Postimmunization Serologic Testing. Postimmunization testing for anti-HAV is not indicated because of the high seroconversion rates in adults and children. In addition, commercially available anti-HAV tests may not detect low but protective concentrations of antibody induced by the first dose of vaccine.

RECOMMENDATIONS FOR IMMUNOPROPHYLAXIS:

Preexposure Prophylaxis (see Table 3.13, p 312).

Foreign Travel. For susceptible people traveling to or working in areas with intermediate or high endemic rates of HAV infection, immunoprophylaxis before departure is indicated. Such areas include countries other than those in western Europe and Scandinavia and Australia, Canada, Japan, and New Zealand. Factors to consider in choosing active and/or passive prophylaxis include the interval before departure, the relative costs and availability of IG and HAV vaccine, the duration of the stay, and the likelihood of repeated exposure during subsequent travel (see Table 3.13, p 312). Regardless of these factors, for people 2 years of age and older, vaccine is always the preference over IG unless there is a specific contraindication.

Immune globulin is considered protective against hepatitis A immediately after administration, whereas the precise time required from receiving 1 dose of vaccine to onset of protection has not been established but likely requires 2 to 4 weeks. To ensure protection in travelers whose departure is imminent, both IG (see Table 3.13, p 312) and the first dose of vaccine (see Effect of IG on Vaccine Immunogenicity, p 313) can be administered simultaneously. However, the additional benefit of administration of IG with the first dose of vaccine has not been evaluated in field trials and may be marginal.

Children younger than 2 years of age should receive only IG, because vaccine is not yet approved for this age group (see Table 3.13, p 312).

Other Indications for Immunization. Hepatitis A immunization is recommended routinely for the following:

- *Children living in US communities with consistently high hepatitis A rates.* Areas with consistently high rates of hepatitis A can be considered to include states, counties, and communities in which the average annual reported hepatitis A incidence during 1987–1997 was equal to or greater than twice the national average, which is approximately 10 cases per 100 000 population. States in this category include Arizona, Alaska, Oregon, New Mexico, Utah, Washington, Oklahoma, South Dakota, Idaho, Nevada, and California. Routine immunization of children living in these areas is recommended to achieve a sustained decrease in HAV infection incidence. In addition, routine immunization can be considered for children living in states, counties, and communities where reported hepatitis A rates were less than twice but at least at the national average during this time (eg, >10 but <20 cases per 100 000 population). These states include Missouri, Texas, Colorado, Arkansas, Montana, and Wyoming. Hepatitis A vaccine is licensed only for children 2 years of age and older. In addition, hepatitis A immunization programs can be considered to control ongoing community-wide epidemics. However, in general, available data suggest the effect of such programs may be limited, and efforts might be better focused on ongoing routine immunization to prevent future epidemics.

  Widespread use of IG during community-wide epidemics, other than for contacts of hepatitis A cases, generally has not been effective, because unrecognized transmission is common and protection is of limited duration.

- *People with chronic liver disease.* Because people with chronic liver disease are at increased risk of fulminant hepatitis A, susceptible patients with chronic liver disease should be immunized. The reported incidence of adverse events after hepatitis A immunization of people with chronic liver disease has not been higher than that reported among healthy adults.

- *Homosexual and bisexual men.* Hepatitis A outbreaks among men who have sex with men have been reported often, including in urban areas in the United States, Canada, and Australia. Therefore, men (adolescents and adults) who have sex with men should be immunized. Preimmunization serologic testing may be warranted for older people in this group.

- *Users of injection and noninjection illegal drugs.* Periodic outbreaks among injection and noninjection drug users have been reported during the past decade in many parts of the United States and in Europe. Adolescents and adults who use illegal drugs should be immunized. Preimmunization serologic testing may be cost-effective for older people in this group.
- *Patients with clotting-factor disorders.* Reported outbreaks of hepatitis A in patients with hemophilia receiving solvent-detergent-treated factor VIII and factor IX concentrates have occurred primarily in Europe, but one instance in the United States has been reported. Therefore, susceptible patients who receive clotting factor concentrates, especially those receiving solvent-detergent-treated preparations, should be immunized. Preimmunization testing for anti-HAV may be cost-effective.
- *People at risk of occupational exposure (eg, handlers of nonhuman primates and people working with HAV in a research laboratory setting).* Outbreaks of hepatitis A have been reported among people working with nonhuman primates that are susceptible to hepatitis A infection. Infected primates were those born in the wild, not those that had been born and raised in captivity.

Hepatitis A Immunization in Other Settings.

- *Child care center staff and attendees.* Hepatitis A outbreaks at child care centers may be the source of outbreaks in a community, but disease in child care centers more commonly reflects extended transmission from the community. In addition to the recommended postexposure prophylaxis (see p 314), hepatitis A immunization of children 2 years of age and older can be considered in child care settings with ongoing or recurrent outbreaks, especially in communities where routine immunization of children is recommended. In the absence of ongoing outbreaks, immunization in child care centers also can be used to implement routine hepatitis A immunization, particularly in communities where cases in the child care centers contribute substantially to the total number of hepatitis A cases and seem to have a role in sustaining community-wide outbreaks.
- *Custodial care institutions.* Epidemic hepatitis A was reported in custodial care institutions during the 1970s and 1980s, but few cases have been reported recently. However, hepatitis A vaccine, in addition to IG as indicated for postexposure prophylaxis (see p 314), may be considered for staff and residents in institutions in which a hepatitis A outbreak is occurring.
- *Hospital personnel.* Usually, nosocomial hepatitis A in hospital personnel has occurred through spread from patients with acute infection in whom the diagnosis of HAV infection was not recognized. Careful hygienic practices should be emphasized when a patient with hepatitis A infection is admitted to the hospital. When outbreaks occur, IG is recommended for people in close contact with infected patients (see p 318). The role of hepatitis A vaccine in these settings has not been studied. Routine preexposure use of hepatitis A vaccine for hospital personnel is not recommended.

- **Food handlers.** Recognized foodborne outbreaks of hepatitis A are relatively uncommon in the United States and usually are associated with contamination of uncooked food during preparation by a food handler who is infected with HAV. The most important means of preventing these outbreaks is using careful hygienic practices during food preparation. Routine hepatitis A immunization of food handlers is not recommended.
- **Other.** In addition, any healthy person 2 years of age and older may receive hepatitis A vaccine at the discretion of the physician and the patient or patient's family.

Postexposure Prophylaxis (see Table 3.14, p 313). Use of IG is recommended as follows (see Table 3.14 for dosages):

- **Household and sexual contacts.** All previously unimmunized people with close personal contact with a hepatitis A case, such as household and sexual contacts, should receive IG within 2 weeks after most recent exposure. Serologic testing of contacts is not recommended, because testing adds unnecessary cost and may delay administration of IG. The use of IG more than 2 weeks after the most recent exposure is not indicated.
- **Newborn infants of HAV-infected mothers.** Perinatal transmission of HAV is rare. Some experts advise giving IG (0.02 mL/kg) to the infant if the mother's symptoms began between 2 weeks before and 1 week after delivery. Efficacy in this circumstance has not been established. Severe disease in healthy infants is rare.
- **Child care center staff, employees, children, and their household contacts.** Serologic testing to confirm HAV infection in suspected cases is indicated. When hepatitis A infection is identified in an employee or child enrolled in a center in which all children are toilet trained, IG is recommended for previously unimmunized employees in contact with the index case and for unimmunized children in the same room as the index case.

  When HAV infection is identified in an employee or a child or in the household contacts of 2 or more of the enrolled children in a child care center in which children are not toilet trained, IG is recommended for all previously unimmunized employees and children in the facility. During the 6 weeks after the last case is identified, unimmunized new employees and children also should receive IG.

  Hepatitis A vaccine can be given with IG to previously unimmunized children if routine immunization is recommended for children in the community (see p 35).

  If recognition of a hepatitis A outbreak in a child care center is delayed by 3 or more weeks from the onset of the index case or if illness has occurred in 3 or more families, the infection is likely to have already spread widely. In these circumstances, IG also should be considered for household members of center attendees.

  Children and adults with acute HAV infection should be excluded from the center until 1 week after onset of the illness, until the IG prophylaxis program has been completed, or until directed by the responsible health department. Although precise data concerning the onset of protection after a dose of IG are not available, allowing IG recipients to return to the child care center setting immediately after receipt of the IG dose seems reasonable.

- **Schools.** Schoolroom exposure generally does not pose an appreciable risk of infection, and IG administration is not indicated when a single case occurs. However, IG could be used if transmission within the school setting is documented. Hepatitis A vaccine can be given in addition to IG if routine immunization of children in the community is recommended.

- **Institutions and hospitals.** In institutions for custodial care with an outbreak of HAV infection, residents and staff in close personal contact with infected patients should receive IG. Administration of IG to hospital personnel caring for patients with hepatitis A is not indicated routinely, unless an outbreak among patients or between patients and staff is documented. The addition of hepatitis A vaccine can be considered if repeated exposure is anticipated.

- **Common-source exposure.** These outbreaks often are recognized too late for IG to be effective in preventing hepatitis A in exposed people, and IG administration usually is not recommended. Immune Globulin can be considered if it can be administered to exposed people within 2 weeks of the last exposure to the HAV-contaminated water or food.

- **Hepatitis A vaccine for postexposure prophylaxis.** Available data are insufficient to recommend hepatitis A vaccine alone for postexposure prophylaxis. Clinical trials are needed to determine the effectiveness of hepatitis A vaccine compared with IG after exposure.

Hepatitis B

CLINICAL MANIFESTATIONS: People with hepatitis B virus (HBV) infection may present with a variety of signs and symptoms, including subacute illness with nonspecific symptoms (eg, anorexia, nausea, or malaise), clinical hepatitis with jaundice, and fulminant fatal hepatitis. Asymptomatic seroconversion is common, and the likelihood of developing symptoms of hepatitis is age dependent. Anicteric or asymptomatic infection is most common in young children. Extrahepatic manifestations, such as arthralgias, arthritis, macular rashes, thrombocytopenia, or papular acrodermatitis (Gianotti-Crosti syndrome), can occur early in the course of the illness and may precede jaundice. Acute hepatitis B cannot be distinguished from other forms of acute viral hepatitis on the basis of clinical signs and symptoms or nonspecific laboratory findings. Chronic HBV infection is defined as the presence of hepatitis B surface antigen (HBsAg) in serum for at least 6 months or by the presence of HBsAg in a person who tests negative for antibody of the immunoglobulin (Ig) M subclass to hepatitis B core antigen (anti-HBc).

Age at the time of acute infection is the primary determinant of the risk of progressing to chronic infection. More than 90% of infants infected perinatally will develop chronic HBV infection. Between 25% and 50% of children infected between 1 and 5 years of age become chronically infected, whereas only 6% to 10% of acutely infected older children and adults develop chronic HBV infections. Patients who develop acute HBV infection while immunosuppressed or with an underlying chronic illness have an increased risk of developing chronic infection. Up to 25% of infants and older children who acquire chronic HBV infection will eventually develop HBV-related hepatocellular carcinoma or cirrhosis.

The clinical outcome of untreated chronic HBV infection varies according to the population studied, reflecting differences in the age of acquisition, the rate of loss of hepatitis B e antigen (HBeAg), and possibly, patient genotype. Perinatally infected children usually have normal alanine transaminase (ALT) concentrations and minimal or mild liver histologic changes for years to decades after initial infection ("tolerant phase"). Chronic HBV infection acquired during later childhood or adolescence usually is accompanied by more active liver disease and increased serum transaminase concentrations. Patients with detectable HBeAg *(HBeAg-positive chronic hepatitis B)* usually have high blood concentrations of HBV DNA and HBsAg and are more likely to transmit infection. Seroconversion to presence of antibody to HBeAg (anti-HBe) is accompanied by decreases in serum HBV DNA and serum transaminase concentrations and may be preceded by a temporary exacerbation of liver disease. Serologic reversion (reappearance of HBeAg) is common if loss of HBeAg is not accompanied by development of anti-HBe; reversion with loss of anti-HBe also can occur.

Over time, some patients develop an *inactive chronic HBV infection* in which HBsAg is present, HBV DNA concentrations decrease, HBeAg disappears, and anti-HBe may appear. Patients with the inactive chronic infection still may have exacerbations of hepatitis. Some patients who lose HBeAg may continue to have ongoing histologic evidence of liver damage and moderate to high concentrations of HBV DNA *(HBeAg-negative chronic hepatitis B)*. In general, patients with histologic evidence of chronic hepatitis B, regardless of HBeAg status, remain at higher risk of death attributable to liver failure compared with HBV-infected people with no histologic evidence of liver inflammation and fibrosis. Other factors that may influence natural history of chronic infection include gender, race, alcohol use, and coinfection with hepatitis A, hepatitis C, or hepatitis D viruses.

Resolved hepatitis B is defined as the clearance of HBsAg and normalization of serum transaminase concentrations; development of antibody to HBsAg (anti-HBs) also may be noted. Chronically infected adults clear HBsAg and develop anti-HBs at the rate of 1% to 2% annually; during childhood, the annual clearance rate is less than 1%. Reactivation of resolved chronic infection is possible with immunosuppression.

ETIOLOGY: Hepatitis B virus is a DNA-containing, 42-nm-diamter hepadnavirus. Important components of the viral particle include HBsAg, hepatitis B core antigen, and HBeAg. Antibody to HBsAg (anti-HBs) provides protection from HBV infection.

EPIDEMIOLOGY: Hepatitis B virus is transmitted through blood or body fluids, including wound exudates, semen, cervical secretions, and saliva. Blood and serum contain the highest concentrations of virus; saliva contains the lowest. People with chronic HBV infection are the primary reservoirs for infection. Common modes of transmission include percutaneous and permucosal exposure to infectious body fluids, sharing or using nonsterilized needles or syringes, sexual contact with an infected person, and perinatal exposure to an infected mother. Transmission by transfusion of contaminated blood or blood products now is rare in the United States because of routine screening of blood donors and viral inactivation of certain blood products (see Blood Safety, p 106). Person-to-person spread of HBV can occur in settings involving interpersonal contact over extended periods, such as when a person with chronic HBV infection resides in a household. In household settings, nonsexual transmission occurs primarily from child to child, and young children are at highest risk of infection. The precise mechanisms of transmission from child to child are unknown; however, frequent interpersonal contact of nonintact skin or mucous membranes with blood-containing secretions or, perhaps, saliva are the most likely means of transmission. Transmission from sharing inanimate objects, such as wash cloths, towels, razors, or toothbrushes, also may occur. Hepatitis B virus can survive in the environment for 1 week or longer but is inactivated by commonly used disinfectants, including household bleach diluted 1:10 with water. Hepatitis B virus is not transmitted by the fecal-oral route.

Perinatal transmission of HBV is highly efficient and usually occurs from blood exposures during labor and delivery. In utero transmission of HBV is rare, accounting for <2% of perinatal infections in most studies. The risk of an infant acquiring HBV from an infected mother is 70% to 90% for infants born to mothers who are HBsAg and HBeAg positive; the risk is 5% to 20% for infants born to HBeAg-negative mothers.

Multiple studies have documented high rates of early childhood (nonperinatal) HBV transmission in the United States. During the 1980s, before implementation of routine childhood hepatitis B immunization, an estimated 16 000 children (younger than 10 years of age) were infected each year. The highest risk of early childhood transmission is among children who immigrated to the United States from countries where HBV infection is highly endemic (eg, Southeast Asia, China).

Other young children at risk of infection include: (1) household contacts of people with chronic HBV infection; (2) residents of institutions for the developmentally disabled; (3) patients undergoing hemodialysis; and (4) patients with clotting disorders and others repeatedly receiving blood products. In child care facilities in the United States, the risk of transmission has become negligible as a result of infant hepatitis B vaccine coverage. Although fewer than 10% of new HBV infections occur in children, approximately one third of the estimated 1.25 million Americans with chronic HBV infection acquired infection as infants or young children.

Acute HBV infection occurs most commonly among adolescents and adults in the United States. Groups at highest risk include users of injection drugs, people with multiple heterosexual partners, and young men who have sex with men. Others at increased risk include people with occupational exposure to blood or body fluids, staff of institutions and nonresidential child care programs for the developmentally disabled, patients undergoing hemodialysis, and sexual or household contacts of people with an acute or chronic infection. Approximately one third of infected people do not have a readily identifiable risk factor. The prevalence of infection among adolescents and adults is 3 to 4 times greater for black individuals than for white individuals. Hepatitis B virus infection in adolescents and adults is associated with other sexually transmitted diseases, including syphilis and infection with human immunodeficiency virus (HIV).

The frequency of HBV infection and patterns of transmission vary markedly throughout the world. Most areas of the United States, Canada, western Europe, Australia, and southern South America have a low endemicity of HBV infection. Infection occurs primarily in adolescents and adults; 5% to 8% of the total population has been infected, and 0.2% to 0.9% of the population has chronic infection. However, within these geographic areas are populations with a high endemicity of infection, including Alaska Natives, Asian-Pacific Islanders, and immigrants from endemic countries. Hepatitis B virus infection is highly endemic in China, Southeast Asia, eastern Europe, the Central Asian republics of the former Soviet Union, most of the Middle East, Africa, the Amazon Basin, and the Pacific Islands. In these areas, most infections occur in infants or children younger than 5 years of age; 70% to 90% of the adult population has been infected, and 8% to 15% of the population has chronic infection. In the rest of the world, HBV infection is of intermediate endemicity, with chronic HBV infection occurring in 2% to 7% of the population.

The **incubation period** for acute infection is 45 to 160 days, with an average of 90 days.

DIAGNOSTIC TESTS: Commercial serologic antigen tests are available to detect HBsAg and HBeAg. Assays also are available for detection of antibody to HBsAg (anti-HBs), total antibody to hepatitis B core antigen (anti-HBc), IgM anti-HBc, and antibody to HBeAg (see Table 3.16, p 322). In addition, hybridization assays and gene amplification techniques (eg, polymerase chain reaction, branched DNA methods) are available to detect and quantitate HBV DNA. Hepatitis B surface antigen is detectable during acute infection. If the infection is self-limited, HBsAg disappears in most patients before serum anti-HBs can be detected (termed the *window phase* of infection). The IgM anti-HBc is highly specific for establishing the diagnosis of acute infection, because it is present early in the infection and during the window phase in older children and adults. However, IgM anti-HBc usually is not present in infants infected perinatally. People with chronic HBV infection have circulating HBsAg and anti-HBc; on rare occasions, anti-HBs also is present. Both anti-HBs and anti-HBc are detected in people with resolved infection, whereas anti-HBs alone is present in people immunized with hepatitis B vaccine. The presence of HBeAg in serum correlates with higher titers of HBV and greater infectivity. Tests for HBeAg and HBV DNA are useful in the selection of candidates to receive antiviral therapy and to monitor the response to therapy.

TREATMENT: No specific therapy for acute HBV infection is available. Hepatitis B Immune Globulin (HBIG) and corticosteroids are not effective. From 25% to 40% of adults with chronic HBV infection and liver disease achieve long-term remission (loss of detectable HBV DNA or loss of HBeAg) after treatment with interferon-alfa. This remission rate is approximately 20% higher than the spontaneous remission rate observed in untreated controls. Adult patients who clear HBeAg have decreases in rates of mortality and clinical complications of cirrhosis. Less data are available for treatment of children, but several studies indicate that approximately 30% of children with increased transaminase concentrations who are treated with interferon alfa-2b for 6 months lose HBeAg, compared with approximately 10% of untreated controls. Interferon-alfa is less effective for chronic infections acquired during early

Table 3.16. **Diagnostic Tests for Hepatitis B Virus (HBV) Antigens and Antibodies**

Factor To Be Tested	Hepatitis B Virus Antigen or Antibody	Use
HBsAg	Hepatitis B surface antigen	Detection of acutely or chronically infected people; antigen used in hepatitis B vaccine
Anti-HBs	Antibody to HBsAg	Identification of people who have resolved infections with HBV; determination of immunity after immunization
HBeAg	Hepatitis B e antigen	Identification of infected people at increased risk of transmitting HBV
Anti-HBe	Antibody to HBe	Identification of infected people with lower risk of transmitting HBV
Anti-HBc	Antibody to HBcAg[1]	Identification of people with acute, resolved, or chronic HBV infection (not present after immunization)
IgM anti-HBc	IgM antibody to HBcAg	Identification of people with acute or recent HBV infections (including HBsAg-negative people during the "window" phase of infection)

Ig indicates immunoglobulin.
[1] No test is available commercially to measure hepatitis B core antigen (HBcAg).

childhood, especially if transaminase concentrations are normal. Lamivudine is licensed for treatment of chronic HBV infection in people 2 years of age and older. Children with chronic hepatitis B infection who were treated with lamivudine had higher rates of virologic response (loss of detectable HBV DNA and loss of HBeAg) after 1 year of treatment than did those who received placebo (23% vs 13%). The FDA has licensed adefovir dipivoxil for treatment of chronic HBV infection in adults, but safety and effectiveness for children has not been established.

Children and adolescents who have chronic HBV infection are at risk of developing serious liver disease, including primary hepatocellular carcinoma (HCC), with advancing age. Although the peak incidence of primary HCC is in the fifth decade of life, HCC occasionally occurs in children who become infected perinatally or in early childhood. The primary risk factor for serious liver disease is acquisition of chronic infection at birth or during early childhood. Children with chronic HBV infection should be screened periodically for hepatic complications using serum liver transaminase tests, α-fetoprotein concentration, and abdominal ultrasonography. Definitive recommendations on the frequency and indications for specific tests are not yet available because of a lack of data on reliability in predicting sequelae. Patients with persistently increased serum ALT concentrations (exceeding twice the upper limits of normal) and patients with an increased serum α-fetoprotein concentration or abnormal findings on abdominal ultrasonography should be referred to a gastroenterologist for further management. All patients with chronic hepatitis B infection who are not immune to hepatitis A should receive hepatitis A vaccine.

ISOLATION OF THE HOSPITALIZED PATIENT: Standard precautions are indicated for patients with acute or chronic HBV infection.

For infants born to HBsAg-positive mothers, no special care other than removal of maternal blood by a gloved attendant and standard precautions is necessary.

CONTROL MEASURES:

Strategy for Prevention of HBV

The primary goal of HBV prevention programs is decreasing the rates of chronic HBV infection and HBV-related chronic liver disease. A secondary goal is the prevention of acute hepatitis B infection. Over the past 2 decades, a comprehensive immunization strategy in the United States has been developed that includes the following 4 components: (1) immunization of infants, children, adolescents, and adults at increased risk of infection (1982); (2) prevention of perinatal HBV infection through routine screening of all pregnant women and appropriate treatment of children born to HBsAg-positive women (1988); (3) routine immunization of infants (1992); and (4) routine immunization of adolescents who previously have not been immunized (1995).

Hepatitis B Immunoprophylaxis. Two types of products are available for immunoprophylaxis. Hepatitis B Immune Globulin provides short-term protection (3–6 months) and is indicated only in specific postexposure circumstances (see Care of Exposed People, p 331). Hepatitis B vaccine is used for preexposure and postexposure protection and provides long-term protection. Preexposure immunization with hepatitis B vaccine is the most effective means to prevent HBV transmission. To decrease the rate of, and eventually eliminate, transmission of HBV as soon as possible, universal immunization is necessary. Accordingly, hepatitis B immunization is recommended for all infants as part of the routine childhood and adolescent immunization schedule, and all children who have not received the vaccine previously should be immunized by or before 11 to 12 years of age. Immunization before 11 years of age (for children not previously immunized) can be advantageous because of better compliance with routine medical visits to complete the 3-dose schedule.

Postexposure immunoprophylaxis with either hepatitis B vaccine and HBIG or hepatitis B vaccine alone effectively prevents infection after exposure to HBV. Serologic testing of all pregnant women for HBsAg is essential for identifying women whose infants will require postexposure immunoprophylaxis beginning at birth (see Care of Exposed People, p 331).

Hepatitis B Immune Globulin. * Hepatitis B Immune Globulin is prepared from hyperimmunized donors whose plasma is known to contain a high concentration of anti-HBs and to be negative for antibodies to HIV and hepatitis C virus (HCV).

---

* Dosages recommended for postexposure prophylaxis are for products licensed in the United States. Because the concentration of anti-HBs in other products may vary, different dosages may be recommended in other countries.

The process used to prepare HBIG inactivates or eliminates HIV and HCV. Standard Immune Globulin is not effective for postexposure prophylaxis against HBV infection, because concentrations of anti-HBs are too low.

Hepatitis B Vaccine

Highly effective and safe hepatitis B vaccines produced by recombinant DNA technology have been licensed in the United States in single-antigen formulations and as components of combination vaccines. Plasma-derived hepatitis B vaccines no longer are available in the United States but are used widely and successfully in other countries. The recombinant vaccines contain 5 to 40 µg of HBsAg protein per mL adsorbed to aluminum hydroxide. All pediatric formulations contain no thimerosal or only trace amounts. Although the concentration of recombinant HBsAg protein differs among vaccine products, rates of seroconversion are equivalent when given to immunocompetent infants, children, adolescents, or young adults in the doses recommended (see Table 3.17, p 325).

Hepatitis B vaccine can be given concurrently with other vaccines (see Simultaneous Administration of Multiple Vaccines, p 33).

Vaccine Interchangeability. The hepatitis B vaccines are interchangeable within an immunization series. The immune response using 1 or 2 doses of a vaccine produced by one manufacturer followed by 1 or more subsequent doses from a different manufacturer is comparable to a full course of immunization with a single product. The interchangeability of the combination diphtheria and tetanus toxoids and acellular pertussis (DTaP), inactivated poliovirus (IPV), and hepatitis B vaccine (Pediarix [GlaxoSmithKline Biologicals, Rixensart, Belgium] with licensed DTaP, IPV, and recombinant hepatitis B vaccines may be limited because of the DTaP component (see Pertussis, p 479).

Routes of Administration. Vaccine is administered intramuscularly in the anterolateral thigh or deltoid area, depending on the age and size of the recipient (see Vaccine Administration, p 17). Administration in the buttocks or intradermally has been associated with decreased immunogenicity and is not recommended. In patients with a bleeding diathesis, the risk of bleeding after intramuscular vaccine injection can be minimized by administration immediately after the patient receives replacement factor, use of a 23-gauge needle (or smaller), and application of direct pressure to the immunization site for at least 2 minutes.

Efficacy and Duration of Protection. Hepatitis B vaccines licensed in the United States have a 90% to 95% efficacy for preventing HBV infection and clinical hepatitis B among susceptible children and adults. Long-term studies of adults and children indicate that immune memory remains intact for 15 years or more and protects against clinical acute infections and chronic HBV infection, even though anti-HBs concentrations may become low or undetectable over time.

Booster Doses. For children and adults with normal immune status, routine booster doses of vaccine are not recommended. For hemodialysis patients and other immunocompromised people at continued risk of infection, the need for booster doses should be assessed by annual anti-HBs testing, and a booster dose should be given when the anti-HBs concentration is less than 10 mIU/mL.

Table 3.17. **Recommended Dosages of Hepatitis B Vaccines**

Patients	Vaccine[1]	
	Recombivax HB[2] Dose, µg (mL)	Engerix-B[3] Dose, µg (mL)
Infants of HBsAg-negative mothers and children and adolescents younger than 20 y of age	5 (0.5)	10 (0.5)
Infants of HBsAg-positive mothers (HBIG [0.5 mL] also is recommended)	5 (0.5)	10 (0.5)
Adults 20 y of age or older	10 (1.0)	20 (1.0)
Patients undergoing dialysis and other immunosuppressed adults	40 (1.0)[4]	40 (2.0)[5]

HBsAg indicates hepatitis B surface antigen; HBIG, Hepatitis B Immune Globulin.

[1] Both vaccines are administered in a 3- or 4-dose schedule; 4 doses may be administered if a birth dose is given and a combination vaccine is used to complete the series. Only single-antigen hepatitis B vaccine can be used for the birth dose. Single-antigen or combination vaccine containing hepatitis B vaccine may be used to complete the series.

[2] Available from Merck & Co Inc, West Point, PA. A 2-dose schedule, administered at 0 mo and then 4 to 6 mo later, is available for adolescents 11 to 15 years of age using the adult dose of Recombivax HB (10 µg). In addition, a combination of hepatitis B (Recombivax, 5 µg) and *Haemophilus influenzae* type b (PRP-OMP) vaccine is licensed for use at 2, 4, and 12 to 15 months of age (Comvax).

[3] Available from GlaxoSmithKline Biologicals, Rixensart, Belgium. The US Food and Drug Administration has licensed this vaccine for use in an optional 4-dose schedule at 0, 1, 2, and 12 mo of age.

a) In addition, a combination of hepatitis B (Engerix-B, 20 µg) and hepatitis A (Havrix, 720 ELU) vaccine (Twinrix) is licensed for use in people 18 years of age and older in a 3-dose schedule administered at 0, 1, and 6 or more months later.

b) Also, a combination of diphtheria and tetanus toxoids and acellular pertussis (DTaP), inactivated poliovirus (IPV), and hepatitis B (Engerix-B 10 µg) is licensed for use in people from 6 weeks through 6 years of age in a 3-dose schedule administered preferably at 2, 4, and 6 months of age (Pediarix [GlaxoSmithKline Biologicals, Rixensart, Belgium]). For additional information, see Pertussis (p 479).

[4] Special formulation for dialysis patients.

[5] Two 1.0-mL doses given in 1 site in a 4-dose schedule at 0, 1, 2, and 6 to 12 mo.

Adverse Reactions. The most commonly reported adverse effects in adults and children are pain at the injection site, reported by 3% to 29% of recipients, and a temperature greater than 37.7°C (99.8°F), reported by 1% to 6%. Anaphylaxis is uncommon, occurring in approximately 1 in 600 000 recipients, according to passive reporting of vaccine adverse events. Large, controlled epidemiologic studies show no association between hepatitis B vaccine and sudden infant death syndrome, diabetes mellitus, or demyelinating disease, including multiple sclerosis.

Immunization During Pregnancy or Lactation. No adverse effect on the developing fetus has been observed when pregnant women have been immunized. Because HBV infection may result in severe disease in the mother and chronic infection in the newborn, pregnancy is not a contraindication to immunization. Lactation is not a contraindication.

Serologic Testing. Susceptibility testing before immunization is not indicated routinely for children or adolescents. Testing for previous infection may be considered for people in risk groups with high rates of HBV infection, such as users of injection drugs, homosexually or bisexually active men, and household contacts of HBsAg-positive people, provided testing does not delay or impede immunization efforts.

Routine postimmunization testing for anti-HBs is not necessary, but is recommended 1 to 2 months after the third vaccine dose for the following specific groups: (1) hemodialysis patients; (2) people with HIV infection; (3) people at occupational risk of exposure from sharps injuries; (4) immunocompromised patients at risk of exposure to HBV; and (5) regular sexual contacts of HBsAg-positive people. In addition, infants born to HBsAg-positive mothers should be tested for HBsAg and anti-HBs at 9 to 15 months of age. Some experts prefer to perform serologic testing 1 to 3 months after completion of the primary series (see Prevention of Perinatal HBV Infection, p 331).

Management of Nonresponders. Vaccine recipients who do not develop a serum anti-HBs response ($\geq$10 mIU/mL) after a primary vaccine series should be reimmunized (unless they are determined to be HBsAg positive) with an additional 3-dose series. People who remain anti-HBs negative after a reimmunization series are unlikely to respond to additional doses of vaccine.

Altered Doses and Schedules. Larger vaccine doses, an increased number of doses, or both may be required to induce protective anti-HBs concentrations in adult hemodialysis patients (Table 3.17, p 325). Additional or larger doses also may be necessary for immunocompromised people, including HIV-seropositive people. However, few data exist for adults, and no data exist for children concerning the response to higher doses of vaccine in these patients, and no specific recommendations can be made. For children with progressive chronic renal failure, hepatitis B vaccine is recommended early in the disease course to provide protection and potentially decrease the need for larger doses once dialysis is initiated. A 2-dose schedule for one vaccine formulation is licensed for 11- to 15-year-olds; the first dose is followed 4 to 6 months later by the second dose.

Preexposure Universal Immunization. Routine preexposure immunization is recommended for all infants. The first dose should be given soon after birth and before hospital discharge. The first dose also may be given by 2 months of age, but only if the infant's mother is HBsAg negative. The hepatitis B vaccine series (3 or 4 doses, see discussion about birth dose, below) for infants born to HBsAg-negative mothers should be completed by 6 to 18 months of age. All children and adolescents who have not been immunized against hepatitis B should begin the series during any visit.

High seroconversion rates and protective concentrations of anti-HBs ($\geq$10 mIU/mL) are achieved when hepatitis B vaccine is administered in any of the various 3- and 4-dose schedules, including those begun soon after birth in term infants. Only single-antigen hepatitis B vaccine can be used for doses given between birth and 6 weeks of age. Single-antigen or combination vaccine may be used to complete the series; 4 doses of vaccine may be administered if a birth dose is given and a combination vaccine containing a hepatitis B component is used to complete the series.* For

---

* Centers for Disease Control and Prevention. Combination vaccines for childhood immunization. Recommendations of the Advisory Committee on Immunization Practices (ACIP), the American Academy of Pediatrics (AAP), and the American Academy of Family Physicians (AAFP). *MMWR Recomm Rep.* 1999;48(RR-05):1–15

guidelines for minimum scheduling time between vaccine doses for infants, see Table 1.7 (p 29). The choice of schedule should be used to facilitate high rates of compliance with the 3- or 4-dose primary vaccine series. For immunization of older children and adolescents, doses may be given in a schedule of 0, 1, and 6 months or of 0, 2, and 4 months; for adolescents, spacing at 0, 12, and 24 months results in equivalent immunogenicity. A 2-dose schedule for one vaccine formulation is licensed for 11- to 15-year-olds; the schedule is 0 and 4 to 6 months.

The recommended schedule for routine hepatitis B immunization of infants born to HBsAg-negative mothers is given in Fig 1.1 (p 24). Age-specific vaccine dosages are given in Table 3.17 (p 325). Combination products containing hepatitis B vaccine may be given in the United States, provided they are approved by the US Food and Drug Administration for the child's current age, and administration of the other vaccine component(s) also is indicated.

Lapsed Immunizations. For infants with lapsed immunizations (ie, the interval between doses is longer than that in one of the recommended schedules), the 3-dose series can be completed, regardless of the interval from the last dose of vaccine (see Lapsed Immunizations, p 33).

SPECIAL CONSIDERATIONS:

Preterm Infants. Studies demonstrate that decreased seroconversion rates might occur among certain preterm infants with low birth weight (ie, <2000 g) after administration of hepatitis B vaccine at birth. However, by the chronologic age of 1 month, all medically stable preterm infants (see Preterm and Low Birth Weight Infants, p 66), regardless of initial birth weight or gestational age, are as likely to respond to hepatitis B immunization as are older and larger infants. All preterm infants who are born to an HBsAg-positive mother should receive immunoprophylaxis with hepatitis B vaccine and HBIG within 12 hours after birth, followed by the remaining doses in the series and postimmunization testing appropriate for term infants (see Table 3.18, p 328). If the preterm infant born to an HBsAg-positive mother weighs less than 2000 g at birth, the birth dose of hepatitis B vaccine should not be counted toward completion of the hepatitis B vaccine series, and 3 doses of hepatitis B vaccine should be administered beginning when the infant is 1 month of age (see Table 3.18, p 328). Only monovalent hepatitis B vaccines should be used from birth to 6 weeks of age.

If the maternal HBsAg status is unknown at birth, the preterm infant should receive hepatitis B vaccine within 12 hours of birth. For preterm infants weighing greater than 2000 g at birth, the mother's HBsAg status should be determined as quickly as possible and if positive, HBIG should be given as soon as possible, but within 7 days of birth, at a separate site from the hepatitis B vaccine. If the infant's birth weight is less than 2000 g and the maternal HBsAg status cannot be determined within 12 hours of life, HBIG should be given, because the less reliable immune response in preterm infants weighing <2000 g precludes the option of the 7-day waiting period acceptable for term and larger preterm infants. Only monovalent hepatitis B vaccine should be used from birth to 6 weeks of life.

Table 3.18. Hepatitis B Immunoprophylaxis Scheme for Preterm and Low Birth Weight Infants[1]

Maternal Status	Infant ≥2000 g	Infant <2000 g
HBsAg positive	Hepatitis B vaccine + HBIG (within 12 h of birth)	Hepatitis B vaccine + HBIG (within 12 h of birth)
	Immunize with 3 vaccine doses at 0, 1, and 6 mo of chronologic age	Immunize with 4 vaccine doses at 0, 1, 2–3, and 6–7 mo of chronologic age
	Check anti-HBs and HBsAg at 9–15 mo of age[2]	Check anti-HBs and HBsAg at 9–15 mo of age[2]
	If infant is HBsAg and anti-HBs negative, reimmunize with 3 doses at 2-mo intervals and retest	If infant is HBsAg and anti-HBs negative, reimmunize with 3 doses at 2-mo intervals and retest
HBsAg status unknown	Hepatitis B vaccine (by 12 h) + HBIG (within 7 days) if mother tests HBsAg positive	Hepatitis B vaccine + HBIG (by 12 h)
	Test mother for HBsAg immediately	Test mother for HBsAg within 12 h of birth and if unavailable, give infant HBIG
HBsAg negative	Hepatitis B vaccine at birth preferred	Hepatitis B vaccine dose 1 at 30 days of chronologic age if medically stable, or at hospital discharge if before 30 days of chronologic age
	Immunize with 3 doses at 0–2, 1–4, and 6–18 mo of chronologic age	Immunize with 3 doses at 1–2, 2–4, and 6–18 mo of chronologic age
	May give hepatitis B-containing combination vaccine beginning at 6–8 wk of chronologic age	May give hepatitis B-containing combination vaccine beginning at 6–8 wk of chronologic age
	Follow-up anti-HBs and HBsAg testing not needed	Follow-up anti-HBs and HBsAg testing not needed

HBsAg indicates hepatitis B surface antigen; HBIG, hepatitis B Immune Globulin; anti-HBs, antibody to hepatitis B surface antigen; Hib, *Haemophilus influenzae* type b.

[1] Extremes of gestational age and birth weight no longer a consideration for timing of HBV doses.

[2] Some experts prefer to perform serologic testing 1 to 3 months after completion of the primary series.

All preterm infants of HBsAg-negative mothers with a birth weight of less than 2000 g can receive the first dose of hepatitis B vaccine series starting at 1 month of chronologic age. Preterm infants weighing more than 2000 g and low birth weight infants who are medically stable and showing consistent weight gain when discharged from the hospital before 1 month of age may receive the first dose of hepatitis B vaccine at the time of discharge. Infants born to HBsAg-negative mothers do not need to have postimmunization serologic testing for anti-HBs. Table 3.18 (above) provides a summary of the recommendations for immunization of PT and

LBW infants on the basis of maternal hepatitis B status and infant birth weight. For information on use of combination vaccines containing hepatitis B as a component to complete the series, see Pertussis (p 479).

Immunization of High-Risk Groups (see Table 3.19, p 330).

Ethnic populations at high risk of HBV infection. Despite initiation of routine immunization of infants, many children and adolescents are unimmunized and remain at risk of HBV infection. In particular, without immunization during early childhood, high rates of HBV infection would be expected to continue to occur among Alaska Native and Asian-Pacific Islander children and among children residing in households of first-generation immigrants from countries where HBV infection is endemic. As a result, targeted efforts are needed to achieve high immunization coverage among these children.

Sexually Active Heterosexual Adolescents and Adults. People diagnosed with a sexually transmitted disease or people who have had more than 1 sexual partner during the previous 6 months should be immunized.

Household Contacts and Sexual Partners of People With Chronic HBV Infection. Household and sexual contacts of people with chronic HBV infection identified through prenatal screening, blood donor screening, or diagnostic or other serologic testing should be immunized.

Health Care Professionals and Others With Occupational Exposure to Blood. The risk of HBV exposure to a health care professional depends on the tasks the person performs. Health care professionals who have contact with blood or blood-contaminated body fluids should be immunized. Because the risks of occupational HBV infection often are highest during the training of health care professionals, immunization should be completed during training and before contact with blood.

Residents and Staff of Institutions for People With Developmental Disabilities. Susceptible children in institutions for people with developmental disabilities and staff who work with the children should be immunized. Children discharged from residential institutions into community programs (eg, schools, sheltered workshops) should be screened for HBsAg to allow appropriate measures to prevent HBV transmission. Susceptible children and staff who live or work in smaller (group) residential settings where other staff members or residents are known to be HBsAg positive and staff of nonresidential child care programs (eg, schools and other group settings) attended by HBsAg-positive developmentally disabled people also should be immunized. Immunization should be considered for all attendees in nonresidential programs attended by HBsAg-positive people and is encouraged strongly if an attendee who is HBsAg-positive behaves aggressively or has special medical problems (eg, exudative dermatitis or open skin lesions) that increase the risk of exposure to that attendee's blood or secretions.

Patients Undergoing Hemodialysis. Immunization is recommended for susceptible hemodialysis patients. Immunization early in the course of renal disease is encouraged, because response is better than in advanced disease.

Adoptees and Their Household Contacts From Countries Where HBV Infection Is Endemic. Adoptees from countries where HBV infection is endemic should be screened for HBsAg at or before the time of adoption. Previously unimmunized family members and other household contacts should be immunized if

Table 3.19. People Who Should Receive Preexposure Hepatitis B Immunization

All infants

All unimmunized children and adolescents 0–18 years of age

Children at high risk of early childhood HBV infection[1]

Adolescents: hepatitis B immunization should be given by or before 11–12 years of age; special efforts should be made to immunize all adolescents, not only those at high risk

Injection drug users

Sexually active heterosexual people with more than one sexual partner during the previous 6 months or who have a sexually transmitted disease

Men who have sex with men

Household contacts and sexual partners of people with chronic HBV infection

Health care professionals and others at occupational risk of exposure to blood or blood-contaminated body fluid

Residents and staff of institutions for developmentally disabled people

Staff of nonresidential child care and school programs for developmentally disabled people if the program is attended by a known HBsAg-positive person

Patients undergoing hemodialysis

Members of households with adoptees who are HBsAg-positive

Inmates of juvenile detention and other corrections facilities

Patients with bleeding disorders who receive clotting factor concentrates

Long-term international travelers to areas where HBV infection is of high or intermediate endemicity

---

HBV indicates hepatitis B virus; HBsAg, hepatitis B surface antigen.

[1] Special efforts should be made to immunize Alaska Native and Asian-Pacific Islander children and children born to first-generation immigrants from HBV-endemic areas.

an adoptee is found to be HBsAg-positive, preferably before adoption. Adoptees found to be HBsAg negative should be immunized.

Inmates in Juvenile Detention and Other Corrections Facilities. Previously unimmunized or underimmunized people in juvenile and adult facilities, including jails, should be immunized appropriately. If the length of stay is not sufficient to complete the immunization series, the series should be initiated and follow-up mechanisms with a health care facility should be established to ensure completion of the series (see Hepatitis and Youth in Corrections Facilities, p 167).

Patients With Bleeding Disorders Who Receive Clotting Factor Concentrates. Although the risk from currently manufactured products is low, the potential risk of HBV transmission remains; thus, immunization is recommended as soon as the specific clotting disorder is diagnosed.

International Travelers. People traveling for 6 months or longer to areas where HBV infection is of high or intermediate endemicity (see Epidemiology, p 319) who will have close contact with the local population should be immunized. People who are traveling for a shorter duration but likely will have contact with blood (eg, in a medical setting or through drug use) or sexual contact with residents also should be immunized. Immunization should begin at least 4 to 6 months before travel so that a 3-dose regimen can be completed (see Preexposure Universal Immunization, p 326). If immunization is initiated fewer than 4 months before departure, the alternative 4-dose schedule of 0, 1, 2, and 12 months (see Table 3.17, p 325) should provide protection if the first 3 doses can be administered before travel. Individual clinicians may choose to use an accelerated schedule (eg, doses at days 0, 7, and 14) for travelers who will depart before an approved immunization schedule can be completed. The FDA has not licensed schedules that involve immunization at more than one time point during a single month for hepatitis B vaccine licensed in the United States. People who receive an immunization on an accelerated schedule that is not FDA-licensed also should receive a booster dose at least 6 months after initiation of the series to promote long-term immunity (see Lapsed Immunizations, p 33).

These and additional indications for immunization of high-risk people are given in Table 3.19, p 330.

Care of Exposed People (Postexposure Immunoprophylaxis) (see also Table 3.20, p 332).

Prevention of Perinatal HBV Infection. Transmission of perinatal HBV infection can be prevented in approximately 95% of infants born to HBsAg-positive mothers by early active and passive immunoprophylaxis of the infant (ie, immunization and HBIG administration). Immunization subsequently should be completed during the first 6 months of life. Hepatitis B immunization alone, initiated at or shortly after birth, also is highly effective for preventing perinatal HBV infections.

Serologic Screening of Pregnant Women. Prenatal HBsAg testing of all pregnant women is recommended to identify newborn infants who require immediate postexposure prophylaxis. All pregnant women should be tested during an early prenatal visit with every pregnancy. Testing should be repeated during late pregnancy for HBsAg-negative women who are at high risk of HBV infection (eg, injection drug users and those with intercurrent sexually transmitted diseases) or who have had clinical hepatitis. Household contacts and sexual partners of HBsAg-positive women should be immunized. Women who are HBsAg positive should be reported to local health departments for appropriate case management to ensure follow-up of their infants and immunization of sexual and household contacts. In populations where HBsAg testing of pregnant women is not feasible, all infants should receive hepatitis B vaccine within 12 hours of birth, the second dose by 2 months of age, and the third dose at 6 months of age.

Management of Infants Born to HBsAg-Positive Women. Infants born to HBsAg-positive mothers, including preterm infants, should receive the initial dose of hepatitis B vaccine within 12 hours of birth (see Table 3.17, p 325, for appropriate dosages), and HBIG (0.5 mL) should be given concurrently but at a different anatomic site. Subsequent doses of vaccine should be given as recommended in Table 3.21 (p 333) and Table 3.18 (p 328). For preterm infants who weigh less than 2000 g at birth, the initial vaccine dose should not be counted in the required 3-dose schedule (a total of 4 doses of hepatitis B vaccine), and the subsequent 3 doses should be given in accordance with the schedule for immunization of preterm infants (see Preterm and Low Birth Weight Infants, p 66).

Table 3.20. Guide to Postexposure Immunoprophylaxis for Hepatitis B Virus Infection

Type of Exposure	Immunoprophylaxis[1]	Refer to:
Percutaneous or permucosal exposure to blood	Immunization ± HBIG	p 335 (see Table 3.22)
Household contact HBsAg-positive person	Immunization	p 329
Household contact acute case with identifiable blood exposure	Immunization + HBIG	p 334
Perinatal	Immunization + HBIG	p 331
Sexual, partner has acute infection	Immunization + HBIG	p 334
Sexual, partner has chronic infection	Immunization	p 329

HBIG indicates Hepatitis B Immune Globulin; HBsAg, hepatitis B surface antigen.
[1] For susceptible patients (eg, previously unimmunized).

Infants born to HBsAg-positive women should be tested for anti-HBs and HBsAg after completion of the immunization series, at 9 to 15 months of age. Testing should not be performed before 9 months of age to avoid detection of anti-HBs from HBIG administered during infancy and to maximize the likelihood of detecting late HBV infections. Testing for HBsAg will identify infants who become chronically infected despite immunization (because of intrauterine infection or vaccine failure) and will aid in their long-term medical management. Infants with anti-HBs concentrations of less than 10 mIU/mL and who are HBsAg-negative should receive 3 additional doses of vaccine in a 0-, 1-, and 6-month schedule followed by testing for anti-HBs 1 month after the third dose. Alternatively, additional doses (1–3) of vaccine can be administered, followed by testing for anti-HBs 1 month after each dose to determine whether subsequent doses are needed.

Term Infants Born to Mothers Not Tested During Pregnancy for HBsAg. Pregnant women whose HBsAg status is unknown at delivery should undergo blood testing as soon as possible to determine her HBsAg status. While awaiting results, the infant should receive the first hepatitis B vaccine dose within 12 hours of birth in the dose recommended for infants born to HBsAg-positive mothers (see Table 3.17, p 325). Because hepatitis B vaccine when given at birth is highly effective for preventing perinatal infection in term infants, the possible added value and the cost of HBIG do not warrant its immediate use in term infants when the mother's HBsAg status is not known. If the woman is found to be HBsAg-positive, term infants should receive HBIG (0.5 mL) as soon as possible, but within 7 days of birth, and should complete the hepatitis B immunization series as recommended (see Table 3.17, p 325, and Table 3.18, p 328). If HBIG is unavailable, the infant still should receive the 2 subsequent doses of hepatitis B vaccine at 1 to 2 and 6 months of age (see Table 3.21, p 333). If the mother is found to be HBsAg-negative, hepatitis B immunization in the dose and routine schedule recommended for term infants born to HBsAg-negative mothers should be completed (see Table 3.17, p 325). If the mother's HBsAg status remains unknown, some experts

Table 3.21. Recommended Schedule of Hepatitis B Immunoprophylaxis to Prevent Perinatal Transmission

Vaccine Dose[1] and HBIG	Age
Infant Born to Mother Known To Be HBsAg Positive[2]	
First dose	Birth (within 12 h)
HBIG[3]	Birth (within 12 h)
Second dose	1–2 mo
Third dose	6 mo
Term Infant Born to Mother Not Screened for HBsAg[4]	
First dose	Birth (within 12 h)
HBIG[3]	If mother found to be HBsAg positive, give 0.5 mL as soon as possible, not later than 1 wk after birth[4]
Second dose	1–2 mo
Third dose	6 mo[5]

HBIG indicates Hepatitis B Immune Globulin; HBsAg, hepatitis B surface antigen.
[1] See Table 3.17 (p 325) for appropriate vaccine dose.
[2] See text (p 331) for recommendations for subsequent serologic testing.
[3] HBIG (0.5 mL) given intramuscularly at a site different from that used for vaccine.
[4] See text (below) for immunization recommendations for preterm infants.
[5] Infants of HBsAg-negative mothers should receive third dose at 6 to 18 months of age.

would administer HBIG within 7 days of birth and complete the hepatitis B immunization series as recommended for infants born to mothers who are HBsAg positive (Table 3.18, p 328).

Preterm Infants Born to Mothers Not Tested During Pregnancy for HBsAg. The maternal HBsAg status should be determined as soon as possible. Preterm infants born to mothers whose HBsAg status is unknown should receive hepatitis B vaccine within the first 12 hours of life. Preterm infants weighing more than 2000 g at birth who are born to mothers whose HBsAg status is unknown should follow recommendations for term infants. Preterm infants weighing less than 2000 g at birth who are born to mothers whose HBsAg status is unknown should receive HBIG (0.5 mL) if the mother's HBsAg status cannot be determined within the initial 12 hours of birth because of the potentially decreased immunogenicity of vaccine in these infants. In these infants, the initial vaccine dose should not be counted toward the 3 doses of hepatitis B vaccine required to complete the immunization series. The subsequent 3 doses (for a total of 4 doses) are given in accordance with recommendations for immunization of preterm infants with a birth weight less than 2000 g according to the HBsAg status of the mother (see Table 3.18, p 328). Follow-up testing on completion of the immunization series is recommended for all preterm infants of HBsAg-positive mothers (see Management of Infants Born to HBsAg-Positive Women, p 331).

Breastfeeding. Breastfeeding of the infant by an HBsAg-positive mother poses no additional risk of acquisition of HBV infection by the infant (see Human Milk, p 117).

Household Contacts of People With Acute HBV Infection. Infants (ie, younger than 12 months of age) who have close contact with primary caregivers with acute infection require immunoprophylaxis. If at the time of exposure, the infant has been immunized fully or has received at least 2 doses of vaccine, the infant should be presumed protected, and HBIG is not required. If only one dose of vaccine has been administered, the second dose should be administered if the interval is appropriate, or HBIG should be administered if immunization is not due. If immunization has not been initiated, the infant should receive HBIG (0.5 mL), and hepatitis B vaccine should be given in accordance with the routinely recommended 3-dose schedule (see Preexposure Universal Immunization, p 326).

Prophylaxis with HBIG for other unimmunized household contacts of people with acute HBV infection is not indicated unless they have identifiable blood exposure to the index patient, such as by sharing of toothbrushes or razors. Such exposures should be treated in the same way as sexual exposures to a person with acute HBV infection. All such people should be immunized as soon as possible against hepatitis B because of the possibility of future household exposures.

Sexual Partners of People With Acute HBV Infection. Susceptible sexual partners should receive a single dose of HBIG (0.06 mL/kg) and should begin the hepatitis B vaccine series. Sexual partners of people with acute HBV infection are at increased risk of infection, and HBIG is 75% effective for preventing these infections. The period after sexual exposure during which HBIG is effective is unknown, but is unlikely to exceed 14 days.

Exposure to Blood That Contains (or Might Contain) HBsAg. For inadvertent percutaneous (eg, needlestick, laceration, or bite) or permucosal (eg, ocular or mucous membrane) exposure to blood, the decision to give HBIG prophylaxis and to immunize the exposed person includes consideration of whether the HBsAg status of the person who was the source of the exposure is known and the hepatitis B immunization and response status of the exposed person. Immunization is recommended for any person who was exposed but not previously immunized. If possible, a blood specimen from the person who was the source of the exposure should be tested for HBsAg and appropriate prophylaxis should be administered according to the hepatitis B immunization status and anti-HBs response status (if known) of the exposed person (see Table 3.22, p 335, and Injuries From Discarded Needles in the Community, p 180).

Detailed guidelines for the management of health care professionals and other people exposed to blood that is or might be HBsAg-positive is provided in the recommendations of the Advisory Committee on Immunization Practices of the Centers for Disease Control and Prevention* (see also Table 3.22, p 335).

Victims of Sexual Assault or Abuse. If previously immunized, sexual assault victims should be assumed to be protected from acute and chronic HBV infection. For unimmunized victims, active postexposure prophylaxis (ie, vaccine alone) should

---

* Centers for Disease Control and Prevention. Hepatitis B virus infection: a comprehensive immunization strategy to eliminate transmission in the United States—2003 update: recommendations of the Advisory Committee on Immunization Practices (ACIP). *MMWR Morb Mortal Wkly Rep.* In press

Table 3.22. Recommendations for Hepatitis B Prophylaxis After Percutaneous Exposure to Blood That Contains or Might Contain HBsAg[1]

Exposed Person	Treatment When Source Is		
	HBsAg-Positive	HBsAg-Negative	Unknown or Not Tested
Unimmunized	Administer HBIG[2] (1 dose), and initiate hepatitis B vaccine series	Initiate hepatitis B vaccine series	Initiate hepatitis B vaccine series
Previously immunized			
Known responder	No treatment	No treatment	No treatment
Known nonresponder	HBIG (1 dose) **and** initiate reimmunization[3] or HBIG (2 doses)	No treatment	If known high-risk source, treat as if source were HBsAg positive
Response unknown	Test exposed person for anti-HBs[4] • If inadequate, HBIG[2] (1 dose) **and** vaccine booster dose[5] • If adequate, no treatment	No treatment	Test exposed person for anti-HBs[4] • If inadequate, vaccine booster dose[5] • If adequate, no treatment

HBsAg indicates hepatitis B surface antigen; HBIG, Hepatitis B Immune Globulin; anti-HBs, antibody to HBsAg.

[1] Centers for Disease Control and Prevention. Updated US Public Health Service guidelines for the management of occupational exposures to HBV, HCV, and HIV and recommendations for postexposure prophylaxis. *MMWR Recomm Rep.* 2001;50(RR-11):1–52.

[2] Dose of HBIG, 0.06 mL/kg, intramuscularly.

[3] The option of giving 1 dose of HBIG (0.06 mL/kg) and reinitiating the vaccine series is preferred for nonresponders who have not completed a second 3-dose vaccine series. For people who previously completed a second vaccine series but failed to respond, 2 doses of HBIG (0.06 mL/kg) are preferred, 1 dose as soon as possible after exposure and the second 1 mo later.

[4] Adequate anti-HBs is ≥10 mIU/mL.

[5] The person should be evaluated for antibody response after the vaccine booster dose. For people who received HBIG, anti-HBs testing should be performed when passively acquired antibody from HBIG no longer is detectable (eg, 4–6 mo); for people who did not receive HBIG, anti-HBs testing should be performed 1 to 2 mo after the vaccine booster dose. If anti-HBs is inadequate (<10 mIU/mL) after the vaccine booster dose, 2 additional doses should be administered to complete a 3-dose reimmunization series.

be initiated, with the first dose of vaccine given as part of the initial clinical evaluation. Unless the offender is known to have acute hepatitis B, HBIG is not required to achieve a high level of postexposure protection. In the case of children, sexual abuse commonly occurs over a prolonged period, often making it difficult to define the last exposure. However, when sexual abuse is identified, hepatitis B immunization should be initiated in previously unimmunized children.

Child Care. All children, including children in child care, should receive hepatitis B vaccine as part of their routine immunization schedule. Immunization not only will decrease the potential for transmission after bites but also will allay anxiety about transmission from attendees who may be HBsAg positive.

Children who are HBsAg-positive and who have no behavioral or medical risk factors, such as unusually aggressive behavior (eg, biting), generalized dermatitis, or a bleeding problem, should be admitted to child care without restrictions. Under these circumstances, the risk of HBV transmission in child care settings is negligible, and routine screening for HBsAg is not warranted. Admission of HBsAg-positive children with behavioral or medical risk factors should be assessed on an individual basis by the child's physician, the program director, and the responsible public health authorities (for further discussion, see Children in Out-of-Home Child Care, p 123).

Effectiveness of Hepatitis B Prevention Programs. Routine hepatitis B immunization programs have resulted in significant decreases in the prevalence of HBV infection among children in populations with a high incidence of HBV infection. There is an association between higher coverage with hepatitis B vaccine and larger decreases in HBsAg prevalence. Demonstration of decreases in areas with lower HBV infection incidence will require longer term and larger studies.

Although the long-term sequelae of chronic HBV infection usually are not seen until adulthood, cirrhosis and HCC do occur in children. In Taiwan, the average annual incidence of HCC among 6- to 14-year-old children decreased significantly within 10 years of routine infant hepatitis B immunization. Worldwide, routine infant immunization programs are expected to decrease significantly the incidence of death from cirrhosis and HCC over the next 30 to 50 years.

The Division of Viral Hepatitis at the CDC maintains a toll-free number for information on viral hepatitis (1-888-4HEPCDC) and maintains a Web site (www.cdc.gov/hepatitis) with information on hepatitis for health care professionals and the public.

Hepatitis C

CLINICAL MANIFESTATIONS: The signs and symptoms of hepatitis C virus (HCV) infection are indistinguishable from those of hepatitis A or B. Acute disease tends to be mild and insidious in onset, and most infections are asymptomatic. Jaundice occurs in <20% of patients, and abnormalities in liver function tests generally are less pronounced than abnormalities in patients with hepatitis B virus infection. Persistent infection with HCV occurs in 50% to 60% of infected children, even in the absence of biochemical evidence of liver disease. Most children with chronic infection are asymptomatic. Although chronic hepatitis develops in approximately 60% to 70% of infected adults, limited data indicate that <10% of infected children develop chronic hepatitis, and <5% develop cirrhosis. Infection with HCV is the leading reason for liver transplantation among adults in the United States.

ETIOLOGY: Hepatitis C virus is a small, single-stranded RNA virus and is a member of the Flavivirus family. Multiple HCV genotypes and subtypes exist.

EPIDEMIOLOGY: The prevalence of HCV infection in the general population of the United States is estimated at 1.8%. The seroprevalence is 0.2% for children younger than 12 years of age and 0.4% for adolescents 12 to 19 years of age. Seroprevalences vary among populations according to their associated risk factors.

Infection is spread primarily by parenteral exposure to blood of HCV-infected people. The current risk of HCV infection after blood transfusion in the United States is estimated to be less than 1 in 1 million units transfused because of the exclusion of high-risk donors and of HCV-positive units by antibody testing and screening of pools of blood units by some form of nucleic acid amplification test (see Blood Safety, p 106). One outbreak of HCV associated with contaminated Immune Globulin Intravenous (IGIV) has occurred in the United States. Currently, all intravenous and intramuscular Immune Globulin products available commercially in the United States undergo an inactivation procedure for HCV or are documented to be HCV RNA negative before release.

The highest seroprevalences of HCV infection (60%–90%) are in people with large or repeated direct percutaneous exposure to blood or blood products, such as injection drug users and people with hemophilia who were treated with clotting factor concentrates produced before 1987. Prevalences are moderately high among people with frequent but smaller direct percutaneous exposures, such as patients receiving hemodialysis (10%–20%). Lower prevalences are found among people with inapparent percutaneous or mucosal exposures, such as people with high-risk sexual behaviors (1%–10%), and among people with sporadic percutaneous exposures, such as health care professionals (1%).

Other body fluids contaminated with infected blood can be sources of infection. Sexual transmission among monogamous couples is uncommon, with infection found only in 1.5% of spouses without other risk factors. Transmission among family contacts also is uncommon but could occur from direct or inapparent percutaneous or mucosal exposure to blood. For most infected children and adolescents, no specific source of infection can be identified.

Seroprevalence among pregnant women in the United States has been estimated at 1% to 2%. The risk of maternal-infant (perinatal) transmission averages 5% to 6%, and transmission occurs only from women who are HCV RNA positive at the time of delivery. Maternal coinfection with human immunodeficiency virus (HIV) has been associated with increased risk of perinatal transmission of HCV, which depends in part on the serum titer of maternal HCV RNA. Serum anti-HCV antibody and HCV RNA have been detected in colostrum, but HCV transmission through breastfeeding has not been demonstrated. The rate of transmission among breastfed infants has been the same as that among bottle-fed infants.

All people with HCV antibody or HCV-RNA in their blood are considered to be infectious.

The **incubation period** for hepatitis C disease averages 6 to 7 weeks, with a range of 2 weeks to 6 months. The time from exposure to development of viremia generally is 1 to 2 weeks.

DIAGNOSTIC TESTS*: The 2 major types of tests available for the laboratory diagnosis of HCV infections are antibody assays for anti-HCV and nucleic acid test (NATs) to detect HCV RNA. Diagnosis by antibody assays involves an initial screening enzyme immunoassay; repeated positive results are confirmed by a recombinant immunoblot assay (RIBA). Both assays detect immunoglobulin (Ig) G antibody; no IgM assays are available. The current enzyme immunoassays are at least 97% sensitive and more than 99% specific. False-negative results early in the course of acute infection result from the prolonged interval between exposure and onset of illness and seroconversion. Within 15 weeks after exposure and within 5 to 6 weeks after the onset of hepatitis, 80% of patients will have positive test results for serum HCV antibody. Among infants born to anti-HCV–positive mothers, passively acquired maternal antibody persists for up to 18 months.

Food and Drug Administration (FDA)-licensed diagnostic NATs for qualitative detection of HCV RNA use reverse transcriptase-polymerase chain reaction (RT-PCR) assays. Hepatitis C virus RNA can be detected in serum or plasma within 1 to 2 weeks after exposure to the virus and weeks before onset of liver enzyme abnormalities or appearance of anti-HCV. Reverse transcriptase-polymerase chain reaction assays for HCV RNA are used commonly in clinical practice in the early diagnosis of infection, for identifying infection in infants early in life (ie, perinatal transmission) when maternal serum antibody interferes with the ability to detect antibody produced by the infant, and for monitoring patients receiving antiviral therapy. However, false-positive and false-negative results can occur from improper handling, storage, and contamination of the test specimens. Viral RNA may be detected intermittently, and thus, a single negative assay result is not conclusive. Quantitative assays for measuring the concentration of HCV RNA are available. The clinical value of these quantitative assays appears to be primarily as a prognostic indicator for patients undergoing or about to undergo antiviral therapy.

TREATMENT: Interferon-alfa or pegylated interferon alfa-2b alone, interferon-alfa in combination with ribavirin, and pegylated interferon alfa-2a are licensed by the FDA for treatment of chronic hepatitis C in adults. Given alone, interferon-alfa results in a sustained response in 10% to 20% of patients treated; pegylated interferons alfa-2a and alfa-2b, which require only 1 dose weekly, result in average sustained response rates of 39% and 25%, respectively. Lower sustained response rates are observed in patients with genotype 1, the most common strain in the United States. Combination therapy with interferon alfa-2b and ribavirin results in a sustained response in 33% of patients infected with genotype 1 and approximately 80% in patients with genotypes 2 or 3. Combination therapy with pegylated interferons results in higher sustained response rates, particularly among patients with genotype 1 (40%). There are no FDA-licensed therapies for people younger than 18 years of age. Limited experience with interferon-alfa therapy in children suggests efficacy

---

* Centers for Disease Control and Prevention. Guidelines for laboratory testing and result reporting of antibody to hepatitis C virus. *MMWR Recomm Rep.* 2003;52(RR-3):1–16

similar to that observed in adults. Children with severe disease or histologically advanced pathologic features (bridging necrosis or active cirrhosis) should be referred to a specialist in the management of chronic hepatitis C.

People with HCV-related chronic liver disease, if susceptible, should be immunized against hepatitis A and B viruses.

Management of Chronic HCV Infection. With advancing age, people who have chronic HCV infection are at risk of developing chronic hepatitis and its complications, including cirrhosis and primary hepatocellular carcinoma. However, primary hepatocellular carcinoma secondary to chronic hepatitis C has been reported only in adults. Children with chronic infection should be screened periodically for chronic hepatitis with serum liver enzyme tests because of potential long-term risk of chronic liver disease. Definitive recommendations on frequency of screening have not been established. Children with persistently increased serum transaminase concentrations should be referred to a gastroenterologist for further management. The need for testing of α-fetoprotein concentration and for abdominal ultrasonography in children has not been determined.

ISOLATION OF THE HOSPITALIZED PATIENT: Standard precautions are recommended.

CONTROL MEASURES:

Care of Exposed People.

Immunoprophylaxis. Immune Globulin is manufactured from plasma that tests negative for anti-HCV antibodies. On the basis of lack of clinical efficacy in humans and on data from studies using animals, the use of Immune Globulin for postexposure prophylaxis against HCV infection is not recommended.

Breastfeeding. Mothers infected with HCV should be advised that transmission of HCV by breastfeeding has not been documented. According to current guidelines of the Centers for Disease Control and Prevention (CDC), maternal HCV infection is not a contraindication to breastfeeding. Mothers who are HCV positive and choose to breastfeed should consider abstaining if their nipples are cracked or bleeding.

Child Care. Exclusion of children with HCV infection from out-of-home child care is not indicated.

Serologic Testing for HCV Infection.

People Who Have Risk Factors for HCV Infection. Routine serologic testing is recommended for current or former injection drug users, recipients of one or more units of blood or blood products before July 1992, recipients of a solid organ transplant before July 1992, patients receiving long-term hemodialysis, people who received clotting factor concentrates produced before 1987, and people with persistently abnormal alanine transaminase (ALT) concentrations.

Pregnant Women. Routine serologic testing of pregnant women for HCV infection is not recommended.

Children Born to Women With HCV Infection. Children born to women previously identified to be HCV-infected should be tested for HCV infection, because approximately 5% will acquire the infection. The duration of passive maternal antibody in infants is approximately 18 months. Therefore, testing for anti-HCV should not be performed until after 18 months of age. If earlier diagnosis is desired, RT-PCR assay for HCV RNA may be performed at or after the infant's first well-child visit at 1 to 2 months of age.

Adoptees. Routine serologic testing of adoptees, either domestic or international, is not recommended. Testing is indicated, however, if the biologic mother has an increased risk of HCV infection (see Medical Evaluation of Internationally Adopted Children for Infectious Diseases, p 173).

Recipients of IGIV. The US Public Health Service recommends that people who received Gammagard (produced by Baxter Healthcare Corporation, Glendale, CA) between April 1, 1993 and February 23, 1994 be offered serologic testing for anti-HCV and determination of ALT concentrations. Because of concerns that anti-HCV may not be detectable in people who are immunocompromised, RT-PCR testing for HCV RNA is recommended for people with increased ALT concentrations who test negative for anti-HCV on repeated testing. Screening of people who have received other IGIV products is not indicated.

Counseling of Patients With HCV Infection. All people with HCV infection should be considered infectious, should be informed of the possibility of transmission to others, and should refrain from donating blood, organs, tissues, or semen and sharing toothbrushes and razors.

Infected people should be counseled to avoid hepatotoxic agents, including medications, and should be informed of the risks of alcohol ingestion. Patients with chronic liver disease, if susceptible, should be immunized against hepatitis A and B viruses.

Changes in sexual practices of infected people with a steady partner are not recommended; however, they should be informed of the possible risks and use of precautions to prevent transmission. People with multiple partners should be advised to decrease the number of partners and to use condoms to prevent transmission. No data exist to support counseling a woman against pregnancy.

The Division of Viral Hepatitis at the CDC has implemented a toll-free number for information on viral hepatitis (1-888-4HEPCDC) and maintains a Web site (www.cdc.gov/hepatitis) with information on hepatitis for health care professionals and the public, which includes specific information for people who have received blood transfusions before 1992. Information also can be obtained from the National Institutes of Health Web site (www.niddk.nih.gov/health/digest/pubs/chrnhepc/chrnhepc.htm).

Hepatitis D

CLINICAL MANIFESTATIONS: Hepatitis D virus (HDV) causes hepatitis only in people with acute or chronic hepatitis B virus (HBV) infection; HDV requires HBV as a helper virus and cannot produce infection in the absence of HBV. The importance of HDV infection lies in its ability to convert an asymptomatic or mild chronic HBV infection into fulminant or more severe or rapidly progressive disease.

Acute coinfection with HBV and HDV usually causes an acute illness indistinguishable from acute HBV infection alone, except that the likelihood of fulminant hepatitis can be as high as 5%.

ETIOLOGY: Hepatitis D virus measures 36- to 43-nm in diameter and consists of an RNA genome and a delta protein antigen, both of which are coated with hepatitis B surface antigen (HBsAg).

EPIDEMIOLOGY: Hepatitis D virus can cause an infection at the same time as the initial HBV infection (coinfection), or it can infect a person already chronically infected (superinfection). Acquisition of HDV is similar to that of HBV (ie, by parenteral, percutaneous, or mucous membrane inoculation). Hepatitis D virus can be transmitted by blood or blood products, injection drug use, or sexual contact as long as HBV also is present in the patient. Transmission from mother to newborn infant is uncommon. Intrafamilial spread can occur among people with chronic HBV infection. High-prevalence areas include southern Italy and parts of eastern Europe, South America, Africa, and the Middle East. In contrast to HBV, HDV infection is uncommon in the Far East. In the United States, HDV infection is found most commonly in parenteral drug abusers, people with hemophilia, and people who have immigrated from endemic areas.

The **incubation period** for HDV superinfection, estimated from inoculation of animals, is approximately 2 to 8 weeks. When HBV and HDV viruses infect simultaneously, the incubation period is similar to that of hepatitis B (45–160 days; average, 90 days).

DIAGNOSTIC TESTS: Radioimmunoassay and enzyme immunoassay for anti-HDV antibody are available commercially. Anti-HDV may not be present until several weeks after onset of illness, and acute and convalescent sera may be required to confirm the diagnosis. Coinfection usually can be differentiated from superinfection with HBV by testing for immunoglobulin (Ig) M hepatitis B core antibody (anti-HBc); absence of IgM anti-HBc suggests that the person with chronic HBV infection has a superinfection. Testing for the IgM anti-HDV response is not useful for distinguishing acute from chronic HDV infection, because IgM anti-HDV persists during chronic infection. Tests for IgM anti-HDV, HDAg, and HDV RNA are research procedures.

TREATMENT: Supportive.

ISOLATION OF THE HOSPITALIZED PATIENT: Standard precautions are recommended.

CONTROL MEASURES: The same control and preventive measures used for HBV infection are indicated. Because HDV cannot be transmitted in the absence of HBV infection, hepatitis B immunization protects against HDV infection. People with chronic HBV infection should take extreme care to avoid exposure to HDV.

Hepatitis E

CLINICAL MANIFESTATIONS: Hepatitis E infection is an acute illness with symptoms including jaundice, malaise, anorexia, fever, abdominal pain, and arthralgia. Subclinical infection also occurs.

ETIOLOGY: The hepatitis E virus (HEV) is a spherical, nonenveloped, positive-strand RNA virus, which is the only known agent of enterically transmitted non-A, non-B hepatitis. Hepatitis E virus formerly was classified in the family Caliciviridae, genus *Calicivirus;* however, HEV has been reassigned to an unassigned genus of "hepatitis E-like" viruses, because certain characteristics distinguish HEV from typical caliciviruses.

EPIDEMIOLOGY: Transmission of HEV is by the fecal-oral route. Disease is more common among adults than among children. It has an unusually high case-fatality rate among pregnant women. Cases have been reported in epidemics or sporadically in parts of Asia, Africa, and Mexico. Outbreaks usually have been associated with contaminated water. Hepatitis E virus infection rarely is reported in the United States, and most reported cases have occurred among travelers to endemic regions. However, acute HEV infection cases, verified by isolation of a "US strain" of HEV, have been reported among people with no recent history of travel outside the United States. The discovery of a swine virus in the United States that is related closely to human HEV raises the possibility of a zoonotic reservoir for HEV. The period of communicability after acute infection is unknown, but fecal shedding of the virus and viremia occur commonly for at least 2 weeks. Chronic infection does not seem to occur.

DIAGNOSTIC TESTS: The diagnosis of acute HEV infection can be made by detecting immunoglobulin (Ig) M antibody to HEV (anti-HEV) in serum or by detecting HEV RNA by reverse-transcriptase polymerase chain reaction assay in serum or fecal specimens. Serologic and reverse transcriptase-polymerase chain reaction-based assays for the diagnosis of acute HEV infection are available in research and commercial laboratories; however, none of these assays are licensed by the US Food and Drug Administration for this purpose. The CDC criteria for considering whether an acute phase serum specimen should be tested for evidence of HEV infection include a discrete onset of illness associated with jaundice or a serum alanine transaminase concentration at least 2.5 times the upper limit of normal and negative results of testing for IgM antibody to hepatitis A virus, IgM antibody to hepatitis B core antigen, and antibody to hepatitis C virus.

TREATMENT: Supportive.

ISOLATION OF THE HOSPITALIZED PATIENT: In addition to standard precautions, contact precautions are recommended.

CONTROL MEASURES: Good sanitation and not ingesting potentially contaminated food and water are the most effective measures. Passive immunoprophylaxis against HEV infection with Immune Globulin prepared in the United States has not proven effective.

Hepatitis G

CLINICAL MANIFESTATIONS: Although hepatitis G virus (HGV), also known as hepatitis GB virus (GBV-C), can cause chronic infection and viremia, studies of this and other putative agents of "non-ABCDE" hepatitis (ie, transfusion-transmitted virus [TTV], SEN viruses [SEN-V]) have failed to show an association with acute, fulminant, or chronic liver disease. Although high concentrations of HGV RNA are found in blood, the liver has not been shown to be a site of replication. Hepatitis G virus coinfection does not seem to affect the course or severity of concurrent infection with hepatitis B virus (HBV) or hepatitis C virus (HCV) but has been associated with decreased mortality among patients with concurrent human immunodeficiency virus infection.

ETIOLOGY: Hepatitis G virus is a single-stranded RNA virus that is included in the Flaviviridae family and shares a 27% homology with HCV. Hepatitis G virus has not yet been isolated.

EPIDEMIOLOGY: Hepatitis G virus has been reported in adults and children throughout the world and is found in approximately 1.5% of blood donors in the United States. Infection has been reported in 10% to 20% of adults with chronic HBV or HCV infection, and coinfection occurs most commonly among injection drug users. The primary route of spread is through direct percutaneous exposure to blood, including transfusions and organ transplants from infected donors, and injection drug use. Transmission also has been documented among hemodialysis patients and from mothers to infants. Sexual transmission may occur. Although infected infants and children may become persistently viremic, no disease association has been observed.

The **incubation period** is unknown.

DIAGNOSTIC TESTS: Among chronically infected people, HGV infection can be diagnosed by detecting HGV RNA by polymerase chain reaction assay. Among people with resolved infection, only antibody to HGV is detectable. Neither nucleic acid nor serologic-based tests are available commercially.

TREATMENT: No treatment is available or indicated.

ISOLATION OF THE HOSPITALIZED PATIENT: Standard precautions are recommended.

CONTROL MEASURES: No method to prevent infection with HGV is known.

Herpes Simplex

CLINICAL MANIFESTATIONS:

Neonatal. In newborns, herpes simplex virus (HSV) infection can manifest as the following: (1) disseminated disease involving multiple organs, most prominently liver and lungs; (2) localized central nervous system (CNS) disease; or (3) disease localized to the skin, eyes, and mouth. Approximately one third of cases are disseminated, one third are CNS disease, and one third affect the skin, eyes, and mouth, although there may be clinical overlap among disease types. In many neonates with disseminated or CNS disease, skin lesions do not develop or the lesions appear late in the course of infection. In the absence of skin lesions, the diagnosis of neonatal HSV infection is difficult. Disseminated infection should be considered in neonates with sepsis syndrome, negative bacteriologic culture results, and severe liver dysfunction. Herpes simplex virus also should be considered as a causative agent in neonates with fever, irritability, and abnormal cerebrospinal fluid (CSF) findings, especially in the presence of seizures. Although asymptomatic HSV infection is common in older children, it rarely, if ever, occurs in neonates.

Neonatal herpetic infections often are severe, with attendant high mortality and morbidity rates, even when antiviral therapy is administered. Recurrent skin lesions are common in surviving infants and may be associated with CNS sequelae if skin lesions occur frequently during the first 6 months of life.

Initial symptoms of HSV infection can occur anytime between birth and approximately 4 weeks of age. Disseminated disease has the earliest age of onset, often during the first week of life; CNS disease manifests latest, usually between the second and third weeks of life.

Children Beyond the Neonatal Period and Adolescents. Most primary HSV infections are asymptomatic. Gingivostomatitis, which is the most common clinical manifestation in this age group, usually is caused by HSV type 1 (HSV-1). Gingivostomatitis is characterized by fever, irritability, tender submandibular adenopathy, and an ulcerative enanthem involving the gingiva and mucous membranes of the mouth, often with perioral vesicular lesions.

Genital herpes, which is the most common manifestation of HSV infection in adolescents and adults, is characterized by vesicular or ulcerative lesions of the male or female genital organs, perineum, or both. Genital herpes usually is caused by HSV type 2 (HSV-2), but HSV type 1 appears to be increasing in frequency.

Eczema herpeticum with vesicular lesions concentrated in the areas of eczematous involvement can develop in patients with dermatitis who are infected with HSV.

In immunocompromised patients, severe local lesions and, less commonly, disseminated HSV infection with generalized vesicular skin lesions and visceral involvement can occur.

After primary infection, HSV persists for life in a latent form. The site of latency for virus causing herpes labialis is the trigeminal ganglion, and the usual site of latency for genital herpes is the sacral ganglia, although any sensory ganglia can be involved, depending on the site of primary infection. Reactivation of latent virus most commonly occurs in the absence of symptoms. When symptomatic, recurrent herpes labialis HSV-1 manifests as single or grouped vesicles in the perioral region, usually on the vermilion border of the lips (cold sores). Symptomatic recurrent genital herpes manifests as vesicular lesions on the penis, scrotum, vulva, cervix, buttocks, perianal areas, thighs, or back.

Conjunctivitis and keratitis can result from primary or recurrent HSV infection. Herpetic whitlow consists of single or multiple vesicular lesions on the distal parts of fingers. Herpes simplex virus infection has been implicated as a precipitating factor in erythema multiforme.

Herpes simplex virus encephalitis can result from primary or recurrent infection and usually is associated with fever, alterations in the state of consciousness, personality changes, seizures, and focal neurologic findings. Encephalitis commonly has an acute onset with a fulminant course, leading to coma and death in untreated patients. Cerebrospinal fluid pleocytosis with a predominance of lymphocytes and some erythrocytes is usual. Herpes simplex virus infection also can cause meningitis with nonspecific clinical manifestations that usually are mild and self-limited. Such episodes of meningitis usually are associated with genital HSV-2 infection. A number of unusual CNS manifestations of HSV have been described, including Bell's palsy, atypical pain syndromes, trigeminal neuralgia, ascending myelitis, and postinfectious encephalomyelitis.

ETIOLOGY: Herpes simplex viruses are enveloped, double-stranded, DNA viruses. Infections with HSV-1 usually involve the face and skin above the waist; however, an increasing number of genital herpes cases are attributable to HSV-1. Infections with HSV-2 usually involve the genitalia and skin below the waist in sexually active adolescents and adults. Either type of virus can be found in either area. Herpes simplex virus type 2 is the most common cause of disease in neonates.

EPIDEMIOLOGY: Herpes simplex virus infections are ubiquitous and are transmitted from people who are symptomatic or asymptomatic with primary or recurrent infections.

Neonatal. The incidence of neonatal HSV infection is estimated to range from 1 in 3000 to 20 000 live births. Infants in whom HSV infection develops are significantly more likely to have been born prematurely. Herpes simplex virus is transmitted to an infant most often during birth through an infected maternal genital tract or by an ascending infection, sometimes through apparently intact membranes. In the United States, approximately 75% of neonatal infections are caused by HSV-2, and 25% are caused by HSV-1. Intrauterine infections causing congenital malformations have been implicated in rare cases. Other less common sources of neonatal infection include postnatal transmission from a parent or other caregiver, most often from a nongenital infection (eg, mouth or hands) or from another infected infant or caregiver in the nursery, probably via the hands of health care professionals attending the infants.

The risk of HSV infection at delivery in an infant born vaginally to a mother with primary genital infection is estimated to be 33% to 50%. The risk to an infant born to a mother shedding HSV as a result of reactivated infection is less than 5%. Distinguishing between primary and recurrent HSV infections in women by history or physical examination may be impossible. Primary and recurrent infections may be asymptomatic or associated with nonspecific findings (eg, vaginal discharge, genital pain, or shallow ulcers). More than three quarters of infants who contract HSV infection have been born to women who had no history or clinical findings suggestive of active HSV infection during pregnancy.

Children Beyond the Neonatal Period and Adolescents. Patients with primary gingivostomatitis or genital herpes usually shed virus for at least 1 week and occasionally for several weeks. Patients with recurrent infection shed virus for a shorter period, typically 3 to 4 days. Intermittent asymptomatic reactivation of oral and genital herpes is common and persists for life, occurring in 1% of days among previously infected people. The greatest concentration of virus is shed during symptomatic primary infections and the least during asymptomatic recurrent infections.

Infection with HSV-1 usually results from direct contact with infected oral secretions or lesions. Infections with HSV-2 usually result from direct contact with infected genital secretions or lesions through sexual activity. Genital infections caused by HSV-1 in children can result from autoinoculation of virus from the mouth, but sexual abuse always should be considered in prepubertal children with genital HSV-2 infections. Therefore, genital HSV isolates from children should be typed to differentiate between HSV-1 and HSV-2.

The incidence of HSV-2 infection correlates with the number of sexual partners and with the acquisition of other sexually transmitted diseases. After primary genital infection, which often is asymptomatic, some people experience frequent clinical recurrences, and others have no recurrences. Genital HSV-2 infection is more likely to recur than is genital infection caused by HSV-1.

Inoculation of skin occurs from direct contact with HSV-containing oral or genital secretions. This contact can result in herpes gladiatorum among wrestlers, herpes rugbiaforum among rugby players, or herpetic whitlow of the fingers in any exposed person.

The **incubation period** for HSV infection occurring beyond the neonatal period ranges from 2 days to 2 weeks.

DIAGNOSTIC TESTS: Herpes simplex virus grows readily in cell culture. Special transport media are available for specimens that cannot be inoculated immediately onto susceptible cell culture media. Cytopathogenic effects typical of HSV infection usually are observed 1 to 3 days after inoculation. Methods of culture confirmation include fluorescent antibody staining and enzyme immunoassays. Cultures that remain negative by day 15 are likely to continue to remain negative. Herpes simplex virus DNA in CSF often can be detected by polymerase chain reaction assay in patients with HSV encephalitis and is the diagnostic method of choice when performed by experienced laboratory personnel. Histologic examination and viral culture of a brain tissue specimen obtained by biopsy is the most definitive method of confirming the diagnosis of encephalitis caused by HSV. Cultures of CSF from a patient with HSV encephalitis usually are negative.

For the diagnosis of neonatal HSV infection, specimens for culture should be obtained from skin vesicles, mouth or nasopharynx, eyes, urine, blood, stool or rectum, and CSF. Positive cultures obtained from any of these sites more than 48 hours after birth indicate viral replication suggestive of infant infection rather than colonization after intrapartum exposure. Rapid diagnostic techniques also are available, such as direct fluorescent antibody staining of vesicle scrapings or enzyme immunoassay detection of HSV antigens. These techniques are as specific but slightly less sensitive than culture. Typing HSV strains differentiates between HSV-1 and HSV-2 isolates. Polymerase chain reaction assay is a sensitive method for detecting HSV DNA and is of particular value for evaluating CSF specimens from people with suspected herpes encephalitis. Histologic examination of lesions for the presence of multinucleated giant cells and eosinophilic intranuclear inclusions typical of HSV (eg, with Tzanck test) has low sensitivity and is not recommended as a rapid diagnostic test.

Both type-specific and nonspecific antibodies to HSV develop during the first several weeks after infection and persist indefinitely. Although type-specific HSV-2 antibody almost always indicates anogenital infection, the presence of HSV-1 antibody does not distinguish anogenital from orolabial infection. Type-specific serologic tests may be useful in confirming a clinical diagnosis of genital herpes. Additionally, they can be used to diagnose people with unrecognized infection and to manage sexual partners of people with genital herpes.

Several glycoprotein G (gG)-based type-specific assays have been approved by the US Food and Drug Administration (FDA), including at least one that can be used as a point-of-care test. The sensitivities of these tests for detection of HSV-2 antibody vary from 80% to 98%, and false-negative results may occur, especially early after infection. The specificities of these assays are >96%; false-positive results can occur, especially in patients with low likelihood of HSV infection. Therefore, repeat testing or a confirmatory test (eg, an immunoblot assay if the initial test was an enzyme-linked immunosorbent assay) may be indicated in some settings.

TREATMENT: For recommended antiviral dosages and duration of therapy with acyclovir, valacyclovir hydrochloride, famciclovir, and penciclovir for different HSV infections, see Antiviral Drugs for Non-Human Immunodeficiency Virus Infections (p 729). Neither valacyclovir nor famciclovir is licensed by the FDA for use in children.

Neonatal. Parenteral acyclovir is the treatment of choice for neonatal HSV infections. Acyclovir should be administered to all neonates with HSV infection, regardless of manifestations and clinical findings. The best outcome in terms of morbidity and mortality is observed among infants with disease limited to the skin, eyes, and mouth. Although most neonates treated for HSV encephalitis survive, most suffer substantial neurologic sequelae. Approximately 25% of neonates with disseminated disease die despite antiviral therapy. The dosage of acyclovir is 60 mg/kg per day in 3 divided doses, given intravenously for 14 days if disease is limited to the skin, eye, and mouth and for 21 days if disease is disseminated or involves the CNS. Relapse of diseases of the skin, eyes, mouth, and CNS can occur after cessation of treatment. The optimal management of these recurrences is not established. The value of long-term suppressive or intermittent acyclovir therapy for neonates with disease of the skin, eyes, and mouth is being evaluated.

Infants with ocular involvement attributable to HSV infection should receive a topical ophthalmic drug (1%–2% trifluridine, 0.1% iododeoxyuridine, or 3% vidarabine) as well as parenteral antiviral therapy.

Genital Infection.

Primary. Many patients with first-episode herpes have mild clinical manifestations but go on to develop severe or prolonged symptoms. Therefore, most patients with initial genital herpes should receive antiviral therapy. In adults, acyclovir and valacyclovir decrease the duration of symptoms and viral shedding in primary genital herpes. Oral acyclovir therapy, initiated within 6 days of onset of disease, shortens the duration of illness and viral shedding by 3 to 5 days. Valacyclovir and famciclovir do not seem to be more effective than acyclovir, but they offer the advantage of less frequent dosing. No pediatric formulations of valacyclovir or famciclovir are available. Intravenous acyclovir is indicated for patients with a severe or complicated primary infection that requires hospitalization. Topical acyclovir (5%) ointment for primary genital herpes infection is not recommended. Systemic or topical treatment of primary herpetic lesions does not affect the subsequent frequency or severity of recurrences.

Recurrent. Antiviral therapy for recurrent genital herpes can be administered either episodically to ameliorate or shorten the duration of lesions or continuously as suppressive therapy to decrease the frequency of recurrences. Many patients benefit from antiviral therapy; therefore, options for treatment should be discussed with all patients. Oral acyclovir therapy initiated within 2 days of the onset of symptoms shortens the mean clinical course by approximately 1 day. Drug or a prescription for the medication should be provided with instructions to initiate treatment immediately when symptoms begin. Valacyclovir and famciclovir are licensed for treatment of adults with recurrent genital herpes; however, no data exist for treatment of pediatric disease. Topical acyclovir is not beneficial for immunocompetent hosts.

In adults with frequent genital HSV recurrences (6 or more episodes per year), daily oral acyclovir suppressive therapy is effective for decreasing the frequency of symptomatic recurrences. After approximately 1 year of continuous daily therapy, acyclovir should be discontinued and the recurrence rate should be assessed. If recurrences are observed, additional suppressive therapy should be considered. Acyclovir seems to be safe for adults receiving the drug for more than 15 years, but long-term effects are unknown. Data also support suppressive therapy in adults with valacyclovir or famciclovir.

Data on the use of acyclovir, valacyclovir, or famciclovir for suppressive therapy in children are not available. The safety of systemic acyclovir, valacyclovir, and famciclovir therapy in pregnant women has not been established. Available data do not indicate an increased risk of major birth defects in comparison with the general population in women treated with acyclovir during the first trimester. Acyclovir may be administered orally to pregnant women with first-episode genital herpes or severe recurrent herpes and should be given intravenously to pregnant women with severe HSV infection.

Mucocutaneous

Immunocompromised Hosts. Intravenous acyclovir is effective for treatment and prevention of mucocutaneous HSV infections. Topical acyclovir also may accelerate healing of lesions in immunocompromised patients.

Acyclovir-resistant strains of HSV have been isolated from immunocompromised people receiving prolonged treatment with acyclovir. Under these circumstances, progressive disease may be observed despite acyclovir therapy. Foscarnet sodium is the drug of choice for disease caused by acyclovir-resistant HSV isolates.

Immunocompetent Hosts. Limited data are available on the effects of acyclovir on the course of primary or recurrent nongenital mucocutaneous HSV infections in immunocompetent hosts. Therapeutic benefit has been noted in a limited number of children with primary gingivostomatitis treated with oral acyclovir. Minimal therapeutic benefit of oral acyclovir therapy has been demonstrated among adults with recurrent herpes labialis. Topical acyclovir is ineffective.

In a small controlled study in adults with recurrent herpes labialis (6 or more episodes per year), prophylactic acyclovir given in a dosage of 400 mg twice a day was effective for decreasing the frequency of recurrent episodes. Although no studies of prophylactic therapy have been performed in children, those with frequent recurrences may benefit from continuous oral acyclovir therapy (80 mg/kg per day in 3 divided doses; maximum 1000 mg/day); reevaluation should be performed after 1 year of continuous therapy.

Other HSV Infections

Central Nervous System. Patients with HSV encephalitis should be treated for 21 days with intravenous acyclovir. Therapy is less effective in older adults than in children. Patients who are comatose or semicomatose at initiation of therapy have a poor outcome. For people with Bell palsy, the combination of acyclovir and prednisone should be considered.

Ocular. Treatment of eye lesions should be undertaken in consultation with an ophthalmologist. Several topical drugs, such as 1% to 2% trifluridine, 0.1% iododeoxyuridine, and 3% vidarabine, have proven efficacy for superficial keratitis. Topical corticosteroids are contraindicated in suspected HSV conjunctivitis; however, ophthalmologists may choose to use corticosteroids in conjunction with antiviral drugs to treat locally invasive infections. For children with recurrent ocular lesions, oral suppressive therapy with acyclovir (80 mg/kg per day in 3 divided doses; maximum 1000 mg/day) may be of benefit.

ISOLATION OF THE HOSPITALIZED PATIENT: In addition to standard precautions, the following recommendations should be followed.

Neonates With HSV Infection. Neonates with HSV infection should be hospitalized and managed with contact precautions if mucocutaneous lesions are present.

Neonates Exposed to HSV During Delivery. Infants born to women with active HSV lesions should be managed with contact precautions during the incubation period. Some experts believe that contact precautions are unnecessary if exposed infants were born by cesarean delivery, provided membranes were ruptured for less than 4 hours. The risk of HSV infection in possibly exposed infants (eg, infants born to a mother with a history of recurrent genital herpes) is low.

One method of infection control for neonates with documented perinatal exposure to HSV is continuous rooming-in with the mother in a private room.

Women in Labor and Postpartum Women With HSV Infection. Women with active HSV lesions should be managed during labor, delivery, and the postpartum period with contact precautions. These women should be instructed about the importance of careful hand hygiene before and after caring for their infants. The mother may wear a clean covering gown to help avoid contact of the infant with lesions or infectious secretions. A mother with herpes labialis or stomatitis should wear a disposable surgical mask when touching her newborn infant until the lesions have crusted and dried. She should not kiss or nuzzle her newborn until the lesions have cleared. Herpetic lesions on other skin sites should be covered.

Breastfeeding is acceptable if no lesions are present on the breasts and if active lesions elsewhere on the mother are covered (see Human Milk, p 117).

Children With Mucocutaneous HSV Infection. Contact precautions are recommended for patients with severe mucocutaneous HSV infection. Patients with localized recurrent lesions should be managed with standard precautions.

Patients With HSV Infection of the CNS. Standard precautions are recommended for patients with infection limited to the CNS.

CONTROL MEASURES:

Prevention of Neonatal Infection. Expert opinion on the appropriate management of pregnant women to minimize the risk of neonatal HSV infection has changed considerably. Cultures for HSV obtained weekly during pregnancy no longer are recommended. Women with a history of genital HSV infection and women whose sexual partners have genital HSV infection are recognized to be at low risk of transmitting HSV to their infants (see Epidemiology, p 345).

Management of infants exposed to HSV during delivery differs according to the status of the mother's infection, mode of delivery, and expert opinion (see Care of Newborn Infants Whose Mothers Have Active Genital Lesions, p 351). Current recommendations for management of pregnant women for prevention of HSV infection include the following:

- **During pregnancy.** During prenatal evaluations, all pregnant women should be asked about past or current signs and symptoms consistent with genital herpes infection in themselves and their sexual partners.
- **Women in labor.** During labor, all women should be asked about recent and current signs and symptoms consistent with genital herpes infection, and they should be examined carefully for evidence of genital infection. Cesarean delivery for women who have clinically apparent HSV infection may decrease the risk of neonatal HSV infection if performed within 4 to 6 hours of membrane rupture but is less likely to decrease neonatal infection if performed later. However, many experts recommend cesarean delivery whenever the birth canal is infected, even if membranes have been ruptured for 6 hours or more. In the absence of genital lesions, a maternal history of genital HSV is not an indication for cesarean delivery. Scalp monitors should be avoided when possible in infants of women suspected of having active genital herpes infection.

  A cesarean delivery should be performed immediately for a woman who has ruptured membranes and active genital lesions at term. The appropriate management of delivery is not established if membranes rupture in the presence of active genital lesions at a time when the fetal lung is immature. Some experts recommend that intravenous acyclovir (15 mg/kg in 3 divided doses, maximum 1200 mg/day) be administered to the mother if labor and delivery are delayed. The value and risks of acyclovir in this situation are unknown. Acyclovir is not licensed by the FDA for this indication.

Care of Newborn Infants Whose Mothers Have Active Genital Lesions.

By Vaginal Delivery. Because the risk to infants exposed to HSV lesions during delivery varies in different circumstances from less than 5% to 50% or more, the decision to treat the asymptomatic exposed infant empirically with intravenous acyclovir is controversial. Because the infection rate of infants born to mothers with active recurrent genital herpes infections is less than 5%, most experts would not treat these infants empirically with acyclovir. The infant's parents or caregivers, however, should be educated about the signs and symptoms of neonatal HSV infection.

For infants born to mothers with a primary genital infection, the risk of infection may exceed 50%. Because of this high infection rate, some experts recommend empiric acyclovir treatment at birth after HSV cultures have been obtained, and others would obtain HSV cultures 24 to 48 hours after delivery and initiate acyclovir therapy only if HSV is recovered from these cultures. However, if the infant has symptoms suggestive of HSV infection, such as skin or scalp rashes (especially vesicular lesions) or unexplained clinical manifestations (such as those of sepsis), cultures should be obtained, regardless of age, and acyclovir therapy should be initiated immediately.

Differentiating primary genital infection from recurrent HSV infection in the mother would be helpful for assessing the risk of HSV infection for the exposed infant, but the distinction may be difficult. First-episode clinical infections are not always primary infections. Often, primary infections are asymptomatic, in which case the first symptomatic episode will represent a reactivated recurrent infection. In selected instances, serologic testing can be useful. For example, if a woman with herpetic lesions has no detectable HSV antibodies, she is experiencing a primary infection. Assessment of seropositive women necessitates differentiation of HSV-1 from HSV-2 antibodies. Currently, only assays based on detection of type-specific glycoprotein G make this distinction reliably.

Recommendations. The management of exposed asymptomatic infants who were born vaginally to mothers with active genital lesions can be categorized according to the type of maternal infection as follows:
- Mother with primary infection
- Mother with known recurrent lesions
- Mother whose status (primary vs recurrent) is unknown

For infants in each category, cultures should be obtained for HSV at 24 to 48 hours after birth. Specimens for cultures should include urine and stool and rectal, mouth, and nasopharynx swabs (see Diagnostic Tests, p 346). For infants whose mothers have presumed or proven primary infection, some experts recommend empiric acyclovir treatment at birth, although no data exist to support the efficacy of such an approach. Other experts would await positive HSV culture results or clinical manifestations of infection before starting therapy.

The infant whose mother has known, recurrent genital lesions should be observed carefully for signs of infection, including vesicular lesions of the skin, respiratory distress, seizures, or signs of sepsis. Education of parents and caregivers about the signs and symptoms of neonatal HSV infection is prudent. An infant with any of these manifestations should be evaluated immediately for possible HSV infection (as well as for bacterial infection). Specimens for HSV culture should be obtained from skin lesions, conjunctiva, nasopharynx, mouth, stool and rectal swabs, urine, stool blood buffy coat, and CSF. Testing of CSF by polymerase chain reaction assay also is recommended. Acyclovir therapy should be initiated if any of the culture results are positive, CSF or polymerase chain reaction assay findings are abnormal, or HSV infection is otherwise strongly suspected.

Infants born by cesarean delivery to mothers with herpetic lesions should be observed carefully, with cultures performed as recommended for potentially exposed infants born by vaginal delivery. Antiviral therapy should be initiated if culture results from the infant are positive or if HSV is suspected strongly for other reasons.

Other Recommendations.

- The length of in-hospital observation for infants at increased risk of neonatal HSV is variable and based on factors specific to the infant and local resources, such as the family's ability to observe the infant at home, availability of follow-up care, and clinical assessment.
- Neonatal HSV infection can occur as late as 6 weeks after delivery, although most infected infants are symptomatic by 4 weeks of age. Parents and physicians must be vigilant, and any rash or other symptoms that may be caused by HSV must be evaluated carefully.

Infected Hospital Personnel. Transmission of HSV in newborn nurseries from infected personnel to newborns rarely has been documented. The risk of transmission to infants by personnel who have herpes labialis or who are asymptomatic oral shedders of virus is low. Compromising patient care by excluding personnel with cold sores who are essential for the operation of the nursery must be weighed against the potential risk of infecting newborns. Personnel with cold sores who have contact with infants should cover and not touch their lesions and should comply with hand hygiene policies. Transmission of HSV infection from personnel with genital lesions is not likely as long as personnel comply with hand hygiene policies. Personnel with an active herpetic whitlow should not have responsibility for direct care of neonates or immunocompromised patients.

Infected Household Contacts of Newborns. Intrafamilial transmission of HSV to newborn infants has been described but is rare. Household members with herpetic skin lesions (eg, herpes labialis or herpetic whitlow) should be counseled about the risk and should avoid contact of their lesions with newborn infants by taking the same measures as recommended for infected hospital personnel as well as avoiding kissing and nuzzling the infant while they have active lip lesions or touching the infant while they have herpetic whitlow.

Care of People With Extensive Dermatitis. Patients with dermatitis are at risk of developing eczema herpeticum. If these patients are hospitalized, special care should be taken to avoid exposure to HSV. They should not be kissed by people with cold sores or touched by people with herpetic whitlow.

Care of Children With Mucocutaneous Infections Who Are in Child Care or School. Oral HSV infections are common among children who are in child care or school. Most of these infections are asymptomatic, with shedding of virus in saliva occurring in the absence of clinical disease. Only children with HSV gingivostomatitis (ie, primary infection) who do not have control of oral secretions should be excluded from child care. Exclusion of children with cold sores (ie, recurrent infection) from child care or school is not indicated.

Children with uncovered lesions on exposed surfaces pose a small potential risk to contacts. If children are certified by a physician to have recurrent HSV infection, covering the active lesions with clothing, a bandage, or an appropriate dressing when they attend child care or school is sufficient.

Herpes Simplex Virus Infections Among Wrestlers and Rugby Players. Infection with HSV-1 has been transmitted during athletic competition involving close physical contact and frequent skin abrasions, such as wrestling (herpes gladiatorum) and rugby (herpes rugbiaforum or scrum pox). Competitors often do not recognize or may deny possible infection. Transmission of these infections can be limited or prevented by the following: (1) examination of wrestlers and rugby players for vesicular or ulcerative lesions on exposed areas of their bodies and around their mouths or eyes before practice or competition by a person familiar with the appearance of mucocutaneous infections (including HSV, herpes zoster, and impetigo); (2) exclusion of athletes with these conditions from competition or practice until healing occurs or a physician's written statement declaring their condition noninfectious is obtained; and (3) cleaning wrestling mats with a freshly prepared solution of household bleach (one quarter cup of bleach in 1 gallon of water) applied for a minimum contact time of 15 seconds at least daily and, preferably, between matches. Despite these precautions, HSV spread during wrestling and other sports involving close personal contact still can occur through contact with asymptomatic infected people.

Histoplasmosis

CLINICAL MANIFESTATIONS: *Histoplasma capsulatum* causes symptoms in fewer than 5% of infected people. Clinical manifestations may be classified according to site (pulmonary, extrapulmonary, or disseminated), duration (acute, chronic), and pattern (primary vs reactivation) of infection. Most symptomatic patients have acute pulmonary histoplasmosis, an influenza-like illness with nonpleuritic chest pain, hilar adenopathy, and mild pulmonary infiltrates; symptoms persist for 2 days to 2 weeks. Intense exposure to spores can cause severe respiratory tract symptoms and diffuse nodular pulmonary infiltrates, prolonged fever, fatigue, and weight loss. Erythema nodosum can occur in adolescents. Primary cutaneous infections can occur after trauma.

Progressive disseminated histoplasmosis (PDH) can develop in otherwise healthy infants younger than 2 years of age. Early manifestations include prolonged fever, failure to thrive, and hepatosplenomegaly; if untreated, malnutrition, diffuse adenopathy, pneumonia, mucosal ulceration, pancytopenia, disseminated intravascular coagulopathy, and gastrointestinal bleeding can ensue. Central nervous system involvement is common. Chronic pulmonary and disseminated infection are rare. Histoplasmosis may reactivate in patients with poor cell-mediated immunity years after primary infection; an early symptom is fever with no apparent focus. Later, diffuse pneumonitis, skin lesions, meningitis, lymphadenopathy, hepatospleno-megaly, pancytopenia, and coagulopathy occur.

ETIOLOGY: *Histoplasma capsulatum* var *capsulatum* is a dimorphic fungus. It grows in soil as a spore-bearing mold with macroconidia but converts to yeast phase at body temperature.

EPIDEMIOLOGY: *Histoplasma capsulatum* is encountered in many parts of the world and is endemic in the eastern and central United States, particularly the Mississippi, Ohio, and Missouri River valleys. Infections occur sporadically, in out-breaks when weather conditions predispose to spread of spores, or in point-source epidemics from exposure to gardening activities; playing in barns, hollow trees, caves, or bird roosts; or excavation, demolition, cleaning, or renovation of contam-inated buildings. The organism grows in moist soil. Its growth is facilitated by bat, bird, and chicken droppings. Spores are spread in dry and windy conditions or when occupational or recreational activities disturb contaminated sites. Infection is acquired when spores (conidia) are inhaled. The inoculum inhaled, strain viru-lence, and immune status of the host affect the degree of illness. Reinfection is possi-ble but requires a large inoculum. Person-to-person transmission does not occur.

The **incubation period** is variable but usually is 1 to 3 weeks.

DIAGNOSTIC TESTS: Culture is the definitive method of diagnosis. *Histoplasma capsulatum* from bone marrow, blood, sputum, and tissue specimens grows on stan-dard mycologic media in 1 to 6 weeks. The lysis-centrifugation method is preferred for blood cultures. A DNA probe for *H capsulatum* permits rapid identification.

Demonstration of typical intracellular yeast forms by examination with Gomori methenamine silver or other stains of tissue, blood, bone marrow, or bronchoalveolar lavage specimens strongly supports the diagnosis of histoplasmosis when clinical, epi-demiologic, and other laboratory studies are compatible.

Detection of *H capsulatum* polysaccharide antigen (HPA) in serum, urine, or bronchoalveolar lavage fluid by radioimmunoassay or enzyme immunoassay is a rapid and specific diagnostic method. It is most sensitive for progressive disseminated infections; a negative test does not exclude infection. If initially positive, the antigen test can be used to monitor treatment response and to identify relapse in human immunodeficiency virus (HIV)-infected patients. Cross reactions occur in patients with blastomycosis, coccidioidomycosis, paracoccidioidomycosis, and *Penicillium marneffei* infection; clinical and epidemiologic circumstances assist in differentiating these infections. The HPA test has low sensitivity for diagnosis of acute pulmonary histoplasmosis in immunocompromised people.

Both mycelial-phase (histoplasmin) and yeast-phase antigens are used in sero-logic testing for complement-fixing antibodies to *H capsulatum*. A fourfold increase in yeast-phase titers or a single titer of 1:32 or greater is presumptive evidence of active infection. Cross-reacting antibodies can result from *Blastomyces dermatitidis* and *Coccidioides immitis* infections. In the immunodiffusion test, H bands, although rarely encountered, are highly suggestive of acute infection. The immunodiffusion test is more specific than the complement fixation test, but the complement fixation test is more sensitive.

The histoplasmin skin test is not useful for diagnostic purposes and is not available in the United States.

TREATMENT: Immunocompetent children with uncomplicated, primary pulmonary histoplasmosis rarely require antifungal therapy. Indications for therapy include PDH in infants and acute infection in immunocompromised patients. Other manifestations of histoplasmosis in immunocompetent children for which antifungal therapy should be considered include pulmonary disease with symptoms persisting more than 4 weeks, serious illness with intense exposures, and granulomatous adenitis that obstructs critical structures (eg, bronchi or blood vessels).

Amphotericin B is recommended for disseminated disease and other serious infections (see Drugs for Invasive and Other Serious Fungal Infections, p 725), because most experts believe clinical improvement occurs more rapidly with it than with the azoles. In other circumstances in which antifungal therapy is warranted, itraconazole and fluconazole also have been effective. The safety and efficacy of itraconazole for use in children have not been established, but in adults, itraconazole is preferred over fluconazole and has negligible toxic effects. Itraconazole also has proven effective in the treatment of mild disseminated histoplasmosis in HIV-infected patients.

The duration of amphotericin B treatment for PDH is 4 to 6 weeks. Although data for children are limited, some experts recommend limiting amphotericin B therapy to 2 to 3 weeks, if substantial clinical improvement has occurred, to be followed by 3 to 6 months of itraconazole. Mild infections in HIV-infected patients can be treated with itraconazole for 3 months. Patients with HIV infection and PDH require lifelong suppressive therapy with itraconazole to prevent relapse; fluconazole can be given if itraconazole is not tolerated.

Erythema nodosum, arthritis syndromes, and pericarditis do not necessitate antifungal therapy. Pericarditis is treated with indomethacin. Dense fibrosis of mediastinal structures without an associated granulomatous inflammatory component does not respond to antifungal therapy.

ISOLATION OF THE HOSPITALIZED PATIENT: Standard precautions are recommended.

CONTROL MEASURES: In outbreaks, investigation for the common source of infection is indicated. Exposure to soil and dust from areas with significant accumulations of bird and bat droppings should be avoided, especially by immunocompromised people, or, if unavoidable, controlled through the use of masks, gloves, and disposable clothing. Guidelines for preventing histoplasmosis designed for health and safety professionals, environmental consultants, and people supervising workers involved in activities in which contaminated materials are disturbed are available. Additional information about the guidelines is available from the National Institute for Occupational Safety and Health (NIOSH; publication No. 97-146), Publications Dissemination, 4676 Columbia Parkway, Cincinnati, OH 45226-1998; telephone

800/356-4674; the National Center for Infectious Diseases, telephone 404/639-3158; and the NIOSH Web site (www.cdc.gov/niosh/97-146.html).

Hookworm Infections
(*Ancylostoma duodenale* and *Necator americanus*)

CLINICAL MANIFESTATIONS: Patients with hookworm infestation most often are asymptomatic; however, chronic hookworm infestation is a common cause of hypochromic microcytic anemia in people living in tropical developing countries, and heavy infestation can cause hypoproteinemia with edema. After contact with contaminated soil, initial skin penetration of larvae usually involving the feet can cause a stinging or burning sensation followed by pruritus and a papulovesicular rash that may persist for 1 to 2 weeks. Pneumonitis associated with migrating larvae is uncommon and usually mild, except in heavy infestations. Disease after oral ingestion of infectious *Ancylostoma duodenale* larvae can manifest with pharyngeal itching, hoarseness, nausea, and vomiting shortly after ingestion. Colicky abdominal pain, nausea, and/or diarrhea and marked eosinophilia can develop 4 to 6 weeks after exposure.

ETIOLOGY: Infestation usually is caused by *A duodenale* or *Necator americanus,* 2 roundworms (nematodes) with similar life cycles.

EPIDEMIOLOGY: Humans are the major reservoir. Hookworms are prominent in rural, tropical, and subtropical areas where soil contamination with human feces is common. Although both hookworm species are equally prevalent in many areas, *A duodenale* is the predominant species in Europe, the Mediterranean region, northern Asia, and the west coast of South America. *Necator americanus* is predominant in the Western hemisphere, sub-Saharan Africa, southeast Asia, and a number of Pacific islands. Larvae and eggs survive in loose, sandy, moist, shady, well-aerated, warm soil (optimal temperature 23°C–33°C [73°F–91°F]). Hookworm eggs from stool hatch in soil in 1 to 2 days as rhabdoid larvae. These larvae develop into infective filariform larvae in soil within 5 to 7 days and can persist for weeks to months. Percutaneous infestation occurs after exposure to infectious larvae. *Ancylostoma duodenale* transmission can occur by oral ingestion and possibly through human milk. Untreated infested patients can harbor worms for 5 to 15 years, but a decrease in worm burden of at least 70% generally occurs within 1 to 2 years.

The time from exposure to development of noncutaneous symptoms is 4 to 12 weeks.

DIAGNOSTIC TESTS: Microscopic demonstration of hookworm eggs in feces is diagnostic. Adult worms or larvae rarely are seen. Approximately 8 to 12 weeks are required after infestation for eggs to appear in feces. A direct stool smear with saline solution or potassium iodide saturated with iodine is adequate for diagnosis of heavy hookworm infestation; light infestations require concentration techniques. Quantification techniques (eg, Kato-Katz, Beaver direct smear, or Stoll egg-counting techniques) to determine the clinical significance of infestation and the response to treatment may be available from state or reference laboratories.

TREATMENT: Albendazole, mebendazole, and pyrantel pamoate all are effective treatments (see Drugs for Parasitic Infections, p 744). In children younger than 2 years of age, in whom experience with these drugs is limited, the World Health Organization (WHO) recommends one half the adult dose of albendazole or mebendazole in heavy hookworm infestations. The dose of pyrantel is determined by weight. In heavy hookworm infestation during pregnancy, deworming treatment is recommended by the WHO during the second or third trimester. Albendazole, mebendazole, or pyrantel may be used. A repeated stool examination, using a concentration technique, should be performed 2 weeks after treatment, and if positive, retreatment is indicated. Nutritional supplementation, including iron, is important when anemia is present. Severely affected children may require blood transfusion.

ISOLATION OF THE HOSPITALIZED PATIENT: Only standard precautions are recommended, because there is no direct person-to-person transmission.

CONTROL MEASURES: Sanitary disposal of feces to prevent contamination of soil, particularly in endemic areas, is necessary but rarely accomplished. Treatment of all known infested people and screening of high-risk groups (ie, children and agricultural workers) in endemic areas can help decrease environmental contamination. Wearing shoes also may be helpful. Despite relatively rapid reinfestation, periodic deworming treatments targeting school-aged children have been advocated to prevent morbidity associated with heavy intestinal helminth infestations.

Human Herpesvirus 6 (Including Roseola) and 7

CLINICAL MANIFESTATIONS: Clinical manifestations of primary infection with human herpesvirus (HHV)-6 include roseola (exanthem subitum, sixth disease) in approximately 20% of infected children, undifferentiated febrile illness without rash or localizing signs, and other acute febrile illnesses, often accompanied by cervical and postoccipital lymphadenopathy, gastrointestinal or respiratory tract signs, and inflamed tympanic membranes. Fever is characteristically high (>39.5°C [>103.0°F]) and persists for 3 to 7 days. In roseola, fever is followed by an erythematous maculopapular rash lasting hours to days. Seizures occur during the febrile period in approximately 10% to 15% of primary infections. A bulging anterior fontanelle and encephalopathy occur occasionally. The virus persists and may reactivate. The clinical circumstances and manifestations of reactivation in healthy people are unclear. Illness associated with reactivation, primarily in immunosuppressed hosts, has been described in association with manifestations such as fever, hepatitis, bone marrow suppression, pneumonia, and encephalitis.

Recognition of the varied clinical manifestations of HHV-7 infection is evolving. Many, if not most, primary infections with HHV-7 may be asymptomatic or mild; some may present as typical roseola and may account for second or recurrent cases of roseola. Febrile illnesses associated with seizures also have been reported. Some investigators suggest that the association of HHV-7 with these clinical manifestations results from the ability of HHV-7 to reactivate HHV-6 from latency.

ETIOLOGY: Human herpesvirus 6 and HHV-7 are closely related members of the Herpesviridae family. Strains of HHV-6 belong to 1 of 2 major groups, variants A and B. Almost all primary infections in children are caused by variant B strains.

EPIDEMIOLOGY: Humans are the only known natural hosts for HHV-6 and HHV-7. Transmission of HHV-6 to an infant most likely results from asymptomatic shedding of persistent virus in secretions of a family member, caregiver, or other close contact. During the febrile phase of primary infection, HHV-6 can be isolated from peripheral blood lymphocytes, saliva, and cerebrospinal fluid. Virus-specific maternal antibody is present uniformly in the serum of infants at birth and provides transient protection. As the concentration of maternal antibody decreases during the first year of life, the rate of infection increases rapidly, peaking between 6 and 24 months of age. Most children are seropositive by 4 years of age. Infections occur throughout the year without a seasonal pattern. Secondary cases rarely are identified. Occasional outbreaks of roseola have been reported.

Human herpesvirus-7 infection occurs somewhat later in life than HHV-6. By adulthood, the seroprevalence of HHV-7 is approximately 85%. Lifelong persistent infection with HHV-6 and HHV-7 is established after primary infection. Infectious virus is present in more than three fourths of saliva specimens obtained from healthy adults. Transmission of HHV-6 and HHV-7 to young children is likely to occur from contact with infected respiratory tract secretions of healthy people.

The mean **incubation period** for HHV-6 is 9 to 10 days. The incubation period for HHV-7 is unknown.

DIAGNOSTIC TESTS: The definitive diagnosis of primary HHV-6 infection currently necessitates use of research techniques to isolate the virus from a peripheral blood specimen as well as to demonstrate seroconversion. A fourfold increase in serum antibody concentration alone does not necessarily indicate new infection, as an increase in titer also may occur with reactivation and in association with other infections. Commercial assays for antibody and antigen detection and polymerase chain reaction assay for detecting HHV-6 DNA are in development, but none of these assays can differentiate reliably between primary infection and viral persistence or reactivation.

Diagnostic tests for HHV-7 also are limited to research laboratories, and reliable differentiation between primary infection and reactivation is problematic. Serodiagnosis of HHV-7 is confounded by serologic cross-reactivity with HHV-6 and by the potential ability of HHV-6 to be reactivated by HHV-7 and possibly other infections.

TREATMENT: Supportive. Some experts recommend therapy with ganciclovir for immunocompromised patients with serious HHV-6 disease.

ISOLATION OF THE HOSPITALIZED PATIENT: Standard precautions are recommended.

CONTROL MEASURES: None.

Human Herpesvirus 8

CLINICAL MANIFESTATIONS: For children, the clinical implications of the most recently discovered member of the herpesvirus family, human herpesvirus (HHV)-8, are unknown. In adults, HHV-8 etiologically is associated with Kaposi sarcoma. The HHV-8 DNA sequences have been detected in all forms of Kaposi sarcoma from all parts of the world in patients with and without human immunodeficiency virus (HIV) infection, with primary effusion lymphomas of the abdominal cavity, with lymphoproliferative syndrome (although less commonly than has Epstein-Barr virus [EBV]), and with multicentric Castleman disease. Evidence of HHV-8 infection in children is rare, and no clinical associations are known.

ETIOLOGY: Human herpesvirus 8 is a member of the family Herpesviridae, the gammaherpesvirus subfamily closely related to herpesvirus saimiri of monkeys and EBV.

EPIDEMIOLOGY: Little is known about the epidemiology and transmission of HHV-8. However, HHV-8 has been reported to be latent in peripheral blood mononuclear cells and lymphoid tissue from immunocompromised patients and some healthy people, suggesting that transmission could be via blood or secretions. In the United States in patients with HIV, HHV-8 infection does not appear to occur until after adolescence.

The **incubation period** of HHV-8 is unknown.

DIAGNOSTIC TESTS: Diagnostic tests for detection of HHV-8 infections are limited to research laboratories, and reliable differentiation of primary versus latent infection is problematic.

TREATMENT: No effective treatment is known for HHV-8.

ISOLATION OF THE HOSPITALIZED PATIENT: Standard precautions are recommended.

CONTROL MEASURES: None.

Human Immunodeficiency Virus Infection*

CLINICAL MANIFESTATIONS: Human immunodeficiency virus (HIV) infection in children and adolescents causes a broad spectrum of disease and a varied clinical course. Acquired immunodeficiency syndrome (AIDS) represents the most severe end of the clinical spectrum. The current surveillance definitions of the Centers for Disease Control and Prevention (CDC) for AIDS in adults and adolescents are listed in Table 3.23 (p 361), and the CDC clinical categories and pediatric classification system for children younger than 13 years of age who are born to HIV-infected mothers or who are known to be infected with HIV are presented in Tables 3.24 (p 362) and 3.25 (p 364).[†‡] This pediatric classification system, which was established for surveillance of HIV infection, emphasizes the importance of the CD4+ T-lymphocyte count as an immunologic surrogate and marker of prognosis but does not use information on viral load as quantitated by RNA polymerase chain reaction (PCR) assay.

The manifestations of pediatric HIV infection include generalized lymphadenopathy, hepatomegaly, splenomegaly, failure to thrive, oral candidiasis, recurrent diarrhea, parotitis, cardiomyopathy, hepatitis, nephropathy, central nervous system (CNS) disease (including developmental delay), lymphoid interstitial pneumonia, recurrent invasive bacterial infections, opportunistic infections,[§] and specific malignant neoplasms.

Pneumocystis pneumonia (PCP) is one of the most commonly reported opportunistic infections in children with AIDS and is associated with a high mortality rate (see *Pneumocystis jiroveci* Infections, p 500). Although PCP occurs most commonly in infants between 3 and 6 months of age who acquired HIV infection before or at birth, PCP can occur in younger infants beginning as early as 4 to 6 weeks of age or in older children whose immunologic status has deteriorated. Other common opportunistic infections in children include *Candida* species esophagitis, disseminated cytomegalovirus (CMV) infection, and chronic or disseminated herpes simplex and varicella-zoster virus infections, and less commonly, *Mycobacterium tuberculosis, Mycobacterium avium* complex (MAC) infection, and chronic enteritis caused by *Cryptosporidium* species, *Isospora* species, or other agents. Rarely, disseminated or CNS cryptococcal or *Toxoplasma gondii* infections occur in children.

---

* For a complete listing of current policy statements from the American Academy of Pediatrics regarding human immunodeficiency virus and acquired immunodeficiency syndrome, see http://aappolicy.aapjournals.org/.
† Centers for Disease Control and Prevention. 1993 revised classification system for HIV infection and expanded surveillance case definition for AIDS among adolescents and adults. *MMWR Recomm Rep.* 1992;41(RR-17):1–19
‡ Centers for Disease Control and Prevention. 1994 revised classification system for human immunodeficiency virus infection in children less than 13 years of age. Official authorized addenda: human immunodeficiency virus infection codes and official guidelines for coding and reporting ICD-9-CM. *MMWR Recomm Rep.* 1994;43(RR-12):1–19
§ Centers for Disease Control and Prevention. Guidelines for preventing opportunistic infections among HIV-infected persons—2002. Recommendations of the US Public Health Service and the Infectious Diseases Society of America. *MMWR Recomm Rep.* 2002;51(RR-8):1–46

Table 3.23. **1993 Revised Case Definition of AIDS-Defining Conditions for Adults and Adolescents 13 Years of Age and Older[1]**

- Candidiasis of bronchi, trachea, or lungs
- Candidiasis, esophageal
- Cervical cancer, invasive
- Coccidioidomycosis, disseminated or extrapulmonary
- Cryptococcosis, extrapulmonary
- Cryptosporidiosis, chronic intestinal (>1 mo duration)
- Cytomegalovirus disease (other than liver, spleen, or nodes)
- Cytomegalovirus retinitis (with loss of vision)
- Encephalopathy, HIV related
- Herpes simplex: chronic ulcer(s) (>1 mo duration) or bronchitis, pneumonitis, or esophagitis
- Histoplasmosis, disseminated or extrapulmonary
- Isosporiasis, chronic intestinal (>1 mo duration)
- Kaposi sarcoma
- Lymphoma, Burkitt (or equivalent term)
- Lymphoma, immunoblastic (or equivalent term)
- Lymphoma, primary or brain
- *Mycobacterium avium* complex or *Mycobacterium kansasii,* disseminated or extrapulmonary
- *Mycobacterium tuberculosis,* any site, pulmonary or extrapulmonary
- *Mycobacterium,* other species or unidentified species, disseminated or extrapulmonary
- *Pneumocystis* pneumonia
- Pneumonia, recurrent
- Progressive multifocal leukoencephalopathy
- *Salmonella* septicemia, recurrent
- Toxoplasmosis of brain
- Wasting syndrome attributable to HIV
- CD4+ T-lymphocyte count less than 200/μL (0.20 × 10^9/L) or CD4+ percentage less than 15%

AIDS indicates acquired immunodeficiency syndrome; HIV, human immunodeficiency virus.
[1] Modified from Centers for Disease Control and Prevention. 1993 revised classification system for HIV infection and expanded surveillance case definition for AIDS among adolescents and adults. *MMWR Recomm Rep.* 1992;41(RR-17):1–19.

The occurrence of malignant neoplasms in children with HIV infection has been relatively uncommon, but leiomyosarcomas and certain lymphomas, including those of the CNS and non-Hodgkin B-cell lymphomas of the Burkitt type, occur more commonly in children with HIV infection than in immunocompetent children. Kaposi sarcoma is rare in children in the United States but occurs commonly among HIV-infected children in highly endemic areas of the world.

The development of opportunistic infections, particularly PCP, progressive neurologic disease, and severe wasting, is associated with a poor prognosis. The prognosis for survival also is poor in perinatally infected infants when viral load exceeds 300 000 copies/mL and the CD4+ T-lymphocyte count is decreased and when symptoms develop during the first year of life. With earlier use of potent combination antiretroviral therapy, prognosis and survival rates have improved.

Table 3.24. Clinical Categories for Children Younger Than 13 Years of Age With Human Immunodeficiency Virus (HIV) Infection[1]

Category N: Not Symptomatic
Children who have no signs or symptoms considered to be the result of HIV infection or have only 1 of the conditions listed in Category A.

Category A: Mildly Symptomatic
Children with 2 or more of the conditions listed but none of the conditions listed in categories B and C.
- Lymphadenopathy (≥0.5 cm at more than 2 sites; bilateral at 1 site)
- Hepatomegaly
- Splenomegaly
- Dermatitis
- Parotitis
- Recurrent or persistent upper respiratory tract infection, sinusitis, or otitis media

Category B: Moderately Symptomatic
Children who have symptomatic conditions other than those listed for category A or C that are attributed to HIV infection.
- Anemia (hemoglobin, <8 g/dL [<80 g/L]), neutropenia (white blood cell count, <1000/μL [<1.0 × 10⁹/L]), and/or thrombocytopenia (platelet count, <100 × 10³/μL [<100 × 10⁹/L]) persisting for ≥30 days
- Bacterial meningitis, pneumonia, or sepsis (single episode)
- Candidiasis, oropharyngeal (thrush), persisting (>2 mo) in children older than 6 mo of age
- Cardiomyopathy
- Cytomegalovirus infection, with onset before 1 mo of age
- Diarrhea, recurrent or chronic
- Hepatitis
- Herpes simplex virus (HSV) stomatitis, recurrent (>2 episodes within 1 year)

Category B: Moderately Symptomatic, continued
- HSV bronchitis, pneumonitis, or esophagitis with onset before 1 mo of age
- Herpes zoster (shingles) involving at least 2 distinct episodes or more than 1 dermatome
- Leiomyosarcoma
- Lymphoid interstitial pneumonia or pulmonary lymphoid hyperplasia complex
- Nephropathy
- Nocardiosis
- Persistent fever (lasting >1 mo)
- Toxoplasmosis, onset before 1 mo of age
- Varicella, disseminated (complicated chickenpox)

Category C: Severely Symptomatic
- Serious bacterial infections, multiple or recurrent (ie, any combination of at least 2 culture-confirmed infections within a 2-y period), of the following types: septicemia, pneumonia, meningitis, bone or joint infection, or abscess of an internal organ or body cavity (excluding otitis media, superficial skin or mucosal abscesses, and indwelling catheter-related infections)
- Candidiasis, esophageal or pulmonary (bronchi, trachea, lungs)
- Coccidioidomycosis, disseminated (at site other than or in addition to lungs or cervical or hilar lymph nodes)
- Cryptococcosis, extrapulmonary
- Cryptosporidiosis or isosporiasis with diarrhea persisting >1 mo
- Cytomegalovirus disease with onset of symptoms after 1 mo of age (at a site other than liver, spleen, or lymph nodes)

Category C: Severely Symptomatic, continued

- Encephalopathy (at least 1 of the following progressive findings present for at least 2 mo in the absence of a concurrent illness other than HIV infection that could explain the findings): (1) failure to attain or loss of developmental milestones or loss of intellectual ability, verified by standard developmental scale or neuropsychologic tests; (2) impaired brain growth or acquired microcephaly demonstrated by head circumference measurements or brain atrophy demonstrated by computed tomography or magnetic resonance imaging (serial imaging required for children younger than 2 y of age); (3) acquired symmetric motor deficit manifested by 2 or more of the following: paresis, pathologic reflexes, ataxia, or gait disturbance
- HSV infection causing a mucocutaneous ulcer that persists for greater than 1 mo or bronchitis, pneumonitis, or esophagitis for any duration affecting a child older than 1 mo of age
- Histoplasmosis, disseminated (at a site other than or in addition to lungs or cervical or hilar lymph nodes)
- Kaposi sarcoma
- Lymphoma, primary, in brain
- Lymphoma, small, noncleaved cell (Burkitt), or immunoblastic; or large-cell lymphoma of B-cell or unknown immunologic phenotype
- *Mycobacterium tuberculosis*, disseminated or extrapulmonary
- *Mycobacterium*, other species or unidentified species, disseminated (at a site other than or in addition to lungs, skin, or cervical or hilar lymph nodes)
- *Pneumocystis* pneumonia
- Progressive multifocal leukoencephalopathy
- *Salmonella* (nontyphoid) septicemia, recurrent
- Toxoplasmosis of the brain with onset at after 1 mo of age
- Wasting syndrome in the absence of a concurrent illness other than HIV infection that could explain the following findings: (1) persistent weight loss >10% of baseline; (2) downward crossing of at least 2 of the following percentile lines on the weight-for-age chart (eg, 95th, 75th, 50th, 25th, 5th) in a child 1 y of age or older; OR (3) <5th percentile on weight-for-height chart on 2 consecutive measurements, ≥30 days apart; PLUS (1) chronic diarrhea (ie, at least 2 loose stools per day for >30 days); OR (2) documented fever (for >30 days, intermittent or constant)

---

[1] Modified from Centers for Disease Control and Prevention. 1994 revised classification system for human immunodeficiency virus infection in children less than 13 years of age. Official authorized addenda: human immunodeficiency virus infection codes and official guidelines for coding and reporting ICD-9-CM. *MMWR Recomm Rep.* 1994;43(RR-12):1–19

Table 3.25. Pediatric Human Immunodeficiency Virus (HIV) Classification for Children Younger Than 13 Years of Age[1]

| Immunologic Definitions | Clinical Classifications[2] | | | | Immunologic Categories — Age-Specific CD4+ T-Lymphocyte Count and Percentage of Total Lymphocytes[3] | | | | | |
	N: No Signs or Symptoms	A: Mild Signs and Symptoms	B: Moderate Signs and Symptoms[4]	C: Severe Signs and Symptoms[4]	<12 mo µL	<12 mo %	1–5 y µL	1–5 y %	6–12 y µL	6–12 y %
1: No evidence of suppression	N1	A1	B1	C1	≥1500	≥25	≥1000	≥25	≥500	≥25
2: Evidence of moderate suppression	N2	A2	B2	C2	750–1499	15–24	500–999	15–24	200–499	15–24
3: Severe suppression	N3	A3	B3	C3	<750	<15	<500	<15	<200	<15

[1] Modified from Centers for Disease Control and Prevention. 1994 revised classification system for human immunodeficiency virus infection in children less than 13 years of age. Official authorized addenda: human immunodeficiency virus infection codes and official guidelines for coding and reporting ICD-9-CM. *MMWR Recomm Rep.* 1994;43(RR-12):1–19

[2] Children whose HIV infection status is not confirmed are classified by using this grid with a letter E (for perinatally exposed) placed before the appropriate classification code (eg, EN2).

[3] To convert values in µL to Système International units (× 10^9/L), multiply by 0.001.

[4] Lymphoid interstitial pneumonitis in category B or category C is reportable to state and local health departments as acquired immunodeficiency syndrome (see Table 3.24, p 362, for further definition of clinical categories).

Data on long-term survival rates of children receiving this combination antiretroviral therapy are being collected. Median survival to 9 years of age was reported before the availability of more potent combination antiretroviral therapy.

ETIOLOGY: Infection is caused by human RNA retroviruses, HIV type 1 (HIV-1) and, less commonly, HIV type 2 (HIV-2), a related virus that is rare in the United States but more common in West Africa.

EPIDEMIOLOGY: Humans are the only known reservoir of HIV, although related viruses, perhaps genetic ancestors, have been identified in chimpanzees and monkeys. Because retroviruses integrate into the target cell genome as proviruses and the viral genome is copied during cell replication, the virus persists in infected people for life. Data demonstrate the persistence of latent virus in peripheral blood mononuclear cells even when the viral RNA is below the limit of detection in blood. Human immunodeficiency virus has been isolated from blood (including lymphocytes, macrophages, and plasma) and from other body fluids, including cerebrospinal fluid, pleural fluid, human milk, semen, cervical secretions, saliva, urine, and tears. Only blood, semen, cervical secretions, and human milk have been implicated epidemiologically in transmission of infection.

The established modes of HIV transmission in the United States are the following: (1) sexual contact (vaginal, anal, or oral); (2) percutaneous (from needles or other sharp instruments) or mucous membrane exposure to contaminated blood or other body fluids with high titers of HIV; (3) mother-to-infant transmission before or around the time of birth; and (4) breastfeeding. Because of exclusion of infected donors, viral inactivation treatment of clotting factor concentrates, and the availability of recombinant clotting factors (see Blood Safety, p 106), transfusion of blood, blood components, or clotting factor concentrates has been a rare source of HIV transmission in the United States. In the absence of documented sexual transmission or parenteral or mucous membrane contact with blood or blood-containing body fluids, transmission of HIV rarely has been demonstrated to occur in families or households or with routine care in hospitals or clinics. Transmission of HIV has not occurred in schools or child care settings.

Cases of AIDS in children have accounted for approximately 1% of all reported cases in the United States. The total number of reported cases of AIDS in children decreased 81% in 2000 compared with 1992 as a result of a dramatic decrease in the rate of perinatal HIV transmission and availability of potent combination antiretroviral therapy.

More than 90% of HIV-infected children younger than 13 years of age in the United States acquired infection from their mothers. Almost all of the remainder, including patients with hemophilia or other coagulation disorders, received contaminated blood, blood components, or clotting factor concentrates. A few cases of HIV infection in children have resulted from sexual abuse by an HIV-seropositive person. Fewer than 5% of cases have been reported to have no identifiable risk factor, and after careful investigation, most are reclassified into one of the established risk factor groups. Perinatally acquired infection now accounts for almost all new infections in preadolescent children.

The rate of acquisition of HIV during adolescence continues to increase and contributes to the large number of cases in young adults. Transmission of HIV among adolescents is attributable primarily to sexual exposure. Approximately 25% of HIV transmission in the United States is estimated to occur among people younger than 21 years of age. Among adolescents, the incidence of HIV infection in females is surpassing that in males. Most HIV-infected adolescents are asymptomatic and are not aware that they are infected.

The risk of infection for an infant born to an HIV-seropositive mother who did not receive antiretroviral therapy during pregnancy is estimated to be between 13% and 39%. Studies on the timing of transmission from an infected mother to her infant suggest that in a nonbreastfeeding population, approximately 25% to 40% of transmission occurs in utero. The absolute risk for in utero transmission is approximately 5% and for intrapartum transmission is approximately 13% to 18%. A number of studies have shown that maternal viral load is a critical determinant of perinatal HIV transmission. Studies with small numbers of pregnant women have suggested higher rates of perinatal transmission by women who seroconvert during pregnancy. Other factors associated with an increased risk of transmission include low CD4+ T-lymphocyte counts, advanced maternal illness, intrapartum events resulting in increased exposure of the fetus to maternal blood, placental membrane inflammation, premature delivery, prolonged labor, and longer duration of rupture of membranes. Prolonged rupture of membranes in the presence of antiretroviral therapy but detectable viral load is associated with an increased risk of transmission and must be considered when evaluating the mode of delivery and transmission.

Postpartum transmission occurs through breastfeeding. Worldwide, an estimated one third to one half of mother-to-child transmission of HIV may occur through breastfeeding. Human immunodeficiency virus genomes have been detected in cellular and cell-free fractions of human milk. In the United States, it is possible to provide safe alternative feeding for infants and, therefore, to avoid human-milk transmission of HIV. A means to diminish HIV transmission and continue safe feeding practices for infants born to HIV-infected women in the developing world is needed (see Human Milk, p 117).

INCUBATION PERIOD: Although the median age of onset of symptoms is approximately 12 to 18 months for untreated perinatally infected infants, some children are identified who have remained asymptomatic for more than 5 years, and some sites are reporting perinatally infected children who are first positively identified as such during adolescence. Two patterns of progression of infection based on symptoms have been recognized. Approximately 15% to 20% of untreated children die before 4 years of age, with a median age at death of 11 months, whereas most children survive beyond 5 years of age. Adults and children develop serum antibody to HIV by 6 to 12 weeks after infection. Infants born to HIV-infected women have transplacentally acquired antibody and, therefore, test seropositive from the time of birth.

DIAGNOSTIC TESTS: The laboratory diagnosis of HIV infection during infancy depends on detection of virus or viral nucleic acid. The transplacental transfer of antibody complicates the use of antibody-based assays (eg, HIV enzyme immunoassay [EIA] and Western blot analysis) for diagnosis of infant infection, because all infants born to HIV-positive mothers infected 6 to 12 weeks or more before delivery have maternal antibodies.

Human immunodeficiency virus nucleic acid detection by PCR assay of DNA extracted from peripheral blood mononuclear cells is the preferred test for diagnosis of HIV infection in infants, and results can be available within 24 hours of obtaining a sample of anticoagulated whole blood (see Table 3.26, p 368). Approximately 30% of infants with HIV infection will have a positive DNA PCR assay result from samples obtained before 48 hours of age. The test routinely can detect 1 to 10 DNA copies. Approximately 93% of infected infants have detectable HIV DNA by 2 weeks of age, and almost all infants are HIV positive by 1 month of age. A single DNA PCR assay has a sensitivity of 95% and a specificity of 97% on samples collected from infants 1 to 36 months of age. The DNA PCR assay is more sensitive on a single assay than is virus culture, and virus need not be replication competent to be detected.

Virus isolation by culture is expensive, is available only in a few laboratories, and requires up to 28 days for positive results. This test essentially has been replaced by DNA PCR assay.

Detection of the p24 antigen (including immune complex dissociated) is substantially less sensitive than are DNA PCR assay or culture. An additional drawback is the occurrence of false-positive test results in samples obtained from infants younger than 1 month of age.

Plasma HIV RNA PCR assay may be used to diagnose HIV infection if the result is positive. However, this test result may be negative in HIV-infected people. The test is licensed by the US Food and Drug Administration only in quantitative format and currently is used for quantifying the amount of virus present as a predictor of disease progression, not routinely for diagnosis of HIV infection in infants.

Infants born to HIV-infected women should be tested by HIV DNA PCR during the first 48 hours of life. Because of possible contamination with maternal blood, umbilical cord blood should not be used for this determination. A second test should be performed at 1 to 2 months of age. Obtaining the sample as early as 14 days of age may enable decisions to be made about antiretroviral therapy at an earlier age. A third test is recommended at 2 to 4 months of age. Any time an infant tests positive, testing should be repeated on a second blood sample as soon as possible to confirm the diagnosis. An infant is considered infected if 2 separate samples are positive.* An HIV antibody test can be performed on samples of blood, oral fluid, or urine. A rapid test for HIV antibodies has been licensed for use in the United States; this test is used widely throughout the world, particularly for screening in maternity settings. Infection can be excluded reasonably when 2 HIV DNA PCR assays performed at or beyond 1 month of age, and a third performed on a sample obtained at 4 months of age or older, are negative. Alternatively, an infant with 2 blood samples negative for HIV antibody obtained after 6 months of age and at an interval of at least 1 month also can be considered not infected.

---

* Centers for Disease Control and Prevention. Guidelines for national human immunodeficiency virus case surveillance, including monitoring for human immunodeficiency virus infection and acquired immunodeficiency syndrome. *MMWR Recomm Rep.* 1999;48(RR-13):1–28

Table 3.26. **Laboratory Diagnosis of HIV Infection**[1]

Test	Comment
HIV DNA PCR	Preferred test to diagnose HIV infection in infants and children younger than 18 months of age; highly sensitive and specific by 2 weeks of age and available; performed on peripheral blood mononuclear cells
HIV p24 Ag	Less sensitive, false-positive results during first month of life, variable results; not recommended
ICD p24 Ag	Commonly available; negative test result does not rule out infection; not recommended
HIV culture	Expensive, not easily available, requires up to 4 weeks to do test
HIV RNA PCR	Not recommended for routine testing of infants and children younger than 18 months of age, because a negative result cannot be used to exclude HIV infection

[1] HIV indicates human immunodeficiency virus; PCR, polymerase chain reaction; Ag, antigen; and ICD, immune complex dissociated.

Enzyme immunoassays are used widely as the initial test for serum HIV antibody. These tests are highly sensitive and specific. Repeated EIA testing of initially reactive specimens is required to decrease the small likelihood of laboratory error. Western blot analysis or indirect immunofluorescence antibody assays should be used for confirmation, which will overcome the problem of a false-positive EIA result. A positive HIV antibody test result in a child 18 months of age or older usually indicates infection.*

Serum antibodies to HIV are present in almost all infected people, with the exception of the rare individual who is hypogammaglobulinemic and the few people with AIDS who become seronegative late in disease. Some infants who receive combination antiretroviral therapy from early infancy also lose detectable antibody but remain infected.

The most notable laboratory finding in perinatally infected infants is a high viral load (as measured by RNA PCR assay) that does not decrease rapidly during the first year of life unless combination antiretroviral therapy is initiated. As the disease progresses, there is an increasing loss of cell-mediated immunity. The peripheral blood lymphocyte count at birth and during the first years of infection can be normal, but eventually lymphopenia, resulting from a decrease in the total number of circulating CD4+ lymphocytes, develops. The T-suppressor CD8+ lymphocyte count usually increases initially, and CD8+ cells are not depleted until late in the course of the infection. These changes in cell populations result in a decrease in the normal CD4+ to CD8+ cell ratio. This nonspecific finding, although characteristic of HIV infection, also occurs with other acute viral infections, including infections caused by CMV and Epstein-Barr virus. The normal values for peripheral CD4+ lymphocyte counts are age related, and the lower limits of normal are given in Table 3.25 (p 364).

---

* Centers for Disease Control and Prevention. Guidelines for national human immunodeficiency virus case surveillance, including monitoring for human immunodeficiency virus infection and acquired immunodeficiency syndrome. *MMWR Recomm Rep.* 1999;48(RR-13):1–28

Although the B-lymphocyte count remains normal or is somewhat increased, humoral immune dysfunction may precede and accompany cellular dysfunction. Increased serum immunoglobulin (Ig) concentrations, particularly IgG and IgA, are manifestations of the humoral immune dysfunction. Specific antibody responses to antigens to which the patient has not been exposed previously can be abnormal, and later in disease, recall antibody responses are slow and diminish in magnitude. A small proportion (<10%) of patients will develop panhypogammaglobulinemia.

Perinatal HIV Serologic Testing. The American Academy of Pediatrics (AAP) and American College of Obstetricians and Gynecologists recommendations include the following*:

- On the basis of recent advances in prophylaxis to decrease the rate of perinatal HIV transmission, the AAP recommends routinely offering counseling and testing with consent to all pregnant women in the United States. Consent for maternal HIV testing may be obtained in a variety of ways, including by right of refusal (ie, with testing to take place unless rejected in writing by the patient). The AAP supports use of consent procedures that facilitate rapid incorporation of HIV education and testing into routine medical care settings. For women who are examined by a health care professional for the first time in labor and have not been tested for HIV infection during the current pregnancy, counseling and immediate testing should be considered, because administration of antiretroviral therapy during labor is recommended and may diminish transmission. Careful attention to further education about HIV infection is recommended during the perinatal period.
- Routine education about HIV infection and testing should be a part of a comprehensive program of health care for women.
- If the mother's HIV antibody status was not determined during pregnancy or the postpartum period, the newborn's health care professional should inform the mother about the potential benefits of HIV testing for her infant and the possible risks and benefits to herself of knowing the child's serostatus and should recommend immediate HIV testing for the newborn.
- In the absence of known maternal HIV antibody status and parental availability for consent to test the newborn for HIV antibody, procedures should be established to facilitate rapid evaluation and testing of the infant.
- The newborn's health care professional should be informed of maternal HIV serostatus so that appropriate care and testing of the newborn can be accomplished. Similarly, if the newborn is found to be seropositive, but maternal HIV infection was unknown, the newborn's health care professional should ensure that this information and its significance is conveyed to the mother and, with her consent, to her health care professional. The mother should be referred to an appropriate HIV-related service for adults.
- Comprehensive HIV-related medical services should be accessible to all infected mothers, their infants, and other family members.
- The AAP supports legislation and public policy directed toward eliminating any form of discrimination on the basis of HIV serostatus.

---

* American Academy of Pediatrics, American College of Obstetricians and Gynecologists. Human Immunodeficiency virus screening. Joint statement of the American Academy of Pediatrics and the American College of Obstetricians and Gynecologists. *Pediatrics.* 1999;104:128

- Routine education about HIV infection and testing should be part of a comprehensive program of health care for adolescents.

Informed Consent for HIV Serologic Testing. Testing for HIV infection is unlike most routine blood testing, because risks of discrimination in jobs, school, child care, and insurance coverage can be incurred. Parents or other primary caregivers and the patient, if old enough to comprehend, should be counseled about the possible risks and benefits of testing a child and the consequences of HIV infection. The necessity of counseling and consent should not deter efforts to undertake appropriate diagnostic testing for HIV infection. Consent should be obtained from the parent or legal guardian and recorded in the patient's medical chart. State and local laws and hospital regulations should be considered when deciding whether written consent is required and under what circumstances testing can be performed without consent. Refusal of parents or patients to give consent does not relieve physicians of professional and legal responsibilities to their patients. If the physician believes that testing is essential to the child's health, authorization for testing may be possible through local laws and can be obtained by other means. The results of serologic tests should be discussed in person with the family, primary caregiver, and if appropriate according to age, the patient. In many states, minor adolescents can provide their own consent for testing, but involvement of a supportive adult should be sought. Appropriate counseling and follow-up care must be provided. Maintaining confidentiality in all cases is essential to preserving patient and parent trust and consent.

TREATMENT: (See Tables 4.9–4.11, pp 733–740, for a list of antiretroviral drugs and their recommended dosages.) Primary care physicians are encouraged to participate actively in the care of HIV-infected patients in consultation with specialists who have expertise in the care of HIV-infected children and adolescents. Current treatment recommendations for HIV-infected children are available online (www.aidsinfo.nih.gov). When possible, enrollment of an HIV-infected child into available clinical trials should be encouraged. Information about trials for adolescents and children can be obtained by contacting the AIDS Clinical Trials Information Service.*

Antiretroviral therapy is indicated for most HIV-infected children. Initiation of antiretroviral therapy depends on virologic, immunologic, and clinical criteria.[†] Because this is a rapidly changing area, consultation with an expert in pediatric HIV infection is suggested. Many experts recommend antiretroviral therapy for all HIV-infected children younger than 12 months of age or when more than 100 000 copies of HIV RNA per mL of plasma are detected, regardless of age. Therapy should consist of at least 3 antiretroviral drugs because of a superior decrease in viral load and the better prognosis associated with lower viral load. Some experts would elect not to initiate therapy for children older than 1 year of age who are at low risk of disease progression (eg, have low viral load, are asymptomatic, and have normal CD4+ T-lymphocyte counts). Adolescent treatment generally follows

---

* See Appendix I, Directory of Resources, p 789: AIDS Clinical Trials Information Service (available at www.aidsinfo.nih.gov)
† Centers for Disease Control and Prevention. Guidelines for the use of antiretroviral agents in pediatric HIV infection. *MMWR Recomm Rep.* 1998;47(RR-4):1–31

adult guidelines, with some variation in dosages depending on physical development (Tanner staging).*

Combination antiretroviral therapy has been shown to be more effective than monotherapy. Data indicate that good HIV suppression can be achieved with triple therapy including a protease inhibitor or a nonnucleoside reverse transcriptase inhibitor, indicating that at least 3 antiretroviral drugs should be given whenever possible. Suppression of virus to undetectable levels is the desired goal. A change in antiretroviral therapy should be considered if there is evidence of disease progression (virologic, immunologic, or clinical), toxic effects or intolerance of drugs, or data suggesting a superior regimen.

Immune Globulin Intravenous (IGIV) therapy is recommended in combination with antiviral agents only for HIV-infected children with one or more of the following: (1) hypogammaglobulinemia (IgG <400 mg/dL [4.0 g/L]); (2) recurrent, serious bacterial infections, defined as 2 or more serious bacterial infections, such as bacteremia, meningitis, or pneumonia, during a 1-year period (although IGIV may not provide additional benefit to children who are receiving trimethoprim-sulfamethoxazole for PCP prophylaxis); (3) failure to form antibodies to common antigens; and (4) chronic parvovirus B19 infections. The dose of IGIV generally is 400 mg/kg per dose, given every 4 weeks. Higher doses may be required for parvovirus B19 infection. Also, Rh_o (D) Immune Globulin or IGIV may be useful for treatment of HIV-associated thrombocytopenia in a dose of 500 to 1000 mg/kg per day for 3 to 5 days. In addition, children with bronchiectasis may benefit from adjunctive IGIV therapy at 600 mg/kg per dose, given monthly.

Early diagnosis and aggressive treatment of opportunistic infections may prolong survival. Children born to women coinfected with HIV and hepatitis C virus should be tested for hepatitis C virus infection. Because PCP can be an early complication of perinatally acquired HIV infection and the mortality rate is high, chemoprophylaxis should be given to HIV-exposed infants. For infants younger than 12 months of age with possible or proven HIV infection, PCP prophylaxis should be administered beginning at 4 to 6 weeks of age and continued for the first year of life unless HIV infection is excluded. The need for PCP prophylaxis for HIV-infected children 1 year of age and older is determined by age-specific CD4+ T-lymphocyte counts (see *Pneumocystis jiroveci* Infections, p 500).

Guidelines for prevention and treatment of opportunistic infections in children, adolescents, and adults provide indications for administration of drugs for infection with MAC, CMV, toxoplasmosis, and other organisms.[†] Of note, potent highly active antiretroviral therapy (HAART) that successfully suppresses HIV replication to undetectable levels has decreased the occurrence of opportunistic infections; PCP, CMV retinitis, MAC infection, toxoplasmosis, and cryptosporidiosis have diminished dramatically. Data on the safety of discontinuing prophylaxis in HIV-infected

---

* Centers for Disease Control and Prevention. Guidelines for using antiretroviral agents among HIV-infected adults and adolescents. Recommendations of the Panel on Clinical Practice for Treatment of HIV. *MMWR Recomm Rep.* 2002;51(RR-7):1–56. See www.aidsinfo.nih.gov for periodic updates of new drugs and new treatment recommendations.

[†] Centers for Disease Control and Prevention. Guidelines for preventing opportunistic infections among HIV-infected persons—2002. Recommendations of the US Public Health Service and the Infectious Diseases Society of America. *MMWR Recomm Rep.* 2002;51(RR-8):1–46

children receiving HAART are not yet available; recommendations are expected to continue to evolve to guide physicians in stopping prophylaxis in children with successful HIV suppression and immune reconstitution as more data become available.

Immunization Recommendations (see also Immunocompromised Children, p 69, and Table 3.27, p 373).

Children with HIV infection should be immunized as soon as is age appropriate with inactivated vaccines (diphtheria and tetanus toxoids and acellular pertussis [DTaP], inactivated poliovirus [IPV], *Haemophilus influenzae* type b, hepatitis B virus, and pneumococcal conjugate vaccine) as well as with an annual influenza vaccine. The suggested schedule for administration of these immunogens is in the Recommended Childhood and Adolescent Immunization Schedule (Fig 1.1, p 24). Oral poliovirus vaccine no longer is recommended routinely for use in any child in the United States, including HIV-infected children or members of their households.

Measles-mumps-rubella (MMR) vaccine should be administered to HIV-infected children at 12 months of age unless the children are severely immunocompromised (category 3, Table 3.25, p 364; see also Measles, p 419).* The second dose of MMR vaccine may be administered as soon as 4 weeks after the first rather than waiting until school entry. Children receiving routine IGIV prophylaxis may not respond to MMR vaccine. During an outbreak of measles, when exposure is likely, immunization should begin as early as 6 to 9 months.

In general, children with symptomatic HIV infection have poor immunologic responses to vaccines. Hence, these children, when exposed to a vaccine-preventable disease such as measles or tetanus, should be considered susceptible regardless of the history of immunization and should receive, if indicated, passive immunoprophylaxis (see Passive Immunization of Children With HIV Infection, p 373). Immune Globulin (IG) also should be given to any unimmunized household member who is exposed to measles infection to decrease the likelihood that the HIV-infected child will be exposed.

Children infected with HIV may be at increased risk of morbidity from varicella and herpes zoster. Limited data on varicella immunization of HIV-infected children in CDC immunologic category 1 indicate that the vaccine is safe, immunogenic, and effective. Weighing potential risks and benefits, varicella vaccine should be considered for HIV-infected children in CDC categories N1 and A1 (ie, having no or mild signs or symptoms of disease).

Hepatitis A vaccine is recommended for children living in states or regions with consistently increased hepatitis A rates and for people with chronic liver disease (see Hepatitis A, p 309).

In the United States and in areas of low prevalence of tuberculosis, bacille Calmette-Guérin (BCG) vaccine is not recommended. However, in developing countries where the prevalence of tuberculosis is high, the World Health Organization recommends that BCG vaccine be given to all infants at birth if they are asymptomatic, regardless of maternal HIV infection. Disseminated BCG infection has occurred in HIV-infected infants immunized with BCG vaccine.

---

* American Academy of Pediatrics, Committee on Infectious Diseases and Committee on Pediatric AIDS. Measles immunization in HIV-infected children. *Pediatrics.* 1999;103:1057–1060

Table 3.27. **Recommendations for Routine Immunization of HIV-Infected Children in the United States[1]**

Vaccines	Known Asymptomatic HIV Infection	Symptomatic HIV Infection
Hepatitis B	Yes	Yes
DTaP	Yes	Yes
IPV[2]	Yes	Yes
MMR	Yes	Yes[3]
Hib	Yes	Yes
Pneumococcal[4]	Yes	Yes
Influenza[5]	Yes	Yes
Varicella[6]	Consider	Consider
BCG	No	No
Hepatitis A[7]	See text	See text

HIV indicates human immunodeficiency virus; DTaP, diphtheria and tetanus toxoids and acellular pertussis; IPV, inactivated poliovirus; MMR, live-virus measles-mumps-rubella; Hib, *Haemophilus influenzae* type b conjugate; and BCG, bacille Calmette-Guérin.

[1] See Fig 1.1 (p 24) and disease-specific chapters for age at which specific vaccines are indicated.

[2] Only IPV vaccine should be used for HIV-infected children, HIV-exposed infants whose status is indeterminate, and household contacts of HIV-infected people.

[3] Severely immunocompromised HIV-infected children should not receive MMR vaccine (see text).

[4] Pneumococcal vaccine should be administered to all age-appropriate HIV-infected children. Children who are older than 2 months of age should receive pneumococcal vaccine at the time of diagnosis. Reimmunization after 3 to 5 years is recommended in either circumstance.

[5] Influenza vaccine should be provided each autumn for HIV-exposed infants 6 months of age and older, HIV-infected children and adolescents, and household contacts of HIV-infected people.

[6] Consider for HIV-infected children in Centers for Disease Control and Prevention class N1 and A1 (see Varicella-Zoster Infections, p 672).

[7] Also see Hepatitis A (p 309).

Seronegative Children Residing in the Household of a Patient With Symptomatic HIV Infection. In a household in which an adult or child is immunocompromised as the result of HIV infection, all children should receive IPV vaccine. Household contacts may receive MMR vaccine, because these vaccine viruses are not transmitted. To decrease the risk of transmission of influenza to patients with symptomatic HIV infection, all household members 6 months or older should receive yearly influenza immunization (see Influenza, p 382). Varicella immunization of siblings and susceptible adult caregivers of patients with HIV infection is encouraged to prevent acquisition of wild-type varicella-zoster infection, which can cause severe disease in immunocompromised hosts. Varicella vaccine virus transmission from an immunocompetent host is rare.

Passive Immunization of Children With HIV Infection.

- **Measles** (see Measles, p 419). Symptomatic HIV-infected children who are exposed to measles should receive intramuscular IG prophylaxis (0.5 mL/kg, maximum 15 mL), regardless of immunization status. Exposed, asymptomatic HIV-infected patients also should receive IG; the recommended dose is 0.25

mL/kg intramuscularly. Children who have received IGIV within 2 weeks of exposure do not require additional passive immunization.

- **Tetanus.** In the management of wounds classified as tetanus prone (see Tetanus, p 611, and Table 3.61, p 614), children with HIV infection should receive Tetanus Immune Globulin regardless of immunization status.
- **Varicella.** Children infected with HIV who are exposed to varicella or zoster should receive Varicella-Zoster Immune Globulin (see Varicella-Zoster Infections, p 672). Children who have received IGIV or Varicella-Zoster Immune Globulin within 2 weeks of exposure do not require additional passive immunization.

ISOLATION OF THE HOSPITALIZED PATIENT: Standard precautions should be followed by all health care personnel. The risk to health care personnel of acquiring HIV infection from a patient is minimal, even after accidental exposure from a needlestick injury (see Epidemiology, p 365). Every effort, nevertheless, should be made to avoid exposures to blood and other body fluids that could contain HIV.

CONTROL MEASURES:

Decrease in Perinatal HIV Transmission.[*] Oral administration of zidovudine to pregnant women with HIV infection beginning at 14 to 34 weeks' gestation and continuing throughout pregnancy, intravenous administration of zidovudine during labor until delivery (ie, intrapartum), and oral administration of zidovudine to the newborn infant for the first 6 weeks of life decreased the risk of perinatal HIV transmission by two thirds (see Table 3.28, p 375) in a controlled clinical trial. Current guidelines for use of antiretroviral drugs in pregnant HIV-infected women are similar to those for nonpregnant adults.[†] Therefore, many HIV-infected pregnant women will be receiving combination antiretroviral therapy for treatment of their HIV disease; use of zidovudine prophylaxis alone would be recommended rarely. However, the potential effect on the fetus and infant of antiretroviral drugs, particularly when used in combination, is unknown, and decisions about use of any antiretroviral drug during pregnancy require a discussion of the known benefits and unknown risks to the woman and her fetus. Long-term follow-up is recommended for all infants born to women who have received antiretroviral drugs during pregnancy. Health care professionals who are treating HIV-1-infected pregnant women and their newborn infants are advised to report instances of prenatal exposure to antiretroviral drugs to the Antiretroviral Pregnancy Registry (1-800-258-4263 or www.apregistry.com).

Several international antiretroviral prophylaxis clinical trials using zidovudine, lamivudine, and nevirapine alone or in combination during various combinations of prepartum, intrapartum, and postpartum periods showed decreases in HIV perinatal

---

[*] Centers for Disease Control and Prevention. US Public Health Service Task Force recommendations for use of antiretroviral drugs in pregnant HIV-1-infected women for maternal health and for interventions to reduce perinatal HIV-1 transmission in the United States. *MMWR Morb Mortal Wkly Rep.* 2002;51(RR-18):1–38. See www.aidsinfo.nih.gov for periodic updates.

[†] Centers for Disease Control and Prevention. Guidelines for using antiretroviral agents among HIV-infected adults and adolescents. Recommendations of the Panel on Clinical Practice for Treatment of HIV. *MMWR Recomm Rep.* 2002;51(RR-7):1–56. See www.aidsinfo.nih.gov for periodic updates of new drugs and new treatment recommendations.

Table 3.28. Zidovudine Regimen for Decreasing the Rate of Perinatal Transmission of Human Immunodeficiency Virus (HIV)[1]

Period of Time	Route	Dosage
During pregnancy, initiate anytime after wk 14 of gestation and continue throughout pregnancy	Oral	200 mg, 3 times per day or 300 mg, 2 times per day
During labor and delivery	Intravenous	2 mg/kg during the first hour, then 1 mg/kg per hour until delivery
For the newborn, within 6–12 h of birth	Oral	2 mg/kg, 4 times per day, for the first 6 wk of life

[1] Centers for Disease Control and Prevention. US Public Health Service Task Force recommendations for use of antiretroviral drugs in pregnant HIV-1-infected women for maternal health and for interventions to reduce perinatal HIV-1 transmission in the United States. *MMWR Morb Mortal Wkly Rep.* 2002;51(RR-18):1–38. Information about other antiretroviral drugs for decreasing the rate of perinatal transmission of HIV can be found online (www.aidsinfo.nih.gov).

transmission.* These "short-course" regimens support administration of antiretroviral agents, even to women diagnosed late in pregnancy or at delivery, although the short-course regimens seem less effective than the full 3-part zidovudine regimen. The goal should be to diagnose HIV infection early in pregnancy to allow initiation of zidovudine prophylaxis and whatever other drugs are needed to treat maternal infection.

In the United States, antiretroviral drugs should be administered to the HIV-infected woman during pregnancy, labor, and delivery. Zidovudine should be given to all newborn infants if exposure is recognized before 7 days of age, even if their mothers did not receive zidovudine. Recommendations for use of antiretroviral drugs to decrease the risk of perinatal HIV-1 transmission for HIV-1-infected women in labor who have not received previous therapy and for infants born to mothers who have received no antiretroviral therapy during pregnancy or intrapartum are available.*

A meta-analysis has shown that the rate of transmission decreased by 50% in the absence of zidovudine when delivery was by elective cesarean section before rupture of membranes and onset of labor. The transmission rate was decreased to 2% if the mother received antiretroviral therapy and underwent elective cesarean delivery before onset of labor and before rupture of membranes. Vaginal delivery and antiretroviral therapy were associated with transmission rates of 7%. However, transmission rates for women receiving combination antiretroviral therapy in whom viral load is decreased to levels below assay detection may be lower than in women receiving zidovudine monotherapy. The additional benefit of cesarean delivery for further decreasing transmission risk in such women is unknown and may not outweigh the potential risk of operative delivery for the infected mother. The American College of Obstetricians and Gynecologists recommends that HIV-infected pregnant

---

* Centers for Disease Control and Prevention. US Public Health Service Task Force recommendations for use of antiretroviral drugs in pregnant HIV-1-infected women for maternal health and for interventions to reduce perinatal HIV-1 transmission in the United States. *MMWR Morb Mortal Wkly Rep.* 2002;51(RR-18):1–38. See www.aidsinfo.nih.gov for periodic updates.

women with viral loads of 1000/mL or greater should be counseled regarding the potential benefit of elective cesarean delivery to further decrease the risk of HIV perinatal transmission.*

Breastfeeding (see also Human Milk, p 117). Transmission of HIV by breast-feeding, especially from mothers who acquire infection during the postpartum period, has been demonstrated. In the United States, where safe alternative sources of feeding are readily available, affordable, and culturally accepted, HIV-infected women should be counseled not to breastfeed their infants or donate to milk banks. The AAP guidelines for women in the United States are as follows[†]:

- Women and their health care professionals need to be aware of the potential risk of transmission of HIV infection to infants during pregnancy and the peripartum period as well as through human milk.
- Routine HIV testing with consent should be part of prenatal care for all women. Each woman should know her HIV status and the methods available to prevent acquisition and transmission of HIV and to determine whether breastfeeding is appropriate.
- During labor, if a woman's HIV status during the current pregnancy is unknown, it is strongly recommended that she be counseled and tested as rapidly as possible. Each woman should understand the benefits to her and her infant of knowing her serostatus. Antiretroviral drugs can be administered during labor and to the infant if the woman is HIV-positive with the hope that transmission of virus will be avoided or decreased. It is important for the mother to know her HIV infection status for subsequent decisions about breastfeeding. Hopefully, education will encourage behaviors that would decrease the likelihood of acquisition and transmission of HIV.
- Women who are known to be HIV infected must be counseled not to breastfeed or provide their milk to milk banks.
- In general, women who are known to be HIV-seronegative should be encouraged to breastfeed. However, women who are HIV-seronegative and known to have HIV-positive sexual partners or to be active drug users should be counseled about the potential risk of transmitting HIV through human milk and about methods to decrease the risk of acquiring HIV infection.
- Each woman whose HIV status is unknown should be informed of the potential for HIV-infected women to transmit HIV during the peripartum period and through human milk. She also should know the potential benefits to her and her infant of knowing her HIV status and understand how HIV is acquired and transmitted. All women are recommended to be tested to learn their HIV status. The health care professional should make an individualized recommendation to assist the woman to decide whether to breastfeed.
- Neonatal intensive care units should develop policies for use of expressed human milk for neonates that are consistent with these recommendations. Current standards of the Occupational Safety and Health Administration do not require use of gloves for routine handling of expressed human milk.

---

* American College of Obstetricians and Gynecologists. Scheduled cesarean delivery and the prevention of vertical transmission of HIV infection. *ACOG Comm Opin.* 2000;234:1–3

† American Academy of Pediatrics, Committee on Pediatric AIDS. Human milk, breastfeeding, and transmission of HIV-1 infection in the United States. *Pediatrics.* In press.

Gloves, however, should be worn by health care personnel when exposure to human milk might be frequent or prolonged, such as in milk banking.

- Human milk banks should follow the guidelines developed by the US Public Health Service, which include screening all donors for HIV infection, assessing risk factors that predispose to infection, and pasteurizing all donated milk.

Adolescent Education. Adolescents who are sexually active or using illicit injection drugs are at risk of HIV infection. All adolescents should be educated about HIV infection and have access to HIV testing and knowledge of their serostatus. Particular efforts should be made to provide access for adolescents who may not have a regular health care professional. Informed consent for testing or release of information about serostatus is necessary.

Specific AAP recommendations for pediatricians caring for adolescents are as follows*:

- Information about HIV infection and AIDS and availability of HIV testing should be regarded as an essential component of the anticipatory guidance provided by pediatricians to all adolescent patients. This guidance should include information about HIV prevention and transmission and implications of infection.
- Preventive guidance should include helping adolescents understand the responsibilities of becoming sexually active. Information should be provided on abstinence from sexual activity and use of safer sexual practices to decrease the risk of unplanned pregnancy and sexually transmitted diseases, including HIV. All adolescents should be counseled about the correct and consistent use of latex condoms to decrease risk of infection.
- Availability of HIV testing should be discussed with all adolescents and should be encouraged with consent for adolescents who are sexually active or use drugs.
- Although parental involvement in adolescent health care is a desirable goal, consent of an adolescent alone should be sufficient to provide evaluation and treatment for suspected or confirmed HIV infection.
- A negative HIV test result can allay anxiety resulting from a high-risk event or high-risk behaviors and is a good opportunity to counsel on decreasing high-risk behaviors to decrease future risk.
- For adolescents with a positive HIV test result, it is important to provide support, address medical and psychosocial needs, and arrange linkages to appropriate care.
- Pediatricians should help adolescents with HIV infection to understand the importance of informing their sexual partners of their potential exposure to HIV. Pediatricians can provide this help directly or via referral to a state or local health department's partner referral program.
- Pediatricians should advocate for the special needs of adolescents for information about HIV, access to HIV testing and counseling, and HIV treatment.

* For further information, see American Academy of Pediatrics, Committee on Pediatric AIDS and Committee on Adolescence. Adolescents and human immunodeficiency virus infection: the role of the pediatrician in prevention and intervention. *Pediatrics.* 2001;107:188–190

School Attendance and Education of Children With HIV Infection.* In the absence of blood exposure, HIV infection is not acquired through the types of contact that usually occur in a school setting, including contact with saliva or tears. Hence, children with HIV infection should not be excluded from school for the protection of other children or personnel, and disclosure of infection should not be required. Specific recommendations about school attendance of children and adolescents with HIV infection are the following:

- Most school-aged children and all adolescents infected with HIV should be allowed to attend school without restrictions, provided the child's physician gives approval. The need for a more restricted school environment for the rare infected child who might have an increased likelihood of exposing others should be evaluated on a case-by-case basis by the physician. Exudative skin lesions or aggressive biting behavior are examples of conditions in which a theoretic increased risk of exposure occurs.
- Only the child's parents, other guardians, and physician have an absolute need to know that the child is HIV-infected. The number of personnel aware of the child's condition should be kept to the minimum needed to ensure proper care of the child. The family has the right, but is not obligated, to inform the school. People involved in the care and education of an infected student must respect the student's right to privacy.
- All schools should adopt routine procedures for handling blood or blood-contaminated fluids, including disposal of sanitary napkins, regardless of whether students with HIV infection are known to be in attendance. School health care professionals, teachers, administrators, and other employees should be educated about procedures (see Housekeeping Procedures for Blood and Body Fluids, p 380).
- Children infected with HIV may be at increased risk of experiencing severe complications from infections, such as varicella, tuberculosis, measles, CMV, and herpes simplex virus. Schools should develop procedures for notification of all parents of communicable diseases, such as varicella or measles.
- Routine screening of school children for HIV infection is not recommended.

As the life expectancy of HIV-infected children and adolescents increases, the school population of children and adolescents with this disease also will increase. An understanding of the effect of chronic illness and the recognition of neurodevelopmental problems in some of these children are essential to provide appropriate educational programs. The AAP recommendations regarding the education of children with HIV infection are as follows[†]:

- All children with HIV infection should receive an appropriate education that is adapted to their evolving special needs. The spectrum of needs differs with the stage of disease and age of the child.
- Infection with HIV should be treated like other chronic illnesses that require special education and other related services.

---

[*] American Academy of Pediatrics, Committee on Pediatric AIDS and Committee on Infectious Diseases. Issues related to human immunodeficiency virus transmission in schools, child care, medical settings, the home, and community. *Pediatrics.* 1999;104:318–324

[†] American Academy of Pediatrics, Committee on Pediatric AIDS. Education of children with human immunodeficiency virus infection. *Pediatrics.* 2000;105:1358–1360

- Continuity of education must be ensured whether at school or at home.
- Because of the stigma associated with this disease, maintaining confidentiality is essential. Disclosure of information should be only with the informed consent of the parents or legal guardians and age-appropriate assent of the student.

Human Immunodeficiency Virus in the Athletic Setting. Athletes and staff of athletic programs can be exposed to blood during athletic activity. Recommendations have been developed by the AAP for prevention of transmission of HIV and other bloodborne pathogens in the athletic setting (see School Health, Infections Spread by Blood and Body Fluids, p 143).

Child Care and Foster Care.[*] Current AAP recommendations are as follows[†‡]:

- No reason exists to restrict foster care or adoptive placement of children who have HIV infection to protect the health of other family members. The risk of transmission of HIV infection in family environments is negligible.
- No need exists to restrict placement of HIV-infected children in child care settings to protect personnel or other children, because the risk of transmission of HIV in these settings is negligible.
- Child care providers need not be informed of the HIV status of a child to protect the health of caregivers or other children in the child care environment. In some jurisdictions, the child's diagnosis cannot be divulged without the written consent of the parent or legal guardian. Parents may choose to inform the child care provider of the child's diagnosis to support a request that the caregiver observe the child closely for signs of illness that may require medical attention and assist the parents with the child's special emotional and social needs.
- Recommended standard precautions should be followed in all child care settings when blood or blood-containing body fluids are handled to minimize transmission of bloodborne disease (see Housekeeping Procedures for Blood and Body Fluids, p 380).
- All preschool child care programs routinely should inform all families whenever a highly contagious illness, such as varicella or measles, occurs in any child in that setting. This process will help families protect their immunocompromised children.
- Ascertainment of HIV status is recommended for all pregnant women and newborn infants. This knowledge may help facilitate foster care or adoptive placement.

Adults With HIV Infection Working in Child Care Settings or Schools. Asymptomatic HIV-infected adults may care for children in school or child care settings provided that they do not have conditions that would allow contact with their body fluids. No data indicate that HIV-infected adults have transmitted HIV during routine child care or school responsibilities. Adults with symptomatic HIV infection

---

[*] For additional discussion of recommendations for child care, see Children in Out-of-Home Child Care, p 123.

[†] American Academy of Pediatrics, Committee on Pediatric AIDS and Committee on Infectious Diseases. Issues related to human immunodeficiency virus transmission in schools, child care, medical settings, the home, and community. *Pediatrics*. 1999;104:318–324

[‡] Adapted from American Academy of Pediatrics, Committee on Pediatric AIDS. Identification and care of HIV-exposed and HIV-infected infants, children, and adolescents in foster care. *Pediatrics*. 2000;106:149–153

are immunocompromised and at increased risk of complications if they acquire infectious diseases of young children. They should consult their physicians about the safety of continuing to work in child care or school settings.

Housekeeping Procedures for Blood and Body Fluids. In general, routine housekeeping procedures using a commercially available cleaner (detergent, disinfectant-detergent, or chemical germicide) compatible with most surfaces is satisfactory for cleaning spills of vomitus, urine, and feces. Nasal secretions can be removed with tissues and discarded in routine waste containers. For spills involving blood or other body fluids, organic material should be removed, and the surface should be disinfected with freshly diluted bleach (1:10). Reusable rubber gloves should be used for cleaning large spills to avoid contamination of the hands of the person cleaning the spill, but gloves are not essential for cleaning small amounts of blood that can be contained easily by the material used for cleaning. People involved in cleaning contaminated surfaces should avoid exposure of open skin lesions or mucous membranes to blood or bloody fluids. Whenever possible, disposable towels or tissues should be used and properly discarded, and mops should be rinsed in disinfectant. After cleanup and after removal of gloves, hands should be washed thoroughly with soap and water. Gloves are not indicated for routine cleaning tasks that do not involve contact with body secretions, such as sweeping floors or dusting.

Management and Counseling of Families.* Serologic screening of siblings and parents for HIV is recommended when HIV is identified in a child. In each case, the physician should provide education and ongoing counseling about HIV and its transmission and outline precautions to be taken within the household and the community to prevent HIV spread.

Women infected with HIV need to be made aware of the risk of having an infected child if they become pregnant, and they should be referred for family planning counseling. Infected people should not donate blood, plasma, sperm, organs, corneas, bone, other tissues, or human milk.

An infected child should be taught appropriate hygiene and behavior. How much the child is told about the illness depends on age and maturity. Older children and adolescents should be made aware that the disease can be transmitted sexually, and they should be counseled appropriately. Many families are not willing to tell others about the diagnosis, because it can result in social isolation.

Sexual Abuse. After sexual abuse, the child should be tested serologically as soon as possible and periodically for 6 months (eg, at 4–6 weeks, 12 weeks, and 6 months after sexual contact) (see Sexually Transmitted Diseases, p 157). Serologic evaluation of the perpetrator for HIV should be attempted but usually cannot be obtained in proximity to the abuse and often is not possible until indictment has occurred. Counseling of the child and family needs to be provided (see Sexually Transmitted Diseases, p 157).

Postexposure Prophylaxis for Possible Sexual or Other Nonoccupational Exposure to HIV. Decisions to provide antiretroviral agents to people after possible nonoccupational HIV exposure must balance the potential benefits and risks. Considerations related to use of antiretroviral prophylaxis in such circumstances

---

* Centers for Disease Control and Prevention. *HIV Counseling, Testing, and Referral Standards and Guidelines.* Atlanta, GA: US Dept of Health and Human Services; 1994. Available at: www.cdc.gov/publications.htm.

include the probability that the source is HIV infected, the likelihood of transmission by the particular exposure, the interval between exposure and initiation of therapy, the efficacy of the drug(s) used, and the patient's adherence to the drug(s).

The estimated risk of transmission per episode of percutaneous exposure (needlestick in a nonoccupational exposure) to HIV-infected blood is 0.49% (upper limit of 95% confidence interval [CI] = 0.8%). The estimated risk of HIV transmission per episode of receptive penile-anal sexual exposure is 0.1% to 3%; the estimated risk per episode of receptive vaginal exposure is 0.1% to 0.2%. The actual risks to an infant or child after a needlestick or sexual abuse are unknown. However, to date, there are no known transmissions of HIV from accidental nonoccupational needlesticks.

In 1995, surveillance data from health care personnel were used in a case-control study that suggested zidovudine use was associated with an 81% (95% CI = 48%–94%) decrease in risk of HIV infection after percutaneous exposure to HIV-infected blood. This may be an overestimate of the benefits because of methodologic constraints.

All antiretroviral agents have adverse effects. Twenty-four percent to 36% of adults discontinued drugs used in combination because of adverse effects. Severe adverse effects, such as nephrolithiasis, nephrotoxicity, pancreatitis, pancytopenia, or hepatotoxicity, have been reported.

Antiretroviral agents generally should not be used if the risk of transmission is low (eg, needlestick from unknown nonoccupational source) or if care is sought more than 72 hours after reported exposure.* The physician and patient or parent should decide when risk of infection is high, intervention is prompt, and adherence is likely. Consultation with an experienced pediatric HIV health care professional is essential.

Blood, Blood Components, and Clotting Factors. Screening blood and plasma for HIV antibody has decreased dramatically the risk of infection through transfusion (see Blood Safety, p 106). Nevertheless, careful scrutiny of the requirements of each patient for blood, its components, or clotting factors is important.

Human Immunodeficiency Virus-Exposed Health Care Personnel. Accidental exposure of health care personnel to HIV, such as from needlestick injuries or HIV-infected blood, rarely has resulted in HIV infection. The risk of infection varies according to the severity and type of exposure. The risk of infection after a percutaneous exposure to HIV-infected blood is 0.3%. The risks after mucous membrane contact and skin exposure to HIV-infected blood are 0.1% and less than 0.1%, respectively. Many of the known cases could have been prevented by careful adherence to infection control measures (see Control Measures, p 374). A health care worker who has had a percutaneous or mucous membrane exposure to blood or bloody secretions from an HIV-seropositive patient should receive counseling and medical evaluation as soon as possible after the exposure. A baseline HIV antibody test should be performed, and the HIV status of the blood source should be investigated. A health care worker who is seronegative should be retested 4 to 6 weeks, 12 weeks, and 6 months after exposure to determine whether transmission has occurred. Most exposed people who have been infected will seroconvert during the first 3 months after exposure.

---

* American Academy of Pediatrics, Committee on Pediatric AIDS. Postexposure prophylaxis in children and adolescents for nonoccupational exposure to human immunodeficiency virus. *Pediatrics.* In press

Revised recommendations for postexposure prophylaxis were issued by the US Public Health Service in 2001.* Recommendations for HIV postexposure prophylaxis include a basic 4-week regimen of 2 drugs (zidovudine plus lamivudine; stavudine plus lamivudine; or stavudine plus didanosine) for most HIV exposures and an expanded regimen that includes addition of a third antiretroviral drug for HIV exposures that pose an increased risk of transmission. When the source person's virus is known or suspected to be resistant to one or more of the drugs considered for prophylaxis, selection of drugs to which the source person's virus is unlikely to be resistant is recommended. Clinicians also can receive assistance and advice by calling the National HIV/AIDS Clinicians' Consulting Center at 888-448-4911.

Reporting of Cases. Cases meeting the criteria for AIDS (see Tables 3.24, p 362, and 3.25, p 364) must be reported to the appropriate public health department in all states. In many states, HIV infection or perinatal exposure to HIV also must be reported. The AAP recommends routine reporting of perinatal HIV exposure, infection, and AIDS.

Influenza

CLINICAL MANIFESTATIONS: Influenza classically is characterized by sudden onset of fever, often with chills or rigors, headache, malaise, diffuse myalgia, and a nonproductive cough. Subsequently, the respiratory tract signs of sore throat, nasal congestion, rhinitis, and cough become more prominent. Conjunctival injection, abdominal pain, nausea, and vomiting can occur. In some children, influenza can appear as an upper respiratory tract infection or as a febrile illness with few respiratory tract signs. In young infants, influenza can produce a sepsis-like picture and occasionally can cause croup, bronchiolitis, or pneumonia. Acute myositis characterized by calf tenderness and refusal to walk may develop after several days of influenza illness, particularly with type B infection. Reye syndrome has been associated with influenza infection, primarily with influenza B. Influenza can alter the metabolism of certain medications, especially theophylline, potentially resulting in the development of toxic effects from high serum concentrations.

ETIOLOGY: Influenza viruses are orthomyxoviruses of 3 antigenic types (A, B, and C). Epidemic disease is caused by influenza virus types A and B. Influenza A viruses are subclassified by 2 surface antigens, hemagglutinin (HA) and neuraminidase (NA). Viruses bearing 3 immunologically distinct hemagglutinin subtypes (H1, H2, and H3) and 2 neuraminidase subtypes (N1 and N2) have been recognized as causing global human epidemics. Specific antibodies to these various antigens, especially hemagglutinin, are important determinants of immunity. Major changes leading to the emergence of a new hemagglutinin, such as H1 to H2, or emergence of a new hemagglutinin or new neuraminidase, are called *antigenic shifts;* minor antigenic variations within the same subtypes are called *antigenic drifts.* Antigenic shift

---

* Centers for Disease Control and Prevention. Updated U.S. Public Health Service guidelines for the management of occupational exposures to HBV, HCV, and HIV and recommendations for postexposure prophylaxis. *MMWR Recomm Rep.* 2001;50(RR-11):1-42

has occurred only with influenza A, usually at irregular intervals of 10 or more years. Antigenic drift occurs continuously and results in variant influenza A and B viruses. Influenza B viruses change more slowly and are not divided into subtypes.

EPIDEMIOLOGY: Influenza is spread from person to person by droplets or by direct contact with articles recently contaminated by nasopharyngeal secretions. During community outbreaks of influenza, the highest attack rates occur among school-aged children. Secondary spread to adults and other children within the family is common. The attack rates depend in part on immunity developed by previous experience (by natural disease or immunization) with the circulating strain or a related strain. Antigenic drift in the circulating strain is associated with seasonal epidemics, and antigenic shift can precipitate global pandemics. In temperate climates, seasonal epidemics usually occur during the winter months. Community outbreaks can peak within 2 weeks of onset and last 4 to 8 weeks or longer. Circulation of 2 or 3 influenza virus strains in a community may be associated with a prolonged influenza season of 3 months or more and bimodal peaks in activity. Influenza is highly contagious, especially among semi-enclosed institutionalized populations. Patients are most infectious during the 24 hours before the onset of symptoms and during the most symptomatic period. Viral shedding in the nasal secretions usually ceases within 7 days of the onset of illness but can be prolonged in young children and immunodeficient patients.

Attack rates in healthy children have been estimated at 10% to 40% each year, with approximately 1% resulting in hospitalization. The risk of lower respiratory tract disease complicating influenza infection in children, primarily pneumonia, croup, wheezing, and bronchiolitis, has ranged from 0.2% to 25%. A wide spectrum of complications, including Reye syndrome, myositis, and central nervous system (CNS) manifestations, can occur. The risk of Reye syndrome, which occurs primarily in school-aged children, has decreased during recent years, probably as a result of decreased use of salicylates. Because other respiratory tract viruses, including respiratory syncytial virus and parainfluenza viruses, also cause substantial disease in young children, precise morbidity and mortality rates attributable to influenza are difficult to determine unless specific etiologic diagnosis is sought for all infections.

Excess rates of hospitalization attributable to influenza virus infections have been documented for otherwise healthy children younger than 5 years of age. Rates of hospitalization and morbidity attributable to complications, such as bronchitis and pneumonia, are even greater in children with hemoglobinopathies, bronchopulmonary dysplasia, asthma, cystic fibrosis, malignancy, diabetes mellitus, chronic renal disease, and congenital heart disease. Influenza virus infection in neonates also has been associated with considerable morbidity, including a sepsis-like syndrome, apnea, and lower respiratory tract disease.

Influenza Pandemics. When a new influenza A virus subtype emerges and spreads widely, global pandemics can occur, leading to substantially increased morbidity and mortality rates. During the 20th century, there were 3 influenza pandemics, including one in 1918 that killed more than 20 million people worldwide, including more than 500 000 people in the United States, many of whom were young adults. Mortality rates with the pandemics of 1957 and 1968 were lower, in part, because of the use of antimicrobial therapy for secondary bacterial infections and more aggressive supportive care. Experience indicates that pandemics occur at irregular and unpredictable intervals. They have the potential to be true public health emergencies. Dealing with the next influenza pandemic will require extensive use of vaccine and antimicrobial agents and development of triage policies for hospital and intensive care utilization. A federal interagency group, which includes members of the American Academy of Pediatrics, is preparing a plan for the public health response to the next pandemic.

The **incubation period** usually is 1 to 3 days.

DIAGNOSTIC TESTS: When viral cultures or rapid diagnostic tests are performed, specimens should be obtained during the first 72 hours of illness, because the quantity of virus shed decreases rapidly from that point. Nasopharyngeal secretion specimens obtained by swab or aspirate should be placed in appropriate transport media for culture. After inoculation into eggs or cell culture, virus usually can be isolated within 2 to 6 days. Rapid diagnostic tests for identification of influenza A and B antigens in nasopharyngeal secretion specimens are available commercially, although their reported sensitivity (45%–90%) and specificity (60%–95%) compared with viral culture are variable and differ by test and specimen type. Serologic diagnosis can be established retrospectively by a fourfold or greater increase in antibody titer in serum specimens obtained during the acute and convalescent stages of illness, as determined by hemagglutination inhibition testing, complement fixation testing, neutralization testing, or enzyme immunoassay; however, serologic testing rarely is useful in patient management.

TREATMENT: Amantadine hydrochloride and rimantadine hydrochloride are licensed for treatment of influenza A in adults, but only amantadine is licensed for treatment in children (Table 3.29, p 385). Studies evaluating the efficacy of amantadine and rimantadine in children are limited, but they indicate that treatment with either drug diminishes the severity of influenza A infection when administered within 48 hours of onset of illness. Neither amantadine nor rimantadine is effective against influenza B infections. Two products from another class of antiviral drugs, the neuraminidase inhibitors, have been approved for treatment of uncomplicated influenza A and B in patients within 2 days of onset of symptoms.* These drugs function by decreasing release of virus from infected cells. Zanamivir is approved for people 7 years of age and older. Zanamivir is an inhaled powder formulation that is administered twice a day for 5 days using a special breath-activated plastic inhaler. Oseltamivir is approved for people 1 year of age and older and is administered orally twice a day for 5 days. In an efficacy trial in children 5 to 12 years of age, when therapy was instituted within 36 hours of onset, Zanamivir decreased the duration of symptoms by one day, compared with placebo. Safety and efficacy have not been established in children with high-risk underlying medical conditions. In children 1 to 12 years of age, oseltamivir decreased the duration of symptoms by 1.5 days. The neuraminidase inhibitors are the only available antiviral agents with

---

* American Academy of Pediatrics, Committee on Infectious Diseases. Policy statement: reduction of the influenza burden in children. *Pediatrics.* 2002;110:1246–1252; and American Academy of Pediatrics, Committee on Infectious Diseases. Technical report: reduction of the influenza burden in children. *Pediatrics.* 2002;110(6). Available at: www.pediatrics.org/cgi/content/full/110/e80

Table 3.29. **Antiviral Drugs for Influenza**

	Amantadine	Rimantadine	Zanamivir	Oseltamivir
Virus	A	A	A and B	A and B
Administration	Oral	Oral	Inhalation	Oral
Treatment indications[1]	≥1 y of age	≥13 y of age	≥7 y of age	≥1 y of age
Prophylaxis indications[1]	≥1 y of age	≥1 y of age	Not licensed	≥13 y of age
Adverse effects	Central nervous system, anxiety	Central nervous system, anxiety	Bronchospasm	Nausea, vomiting

[1] Licensed ages.

activity against influenza B, although their role in treatment of children requires further evaluation.

Therapy for influenza virus infection should be considered for (1) patients in whom shortening or amelioration of clinical symptoms may be particularly benefi-cial, such as children at increased risk of severe or complicated influenza infection; (2) healthy children with severe illness; and (3) people with special environmental, family, or social situations for which ongoing illness would be detrimental. Although influenza A virus rapidly may become resistant to amantadine and rimantadine dur-ing treatment, this does not seem to affect clinical benefits. Resistant virus has not been demonstrated to spread more easily or cause more serious disease and has not been shown to persist in the population in the absence of antiviral drug therapy. Nevertheless, the epidemiologic implications of influenza A anti-viral drug resistance are unclear. Any influenza isolate obtained from a patient while receiving influenza prophylaxis should be submitted for antiviral susceptibility testing to the Centers for Disease Control and Prevention (CDC) through the state health department. Development of resistance to zanamivir and oseltamivir during treatment has been identified but does not appear to be common, but the clinical significance of resis-tance to the neuraminidase inhibitors has not been characterized fully.

If antiviral therapy is prescribed, treatment should be started as soon as possible after the onset of symptoms and discontinued approximately 24 to 48 hours after the symptoms resolve (amantadine or rimantadine) or after a 5-day course (neu-raminidase inhibitors). The recommended dosages for drugs approved for treatment and prophylaxis of influenza are given in Table 4.8 (p 729). Patients with any degree of renal insufficiency should be monitored for adverse events. Only zanamivir does not require adjustment for people with severe renal insufficiency. Both amantadine and rimantadine, but especially amantadine, may cause CNS symptoms, which resolve with discontinuation of the drug. An increased incidence of seizures has been reported in children with epilepsy who receive amantadine and, to a lesser extent, in children who receive rimantadine. The most common adverse effects of oseltamivir are nausea and vomiting. Zanamivir use has been associated with bron-chospasm in some individuals but systemic adverse effects are rare. Zanamivir gener-ally is not recommended for use in patients with underlying airway disease.

Control of fever with acetaminophen or other appropriate antipyretics may be important in young children, because the fever and other symptoms of influenza could exacerbate underlying chronic conditions. Children and adolescents with influenza should not receive salicylates because of the resulting increased risk of developing Reye syndrome.

ISOLATION OF THE HOSPITALIZED PATIENT: In addition to standard precautions, droplet precautions are recommended for children hospitalized with influenza or an influenza-like illness for the duration of the illness. Respiratory tract secretions should be considered infectious, and strict hand hygiene procedures should be used.

CONTROL MEASURES:

Influenza Vaccine. The inactivated influenza vaccines produced in embryonated hen eggs are immunogenic and associated with minimal adverse effects. These multivalent vaccines contain 3 virus strains (usually 2 type A and 1 type B). Typically, 1 or 2 strains are changed each year in anticipation of the predominant influenza strains expected to circulate in the United States in the upcoming winter. Inactivated influenza vaccine distributed in the United States is either subvirion vaccine, prepared by disrupting the lipid-containing membrane of the virus, or purified surface-antigen vaccine. Whole-cell influenza vaccine, available before 2001, no longer is available in the United States. A cold-adapted, trivalent live-attenuated influenza vaccine that is prepared by viral reassortment and is administered intranasally is under consideration for licensure by the US Food and Drug Administration (FDA).

Immunogenicity in Children. Children younger than 9 years of age, because they have had little experience with influenza, require 2 doses of vaccine administered 1 month apart to produce a satisfactory antibody response (see Table 3.30, p 387). Children previously primed with a related strain of influenza by infection or immunization mount a brisk antibody response to 1 dose of the vaccine.

Vaccine Efficacy. The effectiveness of influenza immunization on acute respiratory tract illness is less evident in pediatric than in adult populations because of the frequency of upper respiratory tract infections and influenza-like illness caused by other viral agents in young children. Protection in healthy subjects usually is 70% to 80%, with a range of 50% to 95% varying with the closeness of vaccine strain match to the wild strain. The duration of protection is presumed to be less than 1 year usually. Efficacy has not been evaluated in infants immunized during the first 6 months of life, and the available vaccines have not been licensed by the FDA for people of that age group.

Special Considerations, Inactivated Influenza Virus Vaccine.

- In children receiving immunosuppressive chemotherapy, influenza immunization with a new vaccine antigen results in a poor response. The optimal time to immunize children with malignant neoplasms who must undergo chemotherapy is >3 weeks after chemotherapy has been discontinued, when the peripheral granulocyte and lymphocyte counts are greater than $1000/\mu L$ $(1.0 \times 10^9/L)$. Children who no longer are receiving chemotherapy generally have high rates of seroconversion.

Table 3.30. **Schedule for Inactivated Influenza Vaccine Dosage by Age[1]**

Age	Dose, mL[2]	No. of Doses	Route[3]
6–35 mo	0.25	1–2[4]	Intramuscular
3–8 y	0.5	1–2[4]	Intramuscular
≥9 y	0.5	1	Intramuscular

[1] Manufacturers include Aventis Pasteur (Fluzone, split-virus vaccine licensed for people ≥6 months of age) and Evans Vaccines Ltd (Fluvirin, purified surface antigen, licensed for people ≥4 years of age). Flushield (Wyeth-Lederle) no longer is manufactured.

[2] Dosages are those recommended in recent years. Physicians should refer to the product circular each year to ensure that the appropriate dosage is given.

[3] For adults and older children, the recommended site of immunization is the deltoid muscle. For infants and young children, the preferred site is the anterolateral aspect of the thigh.

[4] Two doses administered at least 1 month apart are recommended for children who are receiving inactivated influenza vaccine for the first time. If possible, the second dose should be administered before December.

- Children with hemodynamically unstable cardiac disease constitute a large group potentially at high risk of complications of influenza. The immune response and safety of inactivated influenza virus vaccine in these children are comparable to the immune response and safety in healthy children.
- Corticosteroids administered for brief periods or every other day seem to have a minimal effect on antibody response to influenza vaccine. Prolonged administration of high doses of corticosteroids (ie, a dose of prednisone of either ≥2 mg/kg or a total of 20 mg/day) may impair antibody response. Influenza immunization can be deferred temporarily during the time of receipt of high-dose corticosteroids, provided deferral does not compromise the likelihood of immunization before the start of the influenza season (see Vaccine Administration, p 389).
- Infants younger than 6 months of age with high-risk conditions (see Recommendations for Influenza Immunization, p 388), especially infants with cardiopulmonary compromise, may have the same or greater risk of serious illness from influenza as older children. However, neither influenza vaccine nor prophylaxis with rimantadine, amantadine, or neuraminidase inhibitors is recommended for this age group. Immunization and chemoprophylaxis of older children and adults who are in close contact with high-risk infants are important means of protection of infants (see Recommendations for Influenza Immunization, p 388, and Indications for Chemoprophylaxis, p 390).
- Some studies indicate that influenza vaccine may decrease the incidence of acute otitis media in children in child care centers.

Recommendations for Influenza Immunization. *

Annual influenza immunization should be encouraged, to the extent feasible, in healthy children 6 to 24 months of age and their household contacts. Children, adolescents, and adults can be immunized to decrease the impact of influenza. Priority should be given to targeted high-risk groups.

Targeted High-Risk Children and Adolescents. Yearly influenza immunization, administered during the autumn (see Vaccine Administration, p 389), is recommended for children 6 months of age and older with one or more of the following specific risk factors:

- Asthma or other chronic pulmonary diseases, such as cystic fibrosis
- Hemodynamically significant cardiac disease
- Immunosuppressive disorders or therapy (see Special Considerations, p 386)
- Human immunodeficiency virus (HIV) infection (see Human Immunodeficiency Virus Infection, p 360)
- Sickle cell anemia and other hemoglobinopathies
- Diseases requiring long-term salicylate therapy, such as rheumatoid arthritis or Kawasaki syndrome, which may increase the risk of developing Reye syndrome after influenza illness
- Chronic renal dysfunction
- Chronic metabolic disease, including diabetes mellitus

Pregnancy. Women who will be in the second or third trimester of pregnancy during influenza season should receive inactivated influenza vaccine during the autumn, because pregnancy increases the risk of complications and hospitalization from influenza. Because the current intramuscularly administered inactivated influenza vaccine is not a live-virus vaccine and only rarely is associated with major systemic reactions, some experts consider the vaccine safe during any stage of pregnancy. However, some other experts prefer immunization only during the second and third trimesters. Because spontaneous abortion is common during the first trimester of pregnancy, unnecessary exposures to antigens during this time generally are avoided.

Close Contacts of High-Risk Patients. Immunization and chemoprophylaxis of people who are in close contact with children with high-risk conditions and children younger than 24 months of age are important means of protection for these children. In addition, immunization of pregnant women may benefit their unborn infants, because transplacentally acquired antibody may protect infants from infection with influenza A virus. Immunization is recommended for the following:

- All health care professionals in contact with pediatric patients in hospitals, outpatient care settings, and chronic care facilities
- Household contacts, including siblings and primary caregivers, of high-risk children
- Children who are members of households with high-risk adults, including children with symptomatic HIV infection
- Providers of home care to children younger than 24 months of age and to high-risk groups of children and adolescents

---

* American Academy of Pediatrics, Committee on Infectious Diseases. Policy statement: reduction of the influenza burden in children. *Pediatrics.* 2002;110:1246–1252; and American Academy of Pediatrics, Committee on Infectious Diseases. Technical report: reduction of the influenza burden in children. *Pediatrics.* 2002;110(6). Available at: www.pediatrics.org/cgi/content/full/110/e80

International Travel. People traveling internationally to areas where influenza outbreaks are or may be occurring should be considered for immunization. The decision to immunize will depend on the person's destination, duration of travel, risk of acquiring influenza (such as the season of the year and immunization history), and potential for severe illness. In temperate climate zones of the northern and southern hemispheres, travelers also can be exposed to influenza during the summer, especially when traveling as part of large organized tourist groups that include people from areas of the world where influenza viruses may be circulating.

Other Children. Immunization should be considered for any child or adolescent with an underlying condition that may compromise the child's resistance to influenza, including young age, and for groups of people whose close contact facilitates rapid transmission and spread of infection that may result in disruption of routine activities. These groups include students in colleges, schools, and other institutions of learning, particularly people who reside in dormitories or who are members of athletic teams, and people living in residential institutions. Inactivated influenza vaccine also may be administered to any immunocompetent child or adolescent who wishes to decrease the chance of becoming infected with influenza. The morbidity from influenza among healthy children can be appreciable.

Breastfeeding. Inactivated influenza virus vaccine does not adversely affect the safety of breastfeeding for mothers or infants; therefore, breastfeeding is not a contraindication for immunization.

Vaccine Administration. Inactivated influenza vaccine should be administered during the autumn of each year before the start of the influenza season, at the time specified in the yearly recommendations of the CDC Advisory Committee on Immunization Practices. The usual recommended time is from the beginning of October through December. However, people may be immunized in September, when the vaccine for the forthcoming influenza season becomes available. Importantly, vaccine should continue to be offered even after December if influenza activity is continuing. The recommended vaccine dose and schedule for different age groups are given in Table 3.30 (p 387).

Annual immunization is recommended, because immunity can decrease during the year after immunization and because in most years, at least one of the vaccine antigens is changed to match ongoing antigenic changes in circulating strains.

Inactivated influenza vaccine may be administered simultaneously (but at a separate site and with a different syringe) with other recommended immunizations for children.

Reactions, Adverse Effects, and Contraindications. Inactivated influenza vaccine contains only noninfectious viruses and cannot cause influenza. In children younger than 13 years of age, febrile reactions are rare. Fever occurs primarily 6 to 24 hours after immunization in children younger than 24 months of age. Local reactions are rare in children younger than 13 years of age. In children 13 years of age or older, local reactions occur in approximately 10% of recipients.

In some years, influenza vaccines have been associated with a slightly increased frequency of Guillain-Barré syndrome (GBS). Estimating the precise risk of a rare condition such as GBS is difficult, but a study conducted during 1992–1994 showed that a small increase may have occurred in the number of GBS cases in immunized adults. This represented an excess rate of approximately 1 GBS case per million

people immunized. Even if GBS were a causally related adverse effect, the low estimated risk of GBS is much less than that of severe influenza that could be prevented
by immunization. Immunization of children who have asthma or cystic fibrosis with
the currently available inactivated influenza vaccines is not associated with a
detectable increase in adverse reactions or exacerbations.

Children demonstrating severe anaphylactic reaction to chickens or egg protein
or other components of the inactivated influenza vaccine can experience, on rare
occasions, a similar type of reaction to inactivated influenza vaccines. Although
inactivated influenza vaccine has been administered safely to such children after
skin testing and, when appropriate, desensitization, these children generally should
not receive inactivated influenza vaccine because of their risk of reactions, the likely
need for yearly immunization, and the availability of chemoprophylaxis against
influenza infection.

Chemoprophylaxis: An Alternative Method of Protecting Children Against Influenza.

Chemoprophylaxis should not be considered a substitute for immunization in most
cases; however, the currently licensed drugs are important adjuvants to inactivated
influenza vaccine for the control and prevention of influenza disease. Amantadine
and rimantadine are approved for prophylaxis of influenza A in children older than
1 year of age. Studies of prophylaxis against influenza A infection in adults have
demonstrated 70% to 90% effectiveness in preventing clinical illness, but asymptomatic infection can occur. Studies in children have indicated a similar beneficial
effect in diminishing spread of influenza A among institutionalized children and
family members and in pediatric hospitals. The usual recommended doses of rimantadine and amantadine for prophylaxis are the same as those for treatment and are
given in Table 4.8 (p 729). Oseltamivir is approved for prophylaxis in children
13 years of age and older. Zanamivir is not approved for chemoprophylaxis.

Indications for Chemoprophylaxis

Chemoprophylaxis may be considered for the following situations:
- Protection of high-risk children during the 2 weeks after immunization
  while an immune response is developing or if the children are immunized
  after influenza circulation has been documented (chemoprophylaxis is not
  recommended if immunization occurs before influenza viruses have begun
  to circulate)
- Protection of children at increased risk of severe infection or complications,
  such as high-risk children for whom the vaccine is contraindicated (ie, children
  with a history of anaphylactic reaction to eggs)
- Protection of nonimmunized close contacts of high-risk children
- Protection of immunocompromised children who may not respond to vaccine
- Control of influenza outbreaks in a closed setting, such as an institution with
  high-risk children
- Protection of immunized high-risk individuals if vaccine strain poorly matches
  circulating influenza strains

Chemoprophylaxis of immunized people does not interfere with the immune
response to the inactivated influenza virus vaccine and may provide additional
protection.

Information about influenza surveillance is available through the CDC Voice Information System (influenza update, 888-232-3228) or through www.cdc.gov/ncidod/diseases/flu/weekly.htm.

Isosporiasis
(Isospora belli)

CLINICAL MANIFESTATIONS: Protracted, foul-smelling, watery diarrhea is the most common symptom. Manifestations are similar to those caused by *Cryptosporidium* and *Cyclospora* organisms and can include abdominal pain, anorexia, and weight loss. Fever, malaise, vomiting, and headache have been reported. Severity of infection ranges from self-limiting in immunocompetent hosts to life threatening in immunocompromised patients, particularly people with human immunodeficiency virus (HIV) infection.

ETIOLOGY: *Isospora belli* is a spore-forming coccidian protozoan.

EPIDEMIOLOGY: Humans are the only known host for *I belli.* The frequency of asymptomatic infection with this parasite is unknown. Infection is more common in tropical and subtropical climates and in areas of poor sanitary conditions. Human infection occurs by the fecal-oral route and has been linked with contaminated food and water. *Isospora belli* has been reported as a cause of traveler's diarrhea in visitors to endemic areas and of institutional outbreaks. Oocysts are passed unsporulated and require exposure to oxygen and temperatures lower than 37°C (98°F) before becoming infectious. Oocysts are resistant to most disinfectants and may remain viable for months in a cool, moist environment.

The **incubation period** is thought to be 8 to 10 days.

DIAGNOSTIC TESTS: Demonstration of oocysts in feces or in duodenal aspirates or finding the parasite in developmental stages in biopsy specimens of the small intestine is diagnostic. Oocysts in stool can be distinguished by their size; they are 5 times larger than *Cryptosporidium* organisms and oval shaped. Oocysts can be detected with modified Kinyoun carbolfuchsin and with auramine-rhodamine stains. Concentration techniques may be needed before staining, because the organisms often are present in small numbers.

TREATMENT: Trimethoprim-sulfamethoxazole is the drug of choice. Pyrimethamine is an alternative treatment for people who cannot tolerate trimethoprim-sulfamethoxazole. Ciprofloxacin also may be effective, although ciprofloxacin is not licensed for use in people younger than 18 years of age (see Antimicrobial Agents and Related Therapies, p 693). Antimicrobial prophylaxis to prevent recurrent disease may be indicated for people infected with HIV.

ISOLATION OF THE HOSPITALIZED PATIENT: In addition to standard precautions, contact precautions are recommended for diapered and incontinent children.

CONTROL MEASURES: None.

Kawasaki Syndrome

CLINICAL MANIFESTATIONS: Kawasaki syndrome is a febrile, exanthematous, multisystem vasculitis of importance, because approximately 20% of untreated children will develop coronary artery abnormalities. Most cases of Kawasaki syndrome occur in children between 1 and 8 years of age. Within several days of onset of fever, characteristic features of illness usually appear, including: (1) bilateral bulbar conjunctival injection without exudate; (2) erythematous mouth and pharynx, strawberry tongue, and red, cracked lips; (3) a polymorphous, generalized, erythematous rash that can be morbilliform, maculopapular, or scarlatiniform or may resemble erythema multiforme; (4) changes in the peripheral extremities consisting of induration of the hands and feet with erythematous palms and soles or periungual desquamation; and (5) acute, nonsuppurative cervical lymphadenopathy with at least one node 1.5 cm in diameter. For diagnosis of classic Kawasaki syndrome, patients should have fever for at least 5 days and at least 4 of these 5 features without another reasonable explanation. Irritability, abdominal pain, diarrhea, and vomiting are commonly associated features. Other findings include urethritis with sterile pyuria (70% of cases), mild hepatic dysfunction (40%), arthritis or arthralgia (10%–20%), aseptic meningitis (25%), pericardial effusion (20%–40%), gallbladder hydrops (<10%), and myocarditis manifested by congestive heart failure (<5%).

Incomplete or atypical Kawasaki syndrome is more common in infants younger than 12 months of age than in older children, and clinical features of Kawasaki syndrome may be particularly subtle in this age group. Infants with Kawasaki syndrome also have a higher risk of developing coronary aneurysms than older children, making diagnosis and timely treatment especially important in these young patients. The laboratory findings of incomplete cases appear to be similar to those of classic cases. Therefore, although laboratory findings in Kawasaki syndrome are nonspecific, they may prove useful in increasing or decreasing suspicion of incomplete Kawasaki syndrome. Early echocardiographic study may be useful in the evaluation of patients with suspected incomplete Kawasaki syndrome. Infants and children with signs and symptoms compatible with incomplete Kawasaki syndrome and with no alternative diagnosis that is more likely should be considered for treatment with IGIV and aspirin within 10 days of the onset of fever.

Without aspirin and Immune Globulin Intravenous (IGIV) therapy, fever may last 2 weeks or longer. After fever resolves, patients can remain anorectic or irritable for 2 to 3 weeks. During this subacute phase, desquamation of the groin and, later, desquamation of the fingers, toes, and other areas may occur. Recurrent disease occurring months to years later develops in fewer than 2% of patients.

Coronary artery aneurysms can be demonstrated with 2-dimensional echocardiography in 20% to 25% of patients who are not treated within 10 days of onset of fever. Patients at increased risk of developing coronary aneurysms include males, infants younger than 12 months of age, children older than 8 years of age, people whose fever persists for more than 10 days, people with higher baseline neutrophil and band counts or lower hemoglobin concentrations (<10 g/dL), and people with thrombocytopenia and fever persisting after IGIV administration. Aneurysms of the coronary arteries have been demonstrated by echocardiography as soon as a few days after onset of illness but more typically occur between 1 to 4 weeks after onset of illness; their appearance later than 6 weeks is uncommon. Giant coronary aneurysms (≥8 mm in diameter) are likely to be associated with long-term complications. Aneurysms occurring in other medium-sized arteries (eg, iliac, femoral, renal, and axillary vessels) are uncommon and generally do not occur in the absence of coronary abnormalities. In addition to coronary artery disease, carditis can involve the pericardium, myocardium, or endocardium, and mitral and aortic regurgitation can develop. Carditis generally resolves when fever resolves.

In children with mild coronary dilation or ectasia, coronary artery dimensions often return to baseline within 6 to 8 weeks after onset of disease. Approximately 50% of nongiant coronary aneurysms regress to normal lumen size within 1 to 2 years, although this process may be accompanied by coronary stenosis. In addition, aneurysm regression may result in a poorly compliant, fibrotic vessel wall.

The current case fatality rate in the United States is less than 0.01%. The principal cause of death is myocardial infarction resulting from coronary occlusion attributable to thrombosis or progressive stenosis. Rarely, a large coronary aneurysm may rupture. Most fatalities occur within 6 weeks of the onset of symptoms, but myocardial infarction and sudden death can occur months to years after the acute episode. The vasculitis of Kawasaki syndrome may be a risk factor for premature atherosclerotic disease.

ETIOLOGY: The cause is unknown. Epidemiologic and clinical features strongly suggest an infectious cause.

EPIDEMIOLOGY: Peak age of occurrence in the United States is between 18 and 24 months. Fifty percent of patients are younger than 2 years of age, and 80% are younger than 5 years of age; children older than 8 years of age rarely develop the disease. In children younger than 6 months of age, the diagnosis often is delayed because of atypical symptoms; the prevalence of coronary artery abnormalities may be especially high when the diagnosis is delayed because symptoms and signs may not suggest Kawasaki syndrome. The male-female ratio is approximately 1.5:1. The incidence is highest in Asians; 3000 to 5000 cases are estimated to occur annually in the United States. Kawasaki syndrome was first described in Japan, where a pattern of endemic occurrence with superimposed epidemic outbreaks was recognized. A similar pattern of steady or increasing endemic disease with occasional sharply defined community-wide epidemics has been recognized in diverse locations in North America and Hawaii. Epidemics generally occur during the winter and spring. No evidence indicates person-to-person or common-source spread, although the incidence is somewhat higher in siblings of children with the disease.

The **incubation period** is unknown.

DIAGNOSTIC TESTS: No specific diagnostic test is available. The diagnosis is established by fulfillment of the syndrome criteria (see Clinical Manifestations, p 392) and exclusion of other possible illnesses, such as measles, streptococcal infection (ie, scarlet fever), viral and rickettsial exanthems, drug reactions (eg, Stevens-Johnson syndrome), staphylococcal scalded skin syndrome, toxic shock syndrome, and juvenile rheumatoid arthritis.* An increased sedimentation rate and serum C-reactive protein concentration during the first 2 weeks of illness and an increased platelet count (>450 000/μL [>450 × 10^9/L]) after the first week of illness are almost universal laboratory features. These values usually normalize within 6 to 8 weeks.

TREATMENT: Management during the acute phase is directed at decreasing inflammation of the myocardium and coronary artery wall and providing supportive care. Anti-inflammatory therapy should be initiated when the diagnosis is established or strongly suspected. Once the acute phase has passed, therapy is directed at prevention of coronary artery thrombosis. Specific recommendations for therapy include the following measures:

Immune Globulin Intravenous. Therapy with high-dose IGIV and aspirin initiated within 10 days of the onset of fever substantially decreases progression to coronary artery dilation and aneurysms at 2 to 7 weeks, compared with treatment with aspirin alone, and results in more rapid resolution of fever and other indicators of acute inflammation. Therapy with IGIV should be initiated as soon as possible; its efficacy when initiated later than the 10th day of illness or after aneurysms have been detected has not been evaluated in controlled trials. However, therapy with IGIV and aspirin should be provided for patients diagnosed after day 10 who have manifestations of continuing inflammation (eg, fever or other symptoms or laboratory abnormalities) or of evolving coronary artery disease. Despite prompt treatment with IGIV and aspirin, 2% to 4% of patients will develop coronary artery abnormalities.

Dose. The optimal therapeutic dose of IGIV is unknown. A dose of 2 g/kg as a single dose, given over 10 to 12 hours, is recommended. Few complications occur from this regimen.

Retreatment. Approximately 5% to 10% of patients who receive IGIV and aspirin therapy will experience persistent fever or recurrence of fever after an initial period of being afebrile for 48 hours or less. Other clinical indications of inflammation, such as conjunctival injection and rash, also may persist or recur. In these situations, retreatment with IGIV (2 g/kg) and continued aspirin therapy may be indicated, because persistent fever may be associated with increased concentrations of inflammatory cytokines and an increased risk of coronary artery abnormalities. At the present time, the use of systemic corticosteroids in the treatment of Kawasaki syndrome is controversial. Several studies have reported that patients treated with corticosteroids alone or in combination with aspirin have a higher frequency of coronary artery abnormalities, and other uncontrolled studies suggest oral or intravenous prednisolone therapy may be useful in some patients who are resistant to repeat doses of IGIV.

Aspirin. Aspirin is used for anti-inflammatory and antithrombotic actions, although convincing data that aspirin decreases coronary artery abnormalities are not available. Aspirin is administered in doses of 80 to 100 mg/kg per day in 4 divided doses during the acute phase. Children with acute Kawasaki syndrome have decreased aspirin absorption and increased clearance, so some children may

---

* For further information on the diagnosis of this disease, see recommendations of the American Heart Association in Dajani AS, Taubert KA, Gerber MA, et al. Diagnosis and therapy of Kawasaki disease in children. *Circulation.* 1993;87:1776–1780

not achieve therapeutic concentrations. In most children, this is not clinically significant, and it is not necessary to monitor aspirin concentrations. After fever is controlled for 4 or 5 days, the aspirin dose is decreased to 3 to 5 mg/kg per day to continue antithrombotic activity. Aspirin is discontinued if no coronary artery abnormalities have been detected by 6 to 8 weeks after onset of illness. Low-dose aspirin therapy should be continued indefinitely for people in whom coronary artery abnormalities are present. Because of the potential risk of Reye syndrome in patients with influenza or varicella receiving salicylates, parents of children receiving aspirin should be instructed to contact their child's physician promptly if the child develops symptoms of or is exposed to either disease.

*Cardiac Care.** An echocardiogram should be obtained early in the acute phase of illness and 6 to 8 weeks after onset. The care of patients with carditis should involve a cardiologist experienced in management of patients with Kawasaki syndrome and in assessing echocardiographic studies of coronary arteries in children. Long-term management of Kawasaki syndrome should be based on the degree of coronary artery involvement. Children should be assessed during the first 2 months to detect evidence of arrhythmias, congestive heart failure, and valvular regurgitation. In addition to prolonged low-dose aspirin therapy to suppress platelet aggregation in patients with persistent coronary artery abnormalities, some experts recommend 4 mg/kg per day of dipyridamole, given in 3 divided doses. Development of giant coronary artery aneurysms (≥8 mm in diameter) may require the addition of anticoagulant therapy, such as warfarin sodium, to prevent thrombosis.

Subsequent Immunization. Measles and varicella immunizations should be deferred for 11 months after IGIV administration in children who have received high-dose IGIV for treatment of Kawasaki syndrome. If the child's risk of exposure to measles is high, the child should be immunized and then reimmunized at least 11 months after administration of IGIV unless serologic testing indicates successful immunization by the earlier dose (see Measles, p 419). The schedule for subsequent administration of other childhood immunizations should not be interrupted. Yearly influenza immunization is indicated for patients 6 months of age and older who require long-term aspirin therapy because of the possible increased risk of developing Reye syndrome (see Influenza, p 382).

ISOLATION OF THE HOSPITALIZED PATIENT: Standard precautions are indicated.

CONTROL MEASURES: None.

---

* For specific recommendations of the American Heart Association, see Dajani AS, Taubert KA, Takahashi M, et al. Guidelines for long-term management of patients with Kawasaki disease: Report from the Committee on Rheumatic Fever, Endocarditis, and Kawasaki Disease, Council on Cardiovascular Disease in the Young, American Heart Association. *Circulation.* 1994;89:916–922

Kingella kingae Infections

CLINICAL MANIFESTATIONS: The most common infections associated with *Kingella kingae* are suppurative arthritis and osteomyelitis. Most of these infections occur in children younger than 5 years of age. Pyogenic arthritis caused by *K kingae* generally is monoarticular, with a knee being the most commonly involved joint, followed in frequency by hips and ankles. Clinical manifestations are similar to those associated with infection attributable to other bacterial pathogens in immunocompetent children. Osteomyelitis caused by *K kingae* has clinical manifestations similar to *Staphylococcus aureus* osteomyelitis. The femur is the most common site of infection. *Kingella kingae* also has been associated with diskitis, meningitis, endocarditis in children with underlying heart disease, and pneumonia.

ETIOLOGY: *Kingella* organisms are fastidious, gram-negative coccobacilli previously classified as *Moraxella*. Of the 3 species in the genus *Kingella*, *K kingae* is the species most commonly associated with infection.

EPIDEMIOLOGY: The human oropharynx is the usual habitat of *K kingae*. The organism more frequently colonizes the respiratory tracts of children than adults and can be transmitted among children in child care centers, generally without causing disease.

The **incubation period** is variable.

DIAGNOSTIC TESTS: *Kingella kingae* can be isolated from blood, joint fluid, bone, cerebrospinal fluid, respiratory tract secretions, and other sites of infection. Organisms grow better in anaerobic conditions with enhanced carbon dioxide. In patients with septic arthritis and osteomyelitis, blood cultures often are negative. Joint fluid and bone aspirates from children 5 years of age or younger with suspected infection should be inoculated into Bactec, BacT/Alert, or similar blood culture systems and held for at least 7 days to maximize recovery.

TREATMENT: Penicillin is the drug of choice for treatment of invasive infections with β-lactamase-negative strains of *K kingae*. Other β-lactam agents also are effective. Strains generally are susceptible to aminoglycosides, ciprofloxacin, erythromycin, trimethoprim-sulfamethoxazole, and oxacillin and exhibit variable resistance to clindamycin and vancomycin hydrochloride. Gentamicin sulfate in combination with pencillin can be useful for the initial treatment of endocarditis.

ISOLATION OF THE HOSPITALIZED PATIENT: Standard precautions are recommended.

CONTROL MEASURES: None.

Legionella pneumophila Infections

CLINICAL MANIFESTATIONS: Legionellosis is associated with 2 clinically and epidemiologically distinct illnesses: legionnaires disease and Pontiac fever. Legionnaires disease varies in severity from mild to severe pneumonia characterized by fever, cough, and progressive respiratory distress. Legionnaires disease can be associated with chills; myalgias; and gastrointestinal tract, central nervous system, and renal manifestations. Respiratory failure and death may occur. Pontiac fever is a milder febrile illness without pneumonia that occurs in epidemics and is characterized by an abrupt onset and a self-limited, influenza-like manifestation.

ETIOLOGY: *Legionella* species are fastidious aerobic bacilli that stain gram-negative after recovery on artificial media. At least 18 different species have been implicated in human disease, but most documented *Legionella* infections in the United States are caused by the *Legionella pneumophila* serogroup 1.

EPIDEMIOLOGY: Legionnaires disease is acquired through inhalation of aerosolized water contaminated with *L pneumophila*. Person-to-person transmission has not been demonstrated. More than 80% of cases are sporadic; the sources of infection may be related to exposure to *L pneumophila*-contaminated water in the patient's home, workplace, or location of medical therapy or to aerosol-producing devices in public places. Outbreaks have been ascribed to common-source exposure to contaminated cooling towers, evaporative condensers, potable water systems, whirlpool spas, humidifiers, and respiratory therapy equipment. Outbreaks have occurred in hospitals, cruise ships, hotels, and other large buildings. Nosocomial infections occur and often have been traced to a hot water supply. The disease occurs most commonly in elderly and immunocompromised people. Infection in children is rare and usually is asymptomatic or mild and unrecognized. Severe disease has occurred in children with malignant neoplasms, severe combined immunodeficiency, chronic granulomatous disease, organ transplantation, end-stage renal disease or underlying pulmonary disease, and immunosuppression with corticosteroids.

The **incubation period** for legionnaires disease (pneumonia) is 2 to 10 days; for Pontiac fever, the incubation period is 1 to 2 days.

DIAGNOSTIC TESTS: Recovery of *L pneumophila* from respiratory tract secretions, lung tissue, pleural fluid, or other normally sterile fluid specimens by using special culture media provides definitive evidence of infection. The bacterium can be demonstrated in these specimens by direct immunofluorescence, but this test is less sensitive and less specific than culture. Detection of *Legionella* antigens in urine by commercially available immunoassays is highly specific and more sensitive than immunofluorescence using respiratory tract secretions. Such tests are most sensitive for *L pneumophilia* serogroup 1 but detect antigen in some patients infected with other *L pneumophilia* serogroups or species. For serologic diagnosis, a fourfold increase in titer of antibodies to *L pneumophila* serogroup 1, measured by indirect immunofluorescence antibody (IFA) assay, also indicates acute infection. Antibody titers usually increase within 1 to 6 weeks after onset of symptoms, but the increase can be delayed for as long as 12 weeks. The positive predictive value of a single titer of ≥1:256 is low and does not provide definitive evidence of infection. Antibodies to several gram-negative organisms, including *Pseudomonas* species, *Bacteroides fragilis,* and *Campylobacter jejuni,* may cause false-positive IFA test results. Newer serologic assays, such as enzyme immunoassay or tests using *Legionella* antigens other than serogroup 1, are available commercially but have not been standardized adequately.

TREATMENT: Intravenous azithromycin dihydrate (10 mg/kg per day as a single dose; maximum 500 mg) has replaced erythromycin as the drug of choice. Once the patient's condition is improving, oral therapy can be substituted. The addition of rifampin is recommended for patients with confirmed disease who are severely ill or immunocompromised or in whom the infection does not respond promptly to intravenous azithromycin. Fluoroquinolones, such as ciprofloxacin and levofloxacin, are bactericidal and effective but are not approved for use in people younger than 18 years of age. Doxycycline and trimethoprim-sulfamethoxazole are alternative drugs. Doxycycline should not be used by pregnant women and children younger than 8 years of age because of the risk of dental staining. Duration of therapy is 5 to 10 days if azithromycin is administered and 14 to 21 days for other drugs; longer courses are recommended for patients who are immunocompromised or have severe disease.

ISOLATION OF THE HOSPITALIZED PATIENT: Standard precautions are recommended.

CONTROL MEASURES: The main methods for decontaminating potable water supplies in common-source outbreaks are hyperchlorination or superheating (to 71°C–76°C [160°F–170°F]) in conjunction with appropriate mechanical cleaning, followed by continuous chlorination or maintenance of a hot water temperature at the faucet of greater than 50°C (122°F). Other disinfection methods, including copper-silver ionization by electrolysis, have limited the growth of *Legionella* organisms under laboratory conditions.

Occurrence of even a single laboratory-confirmed nosocomial case of legionellosis warrants consideration of an epidemiologic and environmental investigation, particularly in facilities serving highly susceptible, immunocompromised patients. All documented cases of legionellosis should be reported to state and local public health departments.

Leishmaniasis

CLINICAL MANIFESTATIONS: The 3 major clinical syndromes are as follows:
- *Cutaneous leishmaniasis.* After inoculation by the bite of an infected sandfly, parasites proliferate locally in mononuclear phagocytes, leading to an erythematous macula or nodule that typically evolves to form a shallow ulcer with raised borders. Lesions commonly are located on exposed areas of the face and extremities and may be accompanied by satellite lesions and regional adenopathy. The clinical manifestations of Old World and New World cutaneous leishmaniasis are similar. Spontaneous resolution of lesions may take weeks to years and usually results in a flat atrophic (cigarette paper) scar.

- *Mucocutaneous leishmaniasis (espundia).* From the initial cutaneous infection caused by *Leishmania braziliensis* or related New World species, parasites may disseminate to the oral and nasopharyngeal mucosa. In some patients, granulomatous ulceration follows, leading to facial disfigurement, secondary infection, and mucosal perforation months to years after the cutaneous lesion heals.
- *Visceral leishmaniasis (kala-azar).* After cutaneous inoculation of parasites, organisms spread throughout the mononuclear macrophage system and are concentrated in the spleen, liver, and bone marrow. The resulting clinical illness is marked by fever, anorexia, weight loss, splenomegaly, hepatomegaly, lymphadenopathy (in some geographic areas), anemia, leukopenia, thrombocytopenia with hemorrhage, hypoalbuminemia, and hypergammaglobulinemia. Secondary pyogenic, gram-negative enteric, and mycobacterial infections are common. Active untreated visceral disease nearly always is fatal. Reactivation of latent visceral leishmaniasis is common in patients with concurrent human immunodeficiency virus (HIV) infection or other immunocompromising conditions.

ETIOLOGY: In the human host, *Leishmania* species are obligate intracellular parasites of mononuclear phagocytes. A single *Leishmania* species can produce different clinical syndromes, and each syndrome can be caused by different species. For example, cutaneous leishmaniasis typically is caused by *Leishmania tropica, Leishmania major,* and *Leishmania aethiopica* (Old World species) and by *Leishmania mexicana, Leishmania amazonensis, L braziliensis, Leishmania panamensis, Leishmania guyanensis, Leishmania peruviana, Leishmania chagasi,* and other New World species. Mucocutaneous leishmaniasis is caused by *L braziliensis, L panamensis, L guyamenis,* and *L amazonensis.* Visceral leishmaniasis is caused by *Leishmania donovani, Leishmania infantum,* and *Leishmania chagasi,* as well as *L tropica* and *L amazonensis. Leishmania donovani* and *L infantum* also can cause Old World cutaneous leishmaniasis.

EPIDEMIOLOGY: Leishmaniasis typically is a zoonosis with a variety of mammalian reservoir hosts, including canines and rodents. The vectors are phlebotomine sandflies. The distribution of Old World cutaneous leishmaniasis includes the Middle East, some Asian and African countries, the Indian subcontinent, countries of the former Soviet Union, and sporadically, southern Europe. New World cutaneous leishmaniasis is found in areas extending from Mexico to northern Argentina, and a few cases have been reported as far north as Texas. Mucocutaneous leishmaniasis occurs primarily in the Amazon basin and the central plains of Brazil but also has been reported in other countries in South and Central America. The distribution of visceral leishmaniasis in the Old World includes southern Europe, the Mediterranean basin, the Middle East, East Africa, China, and the Indian subcontinent. Endemic foci in the New World are found in South and Central America, particularly in Brazil.

The **incubation periods** for the different forms of leishmaniasis range from several days to months. In cutaneous leishmaniasis, primary skin lesions typically appear several weeks after parasite inoculation. In visceral infection, the incubation period can vary from 6 weeks to 6 months. However, incubation periods from

10 days to 10 years have been reported, and reactivation of previously asymptomatic latent infection can occur in immunosuppressed patients.

DIAGNOSTIC TESTS: Definitive diagnosis is made by demonstration of the presence of the parasite. A common way of identifying the parasite is by microscopic identification of intracellular leishmanial organisms on Wright or Giemsa stains of smears or histologic sections of infected tissues. In cutaneous disease, tissue can be obtained by a 3-mm punch biopsy, by lesion scrapings, or by needle aspiration of the raised nonnecrotic edge (not the center) of the lesion. In visceral leishmaniasis, the organisms can be identified in the spleen and, less commonly, in bone marrow and liver; in East Africa, the organisms also can be identified in the lymph nodes. Blood cultures have been positive in some Indian patients, and organisms sometimes may be observed in blood smears or buffy-coat preparations in HIV-infected patients. Isolation of parasites by culture of appropriate tissue specimens in specialized media should be attempted when possible. Culture media and further information can be provided by the Centers for Disease Control and Prevention (CDC).

The diagnosis of some forms of leishmaniasis can be aided by the performance of serologic testing available at the CDC. Serologic test results usually are positive in cases of visceral and mucocutaneous leishmaniasis if the patient is immunocompetent but often are negative in cutaneous leishmaniasis. False-positive serologic test results may occur in patients with other infectious diseases, especially American trypanosomiasis.

TREATMENT: Because cutaneous lesions may heal without specific therapy, treatment is not always necessary. Treatment is indicated when the ulcers are disabling or disfiguring, when healing is delayed, or when the patient may be infected with *L braziliensis* or other *Leishmania* species that can cause mucocutaneous disease. Drug therapy always is indicated when mucocutaneous or visceral infection is present (see Drugs for Parasitic Infections, p 744).

In the United States, the drug of choice for leishmaniasis is sodium stibogluconate, a parenteral pentavalent antimonial compound that usually is given daily for a minimum of 20 days. Sodium stibogluconate is available under an investigational new drug protocol from the CDC Drug Service (see Appendix I, Directory of Resources, p 789). It generally is well tolerated in young, otherwise healthy patients, but reversible cardiac, pancreatic, and hepatotoxic effects can occur. The related antimonial drug meglumine antimonate (which is not available in the United States) is an alternative agent. Liposomal amphotericin B is licensed by the US Food and Drug Administration for treatment of visceral leishmaniasis. For patients with disease refractory to antimonial therapy, amphotericin B, liposomal amphotericin B, pentamidine, or paromomycin should be considered. In some cases of American cutaneous leishmaniasis, ketoconazole and itraconazole as well as local heat have been used successfully. Local therapy is not advisable for infection that could disseminate to cause mucosal leishmaniasis. In selected cases of Old World and New World cutaneous leishmaniasis, various types of local or topical therapy have been used successfully.

ISOLATION OF THE HOSPITALIZED PATIENT: Standard precautions are recommended.

CONTROL MEASURES: Because elimination of infected animal reservoir hosts and/or sandfly populations is unlikely to occur in most regions that are endemic for leishmaniasis, travelers should be advised to minimize their exposure to sandfly bites by using screened accommodations, fine-mesh bed netting impregnated with an insecticide such as permethrin or deltamethrin, protective clothing, and insect repellent and by minimizing outdoor exposures from dusk to dawn. Patients who have been infected with *Leishmania* species should not donate blood or organs.

Leprosy

CLINICAL MANIFESTATIONS: Leprosy (Hansen disease) is a chronic disease mainly involving skin, peripheral nerves, the mucosa of the upper respiratory tract, and testes. The clinical syndromes of leprosy represent a spectrum that reflects the cellular immune response to *Mycobacterium leprae* and the unique tropism for peripheral nerves. The 2 poles of the leprosy spectrum are tuberculoid and lepromatous forms. Characteristic features are the following:
- *Tuberculoid:* one or a few well-demarcated, hypopigmented or erythematous, hypoesthetic or anesthetic skin lesions, often with raised, active, spreading edges and central clearing. Cell-mediated immune responses are intact.
- *Lepromatous:* initial numerous, ill-defined, hypopigmented, or erythematous maculae that progress to papules, nodules, or plaques; and late-occurring hypoesthesia. Dermal infiltration of the face, hands, and feet in a bilateral and symmetric distribution can occur without preceding maculopapular lesions. *Mycobacterium leprae*-specific, cell-mediated immunity is diminished greatly, but serum antibody responses to *M leprae*-derived antigens may occur, or titers of nonspecific antibodies (such as rheumatoid factor or syphilis [on nontreponemal tests]) may be increased.
- *Borderline (dimorphous):* single or multiple well-defined skin lesions similar to tuberculoid lesions but with a raised central area; and delayed development of dysesthesia. Borderline disease often is subdivided into borderline lepromatous, borderline, and borderline tuberculoid.
- *Indeterminate:* an early form of leprosy that may develop into any of the other forms; typified by hypopigmented maculae with indistinct edges and no associated dysesthesia.
   Serious consequences of leprosy occur from immune reactions and nerve involvement with resulting anesthesia, which can lead to repeated unrecognized trauma, ulcerations, fractures, and bone resorption.

ETIOLOGY: Leprosy is caused by *M leprae*, a gram-positive, obligate intracellular, acid-fast bacillus.

EPIDEMIOLOGY: The major mode of transmission is contact with humans who have untreated or drug-resistant lepromatous, borderline lepromatous, or borderline types. A long duration of exposure, such as to a household contact, is common. However, 70% to 80% of cases in endemic areas do not have a history of household exposure or other contact with a known or suspected case of leprosy, suggesting the possibility of other sources of infection. The major source of infectious material probably is nasal secretions from patients with untreated lepromatous, borderline lepromatous, or borderline disease, from whom organisms are excreted in large numbers. Little shedding of *M leprae* from involved intact skin occurs. In the United States, 90% of reported cases are imported, occurring in immigrants and refugees from areas endemic for leprosy, particularly Mexico and Southeast Asia. Indigenous cases continue to occur in Texas, California, Louisiana, and Hawaii. The infectivity of lepromatous patients probably ceases after treatment is instituted, often within a few days or weeks of initiating rifampin therapy or approximately 3 months after initiating therapy with dapsone or clofazimine. Contaminated soil or insect vectors may play a role in disease transmission.

The **incubation period** ranges from 1 to many years but usually is 3 to 5 years. The incubation period of tuberculoid cases tends to be shorter than that for lepromatous cases.

DIAGNOSTIC TESTS: Histopathologic examination by an experienced pathologist is the best method of establishing the diagnosis and is the basis for the classification of leprosy. Acid-fast bacilli may be found in slit-smears or biopsy specimens of skin lesions but rarely from patients with the tuberculoid and indeterminate forms of disease. Organisms have not been cultured successfully in vitro. Drug resistance is tested by the mouse footpad inoculation test, which is performed only in specialized laboratories.

A polymerase chain reaction test for *M leprae* is available on a limited basis after consultation from the National Hansen's Disease Program, Baton Rouge, LA (800-642-2477; www.bphc.hrsa.gov/nhdp).

TREATMENT: Therapy for patients with leprosy should be undertaken in consultation with an expert in leprosy. The National Hansen's Disease Program provides consultation on clinical and pathologic issues and can provide information about local Hansen disease clinics and clinicians who have experience with the disease.

Dapsone, one of the primary drugs used in the treatment of leprosy, usually is administered in a dosage of 100 mg/day for adults and 1 mg/kg per day for children. People in high-risk groups for glucose-6-phosphate dehydrogenase deficiency should be tested for this disorder before administration. Multidrug therapy is necessary for all patients. Rifampin should be given with dapsone for 1 year for paucibacillary (indeterminate, tuberculoid, and borderline tuberculoid) disease, with close follow-up to detect relapses. Clofazimine should be added for multibacillary (borderline, borderline lepromatous, and lepromatous) disease and for facial or major nerve involvement and continued for at least 2 years. Other drugs, including ofloxacin, levofloxacin, minocycline hydrochloride, and clarithromycin, have activity against *M leprae*. All patients with clinically compatible disease who have demonstrable acid-fast bacilli organisms on skin biopsy specimens or smears should be treated for presumptive multibacillary leprosy.

Corticosteroids are used to treat erythema nodosum leprosum (ENL), which commonly occurs in patients with multibacillary disease after drug therapy is initiated. Thalidomide has been licensed by the US Food and Drug Administration for ENL. Thalidomide never should be given to a woman of childbearing age unless she is using 2 reliable means of contraception. Other agents, including clofazimine, also can be used to treat ENL.

The reversal reaction, seen primarily in patients with borderline disease, is characterized by acute neuropathies and delayed-type hypersensitivity reactions at the site of current or former leprosy lesions. These conditions require aggressive treatment with corticosteroids to avoid permanent neurologic sequelae.

Most patients can be treated as outpatients. Rehabilitative measures, including surgery and physical therapy, may be necessary for some patients.

ISOLATION OF THE HOSPITALIZED PATIENT: Standard precautions are indicated.

CONTROL MEASURES: Hand hygiene is recommended for all people in contact with a patient with lepromatous leprosy. Disinfection of nasal secretions, handkerchiefs, and other fomites should be considered until treatment is established. Household contacts, particularly those with multibacillary disease, should be examined initially and then annually for at least 5 years. Chemoprophylaxis is not recommended. Local public health department regulations for leprosy vary and should be consulted.

A single bacille Calmette-Guérin (BCG) immunization is reported to be approximately 50% protective against leprosy, and 1 or 2 additional doses increases the protection further. The first commercially available leprosy vaccine was approved in India in January 1998. This vaccine is not available in the United States. Neither BCG nor the heat-killed leprosy vaccine is recommended for use in household contacts of people with leprosy in the United States.

Newly diagnosed cases of leprosy in the United States should be reported to local and state public health departments, the Centers for Disease Control and Prevention, and the National Hansen's Disease Program.

Leptospirosis

CLINICAL MANIFESTATIONS: Leptospirosis is an acute febrile disease with varied manifestations resulting from generalized vasculitis. The severity of disease ranges from self-limited systemic illness (approximately 90% of patients) to life-threatening illness with jaundice, renal failure, and hemorrhagic pneumonitis. Regardless of its severity, onset usually is characterized by nonspecific symptoms, including fever, chills, headache, nausea, vomiting, and a transient rash. The most distinct clinical findings are conjunctival suffusion without purulent discharge (30%–40% of cases) and myalgias of the calf and lumbar regions (80% of cases). This initial "septicemic" phase usually lasts for 3 to 7 days and can be followed by a second "immune-mediated" phase. In some patients, these 2 phases are separated by a short-lived abatement of fever (1–3 days). Findings commonly associated with the immune-mediated phase include fever, aseptic meningitis, conjunctival suffusion, uveitis, muscle tenderness, adenopathy, and purpuric rash. Approximately 10% of patients have severe illness, including jaundice and renal dysfunction (Weil syndrome), hemorrhagic pneumonitis, cardiac arrhythmias, or circulatory collapse associated with a case fatality rate of 5% to 40%. The overall duration of symptoms for both phases of disease varies from less than 1 week to several months.

ETIOLOGY: Leptospirosis is caused by spirochetes of the genus *Leptospira*. Previously, the many serovariants that cause leptospirosis all were classified under the species *Leptospira interrogans*. However, genetic subtyping now has determined that there are several distinct species within this pathogenic group of leptospires.

EPIDEMIOLOGY: The reservoirs for *Leptospira* species include a wide range of wild and domestic animals that may remain asymptomatic shedders for years. *Leptospira* organisms excreted in animal urine, amniotic fluid, or placenta are viable in soil or water for weeks to months. Humans become infected through contact of mucosal surfaces or abraded skin with contaminated soil, water, or animal tissues. People who are predisposed by occupation include abattoir and sewer workers, veterinarians, farmers, and military personnel. Recreational exposures and clusters of disease have been associated with wading, swimming, or boating in contaminated water, particularly during flooding. Person-to-person transmission is rare.

The **incubation period** usually is 5 to 14 days, with a range of 2 to 30 days.

DIAGNOSTIC TESTS: *Leptospira* organisms may be isolated from blood or cerebrospinal fluid specimens during the early septicemic phase of illness and from urine specimens after day 7 to 10 of illness. However, isolation of the organism can be very difficult, requiring special media and techniques and incubation for up to 16 weeks. In addition, the sensitivity of culture for diagnosis is low. For these reasons, serum specimens always should be obtained to facilitate serologic diagnosis. Antibodies usually develop during the second week of illness and can be measured by commercially available immunoassays; however, increases in antibody titer can be delayed or absent in some patients. Microscopic agglutination, the confirmatory serologic test, is performed only in reference laboratories and requires both acute and convalescent specimens. Immunohistochemical techniques can detect leptospiral antigens in infected tissues. Polymerase chain reaction assay for the detection of *Leptospira* organisms has been developed but is available only in research laboratories.

TREATMENT: Intravenous penicillin is the drug of choice for patients requiring hospitalization. Penicillin G decreases the duration of systemic symptoms and the persistence of associated laboratory abnormalities and may prevent development of leptospiruria. As with other spirochete infections, a Jarisch-Herxheimer reaction (an acute febrile reaction accompanied by headache, myalgia, and an aggravated clinical picture lasting less than 24 hours) can develop after initiation of penicillin therapy. For patients with mild disease, oral doxycycline has been shown to shorten the course of illness and decrease the occurrence of leptospiruria. Doxycycline should not be used in pregnant women or children younger than 8 years of age because of the risk of dental staining. Oral amoxicillin is an alternative therapy for children younger than 8 years of age.

ISOLATION OF THE HOSPITALIZED PATIENT: In addition to standard precautions, contact precautions are recommended for contact with urine.

CONTROL MEASURES:

- Immunization of animals can decrease their severity of disease but does not prevent leptospiruria. Therefore, immunized animals may transmit the organism to humans.
- In known endemic areas, reservoir control programs may be useful.
- Protective clothing, boots, and gloves should be worn to decrease risk to people with occupational exposure.
- Doxycycline, 200 mg, given orally once a week to adults, may provide effective prophylaxis and could be considered for high-risk occupational groups with short-term exposure. However, indications for prophylactic doxycycline use for children have not been established.

Listeria monocytogenes Infections
(Listeriosis)

CLINICAL MANIFESTATIONS: *Listeria monocytogenes* infections are relatively uncommon. Infections in children are categorized as maternal, neonatal, or childhood with or without associated predisposing conditions. Maternal infection can be associated with an influenza-like illness, fever, malaise, headache, gastrointestinal tract symptoms, and back pain. Neonatal illness has early-onset and late-onset syndromes similar to those of group B streptococcal infections. Prematurity, pneumonia, and septicemia are common in early-onset disease. Approximately 65% of women experience a symptomatic prodromal illness before the diagnosis of listeriosis in their fetus or newborn infant. Amnionitis during labor, brown staining of amniotic fluid, or asymptomatic perinatal infection can occur. An erythematous rash with small, pale nodules characterized histologically by granulomas can occur in severe newborn infection and is termed "granulomatosis infantisepticum." Late-onset infection occurs after the first week of life and usually results in meningitis. Infection occurs most commonly in the perinatal period and in patients with decreased cell-mediated immunity resulting from immunocompromising conditions or therapy, hepatic or renal disease, or infection with human immunodeficiency virus. In childhood infections, most patients have meningitis, and almost half have no predisposing condition. *Listeria monocytogenes* rarely causes diffuse encephalitis. Outbreaks caused by contaminated food and characterized clinically by fever and diarrhea have occurred. Severe disease in adults, including pregnant women, associated with contaminated food emphasizes that older children and adults can have systemic disease with mortality.

ETIOLOGY: *Listeria monocytogenes* is an aerobic, nonspore-forming, motile, gram-positive bacillus that produces a narrow zone of hemolysis on blood agar medium.

EPIDEMIOLOGY: *Listeria monocytogenes* is distributed widely in the environment. Foodborne transmission causes outbreaks and sporadic infections. Incriminated foods include unpasteurized milk; soft cheeses; prepared meats, such as hot dogs, deli meat, and pâté; undercooked poultry; and unwashed raw vegetables. Asymptomatic fecal and vaginal carriage in pregnant women can result in sporadic neonatal disease from transplacental or ascending routes of infection or from exposure during delivery. Maternal infection has been associated with abortion, preterm delivery, and fetal death. Late-onset neonatal infection can result from acquisition of the organism during passage through the birth canal or from environmental sources, followed by hematogenous invasion of the organism from intestine. Nosocomial nursery outbreaks also have occurred.

The **incubation period** is variable, ranging from 1 day to more than 3 weeks.

DIAGNOSTIC TESTS: The organism can be recovered on blood agar media from cultures of blood, cerebrospinal fluid (CSF), meconium, gastric washings, placenta, amniotic fluid, and other infected tissue specimens, including joint, pleural, or pericardial fluid. Gram stain of gastric aspirate material, placental tissue, a biopsy specimen of rash of early-onset infection, or CSF from an infected patient may demonstrate the organism. *Listeria monocytogenes* can be mistaken for a contaminant or saprophyte because of morphologic similarity to diphtheroids and streptococci.

TREATMENT:
- Initial therapy with intravenous ampicillin and an aminoglycoside, usually gentamicin sulfate, is recommended for severe infections. This combination is more effective than ampicillin alone in vitro and in animal models of *L monocytogenes* infection. After clinical response occurs or for less severe infections in immunocompetent hosts, ampicillin alone can be given. For the penicillin-allergic patient, the alternative regimen is trimethoprim-sulfamethoxazole. Cephalosporins are not active against *L monocytogenes*.
- For invasive infections without associated meningitis, treatment for 10 to 14 days usually is satisfactory. For *L monocytogenes* meningitis, most experts recommend 14 to 21 days of treatment. Longer courses are needed for patients who are severely ill or who have endocarditis or rhomboencephalitis.

ISOLATION OF THE HOSPITALIZED PATIENT: Standard precautions are recommended.

CONTROL MEASURES:
- Antimicrobial therapy for infection diagnosed during pregnancy may prevent fetal or perinatal infection and its consequences.
- The incidence of listeriosis has decreased substantially since 1989, when US regulatory agencies began enforcing zero-tolerance guidelines for *L monocytogenes* in ready-to-eat foods.
- The general guidelines for preventing listeriosis are similar to those for preventing other foodborne illnesses (thoroughly cook raw food from animal sources, wash raw vegetables, keep uncooked meats separate from vegetables, avoid unpasteurized dairy products, and wash hands, knives, and cutting boards after exposure to uncooked foods). In addition, people at high risk of complications from listeriosis (pregnant women and immunocompromised people) should follow the dietary recommendations in Table 3.31, p 407.
- Listerosis is a nationally notifiable disease in the United States; cases should be reported to the regional health department to facilitate early recognition and control of common-source outbreaks.

Table 3.31. Dietary Recommendations for People at High Risk of Listeriosis[1]

- Avoid soft cheeses (eg, feta, Brie, Camembert, blue-veined, and Mexican queso fresco cheese). Hard cheeses, processed cheeses, cream cheese, including slices and spreads, cottage cheese, or yogurt need not be avoided

- Cook leftover foods or ready-to-eat foods (eg, hot dogs) until steaming hot before eating

- Avoid foods from delicatessen counters (eg, prepared salads, meats, cheeses) or heat/reheat these foods until steaming before eating

- Avoid refrigerated pâtés and other meat spreads, or heat/reheat these foods until steaming if eaten; canned or shelf-stable pâté and meat spreads need not be avoided

- Avoid raw or unpasteurized milk, including goat's milk, or milk products or foods that contain unpasteurized milk or milk products

[1] High-risk patients are those who are immunocompromised by illness or therapies and pregnant women.

Lyme Disease
(*Borrelia burgdorferi* Infection)

CLINICAL MANIFESTATIONS: The clinical manifestations of Lyme disease are divided into 3 stages: early localized, early disseminated, and late disease. Early localized disease is characterized by a distinctive rash, termed *erythema migrans*, at the site of a recent tick bite. Erythema migrans begins as a red macula or papule that usually expands over days to weeks to form a large, annular, erythematous lesion that is 5 cm or more in diameter (median, 15 cm), sometimes with partial central clearing. Localized erythema migrans can vary greatly in size and shape and may have vesicular or necrotic areas in its center. Fever, malaise, headache, mild neck stiffness, myalgia, and arthralgia often accompany the rash. In untreated people, these associated symptoms may be intermittent and variable over a period of several weeks.

The most common manifestation of early disseminated disease is multiple erythema migrans. This rash usually occurs 3 to 5 weeks after an infective tick bite and consists of secondary annular, erythematous lesions similar to, but usually smaller than, the primary lesion. These lesions reflect spirochetemia with cutaneous dissemination. Other common manifestations of early disseminated illness (that may occur with or without rash) are palsies of the cranial nerves (especially cranial nerve VII), meningitis, and conjunctivitis. Systemic symptoms, such as arthralgia, myalgia, headache, and fatigue, also are common during the early disseminated stage. Carditis, which usually is characterized by various degrees of heart block, occurs rarely in children.

Late disease is characterized most commonly by recurrent arthritis that usually is pauciarticular and affects the large joints, particularly the knees. Arthritis may occur without a history of earlier stages of illness (including erythema migrans). Central nervous system manifestations also may occur very rarely during late disease. Late disease is uncommon in children who are treated with antimicrobial agents in the early stage of the disease.

Because congenital infection occurs with other spirochetal infections, there has been concern that an infected pregnant woman could transmit *Borrelia burgdorferi* to her fetus. No causal relationship between maternal Lyme disease and abnormalities of pregnancy or congenital disease caused by *B burgdorferi* has been documented conclusively. No evidence exists that Lyme disease can be transmitted via human milk.

ETIOLOGY: Infection is caused by the spirochete *B burgdorferi*.

EPIDEMIOLOGY: Lyme disease occurs primarily in 3 distinct geographic regions of the United States. Most cases are reported in the Northeast from southern Maine to northern Virginia. The disease also occurs, but with lower frequency, in the upper Midwest, especially Wisconsin and Minnesota, and less commonly, on the West Coast, especially northern California. The occurrence of cases in the United States correlates with the distribution and frequency of infected tick vectors—*Ixodes scapularis* in the East and Midwest and *Ixodes pacificus* in the West. Reported cases from states without known enzootic risks may have been acquired in endemic states or may be misdiagnoses resulting from false-positive serologic test results. Endemic Lyme disease has been reported in Canada, Europe, states of the former Soviet Union, China, and Japan. Most cases occur between April and October. People of all ages may be affected, but incidence in the United States is highest among children 5 to 9 years of age and adults 45 to 54 years of age.

The **incubation period** from tick bite to appearance of erythema migrans ranges from 3 to 31 days and typically is from 7 to 14 days. Late manifestations occur months to years later.

DIAGNOSTIC TESTS: Diagnosis is best made clinically during the early stages of Lyme disease by recognizing the characteristic rash, erythema migrans. Although cultures of a biopsy specimen of the perimeter of this lesion often yield the organism, *Borrelia* species cultures (which require special media) are not available commercially and are not recommended. Diagnosis in patients who possibly have a later stage Lyme disease is difficult and should be based on clinical findings and serologic tests, preferably performed in a reference laboratory.

Immunoglobulin (Ig) M-specific antibody usually peaks between weeks 3 and 6 after the onset of infection; specific IgG antibody usually increases slowly and generally is highest weeks to months later. Localized erythema migrans typically occurs 1 to 2 weeks after the tick bite; therefore, antibodies against *B burgdorferi* will not be detectable in most patients with erythema migrans. Therefore, routine serologic tests for Lyme disease are not recommended in children with typical symptoms. Some patients who are treated early with antimicrobial agents never develop antibodies against *B burgdorferi*. However, most patients with early disseminated disease and virtually all patients with late disease will have antibodies against *B burgdorferi*. As with other infections, once such antibodies develop, they may persist for many years despite cure of the disease. Consequently, tests for antibodies should not be used to assess the success of treatment. The results of serologic tests for Lyme disease should be interpreted with careful consideration of the clinical setting and the quality of the testing laboratory. Physicians unable to locate high-quality laboratories in their area should contact their state health department for information on reference laboratories.

The enzyme immunoassay (EIA) is the most commonly used test for detection of antibodies against *B burgdorferi*. Enzyme immunoassay and immunofluorescence antibody (IFA) assay may give false-positive results because of cross-reactive antibodies in patients with other spirochetal infections (eg, syphilis, leptospirosis, relapsing fever), certain viral infections (eg, varicella and Epstein-Barr virus), and certain autoimmune diseases (eg, systemic lupus erythematosus). Although antibodies to *B burgdorferi* cross-react with other spirochetes, including *Treponema pallidum*, patients with Lyme disease do not have positive nontreponemal syphilis test results (eg, Venereal Disease Research Laboratories test [VDRL] or rapid plasma reagin [RPR] test). In addition, antibodies directed against spirochetes in normal oral flora may cross-react with antigens of *B burgdorferi* and produce a false-positive test result.

Currently, the Western immunoblot test is most useful for corroborating positive or equivocal EIA or IFA test results, and as a result, a 2-test approach is recommended for serologic diagnosis of *B burgdorferi* infection. Serum specimens that give positive or equivocal results by a sensitive EIA or IFA test should be tested by a standardized Western immunoblot for the presence of antibodies against proteins specific for *B burgdorferi;* serum specimens that give negative results by a sensitive EIA or IFA test do not require immunoblot testing. If a patient with suspected early disease has a negative serologic test result, evidence of infection is best obtained by testing of paired acute- and convalescent-phase serum specimens.

Suspected central nervous system involvement with Lyme disease can be confirmed by demonstration of intrathecal production of antibodies against *B burgdorferi*. However, interpretation of antibody tests of cerebrospinal fluid is complex, and physicians should seek the advice of a specialist experienced in the management of patients with Lyme disease to assist in interpreting results.

The widespread practice of ordering serologic tests for patients with nonspecific symptoms such as fatigue or arthralgia who have a low probability of having Lyme disease is not recommended. Almost all positive serologic test results in these patients are false-positive results. Patients with acute Lyme disease almost always have objective signs of infection (eg, erythema migrans, facial nerve palsy, arthritis). Nonspecific symptoms commonly accompany these specific signs but are almost never the only evidence of Lyme disease.

New, more sensitive and more specific diagnostic tests, such as the polymerase chain reaction assay, which may be able to identify the presence of even small quantities of spirochetal DNA, are in development. However, physicians should be cautious when interpreting results of these investigational tests until their clinical usefulness has been proven.

Recipients of the recombinant outer surface protein A (OspA) vaccine have a positive EIA test result, because whole-cell *B burgdorferi* is used as the antigen. The Western immunoblot can identify non-OspA antibodies, and antibody to OspA is not one of the criteria for a positive immunoblot result. Therefore, immunoblot testing for non-OspA antibody reactivity is essential for establishing or excluding the diagnosis of Lyme disease in people who may have received recombinant OspA vaccine.

TREATMENT: See Table 3.32, p 411.

Early Localized Disease. Doxycycline is the drug of choice for children 8 years of age and older. For children younger than 8 years of age, amoxicillin is recommended. For patients who are allergic to penicillin, alternative drugs are cefuroxime axetil and erythromycin, although erythromycin may be less effective. Most experts treat people with early Lyme disease for 14 to 21 days, but data are limited about the optimal duration of treatment.

Treatment of erythema migrans almost always prevents development of later stages of Lyme disease. Clinical response to therapy often is slow, and signs and symptoms may persist for several weeks, even in successfully treated patients, although erythema migrans usually resolves within several days of initiating treatment.

Early Disseminated and Late Disease. Orally administered antimicrobial agents are recommended for treating multiple erythema migrans and uncomplicated Lyme arthritis. Most experts also recommend oral agents for treatment of facial nerve palsy to prevent further sequelae. Some experts recommend a lumbar puncture if central nervous system involvement is suspected. If cerebrospinal fluid pleocytosis is found, parenterally administered antimicrobial therapy is indicated. Recurrent or persistent arthritis and central nervous system infection should be treated with parenterally administered antimicrobial agents. Carditis usually should be treated with parenteral therapy, although some experts treat mild carditis orally with doxycycline or amoxicillin. The optimal duration of therapy for manifestations of early disseminated or late disease is not well established, but there is no evidence that children with any manifestation of Lyme disease benefit from prolonged courses of orally or parenterally administered antimicrobial agents. Accordingly, the maximum duration of a single course of therapy is 4 weeks.

The Jarisch-Herxheimer reaction (an acute febrile reaction accompanied by headache, myalgia, and an aggravated clinical picture lasting less than 24 hours) can occur transiently when therapy is initiated. Nonsteroidal anti-inflammatory agents may be beneficial, and the antimicrobial agent should be continued.

Pregnancy. Tetracyclines are contraindicated. Otherwise, therapy is the same as recommended for nonpregnant people.

ISOLATION OF THE HOSPITALIZED PATIENT: Standard precautions are recommended.

CONTROL MEASURES:

Ticks. See Prevention of Tickborne Infections, p 186.

Chemoprophylaxis. Many people who seek medical attention for a tick bite have been bitten by a tick that does not transmit Lyme disease. The risk of infection with *B burgdorferi* after a recognized deer tick bite, even in highly endemic areas, is sufficiently low that prophylactic antimicrobial treatment is not indicated routinely for most people. Animal studies indicate that transmission of *B burgdorferi* from infected ticks usually requires a prolonged duration (≥36 hours) of attachment. Analysis of ticks to determine whether they are infected is not indicated, because the predictive values of such tests for human disease are unknown. Although a

Table 3.32. Recommended Treatment of Lyme Disease in Children

Disease Category	Drug(s) and Dose[1]
Early localized disease[1]	
8 y of age or older	Doxycycline, 100 mg, orally, twice a day for 14–21 days
All ages	Amoxicillin, 25–50 mg/kg per day, orally, divided into 2 doses (maximum 2 g/day) for 14–21 days
Early disseminated and late disease	
Multiple erythema migrans	Same oral regimen as for early disease but for 21 days
Isolated facial palsy	Same oral regimen as for early disease but for 21–28 days[2,3]
Arthritis	Same oral regimen as for early disease but for 28 days
Persistent or recurrent arthritis[4]	Ceftriaxone sodium, 75–100 mg/kg, IV or IM, once a day (maximum 2 g/day), for 14–21 days; or penicillin, 300 000 U/kg per day, IV, given in divided doses every 4 h (maximum 20 million U/day) for 14–28 days OR same oral regimen as for early disease
Carditis	Ceftriaxone or penicillin: see persistent or recurrent arthritis
Meningitis or encephalitis	Ceftriaxone or penicillin: see persistent or recurrent arthritis, but for 30–60 days

IV indicates intravenously; IM, intramuscularly.

[1] For patients who are allergic to penicillin, cefuroxime axetil and erythromycin are alternative drugs.
[2] Corticosteroids should not be given.
[3] Treatment has no effect on the resolution of facial nerve palsy; its purpose is to prevent late disease.
[4] Arthritis is not considered persistent or recurrent unless objective evidence of synovitis exists at least 2 months after treatment is initiated. Some experts administer a second course of an oral agent before using an IV-administered antimicrobial agent.

single dose of 200 mg of doxycycline is effective in preventing erythema migrans after a deer tick attachment >72 hours for adults who live in hyperendemic areas, this regimen may be associated with more frequent adverse effects and is not recommended. Amoxicillin is not proven to be effective for prophylaxis.

Blood Donation. Patients with active disease should not donate blood, because spirochetemia occurs in early Lyme disease. Patients who have been treated for Lyme disease can be considered for blood donation.

Vaccines. * A Lyme disease vaccine was licensed by the US Food and Drug Administration (FDA) on December 21, 1998, for people 15 to 70 years of age but subsequently was withdrawn in early 2002 because of low market demand and no longer is available.

---

* American Academy of Pediatrics, Committee on Infectious Diseases. Prevention of Lyme disease. *Pediatrics.* 2000;105:142–147

Lymphatic Filariasis
(Bancroftian, Malayan, and Timorian)

CLINICAL MANIFESTATIONS: Most filarial infections are asymptomatic. Early in infection, symptoms often are caused by an acute inflammatory response in the lymphatic vessels, triggered by death of adult worms. Headache, myalgia, and lymphadenitis can develop with acute inflammation. The acute disease may manifest as early as 3 months after acquisition. However, initial damage to the lymphatic system generally remains subclinical for years. Over time, moderate lymphadenopathy occurs, particularly involving the inguinal lymph nodes. Inflammation secondary to adult worm death in the lymphatics of the extremities and genitalia leads to adenolymphangitis that characteristically is retrograde. Epididymitis, orchitis, and funiculitis also can occur in bancroftian filariasis and may be accompanied by fever, chills, and other nonspecific systemic symptoms. Lymphatic dysfunction, with resulting chronically progressive edema of the limbs and genitalia, is rare in children. In a few people, elephantiasis can result from fibrosis caused by chronic dysfunction of the lymphatic channels and recurrent secondary bacterial infections. Chyluria can occur as a manifestation of bancroftian filariasis. Cough, fever, marked eosinophilia, and high serum immunoglobulin E concentrations are the manifestations of the tropical pulmonary eosinophilia syndrome.

ETIOLOGY: Filariasis is caused by the following 3 filarial nematodes: *Wuchereria bancrofti, Brugia malayi,* and *Brugia timori.*

EPIDEMIOLOGY: The parasite is transmitted by the bite of infected species of various genera of mosquitoes, including *Culex, Aedes, Anopheles,* and *Mansonia. Wuchereria bancrofti* is found in Haiti, the Dominican Republic, Guiana, Brazil, sub-Saharan and North Africa, and Asia, extending into a broad zone from India through the Indonesian archipelago into Southern China and Oceania. Humans are the only definitive host for the parasite. *Brugia malayi* is found mostly in India and Southeast Asia. *Brugia timori* is restricted to certain islands at the eastern end of the Indonesian archipelago. Because the adult worms are long-lived (5–8 years on average) and reinfection is common, microfilariae infective for mosquitoes may remain in the patient's blood for decades; individual microfilaria have a life span up to 1.5 years. The adult worm is not transmissible from person to person or by blood transfusion, but microfilariae may be transmitted by transfusion.

The **incubation period** is not well established; the period from acquisition to the appearance of microfilariae in blood can be 3 to 12 months, depending on the species of parasite.

DIAGNOSTIC TESTS: Microfilariae can be detected microscopically on blood smears obtained at night (10 PM– 4 AM). Adult worms or microfilariae can be identified in tissue specimens obtained at biopsy. Serologic enzyme immunoassay tests are available, but interpretation of results is affected by cross-reactions of filarial antibodies with antibodies against other helminths. Assays for circulating parasite antigen of *W bancrofti* are available commercially but are not FDA licensed. Lymphatic filariasis often must be diagnosed clinically, because dependable serologic assays are not uniformly available, and in patients with elephantiasis, the microfilariae may no longer be present.

TREATMENT: Diethylcarbamazine citrate (DEC) is the drug of choice for lymphatic filariasis (see Drugs for Parasitic Infections, p 744). The late phase of chronic disease is not affected by chemotherapy. Ivermectin is effective against the microfilariae of *W bancrofti* but has no effect on the adult parasite. Combination therapy with single-dose DEC-albendazole or ivermectin-albendazole has been shown to be more effective than any one drug alone in suppressing microfilaremia.

Complex decongestive physiotherapy may be effective for treating elephantiasis. Chyluria originating in the bladder responds to fulguration; chyluria originating in the kidney usually cannot be corrected. Prompt identification and treatment of superinfections, particularly streptococcal and staphylococcal infections, and careful treatment of intertriginous and ungual infections are important aspects of therapy.

ISOLATION OF THE HOSPITALIZED PATIENT: Standard precautions are recommended.

CONTROL MEASURES: Control measures have been instituted based on annual community-wide single-dose DEC (or combinations of DEC and ivermectin or albendazole and ivermectin) to decrease transmission in high-risk areas.

Lymphocytic Choriomeningitis

CLINICAL MANIFESTATIONS: Postnatal infection is asymptomatic in approximately one third of cases. Symptomatic infection may result in a mild to severe influenza-like illness, which includes fever, malaise, myalgia, retro-orbital headache, photophobia, anorexia, and nausea. Fever usually lasts 1 to 3 weeks, and rash is rare. A biphasic febrile course is common. Up to half of symptomatic patients will develop neurologic manifestations varying from aseptic meningitis to severe encephalitis. Arthralgia or arthritis, respiratory tract symptoms, orchitis, and leukopenia occasionally develop. Recovery without sequelae is the usual outcome. Infection during pregnancy has been associated with abortion. Congenital infection may cause hydrocephalus, chorioretinitis, intracranial calcifications, microcephaly, and mental retardation. Congenital lymphocytic choriomeningitis may be difficult to differentiate from congenital infection attributable to cytomegalovirus (CMV), toxoplasmosis, or rubella.

ETIOLOGY: Lymphocytic choriomeningitis virus is an arenavirus.

EPIDEMIOLOGY: Lymphocytic choriomeningitis is a chronic infection of the common house mouse and pet hamsters, which often are infected asymptomatically and chronically shed virus in urine and other excretions. In addition, laboratory mice and colonized golden hamsters can be chronically infected and can be sources of human infection. Humans are infected by aerosol or by ingestion of dust or food contaminated with the virus from the urine, feces, blood, or nasopharyngeal secretions of infected rodents. The disease is most prevalent in young adults. Human-to-human spread, other than transplacental passage of the virus, has not been reported.

The **incubation period** usually is 6 to 13 days and occasionally as long as 3 weeks.

DIAGNOSTIC TESTS: In patients with central nervous system disease, mononuclear pleocytosis occasionally exceeding several thousand cells is present in the cerebrospinal fluid (CSF). Hypoglycorrhachia also can occur. Lymphocytic choriomeningitis virus can be isolated from blood, CSF, urine, and rarely, nasopharyngeal secretion specimens. Acute and convalescent serum specimens can be tested for increases in antibody titers by immunofluorescence or enzyme immunoassay demonstration of virus-specific immunoglobulin M antibodies in serum or CSF specimens is useful. Infection of mice trapped in or around houses may be identified by demonstrating serum antibody or viral antigen in liver impression smears.

TREATMENT: Supportive.

ISOLATION OF THE HOSPITALIZED PATIENT: Standard precautions are recommended.

CONTROL MEASURES: Infection can be controlled by preventing rodent infestation in animal and food storage areas. Because the virus is excreted for long periods of time by rodent hosts, attempts should be made to monitor laboratory and wholesale colonies of mice and hamsters for infection. Pet rodents or wild mice in a patient's home should be considered likely sources of infection. Pregnant women should avoid exposure to rodents and their aerosolized excreta.

Malaria

CLINICAL MANIFESTATIONS: The classic symptoms of malaria are high fever with chills, rigor, sweats, and headache, which may be paroxysmal. If appropriate treatment is not administered, fever and paroxysms may occur in a cyclic pattern. Depending on the infecting species, fever appears every other or every third day. Other manifestations can include nausea, vomiting, diarrhea, cough, arthralgia, and abdominal and back pain. Anemia and thrombocytopenia are common, and pallor and jaundice caused by hemolysis may occur. Hepatosplenomegaly may be present.

Infection by *Plasmodium falciparum* potentially is fatal and most commonly manifests as a febrile nonspecific influenza-like illness without localizing signs. With more severe disease, however, *P falciparum* infection may manifest as one of the following clinical syndromes:

- *Cerebral malaria,* which may have variable neurologic manifestations, including seizures, signs of increased intracranial pressure, confusion, and progression to stupor, coma, and death
- *Hypoglycemia,* sometimes associated with quinine treatment, requiring urgent correction

- *Noncardiogenic pulmonary edema,* which is difficult to manage and may be fatal (rare in children)
- *Renal failure* caused by acute tubular necrosis (rare in children younger than 8 years of age)
- *Respiratory failure and metabolic acidosis,* without pulmonary edema
- *Severe anemia* attributable to high parasitemia and consequent hemolysis
- *Vascular collapse and shock* associated with hypothermia and adrenal insufficiency

Individuals with asplenia who become infected are at high risk of death.

Syndromes primarily associated with *Plasmodium vivax* and *Plasmodium ovale* infection are as follows:

- *Anemia* attributable to acute parasitemia
- *Hypersplenism* with danger of late splenic rupture
- *Relapse,* for as long as 3 to 5 years after the primary infection, attributable to latent hepatic stages

Syndromes associated with *Plasmodium malariae* infection include:

- *Chronic asymptomatic parasitemia* for as long as several years after the last exposure
- *Nephrotic syndrome* from deposition of immune complexes in the kidney

Congenital malaria secondary to perinatal transmission rarely may occur. Most congenital cases have been caused by *P vivax* and *P falciparum; P malariae* and *P ovale* account for fewer than 20% of such cases. Manifestations can resemble those of neonatal sepsis, including fever and nonspecific symptoms of poor appetite, irritability, and lethargy.

ETIOLOGY: The genus *Plasmodium* includes species of intraerythrocytic parasites that infect a wide range of mammals, birds, and reptiles. The 4 species that infect humans are *P falciparum, P vivax, P ovale,* and *P malariae.*

EPIDEMIOLOGY: Malaria is endemic throughout the tropical areas of the world and is acquired from the bite of the female nocturnal-feeding *Anopheles* species of mosquito. One half of the world's population lives in areas where transmission occurs. Worldwide, there are 300 to 500 million cases annually and 1.5 to 2.7 million deaths. Most deaths occur in young children. Malarial infection poses substantial risks to pregnant women and their fetuses and may result in spontaneous abortion and stillbirth. The risk of malaria is highest for travelers to sub-Saharan Africa, Papua New Guinea, the Solomon Islands, and Vanuatu; the risk is intermediate in Haiti and the Indian subcontinent and is low in most of Southeast Asia and Latin America. Transmission is possible in more temperate climates, including areas in the United States where *Anopheles* species mosquitoes are present. Mosquitoes in airplanes flying from tropical climates have been the source of occasional cases in people working or residing near international airports. However, nearly all of the approximately 1200 annual reported cases in the United States result from infection acquired abroad. Other less common modes of malaria transmission are congenital, through transfusions, or through the use of contaminated needles or syringes.

Plasmodium vivax and *P falciparum* are the most common species worldwide. *Plasmodium vivax* malaria is prevalent on the Indian subcontinent and in Central America. *Plasmodium falciparum* malaria is prevalent in Africa, Haiti, and Papua New Guinea. Malaria attributable to *P vivax* and *P falciparum* is common in southern and Southeast Asia, Oceania, and South America. *Plasmodium malariae*, although much less common, has a wide distribution. *Plasmodium ovale* malaria occurs most often in West Africa but has been reported in other areas.

Relapses may occur in *P vivax* and *P ovale* malaria because of a persistent hepatic (hypnozoite) stage of infection. Recrudescence of *P falciparum* and *P malariae* infection occurs when a persistent low-concentration parasitemia causes recurrence of symptoms of the disease. In hyperendemic areas of Africa and Asia, reinfection in people with partial immunity results in a high prevalence of asymptomatic parasitemia.

The spread of chloroquine-resistant *P falciparum* strains throughout the world is of increasing importance. Resistance to other antimalarial drugs is now occurring in many areas where the drugs are used widely. Chloroquine-resistant *P vivax* has been reported in Indonesia, Papua New Guinea, Solomon Islands, Myanmar, India, and Guyana.

DIAGNOSTIC TESTS: Definitive diagnosis relies on identification of the parasite on stained blood films. Both thick and thin blood films should be examined. The thick film allows for concentration of the blood to find parasites that may be present in small numbers, whereas the thin film is most useful for species identification and determination of the degree of parasitemia (the percentage of erythrocytes harboring parasites). If initial blood smears test negative for *Plasmodium* species but malaria remains a possibility, the smear should be repeated every 12 to 24 hours during a 72-hour period.

In hyperendemic areas, the presence of malaria on a blood smear is not conclusive evidence of malaria as a cause of the manifesting illness, because other infections often are superimposed on low-concentration parasitemia in children with partial immunity.

Confirmation and identification of the species of malaria parasites on the blood smear is important in guiding therapy. Serologic testing generally is not helpful, except in epidemiologic surveys. New diagnostic tests in development, including those using polymerase chain reaction assay, DNA probes, and malarial ribosomal RNA testing, may provide rapid and accurate diagnosis in the future.

TREATMENT: The choice of malaria chemotherapy is based on the infecting species, possible drug resistance, and the severity of disease (see Drugs for Parasitic Infections, p 744). Severe malaria is defined as a parasitemia greater than 5% of red blood cells, signs of central nervous system or other end-organ involvement, shock, acidosis, and/or hypoglycemia. Patients with severe malaria require intensive care and parenteral treatment until the parasite density decreases to less than 1% and they are able to tolerate oral therapy. Exchange transfusion may be warranted when parasitemia exceeds 10% or if there is evidence of complications (eg, cerebral malaria) at lower parasite densities. Other adjunctive therapies, such as iron chelation, are under investigation but are not recommended. For patients with *P falciparum* malaria, sequential blood smears for percent parasitemia are indicated to monitor treatment. New antimalarial drugs are undergoing clinical trials for treatment and chemoprophylaxis of malaria.

ISOLATION OF THE HOSPITALIZED PATIENT: Standard precautions are recommended.

CONTROL MEASURES: Control of the *Anopheles* species mosquito population, treatment of infected people, and chemoprophylaxis of travelers in endemic areas are effective. Measures to prevent contact with mosquitoes, especially from dusk to dawn (because of the nocturnal biting habits of the female *Anopheles* mosquito), through use of bed nets impregnated with insecticide, mosquito repellents containing diethyltoluamide (DEET), and protective clothing also are beneficial and should be optimized. The most current information on country-specific risks, drug resistance, and resulting recommendations for travelers can be obtained by contacting the Centers for Disease Control and Prevention (CDC) Malaria Hotline (770-488-7788).

Chemoprophylaxis for Travelers to Endemic Areas. * The appropriate chemoprophylactic regimen is determined by the traveler's risk of acquiring malaria in the area(s) to be visited and by the risk of exposure to chloroquine-resistant *P falciparum*. Indications for prophylaxis for children are identical to those for adults.

Chemoprophylaxis should begin 1 week before arrival in the endemic area (except doxycycline and atovaquone-proguanil, which should be started 1–2 days before arrival), allowing time for development of adequate blood concentration of the drug and evaluation of any adverse reactions.

Travelers to areas where chloroquine-resistant malaria species have not been reported should take chloroquine, once weekly, starting 1 week before exposure for the duration of exposure and for 4 weeks after departure from the endemic area.

Travelers to areas where chloroquine-resistant *P falciparum* exists should take mefloquine hydrochloride, doxycycline, or atovaquone-proguanil.

- Mefloquine is taken once weekly, starting 1 week before travel, continuing weekly during travel, and for 4 weeks after travel has concluded (see Drugs for Parasitic Infections, p 744). Mefloquine is not licensed by the US Food and Drug Administration (FDA) for children who weigh less than 5 kg or are younger than 6 months of age. However, recent recommendations of the World Health Organization and the CDC suggest that mefloquine be considered for use in children, regardless of weight or age restrictions, when travel to areas of chloroquine-resistant *P falciparum* cannot be avoided. Mefloquine is contraindicated for use by travelers with a known hypersensitivity to mefloquine or people with depression or history of psychosis or convulsions. Although a warning about concurrent use with β-blockers is given in the product labeling, a review of available data suggests that mefloquine may be used by people concurrently receiving β-blockers if they have no underlying arrhythmia. Mefloquine is not recommended for use by people with cardiac conduction abnormalities. Caution should be advised for travelers

---

* For further information on prevention of malaria in travelers, see the annual publication of the US Public Health Service, *Health Information for International Travel*, 2001–2002. Atlanta, GA: US Dept of Health and Human Services, Public Health Service, Centers for Disease Control and Prevention, National Center for Infectious Diseases, Division of Quarantine; 2001 or visit the CDC Web site (www.cdc.gov/travel/malinfo.htm).

involved in tasks requiring fine motor coordination and spatial discrimination. Patients in whom mefloquine prophylaxis fails should be monitored closely if they are treated with quinidine or quinine sulfate, because either drug may exacerbate the known adverse effects of mefloquine.

- Doxycycline is taken daily, starting 1 to 2 days before exposure, for the duration of exposure and for 4 weeks after departure from the endemic area. Travelers taking doxycycline should be advised of the need for strict compliance with daily dosing, the advisability of always taking the drug on a full stomach, and the possible adverse effects, including diarrhea, photosensitivity, and increased risk of monilial vaginitis. Use of doxycycline should be avoided for pregnant women and for children younger than 8 years of age because of the risk of dental staining (see Antimicrobial Agents and Related Therapy, p 693).

- Atovaquone-proguanil is licensed for prevention and treatment of chloroquine-resistant *P falciparum* malaria. Atovaquone-proguanil is taken daily, starting 1 day before exposure and continuing for the duration of exposure and for 1 week after departure from the endemic area. A pediatric formulation is available in the United States but is not licensed for use in children weighing less than 11 kg. Atovaquone-proguanil is contraindicated for pregnant women.

Children who cannot take mefloquine or doxycycline can be given atovaquone-proguanil. Children should avoid travel to areas with chloroquine-resistant *P falciparum* unless they can take a highly effective drug, such as mefloquine, doxycycline, or atovaquone-proguanil.

Prophylaxis During Pregnancy. Malaria infection in pregnant women may be more severe than in nonpregnant women. Malaria may increase the risk of adverse outcomes in pregnancy, including prematurity, abortion, and stillbirth. For these reasons and because no chemoprophylactic regimen is completely effective, women who are pregnant or likely to become pregnant should try to avoid travel to areas where they could contract malaria. Women traveling to areas where drug-resistant *P falciparum* has not been reported may take chloroquine prophylaxis. Harmful effects on the fetus have not been demonstrated when chloroquine is given in the recommended doses for malaria prophylaxis. Pregnancy, therefore, is not a contraindication for malaria prophylaxis with chloroquine.

Mefloquine, according to the product labeling, is not recommended for use during pregnancy. However, a review of data from clinical trials and reports of inadvertent use of mefloquine during pregnancy suggest that its use is not associated with adverse fetal or pregnancy outcomes, such as birth defects, stillbirths, and spontaneous abortions, when taken in prophylactic doses throughout pregnancy. Consequently, mefloquine is the drug of choice for prophylactic use for women who are pregnant or likely to become pregnant when exposure to chloroquine-resistant *P falciparum* is unavoidable.

The combination of chloroquine plus azithromycin dihydrate, which is safe for use during pregnancy, can be used by travelers unable to take mefloquine, doxycycline, or atovaquone-proguanil. However, these agents are less effective than standard therapy for chloroquine-resistant malaria. Consideration should be given for travelers to carry atovaquone-proguanil or sulfadoxine-pyrimethamine (Fansidar, Roche Pharmaceuticals, Nutley, NJ) for use as presumptive self-treatment if a febrile illness develops while taking chemoprophylaxis with recognized decreased effectiveness. Resistance to sulfadoxine-pyrimethamine has been reported from Southeast Asia and the Amazon Basin, and therefore, it should not be used for treatment of malaria acquired in these areas. The CDC also lists several countries in East Africa with malaria resistant to sulfadoxine-pyrimethamine (Kenya, Uganda, Malawi, South Africa, Mozambique, Tanzania) on its Web site (www.cdc.gov/travel). Travelers should be advised that self-treatment is not considered a replacement for seeking prompt medical help. Sulfadoxine-pyrimethamine should not be taken for routine prophylaxis or by patients with known intolerance to either drug or to other sulfonamide drugs or by infants younger than 2 months of age or pregnant women at term, unless circumstances suggest the potential benefit outweighs the possible risk of hyperbilirubinemia in the infant.

Travelers should be advised that any fever or influenza-like illness that develops within 3 months of departure from a malaria-endemic area requires immediate medical evaluation, including blood films to rule out malaria.

Prevention of Relapses. To prevent relapses of *P vivax* or *P ovale* infection after departure from areas where these species are endemic, use of primaquine phosphate should be considered. Primaquine can cause hemolysis in patients with glucose-6-phosphate dehydrogenase deficiency; thus, all patients should be screened for this condition before primaquine therapy is initiated.

Personal Protective Measures. All travelers to areas where malaria is endemic should be advised to use personal protective measures, including the following: (1) using insecticide-impregnated mosquito nets while sleeping; (2) remaining in well-screened areas; (3) wearing protective clothing; and (4) using mosquito repellents containing DEET. To be effective, most of these repellents require frequent reapplications. Because adverse reactions, including toxic encephalopathy, seizures, and rashes have been reported with the use of high concentrations of DEET in children, DEET should be used according to the product label. Travelers, particularly children, should be advised against using products containing high concentrations of DEET (>35%) directly on skin. The risk of serious adverse effects is exceedingly low when used according to FDA-approved product label instructions.

Measles

CLINICAL MANIFESTATIONS: Measles is an acute disease characterized by fever, cough, coryza, conjunctivitis, an erythematous maculopapular rash, and pathognomonic enanthemas (Koplik spots). Complications such as otitis media, bronchopneumonia, laryngotracheobronchitis (croup), and diarrhea occur commonly in young children. Acute encephalitis, which often results in permanent brain damage, occurs in approximately 1 of every 1000 cases. Death, predominantly resulting from respiratory and neurologic complications, occurs in 1 to 3 of every 1000 cases reported in the United States. Case fatality rates are increased in children younger than 5 years of age and immunocompromised children, including children with leukemia, human immunodeficiency virus (HIV) infection, and severe malnutrition. Sometimes the characteristic rash does not develop in immunocompromised patients.

Subacute sclerosing panencephalitis (SSPE), a rare degenerative central nervous system disease characterized by behavioral and intellectual deterioration and seizures that develop years after the original infection, is a result of a persistent measles virus infection. Widespread measles immunization has led to the virtual disappearance of SSPE in the United States.

ETIOLOGY: Measles virus is an RNA virus with 1 serotype, classified as a member of the genus *Morbillivirus* in the Paramyxoviridae family.

EPIDEMIOLOGY: The only natural hosts of measles virus are humans. Measles is transmitted by direct contact with infectious droplets or, less commonly, by airborne spread. In temperate areas, the peak incidence of infection usually occurs during late winter and spring. In the prevaccine era, most cases of measles in the United States occurred in preschool and young school-aged children, and few people remained susceptible by age 20 years. The childhood and adolescent immunization program in the United States has resulted in a greater than 99% decrease in the reported incidence of measles since measles vaccine was first licensed in 1963.

From 1989 to 1991, the incidence of measles in the United States increased because of low immunization rates in preschool-aged children, especially in urban areas. Since 1992, the incidence of measles in the United States has been low (<1000 reported cases per year), and indigenous cases are uncommon. Cases of measles continue to occur from importation of the virus from other countries. Cases are considered imported from another country if the rash onset occurs within 18 days after entering the United States and illness cannot be linked to local transmission.

Vaccine failure occurs in as many as 5% of people who have received a single dose of vaccine at 12 months of age or older. Although waning immunity after immunization may be a factor in some cases, most cases of measles in previously immunized children seem to occur in people in whom response to the vaccine was inadequate (ie, primary vaccine failures).

Patients are contagious from 1 to 2 days before onset of symptoms (3–5 days before the rash) to 4 days after appearance of the rash. Immunocompromised patients who may have prolonged excretion of the virus in respiratory tract secretions can be contagious for the duration of the illness. Patients with SSPE are not contagious.

The **incubation period** generally is 8 to 12 days from exposure to onset of symptoms. In family studies, the average interval between appearance of rash in the source case and subsequent cases is 14 days, with a range of 7 to 18 days. In SSPE, the mean incubation period of 84 cases reported between 1976 and 1983 was 10.8 years.

DIAGNOSTIC TESTS: Measles virus infection can be diagnosed by a positive serologic test result for measles immunoglobulin (Ig) M antibody, a significant increase in measles IgG antibody concentration in paired acute and convalescent serum specimens by any standard serologic assay, or isolation of measles virus from clinical specimens, such as urine, blood, or nasopharyngeal secretions. The state public health laboratory or the Centers for Disease Control and Prevention Measles Laboratory will process these viral specimens. The simplest method of establishing the diagnosis of measles is testing for IgM antibody on a single serum specimen obtained during the first encounter with a person suspected of having disease. The sensitivity of measles IgM assays varies and may be diminished during the first 72 hours after rash onset. If the result is negative for measles IgM and the patient has a generalized rash lasting more than 72 hours, the measles IgM test should be repeated. Measles IgM is detectable for at least 1 month after rash onset. People with febrile rash illness who are seronegative for measles IgM should be tested for rubella using the same specimens. Genotyping of viral isolates allows determination of patterns of importation and transmission. All cases of suspected measles should be reported immediately to the local or state health department, without waiting for the results of diagnostic tests.

TREATMENT: No specific antiviral therapy is available. Measles virus is susceptible in vitro to ribavirin, which has been given by the intravenous and aerosol routes to treat severely affected and immunocompromised children with measles. However, no controlled trials have been conducted, and ribavirin is not licensed by the US Food and Drug Administration for treatment of measles.

Vitamin A. The World Health Organization and the United Nations International Children's Emergency Fund recommend administration of vitamin A to all children diagnosed with measles in communities where vitamin A deficiency is a recognized problem or where the measles case fatality rate is 1% or greater. Vitamin A treatment of children with measles in developing countries has been associated with decreased morbidity and mortality rates. Although vitamin A deficiency is not recognized as a major problem in the United States, low serum concentrations of vitamin A have been found in children with severe measles. Hence, vitamin A supplementation should be considered in the following patients:

- Children 6 months to 2 years of age hospitalized with measles and its complications (eg, croup, pneumonia, and diarrhea). Limited data are available about the safety and need for vitamin A supplementation for infants younger than 6 months of age.
- Children older than 6 months of age with measles who are not already receiving vitamin A supplementation and who have any of the following risk factors: immunodeficiency, clinical evidence of vitamin A deficiency, impaired intestinal absorption, moderate to severe malnutrition, and recent immigration from areas where high mortality rates attributable to measles have been observed.

Parenteral and oral formulations of vitamin A are available in the United States. The recommended dosage, administered as a capsule, is:

- Single dose of 200 000 IU, orally, for children 1 year of age and older (100 000 IU for children 6 months–1 year of age).
- The dose should be repeated the next day and again 4 weeks later for children with ophthalmologic evidence of vitamin A deficiency.

ISOLATION OF THE HOSPITALIZED PATIENT: In addition to standard precautions, airborne transmission precautions are indicated for 4 days after the onset of the rash in otherwise healthy children and for the duration of illness in immunocompromised patients.

CONTROL MEASURES:

Care of Exposed People.

Use of Vaccine. Exposure to measles is not a contraindication to immunization. Available data suggest that live-virus measles vaccine, if given within 72 hours of measles exposure, will provide protection in some cases. If the exposure does not result in infection, the vaccine should induce protection against subsequent measles exposures. Immunization is the intervention of choice for control of measles outbreaks in schools and child care centers.

Use of Immune Globulin. Immune Globulin (IG) can be given to prevent or modify measles in a susceptible person within 6 days of exposure. The usual recommended dose is 0.25 mL/kg given intramuscularly; immunocompromised children should receive 0.5 mL/kg (the maximum dose in either instance is 15 mL). Immune Globulin is indicated for susceptible household contacts of patients with measles, particularly contacts younger than 1 year of age, pregnant women, and immunocompromised people for whom the risk of complications is highest. Immune Globulin is not indicated for household contacts who have received 1 dose of vaccine at 12 months of age or older unless they are immunocompromised.

Immune Globulin Intravenous (IGIV) preparations generally contain measles antibodies at approximately the same concentration per gram of protein as IG, although the concentration may vary by lot and manufacturer. For patients who regularly receive IGIV, the usual dose of 100 to 400 mg/kg should be adequate for measles prophylaxis after exposures occurring within 3 weeks of receiving IGIV.

For children who receive IG for modification or prevention of measles after exposure, measles vaccine (if not contraindicated) should be given 5 months (if the dose was 0.25 mL/kg) or 6 months (if the dose was 0.5 mL/kg) after IG administration, provided that the child is at least 12 months of age. Longer intervals are required after larger doses of IGIV (see Table 3.33, p 423).

HIV Infection. * All children and adolescents with HIV infection and children of unknown infection status born to HIV-infected women who are exposed to wild-type measles should receive IG prophylaxis (0.5 mL/kg, IM, maximum dose 15 mL), regardless of their immunization status (see Human Immunodeficiency Virus Infection, p 360). An exception is the patient receiving IGIV (400 mg/kg) at regular intervals whose last dose was received within 3 weeks of exposure. Because of the rapid metabolism of IGIV, some experts recommend administration of an additional dose of IGIV if exposure to measles occurs 2 or more weeks after the last regular dose of IGIV.

Hospital Personnel. To decrease nosocomial infection, immunization programs should be established to ensure that health care professionals who may be in contact with patients with measles are immune to the disease (see Health Care Personnel, p 90).

Measles Vaccine. The only measles vaccine currently licensed in the United States is a live further-attenuated strain prepared in chicken embryo cell culture. Measles vaccines provided through the Expanded Programme on Immunization

---

* American Academy of Pediatrics, Committee on Infectious Diseases and Committee on Pediatric AIDS. Measles immunization in HIV-infected children. *Pediatrics.* 1999;103:1057–1060

Table 3.33. Suggested Intervals Between Immune Globulin Administration and Measles Immunization (MMR or Monovalent Measles Vaccine)

Indication for Immunoglobulin	Route	Dose		Interval, mo[1]
		U or mL	mg IgG/kg	
Tetanus (as TIG)	IM	250 U	approx 10	3
Hepatitis A prophylaxis (as IG)				
Contact prophylaxis	IM	0.02 mL/kg	3.3	3
International travel	IM	0.06 mL/kg	10	3
Hepatitis B prophylaxis (as HBIG)	IM	0.06 mL/kg	10	3
Rabies prophylaxis (as RIG)	IM	20 IU/kg	22	4
Measles prophylaxis (as IG)				
Standard	IM	0.25 mL/kg	40	5
Immunocompromised host	IM	0.50 mL/kg	80	6
Varicella prophylaxis (as VZIG)	IM	125 U/10 kg (maximum 625 U)	20–39	5
RSV prophylaxis (palivizumab monoclonal antibody)	IM	...	15 mg/kg	None
Blood transfusion				
Washed RBCs	IV	10 mL/kg	Negligible	0
RBCs, adenine-saline added	IV	10 mL/kg	10	3
Packed RBCs	IV	10 mL/kg	20–60	5
Whole blood	IV	10 mL/kg	80–100	6
Plasma or platelet products	IV	10 mL/kg	160	7
Replacement (or therapy) of immune deficiencies (as IGIV)	IV	...	300–400	8
ITP (as IGIV)	IV	...	400	8
RSV-IGIV	IV	...	750	9
ITP	IV	...	1000	10
ITP or Kawasaki syndrome	IV	...	1600–2000	11

MMR indicates measles-mumps-rubella; IgG, immunoglobulin G; TIG, Tetanus Immune Globulin; IG, Immune Globulin; IM, intramuscular; HBIG, Hepatitis B IG; RIG, Rabies IG; VZIG, Varicella-Zoster IG; RBCs, Red Blood Cells; IV, intravenous; IGIV, IG intravenous; ITP, immune (formerly termed "idiopathic") thrombocytopenic purpura; RSV-IGIV, Respiratory Syncytial Virus IGIV.

[1] These intervals should provide sufficient time for decreases in passive antibodies in all children to allow for an adequate response to measles vaccine. Physicians should not assume that children are fully protected against measles during these intervals. Additional doses of IG or measles vaccine may be indicated after exposure to measles (see text).

in developing countries meet the World Health Organization standards and usually are comparable to the vaccine available in the United States. Measles vaccine is available in monovalent (measles only) formulation and in combination formulations, such as measles-rubella (MR) and measles-mumps-rubella (MMR) vaccines. The MMR vaccine is the recommended product of choice in most circumstances.

Vaccine (as a combination or monovalent product) in a dose of 0.5 mL is given subcutaneously. Measles and measles-containing vaccines can be given simultaneously with other immunizations in a separate syringe at a separate site (see Simultaneous Administration of Multiple Vaccines, p 33).

Serum measles antibodies develop in approximately 95% of children immunized at 12 months of age and 98% of people immunized at 15 months of age. Protection conferred by a single dose is durable in most people. However, a small proportion of immunized people may lose protection after several years. More than 99% of people who receive 2 doses separated by at least 1 month (4 weeks), with the first dose administered on or after their first birthday, develop serologic evidence of measles immunity. Immunization is not deleterious for people who already are immune.

Improperly stored vaccine may fail to protect against measles. Since 1979, an improved stabilizer has been added to the vaccine that makes it more resistant to heat inactivation. However, during storage and before reconstitution, measles vaccine should be kept at 2°C to 8°C (36°F–46°F) or colder. Freezing is not harmful to the lyophilized vaccine. The vaccine diluent is sterile water and, when provided in glass vials, should not be frozen, because the vials may break. Measles vaccine must be protected from ultraviolet light (especially after reconstitution), because ultraviolet light can inactivate the virus. Vaccine should be shipped at 10°C (50°F) or colder and may be shipped on dry ice. Reconstituted vaccine should be stored in a refrigerator and discarded if not used within 8 hours.

Vaccine Recommendations (see Table 3.34, p 425, for summary).

Age of Routine Immunization. The first dose of measles vaccine should be given at 12 to 15 months of age. Delays in administering the first dose contributed to large outbreaks from 1989 to 1991. Initial immunization at 12 months of age is recommended for preschool-aged children in high-risk areas, especially large urban areas. The second dose is recommended routinely at school entry (ie, 4–6 years of age) but can be given at any earlier age (eg, during an outbreak or before international travel), provided the interval between the first and second doses is at least 4 weeks. Children who were not reimmunized at school entry should receive the second dose by 11 to 12 years of age. If the child receives a dose of measles vaccine before 12 months of age, 2 additional doses are required beginning at 12 to 15 months of age and separated by at least 4 weeks. As of 2001, all school-aged children should have received 2 doses of measles-containing vaccine.

High School Students and Older People. Because of the continuing occurrence of measles cases in older children and young adults, emphasis must be placed on identifying and appropriately immunizing potentially susceptible adolescents and young adults in high school, college, and health care settings. People should be considered susceptible unless they have documentation of 2 doses of measles vaccine administered at least 1 month apart, physician-diagnosed measles, or laboratory evidence of immunity to measles or were born before 1957. For children, adolescents, and adults born in 1957 or after, 2 doses of measles vaccine are required for evidence of immunity. A parental report of immunization is not considered adequate documentation. Physicians should provide an immunization record for patients only if they have administered the vaccine or have seen a record documenting immunization.

Table 3.34. **Recommendations for Measles Immunization**[1]

Category	Recommendations
Unimmunized, no history of measles (12–15 mo of age)	A 2-dose schedule (with MMR) is recommended. The first dose is recommended at 12–15 mo of age; the second is recommended at 4–6 y of age
Children 6–11 mo of age in epidemic situations[2]	Immunize (with monovalent measles vaccine or, if not available, MMR); reimmunization (with MMR) at 12–15 mo of age is necessary, and a third dose is indicated at 4–6 y of age
Children 4–12 y of age who have received 1 dose of measles vaccine at ≥12 mo of age	Reimmunize (1 dose)
Students in college and other post-high school institutions who have received 1 dose of measles vaccine at ≥12 mo of age	Reimmunize (1 dose)
History of immunization before the first birthday	Consider susceptible and immunize (2 doses)
History of receipt of inactivated measles vaccine or unknown type of vaccine, 1963–1967	Consider susceptible and immunize (2 doses)
Further attenuated or unknown vaccine given with IG	Consider susceptible and immunize (2 doses)
Allergy to eggs	Immunize; no reactions likely (see text for details)
Neomycin allergy, nonanaphylactic	Immunize; no reactions likely (see text for details)
Severe hypersensitivity (anaphylaxis) to neomycin or gelatin	Avoid immunization
Tuberculosis	Immunize (see Tuberculosis, p 642); vaccine does not exacerbate infection
Measles exposure	Immunize and/or give IG, depending on circumstances (see text, p 422)
HIV-infected	Immunize (2 doses) unless severely immunocompromised (see text, p 428)
Personal or family history of seizures	Immunize; advise parents of slightly increased risk of seizures
Immunoglobulin or blood recipient	Immunize at the appropriate interval (see Table 3.33, p 423)

MMR indicates measles-mumps-rubella vaccine; IG, Immune Globulin; HIV, human immunodeficiency virus.

[1] See text for details.

[2] See Outbreak Control (p 429).

Colleges and Other Institutions for Education Beyond High School. Colleges and other institutions should require that all entering students have documentation of physician-diagnosed measles, serologic evidence of immunity, or receipt of 2 doses of measles-containing vaccines. Students without documentation of any measles immunization or immunity should receive a dose on entry, followed by a second dose 4 weeks later.

Immunization During an Outbreak. During an outbreak, monovalent measles vaccine may be given to infants as young as 6 months of age (see Outbreak Control, p 429). If monovalent vaccine is not available, MMR may be given. However, seroconversion rates after MMR immunization are significantly lower in children immunized before the first birthday than are seroconversion rates in children immunized after the first birthday. Therefore, children immunized before their first birthday should be immunized with MMR vaccine at 12 to 15 months of age (at least 4 weeks after the initial measles immunization) and again at school entry (4–6 years).

International Travel. People traveling internationally should be immune to measles. For young children traveling to areas where measles is endemic or epidemic, the age for initial measles immunization may need to be lowered. Infants 6 to 11 months of age should receive a dose of monovalent measles vaccine before departure, and then they should receive MMR vaccine at 12 to 15 months of age (at least 4 weeks after the initial measles immunization) and again at 4 to 6 years of age. Children 12 to 15 months of age should be given their first dose of MMR vaccine before departure. Children who have received 1 dose and are traveling to areas where measles is endemic or epidemic should receive their second dose before departure, provided the interval between doses is 4 weeks or more.

Health Care Facilities. Evidence of having had measles, of measles immunity, or of receipt of 2 measles immunizations is recommended before beginning employment for all health care professionals born in 1957 or after (see Health Care Personnel, p 90). For recommendations during an outbreak, see Outbreak Control (p 429).

Adverse Events. A temperature of 39.4°C (103°F) or higher develops in approximately 5% to 15% of susceptible vaccine recipients, usually between 6 and 12 days after MMR immunization; fever generally lasts 1 to 2 days but may last as long as 5 days. Most people with fever are otherwise asymptomatic. Transient rashes have been reported in approximately 5% of vaccine recipients. Transient thrombocytopenia occurs in 1 in 25 000 to 1 in 2 million people after administration of measles-containing vaccines, specifically MMR (see Thrombocytopenia, p 427). The reported frequency of central nervous system conditions after measles immunization, including encephalitis and encephalopathy, is less than 1 per million doses administered in the United States. Because the incidence of encephalitis or encephalopathy after measles immunization in the United States is lower than the observed incidence of encephalitis of unknown cause, some or most of the rare reported severe neurologic disorders may be related coincidentally, rather than causally, to measles immunization. Although cases of autism and inflammatory bowel disease have been reported subsequent to measles immunization, multiple studies refute a causal relationship between these diseases and MMR vaccine. After reimmunization, reactions are expected to be similar clinically but much less common in occurrence, because most of these vaccine recipients are immune.

Seizures. Children predisposed to febrile seizures can experience seizures after measles immunization. Children with histories of seizures or children whose first-degree relatives have histories of seizures may be at a slightly increased risk of a seizure but should be immunized, because the benefits greatly outweigh the risks.

Subacute Sclerosing Panencephalitis. Measles vaccine, by protecting against measles, significantly decreases the possibility of developing SSPE.

Precautions and Contraindications (see also Table 3.33, p 423).

Febrile Illnesses. Children with minor illnesses, such as upper respiratory tract infections, may be immunized (see Vaccine Safety and Contraindications, p 37). Fever is not a contraindication to immunization. However, if other manifestations suggest a more serious illness, the child should not be immunized until recovered.

Allergic Reactions. Hypersensitivity reactions occur rarely and usually are minor, consisting of wheal and flare reactions or urticaria at the injection site. Reactions have been attributed to trace amounts of neomycin or gelatin or some other component in the vaccine formulation. Anaphylaxis is rare. Measles vaccine is produced in chicken embryo cell culture and does not contain significant amounts of egg white (ovalbumin) cross-reacting proteins. Children with egg allergy are at low risk of anaphylactic reactions to measles-containing vaccines (including MMR). Skin testing of children for egg allergy is not predictive of reactions to MMR vaccine and is not required before administering MMR or other measles-containing vaccines. People with allergies to chickens or feathers are not at increased risk of reaction to the vaccine.

People who have had a significant hypersensitivity reaction after the first dose of measles vaccine should: (1) be tested for measles immunity and, if immune, should not be given a second dose; or (2) receive evaluation and possible skin testing before receiving a second dose. People who have had an immediate anaphylactic reaction to previous measles immunization should not be reimmunized but require testing to determine whether they are immune.

People who have experienced anaphylactic reactions to gelatin or topically or systemically administered neomycin should receive measles vaccine only in settings where such reactions could be managed and after consultation with an allergist or immunologist. Most often, however, neomycin allergy manifests as contact dermatitis, which is not a contraindication to receiving measles vaccine.

Thrombocytopenia. Rarely, MMR vaccine can be associated with thrombocytopenia within 2 months of immunization, with a temporal clustering 2 to 3 weeks after immunization. On the basis of case reports, the risk of vaccine-associated thrombocytopenia may be higher for people who previously experienced thrombocytopenia, especially when it occurred in temporal association with earlier MMR immunization. The decision to immunize these children should be based on the benefits of protection against measles, mumps, and rubella in comparison with the risks of recurrence of thrombocytopenia after immunization. There have been no reported cases of thrombocytopenia associated with receipt of MMR vaccine that have resulted in death.

Recent Administration of IG. Immune Globulin preparations interfere with the serologic response to measles vaccine for variable periods, depending on the dose of IG administered. Suggested intervals between IG or blood product administration and measles immunization are given in Table 3.33 (p 423). If vaccine is given at intervals shorter than those indicated, as may be warranted if the risk of exposure to measles is imminent, the child should be reimmunized at or after the appropriate interval for immunization (and at least 4 weeks after the earlier immunization) unless serologic testing indicates that measles-specific antibodies were produced.

If IG is to be administered in preparation for international travel, administration of vaccine should precede receipt of IG by at least 2 weeks to preclude interference with replication of the vaccine virus.

Tuberculosis. Tuberculin skin testing is not a prerequisite for measles immunization. Because of a theoretical concern that measles vaccine might exacerbate tuberculosis, antituberculosis therapy should be initiated before administering MMR to people with untreated active tuberculosis. If tuberculin skin testing is otherwise indicated, it can be done on the day of immunization. Otherwise, testing should be postponed for 4 to 6 weeks, because measles immunization temporarily may suppress tuberculin skin test reactivity.

Altered Immunity. Immunocompromised patients with disorders associated with increased severity of viral infections should not be given live measles virus vaccine (see Immunocompromised Children, p 69). The risk of exposure to measles for immunocompromised patients can be decreased by immunizing their close susceptible contacts. Management of immunodeficient and immunosuppressed patients exposed to measles can be facilitated by previous knowledge of their immune status. Susceptible patients with immunodeficiencies should receive IG after measles exposure (see Care of Exposed People, p 422).

Corticosteroids. For patients who have received high doses of corticosteroids for 14 days or more and who are not otherwise immunocompromised, the recommended interval before immunization is at least 1 month (see Immunocompromised Children, p 69).

HIV Infection. Measles immunization (given as MMR vaccine) is recommended at the usual ages for people with asymptomatic HIV infection and for people with symptomatic infection who are not severely immunocompromised, because measles can be severe and often fatal in patients with HIV infection (see Human Immunodeficiency Virus Infection, p 360). Severely immunocompromised HIV-infected infants, children, adolescents, and young adults, as defined by low CD4+ T-lymphocyte counts or percentage of total lymphocytes, should not receive measles virus-containing vaccine, because vaccine-related pneumonia has been reported (see Human Immunodeficiency Virus Infection, p 360).* All members of the household of an HIV-infected person should receive measles vaccine (preferably as MMR) *unless* they are HIV-infected and severely immunosuppressed, were born before 1957, have had physician-diagnosed measles, have laboratory evidence of measles immunity, have had age-appropriate immunizations, or have a contraindication to measles vaccine.

---

* American Academy of Pediatrics, Committee on Infectious Diseases and Committee on Pediatric AIDS. Measles immunization in HIV-infected children. *Pediatrics.* 1999;103:1057–1060

Regardless of immunization status, symptomatic HIV-infected patients who are exposed to measles should receive IG prophylaxis, because immunization may not provide protection (see Care of Exposed People, p 422).

Personal or Family History of Seizures. Children with this history should be immunized after advising the parents or guardians that the risk of seizures after measles immunization is increased slightly (see Adverse Events, p 426). Because fever induced by measles vaccine usually occurs between 6 and 12 days after immunization, prevention of vaccine-related febrile seizures is difficult. Children receiving anticonvulsants should continue such therapy after measles immunization.

Pregnancy. Live-virus measles vaccine, when given as monovalent vaccine or as a component of MR or MMR, should not be given to women known to be pregnant. Women who are given MMR should not become pregnant for at least 28 days. This precaution is based on the theoretic risk of fetal infection, which applies to the administration of any live-virus vaccine to women who might be pregnant or who might become pregnant shortly after immunization. No evidence, however, substantiates this theoretic risk. In the immunization of adolescents and young adults against measles, asking women if they are pregnant, excluding women who are, and explaining the theoretic risks to the others are recommended precautions.

Outbreak Control. Every suspected measles case should be reported immediately to the local health department, and every effort must be made to verify that the illness is measles, especially if the illness may be the first case in the community. Subsequent prevention of the spread of measles depends on prompt immunization of people at risk of exposure or already exposed who cannot readily provide documentation of measles immunity, including the date of immunization. Unimmunized people who have been exempted from measles immunization for medical, religious, or other reasons, if not immunized within 72 hours of exposure, should be excluded from school, child care, and health care settings until at least 2 weeks after the onset of rash in the last case of measles.

Schools and Child Care Facilities. During measles outbreaks in child care facilities, schools, and colleges and other institutions of higher education, all students, their siblings, and personnel born in 1957 or after who cannot provide documentation that they received 2 doses of measles-containing vaccine on or after their first birthday or other evidence of measles immunity should be immunized. People receiving their second dose, as well as unimmunized people receiving their first dose as part of the outbreak control program, may be readmitted immediately to school.

Health Care Facilities. If an outbreak occurs in an area served by a hospital or within a hospital, all employees with direct patient contact who were born in 1957 or after who cannot provide documentation that they have received 2 doses of measles vaccine on or after their first birthday or other evidence of immunity to measles should receive a dose of measles vaccine. Because some health care professionals who have acquired measles in health care facilities were born before 1957, immunization of older employees who may have occupational exposure to measles also should be considered. Susceptible personnel who have been exposed should be relieved from direct patient contact from the fifth to the 21st day after exposure, regardless of whether they received vaccine or IG after the exposure. Personnel who become ill should be relieved from patient contact for 4 days after rash develops.

Meningococcal Infections

CLINICAL MANIFESTATIONS: Invasive infection usually results in meningococcemia, meningitis, or both. Onset often is abrupt in meningococcemia with fever, chills, malaise, prostration, and a rash that initially may be macular, maculopapular, or petechial. In fulminant cases (Waterhouse-Friderichsen syndrome), purpura, disseminated intravascular coagulation, shock, coma, and death can ensue within several hours despite appropriate therapy. The signs and symptoms of meningococcal meningitis are indistinguishable from signs and symptoms of acute meningitis caused by *Streptococcus pneumoniae* or other meningeal pathogens. Less common manifestations include pneumonia, febrile occult bacteremia, conjunctivitis, and chronic meningococcemia. Invasive meningococcal infections can be complicated by arthritis, myocarditis, pericarditis, and endophthalmitis.

ETIOLOGY: *Neisseria meningitidis* is a gram-negative diplococcus with at least 13 serogroups. Strains belonging to groups A, B, C, Y, and W-135 are implicated most commonly in systemic disease. The distribution of meningococcal serogroups in the United States has shifted in recent years. Serogroups B, C, and Y each account for approximately 30% of reported cases, but serogroup distribution may vary by location and time. Serogroup A has been associated frequently with epidemics elsewhere in the world, primarily in sub-Saharan Africa. Worldwide, serogroup W-135 causes less than 5% of reported cases. In 2000, the first epidemic of serogroup W-135 was reported in association with the Hajj in Saudi Arabia, and in 2002, a serogroup W-135 epidemic was reported in sub-Saharan Africa.

EPIDEMIOLOGY: Asymptomatic colonization of the upper respiratory tract provides the source from which the organism is spread. Transmission occurs from person to person through respiratory tract droplets. Since introduction of *Haemophilus influenzae* type b immunization for infants, *N meningitidis* has become one of the 2 leading causes of bacterial meningitis in young children and remains an important cause of septicemia. Disease most often occurs in children younger than 5 years of age; the peak attack rate occurs in 3- to 5-month-olds. Approximately half of the cases occur in people 16 years of age or older. Close contacts of patients with meningococcal disease are at increased risk of developing infection. Outbreaks have occurred in semiclosed communities, including child care centers, schools, colleges, and military recruit camps. An increased number of meningococcal serogroup C outbreaks in the United States were reported during the 1990s. However, most cases are sporadic, with fewer than 5% associated with outbreaks. Outbreaks often are heralded by a shift in the distribution of cases to an older age group. Multilocus enzyme electrophoresis and pulsed-field gel electrophoresis of enzyme-restricted DNA fragments can be used as epidemiologic tools during a suspected outbreak to detect divergence among strains. Patients with deficiency of a terminal complement component (C5–C9), C3 or properdin deficiencies, or anatomic or functional asplenia are at increased risk of invasive and recurrent meningococcal disease. Patients are considered capable of transmitting the organism for up to 24 hours after initiation of effective antimicrobial treatment.

The **incubation period** is from 1 to 10 days, usually less than 4 days.

DIAGNOSTIC TESTS: Cultures of blood and cerebrospinal fluid (CSF) are indicated for patients with suspected invasive meningococcal disease. Cultures of a petechial or purpuric scraping, synovial fluid, sputum, and other body fluid specimens yield the organism in some patients. A Gram stain of a petechial or purpuric scraping, CSF specimen, and buffy coat smear of blood can be helpful. Because *N meningitidis* can be a component of the nasopharyngeal flora, isolation of *N meningitidis* from this site is not helpful. Bacterial antigen detection in CSF supports the diagnosis of a probable case if the clinical illness is consistent with meningococcal disease; use of latex agglutination assays for detection of meningococcal polysaccharide antigen in serum or urine specimens is not recommended. A serogroup-specific polymerase chain reaction test to detect *N meningitidis* from clinical specimens is used routinely in the United Kingdom, where 30% to 50% of cases are confirmed by polymerase chain reaction assay alone.

Case definitions for invasive disease are given in Table 3.35 (p 432).

SUSCEPTIBILITY TESTING: Routine susceptibility testing of meningococcal isolates is not recommended. However, *N meningitidis* strains with resistance to penicillin have been identified sporadically from several regions of the United States and have been reported widely from Spain, Italy, and parts of Africa. Resistant meningococcal strains for which the minimum inhibitory concentration to penicillin is more than 1 µg/mL are rare. Most reported isolates are moderately susceptible, with a minimum inhibitory concentration to penicillin of between 0.12 µg/mL and 1.0 µg/mL. Treatment with high-dose penicillin is effective against moderately susceptible strains. Cefotaxime sodium and ceftriaxone sodium show a high degree of in vitro activity against moderately susceptible meningococci. Continued surveillance is necessary to monitor trends in the antimicrobial susceptibility of meningococci in the United States.

TREATMENT:
- Penicillin G should be administered intravenously (250 000 U/kg per day, maximum 12 million U/day, divided every 4–6 hours) for patients with invasive meningococcal disease including meningitis. Cefotaxime, ceftriaxone, and ampicillin are acceptable alternatives. In a patient with penicillin allergy characterized by anaphylaxis, chloramphenicol is recommended. For travelers from areas such as Spain, where penicillin resistance has been reported, cefotaxime, ceftriaxone, or chloramphenicol is recommended. Five to 7 days of antimicrobial therapy is adequate for most cases of invasive meningococcal disease.

ISOLATION OF THE HOSPITALIZED PATIENT: In addition to standard precautions, droplet precautions are recommended until 24 hours after initiation of effective antimicrobial therapy.

Table 3.35. **Case Definitions for Invasive Meningococcal Disease**

Confirmed
- Isolation of *Neisseria meningitidis* from a usually sterile site, for example:
  Blood
  Cerebrospinal fluid
  Synovial fluid
  Pleural fluid
  Pericardial fluid
  Petechial or purpuric lesion in a person with a clinically compatible illness

Presumptive
- Gram-negative diplococci in any sterile fluid, such as cerebrospinal fluid, synovial fluid, or scraping from a petechial or purpuric lesion

Probable
- A positive antigen test for *N meningitidis* in cerebrospinal fluid in the absence of a positive sterile site culture in a person with clinical illness consistent with meningococcal disease or purpura fulminans in the absence of a positive blood culture

CONTROL MEASURES:

Care of Exposed People.

Careful observation. Exposed household, school, or child care contacts must be observed carefully. Exposed people in whom a febrile illness develops should receive prompt medical evaluation and, if indicated, antimicrobial therapy appropriate for invasive meningococcal infection.

Chemoprophylaxis. The risk of contracting invasive meningococcal disease among contacts of infected individuals is the determining factor in the decision to give chemoprophylaxis (see Table 3.36, p 433). Close contacts of all people with invasive disease (see Table 3.36), whether sporadic or in an outbreak, are at high risk and should receive prophylaxis ideally within 24 hours of diagnosis of the primary case. Throat and nasopharyngeal cultures are of no value in deciding who should receive prophylaxis.

Household, child care facility, and nursery school contacts. Household, child care, and nursery school contacts are at high risk and are considered close contacts. The attack rate for household contacts is more than 300 times the rate in the general population.

Other contacts. Prophylaxis is warranted for people who have had contact with the patient's oral secretions through kissing or through sharing of toothbrushes or eating utensils, markers of close social contact, during the 7 days before onset of disease in the index case. In addition, people who frequently ate or slept in the same dwelling as the infected individual within this period should receive chemoprophylaxis. For airline flights lasting more than 8 hours, passengers who are seated directly next to an infected individual should be considered candidates for prophylaxis. Routine prophylaxis is not recommended for health care professionals (Table 3.36) unless they have had intimate exposure, such as occurs with unprotected

Table 3.36. **Disease Risk for Contacts of Individuals With Meningococcal Disease**

High risk: chemoprophylaxis recommended (close contact)
- Household contact: especially young children
- Child care or nursery school contact during 7 days before onset of illness
- Direct exposure to index patient's secretions through kissing or through sharing toothbrushes or eating utensils, markers of close social contact during 7 days before onset of illness
- Mouth-to-mouth resuscitation, unprotected contact during endotracheal intubation during 7 days before onset of illness
- Frequently slept or ate in same dwelling as index patient during 7 days before onset of illness

Low risk: chemoprophylaxis not recommended
- Casual contact: no history of direct exposure to index patient's oral secretions (eg, school or work mate)
- Indirect contact: only contact is with a high-risk contact, no direct contact with the index patient
- Health care professionals without direct exposure to patient's oral secretions

In outbreak or cluster
- Chemoprophylaxis for people other than those at high risk should be administered only after consultation with the local public health authorities

---

mouth-to-mouth resuscitation, intubation, or suctioning, before antimicrobial therapy was initiated.

Antimicrobial regimens for prophylaxis (see Table 3.37, p 434). Rifampin, ceftriaxone, and ciprofloxacin are appropriate drugs for chemoprophylaxis in adults. The drug of choice for most children is rifampin. The recommended regimen for rifampin is listed in Table 3.37. Some experts recommend azithromycin dihydrate, which has been shown to be effective for eradication.

Ceftriaxone given in a single intramuscular dose has been demonstrated to be as effective as oral rifampin in eradicating pharyngeal carriage of group A meningococci. The efficacy of ceftriaxone has been confirmed only for group A strains, but its effect is likely to be similar for other serogroups. Ceftriaxone has the advantage of ease of administration, which increases compliance, and is safe for use during pregnancy. Rifampin is not recommended for pregnant women.

Ciprofloxacin administered to adults in a single oral dose also is effective in eradicating meningococcal carriage. At present, ciprofloxacin is not recommended for people younger than 18 years of age or for pregnant women (see Antimicrobial Agents and Related Therapy, p 693).

The index case also should receive chemoprophylaxis before hospital discharge unless the infection was treated with ceftriaxone or cefotaxime, both of which are effective in nasopharyngeal eradication of *N meningitidis*.

Immunoprophylaxis. Because secondary cases can occur several weeks or more after onset of disease in the index case, meningococcal vaccine is a possible adjunct to chemoprophylaxis when an outbreak is caused by a serogroup contained in the vaccine.

Table 3.37. **Recommended Chemoprophylaxis Regimens for High-Risk Contacts and People With Invasive Meningococcal Disease**

Age of Infants, Children, and Adults	Dose	Duration	Efficacy, %	Cautions
Rifampin[1]				
≤1 mo	5 mg/kg, orally, every 12 h	2 days		
>1 mo	10 mg/kg (maximum 600 mg), orally, every 12 h	2 days	72–90	May interfere with efficacy of oral contraceptives and some seizure prevention and anticoagulant medications; may stain soft contact lenses
Ceftriaxone				
≤15 y	125 mg, intramuscularly	Single dose	97	To decrease pain at injection site, dilute with 1% lidocaine
>15 y	250 mg, intramuscularly	Single dose		
Ciprofloxacin[1]				
≥18 y	500 mg, orally	Single dose	90–95	Not licensed for people <18 years of age

[1] Not recommended for use in pregnant women.

Meningococcal Vaccine. A serogroup-specific quadrivalent meningococcal vaccine against serogroups A, C, Y, and W-135 *N meningitidis* is available in the United States for use in children 2 years of age and older. The vaccine is administered subcutaneously as a single 0.5-mL dose and can be given concurrently with other vaccines but at a different site. No vaccine currently is available in the United States for the prevention of group B disease.

Serogroup A meningococcal polysaccharide vaccine is immunogenic in children 3 months of age and older, although a response comparable to that seen in adults is not achieved until 4 or 5 years of age. For children younger than 18 months of age, 2 doses 3 months apart have been given for control of epidemics, although data regarding the efficacy of this schedule are not available. When the quadrivalent A, C, Y, and W-135 vaccine is given to infants during a group A outbreak, response to the other meningococcal polysaccharides usually is poor. The serogroup C polysaccharide is poorly immunogenic in recipients younger than 24 months of age. Serogroups Y and W135 polysaccharides have been demonstrated to be immunogenic and safe for children 2 years of age and older.

Serogroup C polysaccharide conjugate vaccines are licensed in Europe and Canada for use in infants and children.

Indications. Routine childhood immunization with meningococcal polysaccharide vaccine is not recommended, because the infection rate in the general population is low, response is poor in young children, immunity is relatively short-lived, and the response to subsequent vaccine doses is impaired for some serogroups. However, immunization is recommended for children 2 years of age and older in high-risk groups, including people with functional or anatomic asplenia (see Asplenic Children, p 80) and people with terminal complement component or properdin deficiencies. College students who will be living in dormitories for the first time are at increased risk of invasive meningococcal disease. Pediatricians should educate college students and their parents about the risk of vaccine-preventable meningococcal disease for students living in dormitories for the first time and the existence of a safe and effective vaccine. Physicians should immunize students if requested by them or their parents, if required by the educational institution, or if mandated by state law (www.immunize.org/laws). At present, there are no data suggesting that children and adolescents living in noncollege dormitory settings are at increased risk of invasive meningococcal disease.

Immunization may be beneficial for travelers to countries recognized to have hyperendemic or epidemic meningococcal disease caused by a vaccine-preventable serogroup. The vaccine currently is given to all military recruits in the United States. Data suggest that *N meningitidis* isolates pose a potential risk for microbiologists, and these isolates should be handled in a manner that minimizes risk of exposure to aerosols or droplets. Scientists who are exposed routinely to *N meningitidis* in solution should consider immunization.

Reimmunization. Little information is available to determine the need for or timing of reimmunization when the risk of disease continues or recurs. In children, especially children initially immunized when younger than 5 years of age, antibody concentrations decrease markedly during the first 3 years after immunization. Reimmunization may be indicated for people at high risk of infection (eg, people residing in areas in which disease is epidemic), particularly for children who were first immunized when they were younger than 4 years of age; such children should be considered for reimmunization after 2 to 3 years if they remain at high risk. Although the need for reimmunization of older children and adults has not been determined, antibody concentrations rapidly decrease over 2 to 3 years, and if indications still exist for immunization, reimmunization may be considered 3 to 5 years after receipt of the initial dose.

Adverse reactions and precautions. Rare and mild adverse reactions occur, the most common of which is localized pain and erythema for 1 to 2 days. Studies suggest that meningococcal immunization recommendations should not be altered because of pregnancy.

Reporting. All confirmed, presumptive, and probable cases of invasive meningococcal disease must be reported to the regional health department (see Table 3.35, p 432). Timely reporting can facilitate early recognition of outbreaks so that appropriate prevention programs can be implemented rapidly.

Counseling and Public Education. When a case of invasive meningococcal disease is detected, the physician should provide accurate and timely information about meningococcal disease and the risk of transmission to families and contacts of the infected individual. Public health questions, such as whether a mass immunization program is needed, should be referred to the local health department. In appropriate situations, early provision of information in collaboration with the local health department to schools or other groups at increased risk and to the media may help minimize public anxiety and unrealistic or inappropriate demands for intervention.

Microsporidia Infections
(Microsporidiosis)

CLINICAL MANIFESTATIONS: Patients with intestinal infection have watery non-bloody diarrhea. Fever is uncommon. Intestinal infection, often resulting in chronic diarrhea, is most common in immunocompromised people, especially people who are infected with human immunodeficiency virus (HIV). The clinical course is complicated by malnutrition and progressive weight loss. Chronic infection in immunocompetent people is rare. Other clinical syndromes that can occur in HIV-infected and immunocompetent patients include keratoconjunctivitis, myositis, nephritis, hepatitis, cholangitis, peritonitis, and disseminated disease, but they occur rarely.

ETIOLOGY: Microsporidia are obligate, intracellular, spore-forming protozoa. The genera *Encephalitozoon, Enterocytozoon, Nosema, Pleistophora, Trachipleistophora, Brachiola,* and *Vittaforma* have been implicated in human infection, as have unclassified *"Microsporidium"* species. *Enterocytozoon bieneusi* and *Enterocytozoon (Septata) intestinalis* are important causes of chronic diarrhea in HIV-infected people.

EPIDEMIOLOGY: Several studies indicate that waterborne transmission occurs. Person-to-person spread by fecal-oral route also occurs. Spores also have been detected in other body fluids, but their role in transmission is unknown.

The **incubation period** is unknown.

DIAGNOSTIC TESTS: Infection with microsporidia species can be documented by identification of organisms in biopsy specimens from the small intestine. Microsporidia species spores also can be detected in formalin-fixed stool specimens or duodenal aspirates stained with a chromotrope-based stain (a modification of the trichrome stain) and examined by an experienced microscopist. Gram, acid-fast, periodic acid-Schiff, and Giemsa stains also can be used to detect organisms in tissue sections. The organisms often are not noticed, because they are small, stain poorly, and evoke minimal inflammatory response. Use of stool concentration techniques does not seem to improve the ability to detect *E bieneusi* spores. Polymerase chain reaction assay also can be used for diagnosis. Identification for classification purposes and diagnostic confirmation of species requires electron microscopy or molecular techniques. Reliable serologic tests for the diagnosis of human microsporidiosis are lacking.

TREATMENT: No effective therapy is known. For a limited number of patients, albendazole, metronidazole, atovaquone, nitazoxanide, and fumagillin have been reported to decrease diarrhea but without eradication of the organism. Albendazole is the drug of choice for infections caused by *E intestinalis* but is not effective for *E bieneusi* infections, which may respond to fumagillin. Recurrence of diarrhea is common after therapy is discontinued. In HIV-infected patients, highly active antiretroviral therapy-associated improvement in CD4+ T-lymphocyte cell count can favorably modify the course of disease.

ISOLATION OF THE HOSPITALIZED PATIENT: In addition to standard precautions, contact precautions are recommended for diapered and incontinent children for the duration of illness.

CONTROL MEASURES: None have been documented. In HIV-infected people, decreased exposure may result from attention to hand hygiene, drinking bottled or boiled water, and thorough cooking of meat.

Molluscum Contagiosum

CLINICAL MANIFESTATIONS: Molluscum contagiosum is a benign, usually asymptomatic viral infection of the skin with no systemic manifestations. It is characterized by relatively few (usually 2–20) discrete, 5-mm-diameter, flesh-colored to translucent, dome-shaped papules, some with central umbilication. Lesions commonly occur on the trunk, face, and extremities but rarely are generalized. An eczematous reaction encircles the lesions in approximately 10% of patients. Patients with eczema and immunocompromised people, including people with human immunodeficiency virus infection, tend to have more intense and widespread eruptions.

ETIOLOGY: The cause is a poxvirus, which is the sole member of the genus *Molluscipoxvirus.* At least 4 DNA sequence subtypes can be differentiated by polymerase chain reaction assay and restriction enzyme assay, but DNA subtype is not significant in pathogenesis.

EPIDEMIOLOGY: Humans are the only known source of the virus, which is spread by direct contact, including sexual contact, or by fomites, such as towels. Lesions may disseminate by autoinoculation. Infectivity generally is low, but occasional outbreaks have been reported, including in child care centers. The period of communicability is unknown.

The **incubation period** seems to vary between 2 and 7 weeks but may be as long as 6 months.

DIAGNOSTIC TESTS: The diagnosis usually can be made clinically from the characteristic appearance of the lesions. Wright or Giemsa staining of cells expressed from the central core of a lesion reveals characteristic intracytoplasmic inclusions. Electron microscopic examination of these cells will identify the typical poxvirus particles.

TREATMENT: Lesions usually regress spontaneously, but mechanical removal (curettage) of the central core of each lesion may result in more rapid resolution. Children with single or widely scattered lesions need not be treated. A topical anesthetic, such as eutectic mixture of local anesthetics (EMLA) cream, may be applied 30 minutes to 2 hours before the procedure. Alternatively, topical application of cantharidin (0.7% in collodion); peeling agents, such as salicylic and lactic acid preparations; electrocautery; or liquid nitrogen may be successful in removal of lesions. Although lesions can regress spontaneously, treatment may prevent auto-inoculation and spread to other people. Scarring is a rare occurrence.

ISOLATION OF THE HOSPITALIZED PATIENT: Standard precautions are recommended.

CONTROL MEASURES: No control measures are known for isolated cases. For outbreaks, which are common in the tropics, restricting direct person-to-person contact and sharing of potentially contaminated fomites may decrease spread.

Moraxella catarrhalis Infections

CLINICAL MANIFESTATIONS: Common infections include acute otitis media and sinusitis. Bronchopulmonary infection, often in patients with chronic lung disease, can occur. The role of *Moraxella catarrhalis* in children with persistent cough is controversial. Rare manifestations are bacteremia (sometimes associated with focal infections, such as preseptal cellulitis, osteomyelitis, septic arthritis, abscesses, or a rash indistinguishable from that observed in meningococcemia) and conjunctivitis or meningitis in neonates. Other unusual manifestations include endocarditis, shunt-associated ventriculitis, and urinary tract infections.

ETIOLOGY: *Moraxella catarrhalis* is a gram-negative aerobic diplococcus. Almost 100% of strains produce β-lactamase that mediates resistance to penicillins.

EPIDEMIOLOGY: *Moraxella catarrhalis* is part of the normal flora of the upper respiratory tract of humans. The mode of transmission is presumed to be direct contact with contaminated respiratory tract secretions or droplet spread. Infection is most common in infants and young children, but it occurs at all ages. Transmission within families, schools, and child care centers has not been studied. The duration of carriage by infected and colonized children and the period of communicability are unknown.

The **incubation period** is unknown.

DIAGNOSTIC TESTS: The organism can be isolated on blood and chocolate agar culture media after incubation in air or with increased carbon dioxide. Culture of middle ear or sinus aspirates is indicated for patients with unusually severe infection, patients in whom infection fails to respond to treatment, and immuno-compromised children. Concomitant recovery of *M catarrhalis* with other pathogens (*Streptococcus pneumoniae* or *Haemophilus influenzae*) can occur and may indicate mixed infection.

TREATMENT: Although most strains of *Moraxella* species produce β-lactamase and are resistant to amoxicillin in vitro, this agent remains effective as empiric therapy for otitis media and other respiratory tract infections. When *M catarrhalis* is isolated from appropriately obtained specimens (middle ear fluid, sinus aspirates, or lower respiratory tract secretions) or when initial therapy has been unsuccessful, appropriate antimicrobial agents include amoxicillin-clavulanate potassium, cefuroxime, cefprozil, erythromycin, clarithromycin, azithromycin dihydrate, and trimethoprim-sulfamethoxazole. If parenteral antimicrobial therapy is needed to treat *M catarrhalis* infection, in vitro data indicate that the following drugs are effective: cefuroxime, cefotaxime sodium, ceftriaxone sodium, ceftazidime, and trimethoprim-sulfamethoxazole.

ISOLATION OF THE HOSPITALIZED PATIENT: Standard precautions are recommended.

CONTROL MEASURES: None.

Mumps

CLINICAL MANIFESTATIONS: Mumps is a systemic disease characterized by swelling of one or more of the salivary glands, usually the parotid glands. Approximately one third of infections do not cause clinically apparent salivary gland swelling. More than 50% of people with mumps have cerebrospinal fluid pleocytosis, but fewer than 10% have symptoms of central nervous system infection. Orchitis is a common complication after puberty, but sterility rarely occurs. Other rare complications include arthritis, thyroiditis, mastitis, glomerulonephritis, myocarditis, endocardial fibroelastosis, thrombocytopenia, cerebellar ataxia, transverse myelitis, ascending polyradiculitis, pancreatitis, oophoritis, and hearing impairment.

ETIOLOGY: Mumps is caused by an RNA virus classified as a Rubulavirus in the Paramyxoviridae family. Other causes of parotitis include infection with cytomegalovirus, parainfluenza virus types 1 and 3, influenza A virus, coxsackieviruses, lymphocytic choriomeningitis virus, enteroviruses, human immunodeficiency virus (HIV), *Staphylococcus aureus*, and nontuberculous mycobacterium; starch ingestion; drug reactions (eg, phenylbutazone, thiouracil, iodides); and metabolic disorders (diabetes mellitus, cirrhosis, and malnutrition).

EPIDEMIOLOGY: Humans are the only known natural hosts. The virus is spread by contact with infected respiratory tract secretions. Infection can occur throughout childhood. During adulthood, infection is likely to produce more severe disease, including orchitis. Death attributable to mumps is rare; the estimated case fatality rate is 1.6 to 3.8 per 10 000. More than half of the fatalities occur in people older than 19 years of age. Mumps infection during the first trimester of pregnancy is associated with an increased rate of spontaneous abortion. Although mumps virus can cross the placenta, no evidence exists that mumps infection during pregnancy causes congenital malformations. Historically, the peak incidence was between January and May; however, seasonality no longer is evident. The incidence in the United States, which has decreased markedly since introduction of the mumps vaccine, is now fewer than 500 reported cases per year. Most of the reported cases of mumps are in children 5 to 14 years of age. In immunized children, most cases of parotitis are not caused by mumps infection. Outbreaks can occur in highly immunized populations. Like measles vaccine, a single dose of mumps-containing vaccine does not always induce protection. The period of maximum communicability is from 1 to 2 days before onset of parotid swelling to 5 days after onset of parotid swelling. Virus has been isolated from saliva from 7 days before through 9 days after onset of swelling.

The **incubation period** usually is 16 to 18 days, but cases may occur from 12 to 25 days after exposure.

DIAGNOSTIC TESTS: Children with parotitis lasting 2 days or more without other apparent cause should undergo diagnostic testing to confirm mumps virus as the cause, because mumps is now an uncommon infection and parotitis has other etiologies, including other infectious agents. Mumps can be confirmed by isolating the virus in cell culture inoculated with throat washing, urine, or spinal fluid specimens or by a significant increase between acute and convalescent titers in serum mumps immunoglobulin (Ig) G antibody titer determined by any standard serologic assay (eg, complement fixation, neutralization, hemagglutination inhibition test, or enzyme immunoassay or mumps IgM antibody test [past infection is best assessed by enzyme immunoassay or a neutralization test; complement fixation and hemagglutination inhibition tests are unreliable for this purpose]). Skin tests also are unreliable and should not be used to test immune status.

TREATMENT: Supportive.

ISOLATION OF THE HOSPITALIZED PATIENT: In addition to standard precautions, droplet precautions are recommended until 9 days after onset of parotid swelling.

CONTROL MEASURES:

School and Child Care. Children should be excluded for 9 days from onset of parotid gland swelling. For control measures during an outbreak, see Outbreak Control, p 442.

Care of Exposed People. Mumps vaccine has not been demonstrated to be effective in preventing infection after exposure. However, mumps vaccine can be given after exposure, because immunization will provide protection against subsequent exposures. Immunization during the incubation period has no increased risk. The routine use of mumps vaccine is not advised for people born before 1957, because most of these people are immune. Mumps Immune Globulin is of no value and no longer is manufactured or licensed in the United States.

Mumps Vaccine. Live-virus mumps vaccine is prepared in chicken embryo cell cultures. Vaccine is administered by subcutaneous injection of 0.5 mL, alone as a monovalent vaccine or, preferably, as the combined measles-mumps-rubella (MMR) vaccine. Antibody develops in more than 95% of all susceptible people after a single dose. Serologic and epidemiologic evidence extending for more than 25 years indicates that vaccine-induced immunity is long lasting.

Vaccine Recommendations.

- Mumps vaccine should be given as MMR routinely to children at 12 to 15 months of age, with a second dose of MMR at 4 to 6 years of age. Reimmunization for mumps is important, because mumps can occur in highly immunized populations, including people with a history of mumps immunization. Administration of MMR is not harmful if given to a person already immune to one or more of the viruses (from previous infection or immunization).
- Mumps immunization is of particular importance for children approaching puberty, adolescents, and adults who have not had mumps or mumps vaccine. At office visits of prepubertal children and adolescents, the status of immunity to mumps should be assessed. People should be considered susceptible unless they have documentation of at least 1 dose of vaccine on or after their first birthday, documentation of physician-diagnosed mumps, or serologic evidence of immunity or were born before 1957.
- Susceptible children, adolescents, and adults born during or after 1957 should be offered mumps immunization (usually as MMR) before beginning travel, because mumps is still endemic throughout most of the world. Because of concern about inadequate seroconversion related to persisting maternal antibodies and because the risk of serious disease from mumps infection is relatively low, people younger than 12 months of age need not be given mumps vaccine before travel.
- The routine use of mumps vaccine is not advised for people born before 1957 unless they are considered susceptible, as defined by seronegativity. However, immunization is not contraindicated in these people if their serologic status is unknown.
- The MMR vaccine may be given with other vaccines at different injection sites and with separate syringes (see Simultaneous Administration of Multiple Vaccines, p 33).

Adverse Reactions. Adverse reactions attributed to live-virus mumps vaccine are rare. Temporally related reactions, including febrile seizures, nerve deafness, meningitis, encephalitis, rash, pruritus, and purpura, may not be related causally. Orchitis and parotitis have been reported rarely. Allergic reactions also are rare (see Precautions and Contraindications). Other reactions that occur after immunization with MMR are attributable to the measles and rubella components of the vaccine (see Measles, p 419, and Rubella, p 536).

Reimmunization with mumps vaccine (monovalent or MMR) is not associated with an increased incidence of reactions. Reactions might be expected only among people not protected by the first dose.

Precautions and Contraindications.

Febrile Illness. Children with minor illnesses with or without fever, such as upper respiratory tract infections, may be immunized (see Vaccine Safety and Contraindications, p 37). Fever is not a contraindication to immunization. However, if other manifestations suggest a more serious illness, the child should not be immunized until recovered.

Allergies. The widespread use of the mumps vaccine since 1967 has resulted in only rare isolated reports of allergic reactions. Allergic reactions to components of the vaccine (eg, neomycin or gelatin) occasionally may occur. Severe allergic reactions, such as anaphylaxis, rarely are reported. Most children with egg hypersensitivity can be immunized safely with MMR vaccine (see Measles, p 419). People with a history of anaphylactic, anaphylactoid, or other immediate reactions subsequent to egg ingestion may be at an increased risk of immediate-type hypersensitivity reactions after immunization.

Recent Administration of Immune Globulin. Live-virus mumps vaccine should be given at least 2 weeks before or at least 3 months after administration of Immune Globulin (IG) or blood transfusion because of the theoretic possibility that antibody will neutralize vaccine virus and interfere with a successful immunization. Because high doses of IG (such as those given for treatment of Kawasaki syndrome) can inhibit the response to measles vaccine for longer intervals, MMR immunization should be deferred for a longer period after administration of IG (see Measles, p 419).

Altered Immunity. Patients with immunodeficiency diseases and people receiving immunosuppressive therapy (eg, patients with leukemia, lymphoma, or generalized malignant disease), including high doses of systemically administered corticosteroids, alkylating agents, antimetabolites, or radiation or who are otherwise immunocompromised should not receive mumps vaccine (see Immunocompromised Children, p 69). The exceptions are patients with HIV infection who are not severely immunocompromised; these patients should be immunized against mumps with MMR vaccine (see Human Immunodeficiency Virus Infection, p 360). The risk of mumps exposure for patients with altered immunity can be decreased by immunizing their close susceptible contacts. Immunized people do not transmit mumps vaccine virus.

After cessation of immunosuppressive therapy, mumps vaccine usually should be withheld for an interval of at least 3 months (with the exception of corticosteroid recipients, see the next paragraph). This interval is based on the assumptions that immunologic responsiveness will have been restored in 3 months and the underlying disease for which immunosuppressive therapy was given is in remission or under control. However, because the interval can vary with the intensity and type of immunosuppressive therapy, radiation therapy, underlying disease, and other factors, a definitive recommendation for an interval after cessation of immunosuppressive therapy when mumps vaccine can be administered safely and effectively often is not possible.

Corticosteroids. For patients who have received high doses of corticosteroids for 14 days or more and who are not otherwise immunocompromised, the recommended interval is at least 1 month after steroids are discontinued (see Immunocompromised Children, p 69).

Pregnancy. Susceptible postpubertal females should not be immunized if they are known to be pregnant. Live-virus mumps vaccine can infect the placenta, but the virus has not been isolated from fetal tissues of susceptible females who received vaccine and underwent elective abortions. In view of the theoretic risk, however, conception should be avoided for 28 days after mumps immunization.

Outbreak Control. When determining means to control outbreaks, exclusion of susceptible students from affected schools and schools judged by local public health authorities to be at risk of transmission should be considered. Such exclusion should be an effective means of terminating school outbreaks and rapidly increasing rates of immunization. Excluded students can be readmitted immediately after immunization. Pupils who continue to be exempted from mumps immunization because of medical, religious, or other reasons should be excluded until at least 26 days after the onset of parotitis in the last person with mumps in the affected school. Experience with outbreak control for other vaccine-preventable diseases indicates that this strategy is effective.

Mycoplasma pneumoniae Infections

CLINICAL MANIFESTATIONS: The most common clinical syndromes are acute bronchitis and upper respiratory tract infections, including pharyngitis and, occasionally, otitis media or myringitis, which may be bullous. Coryza, sinusitis, and croup are rare. Malaise, fever, and occasionally, headache are nonspecific manifestations of infection. In approximately 10% of patients in whom pneumonia develops, cough, usually with widespread rales on physical examination, develops within a few days and lasts for 3 to 4 weeks. The cough is nonproductive initially but later may become productive, particularly in older children and adolescents. Approximately 10% of children with pneumonia exhibit a rash, most often maculopapular. Abnormalities detected on radiography vary, but bilateral, diffuse infiltrates are common, and focal abnormalities, such as consolidation, effusion, and hilar adenopathy may occur.

Unusual manifestations include nervous system disease (eg, aseptic meningitis, encephalitis, cerebellar ataxia, transverse myelitis, peripheral neuropathy) as well as myocarditis, pericarditis, polymorphous mucocutaneous eruptions (including Stevens-Johnson syndrome), hemolytic anemia, and arthritis. In patients with sickle cell disease, Down syndrome, immunodeficiencies, and chronic cardiorespiratory disease, severe pneumonia with pleural effusion can develop.

ETIOLOGY: Mycoplasmas, including *Mycoplasma pneumoniae,* are the smallest free-living microorganisms; they lack a cell wall and are pleomorphic.

EPIDEMIOLOGY: Mycoplasmas are ubiquitous in animals and plants, but *M pneumoniae* causes disease only in humans. It is highly transmissible by respiratory droplets during close contact with a symptomatic person. Outbreaks have been described in hospitals, military bases, colleges, and summer camps. People of any age can be infected, but specific disease syndromes are age related. *Mycoplasma pneumoniae* is an uncommon cause of pneumonia in children younger than 5 years of age but is a leading cause of pneumonia in school-aged children and young adults. Infections occur throughout the world, in any season, and in all geographic settings. Community-wide epidemics occur every 4 to 7 years. Because of a long incubation period, familial spread may continue for many months. Clinical illness within a group or family ranges from mild upper respiratory tract infection to tracheobronchitis or pharyngitis to pneumonia. Asymptomatic carriage after infection may occur for weeks to months. Immunity after infection is not long lasting.

The **incubation period** is 2 to 3 weeks (range, 1–4 weeks).

DIAGNOSTIC TESTS: Recovery of *M pneumoniae* in cultures requires special enriched broth or agar media, is successful in 40% to 90% of cases, and takes up to 21 days. Isolation of *M pneumoniae* in a patient with compatible clinical manifestations suggests causation. Because this organism can be excreted from the respiratory tract for several weeks after an acute infection despite appropriate therapy, isolation of the organism may not indicate acute infection. A sensitive and specific polymerase chain reaction test for *M pneumoniae* has been developed but is not available in most clinical microbiologic laboratories.

The complement fixation test previously had been the serologic assay of choice but has been replaced by more specific immunofluorescence and enzyme immunoassay methods, which are available commercially. The immunofluorescence test and enzyme immunoassay are capable of detecting *M pneumoniae*-specific immunoglobulin (Ig) M and IgG antibodies. Although the presence of IgM antibodies confirms recent *M pneumoniae* infection, they persist in serum for several months and, in adults, may remain increased indefinitely; therefore, IgM antibodies may not necessarily indicate current infection. However, an increased specific IgM against *M pneumoniae* in a pediatric or college-aged young adult during compatible acute respiratory tract illness suggests *M pneumoniae* infection. Serologic diagnosis can be made by demonstrating a fourfold or greater increase in antibody titer between acute and convalescent serum specimens when the complement fixation assay is used. The antibody titer peaks at approximately 3 to 6 weeks and persists for 2 to 3 months after infection. Because *M pneumoniae* antibodies may cross-react with some other antigens, results of these tests should be interpreted cautiously when evaluating febrile illnesses of unknown origin. However, *M pneumoniae* antibodies do not cross-react with other respiratory tract pathogens causing diseases clinically similar to those caused by *M pneumoniae*. False-negative results may occur with all serologic assays.

Serum cold hemagglutinin titers of ≥1:32 are present in approximately 50% of patients with pneumonia caused by *M pneumoniae* by the beginning of the second week of illness. Fourfold increases in cold hemagglutinin titer between acute and convalescent serum specimens occur more often in patients with severe *M pneumoniae* than in people with less severe disease. This test has low specificity for *Mycoplasma* infection, however, and other agents, including adenoviruses, Epstein-Barr virus, and measles, can cause illnesses in infants or children associated with an increase in titer of cold hemagglutinins. A negative test result for cold agglutinins does not exclude the diagnosis of mycoplasmal infection. With the wide availability of specific antibody tests, use of this test has been deemphasized.

TREATMENT: Acute bronchitis and upper respiratory tract illness caused by *M pneumoniae* generally are mild and resolve without antimicrobial therapy. Macrolides, including erythromycin, are the preferred antimicrobial agents for treatment of pneumonia and otitis media in children younger than 8 years of age; clarithromycin and azithromycin dihydrate are equally effective. Tetracycline and doxycycline also are effective and may be used for children 8 years of age and older. Fluoroquinolones are effective but are not recommended as first-choice agents.

ISOLATION OF THE HOSPITALIZED PATIENT: In addition to standard precautions, droplet precautions are recommended for the duration of symptomatic illness.

CONTROL MEASURES: Diagnosis of an infected patient should lead to an increased index of suspicion for *M pneumoniae* infection in household members and close contacts, and therapy should be given if a contact develops compatible lower respiratory tract illness occurs.

Antimicrobial prophylaxis for exposed contacts is not recommended routinely. Tetracycline and azithromycin for prophylaxis have been shown to decrease symptomatic diseases and reduce rates of transmission within families and institutions. People who are exposed intimately to a person infected with *M pneumoniae* or who live in a house with a person who has an underlying condition that predisposes to severe *M pneumoniae* infection, such as children with sickle cell disease, may be considered for prophylactic treatment with erythromycin (or another macrolide) or tetracycline during the acute phase of the index patient's illness.

Nocardiosis

CLINICAL MANIFESTATIONS: Immunocompetent children typically have cutaneous or lymphocutaneous disease with pustular or ulcerative lesions that remain localized after soil contamination of a skin injury. Invasive disease occurs most commonly in immunocompromised patients, particularly people with chronic granulomatous disease, human immunodeficiency virus infection, or disease requiring long-term systemic corticosteroid therapy. In these children, infection characteristically begins in the lungs, and the illness can be acute, subacute, or chronic. Pulmonary disease commonly manifests as rounded nodular infiltrates that can undergo cavitation. Hematogenous spread may occur from lungs to the brain (single or multiple abscesses), skin (pustules, pyoderma, abscesses, mycetoma), and occasionally other organs.

ETIOLOGY: *Nocardia* species are aerobic actinomycetes. Pulmonary or disseminated disease is caused most commonly by the *Nocardia asteroides* complex, which includes *Nocardia farcinica* and *Nocardia nova*. Cutaneous disease is caused most commonly by *Nocardia brasiliensis*. *Nocardia pseudobrasiliensis* is associated with pulmonary, central nervous system (CNS), and systemic nocardiosis.

EPIDEMIOLOGY: *Nocardia* species are saprophytic soil organisms that are found worldwide. The lungs are the probable portal of entry for pulmonary or disseminated disease. Direct skin inoculation occurs, often as the result of contact with contaminated soil after minor trauma. Person-to-person transmission does not occur.

The **incubation period** is unknown.

DIAGNOSTIC TESTS: Isolation of *Nocardia* organisms from body fluid, abscess material, or tissue specimens provides a definitive diagnosis. Stained smears of sputum, body fluids, or pus demonstrating beaded, branched, weakly gram-positive, variably acid-fast rods suggest the diagnosis. The Brown and Brenn and methenamine silver stains are recommended to demonstrate microorganisms in tissue specimens. *Nocardia* organisms are slow growing; cultures from normally sterile sites should be maintained for 3 weeks in a liquid medium, such as Bactec 12B. Serologic tests for *Nocardia* species are not useful.

TREATMENT: Trimethoprim-sulfamethoxazole or a sulfonamide alone (eg, sulfisoxazole acetyl or sulfamethoxazole) is the drug of choice. Preparations that are less urine soluble, such as sulfadiazine, should be avoided. Immunocompetent patients with lymphocutaneous disease usually respond after 6 to 12 weeks of therapy. Immunocompromised patients and patients with invasive disease should be treated for 6 to 12 months and for at least 3 months after apparent cure because of the tendency for relapse. Patients with acquired immunodeficiency syndrome may need even longer therapy. For patients with central nervous system disease, disseminated disease, or overwhelming infection, amikacin sulfate should be included for the first 4 to 12 weeks of treatment or until the patient's condition is improved clinically. Patients with meningitis or brain abscess should be monitored with serial neuroimaging studies. If response to trimethoprim-sulfamethoxazole does not occur, other agents, such as a tetracycline, amoxicillin-clavulanate potassium, imipenem, or meropenem may be beneficial. Linezolid is highly active against all *Nocardia* species in vitro; anecdotal evidence suggests that it may be effective for the treatment of invasive infections. Drug susceptibility testing, if available, is recommended by some experts for isolates from patients with invasive disease and patients who are unable to tolerate a sulfonamide. Drainage of abscesses is beneficial, especially for immunocompromised patients.

ISOLATION OF THE HOSPITALIZED PATIENT: Standard precautions are recommended.

CONTROL MEASURES: None.

Onchocerciasis
(River Blindness, Filariasis)

CLINICAL MANIFESTATIONS: The disease involves skin, subcutaneous tissues, lymphatic vessels, and eyes. Subcutaneous nodules of varying sizes containing adult worms develop 6 to 12 months after initial infection. In patients in Africa, the nodules tend to be found on the lower torso, pelvis, and lower extremities, whereas in patients in Central America, the nodules more often are located on the upper body (the head and trunk) but may occur on the extremities. After the worms mature, microfilariae are produced and migrate in the tissues and may cause a chronic, pruritic dermatitis. After a period of years, the skin can become lichenified and hypopigmented or hyperpigmented. The presence of living or dead microfilariae in the ocular structures leads to photophobia and inflammation of the cornea, iris, ciliary body, retina, choroid, and optic nerve. Blindness can result if the disease is untreated.

ETIOLOGY: *Onchocerca volvulus* is a filarial nematode.

EPIDEMIOLOGY: Larvae are transmitted by the bite of an infected *Simulium* species black fly that breeds in fast-flowing streams and rivers (hence the colloquial name of the disease, "river blindness"). The disease occurs primarily in equatorial Africa, but small foci are found in southern Mexico, Guatemala, northern South America, and Yemen. Prevalence is greatest among people who live near vector breeding areas. Adult worms continue to produce microfilariae capable of infecting flies for more than a decade. The infection is not transmissible by person-to-person contact or blood transfusion.

The **incubation period** from larval inoculation to microfilariae in the skin usually is 6 to 12 months but can be as long as 3 years.

DIAGNOSTIC TESTS: Direct examination of a 1- to 2-mg shaving or biopsy specimen of the epidermis and upper dermis (taken from the scapular or iliac crest area) can reveal microfilariae. Adult worms may be demonstrated in excised nodules that have been sectioned and stained. A slit-lamp examination of the anterior chamber of an involved eye may reveal motile microfilariae or corneal lesions typical of onchocerciasis. Microfilariae rarely are found in blood. Eosinophilia is common. Specific serologic tests and polymerase chain reaction techniques for detection of microfilariae in skin are available only in research laboratories.

TREATMENT: Ivermectin, a microfilaricidal agent, is the drug of choice for treatment of onchocerciasis. Treatment decreases dermatitis and the risk of developing severe ocular disease, but treatment does not kill the adult worms and, thus, is not curative. One single oral dose of ivermectin (150 µg/kg) should be given every 6 to 12 months until asymptomatic. Adverse reactions caused by the death of microfilariae include rash, edema, fever, myalgia, and hypotension (which rarely is severe). Precautions to ivermectin treatment include pregnancy, breastfeeding, central nervous system disorders that may increase the penetration of drug into the CNS, and body weight less than 15 kg. Safety and effectiveness in pediatric patients weighing less than 15 kg have not been established.

ISOLATION OF THE HOSPITALIZED PATIENT: Standard precautions are recommended.

CONTROL MEASURES: Repellents and protective clothing (long sleeves and pants) can decrease exposure to bites from black flies, which bite by day. Treatment of vector breeding sites with larvicides has been effective for controlling black fly populations, particularly in West Africa. A major initiative led by the World Health Organization to distribute ivermectin to all disease-endemic communities to prevent severe morbidity from onchocerciasis has been highly successful.

Human Papillomavirus

CLINICAL MANIFESTATIONS: Most human papillomavirus (HPV) infections produce no lesions and are inapparent clinically. However, HPVs can produce epithelial tumors (warts) of the skin and mucous membranes and are associated with anogenital dysplasia and cancer. Cutaneous nongenital warts include common skin warts, plantar warts, flat warts, thread-like (filiform) warts, and epidermodysplasia verruciformis. Warts also occur on the mucous membranes, including the anogenital, oral, nasal, and conjunctival areas and the respiratory tract, where papillomatosis occurs.

Common **skin warts** are dome-shaped with conical projections that give the surface a rough appearance. They usually are asymptomatic and multiple, occurring commonly on the hands and around or under the nails. When small dermal vessels become thrombosed, black dots appear in the warts. Plantar warts on the foot may be painful and are characterized by marked hyperkeratosis, sometimes with black dots.

Flat warts ("juvenile warts") commonly are found on the face and extremities of children and adolescents. They usually are small, multiple, and flat topped; seldom exhibit papillomatosis; and rarely cause pain. Filiform warts occur on the face and neck. Cutaneous warts are benign.

Anogenital warts, also called **condylomata acuminata,** are skin-colored warts with a cauliflower-like surface that range in size from a few millimeters to several centimeters. In males, these warts may be found on the penis, scrotum, or anal and perianal area. In females, these lesions may occur on the vulva or perianal areas and less commonly in the vagina or on the cervix. Anogenital warts are often multiple and attract attention because of their appearance. Warts usually are painless, although they may cause itching, burning, local pain, or bleeding.

Anogenital HPV infection may be associated with clinically inapparent dysplastic lesions, particularly in the female genital tract (cervix and vagina). These lesions may be made more apparent by applying 3% to 5% acetic acid to the mucosal surface and examining it by magnification. The HPV types associated with these dysplasias also are associated with cancers that occur in the anogenital tract. Human papillomavirus is involved etiologically in 90% of cervical cancers and a substantial proportion of vulvar, anal, and penile cancers.

Respiratory papillomatosis is a rare condition characterized by papillomas in the larynx or other areas of the upper respiratory tract. This condition is diagnosed most commonly in children between 2 and 5 years of age and manifests as a voice change, stridor, or abnormal cry. Respiratory papillomas have been associated with respiratory tract obstruction in young children. Adult onset also has been described.

Epidermodysplasia verruciformis is a rare, lifelong, severe papillomavirus infection believed to be a consequence of an inherited deficiency of cell-mediated immunity. The lesions may resemble flat warts but often are similar to tinea versicolor, covering the torso and upper extremities. Most appear during the first decade of life, but malignant transformation, which occurs in approximately one third of affected people, usually is delayed until adulthood.

ETIOLOGY: Human papillomaviruses are members of the family Papovaviridae and are DNA viruses. More than 100 types have been identified. These viruses are grouped into cutaneous and mucosal types on the basis of their tendency to infect particular types of epithelium. Most often, the HPV types found in nongenital warts will be cutaneous types, and those in respiratory papillomatosis, anogenital warts, dysplasias, or cancers will be mucosal types. Although more than 30 HPV types can infect the genital tract, several found in the anogenital region (types 16, 18, 31, and 45) have been associated with cervical neoplasia.

EPIDEMIOLOGY: Papillomaviruses are distributed widely among mammals and are species-specific. Cutaneous warts occur commonly among school-aged children; the prevalence rate is as high as 50%. Human papillomavirus infections are transmitted from person to person by close contact. Nongenital warts are acquired through minor trauma to the skin. An increase in the incidence of plantar warts has been associated with swimming in public pools. The intense and often widespread appearance of warts in patients with compromised cellular immunity (particularly patients who have undergone transplantation and people with human immunodeficiency virus infection) suggests that alterations in immunity predispose to reactivation of latent intraepithelial infection.

Anogenital HPV infection is the most common sexually transmitted infection in the United States, occurring in more than 40% of sexually active adolescent females. Anogenital HPV infections are transmitted primarily by sexual contact. Infection rarely is transmitted to a child through the birth canal during delivery or transmitted from nongenital sites. When anogenital warts are found in a child who is beyond infancy but prepubertal, sexual abuse must be considered.

Respiratory papillomatosis is believed to be acquired by aspiration of infectious secretions during passage through the infected birth canal.

The **incubation period** is unknown but is estimated to range from 3 months to several years. Papillomavirus acquired by a neonate at the time of birth may not cause clinical manifestations for several years.

DIAGNOSTIC TESTS: Most cutaneous and anogenital warts are diagnosed through clinical inspection. Respiratory papillomatosis is diagnosed using endoscopy and biopsy. Cervical dysplasias may be detected via cytologic examination of a Papanicolaou smear, and biopsy specimens of any tissue may display cytohistologic characteristics of HPV infection.

Human papillomavirus cannot be cultured easily. A definitive diagnosis of HPV infection is based on detection of viral nucleic acid (DNA or RNA) or capsid protein. Papanicolaou-test diagnosis of HPV does not always correlate with detection of HPV DNA in cervical cells. Tests that detect several types of HPV DNA in cells scraped from the cervix are available and may be useful in the triage of women with atypical squamous cells of undetermined significance but not other types of cytologic abnormalities. Screening for clinically inapparent HPV infection or evaluating anogenital warts using HPV DNA or RNA tests is not recommended.

TREATMENT*: Treatment of HPV infection is directed toward eliminating the lesions that result from the infection rather than HPV itself. Most nongenital warts eventually regress spontaneously but may persist for months or years. The optimal treatment for warts that do not resolve spontaneously has not been iden-

---

* Centers for Disease Control and Prevention. Sexually transmitted diseases treatment guidelines— 2002. *MMWR Recomm Rep.* 2002;51(RR-6):1–80

tified. Most methods of treatment rely on chemical or physical destruction of the infected epithelium, such as application of salicylic acid products or cryotherapy with liquid nitrogen. Daily treatment with tretinoin has been useful for widespread flat warts in children. Care must be taken to avoid a deleterious cosmetic result with therapy. Pharmacologic treatments for refractory warts, including cimetidine, have been used with varied success.

The optimal treatment for anogenital warts has not been identified. Spontaneous regression occurs within months in some cases. The application of podophyllum resin or patient-applied podofilox solution or gel (the major cytotoxic ingredient of podo-phyllum resin) often is the initial therapy of choice. These agents have not been tested for safety and efficacy in children, and their use is contraindicated in preg-nancy. Other treatment modalities are cryotherapy, trichloroacetic acid or bichloro-acetic acid, imiquimod (patient-applied), electrocautery, laser surgery, and surgical excision (see Table 4.3, p 713). Although most forms of therapy are successful for the initial removal of warts, treatment may not eradicate HPV infection from the surrounding normal tissue. Therefore, recurrences are common and probably attri-butable to reactivation rather than reinfection. Many unproven compounds are being used to treat HPV. Agents associated with local tissue damage can be harmful.

Human papillomavirus infection of the cervix is common in sexually active adolescents and can be associated with epithelial dysplasia. Cytologic screening of cervical cells should be initiated at the onset of sexual activity. The presence of anogenital warts in an adolescent warrants cytologic screening of cervical cells. Adolescents with cervical dysplasia should be cared for by a physician who is knowledgeable in the management of cervical dysplasia.

Respiratory papillomatosis is difficult to treat and is best managed by an oto-laryngologist. Local recurrence is common, and repeated surgical procedures for removal are often necessary. Extension or dissemination of respiratory papillomas from the larynx into the trachea, bronchi, or lung parenchyma is a rare complica-tion that can result in increased morbidity and mortality. Intralesional interferon, indole-3-carbinole, photodynamic therapy, and intralesional cidofovir have been used as investigational treatments and may be of benefit for patients with frequent recurrences.

Oral warts can be removed through cryotherapy, electrocautery, or surgical excision.

ISOLATION OF THE HOSPITALIZED PATIENT: Standard precautions are recommended.

CONTROL MEASURES: Suspected child abuse should be reported to the appro-priate local agency if anogenital warts are found in a child who is beyond infancy but prepubertal.

Latex condoms, when used consistently and correctly, can decrease the risk of anogenital HPV infection when the infected areas are covered or protected by the condom. In addition, the use of latex condoms has been associated with a decrease in the risk of genital warts and cervical cancer. Although HPV infection may persist for life, the degree and duration of contagiousness in patients with a history of geni-tal infection is unknown.

VACCINE PREVENTABLE DISEASES

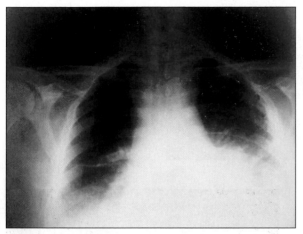

ANTHRAX. Chest radiograph showing widened mediastinum and bilateral pneumonia due to inhalation of anthrax bacilli.

© CDC

ANTHRAX. Cutaneous anthrax lesion on the volar surface of the right forearm.

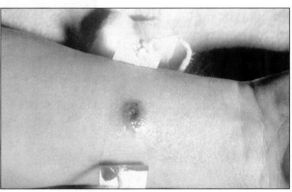

© CDC

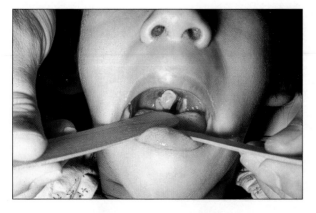

DIPHTHERIA. Pharyngeal diphtheria with membranes covering the tonsils and uvula in a 15-year-old girl.

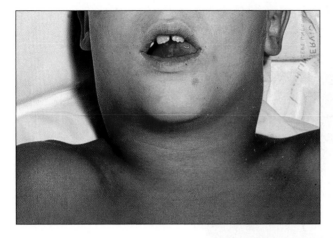

DIPHTHERIA. Bull neck appearance of diphtheritic cervical lymphadenopathy in a 13-year-old boy.

DIPHTHERIA. Diphtheritic pneumonia 3 days after admission following a tracheostomy complicated by early pneumothorax.

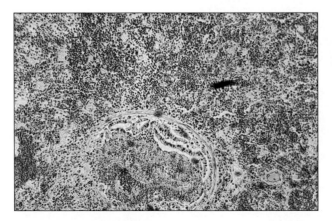

DIPHTHERIA. Diphtheria pneumonia (hemorrhagic) with bronchiolar membranes (hematoxylin-eosin stain).

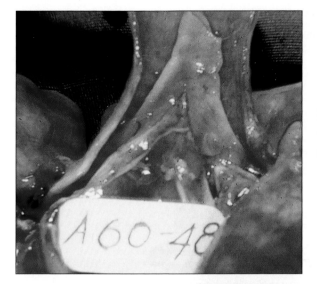

DIPHTHERIA. Diphtheritic tracheobronchial membranes at autopsy.

DIPHTHERIA. Diphtheritic pneumonia 3 days after the admission x-ray following a tracheostomy complicated by early pneumothorax.

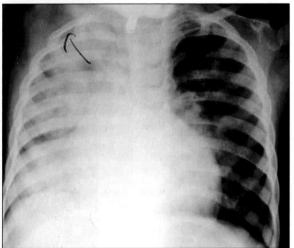

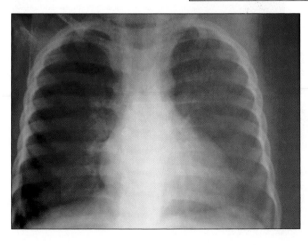

DIPHTHERIA. Chest radiograph of a 2-year-old boy with laryngotracheal diphtheria.

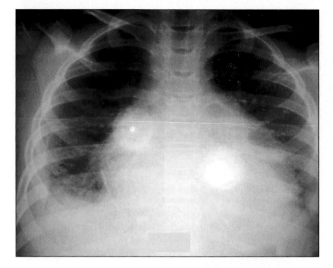

HAEMOPHILUS INFLUENZAE INFECTIONS. *H influenzae* type b bilateral pneumonia, empyema, and purulent pericarditis. Pericardiostomy drainage is important in preventing cardiac restriction.

HAEMOPHILUS INFLUENZAE INFECTIONS. *H influenzae* type b pneumonia with left pleural effusion. Pleural fluid culture and blood culture were positive for *H influenzae* type b.

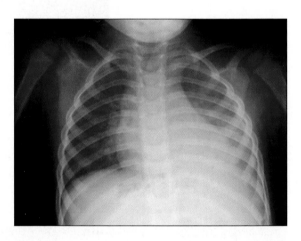

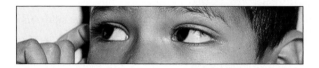

HEPATITIS A. Acute hepatitis A infection with scleral icterus in a 10-year-old boy.

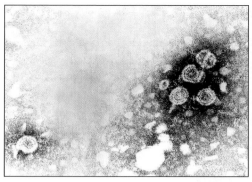

HEPATITIS B. Transmission electron micrograph of hepatitis B virions, also known as Dane particles.

INFLUENZA. Transmission electron micrograph of influenza A virus, late passage.

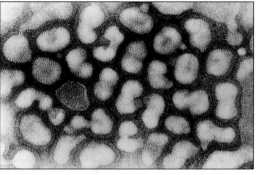

MEASLES. Close-up view of measles rash showing petechiae.

MEASLES. Measles (rubeola) with Koplik spots on fifth day of rash.

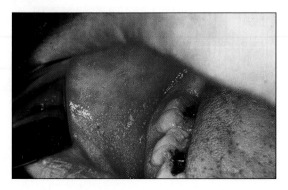

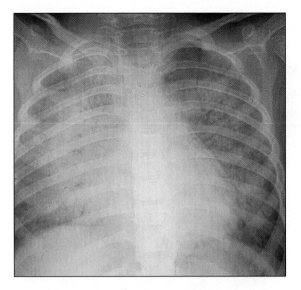

MEASLES. Measles (rubeola) pneumonia in a 6-year-old child with acute lymphoblastic leukemia.

MEASLES. Measles (rubeola) pneumonia with multinucleated giant cells and hyaline membranes (hematoxylin-eosin stain, original magnification ×250).

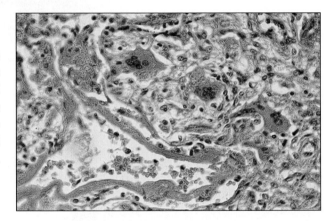

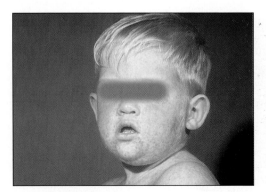

MEASLES. Face of a boy with measles, characteristic of the third day of the rash.

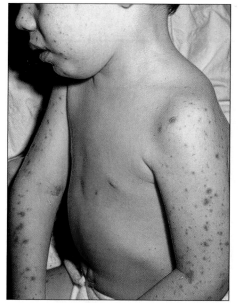

MENINGOCOCCAL INFECTIONS. Meningococcemia showing striking involvement of the extremities with relative sparing of the skin of the child's body surface.

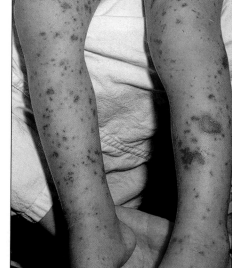

MENINGOCOCCAL INFECTIONS. Meningococcemia. This image shows the lower extremities of the patient in the previous image.

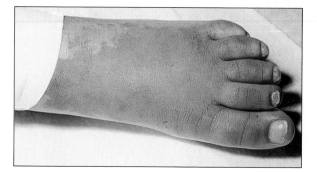

MENINGOCOCCAL INFECTIONS. Patient with marked purpura of the left foot.

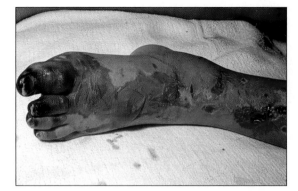

MENINGOCOCCAL INFECTIONS.
Patient shown in the previous
image with gangrene of the toes.

MENINGOCOCCAL INFECTIONS.
Preschool-aged girl with
meningococcal panophthalmitis.

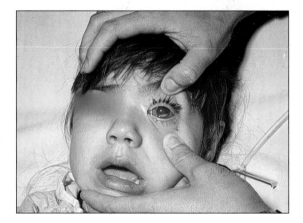

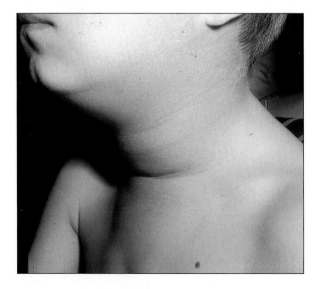

MUMPS. Mumps parotitis
with cervical and presternal
edema and erythema that
resolved spontaneously.

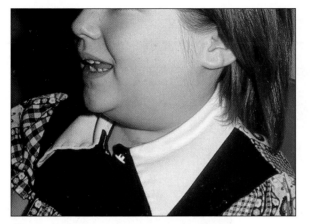

MUMPS. Characteristic appearance of mumps parotitis in an 8-year-old female.

PERTUSSIS. A 4-week-old neonate with pertussis pneumonia with pulmonary air trapping and progressive atelectasis.

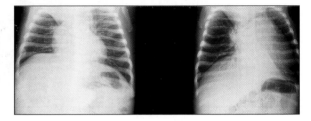

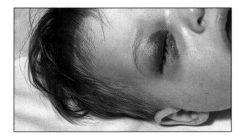

PNEUMOCOCCAL INFECTIONS. Periorbital cellulitis with purulent exudate from which *Streptococcus pneumoniae* and *Haemophilus influenzae* type b were grown on culture. *S pneumoniae* was isolated on blood culture. The cerebrospinal fluid culture was negative.

PNEUMOCOCCAL INFECTIONS. Child with acute mastoiditis due to *Streptococcus pneumoniae*.

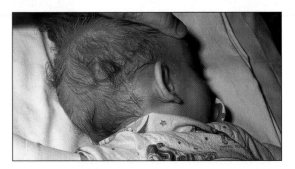

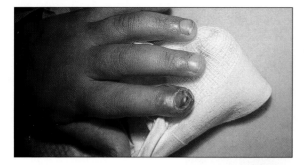

PNEUMOCOCCAL INFECTIONS.
Perionychial abscess caused by
Streptococcus pneumoniae
in a child with acute
lymphoblastic leukemia.

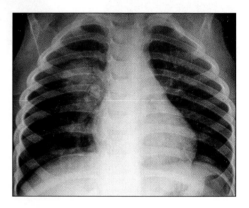

PNEUMOCOCCAL INFECTIONS.
Segmental (nodular) pneumonia due to
Streptococcus pneumoniae.

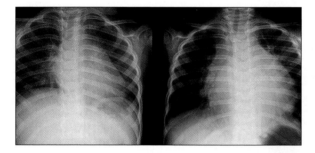

**PNEUMOCOCCAL
INFECTIONS.** Pneumonia
and pericarditis due to
Streptococcus pneumoniae.

PNEUMOCOCCAL INFECTIONS.
Acute pneumococcal pneumonia
of the left upper lobe proven by a
positive blood culture. The upper
left lobe normally appears to
involve entire left lung on the
anteroposterior view.

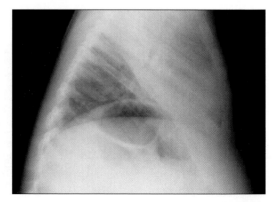

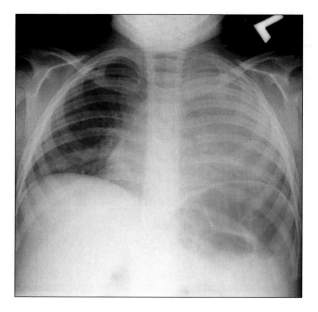

PNEUMOCOCCAL INFECTIONS. Acute pneumococcal pneumonia of the left upper lobe proven by a positive blood culture.

RUBELLA. Rubella rash of a previously unimmunized adolescent girl.

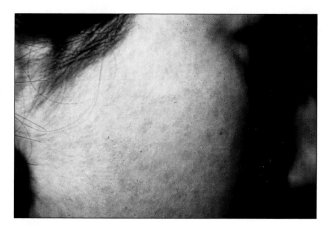

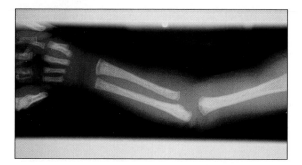

RUBELLA. Radiolucent long bone changes in metaphyses of an infant with congenital rubella.

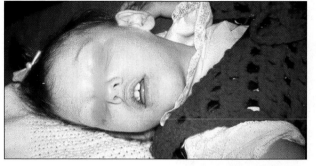

RUBELLA. A 4-year-old girl with congenital rubella with microcephaly.

RUBELLA. A 4-year-old boy with congenital rubella syndrome with unilateral microphthalmos and cataract formation in the left eye.

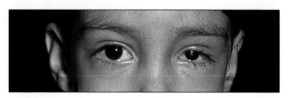

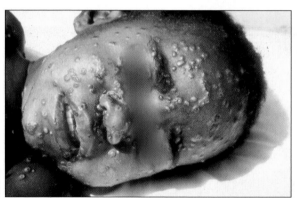

SMALLPOX (VARIOLA). Day 8. Confluence of smallpox lesions on the face and upper trunk.

SMALLPOX (VARIOLA). Posterolateral view of a child showing primary vaccination site and hypersensitivity rash.

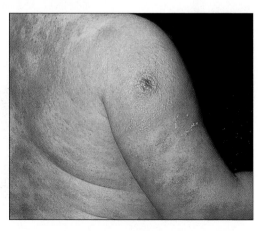

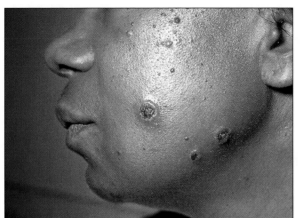

© CDC

SMALLPOX (VARIOLA).
Accidental inoculation of
vaccinia virus on the face after
a grandchild's immunization.

SMALLPOX (VARIOLA). Early smallpox
pustules on the face of an infant.

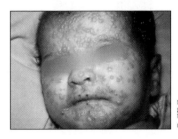

© CDC

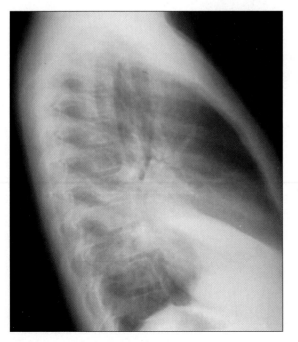

**GROUP A STREPTOCOCCAL
INFECTIONS.** Group A streptococcal pneumonia.

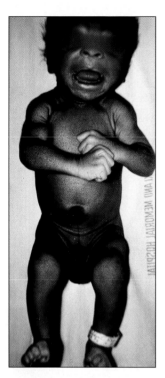

TETANUS. Neonatal tetanus. Note severe muscle spasm, generalized, and rhisus sardonicus.

VARICELLA-ZOSTER INFECTIONS. Varicella with scleral lesions and bulbar conjunctivitis.

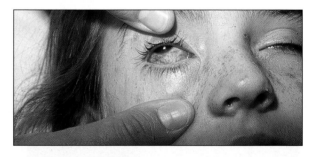

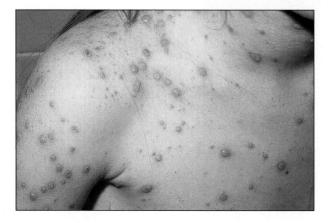

VARICELLA-ZOSTER INFECTIONS. Adolescent girl with varicella lesions in various stages.

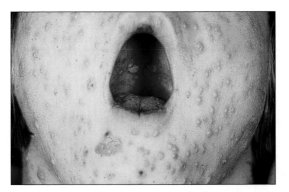

VARICELLA-ZOSTER INFECTIONS.
This child acquired her infection
from a younger sibling.

VARICELLA-ZOSTER INFECTIONS.
School-aged child with varicella who
acquired it from a younger sibling.

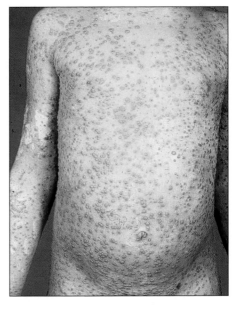

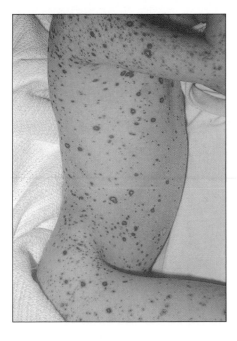

VARICELLA-ZOSTER INFECTIONS.
Hemorrhagic varicella in a 6-year-old
boy with eczema.

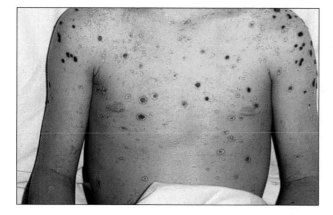

VARICELLA-ZOSTER INFECTIONS. Healing varicella in a child with eczema.

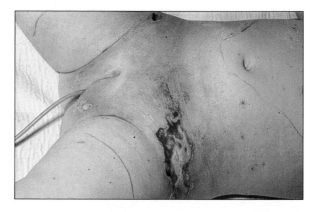

VARICELLA-ZOSTER INFECTIONS. Varicella and necrotizing fasciitis. The blood culture was positive for group A streptococcus.

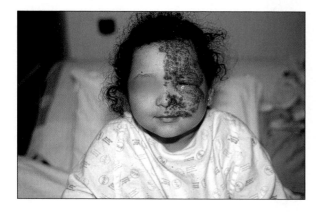

VARICELLA-ZOSTER INFECTIONS. Varicella zoster in a 7-year-old girl.

PEDIATRIC INFECTIOUS DISEASES (OTHER)

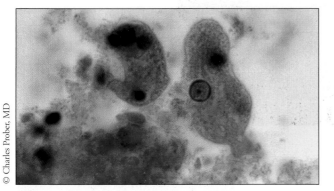

© Charles Prober, MD

AMEBIASIS. Trophozoite of *Entamoeba histolytica.*

HAEMOPHILUS INFLUENZAE **INFECTIONS.** Acute epiglottitis due to *H influenzae* type b proven by blood culture.

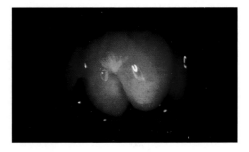

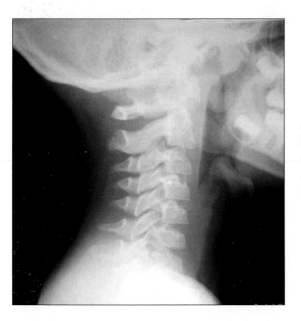

HAEMOPHILUS INFLUENZAE **INFECTIONS.** Acute *H influenzae* type b epiglottitis with striking erythema and swelling of the epiglottis.

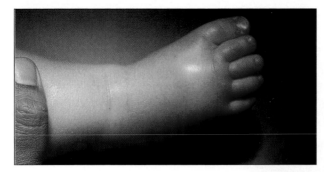

HAEMOPHILUS INFLUENZAE INFECTIONS. _H influenzae_ type b cellulitis of the foot proven by blood culture.

HAEMOPHILUS INFLUENZAE INFECTIONS. _H influenzae_ type b osteomyelitis of the distal humerus with septic arthritis of the elbow. Blood and joint fluid positive for _H influenzae_ type b.

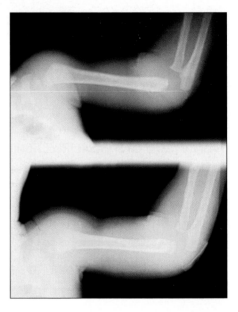

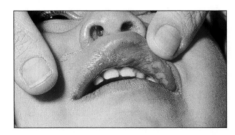

HERPES SIMPLEX. Herpes simplex stomatitis, primary infection.

HERPES SIMPLEX. Herpes simplex stomatitis, primary infection with extension to the face.

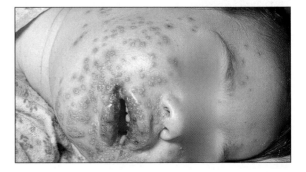

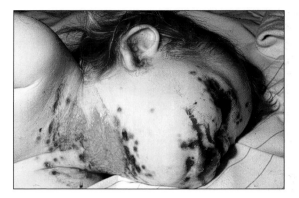

HERPES SIMPLEX. Herpes simplex infection in a child with eczema with Kaposi varicelliform eruption and Stevens-Johnson syndrome.

HERPES SIMPLEX. Neonatal herpes simplex infection with disseminated vesicular lesions.

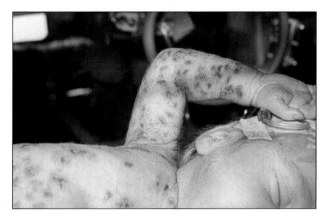

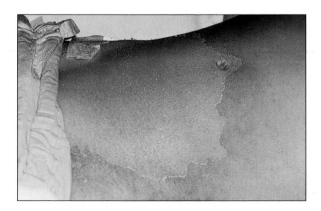

KAWASAKI SYNDROME. Characteristic desquamation of the skin over the abdomen.

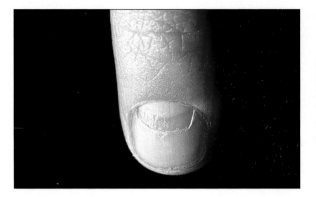

KAWASAKI SYNDROME. Periungual desquamation of a patient with Kawasaki syndrome. This is the same child as in the previous image.

LEISHMANIASIS. Cutaneous leishmaniasis. Infected sandfly inoculation site with satellite lesions.

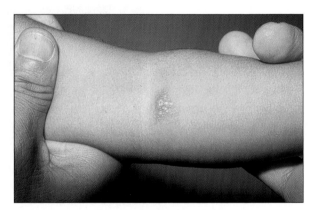

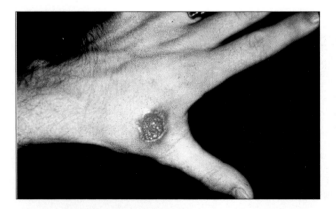

LEISHMANIASIS. Crater lesion of leishmaniasis in the skin.

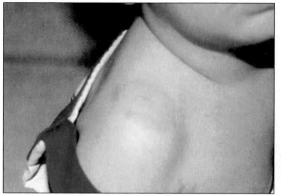

© Richard F. Jacobs, MD

LYME DISEASE. The rash of erythema migrans in a 4-year-old boy with infection due to *Borrelia burgdorferi.*

PARVOVIRUS B19. Parvovirus B19 infection (erythema infectiosum, fifth disease) in a 5-year-old girl.

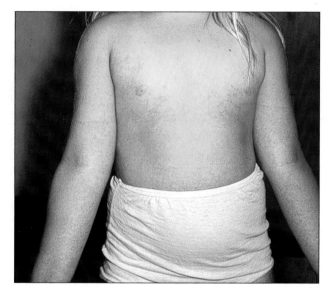

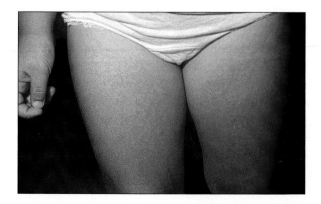

PARVOVIRUS B19. Parvovirus B19 infection (erythema infectiosum, fifth disease). This is the same child as in the previous image.

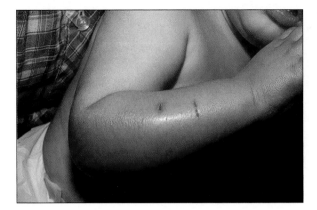

PASTEURELLA MULTOCIDA INFECTIONS. Right forearm of a 1-year-old boy bitten by a stray cat.

PNEUMOCYSTIS JIROVECI INFECTION. *P jiroveci* pneumonia with hyperaeration in an infant with congenital agammaglobulinemia.

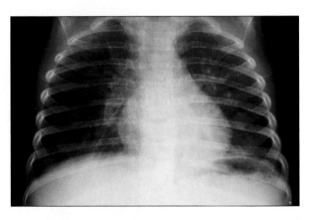

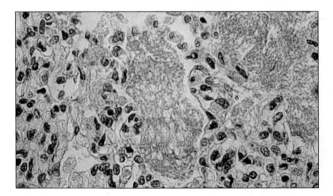

PNEUMOCYSTIS JIROVECI INFECTION. Foamy alveolar exudate in lung biopsy specimen from a patient with *P jiroveci* pneumonia (hematoxylineosin stain).

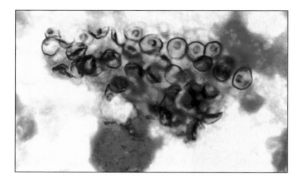

PNEUMOCYSTIS JIROVECI INFECTION. Cysts of *P jiroveci* in smear from bronchoalveolar lavage (methenamine silver stain).

ROCKY MOUNTAIN SPOTTED FEVER. Sixth day of rash without treatment.

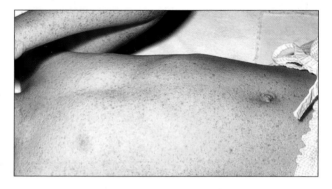

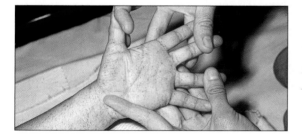

ROCKY MOUNTAIN SPOTTED FEVER. Sixth day of rash without treatment. This is the same patient as in the previous image.

ROCKY MOUNTAIN SPOTTED FEVER. This is a patient with Rocky Mountain spotted fever showing petechial rash and edema of the upper extremity.

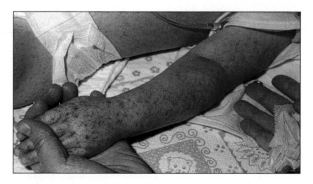

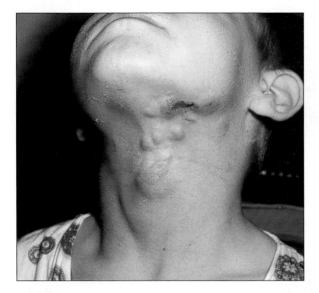

SPOROTRICHOSIS. *Sporothrix schenckii* was cultured from the biopsy specimen from an abscessed cervical lymph node of this 10-year-old boy.

SPOROTRICHOSIS. Linear lymphadenitis secondary to sporotrichosis infection of the foot.

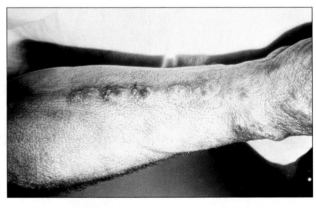

© Charles Prober, MD

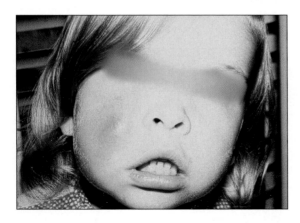

STAPHYLOCOCCAL INFECTIONS. Abscess of the face due to *Staphylococcus aureus* in an 8-year-old girl.

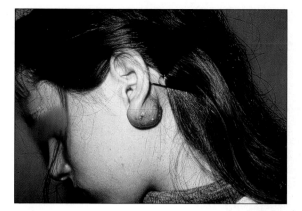

STAPHYLOCOCCAL INFECTIONS. *Staphylococcus aureus* abscess of the lobe of the left ear secondary to ear piercing in an adolescent girl.

STAPHYLOCOCCAL INFECTIONS. Orbital abscess with proptosis of the globe due to *Staphylococcus aureus* in a 12-year-old boy.

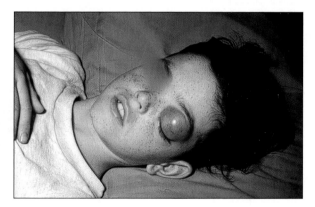

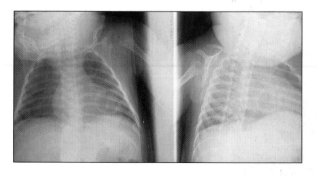

STAPHYLOCOCCAL INFECTIONS. Staphylococcal pneumonia, primary, with pneumatoceles.

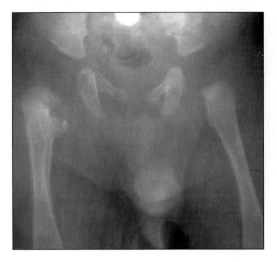

STAPHYLOCOCCAL INFECTIONS.
Osteomyelitis of right proximal femur due to *Staphylococcus aureus* with dislocation of the hip secondary to septic arthritis.

GROUP A STREPTOCOCCAL INFECTIONS. Group A streptococcal pharyngitis with petechiae on the soft palate.

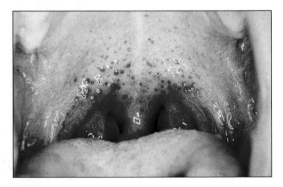

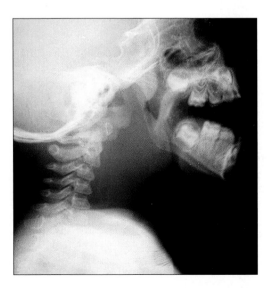

GROUP A STREPTOCOCCAL INFECTIONS. Retropharyngeal abscess on lateral neck radiograph secondary to pharyngeal infection.

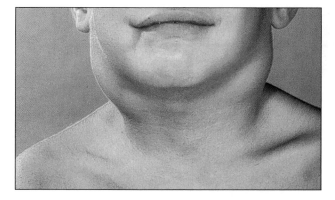

GROUP A STREPTOCOCCAL INFECTIONS. Bilateral cervical lymphadenitis.

GROUP A STREPTOCOCCAL INFECTIONS. Group A streptococcal impetigo.

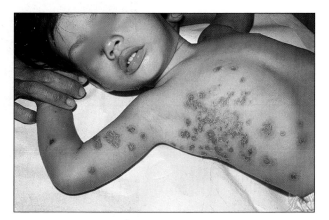

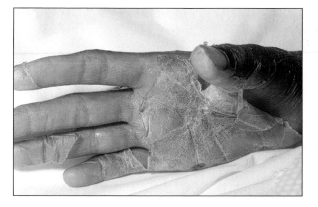

GROUP A STREPTOCOCCAL INFECTIONS. Hand of a 14-year-old boy with group A streptococcal sepsis who had hypotension, azotemia, and oliguria when first examined.

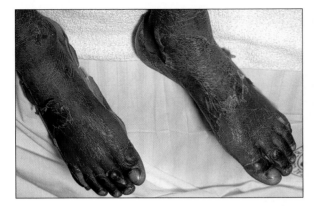

GROUP A STREPTOCOCCAL INFECTIONS. Feet of a 14-year-old boy with group A streptococcal sepsis.

GROUP A STREPTOCOCCAL INFECTIONS. Group A streptococcal pneumonia in an 8-year-old girl.

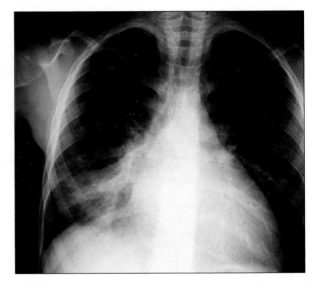

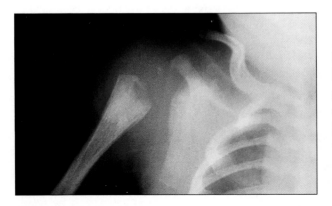

GROUP B STREPTOCOCCAL INFECTIONS. Neonatal group B streptococcal septic arthritis (right shoulder joint) and osteomyelitis (right proximal humerus).

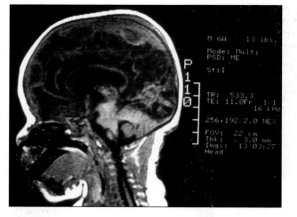

GROUP B STREPTOCOCCAL INFECTIONS. Magnetic resonance imaging after group B streptococcal meningitis.

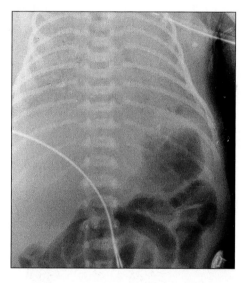

GROUP B STREPTOCOCCAL INFECTIONS. Bilateral, severe group B streptococcal pneumonia in a neonate.

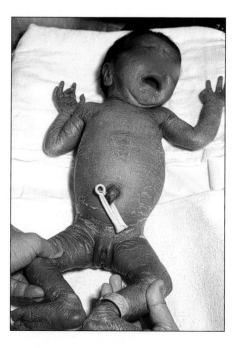

SYPHILIS. Newborn with congenital syphilis. Note the marked generalized desquamation.

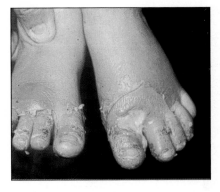

SYPHILIS. Newborn with congenital syphilis with cutaneous ulceration (luetic gumma).

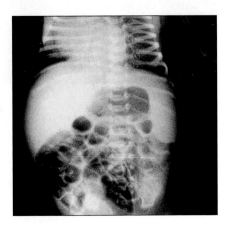

SYPHILIS. Newborn with congenital syphilis with striking hepatosplenomegaly.

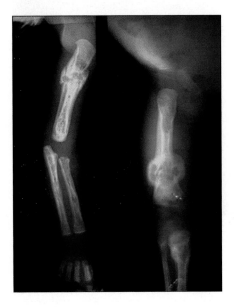

SYPHILIS. Congenital syphilis with a pathologic fracture of the proximal humerus and the distal femur.

SYPHILIS. Congenital syphilis in a 2-week-old infant boy with marked hepatosplenomegaly.

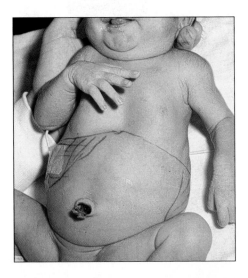

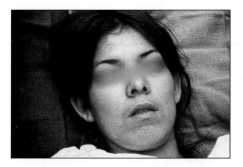

TRICHINOSIS. Striking edema of the face of a 22-year-old woman with trichinosis.

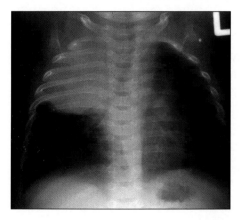

TRICHINOSIS. Striking edema of the feet of the same patient as in the previous image.

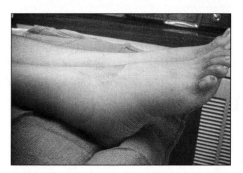

TUBERCULOSIS. A 3-month-old infant with tuberculosis. *Mycobacterium tuberculosis* grew from gastric aspirate culture.

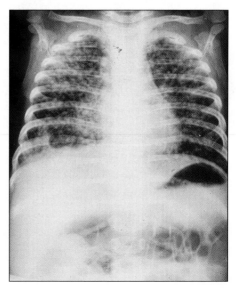

TUBERCULOSIS. Miliary tuberculosis with pulmonary cavitation (right lung).

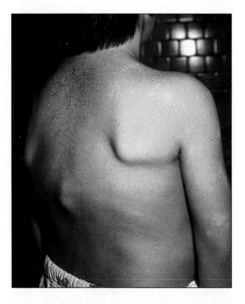

TUBERCULOSIS. Tuberculosis of the spine with paravertebral abscess (Pott disease).

TULAREMIA. *Francisella tularensis* is gram-negative in its staining morphology.

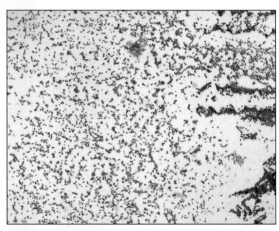

© CDC

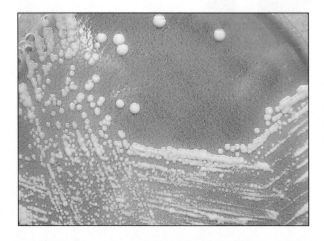

TULAREMIA. *Francisella tularensis* colonization on cysteine heart agar after 72 hours.

Examination of sexual partners is unnecessary for management of anogenital warts, because the role of reinfection probably is minimal, and treatment will not decrease transmission, because therapy usually is not curative. However, sexual partners may benefit from examination to assess for the presence of anogenital warts or other sexually transmitted diseases. Female sexual partners of patients with genital warts should be informed that cytologic screening for cervical cancer is recommended for all sexually active women.

Although respiratory papillomatosis is believed usually to be acquired during passage through the birth canal, this condition has occurred in infants delivered by cesarean section. Because the preventive value of cesarean delivery is unknown, it should not be performed to prevent transmission of HPV to the newborn.

For a report of an expert panel on prevention of genital HPV infection and sequelae, see the Centers for Disease Control and Prevention Web site (www.cdc.gov/nchstp/dstd/Reports_Publications/99HPVReport.htm). For more information on HPV, see the American Social Health Association Web site (www.ashastd.org/stdfaqs/hpv.html).

Paracoccidioidomycosis
(South American Blastomycosis)

CLINICAL MANIFESTATIONS: Disease occurs primarily in adults and is rare in children. The site of primary infection is the lungs. Clinical patterns include acute pneumonia, chronic pneumonia, and disseminated disease. Dissemination to skin, mucous membranes, lymph nodes, liver, spleen, bone, central nervous system, gastrointestinal tract, and adrenals is common in children. Chronic granulomatous lesions of the mucous membranes, especially of the mouth and palate, are typical but rare findings in adults and occur more often in children in association with enlarged, draining lymph nodes. Infection may be latent for years before causing illness.

ETIOLOGY: *Paracoccidioides brasiliensis* is a dimorphic fungus with a yeast and a mycelial phase.

EPIDEMIOLOGY: The infection occurs primarily in South America, where it is endemic. Cases also have been reported in Central America and Mexico. The natural reservoir is unknown, although soil is suspected. The mode of transmission is unknown; person-to-person transmission does not occur.

The **incubation period** is highly variable, ranging from 1 month to many years.

DIAGNOSTIC TESTS: Round, multiple-budding cells with a distinguishing pilot's wheel appearance may be seen in 10% potassium hydroxide preparations of sputum specimens, bronchoalveolar lavage specimens, scrapings from ulcers, and material from lesions or in tissue biopsy specimens. The organism can be cultured easily on most enriched media, including blood agar at 37°C (98°F) and Sabouraud dextrose agar (with cycloheximide) at 24°C (75°F). Complement fixation, enzyme immunoassay, and immunodiffusion methods are useful for detecting specific antibodies. Skin testing is not reliable for diagnosis.

TREATMENT: Amphotericin B is preferred by many experts for treatment of people with severe paracoccidioidomycosis, but amphotericin B is not curative (see Drugs for Invasive and Other Serious Fungal Infections, p 725). Itraconazole is the drug of choice for less severe or localized infection. For adults, most experts recommend itraconazole over ketoconazole; itraconazole is associated with fewer adverse effects and has a lower relapse rate. The safety and efficacy of itraconazole for treatment of children with paracoccidioidomycosis have not been established. However, treated children should receive maintenance therapy with itraconazole (4–10 mg/kg daily; maximum 200 mg, twice daily) or a sulfonamide (trimethoprim-sulfamethoxazole [trimethoprim, 8–10 mg/kg daily]). Prolonged therapy for at least 6 months is necessary to minimize the relapse rate.

ISOLATION OF THE HOSPITALIZED PATIENT: Standard precautions are recommended.

CONTROL MEASURES: None.

Paragonimiasis

CLINICAL MANIFESTATIONS: The disease has an insidious onset and a chronic course. The 2 major forms of paragonimiasis described are (1) classical paragonimiasis, which involves the lungs, and (2) nonclassical paragonimiasis, which results in a larval migrans syndrome. In classical infections, pulmonary disease is associated with chronic cough and dyspnea, but most infections probably are inapparent or result in mild symptoms. Heavy infestations cause paroxysms of coughing, which often produce blood-tinged sputum that is brown because of the presence of *Paragonimus* species eggs. Hemoptysis can be severe. Pleural effusion, pneumothorax, bronchiectasis, and pulmonary fibrosis with clubbing can develop. Extrapulmonary manifestations also may involve the abdominal cavity, skin, and uncommonly, the central nervous system, with meningoencephalitis and seizures attributable to invasion of the brain by adult flukes. Symptoms tend to subside after approximately 5 years but can persist for as many as 20 years.

Nonclassical paragonimiasis is associated with migratory subcutaneous nodules containing juvenile worms, but hemoptysis does not occur. Pleural effusion is common, as is invasion of the brain.

ETIOLOGY: In Asia, classical paragonimiasis is caused by *Paragonimus westermani* and *Paragonimus heterotremus* adult flukes and their eggs. The adult flukes of *P westermani* are up to 12 mm long and 7 mm wide and occur throughout the Far East. A triploid parthenogenetic form of *P westermani,* which is larger, produces more eggs, and elicits greater disease, has been described in Japan, Korea, Taiwan, and parts of eastern China. *Paragonimus heterotremus* occurs in southeast Asia and adjacent parts of China. Nonclassical paragonimiasis is caused by larval stages of *Paragonimus skrjabini* and *Paragonimus miyazakii.* The worms rarely mature. *Paragonimus skrjabini* occurs in China, and *P miyazakii* occurs in Japan. African forms causing classical paragonimiasis include *Paragonimus africanus* (Nigeria, Cameroon) and *Paragonimus uterobilateralis* (Liberia, Guinea, Nigeria, Gabon). *Paragonimus mexicanus* and *Paragonimus ecuadoriensis* occur in Mexico, Costa Rica, Ecuador, and Peru. *Paragonimus kellicotti*, a lung fluke of mink and opossums in the United States, also can cause a zoonotic infection in humans.

EPIDEMIOLOGY: Transmission occurs when raw or undercooked freshwater crabs or crayfish containing larvae (metacercariae) are ingested. The metacercariae excyst in the small intestine and penetrate the abdominal cavity, where they remain for a few days before migrating to the lungs. *Paragonimus westermani* and *P heterotremus* mature within the lungs over 6 to 10 weeks, when they then begin egg production. Eggs escape from pulmonary capsules into the bronchi and exit from the human host in sputum or feces. Eggs hatch in freshwater within 3 weeks, giving rise to miracidia. Miracidia penetrate freshwater snails and emerge several weeks later as cercariae, which encyst within the muscles and viscera of freshwater crustaceans before maturing into infective metacercariae. Transmission also occurs when humans ingest raw pork, usually from wild pigs, containing the juvenile stages of *Paragonimus* species (described as occurring in Japan).

Humans are accidental ("dead-end") hosts for *P skrjabini* and *P miyazakii*. These flukes cannot mature in humans and, hence, do not produce eggs.

Paragonimus species also infect a variety of other mammals, such as canids, mustelids, felids, and rodents, which can serve as animal reservoir hosts.

The **incubation period** is variable; egg production begins approximately 8 weeks after ingestion of *P westermani* metacercariae.

DIAGNOSTIC TESTS: Microscopic examination of stool, sputum, pleural effusion, cerebrospinal fluid, and other tissue specimens may reveal eggs. A Western blot serologic antibody test, available at the Centers for Disease Control and Prevention (CDC), is sensitive and specific but does not distinguish active from past infection. Charcot-Leyden crystals and eosinophils in sputum are useful diagnostic elements. Chest radiographs may appear normal or resemble those from patients with tuberculosis. Misdiagnosis is likely unless paragonimiasis is suspected.

TREATMENT: Praziquantel in a 2-day course is the drug of choice and is associated with high cure rates as demonstrated by the disappearance of egg production and radiographic lesions in the lungs. The drug also is effective for some extrapulmonary manifestations. Bithionol, available from the CDC, is an alternative drug (see Drugs for Parasitic Infections, p 744).

ISOLATION OF THE HOSPITALIZED PATIENT: Standard precautions are recommended.

CONTROL MEASURES: Cooking of crabs and crayfish for several minutes until the meat has congealed and turned opaque kills metacercariae. Similarly, meat from wild pigs should be well cooked before eating. Control of the animal reservoirs is not possible.

Parainfluenza Viral Infections

CLINICAL MANIFESTATIONS: Parainfluenza viruses are the major cause of laryngotracheobronchitis (croup), but they also commonly cause upper respiratory tract infection, pneumonia, or bronchiolitis. Types 1 and 2 viruses are the most common pathogens associated with croup, and type 3 viruses are associated with bronchiolitis and pneumonia in infants and young children. Because type 4 viruses are not detected as often as the other serotypes, infections with type 4 viruses are not as well characterized. Rarely, parotitis, aseptic meningitis, and encephalitis have been associated with type 3 infections. Parainfluenza virus infections can exacerbate symptoms of chronic lung disease in children and adults. Infections can be particularly severe and persistent in immunodeficient children and are associated most commonly with type 3 viruses. Parainfluenza infections do not confer complete protective immunity; therefore, reinfections can occur with all serotypes and at any age, but reinfections usually cause a mild illness limited to the upper respiratory tract.

ETIOLOGY: Parainfluenza viruses are enveloped RNA viruses classified as paramyxoviruses. Four antigenically distinct types—1, 2, 3, and 4 (with 2 subtypes, 4A and 4B)—have been identified.

EPIDEMIOLOGY: Parainfluenza viruses are transmitted from person to person by direct contact and exposure to contaminated nasopharyngeal secretions through respiratory tract droplets and fomites. Parainfluenza viral infections produce sporadic infections as well as epidemics of disease. Seasonal patterns of infection are distinctive, predictable, and cyclic. Different serotypes have distinct epidemiologic patterns. Type 1 virus tends to produce outbreaks of respiratory tract illness, usually croup, in the autumn of every other year. A major increase in the number of cases of croup in the autumn indicates a parainfluenza type 1 outbreak. Type 2 virus also can cause outbreaks of respiratory tract illness in the autumn, often in conjunction with type 1 outbreaks, but type 2 outbreaks tend to be less severe, irregular, and less common. Parainfluenza type 3 virus usually is prominent during spring and summer in temperate climates but often continues into autumn, especially in years when autumn outbreaks of parainfluenza types 1 or 2 are absent. Infections with type 4 virus are recognized less commonly, are sporadic, and generally are associated with mild illnesses.

The age of primary infection varies with serotype. Primary infection with all types usually occurs by 5 years of age. Infection with type 3 virus more often occurs in infants and is a prominent cause of lower respiratory tract illnesses. By 12 months of age, 50% of infants have acquired type 3 infection. Infections between 1 and 5 years of age are associated most commonly with type 1 and less so with type 2. Type 4 infections are not as well understood.

Immunocompetent children with primary parainfluenza infection may shed virus for up to 1 week before the onset of clinical symptoms until 1 to 3 weeks after symptoms have disappeared, depending on serotype. Severe lower respiratory tract disease with prolonged shedding of the virus can develop in immunodeficient people. In these patients, infection may spread beyond the respiratory tract to the liver and lymph nodes.

The **incubation period** ranges from 2 to 6 days.

DIAGNOSTIC TESTS: Virus may be isolated from nasopharyngeal secretions usually within 4 to 7 days of culture inoculation or earlier by using centrifugation of a specimen onto a monolayer of susceptible cells with subsequent staining for viral antigen (shell viral assay). Confirmation is made by rapid antigen detection, usually immunofluorescence. Rapid antigen identification techniques, including immunofluorescence assays, enzyme immunoassays, radioimmunoassays, and fluoroimmunoassays, can be used to detect the virus in nasopharyngeal secretions, but the sensitivities of the tests vary. Multiplex reverse transcriptase-polymerase chain reaction assay, with high sensitivity and specificity, is available for detection and differentiation of parainfluenza viruses. Serologic diagnosis, made retrospectively by a significant increase in antibody titer between serum specimens obtained during acute infection and convalescence, may be confusing, because increases in heterotypic antibody concentrations attributable to infections caused by other serotypes of parainfluenza and mumps viruses are common. Furthermore, infection may not always be accompanied by a significant homotypic antibody response. Less is known about the antibody response to type 4 infection, but homotypic response is usual in primary infection.

TREATMENT: Specific antiviral therapy is not available. Most infections are self-limited and require no treatment. Monitoring for oxygenation and hypercapnia for more severely affected children with lower respiratory tract disease may be helpful. Epinephrine aerosol commonly is given to severely affected, hospitalized patients with laryngotracheobronchitis to decrease airway obstruction. Parenteral dexamethasone in high doses (>0.3 mg/kg), oral dexamethasone (0.15–0.6 mg/kg), and nebulized corticosteroids have been demonstrated to lessen the severity and duration of symptoms and hospitalization in patients with moderate to severe laryngotracheobronchitis. Oral dexamethasone (0.15 mg/kg) also is effective for outpatients with less severe croup. Management otherwise is supportive. Antimicrobial agents should be reserved for documented secondary bacterial infections.

ISOLATION OF THE HOSPITALIZED PATIENT: In addition to standard precautions, contact precautions are recommended for hospitalized infants and young children for the duration of illness. Strict adherence to infection control procedures, including prevention of environmental contamination by respiratory tract secretions and careful hand hygiene, should control nosocomial spread. Immunocompromised patients with type 3 infection should be isolated to prevent nosocomial spread.

CONTROL MEASURES: Efforts should be aimed at decreasing nosocomial infection. Hand hygiene should be emphasized.

Parasitic Diseases

Many parasitic diseases traditionally have been considered exotic and, therefore, frequently are not included in differential diagnoses of patients in the United States, Canada, and Europe. Nevertheless, a number of these organisms are endemic in industrialized countries, and overall, parasites are among the most common causes of morbidity and mortality in various and diverse geographic locations worldwide. Outside the tropics and subtropics, parasite diseases are most common among tourists returning to their own countries, immigrants from highly endemic areas, and immunocompromised people. Physicians and clinical laboratory personnel need to be aware of where these infections may be acquired, their clinical presentations, and methods of diagnosis and should advise travelers how to prevent infection. Table 3.38 (p 457) gives details on some infrequently encountered parasitic diseases.

Consultation and assistance in diagnosis and management of parasitic diseases are available from government agencies (eg, Centers for Disease Control and Prevention [CDC] and state health departments) and university departments or divisions of geographic medicine, tropical medicine, pediatric infectious disease, international health, and public health.

The CDC distributes several drugs that are not available commercially in the United States for treatment of parasitic diseases. These drugs are indicated by footnotes in Table 4.14, Drugs for Treatment of Parasitic Infections (p 744). To request these drugs, a physician must contact the CDC Drug Service (see Appendix I, Directory of Resources, p 789) and provide the following information: (1) the physician's name, address, and telephone number; (2) the type of infection to be treated and the method by which the infection was diagnosed; (3) the patient's name, age, weight, sex, and if the patient is female, whether she is pregnant; and (4) basic demographic, clinical, and epidemiologic, information. Consultation with a medical officer from the CDC may be required before a drug is distributed.

Important human parasitic infections are discussed in individual chapters in Section 3; the diseases are arranged alphabetically, and the discussions include recommendations for drug treatment. Tables 4.13 (p 745) and 4.14 (p 770), reproduced from *The Medical Letter* (see Drugs for Treatment of Parasitic Infections, p 744), provide dosage recommendations and other relevant information for specific antiparasitic drugs. Although the recommendations for administration of these drugs given in the disease-specific chapters are similar, they may not be identical in all instances because of differences of opinion among experts. Both sources should be consulted.

Table 3.38. **Additional Parasitic Diseases**[1]

Disease and/or Agent	Where Infection May Be Acquired	Definitive Host	Intermediate Host	Modes of Human Infection	Directly Communicable (Person to Person)	Diagnostic Laboratory Tests in Humans	Causative Form of Parasite	Manifestations in Humans
Angiostrongylus cantonensis	Widespread in the tropics, particularly Pacific Islands, Southeast Asia, and Central America	Rats	Snails and slugs	Eating improperly cooked infected mollusks	No	Eosinophils in CSF; rarely, identification of larvae in CSF or at autopsy	Larval worms	Eosinophilia, meningoencephalitis
Angiostrongylus costaricensis	Central and South America	Rodents	Snails and slugs	Eating poorly cooked infected mollusks or food contaminated by mollusk secretions containing larvae	No	Gel diffusion; identification of larvae and eggs in tissue	Larval worms	Abdominal pain, eosinophilia
Anisakiasis	Cosmopolitan, mainly Japan	Marine mammals	Certain saltwater fish, squid, and octopus	Eating uncooked infected fish	No	Identification of recovered larvae in granulomas or vomitus	Larval worms	Acute gastrointestinal disease
Baylisascaris procyonis (raccoon roundworm)	North America	Raccoon	None	Exposure to raccoon feces (pica, geophagia)	No	Eosinophils in blood and cerebrospinal fluid; identification of larvae in eye or brain; serologic testing	Larval worms	Ocular and neural larval migrans, encephalitis
Clonorchis sinensis, Opisthorchis viverrini, Opisthorchis felineus	Far East, Eastern Europe, Russian Federation	Humans, cats, dogs, other mammals	Certain freshwater snails	Eating uncooked infected freshwater fish	No	Eggs in stool or duodenal fluid	Larvae and mature flukes	Abdominal pain; hepatobiliary disease

Table 3.38. Additional Parasitic Diseases, [1] continued

Diseases and/or Agent	Where Infection May Be Acquired	Definitive Host	Intermediate Host	Modes of Human Infection	Directly Communicable (Person to Person)	Diagnostic Laboratory Tests in Humans	Causative Form of Parasite	Manifestations in Humans
Dracunculiasis (*Dracunculus medinensis*)	Foci in Africa	Humans	Crustacea (copepods)	Drinking infested water	No	Identification of emerging or adult worm in subcutaneous tissues	Adult female worm	Emerging roundworm; inflammatory response; systemic and local blister or ulcer in skin
Fascioliasis (*Fasciola hepatica*)	Foci throughout tropics and temperate areas	Humans, sheep, other herbivores	Certain freshwater snails and vegetation	Eating uncooked infected plants, such as watercress	No	Eggs in feces, duodenal fluid, or bile; serologic tests	Larvae and mature worms	Disease of liver and biliary tree; acute gastrointestinal disease
Fasciolopsiasis (*Fasciolopsis buski*)	Far East	Humans, pigs, dogs	Certain freshwater snails, plants	Eating uncooked infected plants	No	Eggs or worm in feces or duodenal fluid	Larvae and mature worms	Diarrhea, constipation, vomiting, anorexia, edema of face and legs, ascites
Intestinal capillariasis (*Capillaria philippinensis*)	Philippines, Thailand	Humans, fish-eating birds	Fish	Ingestion of uncooked infected fish	Uncertain	Eggs and parasite in feces	Larvae and mature worms	Protein-losing enteropathy, diarrhea, malabsorption, ascites, emaciation

CSF indicates cerebrospinal fluid.
[1] For recommended drug treatment, see Drugs for Treatment of Parasitic Infections (p 744).

Parvovirus B19
(Erythema Infectiosum, Fifth Disease)

CLINICAL MANIFESTATIONS: Infection with parvovirus B19 is recognized most often as erythema infectiosum (EI), which is characterized by mild systemic symptoms, fever in 15% to 30% of patients, and commonly, a distinctive rash. The facial rash is intensely red with a "slapped cheek" appearance that often is accompanied by circumoral pallor. A symmetric, maculopapular, lace-like, and often pruritic rash also occurs on the trunk, moving peripherally to involve the arms, buttocks, and thighs. The rash can fluctuate in intensity and recur with environmental changes, such as temperature and exposure to sunlight, for weeks to months. A brief, mild, nonspecific illness consisting of fever, malaise, myalgias, and headache often precedes the characteristic exanthema by approximately 7 to 10 days. Arthralgia and arthritis occur rarely among infected children but commonly among adults, especially women.

Human parvovirus B19 also can cause other manifestations (Table 3.39, p 460), including asymptomatic infection, a mild respiratory tract illness with no rash, a rash atypical for EI that may be rubelliform or petechial, polyarthropathy syndrome (arthralgia and arthritis in adults in the absence of other manifestations of EI), chronic erythroid hypoplasia in immunodeficient patients, and transient aplastic crisis lasting 7 to 10 days in patients with hemolytic anemias (eg, sickle cell disease and auto-immune hemolytic anemia) and other conditions associated with low hemoglobin concentrations, including hemorrhage, severe anemia, and thalassemia. Chronic parvovirus B19 infection may cause severe anemia in patients infected with human immunodeficiency virus (HIV). In addition, parvovirus B19 infection sometimes has been associated with thrombocytopenia and neutropenia. Patients with aplastic crisis may have a prodromal illness with fever, malaise, and myalgia, but rash usually is absent. Red blood cell aplasia is related to lytic infection in erythrocyte precursors.

Parvovirus B19 infection occurring during pregnancy can cause fetal hydrops and death but is not a proven cause of congenital anomalies. The risk of fetal death is between 2% and 6%, with the greatest risk occurring during the first half of pregnancy.

ETIOLOGY: Human parvovirus B19 is a nonenveloped, single-stranded DNA virus that replicates only in human erythrocyte precursors.

EPIDEMIOLOGY: Parvovirus B19 is distributed worldwide and is a common cause of infection in humans, who are the only known hosts. Modes of transmission include contact with respiratory tract secretions, percutaneous exposure to blood or blood products, and vertical transmission from mother to fetus. Parvovirus B19 infections are ubiquitous, and cases of EI can occur sporadically or in outbreaks in elementary or junior high schools during late winter and early spring. Secondary spread among susceptible household members is common and occurs in approximately 50% of susceptible contacts. The transmission rate in schools is less, but infection can be an occupational risk for school and child care personnel, with approximately 20% of susceptible people becoming infected. In young children, antibody seroprevalence generally is 5% to 10%. In most communities, approxi-

Table 3.39. **Clinical Manifestations of Human Parvovirus B19 Infection**

Conditions	Usual hosts
Erythema infectiosum (fifth disease)	Immunocompetent children
Polyarthropathy syndrome	Immunocompetent adults (more common in women)
Chronic anemia/pure red cell aplasia	Immunocompromised hosts
Transient aplastic crisis	People with hemolytic anemia (ie, sickle cell anemia)
Hydrops fetalis/congenital anemia	Fetus (first 20 weeks of pregnancy)

mately 50% of young adults and often more than 90% of elderly people are seropositive. The annual seroconversion rate in women of childbearing age has been reported to be approximately 1.5%. The timing of the presence of parvovirus B19 DNA in serum and respiratory tract secretions indicates that people with EI are most infectious before onset of the rash and are unlikely to be infectious after onset of the rash. In contrast, patients with aplastic crises are contagious from before the onset of symptoms through at least the week after onset. Transmission from patients with aplastic crisis to hospital personnel can occur.

The **incubation period** from acquisition of parvovirus B19 to onset of initial symptoms usually is between 4 and 14 days but can be as long as 21 days. Rash and joint symptoms occur 2 to 3 weeks after infection.

DIAGNOSTIC TESTS: In the immunocompetent host, detection of serum parvovirus B19-specific immunoglobulin (Ig) M antibody is the preferred diagnostic test. A positive IgM test result indicates that infection probably occurred within the previous 2 to 4 months. On the basis of radioimmunoassay or enzyme immunoassay results, antibody may be detected in 90% or more of patients at the time of the EI rash and by the third day of illness in patients with transient aplastic crisis. Serum IgG antibody indicates previous infection and immunity. These assays are available through commercial laboratories and through some state health department and research laboratories. However, their sensitivity and specificity may vary, particularly for IgM antibody. The optimal method for detecting chronic infection in the immunocompromised patient is demonstration of virus by nucleic acid hybridization or polymerase chain reaction (PCR) assays, because parvovirus B19 antibody is variably present in persistent infection. Because parvovirus B19 DNA can be detected by PCR assay in serum for up to 9 months after the acute viremic phase, detection of parvovirus B19 DNA by PCR assay does not necessarily indicate acute infection. The less sensitive nucleic acid hybridization assays usually are positive for only 2 to 4 days after onset of illness. For HIV-infected patients with severe anemia associated with chronic infection, dot blot hybridization of serum specimens may have adequate sensitivity. Parvovirus B19 has not been grown in standard cell culture, but the virus has been cultivated in experimental cell culture.

TREATMENT: For most patients, only supportive care is indicated. Patients with aplastic crises may require transfusion. For treatment of chronic infection in immunodeficient patients, Immune Globulin Intravenous therapy is often effective and should be considered. Some cases of parvovirus B19 infection concurrent with hydrops fetalis have been treated successfully with intrauterine blood transfusions.

ISOLATION OF THE HOSPITALIZED PATIENT: In addition to standard precautions, droplet precautions are recommended for hospitalized children with aplastic crises or immunosuppressed patients with chronic infection and anemia for the duration of hospitalization. For patients with transient aplastic or erythrocyte crisis, these precautions should be maintained for 7 days.

Pregnant health care professionals should be informed of the potential risks to the fetus from parvovirus B19 infections and about preventive measures that may decrease these risks, for example, attention to strict infection control procedures and not caring for immunocompromised patients with chronic parvovirus infection or patients with parvovirus B19-associated aplastic crises, because patients in both groups are likely to be contagious.

CONTROL MEASURES:
- Women who are exposed to children at home or at work (eg, teachers or child care workers) are at increased risk of infection with parvovirus B19. However, because school or child care center outbreaks often indicate wider spread in the community that includes inapparent infection, women are at some degree of risk of exposure from other sources at home or in the community. In view of the high prevalence of parvovirus B19 infection, the low incidence of ill effects on the fetus, and the fact that avoidance of child care or classroom teaching can decrease but not eliminate the risk of exposure, routine exclusion of pregnant women from the workplace where EI is occurring is not recommended. Women of childbearing age who are concerned can undergo serologic testing for IgG antibody to parvovirus B19 to determine their susceptibility to infection.
- Pregnant women who find that they have been in contact with children who were in the incubation period of EI or with children who were in aplastic crisis should have the relatively low potential risk of infection explained to them, and the option of serologic testing should be offered. Fetal ultrasonography may prove useful in these situations.
- Children with EI may attend child care or school, because they are no longer contagious.
- Transmission of parvovirus B19 is likely to be decreased through use of routine infection control practices, including hand hygiene and proper disposal of used facial tissues.

Pasteurella Infections

CLINICAL MANIFESTATIONS: The most common manifestation in children is cellulitis at the site of a scratch or bite of a cat, dog, or other animal. This usually occurs within 24 hours and includes swelling, erythema, tenderness, and serous or sanguinopurulent discharge at the site. Regional lymphadenopathy, chills, and fever can occur. Local complications, such as septic arthritis, osteomyelitis, and tenosynovitis, are common. Less common manifestations of infection include septicemia, meningitis, respiratory tract infections (eg, pneumonia, pulmonary abscesses, and empyema), appendicitis, hepatic abscess, peritonitis, urinary tract infection, and ocular infections, including conjunctivitis, corneal ulcer, and endophthalmitis. People with underlying abnormalities with host defense, especially liver disease, are predisposed to bacteremia attributable to *Pasteurella multocida* infection.

ETIOLOGY: Species of the genus *Pasteurella* are facultatively anaerobic, saccharolytic, gram-negative coccobacilli or rods that are primary pathogens in animals. The most common human pathogen is *P multocida.* Most human infections are caused by the following species or subspecies: *P multocida* subspecies *multocida, P multocida* subspecies *septica, Pasteurella canis, Pasteurella stomatis, Pasteurella dagmatis,* and *Pasteurella haemolytica.*

EPIDEMIOLOGY: *Pasteurella* species are found in the oral flora of 70% to 90% of cats, 25% to 50% of dogs, and many other animals. Transmission occurs from the bite or scratch of a cat or dog or, less commonly, from another animal. Respiratory tract spread from animals to humans also occurs. In a significant proportion of cases, no animal exposure can be identified. Human-to-human spread has not been documented.

The **incubation period** usually is less than 24 hours.

DIAGNOSTIC TESTS: The isolation of *Pasteurella* species from skin lesion drainage or other sites of infection (eg, joint fluid, cerebrospinal fluid, sputum, pleural fluid, or suppurative lymph nodes) is diagnostic. Although *Pasteurella* species resemble several other organisms morphologically and grow on many culture media at 37°C (98°F), laboratory differentiation is not difficult.

TREATMENT: The drug of choice is penicillin. Other effective oral agents include ampicillin, amoxicillin-clavulanate potassium, cefuroxime, cefpodoxime proxetil, trimethoprim-sulfamethoxazole, doxycycline, and quinolones. Erythromycin, clindamycin, cephalexin, cefadroxil, cefaclor, and dicloxacillin are not as active and should not be used. For patients allergic to β-lactam agents, azithromycin dihydrate or trimethoprim-sulfamethoxazole are alternative choices, but clinical experience with these agents is limited, and there are clinical reports of treatment failure with macrolides. Doxycycline is effective but should be given to children younger than 8 years of age only after assessment of the risk-benefit ratio. Quinolones are not recommended for patients younger than 18 years of age. For polymicrobial infection, which often includes *Staphylococcus aureus,* oral amoxicillin-clavulanate or, for severe infection, intravenous ampicillin-sulbactam sodium or ticarcillin disodium-clavulanate can be given. Parenterally administered, broad-spectrum cephalosporins, such as cefotaxime sodium or cefoxitin sodium, are active against *Pasteurella* species in vitro, but experience with these drugs for treatment is limited. The duration of therapy usually is 7 to 10 days for local infections and 10 to 14 days for more severe infections. Wound drainage or débridement may be necessary.

ISOLATION OF THE HOSPITALIZED PATIENT: Standard precautions are recommended.

CONTROL MEASURES: Education and limiting contact with wild and domestic animals can help to prevent *Pasteurella* infections (see Bite Wounds, p 182). Animal bites and scratches should be irrigated, cleansed, and débrided promptly. Minimal data exist about advisability of surgical closure of the wounds. Antimicrobial prophylaxis with penicillin or amoxicillin-clavulanate may be given, but data supporting efficacy are limited (see Table 2.19, p 183).

Pediculosis Capitis*
(Head Lice)

CLINICAL MANIFESTATIONS: Itching is the most common symptom of head lice infestation, but many children are asymptomatic. Adult lice or eggs (nits) are found in the hair, usually behind the ears and near the nape of the neck. Excoriations and crusting caused by secondary bacterial infection may occur and often are associated with regional lymphadenopathy. In temperate climates, head lice deposit their eggs on a hair shaft 3 to 4 mm from the scalp. Because hair grows at a rate of approximately 1 cm per month, the duration of infestation can be estimated by the distance of the nit from the scalp.

ETIOLOGY: *Pediculus humanus capitis* is the head louse. Both nymphs and adult lice feed on human blood.

EPIDEMIOLOGY: Head lice infestation in children attending child care and school is common in the United States. Head lice are not a sign of poor hygiene, and all socioeconomic groups are affected. Infestations are less common in black children than in children of other races. Head lice infestation is not influenced by hair length or frequency of shampooing or brushing. Head lice are not a health hazard, because they are not responsible for spread of any disease. Transmission occurs by direct contact with hair of infested people and, less commonly, by contact with personal belongings, such as combs, hair brushes, and hats. Head lice can survive only 1 to 2 days away from the scalp, and their eggs cannot hatch at a lower ambient temperature than that close to the scalp.

The **incubation period** from the laying of eggs to the hatching of the first nymph is 6 to 10 days. Mature adult lice capable of reproducing do not appear until 2 to 3 weeks later.

---

* American Academy of Pediatrics, Committee on School Health and Committee on Infectious Diseases. Clinical report: head lice. *Pediatrics.* 2002;110:638–643

DIAGNOSTIC TESTS: Identification of eggs, nymphs, and lice with the naked eye is possible; the diagnosis can be confirmed by using a hand lens or microscope. Adult lice seldom are seen, because they move rapidly and conceal themselves effectively.

TREATMENT: The following agents are effective for treating pediculosis of the scalp (see Drugs for Treatment of Parasitic Infections, p 744). Safety is a major concern with pediculicides, because the infestation itself does not present a risk to the host. Pediculicides should be used only as directed and with care. Instructions on proper use of any product should be explained carefully.

- *Permethrin (1%).* Permethrin is available without a prescription in a 1% cream rinse that is applied to the scalp and hair for 10 minutes. Permethrin has several advantages over other pediculicides: a low potential for toxic effects, a high cure rate, and possible ovicidal activity. Although activity continues for 2 weeks or more after application, most experts advise a second treatment 7 to 10 days after the first. Widespread resistance to permethrin has been reported in other countries. Although resistance to permethrin has been documented in the United States, the prevalence of resistance is not known.

- *Pyrethrin-based products.* Ten-minute shampoos are available without prescription. Ovicidal activity is low, there is no residual activity, and repeated application 7 to 10 days later is necessary to kill newly hatched lice. Resistance to these compounds has not been documented in the United States but has been reported in other countries. These products are contraindicated in people who are allergic to chrysanthemums.

- *Lindane (1%).* This 4-minute shampoo requires a prescription in the United States and is indicated primarily for people who have not responded to or are intolerant of other approved therapies. Ovicidal activity is low, and repeated application 7 to 10 days later often is recommended. Lindane resistance in a number of countries has been reported. Lindane is contraindicated for use in premature infants, people with known seizure disorders, and people with hypersensitivity to the product; lindane should be used with caution in patients with inflamed or traumatized skin, in children younger than 2 years of age, and in pregnant or nursing women. Although lindane has the highest potential for toxic effects of all pediculicides, serious adverse effects rarely have been reported when used according to product instructions. Toxic effects with lindane usually have been associated with misuse, such as ingestion, excessive doses, or prolonged or repeated administration.

- *Malathion (0.5%).* This pesticide requires a prescription, is highly effective for treatment of head lice, and is safe when used as directed. The only preparation currently available in the United States is a 0.5% lotion, recommended for use in an 8- to 12-hour application that is to be repeated in 7 to 9 days if lice are still present at that time. Malathion lotion is flammable and, if ingested, can cause severe respiratory distress. Malathion is contraindicated in neonates and infants because of increased scalp permeability and higher malathion absorption.

Because pediculicides kill lice shortly after application, detection of living lice on scalp inspection 24 hours or more after treatment suggests incorrect use of pediculicide, a very heavy infestation, reinfestation, or resistance to therapy. In such situations, after excluding incorrect use, immediate retreatment with a different pediculicide followed by a second application 7 days later is recommended. Itching or mild burning of the scalp caused by inflammation of the skin in response to topical therapeutic agents can persist for many days after lice are killed and is not a reason for retreatment. Topical corticosteroids and oral antihistamines may be beneficial for relieving these signs and symptoms.

Removal of nits after treatment with a pediculicide is not necessary to prevent spread. Removal of nits may be attempted for aesthetic reasons or to decrease diagnostic confusion, but the process is tedious. Trimethoprim-sulfamethoxazole and ivermectin have been shown to be effective, but neither is licensed by the US Food and Drug Administration for use as a pediculicide. Data are needed to determine whether suffocation of lice by application of occlusive agents, such as petroleum jelly, olive oil, or mayonnaise, is effective as a method of treatment.

ISOLATION OF THE HOSPITALIZED PATIENT: In addition to standard precautions, contact precautions are recommended until the patient has been treated with an appropriate pediculicide.

CONTROL MEASURES: Household and other close contacts should be examined and treated if infested. Differentiation of nits from benign hair casts (a layer of follicular cells that easily slides off the hair shaft), plugs of desquamated epithelial cells, and external debris can be difficult. Bedmates should be treated prophylactically. Children should not be excluded or sent home early from school because of head lice. Parents of affected children should be notified and informed that their child must be properly treated before returning to school on the day after treatment. After proper application of an appropriate pediculicide, reinfestation of children from an untreated infested contact is more common than treatment failure.

"No-nit" policies requiring that children be free of nits before they return to child care or school have not been effective in controlling head lice transmission and are not recommended. Lice incubating in egg cases (nits) are so close to the scalp that they are difficult to remove with nit combs. Egg cases further from the scalp are easier to remove but are empty and, thus, are of no consequence.

Most children can be treated effectively without extra efforts to treat their clothing or bedding. Although fomites do not have a major role in transmission of head lice, some parents may wish to disinfest headgear, pillow cases, and towels by washing them in hot water and machine drying (using a hot cycle). Combs and hair brushes can be washed with a pediculicide shampoo or soaked in hot water. Temperatures exceeding 53.5°C (128.3°F) for 5 minutes are lethal to lice and eggs. Although rarely necessary, dry cleaning clothing or simply storing contaminated items in well-sealed plastic bags for 10 days also is effective. Disinfesting furniture, such as chairs and sofas, is not necessary. Environmental insecticide sprays increase chemical exposure of household members and have not been helpful in the control of head lice. Vacuuming is a safe and effective alternative to spraying. Treatment of dogs, cats, or other pets is not indicated.

Pediculosis Corporis
(Body Lice)

CLINICAL MANIFESTATIONS: Intense itching, particularly at night, is common with body lice infestations. Body lice and their eggs live in the seams of clothing. Rarely, a louse can be seen feeding on the skin. Secondary bacterial infection of the skin caused by scratching is common.

ETIOLOGY: *Pediculus humanus corporis* (or *humanus*) is the body louse. Nymphs and adult lice feed on human blood.

EPIDEMIOLOGY: Body lice generally are found on people with poor hygiene. Fomites have a role in transmission. Body lice cannot survive away from a blood source for longer than 10 days. In contrast with head lice, body lice are well-recognized vectors of disease (eg, epidemic typhus, trench fever, and relapsing fever).

The **incubation period** from laying eggs to hatching of the first nymph is 6 to 10 days. Mature adult lice capable of reproducing do not appear until 2 to 3 weeks later.

DIAGNOSTIC TESTS: Identification of eggs, nymphs, and lice with the naked eye is possible; the diagnosis can be confirmed by using a hand lens or microscope. Adult lice seldom are seen, because they move rapidly and conceal themselves effectively.

TREATMENT: Treatment consists of improving hygiene and cleaning clothes and bedding. Infested materials can be washed and dried at hot temperatures to kill lice. Pediculicides are not necessary if materials are laundered at least weekly.

ISOLATION OF THE HOSPITALIZED PATIENT: In addition to standard precautions, contact precautions are recommended until the patient has been treated.

CONTROL MEASURES: The most important factor in the control of body lice infestation is the ability to change and wash clothing. Close contacts should be examined and treated appropriately; clothing and bedding should be laundered.

Pediculosis Pubis
(Pubic Lice)

CLINICAL MANIFESTATIONS: Pruritus of the anogenital area is a common symptom in pubic lice infestations ("crabs"). Many hairy areas of the body can be infested, including the eyelashes, eyebrows, beard, axilla, perianal area, and rarely, the scalp. A characteristic sign of heavy pubic lice infestation is the presence of bluish or slate-colored maculae on the chest, abdomen, or thighs, known as maculae ceruleae.

ETIOLOGY: *Phthirus pubis* is the pubic or crab louse. Nymphs and adult lice feed on human blood.

EPIDEMIOLOGY: Pubic lice infestations are common in adolescents and young adults and usually are transmitted through sexual contact. The pubic louse also can be transferred by contaminated items, such as towels. Pubic lice can be found on the eyelashes of younger children and, although other modes of transmission are possible, may be evidence of sexual abuse. Infested people should be examined for other sexually transmitted diseases, including syphilis and infection with *Neisseria gonorrhoeae, Chlamydia trachomatis,* hepatitis B virus, and human immunodeficiency virus.

The **incubation period** from the laying of eggs to the hatching of the first nymph is 6 to 10 days. Mature adult lice capable of reproducing do not appear until 2 to 3 weeks later.

DIAGNOSTIC TESTS: Identification of eggs, nymphs, and lice with the naked eye is possible; the diagnosis can be confirmed by using a hand lens or microscope. Adult lice seldom are seen, because they move rapidly and conceal themselves effectively.

TREATMENT: The pediculicides used to treat pediculosis capitis are effective for treatment of pubic lice (see Pediculosis Capitis, p 463). Retreatment is recommended 7 to 10 days later. For infestation of eyelashes by pubic lice, petrolatum ointment applied 3 to 4 times daily for 8 to 10 days is effective. Nits should be removed by hand from the eyelashes.

ISOLATION OF THE HOSPITALIZED PATIENT: In addition to standard precautions, contact precautions are recommended until the patient has been treated with an appropriate pediculicide.

CONTROL MEASURES: All sexual contacts should be treated.

Pelvic Inflammatory Disease*

CLINICAL MANIFESTATIONS: Pelvic inflammatory disease (PID) comprises a spectrum of inflammatory disorders of the female upper genital tract, including any combination of endometritis, parametritis, salpingitis, oophoritis, tubo-ovarian abscess, and pelvic peritonitis. Pelvic inflammatory disease typically manifests as dull, continuous, bilateral lower abdominal or pelvic pain that may range from indolent to severe. Additional symptoms can include fever, vomiting, an abnormal vaginal discharge, and irregular vaginal bleeding (signaling endometritis). Some patients have sharp right upper abdominal quadrant pain as a result of perihepatitis. Symptoms often begin within a week after the onset of menses, depending on the etiologic agent.

Examination findings variably include fever, lower abdominal tenderness, tenderness on lateral motion of the cervix, adnexal tenderness that is generally but not always bilateral, and adnexal fullness. Leukocytosis, an erythrocyte sedimentation rate more than 15 mm per hour, and an adnexal mass demonstrated by abdominal or transvaginal ultrasonography are typical findings.

No single symptom, sign, or laboratory finding is sensitive and specific for the diagnosis of acute PID. Many episodes of PID go unrecognized, some because patients are asymptomatic ("silent PID") and others because the symptoms are mild and nonspecific, so the diagnosis is not considered. Combinations of findings that improve sensitivity (ie, correctly detect women who have PID) do so only while decreasing specificity (ie, incorrectly including women who do not have PID). The diagnostic criteria currently recommended by the Centers for Disease Control and Prevention are presented in Table 3.40 (p 469).

Complications of PID may include perihepatitis (Fitz-Hugh-Curtis syndrome) and tubo-ovarian abscess. Important long-term sequelae are recurrent infection, chronic pelvic pain, a sixfold increase in incidence of ectopic pregnancy, and infertility resulting from tubal occlusion. Risk of tubal infertility is estimated to be 10% after a single episode of PID and more than 50% after 3 or more episodes. Factors that may increase the likelihood of infertility are older age at time of infection, chlamydial disease, PID determined to be severe by laparoscopic examination, and delayed antimicrobial treatment.

ETIOLOGY: Sexually transmitted organisms, especially *Neisseria gonorrhoeae* and *Chlamydia trachomatis,* are implicated in most cases of PID. However, other organisms, such as anaerobes, including *Bacteroides* and *Peptostreptococcus* species; facultative anaerobes, including *Gardnerella vaginalis, Haemophilus influenzae, Streptococcus* species, and enteric gram-negative bacilli; genital tract mycoplasmas, including *Mycoplasma hominis* and *Ureaplasma urealyticum;* and cytomegalovirus, also are associated with PID.

EPIDEMIOLOGY: As is true for other sexually transmitted diseases (STDs), the incidence of PID is highest among adolescents and young adults. Other risk factors for PID include numerous sexual partners, use of an intrauterine device in the pres-

---

* Centers for Disease Control and Prevention. Sexually transmitted diseases treatment guidelines—2002. *MMWR Recomm Rep.* 2002;51(RR-6):1–80

Table 3.40. Criteria for Clinical Diagnosis of Pelvic Inflammatory Disease (PID)

Minimum Criteria

Empiric treatment of PID should be initiated in sexually active young women and others at risk of STDs if the following **minimum criteria** are present and no other cause(s) for the illness can be identified:

- Uterine or adnexal tenderness
                OR
- Cervical motion tenderness

Additional Criteria

More elaborate diagnostic evaluation often is needed, because incorrect diagnosis and management might cause unnecessary morbidity. These additional criteria may be used to enhance the specificity of the minimum criteria listed previously. Additional criteria that support a diagnosis of PID include the following:

- Oral temperature >38.3°C (>101°F)
- Abnormal cervical or vaginal mucopurulent discharge
- Presence of white blood cells (WBCs) on saline microscopy of vaginal secretions
- Increased erythrocyte sedimentation rate
- Increased C-reactive protein
- Laboratory documentation of cervical infection with *Neisseria gonorrhoeae* or *Chlamydia trachomatis*

Most women with PID have mucopurulent cervical discharge OR evidence of WBCs on a microscopic evaluation of a saline preparation of vaginal fluid. If the cervical discharge appears normal AND no WBCs are found on the wet preparation, the diagnosis of PID is unlikely, and alternative causes of pain should be sought.

The **most specific criteria** for diagnosing PID include the following:

- Endometrial biopsy with histopathologic evidence of endometritis;
- Transvaginal sonography or magnetic resonance imaging techniques showing thickened, fluid-filled tubes with or without free pelvic fluid or tubo-ovarian complex; and
- Laparoscopic abnormalities consistent with PID.

A diagnostic evaluation that includes some of these more extensive studies may be warranted in selected cases.

STDs indicates sexually transmitted diseases.
Adapted from the Centers for Disease Control and Prevention. Sexually transmitted diseases treatment guidelines—2002. *MMWR Recomm Rep.* 2002;51(RR-6):1–80.

ence of an existing infection or multiple sexual partners after insertion, douching, and previous episodes of PID. Latex condoms, when used consistently and correctly, are highly effective in preventing sexual transmission of gonorrhea, chlamydia, trichomoniasis, and human immunodeficiency virus (HIV). Condom use has been associated with a lower rate of cervical cancer, a human papilloma virus-associated disease. Other barrier contraceptive methods, such as the contraceptive sponge and diaphragm, also have been shown to be effective in preventing transmission of STDs. Oral contraceptive pills decrease the likelihood of PID in the face of gonococcal or chlamydial cervicitis. Ascending pelvic infection is a rare complication of gonococcal vaginitis in prepubertal girls.

An **incubation period** for PID is undefined. In women with gonococcal cervicitis, symptoms of PID generally appear during the first half of the menstrual cycle.

DIAGNOSTIC TESTS: The diagnosis of PID usually is made on the basis of clinical findings (see Table 3.40, p 469) and is supported by findings of a preponderance of leukocytes in cervical secretions, leukocytosis, an increased C-reactive protein concentration or erythrocyte sedimentation rate, identification of *N gonorrhoeae* in an endocervical culture, or presence of *C trachomatis* in a rapid detection test of endocervical secretions (see *Chlamydia trachomatis,* p 238, and Gonococcal Infections p 285). An endocervical culture for *N gonorrhoeae* and an endocervical test for *C trachomatis* should be obtained before treatment is begun. Ultrasonography and laparoscopy are useful when appendicitis, ruptured ovarian cyst, or ectopic pregnancy are possible differential diagnoses. Laparoscopy also permits bacteriologic specimens to be obtained directly from tubal exudate or the cul-de-sac. However, laparoscopy cannot detect endometritis and is not indicated in most cases. Because an adolescent's recollection of her menstrual history is not always reliable and because PID and ectopic pregnancy both can produce abdominal pain and irregular bleeding, a pregnancy test is indicated in the diagnostic evaluation of the adolescent with suspected PID or lower abdominal pain.

TREATMENT: Because the clinical diagnosis of PID, even in the most experienced hands, is imprecise and because the consequences of untreated infection are substantial, most experts provide antimicrobial therapy to patients who fulfill minimum criteria rather than limiting therapy to patients who fulfill additional criteria for the diagnosis of PID (Table 3.40, p 469). To minimize the risks of progressive infection and subsequent infertility, treatment should not await culture results but should be instituted as soon as the clinical diagnosis is made.

Observation and treatment in the hospital are suggested in the following circumstances: (1) a surgical emergency, such as ectopic pregnancy or appendicitis, cannot be excluded; (2) compliance with or tolerance of an outpatient treatment regimen and follow-up within 72 hours cannot be ensured; (3) the patient's illness is severe (eg, nausea, vomiting, severe pain, overt peritonitis, or high fever); (4) a tubo-ovarian abscess is present; (5) the patient is pregnant; or (6) the patient has failed to respond clinically to outpatient therapy. Although in the past, many experts have recommended hospitalization for all adolescent patients with PID, data to support this recommendation are lacking. Current data are insufficient to determine whether hospitalization is indicated for women with PID and HIV infection.

The choice of an antimicrobial regimen for PID is empiric, broad spectrum, and directed against the most common causative agents. Antimicrobial regimens consistent with those recommended by the Centers for Disease Control and Prevention (2002) are summarized in Table 3.41 (p 471). Clinical outcome data are lacking about the use of other cephalosporin antimicrobial agents, such as ceftizoxime sodium, cefotaxime sodium, and ceftriaxone sodium. Some experts believe that these agents can be used to replace cefoxitin sodium or cefotetan disodium for PID treatment; however, cefoxitin and cefotetan are more active against anaerobes. Fluoroquinolones are not licensed by the US Food and Drug Administration for use in patients younger than 18 years of age. Consideration should be given to

Table 3.41. Recommended Treatment of Pelvic Inflammatory Disease (PID)[1]

Parenteral: Regimen A[2]

Cefotetan, 2 g, IV, every 12 h

OR

Cefoxitin, 2 g, IV, every 6 h

PLUS

Doxycycline, 100 mg, orally or IV, every 12 h

OR

Parenteral: Regimen B[5]

Clindamycin, 900 mg, IV, every 8 h

PLUS

Gentamicin: loading dose, IV or IM (2 mg/kg), followed by maintenance dose (1.5 mg/kg) every 8 h. Single daily dosing may be substituted.

NOTE

Parenteral therapy may be discontinued 24 hours after a patient improves clinically; continuing oral therapy should consist of doxycycline (100 mg, orally, twice a day) or clindamycin (450 mg, orally, 4 times a day) to complete a total of 14 days of therapy.

Ambulatory: Regimen A[3] (all oral)

Ofloxacin,[4] 400 mg, orally, twice a day for 14 days

OR

Levofloxacin[4] 500 mg, orally, once daily for 14 days,

WITH or WITHOUT

Metronidazole, 500 mg, orally, twice a day for 14 days

OR

Ambulatory: Regimen B

Ceftriaxone, 250 mg, IM, once

OR

Cefoxitin, 2 g, IM, plus **probenecid,** 1 g, orally, in a single dose concurrently once

OR

Other parenteral third-generation **cephalosporin[6]** (eg, **ceftizoxime** or **cefotaxime**),

PLUS

Doxycycline, 100 mg, orally, twice a day for 14 days

WITH or WITHOUT

Metronidazole, 500 mg, orally, twice a day for 14 days

IV indicates intravenous; IM, intramuscular.

[1] For further alternative treatment regimens, see Centers for Disease Control and Prevention. Sexually transmitted diseases treatment guidelines—2002. *MMWR Recomm Rep.* 2002;51(RR-6):1–80

[2] Many experts recommend hospitalization for all patients with PID, particularly adolescents.

[3] Patients with inadequate response to outpatient therapy after 72 hours should be reevaluated for possible misdiagnosis and should receive parenteral therapy.

[4] Fluoroquinolones are contraindicated for patients younger than 18 years of age, for pregnant women, and during lactation (see Antimicrobial Agents and Related Therapy, p 693).

[5] Alternative parenteral regimens include ofloxacin or levofloxacin plus metronidazole; and ampicillin-subactam sodium plus doxycycline.

[6] Data to indicate whether expanded-spectrum cephalosporins (ceftizoxime, cefotaxime, ceftriaxone) can replace cefoxitin or cefotetan are limited. Many authorities believe they also are effective therapy for PID, but they are less active against anaerobes.

selecting an antimicrobial regimen that is effective against *N gonorrhoeae* and *C trachomatis*. Broad anaerobic coverage (clindamycin or metronidazole) should be provided for patients with tubo-ovarian abscess, recurrent PID, or recent pelvic surgery. If the patient has an intrauterine device in place, the device should be removed immediately. In patients treated orally or parenterally, clinical improvement can be expected within 72 hours after initiation of treatment. Accordingly, outpatients should be reevaluated routinely on the third or fourth day of treatment.

ISOLATION OF THE HOSPITALIZED PATIENT: Standard precautions are recommended.

CONTROL MEASURES:
- Male sexual partners of patients with PID should receive diagnostic evaluation for gonococcal and chlamydial urethritis and then should be treated presumptively for both infections if they had sexual contact with the patient during the 60 days preceding onset of symptoms in the patient. A large proportion of these males will be asymptomatic.
- The patient should abstain from sexual intercourse until she and her partner(s) have completed treatment.
- The patient and her partner(s) should be encouraged to use condoms consistently.
- The patient should be tested for syphilis and HIV infection, and a Papanicolaou smear should be performed.
- Unimmunized or incompletely immunized patients should begin or complete hepatitis B immunization (see Recommended Childhood and Adolescent Immunization Schedule, p 24).
- Because of the high risk of reinfection, some experts recommend that patients with PID whose initial test for *N gonorrhoeae* and *C trachomatis* was positive be retested 4 to 6 weeks after completing treatment.
- The diagnosis of PID provides an opportune time to educate the adolescent about prevention of STDs, including abstinence, consistent use of barrier methods of protection, and the importance of receiving periodic screening for STDs.

Pertussis

CLINICAL MANIFESTATIONS: Pertussis begins with mild upper respiratory tract symptoms (catarrhal stage) and progresses to cough and then usually to paroxysms of cough (paroxysmal stage), often with a characteristic inspiratory whoop and commonly followed by vomiting. Fever is absent or minimal. Symptoms wane gradually over weeks to months (convalescent stage). Disease in infants younger than 6 months of age may be atypical; apnea is a common manifestation, and whoop often is absent. Similarly, older children and adults can have atypical manifestations, with prolonged cough with or without paroxysms and no whoop. The duration of classic pertussis is 6 to 10 weeks. Complications include seizures, pneumonia, encephalopathy, and death. Pertussis is most severe when it occurs during the first 6 months of life, particularly for preterm and unimmunized infants. On the basis of cases reported to local and state health departments (1990–1999), pneumonia, seizures, and encephalopathy occurred in 22%, 2%, and <0.5%, respectively, of infants younger than 12 months of age with pertussis. The case fatality rate was approximately 1% in infants younger than 2 months of age and <0.5% in infants 2 to 11 months of age. However, because most infants reported to have pertussis are hospitalized, complication rates are likely to be representative of more severe illness.

ETIOLOGY: *Bordetella pertussis* is a fastidious, gram-negative, pleomorphic bacillus. Other infectious agents may cause a similar cough illness: *Bordetella parapertussis, Mycoplasma pneumoniae, Chlamydia trachomatis, Chlamydia pneumoniae, Bordetella bronchiseptica,* and certain adenoviruses.

EPIDEMIOLOGY: Humans are the only known hosts of *B pertussis.* Transmission occurs by close contact via aerosolized droplets from patients with disease. Pertussis occurs endemically with 3- to 5-year cycles of increased disease. As many as 80% of nonimmune household contacts acquire the disease. Older siblings (including adolescents) and adults may be an important source of pertussis for infants and young children and may have only mild or atypical disease. Patients are most contagious during the catarrhal stage and the first 2 weeks after cough onset. Factors affecting the length of communicability include age, immunization status or previous episode of pertussis, and appropriate antimicrobial therapy. For example, a young unimmunized and untreated infant may be infectious for 6 or more weeks after cough onset; an untreated immunized adolescent may be infectious for only 2 weeks after cough onset. Erythromycin therapy decreases infectivity and limits spread. Nasopharyngeal cultures usually test negative for *B pertussis* within 5 days after initiating therapy.

The **incubation period** is from 6 to 21 days, usually 7 to 10 days.

DIAGNOSTIC TESTS: Culture of *B pertussis* requires inoculation of a specimen of nasopharyngeal secretions, obtained by aspiration or with a Dacron (polyethylene terephthalate) or calcium alginate swab, on special media (such as Regan-Lowe or fresh Bordet-Gengou), with incubation for 10 to 14 days. Because these media may not be available routinely, laboratory personnel should be informed when *B pertussis* is suspected. Specimens should be inoculated into special transport media (Regan-Lowe) and transported promptly to the laboratory; for the highest yield, the plate can be inoculated at the bedside. Negative cultures are common even in the early phase of the illness, because the organism is fastidious; and cultures usually test negative after the fourth week of illness, when patients have been immunized previously, or when patients have received antimicrobial agents. The direct immunofluorescence assay (DFA) of nasopharyngeal secretions has variable sensitivity and low specificity, requires experienced personnel for interpretation, and is not a reliable criterion for laboratory confirmation of the diagnosis. Because false-positive and false-negative DFA results occur, culture confirmation of all suspected pertussis cases should be attempted. If validated, DNA amplification methods, such as polymerase chain reaction assay of nasopharyngeal specimens and cultures, could provide a sensitive and rapid means for the diagnosis of infection with *B pertussis* and *B parapertussis* while waiting for results of cultures but may not be available widely.

No single serologic test is diagnostic of pertussis. *Bordetella pertussis* infections stimulate a heterogeneous antibody response that differs among individuals, depending on age and previous exposure to the organism or to its antigens by immunization. In research laboratories, the serologic diagnosis of pertussis has good sensitivity and specificity when an acute serum specimen is collected early in the illness and tested with a paired convalescent-phase specimen. Measurement of immunoglobulin (Ig) G antibody to pertussis toxin and other less specific antigens generally is available. However, these tests must be interpreted with caution, because they are not standardized, often not validated, and not licensed by the US Food and Drug Administration (FDA).

An increased white blood cell count with absolute lymphocytosis often is present in patients with *B pertussis* but not *B parapertussis* infection, particularly infants and patients who are unimmunized. The degree of increase of the white blood cell count and lymphocytosis often parallels the severity of the patient's cough.

Because laboratory confirmation of pertussis may not be achieved, clinicians often make the diagnosis on the basis of clinical characteristics, such as apnea (in infants), prolonged cough, inspiratory whoop, post-tussive vomiting or cyanosis, and lymphocytosis.

TREATMENT:

- Infants younger than 6 months of age and other patients with severe disease commonly require hospitalization for supportive care to manage apnea, hypoxia, feeding difficulties, and other complications. Intensive care facilities may be required.
- Antimicrobial agents given during the catarrhal stage may ameliorate the disease. After the cough is established, antimicrobial agents may have no discernible effect on the course of illness but are recommended to limit the spread of organisms to others. The drug of choice is erythromycin estolate (40–50 mg/kg per day, orally, in 4 divided doses; maximum 2 g/day). The recommended duration of therapy to prevent bacteriologic relapse is 14 days. Studies have documented that the newer macrolides, azithromycin dihydrate (10–12 mg/kg per day, orally, in 1 dose for 5 days; maximum 600 mg/day) or clarithromycin (15–20 mg/kg per day, orally, in 2 divided doses; maximum 1 g/day for 7 days), may be as effective as erythromycin and have fewer adverse effects and better compliance. Resistance to erythromycin (and other macrolide antimicrobial agents) by *B pertussis* has been reported rarely. Penicillins and first- and second-generation cephalosporins are not effective against *B pertussis*.
- An association between orally administered erythromycin and infantile hypertrophic pyloric stenosis (IHPS) has been reported in infants younger than 2 weeks of age. The risk of IHPS after treatment with other macrolides (eg, azithromycin and clarithromycin) is unknown. Because pertussis can be life threatening in neonates and because alternative therapies are not well studied, the American Academy of Pediatrics continues to recommend use of erythromycin for prophylaxis and treatment of disease caused by *B pertussis*. Physicians who prescribe erythromycin to newborn infants should inform parents about the potential risks of developing IHPS and signs of IHPS.

Cases of pyloric stenosis after use of oral erythromycin should be reported to MEDWATCH (see MEDWATCH, p 771).

- Trimethoprim-sulfamethoxazole is an alternative for patients who cannot tolerate erythromycin or who are infected with an erythromycin-resistant strain. The dosage in children is trimethoprim, 8 mg/kg per day, and sulfamethoxazole, 40 mg/kg per day, in 2 divided doses.
- Pertussis-Specific Immune Globulin is an investigational product that may be effective in decreasing paroxysms of coughing, but further evaluation is required. Controlled, prospective data are not available for corticosteroids, albuterol, and other β_2-adrenergic agents in the treatment of pertussis.

ISOLATION OF THE HOSPITALIZED PATIENT: In addition to standard precautions, droplet precautions are recommended for 5 days after initiation of effective therapy or until 3 weeks after the onset of paroxysms if appropriate antimicrobial therapy is not given.

CONTROL MEASURES:

Care of Exposed People.

Household and Other Close Contacts.
Immunization. Close contacts younger than 7 years of age who are unimmunized or who have received fewer than 4 doses of pertussis vaccine (diphtheria and tetanus toxoids and acellular pertussis [DTaP] or diphtheria and tetanus toxoids and pertussis [DTP]) should have pertussis immunization initiated or continued according to the recommended schedule. Children who received their third dose 6 months or more before exposure should be given a fourth dose at this time. Children who have had 4 doses of pertussis vaccine should receive a booster dose of DTaP unless a dose has been given within the last 3 years or they are 7 years of age or older.

Chemoprophylaxis. Erythromycin (40–50 mg/kg per day, orally, in 4 divided doses; maximum 2 g/day) for 14 days is recommended for all household contacts and other close contacts, such as those in child care, regardless of age and immunization status. Some experts recommend the estolate preparation. For erythromycin use in infants younger than 3 weeks of age, see Treatment, p 474. The newer macrolides, clarithromycin and azithromycin, are potential alternatives for patients who cannot tolerate erythromycin (see Treatment, p 474). Prompt use of chemoprophylaxis in household contacts can limit secondary transmission. The rationale for administering chemoprophylaxis to all household and other close contacts regardless of age or immunization status is that pertussis immunity is not absolute and immunization may not prevent infection. People with mild illness that may not be recognized as pertussis can transmit the infection.

People who have been in contact with an infected person should be monitored closely for respiratory tract symptoms for 21 days after last contact with the infected person.

Child Care. Exposed children, especially incompletely immunized children, should be observed for respiratory tract symptoms for 21 days after contact has been terminated. Pertussis immunization and chemoprophylaxis should be given as recommended for household and other close contacts. Symptomatic children and children with confirmed pertussis should be excluded from child care pending physician evaluation or until completion of 5 days of erythromycin (or other recommended antimicrobial therapy), which is to be given for 14 days, or until 21 days has elapsed from cough onset. Chemoprophylaxis should be considered for adult staff with close or extensive contact. Staff members should be monitored for respiratory tract symptoms, should undergo culture for pertussis if symptoms develop, and should be given antimicrobial therapy if cough develops within 21 days of exposure (see Treatment, p 474).

Schools. Students and staff with pertussis should be excluded from school; if their medical condition allows, they may return 5 days after initiation of the 14-day course of erythromycin or other recommended therapy. People who do not receive appropriate antimicrobial therapy should be excluded from school for 21 days after onset of symptoms. Other public health recommendations to control pertussis transmission have not been established. Schoolwide or classroom chemoprophylaxis generally has not been recommended usually because of the delay in recognition of outbreaks and difficulties of implementation. The immunization status of children younger than 7 years of age should be reviewed and vaccine should be given, if indicated, as for household and other close contacts. Pertussis should be considered in the differential diagnosis of people with cough illness who may have been exposed. Parents and employees should be notified about possible exposures to pertussis. Exclusion of exposed people with cough illness, pending physician evaluation, should be considered. The local health department should be consulted about the possible implementation of this and other control measures.

Immunization. Universal immunization with pertussis vaccine for children younger than 7 years of age is recommended. The pertussis vaccines used in the United States are acellular vaccines in combination with diphtheria and tetanus toxoids. Recommendations for use of DTaP are similar to recommendations for use of DTP, which continues to be given to infants and children in many countries in the world. Acellular vaccines are adsorbed onto an aluminum salt and must be administered intramuscularly. Acellular vaccines contain one or more immunogens derived from *B pertussis* organisms. These antigens include detoxified pertussis toxin (ie, pertussis toxoid, also termed lymphocytosis-promoting factor), filamentous hemagglutinin, fimbrial proteins (agglutinogens), and pertactin (an outer membrane 69-kd protein). As of January 2003, 4 acellular pertussis-containing vaccines (DTaP) are licensed in the United States, and all have been licensed by the US Food and Drug Administration (FDA) for use in infants and for primary immunization. These vaccines include 3 DTaP preparations and 1 combined vaccine that includes DTaP, hepatitis B (HepB), and inactivated poliovirus (IPV). In addition, a combination of DTaP and *Haemophilus influenzae* type b conjugate vaccine is licensed for the dose given at 15 to 18 months of age (see Table 3.42, p 477). Although licensed vaccines differ in their formulation of pertussis antigens, their efficacy seems similar. All DTaP vaccines currently contain pertussis toxoid. Vaccine recommendations are updated and published each January in *Pediatrics*.

The rates of local reactions (erythema and induration at the injection site), fever, and other common systemic symptoms (drowsiness, fretfulness, and anorexia) are substantially lower with acellular pertussis vaccines than with whole-cell pertussis vaccines. Rare, potentially more serious adverse events associated with DTP, such

Table 3.42. Licensed DTaP-Containing Vaccines[1]

Pharmaceutical[2]	Manufacturer	Antigens	Recommended Use
Tripedia (DTaP)	Aventis Pasteur, Swiftwater, PA	PT, FHA	**All 5 doses,** children 6 wk through 6 y of age
Infanrix (DTaP)	GlaxoSmithKline Biologicals, Rixensart, Belgium	PT, FHA, pertactin	**First 4 doses,** children 6 wk to 6 y of age; can be used for the fifth dose for a child who has received 1 or more doses of whole-cell DTP
TriHIBit[3] (DTaP-Hib)	Aventis Pasteur, Swiftwater, PA	PT, FHA	Only fourth dose; TriHIBit can be used for the fourth dose after 3 doses of DTaP or whole-cell DTP and a primary series of any Hib vaccine
DAPTACEL (DTaP)	Aventis Pasteur, Swiftwater, PA	PT, FHA, pertactin, fimbriae types 2 and 3	**First 4 doses,** children 6 wk through 6 y of age; can be used for the fifth dose for a child who has received 1 or more doses of whole-cell DTP
Pediarix (DTaP-hepatitis B-IPV)	GlaxoSmithKline Biologicals, Rixensart, Belgium	PT, FHA, pertactin	**3 doses** at 6- to 8-week intervals beginning at 2 months of age

DTaP indicates diphtheria and tetanus toxoids and acellular pertussis vaccine; Hib, *Haemophilus influenzae* type b vaccine; PT, pertussis toxoid; FHA, filamentous hemagglutinin; DTP, diphtheria and tetanus toxoids and pertussis vaccine; IPV, inactivated poliovirus.

[1] DTaP recommended schedule is 2, 4, 6, and 15 to 18 months and 4 to 6 years of age. The fourth dose can be given as early as 12 months of age, provided 6 months have elapsed since the third dose was given. The fifth dose is not necessary if the fourth dose was given on or after the fourth birthday. Refer to manufacturers' package inserts for comprehensive product information regarding indications and use of the vaccines listed.

[2] ACEL-IMUNE and Certiva no longer are distributed.

[3] TriHIBit is ActHIB (lyophilized) reconstituted with Tripedia.

as seizures, have been found to occur less frequently after acellular pertussis vaccine (see Adverse Events After Pertussis Immunization, p 480).

Dose and Route. Each dose of DTaP is 0.5 mL, given intramuscularly. The use of a decreased volume of individual doses of pertussis vaccines or multiple doses of decreased-volume (fractional) doses is not recommended. The effect of such practices on the frequency of serious adverse events and on protection against disease has not been determined.

Interchangeability of Acellular Pertussis Vaccines. When feasible, the same DTaP vaccine product should be used for all doses of the pertussis immunization series. Insufficient data exist on the safety, immunogenicity, or efficacy of different DTaP vaccines when administered interchangeably in the primary series to make recommendations. However, in circumstances in which the type of DTaP product(s) received previously is not known, or the previously administered product(s) is not readily available, any DTaP vaccine licensed for use in the primary series may be used.

Antipyretic Prophylaxis. Elective administration of acetaminophen or other appropriate antipyretic at the time of immunization with DTaP and at 4 and 8 hours after immunization may decrease the subsequent incidence of fever and local reactions.

Recommendations for Routine Childhood Immunization. A total of 5 doses of pertussis vaccine is recommended before school entry, unless contraindicated (see Contraindications to Pertussis Immunization, p 483, and Precautions for Pertussis Immunization, p 484). If the fourth dose of pertussis vaccine is given after the fourth birthday because of delays in completing the immunization schedule, the fifth dose is not indicated. The first dose is given at 2 months of age, followed by 2 additional doses at intervals of approximately 2 months. The fourth dose is recommended at 15 to 18 months of age. The fifth dose is given before school entry (kindergarten or elementary school) at 4 to 6 years of age to protect these children from pertussis in ensuing years and to decrease transmission of disease to younger children.

In the United States, DTaP is preferred for all doses because of vaccine-associated adverse events such as fever and local reactions. Combination products containing an acellular pertussis vaccine component may be given, provided they are licensed by the FDA for the child's current age and administration of the other components of the vaccine is justified.

Other recommendations are as follows:

- For the fourth dose, DTaP may be given as early as 12 months of age if the interval between the third and fourth doses is at least 6 months and the child is considered unlikely to return for a visit at the recommended age of 15 to 18 months for this dose.
- Simultaneous administration of DTaP and other recommended vaccines is acceptable. Vaccines should not be mixed in the same syringe unless the specific combination is licensed by the FDA (see Simultaneous Administration of Multiple Vaccines, p 33, and *Haemophilus influenzae* Infections, p 293).
- If pertussis is prevalent in the community, immunization can be started as early as 6 weeks of age, and doses 2 and 3 in the primary series can be given at intervals of 4 weeks.
- Pertussis immunization is not recommended for people 7 years of age or older.

- For children who have begun but not completed their primary immunization schedule with DTP, an FDA-licensed DTaP vaccine should be used to complete the pertussis immunization schedule.
- Children who have a contraindication to pertussis immunization should receive no further doses of pertussis-containing vaccine (see Contraindications to Pertussis Immunization, p 483, and Precautions for Pertussis Immunization, p 484).

Combined vaccine. The US Food and Drug Administration in December 2002 licensed a combined DTaP, HepB recombinant, and IPV vaccine (Pediarix, Glaxo-SmithKline Biologicals, Rixensart, Belgium) for use in infants. The DTaP-HepB-IPV combination vaccine may be used as a 3-dose series administered intramuscularly at 6- to 8-week intervals (preferably 8 weeks) to infants at 2, 4, and 6 months of age. The DTaP-HepB-IPV combination vaccine should not be given to people 7 years of age or older or to infants before 6 weeks of age and, therefore, cannot be used for the birth dose of hepatitis B vaccine for any infant. Only a monovalent hepatitis B vaccine should be administered to infants before 6 weeks of age. The DTaP-HepB-IPV combination vaccine also may be used to complete the primary DTaP immunization series in infants born to HBsAg-negative or HBsAg-positive women who have received 1 or more doses of monovalent hepatitis B vaccine and/or combination vaccine containing hepatitis B vaccine and who are scheduled to receive the other components of the combination vaccine. This may require that an extra dose of hepatitis B vaccine be given, which is acceptable.* If the DTaP-HepB-IPV combination vaccine is given as the third dose in the hepatitis B series, it should be given at 6 months of age or older to induce a satisfactory response to the hepatitis B vaccine component. Some experts prefer to complete the hepatitis B vaccine series with monovalent hepatitis B vaccine in infants born to HBsAg-positive women because of a lack of efficacy data for the DTaP-HepB-IPV combination vaccine in these infants.

The DTaP-HepB-IPV combination vaccine may be used interchangeably with the DTaP component from the same manufacturer (Infanrix [GlaxoSmithKline Biologicals, Rixensart, Belgium]) to complete the primary DTaP series among infants and children who are scheduled to receive the other vaccine components. The DTaP-HepB-IPV combination vaccine may be used to complete the primary DTaP series in infants and children who have received another brand of DTaP if the provider does not know or have available the brand of DTaP previously administered and if the infants and children also are scheduled to receive the other vaccine components. Whenever feasible, the same brand of DTaP should be used for all doses of the primary series. The DTaP-HepB-IPV combination vaccine may be used to complete the first 3 doses of the recommended 4-dose IPV series in infants and children who receive 1 or 2 doses of IPV from another manufacturer and who are scheduled to receive the other vaccine components. Administration must take into account the minimum interval between doses for each of the components (see Table 1.7, p 29). The DTaP-HepB-IPV combination vaccine may be given concurrently with a *Haemophilus influenzae* type b vaccine or pneumococcal conjugate

---

* American Academy of Pediatrics, Committee on Infectious Diseases. Combination vaccines for childhood immunization: recommendations of the Advisory Committee on Immunization Practices (ACIP), the American Academy of Pediatrics (AAP), and the American Academy of Family Physicians (AAFP). *Pediatrics.* 1999;103:1064–1077

vaccine at separate injection sites. Higher rates of low-grade fever are observed in children receiving the DTaP-HepB-IPV combination vaccine compared with children receiving the 3 vaccines separately. The DTaP-HepB-IPV combination vaccine should not be given as a booster dose following the 3-dose primary DTaP series, because data are not available regarding safety and efficacy when given as a booster dose.

Recommendations for Scheduling Pertussis Immunization in Special Circumstances.

- For the child whose pertussis immunization schedule is resumed after deferral or interruption of the recommended schedule, the next dose in the sequence should be given, regardless of the interval since the last dose—that is, the schedule is not reinitiated (see Lapsed Immunizations, p 33).
- For children who have received fewer than the recommended number of doses of pertussis vaccine but who have received the recommended number of DT doses for their age (ie, those started on DT, then given DTaP or DTP), DTaP should be given to complete the recommended pertussis immunization schedule. However, the total number of doses of diphtheria and tetanus toxoids (as DT, DTaP, or DTP) should not exceed 6 before the seventh birthday.
- Children who have had well-documented pertussis disease (eg, positive culture for *B pertussis* or epidemiologic linkage to a culture-positive case) should complete the immunization series with at least DT; some experts recommend including the pertussis component as well (ie, administration of DTaP). Although well-documented pertussis disease is likely to confer immunity against pertussis, the duration of such immunity is unknown.
- During pertussis outbreaks, such as in a hospital, immunization with an acellular pertussis-containing vaccine usually is not recommended for adult contacts. Evaluation of decreased-antigen acellular pertussis vaccine for use in adolescents and adults is in progress, and these vaccines should be used only under appropriate research protocols until they are licensed for use in people 7 years of age and older.

Medical Records. Charts of children for whom pertussis immunization has been deferred should be flagged, and the immunization status of these children should be assessed periodically to ensure that they are immunized appropriately.

Adverse Events After Pertussis Immunization.

- *Local and febrile reactions.* Reactions to DTaP vaccine most commonly include redness, edema, induration, and tenderness at the injection site; drowsiness; fretfulness; anorexia; vomiting; crying; and slight to moderate fever. These local and systemic manifestations after pertussis immunization occur within several hours of immunization and subside spontaneously without sequelae. Swelling involving the entire thigh or upper arm has been reported after administration of booster doses of different acellular pertussis vaccines. Because reports of these reactions generally were not solicited during safety studies, their frequency is unknown but has been estimated to range from 1% to 4% after the fifth dose of DTaP. Limb swelling may be accompanied by erythema, pain, and fever. Although swelling may interfere with walking, most children have no limitation of activity. The pathogenesis and frequency of substantial reactions and limb swelling is not known, but these conditions appear to be self-limited and resolve without sequelae.

Whether children who experience entire limb swelling after a fourth dose of DTaP are at increased risk of this reaction after the fifth dose is unknown. Because of the importance of the fifth dose in protecting a child during school years, a history of extensive swelling after the fourth dose should not be considered a contraindication to receipt of a fifth dose at school entry. Parents should be informed of the increase in reactogenicity that has been reported after the fourth and fifth doses of DTaP.

Overall, systemic and local reactions are significantly less common with DTaP than with DTP. Children with such reactions should receive subsequent doses of pertussis vaccine as scheduled.

Bacterial or sterile abscesses at the site of the injection are rare. Bacterial abscesses indicate contamination of the product or nonsterile technique and should be reported (see Reporting of Adverse Events, p 40). The causes of sterile abscesses are unknown. Their occurrence does not contraindicate further doses of DTaP.

- **Allergic reactions.** The rate of anaphylaxis to DTP is estimated to be approximately 2 cases per 100 000 injections; the incidence of allergic reactions after immunization with DTaP is unknown. Severe anaphylactic reactions and resulting deaths, if any, are rare after pertussis immunization. The transient urticarial rashes that occasionally occur after pertussis immunization, unless appearing immediately (ie, within minutes), are unlikely to be anaphylactic (IgE-mediated) in origin. These rashes probably represent a reaction caused by circulating antigen-antibody complexes to antigens in pertussis vaccine and corresponding antibody acquired from an earlier dose or an antibody acquired transplacentally. Because formation of such complexes depends on a precise balance between concentrations of circulating antigen and antibody, such reactions are unlikely to recur after a subsequent dose and are not contraindications to further doses.

- **Seizures.** The incidence of seizures occurring within 48 hours of administration of whole-cell pertussis (ie, DTP) vaccine has been estimated to be 1 case per 1750 doses administered. In clinical trials of DTaP vaccine in Europe and postlicensure surveillance of adverse events associated with DTaP in the United States, the reported incidence of seizures has been substantially less than that associated with DTP.

Most seizures occurring after immunization with DTP are brief, self-limited, and generalized. They usually occur in febrile children after the third or fourth dose of the vaccine series. These characteristics suggest that seizures associated with pertussis vaccine usually are febrile seizures. These seizures have not been demonstrated to result in the subsequent development of recurrent afebrile seizures (ie, epilepsy) or other neurologic sequelae. Predisposing factors to seizures occurring within 48 hours include underlying convulsive disorder, personal history of seizures, and family history of seizures (see Infants and Children With Underlying Neurologic Disorders, p 484, and Children With a Personal or Family History of Seizures, p 81).

- *Hypotonic-hyporesponsive episodes.* These episodes (also termed *collapse* or *shock-like state*) have been reported to occur at a frequency of 1 per 1750 doses of DTP vaccine administered. However, rates seem to vary widely, ranging from 3.5 to 291 cases per 100 000 immunizations in other observations. The rate after immunization with DTaP is unknown. However, in DTaP efficacy trials, these episodes occurred significantly less often after immunization with DTaP than with DTP. A follow-up study of a group of children who experienced hypotonic-hyporesponsive episode (HHE) after immunization with DTP demonstrated no evidence of subsequent serious neurologic damage or intellectual impairment.
- *Temperature of ≥40.5°C (≥104.8°F).* After administration of DTP vaccine, approximately 0.3% of recipients have been reported to develop temperature of ≥40.5°C (≥104.8°F) within 48 hours. The rate after DTaP is significantly less.
- *Prolonged crying.* Persistent, severe, inconsolable screaming or crying for 3 or more hours sometimes is observed within 48 hours of immunization with DTP (1 of 100 doses administered). The frequency of inconsolable crying for 3 or more hours is significantly less after immunization with DTaP. The significance of persistent crying is unknown. It has been noted after receipt of immunizations other than pertussis vaccine and is not known to be associated with sequelae.

Frequency of Adverse Events After Immunization With DTaP. Moderate to severe systemic reactions, including temperature of ≥40.5°C (≥104.8°F), persistent inconsolable crying lasting 3 hours or more, and HHE rarely have been reported after immunization with DTaP, but each of these reactions occurs less often than after immunization with DTP. When these reactions occur after the administration of DTP, they seem to be without sequelae; the limited experience with DTaP suggests a similar outcome. Because DTaP causes high fever less often than DTP, seizures are anticipated to be much less likely after receipt of DTaP than after DTP and have been reported after DTaP immunization at a rate substantially lower than that seen with DTP.

Alleged Reactions to Pertussis Immunization. The temporal association of DTP immunization and severe adverse events such as death, encephalopathy, onset of a seizure disorder, developmental delay, or learning or behavioral problems, does not establish causation. Many manifestations of alleged vaccine reactions have other causes, such as viral encephalitis, concurrent infections, preexisting neurologic disorders, and metabolic and other congenital abnormalities. For example, whereas infantile spasms commonly have their onset during the first 6 months of life and, in some cases, have been related temporally to administration of pertussis vaccine, epidemiologic data demonstrate that pertussis vaccine does not cause infantile spasms. Sudden infant death syndrome (SIDS) has occurred after DTP immunization, but several studies provide evidence that DTP immunization is not associated causally with SIDS. A large case-control study of SIDS in the United States demonstrated that SIDS victims were no more likely to have recently received DTP immunization than were control children. Because SIDS occurs most commonly at the age when DTP immunization is recommended, coincidental (by chance alone) temporal associations between SIDS and immunization are expected.

Evaluation of Adverse Events Temporally Associated With Pertussis Immunization. Appropriate diagnostic studies should be undertaken to establish the cause of serious adverse events occurring temporally with immunization rather than assuming that they are caused by the vaccine. The Centers for Disease Control and Prevention has established independent Clinical Immunization Safety Assessment (CISA) centers to assess individuals with selected adverse events and offer recommendations for management. However, the cause of events temporally related to immunization cannot always be established, even after diagnostic studies.

Severe Acute Neurologic Illness and Permanent Brain Damage. Permanent neurologic disability (brain damage) and even death previously have been considered uncommon sequelae of rare, severe, adverse neurologic events temporally related to whole-cell pertussis vaccine (DTP). Because no specific clinical syndromes or neuropathologic findings have been recognized in these cases, determination of whether pertussis vaccine is the cause of a specific child's deficit is not possible. Such adverse events can occur in immunized and unimmunized children, particularly during the first year of life. Hence, epidemiologic studies have been necessary to determine the risk of severe sequelae after acute events temporally related to pertussis immunization.

The only case-control study that addressed the issue of whether acute neurologic illness associated with DTP immunization results in permanent brain damage is the National Childhood Encephalopathy Study in England, conducted from 1976 to 1979.

The results of this study and the 10-year follow-up study do not establish a causal relationship between whole-cell pertussis immunization and chronic neurologic disorders. Other studies also have not provided evidence to support a causal relationship between DTP immunization and serious acute neurologic illness resulting in permanent neurologic injury. Limited experience with acellular pertussis vaccine does not allow conclusions about the frequency of rare, serious, adverse effects temporally associated with its administration.

Contraindications to Pertussis Immunization. Adverse events after pertussis immunization that contraindicate further administration of DTaP are as follows:

- ***An immediate anaphylactic reaction.*** Further immunization with any of the 3 vaccine components in DTaP or DTP should be deferred because of uncertainty about which antigen may be responsible. People who experience anaphylactic reactions may be referred to an allergist for evaluation and desensitization to tetanus toxoid if a specific allergy can be demonstrated.

- ***Encephalopathy within 7 days.*** This syndrome has been defined as a severe, acute central nervous system disorder unexplained by another cause, which may be manifested by major alterations of consciousness or by generalized or focal seizures that persists for more than a few hours without recovery within 24 hours. Prudence justifies considering such an illness occurring within 7 days of DTP as a possible contraindication to further doses of pertussis vaccine, and DT should be substituted for each of the recommended subsequent doses of diphtheria and tetanus toxoid.

Precautions for Pertussis Immunization. If the following adverse events occur in temporal relation to immunization with DTaP, the decision to administer additional doses of pertussis vaccine should be considered carefully. Although these events once were regarded as contraindications, they now are considered precautions, because they have not been proven to cause permanent sequelae:

- A seizure, with or without fever, occurring within 3 days of immunization with DTP or DTaP
- Persistent, severe, inconsolable screaming or crying for 3 or more hours within 48 hours of immunization
- Collapse or shock-like state (HHE) within 48 hours of immunization
- Temperature of ≥40.5°C (≥104.8°F), unexplained by another cause, within 48 hours of immunization

Before administration of each dose of pertussis vaccine, the child's parent or guardian should be asked about possible adverse events after previous doses.

Although the risks of giving subsequent doses of pertussis vaccine to a child who has experienced one of these events are unknown, the possibility of another reaction of similar or greater severity may justify discontinuing pertussis immunization. However, in circumstances of increased risk, such as during a community outbreak of pertussis, the potential benefit of pertussis immunization may outweigh the risk of another reaction. The decision to give or withhold immunization should be made on the basis of the clinical assessment of the earlier reaction, the likelihood of pertussis exposure in the child's community, and the potential benefits and risks of pertussis vaccine.

Infants and Children With Underlying Neurologic Disorders. The decision to give pertussis vaccine to infants and children with underlying neurologic disorders can be difficult and must be made on an individual basis after careful and continuing consideration of the risks and benefits (see also Children With a Personal or Family History of Seizures, p 81). Rarely, these disorders may constitute a cause for deferring pertussis immunization and, on the basis of the medical history of the child, subsequent administration of pertussis vaccine. Because outbreaks of pertussis continue to occur in the United States, the decision to defer immunization should be reassessed at each subsequent immunization visit, and the decision to give pertussis vaccine should be made on the basis of the risks and consequences of a seizure after DTaP immunization in comparison with the risk of pertussis and its complications. Children with associated neurologic deficits may be at increased risk of complications if infected with *B pertussis*. Children traveling to or residing in areas where pertussis is endemic or epidemic are at increased risk of developing pertussis. Efforts should be undertaken to ensure pertussis immunization of children attending child care centers, special clinics, or residential care institutions.

The different categories of neurologic disorders and the relevant recommendations are as follows:

- ***A progressive neurologic disorder characterized by developmental delay or neurologic findings.*** These conditions are reason for indefinite deferral of pertussis immunization. Administration of DTaP may coincide with or hasten recognition of inevitable manifestations of the disorder, with resulting confusion about causation. Examples include infantile spasms and other epilepsies beginning in infancy. Such disorders should be differentiated from those that are nonprogressive with symptoms that may change as the child matures.

- **Infants and children with a history of previous seizures.** Children with a history of seizures have an increased risk of seizures after receipt of DTP. No evidence indicates that these vaccine-associated seizures induce permanent brain damage, cause epilepsy, aggravate neurologic disorders, or affect the prognosis for children with underlying disorders. However, because the risk of a postimmunization seizure is increased, pertussis immunization of children with recent seizures should be deferred until a progressive neurologic disorder is excluded. Infants and children with well-controlled seizures or those in whom a seizure is unlikely to recur may be immunized with DTaP. Administration of acetaminophen or another appropriate antipyretic agent also should be considered at the time of immunization and every 4 hours for the ensuing 24 hours.

- **Infants and children known to have, or suspected of having, neurologic conditions that predispose to seizures or neurologic deterioration.** Such conditions include tuberous sclerosis and certain inherited metabolic or degenerative diseases. Deferral of pertussis immunization should be considered for these patients. Seizures or encephalopathy can occur in the normal course of these disorders and, thus, may occur after any immunization. Immunization with DTaP may be associated with the occurrence of overt manifestations of the disorders with resulting confusion about causation. Hence, children with unstable or evolving neurologic disorders that may predispose to seizures or neurologic deterioration should be observed before immunization to ascertain the diagnosis and prognosis of the primary neurologic disorder. Pertussis immunization with DTaP should be reconsidered at each visit. Children whose condition is resolved, corrected, or controlled can be immunized.

- **Prematurity.** No evidence indicates that prematurity in the absence of other factors increases the risk of seizures after immunization, and prematurity is not a reason to defer immunization (see Preterm and Low Birth Weight Infants, p 66). Similarly, stable neurologic conditions, such as developmental delay or cerebral palsy, are not contraindications to pertussis immunization.

- **Temporary deferment of pertussis immunization.** Children in the first year of life with neurologic disorders that necessitate temporary deferment of pertussis immunization should not receive DTaP or DT, because in the United States, the risk of acquiring diphtheria or tetanus by children younger than 1 year of age is remote. At or before the first birthday, the decision to give vaccine as DTaP or DT should be made to ensure that the child is at least immunized against diphtheria and tetanus; as children become ambulatory, their risk of tetanus-prone wounds increases.

Children with neurologic disorders that are recognized after the first birthday commonly will have received one or more doses of pertussis-containing vaccine. The physician may temporarily defer additional doses of DTaP in anticipation of clarification of the child's neurologic status. If the physician determines that the child probably should not receive further pertussis immunizations, DT immunization should be completed according to the recommended schedule (see Diphtheria, p 263, and/or Tetanus, p 611).

Children With a Family History of Seizures (see also Children With a Personal or Family History of Seizures, p 81). A history of seizure disorders or adverse events after receipt of a pertussis-containing vaccine in a family member is not a contraindication to pertussis immunization. Although the risk of seizures after immunization with DTP in children with a family history of seizures is increased, these seizures usually are febrile in origin and generally have a benign outcome. In addition, the risk of fever is less with DTaP immunization, and any risk of resulting febrile seizure is outweighed considerably by the continuing risk of pertussis in the United States. Because of the substantial number of children with a family history of seizures who, if not immunized, would remain susceptible to pertussis, DTaP is recommended for these children.

Advice to Parents of Children at Increased Risk of Seizures. Parents of children such as those with a personal or family history of seizures who may be at increased risk of seizure after pertussis immunization should be informed of the risks and benefits of pertussis immunization in these circumstances. Advice should be provided about fever and fever control (see Antipyretic Prophylaxis, p 478) and appropriate medical care in the unlikely event of a seizure.

Pinworm Infection
(Enterobius vermicularis)

CLINICAL MANIFESTATIONS: Although some people are asymptomatic, pinworm infection (enterobiasis) may cause pruritus ani and, rarely, pruritus vulvae. Although pinworms have been found in the lumen of the appendix, most evidence indicates that they are not related causally to acute appendicitis. Many clinical findings, such as grinding of the teeth at night, weight loss, and enuresis, have been attributed to pinworm infections, but proof of a causal relationship has not been established. Urethritis, vaginitis, salpingitis, or pelvic peritonitis may occur from aberrant migration of the adult worm from the perineum.

ETIOLOGY: *Enterobius vermicularis* is a nematode or roundworm.

EPIDEMIOLOGY: Enterobiasis occurs worldwide and commonly clusters within families. In the past, 5% to 15% of the population in the United States was estimated to be infected, but the incidence seems to have decreased. Prevalence rates are higher in preschool- and school-aged children, in primary caregivers for infected children, and in institutionalized people; up to 50% of these populations may be infected.

Egg transmission occurs by the fecal-oral route directly, indirectly, or inadvertently by contaminated hands or fomites, such as shared toys, bedding, clothing, toilet seats, and baths. Female pinworms usually die after depositing eggs on the perianal skin. Reinfection occurs by reingestion of eggs (ie, autoinfection) or acquisition from a new source. A person remains infectious as long as female nematodes are discharging eggs on perianal skin. Eggs remain infective in an indoor environment usually for 2 to 3 weeks. Humans are the only known natural hosts; dogs and cats do not harbor *E vermicularis*.

The **incubation period** from ingestion of an egg until an adult gravid female migrates to the perianal region is 1 to 2 months or longer.

DIAGNOSTIC TESTS: Diagnosis usually is made when adult worms are visualized in the perianal region, which is best examined 2 to 3 hours after the child is asleep. Very few ova are present in stool; therefore, examination of stool specimens for ova and parasites is not recommended. Alternatively, transparent (not translucent) adhesive tape can be applied to the perianal skin to collect any eggs that may be present; the tape is then applied to a glass slide and examined under a low-power microscopic lens. Three consecutive specimens should be obtained when the patient first awakens in the morning before washing.

TREATMENT: The drugs of choice are mebendazole, pyrantel pamoate, and albendazole, usually given in a single dose and repeated in 2 weeks. For children younger than 2 years of age, in whom experience with these drugs is limited, risks and benefits should be considered before drug administration. Other alternatives include piperazine and pyrvinium pamoate, but both drugs are less effective and more cumbersome to use. Reinfection with pinworms occurs easily; prevention should be discussed when treatment is given. Infected people should bathe in the morning; bathing removes a large proportion of eggs. Frequently changing the infected person's underclothes, bedclothes, and bedsheets may decrease the egg contamination of the local environment and decrease risk of reinfection. Specific personal hygiene measures (eg, exercising hand hygiene before eating or preparing food, keeping fingernails short, avoiding scratching of the perianal region, and avoiding nail biting) may decrease risk of autoinfection and continued transmission. Measures such as cleaning or vacuuming the entire house or washing bedclothes and bed sheets daily are not necessary. Repeated infections should be treated by the same method as the first infection. All family members should be treated as a group in situations in which multiple or repeated symptomatic infections occur. Vaginitis is self-limited and does not require separate treatment.

ISOLATION OF THE HOSPITALIZED PATIENT: Standard precautions are indicated.

CONTROL MEASURES: Control is difficult in child care centers and schools, because the rate of reinfection is high. In institutions, mass and simultaneous treatment, repeated in 2 weeks, can be effective. Good hand hygiene is the most effective method of prevention.

Plague

CLINICAL MANIFESTATIONS: Plague most commonly manifests in the bubonic form, with acute onset of fever and painful swollen regional lymph nodes (buboes). Buboes develop most commonly in the inguinal region but also occur in axillary or cervical areas. Less commonly, plague manifests in the septicemic form (hypotension, acute respiratory distress, intravascular coagulopathy) or as pneumonic plague (cough, fever, dyspnea, and hemoptysis) and, rarely, as meningeal plague. Fever, chills, headache, and rapidly progressive weakness are characteristic in all cases. Occasionally, patients have symptoms of mild lymphadenitis or prominent gastrointestinal tract symptoms, which may obscure the correct diagnosis.

ETIOLOGY: Plague is caused by *Yersinia pestis,* a pleomorphic, bipolar-staining, gram-negative coccobacillus.

EPIDEMIOLOGY: Plague is a zoonotic infection of rodents, carnivores, and their fleas that occurs in many areas of the world. Plague has been reported throughout the western United States, but most human cases occur in New Mexico, Arizona, California, and Colorado as isolated cases or in small clusters. There are more cases during summers that follow mild winters and wet springs. In the United States, human plague is a rural disease, usually associated with epizootic infections in ground squirrels, prairie dogs, and other wild rodents. Bubonic plague usually is transmitted by bites of infected rodent fleas and uncommonly by direct contact with tissues and fluids of infected rodents or other mammals, including domestic cats. Septicemic plague occurs most often as a complication of bubonic plague but may result from direct contact with infectious materials or the bite of an infected flea. Primary pneumonic plague is acquired by inhalation of respiratory droplets from a human or animal with respiratory plague or from exposure to laboratory aerosols. Secondary pneumonic plague arises from hematogenous seeding of the lungs with *Y pestis* in patients with bubonic or septicemic plague. Epidemics of human plague occur usually as a consequence of epizootics in domestic rodents or after exposures to pneumonic plague.

The **incubation period** is 2 to 6 days for bubonic plague and 2 to 4 days for primary pneumonic plague.

DIAGNOSTIC TESTS: Plague is characterized by massive growth of *Y pestis* in affected tissues, especially lymph nodes, spleen, and liver. The organism has a bipolar (safety-pin) appearance when viewed with Wayson or Gram stains. The microbiology laboratory examining specimens should be informed when plague organisms are suspected to minimize risks of transmission to laboratory personnel. A positive fluorescent antibody test result for the presence of *Y pestis* in direct smears or cultures of a bubo aspirate, sputum, cerebrospinal fluid, or blood specimen provides presumptive evidence of *Y pestis* infection. A single positive serologic test result by passive hemagglutination assay or enzyme immunoassay in an unimmunized patient who has not had plague previously also provides presumptive evidence of infection. Seroconversion and/or a fourfold difference in antibody titer between 2 serum specimens obtained 4 weeks to 3 months apart provides serologic confirmation. The diagnosis of plague usually is confirmed by culture of *Y pestis* from blood, bubo aspirate, or another clinical specimen. Polymerase chain reaction assay or immunohistochemical staining for rapid diagnosis of *Y pestis* are available in some reference or public health laboratories. Isolates suspected as *Y pestis* should be reported immediately to the state health department and submitted to the Division of Vector-Borne Infectious Diseases of the Centers for Disease Control and Prevention (CDC).

TREATMENT: For children, streptomycin sulfate (30 mg/kg per day in 2 or 3 divided doses, given intramuscularly) is the treatment of choice in most cases. Gentamicin sulfate in standard doses for age given intramuscularly or intravenously is an equally effective alternative to streptomycin. Tetracycline, doxycycline, or chloramphenicol also are effective. Doxycycline or tetracycline should not be given to children younger than 8 years of age unless the benefits of its use outweigh the risks of dental staining (see Antimicrobial Agents and Related Therapy, p 693). Chloramphenicol is the preferred treatment for plague meningitis. The usual duration of antimicrobial treatment is 7 to 10 days or until several days after lysis of fever.

Drainage of abscessed buboes may be necessary; drainage material is infectious until effective antimicrobial therapy has been given.

ISOLATION OF THE HOSPITALIZED PATIENT: For patients with bubonic plague, standard precautions are recommended. Droplet precautions are indicated for all patients until pneumonia is excluded and appropriate therapy has been initiated. In patients with pneumonic plague, droplet precautions should be continued for 48 hours after initiation of appropriate treatment.

CONTROL MEASURES:

Care of Exposed People. Household members and other people with intimate exposure to a patient with plague should report any fever or other illness to their physician. People with close exposure to a patient with pneumonic plague should receive antimicrobial prophylaxis. Previously, for children younger than 8 years of age, prophylactic trimethoprim-sulfamethoxazole has been recommended, but its efficacy is unknown. For adults and children 8 years of age and older and for children younger than 8 years of age at high risk, doxycycline is recommended. Prophylaxis is given for 7 days in the usual therapeutic doses.

Other Measures. State public health authorities should be notified immediately of any suspected cases of human plague. The public should be educated about risk factors for plague, measures to prevent disease, and the signs and symptoms of infection. People living in plague-endemic areas should be informed about the role of dogs and cats in bringing plague-infected rodents and fleas into peridomestic environments, the need for control of fleas and confinement of pets, and the importance of avoiding contact with sick and dead animals. Other preventive measures include surveillance of rodent populations and the use of insecticides and rodent control measures by health authorities when surveillance indicates the occurrence of plague epizootics.

Vaccine. Previously, an inactivated whole-cell *Y pestis* vaccine was available and recommended for people whose occupation regularly placed them at high risk of exposure to *Y pestis* or plague-infected rodents (eg, some field biologists and laboratory workers). Currently, there is no commercially available vaccine for plague in the United States. Information concerning the availability of plague vaccines is available from the CDC Division of Vector-Borne Infectious Diseases.

Pneumococcal Infections*

CLINICAL MANIFESTATIONS: Pneumococcus is the most common bacterial cause of acute otitis media and of invasive bacterial infections in children. Many children with bacteremia have no identifiable primary focus of infection. Pneumococci also are a common cause of sinusitis, community-acquired pneumonia, and conjunctivitis. Pneumococci and meningococci are the 2 most common causes of bacterial meningitis in infants and young children. Pneumococcus occasionally causes endocarditis, osteomyelitis, pericarditis, pyogenic arthritis, soft tissue infection, and early-onset neonatal septicemia.

ETIOLOGY: *Streptococcus pneumoniae* (pneumococci) are lancet-shaped, gram-positive diplococci. Ninety pneumococcal serotypes have been identified. Serotypes 4, 6B, 9V, 14, 18C, 19F, and 23F (Danish serotyping system) cause most invasive childhood pneumococcal infections in the United States and are the 7 types contained in the licensed heptavalent pneumococcal conjugate vaccine. Serotypes 6B, 9V, 14, 19A, 19F, and 23F are the most common isolates associated with resistance to penicillin.

EPIDEMIOLOGY: Pneumococci are ubiquitous, with many people having colonization in their upper respiratory tracts. Transmission is from person to person, presumably by respiratory droplet contact. The period of communicability is unknown and may be as long as the organism is present in respiratory tract secretions but probably is less than 24 hours after effective antimicrobial therapy is begun. Among young children who acquire a new pneumococcal serotype in the nasopharynx, illness (eg, otitis media) occurs in approximately 15%, usually within 1 month of acquisition. Viral upper respiratory tract infections, including influenza, may predispose to pneumococcal infections. Pneumococcal infections are most prevalent during winter months; most common in infants, young children, and the elderly; and more common in black individuals and some American Indian populations than in other racial and ethnic groups. Also, these infections are increased in incidence and severity in people with congenital or acquired humoral immunodeficiency (eg, agammaglobulinemia), human immunodeficiency virus (HIV) infection, or absent or deficient splenic function (eg, sickle cell disease, congenital or surgical asplenia). Other categories at presumed high risk or at moderate risk are outlined in Table 3.43 (p 492).

The **incubation period** varies by type of infection and can be as short as 1 to 3 days.

DIAGNOSTIC TESTS: Material obtained from a suppurative focus should be Gram stained and cultured by appropriate microbiologic techniques. Blood cultures should be obtained from all patients with suspected invasive pneumococcal disease; cultures of CSF and other (eg, pleural fluid) specimens also may be indicated. The white blood cell (WBC) count may be helpful in patients with suspected bacteremia

---

* American Academy of Pediatrics, Committee on Infectious Diseases. Recommendations for the prevention of pneumococcal infections, including the use of pneumococcal conjugate vaccine (Prevnar), pneumococcal polysaccharide vaccine, and antibiotic prophylaxis. *Pediatrics.* 2000;106:362–366.

caused by *S pneumoniae;* young children with high temperatures and leukocytosis (particularly a WBC count of >15 000 cells/mL [>15.0 × 10^9/L]) have an increased likelihood of bacteremia. Although the predictive value of an increased WBC count for pneumococcal bacteremia is not high, a normal WBC count is highly predictive of the absence of bacteremia. Recovery of pneumococci from an upper respiratory tract culture is not indicative of the etiologic diagnosis of pneumococcal disease in the middle ear, lower respiratory tract, or sinus. Rapid methods to detect pneumococcal capsular antigen in CSF, pleural and joint fluid, and concentrated urine usually lack sufficient sensitivity or specificity to be of value clinically.

Susceptibility Testing.* All *S pneumoniae* isolates from normally sterile body fluids (ie, CSF, blood, middle ear, or pleural or joint fluid) should be tested for in vitro antimicrobial susceptibility to determine the minimum inhibitory concentration (MIC) to penicillin and to cefotaxime sodium or ceftriaxone sodium. *Nonsusceptible* is defined to include both *intermediately resistant* and *highly resistant* isolates. Accordingly, current definitions of in vitro susceptibility and nonsusceptibility are as follows for nonmeningeal and meningeal isolates:

Drug and Isolate Location	Susceptible, µg/mL	Nonsusceptible, µg/mL	
		Intermediately Susceptible	Resistant
Penicillin/amoxicillin	≤0.06	0.1–1.0	≥2.0
Cefotaxime **OR** Ceftriaxone			
Nonmeningeal	≤1.0	2.0	≥4.0
Meningeal	≤0.5	1.0	≥2.0

For patients with meningitis whose organism is *nonsusceptible* to penicillin, cefotaxime, and ceftriaxone, susceptibility testing to vancomycin hydrochloride, rifampin, and possibly, meropenem should be performed. If the patient has a nonmeningeal infection caused by an isolate that is *nonsusceptible* to penicillin, cefotaxime, and ceftriaxone; susceptibility testing to clindamycin, erythromycin, rifampin, trimethoprim-sulfamethoxazole, meropenem, and vancomycin should be considered, depending on the patient's response to antimicrobial therapy.

Quantitative MIC testing using reliable methods, such as broth microdilution or antimicrobial gradient strips, should be performed on isolates from children with life-threatening infections. When quantitative testing methods are not available, the qualitative screening test using a 1-µg oxacillin disk on an agar plate reliably identifies all penicillin-*susceptible* pneumococci on the basis of the criterion of a disk-zone diameter of 20 mm or greater. Organisms with an oxacillin disk-zone size of less than 20 mm potentially are *nonsusceptible* and require quantitative susceptibility testing. The oxacillin disk test is used as a screening test for resistance to β-lactam drugs (ie, penicillins and cephalosporins).

---

* For further information, see American Academy of Pediatrics, Committee on Infectious Diseases. Therapy for children with invasive pneumococcal infections. *Pediatrics.* 1997;99:289–299.

Table 3.43. **Children at High and Moderate Risk of Invasive Pneumococcal Infection**

High risk (attack rate of invasive pneumococcal disease ≥150/100 000 people annually)
• Sickle cell disease, congenital or acquired asplenia, or splenic dysfunction
• Infection with human immunodeficiency virus

Presumed high risk (attack rates not calculated)
• Congenital immune deficiency; some B-(humoral) or T-lymphocyte deficiencies, complement deficiencies (particularly C1, C2, C3, and C4), or phagocytic disorders (excluding chronic granulomatous disease)
• Chronic cardiac disease (particularly cyanotic congenital heart disease and cardiac failure)
• Chronic pulmonary disease (including asthma treated with high-dose oral corticosteroid therapy)
• Cerebrospinal leaks from a congenital malformation, skull fracture, or neurological procedure
• Chronic renal insufficiency, including nephrotic syndrome
• Diseases associated with immunosuppressive therapy or radiation therapy (including malignant neoplasms, leukemias, lymphomas, and Hodgkin disease) and solid organ transplantation
• Diabetes mellitus
• Cochlear implants

Moderate risk (attack rate of invasive pneumococcal disease ≥20 cases/100 000 people annually).
• All children 24–35 mo of age
• Children 36–59 mo of age attending out-of-home child care
• Children 36–59 mo of age who are black or of American Indian/Alaska Native descent

TREATMENT: *Streptococcus pneumoniae* strains that are nonsusceptible to penicillin G, cefotaxime, ceftriaxone, and other antimicrobial agents have been identified throughout the United States and worldwide. Among children in some geographic areas of the United States, more than 40% of isolates from sterile body sites are nonsusceptible to penicillin G, and as many as 50% of these isolates are highly resistant. Approximately 50% of penicillin-nonsusceptible strains also are nonsusceptible to cefotaxime or ceftriaxone. Penicillin-nonsusceptible strains also have increased rates of resistance to trimethoprim-sulfamethoxazole, macrolides, and clindamycin.

Vancomycin resistance has not been reported in the United States. If a strain with an in vitro MIC greater than 1.0 µg/mL to vancomycin is isolated, the state health department should be notified promptly and arrangements should be made for confirmatory testing.

Recommendations for treatment of pneumococcal infections are as follows.
***Bacterial Meningitis Possibly or Proven to Be Caused by* S pneumoniae.**
Combination therapy with vancomycin and cefotaxime or ceftriaxone should be administered initially to all children 1 month of age or older with definite or probable bacterial meningitis because of the increased prevalence of *S pneumoniae* resistant to penicillin, cefotaxime, and ceftriaxone. Some experts recommend that

vancomycin not be used if compelling evidence indicates that the cause is an organism other than *S pneumoniae* (eg, gram-negative diplococci on a CSF smear during an outbreak of meningococcal disease).

For children with hypersensitivity to β-lactam antimicrobial agents (ie, penicillins and cephalosporins), the combination of vancomycin and rifampin should be considered. Vancomycin should not be given alone, because bactericidal concentrations in CSF are difficult to sustain, and clinical experience to support use of vancomycin as monotherapy is minimal. Rifampin also should not be given as monotherapy, because resistance may develop during therapy. Other possible antimicrobial agents for treatment of pneumococcal meningitis include meropenem or chloramphenicol (which only should be used for pneumococcal meningitis if the minimal bactericidal concentration is ≤4 µg/mL).

A lumbar puncture should be considered after 24 to 48 hours of therapy in the following circumstances: (1) the organism is penicillin-*nonsusceptible* by oxacillin disk or quantitative (MIC) testing, results from cefotaxime and ceftriaxone quantitative susceptibility testing are not yet available, and the patient's condition has not improved or has worsened; or (2) the child has received dexamethasone, which might interfere with the ability to interpret clinical response, such as resolution of fever.

On the basis of available results of susceptibility testing of the pneumococcal isolate, therapy should be modified according to the guidelines in Table 3.44 (p 494). If the organism is susceptible to penicillin or cefotaxime or ceftriaxone, vancomycin should be discontinued and penicillin or cefotaxime or ceftriaxone should be continued. Vancomycin should be continued only if the organism is nonsusceptible to penicillin and to cefotaxime or ceftriaxone.

Addition of rifampin to vancomycin after 24 to 48 hours of therapy should be considered if the organism is susceptible to rifampin and (1) after 24 to 48 hours, despite therapy with vancomycin and cefotaxime or ceftriaxone, the clinical condition has worsened; (2) the subsequent culture of CSF indicates failure to eradicate or to decrease substantially the number of organisms; or (3) the organism has an unusually high cefotaxime or ceftriaxone MIC (≥4 µg/mL). Consultation with an infectious disease specialist should be considered in such circumstances.

Dexamethasone. For infants and children 6 weeks of age and older, adjunctive therapy with dexamethasone may be considered after weighing the potential benefits and possible risks. Experts vary in recommending the use of corticosteroids in pneumococcal meningitis; data are not sufficient to demonstrate a clear benefit in children.

Nonmeningeal Invasive Pneumococcal Infections Requiring Hospitalization.
For nonmeningeal invasive infections in previously well children who are not critically ill, antimicrobial agents currently in use to treat *S pneumoniae* and other potential pathogens should be initiated at the usually recommended dosages (see Table 3.45, p 495).

For critically ill infants and children with invasive infections potentially attributable to *S pneumoniae*, additional initial antimicrobial therapy may be considered for strains that possibly are nonsusceptible to penicillin, cefotaxime, or ceftriaxone. Such patients include those with myopericarditis or severe multilobar pneumonia with hypoxia or hypotension. If vancomycin is administered, it should be discontinued as soon as antimicrobial susceptibility test results demonstrate effective alternative agents.

Table 3.44. Antimicrobial Therapy for Infants and Children With Meningitis Caused by *Streptococcus pneumoniae* on the Basis of Susceptibility Test Results

Susceptibility Test Results	Antimicrobial Management[1]
Susceptible to penicillin	**Discontinue vancomycin** **AND** Begin penicillin **OR** Continue cefotaxime or ceftriaxone alone[2]
Nonsusceptible to penicillin *(intermediately susceptible* or *resistant)* **AND** *Susceptible* to cefotaxime and ceftriaxone	**Discontinue vancomycin** **AND** Continue cefotaxime or ceftriaxone
Nonsusceptible to penicillin *(intermediately susceptible* or *resistant)* **AND** *Nonsusceptible* to cefotaxime and ceftriaxone *(intermediately susceptible* or *resistant)* **AND** *Susceptible* to rifampin	Continue vancomycin and cefotaxime or ceftriaxone. Rifampin may be added to vancomycin in selected circumstances (see text).

[1] See Table 3.45, p 495 for dosage. Some experts recommend the maximum dosages. For initial therapy, see Bacterial Meningitis Possibly or Proven to Be Caused by *S pneumoniae*, p 492.
[2] Some physicians may choose this alternative for convenience and cost savings.

If the organism is highly resistant to penicillin, cefotaxime, and ceftriaxone, therapy should be modified on the basis of clinical response, susceptibility to other antimicrobial agents, and results of follow-up cultures of blood and other body fluids. Consultation with an infectious disease specialist should be considered.

For children with severe hypersensitivity to the β-lactam antimicrobial agents (ie, penicillins and cephalosporins), initial management for a potential pneumococcal infection should include clindamycin or vancomycin, in addition to antimicrobial drugs for other potential pathogens as indicated. Vancomycin should not be continued if the organism is susceptible to other appropriate non–β-lactam antimicrobial agents. Consultation with an infectious disease specialist should be considered.

Nonmeningeal Invasive Pneumococcal Infections in the Immunocompromised Host. The preceding recommendations for management of possible pneumococcal infections requiring hospitalization also apply to immunocompromised children, provided they are not critically ill. For critically ill patients, consideration should be given to initiating therapy with vancomycin and cefotaxime or ceftriaxone. Vancomycin should be discontinued as soon as antimicrobial susceptibility test results indicate that effective alternative antimicrobial agents are available.

Dosages. The recommended dosages of intravenous antimicrobial agents for treatment of invasive pneumococcal infections are given in Table 3.45 (p 495).

Otitis Media. Most experts recommend empiric initial treatment of acute otitis media (AOM) with high-dose oral amoxicillin (80 mg/kg per day). Standard

Table 3.45. **Dosages of Intravenous Antimicrobial Agents for Invasive Pneumococcal Infections in Infants and Children[1]**

Antimicrobial Agent	Meningitis		Nonmeningeal Infections	
	Dose, kg/day	Dose Interval	Dose, kg/day	Dose Interval
Penicillin G	250 000–400 000 U[2]	4–6 h	250 000–400 000 U[2]	4–6 h
Cefotaxime	225–300 mg	8 h	75–100 mg	8 h
Ceftriaxone	100 mg	12–24 h	50–75 mg	12–24 h
Vancomycin	60 mg	6 h	40–45 mg	6 h
Rifampin[3]	20 mg	12 h	Not indicated	...
Chloramphenicol[4]	75–100 mg	6 h	75–100 mg	6 h
Clindamycin[4]	Not indicated	...	25–40 mg	6–8 h
Meropenem[5]	120 mg	8 h	60 mg	8 h
Imipenem-cilastatin[6]	...	...	60 mg	6 h

[1] Doses are for children 1 month of age or older.
[2] Because 1 U = 0.6 μg/mL, this range is equal to 150 to 240 mg/kg per day.
[3] Indications for use are not defined completely.
[4] Drug should be considered only for patients with life-threatening allergic response after administration of β-lactam antimicrobial agents.
[5] Drug is approved for pediatric patients 3 months of age and older.
[6] Drug is not approved for use in patients younger than 12 years of age and is not recommended in patients with meningitis because of its potential epileptogenic properties.

duration of therapy is 10 days, but uncomplicated cases among children older than 2 years of age can be treated for 5 days. On the basis of concentrations in middle ear fluid and in vitro activity, no currently available oral antimicrobial agent has better activity than amoxicillin against nonsusceptible *S pneumoniae.*

For patients with clinically defined treatment failures when assessed after 3 to 5 days of initial therapy, suitable alternative agents should be active against penicillin-nonsusceptible pneumococci as well as β-lactamase–producing *Haemophilus influenzae* and *Moraxella catarrhalis.* Such agents include oral cefdinir, cefuroxime axetil, intramuscular ceftriaxone, and high-dose oral amoxicillin-clavulanate potassium. Amoxicillin-clavulanate should be given at 80 mg/kg per day of the amoxicillin component (eg, the 7:1 formulation) to decrease the incidence of diarrhea. Erythromycin-sulfisoxazole acetyl, clarithromycin, and azithromycin dihydrate are appropriate alternatives for penicillin-allergic patients.

Myringotomy should be considered for recurrent treatment failures or severe cases to obtain cultures to guide therapy. For multidrug-resistant strains of *S pneumoniae,* the use of clindamycin, rifampin, or other agents in consultation with an expert in infectious diseases should be considered.

Sinusitis. Antimicrobial agents effective for the treatment of acute otitis media also are likely to be effective for acute sinusitis and are recommended.

ISOLATION OF THE HOSPITALIZED PATIENT: Standard precautions are recommended, including for patients with infections caused by drug-resistant *S pneumoniae.*

CONTROL MEASURES:

Active Immunization. Two pneumococcal vaccines are available for use in children, the heptavalent pneumococcal conjugate vaccines (PCV7 [Prevnar, Lederle Laboratories, Pearl River, NY, distributed by Wyeth-Ayerst Pharmaceuticals, Philadelphia, PA]) composed of purified polysaccharides of 7 serotypes (4, 6B, 9V, 14, 18C, 19F, and 23F) conjugated to a diphtheria protein (CRM_{197}) and the 23-valent pneumococcal polysaccharide vaccine (PS23) composed of 23 purified capsular polysaccharides (Pneumovax [Merck & Co Inc, West Point, PA). Prevnar and Pneumovax contain no thimerosal. Each vaccine is recommended in a dose of 0.5 mL to be given intramuscularly. The PS23 vaccine induces protective antibody responses to the most common pneumococcal serotypes in children 2 years of age or older, and the PCV7 vaccine also induces protective antibody responses in children younger than 2 years of age. The 7 serotypes of the PCV7 vaccine account for approximately 88% of the cases of bacteremia, 82% of the cases of meningitis, and 70% of the cases of pneumococcal otitis media in US children younger than 6 years of age in the United States. Eighty percent of penicillin-nonsusceptible strains are one of these 7 serotypes.

Routine Immunization With Pneumococcal Conjugate Vaccine. The PCV7 vaccine is recommended for routine administration as a 4-dose series for all children 23 months of age and younger at 2, 4, 6, and 12 to 15 months of age (Table 3.46, p 497). Each 0.5-mL dose of PCV7 should be administered intramuscularly. Infants should begin the PCV7 immunization series in conjunction with other recommended vaccines at the time of the first regularly scheduled health maintenance visit after at least 6 weeks of age. Infants of very low birth weight (≤1500 g) should be immunized at the time that they attain a chronologic age of 6 to 8 weeks, regardless of their calculated gestational age. All doses of PCV7 may be administered concurrently with all other childhood immunizations, including diphtheria and tetanus toxoids and acellular pertussis (DTaP) vaccines, all *H influenzae* type b vaccines, hepatitis B vaccines, inactivated (or oral) poliovirus vaccines, measles-mumps-rubella vaccine, and varicella vaccine using a separate syringe for the injection of each vaccine and administering each vaccine at a separate site. For children 23 months of age and younger who have not received the first PCV7 dose before 6 months of age, a schedule of a decreased number of doses should be given in accord with Table 3.46. Children 23 months of age or younger who begin catch-up PCV7 immunization series at 7 months of age or older should do so at the first opportunity.

Immunization of Children 24 to 59 Months of Age at High Risk of Invasive Pneumococcal Disease. The PCV7 vaccine is recommended for all children younger than 60 months of age who are at high risk of invasive pneumococcal infection, as defined in Table 3.43. For some high-risk children, supplemental protection should be given with administration of PS23 vaccine. Most high-risk children will have received a series of 4 injections of PCV7 before 24 months of age, and for these children, a dose of PS23 is recommended to be given at 24 months

Table 3.46. **Recommended Schedule for Doses of PCV7, Including Catch-up Immunizations in Previously Unimmunized Children**

Age at First Dose	Timing of Immunization Series
2–6 mo	3 doses, 6–8 wk apart, then 1 dose at 12–15 mo of age
7–11 mo	2 doses, 6–8 wk apart, then 1 dose at 12–15 mo
12–23 mo	2 doses, 6–8 wk apart
24–59 mo	
Immunocompetent	1 dose
High risk, including immunocompromised	2 doses, 6–8 wk apart

PCV7 indicates heptavalent pneumococcal conjugate vaccine

of age and an additional dose of PS23 is recommended to be given 3 to 5 years after the first dose. The recommendations for high-risk children who are 24 to 59 months of age who may have received previous doses of either PS23 or PCV7 vaccines are summarized in Table 3.47 (p 498). All high-risk children who have not previously received doses of PCV7 as infants younger than 24 months of age should receive a series of 2 doses of PCV7 and 1 dose of PS23 given at a 6- to 8-week interval between each dose, followed by another dose of PS23 at 3 to 5 years after the first dose.

Immunization of Children 24 to 59 Months of Age at Moderate or Low Risk of Invasive Pneumococcal Disease. Recommendations for children 24 to 59 months of age who are at moderate risk (Table 3.43, p 492) of pneumococcal disease are listed in Table 3.46 (above). Risk factors other than those listed in Table 3.43 include social or economic disadvantage, residence in crowded or substandard housing, homelessness, chronic exposure to tobacco smoke, or a history of severe or recurrent otitis media within the year before immunization or before placement of tympanostomy tubes.

The relative merits of PCV7 or PS23 given as a single dose in children 24 months of age or older have not been studied. In addition to its impact on invasive infections, use of PCV7 has resulted in a modest decrease in the incidence of otitis media and nasopharyngeal carriage. Furthermore, the duration of antibody responses is greater after PCV7, and this vaccine induces immunologic memory. The preferred vaccine for most children is PCV7. If PCV7 is given, a single dose of PS23 after administration of PCV7 is recommended, particularly for children of American Indian descent. Use of PS23 provides a broader pneumococcal coverage against serotypes not contained within PCV7, because the conjugate vaccine may provide coverage against 75% or fewer of disease-associated serotypes in children older than 24 months of age. However, either PCV7 or PS23 can be used for elective administration to children 24 to 59 months of age who are at moderate risk.

Immunization of Children 5 Years of Age and Older. Immunization at 5 years of age or older may be appropriate for certain children who remain at high risk because of chronic underlying disease. Limited safety and efficacy data are available for PCV7 or PS23 in children who are 60 months of age or older. Studies of small numbers of children with sickle cell disease and HIV infection suggest that PCV7 is

Table 3.47. **Recommendations for Pneumococcal Immunization With PCV7 or PS23 Vaccine for Children at High Risk of Pneumococcal Disease, as Defined in Table 3.43 (p 492)**

Age	Previous Dose(s) of Any Pneumococcal Vaccine	Recommendations
≤23 mo	None	PCV7, as in Table 3.46 (p 497)
24–59 mo	4 doses of PCV7	1 dose of PS23 vaccine at 24 mo of age, at least 6–8 wk after last dose of PCV7. 1 dose of PS23, 3–5 y after the first dose of PS23.
24–59 mo	1–3 previous doses of PCV7	1 dose of PCV7. 1 dose of PS23, 6–8 wk after the last dose of PCV7. 1 dose of PS23, 3–5 y after the first dose of PS23.
24–59 mo	1 dose of PS23	2 doses of PCV7, 6–8 wk apart, beginning at 6–8 wk after last dose of PS23. 1 dose of PS23 vaccine, 3–5 y after the last dose of PS23.
24–59 mo	No previous dose of PS23 or PCV7	2 doses of PCV7, 6–8 wk apart. 1 dose of PS23 vaccine, 6–8 wk after the last dose of PCV7. 1 dose of PS23 vaccine, 3–5 y after the first dose of PS23 vaccine.

safe and immunogenic when administered to children up to 13 years of age. Therefore, administration of a single dose of PCV7 to children of any age, particularly children who are at high risk of invasive pneumococcal disease, is not contraindicated. However, PS23 also may be effective and immunogenic in older children, and therefore, immunization with a single dose of PCV7 or PS23 is acceptable. If both vaccines are used, PCV7 should be administered first and the administration of PS23 should follow at an interval of at least 6 to 8 weeks.

Immunization of Children With Severe or Recurrent Otitis Media. Pneumococcal polysaccharide vaccines have not decreased the incidence of AOM in children of any age; therefore, PS23 is not recommended for prevention of AOM. The PCV7 vaccine provides a modest decrease in recurrent AOM (as defined by 3 or more episodes in 6 months or 4 or more episodes in a year). The PCV7 may be beneficial in children 24 to 59 months of age who previously have not received pneumococcal vaccines and who have a history of recurrent AOM or who have AOM complicated by placement of tympanostomy tubes.

Control of Transmission of Pneumococcal Infection and Invasive Disease Among Children Attending Out-of-Home Care. Rates of invasive pneumococcal infection among children attending out-of-home care are twofold to threefold higher than among healthy children of the same age not enrolled in out-of-home care. The PS23 vaccine does not decrease nasopharyngeal carriage of pneumococci, but limited data suggest a >50% decrease in nasopharyngeal carriage of vaccine serotype among children receiving conjugate pneumococcal vaccine. Available data are insufficient to recommend any antimicrobial regimen for preventing or interrupting the carriage or transmission of pneumococcal infection in these settings, and therefore, antimicrobial chemoprophylaxis is not recommended for contacts of children with invasive pneumococcal disease, regardless of their immunization status.

General Recommendations for Use of Pneumococcal Vaccines.

- Either PS23 or PCV7 may be given concurrently with other vaccines. Pneumococcal vaccine should be injected with a separate syringe in a separate site.
- When elective splenectomy is performed for any reason, immunization with PCV7 or PS23 should be completed at least 2 weeks before splenectomy. Immunization with either vaccine should precede the initiation of immune-compromising therapy by at least 2 weeks.
- Generally, pneumococcal vaccines should be deferred during pregnancy, because it is not known whether pneumococcal vaccines can cause fetal harm when administered to a pregnant woman. However, inactivated or killed vaccines, including other experimental and licensed polysaccharide vaccines, have been administered safely during pregnancy. The risk of severe pneumococcal disease in a pregnant woman should be considered when making decisions regarding the need for pneumococcal immunization.
- Children who have experienced invasive pneumococcal disease should receive all recommended doses of pneumococcal vaccines (PCV7 or 23PS) appropriate for age and underlying condition. The full series of scheduled doses should be completed even if the series is interrupted by an episode of invasive pneumococcal disease.

Adverse Reactions to Pneumococcal Vaccines. Adverse reactions after administration of polysaccharide or conjugate vaccines generally are mild and limited to local reactions of redness or swelling. Fever may occur within the first 1 to 2 days after injections, particularly after use of conjugate vaccine.

Passive Immunization. Immune Globulin Intravenous administration is recommended for preventing pneumococcal infection in patients with congenital or acquired immunodeficiency diseases, including people with HIV infection who have recurrent pneumococcal infections (see Human Immunodeficiency Virus Infection, p 360).

Chemoprophylaxis. Daily antimicrobial prophylaxis is recommended for children with functional or anatomic asplenia, regardless of their immunization status, for prevention of pneumococcal disease (see Asplenic Children, p 80). Oral penicillin V (125 mg twice a day for children younger than 5 years of age; 250 mg twice a day for children 5 years of age and older) is recommended. The results of a multicenter study demonstrated that oral penicillin V (125 mg twice a day) given to infants and young children with sickle cell anemia decreased the incidence of pneumococcal bacteremia by 84% compared with the placebo control group. On the basis of this study, daily penicillin prophylaxis for children with sickle cell anemia beginning before 2 months of age is recommended. The number of cases of penicillin-resistant invasive pneumococcal infections and the prevalence of nasopharyngeal carriage of penicillin-resistant strains in patients with sickle cell disease have increased in recent years. Parents, thus, should be informed that penicillin prophylaxis no longer may be as effective at preventing invasive pneumococcal infections as in the past.

The age at which prophylaxis is discontinued often is an empiric decision. Most children with sickle cell anemia who had received penicillin prophylaxis for prolonged periods, who are receiving regular medical attention, and who have not had a previous severe pneumococcal infection or a surgical splenectomy safely may discontinue prophylactic penicillin at 5 years of age. However, they must be counseled to seek medical attention for all febrile events. The duration of prophylaxis for children with asplenia attributable to other causes is unknown. Some experts continue prophylaxis throughout childhood.

Pneumocystis jiroveci Infections

CLINICAL MANIFESTATIONS: Infants and children develop a characteristic syndrome of subacute diffuse pneumonitis with dyspnea at rest, tachypnea, oxygen desaturation, nonproductive cough, and fever. However, the intensity of these signs and symptoms may vary, and in some immunocompromised children and adults, onset can be acute and fulminant. The chest radiograph often shows bilateral diffuse interstitial or alveolar disease; rarely, lobar, miliary, and nodular lesions occur as well. Rarely, the chest radiograph at the time of diagnosis appears normal. The mortality rate in immunocompromised patients ranges from 5% to 40% if treated and approaches 100% if untreated.

ETIOLOGY: *Pneumocystis jiroveci* (previously *Pneumocystis carinii*) is classified as a fungus on the basis of DNA sequence analysis. However, *P jiroveci* retains several morphologic and biologic similarities to protozoa, including being susceptible to a number of antiprotozoal agents but resistant to most antifungal agents. The 5- to 7-μm-diameter cysts contain up to 8 sporozoites. The acronym PCP will be retained and will refer to *Pneumocystis* pneumonia.

EPIDEMIOLOGY: *Pneumocystis jiroveci* is ubiquitous in mammals worldwide, particularly rodents, and has a tropism for growth on respiratory tract surfaces. *Pneumocystis jiroveci* isolates recovered from mice, rats, and ferrets are diverse genetically from each other and from human *P jiroveci;* isolates from one animal species do not cross-infect other animal species. Asymptomatic infection occurs early in life, with more than 75% of healthy people acquiring antibody by 4 years of age. In resource-limited countries and in times of famine, PCP has occurred in epidemics, primarily affecting malnourished infants and children. Epidemics also have occurred in premature infants. In industrialized countries, PCP occurs almost entirely in immunocompromised people with deficient cell-mediated immunity, particularly people with human immunodefociency virus (HIV) infection, recipients of immunosuppressive therapy after organ transplantation or treatment for malignant neoplasm, and children with congenital immunodeficiency syndromes. Although decreasing in frequency because of effective prophylaxis and antiretroviral therapy, PCP remains one of the most common serious opportunistic infections in infants and children with perinatally acquired HIV infection. Although onset of disease can occur at any age, including rare instances during the first month of life, PCP most commonly occurs in HIV-infected children between 3 and 6 months of age. The mode of transmission is unknown. Hypotheses include person-to-person transmission by the respiratory route and acquisition from the environment. Circumstantial evidence suggests that person-to-person transmission can occur. Primary infection probably accounts for disease during infancy. Although reactivation of latent infection with immunosuppression has been proposed as an explanation for disease after the first 2 years of life, animal models of PCP do not support the existence of latency. In patients with lymphoma or leukemia, the disease can occur during remission or relapse. The period of communicability is unknown.

The **incubation period** is unknown, but animal models suggest 4 to 8 weeks from exposure to clinically apparent infection.

DIAGNOSTIC TESTS: A definitive diagnosis of PCP is made by demonstration of organisms in lung tissue or respiratory tract secretion specimens. The most sensitive and specific diagnostic procedures are open lung biopsy and, in older children, transbronchial biopsy. However, bronchoscopy with bronchoalveolar lavage, induction of sputum in older children and adolescents, and intubation with deep endotracheal aspiration are less invasive and often diagnostic and are sensitive in patients with HIV infection who have an increased number of organisms. Methenamine silver, toluidine blue O, calcofluor white, and fluorescein-conjugated monoclonal antibody are the most useful stains for identifying the thick-walled cysts of *P jiroveci*. Extracystic trophozoite forms are identified with Giemsa stain, modified Wright-Giemsa stain, and fluorescein-conjugated monoclonal antibody stain. Polymerase chain reaction assays for detecting *P jiroveci* infection are experimental and are not recommended for diagnosis. Serologic tests are not useful.

TREATMENT: The drug of choice is intravenous trimethoprim-sulfamethoxazole (trimethoprim, 15–20 mg/kg per day and sulfamethoxazole, 75–100 mg/kg daily, in divided doses every 6 hours). Oral therapy should be reserved for patients with mild disease who do not have malabsorption or diarrhea. The rate of adverse reactions (rash, neutropenia, anemia, renal dysfunction, nausea, vomiting, and diarrhea) to trimethoprim-sulfamethoxazole is higher in HIV-infected children (estimated at 15%) than in other patients. If the adverse reaction is not severe, continuation of therapy is recommended. Half of the patients with adverse reactions subsequently have been treated successfully with trimethoprim-sulfamethoxazole.

Intravenously administered pentamidine (4 mg/kg per day of salt, once daily) is an alternative drug for children and adults who cannot tolerate trimethoprim-sulfamethoxazole or who have severe disease and have not responded to trimethoprim-sulfamethoxazole after 5 to 7 days of therapy. The therapeutic efficacy of parenteral pentamidine in adults with PCP has been similar to that of trimethoprim-sulfamethoxazole. Pentamidine is associated with a high incidence of adverse reactions, including pancreatitis, renal dysfunction, hypoglycemia, hyperglycemia, hypotension, fever, and neutropenia. Pentamidine should not be administered concomitantly with didanosine, because both drugs cause pancreatitis. If a recipient of didanosine develops PCP and requires pentamidine, didanosine should be discontinued until 1 week after pentamidine therapy has been completed.

Atovaquone is approved for the oral treatment of mild to moderate PCP in adults who are intolerant of trimethoprim-sulfamethoxazole. Experience with the use of atovaquone in children is limited. Other potentially useful drugs in adults include dapsone with trimethoprim, trimetrexate glucuronate with leucovorin calcium, and clindamycin with primaquine phosphate. Experience with the use of these combinations in children is limited.

A minimum duration of 2 weeks of therapy is recommended; many experts advise 3 weeks of therapy for patients with acquired immunodeficiency syndrome (AIDS). In patients with AIDS, prophylaxis should be initiated at the end of therapy for acute infection and should be continued until CD4+ T-lymphocyte counts exceed the concentration no longer requiring prophylaxis (see Table 3.48, p 503) or lifelong if CD4+ T-lymphocyte cells do not respond to antiretroviral therapy. Children with PCP infection should be given lifelong prophylaxis to prevent recurrence.

Corticosteroids appear to be beneficial in the treatment of HIV-infected adults with moderate to severe PCP (as defined by an arterial oxygen pressure [PaO_2] of less than 70 mm Hg in room air or an arterial-alveolar gradient of more than 35 mm Hg). For adolescents older than 13 years of age and adults, 80 mg/day of oral prednisone in 2 divided doses for the first 5 days of therapy, 40 mg once a day on days 6 through 10, and 20 mg once a day on days 11 through 21 is recommended. Although no controlled studies of the use of corticosteroids in young children have been performed, most experts would include corticosteroids as part of therapy for children with moderate to severe PCP. The optimal dose and duration of corticosteroid therapy for children have not been determined, but most experts suggest 2 mg/kg per day of prednisone or its equivalent for 7 to 10 days, followed by a tapering dose during the next 10 to 14 days.

Chemoprophylaxis. Prophylaxis against a first episode of PCP is indicated for many patients with significant immunocompromise, including people with HIV infection (see Human Immunodeficiency Virus Infection, p 360) and people with primary or acquired immunodeficiency.

Because half of all cases of PCP in children with perinatally acquired HIV occur in infants 3 to 6 months of age, early identification of infants who have been exposed perinatally to HIV is essential for prophylaxis to be initiated before these infants are at risk. Prophylaxis for PCP is recommended for all infants born to HIV-infected women beginning at 4 to 6 weeks of age (see Table 3.48, p 503). Prophylaxis for PCP should be discontinued in children in whom HIV infection has been excluded unless another immunocompromising condition exists. Children whose HIV infection status is indeterminate should continue prophylaxis throughout the first year of life.

For HIV-infected infants and children, PCP prophylaxis should be continued or administered in the following situations: (1) any CD4+ T-lymphocyte count that indicates severe immunosuppression for age (see Table 3.48, p 503); (2) a rapidly decreasing CD4+ T-lymphocyte count; or (3) severely symptomatic HIV disease (category C) (see Human Immunodeficiency Virus Infection, p 360, and Table 3.48, p 503). Criteria are the same for older children and adolescents, except for different age-specific definitions of low absolute CD4+ T-lymphocyte counts. For adolescents or adults, PCP prophylaxis has been recommended if the patient has a history of oropharyngeal candidiasis. On the basis of experience with discontinuing primary

Table 3.48. **Recommendations for** *Pneumocystis* **Pneumonia (PCP) Prophylaxis for Human Immunodeficiency Virus (HIV)-Exposed Infants and Children, by Age and HIV Infection Status[1]**

Age and HIV Infection Status	PCP Prophylaxis[2]
Birth to 4–6 wk, HIV exposed	No prophylaxis
4–6 wk to 4 mo, HIV exposed	Prophylaxis
4–12 mo	
HIV infected or indeterminate	Prophylaxis
HIV infection excluded[3]	No prophylaxis
1–5 y, HIV-infected	Prophylaxis if: CD4+ T-lymphocyte count is <500 cells/μL or percentage is <15%[4,5]
≥5 y, HIV-infected	Prophylaxis if: CD4+ T-lymphocyte count is <200 cells/μL or percentage is <15%[5]

[1] Modified from Centers for Disease Control and Prevention. 2002 USPHS/IDSA guidelines for preventing opportunistic infections among HIV-infected persons—2002. Recommendations of the US Public Health Service and the Infectious Diseases Society of America. *MMWR Recomm Rep.* 2002;51(RR-8):1–46

[2] Children who have had PCP should receive lifelong PCP prophylaxis.

[3] HIV infection can be excluded reasonably among children who have had 2 or more negative results of HIV diagnostic tests, both of which are performed at ≥1 month of age and 1 of which is performed at ≥4 months of age; or 2 or more negative results of HIV immunoglobulin G antibody tests performed at ≥6 months of age among children who have no clinical evidence of HIV disease (see Human Immunodeficiency Virus Infection, p 360).

[4] Children 1 to 2 years of age who were receiving PCP prophylaxis and had a CD4+ T-lymphocyte count of less than 750/μL or percentage of <15% at younger than 12 months of age should continue prophylaxis.

[5] Prophylaxis should be considered on a case-by-case basis for children who might otherwise be at risk of PCP, such as children with rapidly declining CD4+ T-lymphocyte counts or percentages or children with category C status of HIV infection.

or secondary (after a case of PCP) prophylaxis for PCP in adolescents and adults after an adequate CD4+ T-lymphocyte response to antiretroviral therapy, cessation of prophylaxis also should be considered for patients whose CD4+ T-lymphocyte counts are adequate. Children who have a history of PCP should receive lifelong PCP chemoprophylaxis. The safety of discontinuing secondary prophylaxis among HIV-infected children has not been studied extensively.

Children older than 1 year of age with HIV infection who are not receiving PCP prophylaxis (eg, children not previously identified or children whose PCP prophylaxis was discontinued) should begin prophylaxis if the CD4+ T-lymphocyte cell count indicates severe immunosuppression (see Table 3.48, above).

For PCP, prophylaxis is recommended* for children who have received hematopoietic stem cell transplants (HSCT), all HSCT recipients with hematologic malig-

* Centers for Disease Control and Prevention. Guidelines for preventing opportunistic infections among hematopoietic stem cell transplant recipients. Recommendations of the CDC, the Infectious Diseases Society of America, and the American Society of Blood and Barrow Transplantation. *MMWR Recomm Rep.* 2000;49(RR-10):1–128. See also www.hivatis.org.

nancies (eg, leukemia or lymphoma), and HSCT recipients receiving intense conditioning regimens or graft manipulation. Prophylaxis should be initiated at engraftment and administered for 6 months. Prophylaxis should be continued for more than 6 months in all children receiving immunosuppressive therapy (eg, prednisone or cyclosporin) or in those with chronic graft-versus-host disease.

The recommended drug regimen for PCP prophylaxis for all immunocompromised patients is trimethoprim-sulfamethoxazole administered for 3 consecutive days each week (see Table 3.49, below, for dosage). For patients who cannot tolerate the drug, aerosolized pentamidine administered by the Respirgard II (VitalSigns Inc, Totowa, NJ) nebulizer for people 5 years of age or older is an alternative. Daily oral dapsone is another alternative drug for prophylaxis in children, especially children younger than 5 years of age (see Table 3.49, below). Intravenous pentamidine has been used but is more toxic than other prophylactic regimens.

Other drugs with potential for prophylaxis include pyrimethamine plus dapsone plus leucovorin, pyrimethamine-sulfadoxine, and oral atovaquone.

Table 3.49. Drug Regimens for *Pneumocystis* Pneumonia Prophylaxis for Children 4 Weeks of Age or Older[1]

Recommended regimen:

Trimethoprim-sulfamethoxazole (trimethoprim, 150 mg/m^2 per day with sulfamethoxazole, 750 mg/m^2 per day), orally, in divided doses twice a day, 3 times per week on consecutive days (eg, Monday-Tuesday-Wednesday).

Acceptable alternative trimethoprim-sulfamethoxazole dosage schedules:

- Trimethoprim (150 mg/m^2 per day) with sulfamethoxazole (750 mg/m^2 per day), orally, **as a single daily dose,** 3 times per week on consecutive days (eg, Monday-Tuesday-Wednesday).
- Trimethoprim (150 mg/m^2 per day) with sulfamethoxazole (750 mg/m^2 per day), orally, in divided doses, twice a day, and **administered 7 days per week.**
- Trimethoprim (150 mg/m^2 per day) with sulfamethoxazole (750 mg/m^2 per day), orally, in divided doses twice a day, and administered 3 times per week on alternate days (eg, Monday-Wednesday-Friday).

Alternative regimens if trimethoprim-sulfamethoxazole is not tolerated[2]:

- **Dapsone (children ≥1 mo of age)**
  2 mg/kg (maximum 100 mg), orally, once a day or 4 mg/kg (maximum 200 mg), orally, every week
- **Aerosolized pentamidine (children ≥5 y of age)**
  300 mg, administered via Respirgard II inhaler monthly
- **Atovaquone (children 1–3 mo of age and >24 mo of age)**
  30 mg/kg, orally, once a day
  (children 4–24 mo of age)
  45 mg/kg, orally, once a day

---

[1] Modified from Centers for Disease Control and Prevention. 2002 USPHS/IDSA guidelines for preventing opportunistic infections among HIV-infected persons—2002. Recommendations of the US Public Health Service and the Infectious Diseases Society of America. *MMWR Recomm Rep.* 2002;51(RR-8):1–46

[2] If dapsone, aerosolized pentamidine, and atovaquone are not tolerated, some clinicians use intravenous pentamidine (4 mg/kg) administered every 2 to 4 weeks.

Experience with these drugs in adults and children is limited. These agents should be considered only in situations in which the recommended regimens are not tolerated or cannot be used.

Although prophylaxis substantially decreases the risk of PCP, pulmonary and extrapulmonary *P jiroveci* infections have occurred in HIV-infected adults and children receiving prophylaxis.

ISOLATION OF THE HOSPITALIZED PATIENT: Standard precautions are recommended. Some experts recommend that patients with PCP not share a room with immunocompromised patients, although data are insufficient to support this recommendation as standard practice.

CONTROL MEASURES: Appropriate therapy for infected patients and prophylaxis in immunocompromised patients are the only available means of control. Detailed guidelines recently have been issued by the Centers for Disease Control and Prevention and the Infectious Diseases Society of America and endorsed by the American Academy of Pediatrics.*

Poliovirus Infections

CLINICAL MANIFESTATIONS: Approximately 95% of poliovirus infections are asymptomatic. Nonspecific illness with low-grade fever and sore throat (minor illness) occurs in 4% to 8% of people who become infected. Aseptic meningitis, sometimes with paresthesias, occurs in 1% to 5% of patients a few days after the minor illness has resolved. Rapid onset of asymmetric acute flaccid paralysis with areflexia of the involved limb occurs in 0.1% to 2% of infections, and residual paralytic disease involving the motor neurons (paralytic poliomyelitis) occurs in approximately two thirds of people with acute motor neuron disease. Cranial nerve involvement and paralysis of respiratory muscles can occur. Findings in cerebrospinal fluid (CSF) are characteristic of viral meningitis with mild pleocytosis and lymphocytic predominance.

Adults who contracted paralytic poliomyelitis during childhood may develop the postpolio syndrome 30 to 40 years later. Postpolio syndrome is characterized by slow onset of muscle pain and exacerbation of weakness.

ETIOLOGY: Polioviruses are enteroviruses and consist of 3 serotypes: 1, 2, and 3.

EPIDEMIOLOGY: Poliovirus infections occur only in humans. Spread is by the fecal-oral and respiratory routes. Infection is more common in infants and young children and occurs at an earlier age among children living in poor hygienic conditions. The risk of paralytic disease after infection increases with age. In temperate climates, poliovirus infections are most common during summer and autumn; in the tropics, the seasonal pattern is variable with a less pronounced peak of activity.

---

* Centers for Disease Control and Prevention. Guidelines for preventing opportunistic infections among HIV-infected persons—2002. Recommendations of the US Public Health Service and the Infectious Diseases Society of America. *MMWR Recomm Rep.* 2002;51(RR-8):1–46

The last reported case of poliomyelitis attributable to indigenously acquired, wild-type poliovirus in the United States occurred in 1979. The only identified imported case of paralytic poliomyelitis since 1986 occurred in 1993 in a child transported to the United States for medical care. Since 1979, all other cases have been vaccine-associated paralytic poliomyelitis (VAPP) occurring in vaccine recipients or their contacts and attributable to oral poliovirus (OPV) vaccine. An average of 8 cases of VAPP were reported annually in the United States from 1980 to 1996. Fewer VAPP cases have been reported since 1997 after a shift of US immunization policy toward use of only inactivated poliovirus (IPV) vaccine. Implementation of the all-IVP vaccine schedule in 2000 has ended the occurrence of new VAPP cases in the United States. Circulation of wild-type polioviruses has ceased in the United States, and the risk of contact with imported wild-type polioviruses is decreasing rapidly, parallel with the success of the ongoing global eradication program of the World Health Organization.

Communicability of poliovirus is greatest shortly before and after onset of clinical illness when the virus is present in the throat and excreted in high concentration in feces. The virus persists in the throat for approximately 1 week after onset of illness and is excreted in feces for several weeks. Patients potentially are contagious as long as fecal excretion persists. In recipients of OPV vaccine, the virus persists in the throat for 1 to 2 weeks and is excreted in feces for several weeks, although in rare cases, excretion for more than 2 months can occur. Immunodeficient patients have excreted virus for periods of more than 10 years.

The **incubation period** of asymptomatic or mild poliomyelitis is 3 to 6 days. For the onset of paralysis in paralytic poliomyelitis, the incubation period usually is 7 to 21 days.

DIAGNOSTIC TESTS: Poliovirus can be recovered from the pharynx, feces, urine, and rarely, CSF by isolation in cell culture. Two or more stool and throat swab specimens for enterovirus isolation should be obtained at least 24 hours apart from patients with suspected paralytic poliomyelitis as early in the course of the illness as possible, ideally within 14 days of onset of symptoms. Fecal material is most likely to yield virus.

Because OPV vaccine no longer is available in the United States, the chance of exposure to vaccine-type polioviruses has become remote. Therefore, if a poliovirus is isolated in the United States, the isolate should be sent to the Centers for Disease Control and Prevention through the state health department for further testing. Serologic testing of acute and convalescent serum specimens should be performed when paralytic poliomyelitis is suspected, but interpretation of serologic test results can be difficult. Hence, the diagnostic test of choice for confirming poliovirus disease is viral culture of stool specimens and throat swab specimens obtained as early in the course of illness as possible.

TREATMENT: Supportive.

ISOLATION OF THE HOSPITALIZED PATIENT: In addition to standard precautions, contact precautions are indicated for infants and young children for the duration of hospitalization.

CONTROL MEASURES:

Immunization of Infants and Children.

Vaccines. The 2 types of poliovirus vaccines are inactivated vaccine given parenterally (subcutaneously or intramuscularly) and live-virus vaccine given orally. Inactivated poliovirus vaccine is now the only poliovirus vaccine available in the United States. Inactivated poliovirus vaccine contains the 3 types of poliovirus grown in Vero cells and inactivated with formaldehyde. The IPV vaccine in use in the United States since 1987 has higher potency (enhanced) than earlier formulations. Trace amounts of streptomycin sulfate, neomycin, and polymyxin B sulfate may be present in IPV vaccine. Oral poliovirus vaccine contains attenuated poliovirus types 1, 2, and 3 produced in monkey kidney cells or cell cultures. Inactivated poliovirus also is available in a combined vaccine that contains DTaP, hepatitis B, and IPV (see Pertussis, p 472).

Immunogenicity and Efficacy. Both IPV and OPV vaccines in their recommended schedules are highly immunogenic and effective in preventing poliomyelitis. Administration of IPV vaccine results in seroconversion in 95% or more of vaccine recipients to each of the 3 serotypes after 2 doses and in 99% to 100% of recipients after 3 doses. Immunity is prolonged, perhaps lifelong. Mucosal immunity is induced by enhanced-potency IPV vaccine but to a lesser extent than that with OPV vaccine. After poliovirus infection, IPV-immunized children excrete polioviruses from stool but not from the oropharynx. A 3-dose series of OPV vaccine, as formerly used in the United States, results in sustained, probably lifelong immunity. Immunization with 2 or more doses of OPV vaccine induces excellent serum antibody responses and a high degree of intestinal immunity against poliovirus reinfection, which explains its effectiveness in controlling wild-virus circulation.

Administration With Other Vaccines. Either IPV or OPV vaccine may be given concurrently with other routinely recommended childhood vaccines (see Simultaneous Administration of Multiple Vaccines, p 33). For administration of the combined DTaP, hepatitis B, and IPV vaccine with other vaccines and the interchangeability of the combined vaccine with other vaccine products, see Pertussis (p 472).

Adverse Reactions. No serious adverse events have been associated with use of the currently available IPV vaccine. Because IPV vaccine may contain trace amounts of streptomycin, neomycin, and polymyxin B, allergic reactions are possible in recipients with hypersensitivity to one or more of these antimicrobial agents.

Oral poliovirus vaccine can cause VAPP. Before the expanded use of IPV vaccine in the United States, the overall risk of VAPP was approximately 1 case per 2.4 million doses of OPV vaccine distributed. The rate after the first dose, including vaccine recipient and contact cases, was approximately 1 case per 750 000 doses.

Schedule. The American Academy of Pediatrics recommends a 4-dose all-IPV vaccine schedule for routine immunization of all infants and children in the United States. The first 2 doses should be given at 2-month intervals beginning at 2 months of age (minimum age 6 weeks), and a third dose is recommended at 6 to 18 months of age. Doses may be given at 4-week intervals when accelerated protection is indicated. Administration of the third dose at 6 months of age has the potential advantage of enhancing the likelihood of completion of the primary series and does not compromise seroconversion. A supplemental dose of IPV vaccine should be given before the child enters school (ie, at 4 to 6 years of age). A fourth dose is not necessary if the third dose was given on or after the child's fourth birthday.

Oral poliovirus vaccine is the vaccine of choice for global eradication. It is recommended in the following areas: (1) locations with continued or recent circulation of wild-type poliovirus; (2) most developing countries where the higher cost of IPV vaccine prohibits its use; and (3) where inadequate sanitation necessitates an optimal mucosal barrier to wild-type virus circulation.

Oral poliovirus vaccine no longer is distributed within the United States. However, the potential use of OPV to control a future outbreak of paralytic poliomyelitis remains a public health option. Whenever OPV vaccine is administered, the risk of VAPP in recipients and contacts should be discussed with parents or caregivers.

Children Incompletely Immunized. Children who have not received the recommended doses of poliovirus vaccines on schedule should receive sufficient doses of IPV vaccine to complete the immunization series for their age (see Table 1.6, p 26).

Vaccine Recommendations for Adults. Most adults residing in the United States are immune as a result of immunization received during childhood and have a small risk of exposure to wild-type poliovirus in the United States. Immunization is recommended only for certain adults who are at a greater risk of exposure to wild-type polioviruses than the general population, including the following:

- Travelers to areas or countries where poliomyelitis is or may be epidemic or endemic
- Members of communities or specific population groups with disease caused by wild-type polioviruses
- Laboratory workers handling specimens that may contain wild-type polioviruses
- Health care professionals in close contact with patients who may be excreting wild-type polioviruses

For unimmunized adults, primary immunization with IPV vaccine is recommended. Two doses of IPV vaccine should be given at intervals of 1 to 2 months (4–8 weeks); a third dose is given 6 to 12 months after the second unless the risk of exposure is increased, such as when traveling to areas where wild-type poliovirus is known to be circulating. If time does not allow 3 doses of IPV vaccine to be given according to the recommended schedule before protection is required, the following alternatives are recommended:

- If protection is not needed until 8 weeks or more, 3 doses of IPV vaccine should be given at least 4 weeks apart.
- If protection is not needed for 4 to 8 weeks, 2 doses of IPV vaccine should be given at least 4 weeks apart.
- If protection is needed in fewer than 4 weeks, a single dose of IPV vaccine should be given.

The remaining doses of vaccine to complete the primary immunization schedule should be given subsequently at the recommended intervals if the person remains at an increased risk.

Recommendations in other circumstances are as follows:

- *Incompletely immunized adults.* Adults who previously received less than a full primary course of OPV or IPV vaccine should be given the remaining required doses of IPV vaccine regardless of the interval since the last dose and the type of vaccine that was received previously.

- *Adults who are at an increased risk of exposure to wild-type poliovirus and who previously completed primary immunization with OPV or IPV vaccine.* These adults can receive a single dose of IPV vaccine.

Precautions and Contraindications to Immunization.

Immunodeficiency Disorders. Patients with immunodeficiency disorders, including HIV infection, combined immunodeficiency, abnormalities of immunoglobulin synthesis (ie, antibody deficiency syndromes), leukemia, lymphoma, or generalized malignant neoplasm, or those being given immunosuppressive therapy with pharmacologic agents (see Immunocompromised Children, p 69) or radiation therapy should receive IPV vaccine. A protective immune response to IPV vaccine in an immunodeficient patient cannot be ensured.

Household Contacts of People With Immunodeficiency Disease, Altered Immune States, Immunosuppression Attributable to Therapy for Other Disease, or Known HIV Infection. The IPV vaccine is recommended for these people and OPV vaccine should not be used. If OPV vaccine inadvertently is introduced into a household of an immunodeficient or HIV-infected person, close contact between the patient and the OPV vaccine recipient should be minimized for approximately 4 to 6 weeks after immunization. Household members should be counseled on practices that will minimize exposure of the immunodeficient or HIV-infected person to excreted poliovirus vaccine. These practices include exercising hand hygiene after contact with the child by all and avoiding diaper changing by the immunosuppressed person.

Pregnancy. Immunization during pregnancy generally should be avoided for reasons of theoretic risk, although no convincing evidence indicates that the rates of adverse reactions to IPV vaccine are increased in pregnant women or in their developing fetuses. If immediate protection against poliomyelitis is needed, IPV is recommended (see Vaccine Recommendations for Adults, p 508).

Hypersensitivity or Anaphylactic Reactions to IPV Vaccine, OPV Vaccine, or Antimicrobial Agents Contained in These Vaccines. The IPV vaccine is contraindicated for people who have experienced an anaphylactic reaction after a previous dose of IPV vaccine or to one of the following antimicrobial agents: streptomycin, neomycin, and polymyxin B.

Breastfeeding and mild diarrhea are not contraindications to IPV or OPV vaccine administration.

Reporting of Adverse Events After Immunization. All cases of VAPP and other serious adverse events associated temporally with poliomyelitis vaccine should be reported (see Reporting of Adverse Events, p 40).

Case Reporting and Investigation. A suspected case of poliomyelitis should be reported promptly to the state health department and result in an immediate epidemiologic investigation. Poliomyelitis should be considered in the differential diagnosis of all cases of acute flaccid paralysis, including Guillain-Barré syndrome and transverse myelitis. If the course is compatible clinically with poliomyelitis, specimens should be obtained for viral studies (see Diagnostic Tests, p 506). If the evidence implicates wild-type poliovirus infection, an intensive investigation will be conducted, and a public health decision will be made about the need for supplementary immunizations, choice of vaccine, and other action.

PRION DISEASES

Transmissible Spongiform Encephalopathies*

CLINICAL MANIFESTATIONS: Transmissible spongiform encephalopathies (TSEs), or prion diseases, constitute a group of rare, rapidly progressive, universally fatal neurodegenerative syndromes of humans and animals that are characterized by neuronal degeneration, spongiform change, gliosis, and accumulation of an abnormal protease-resistant amyloid protein (protease-resistant prion protein [PrP^{res}] or scrapie prion protein [PrP^{sc}]) distributed diffusely throughout the brain and sometimes also in discrete plaques. Pathologic involvement of other organ systems has been reported in animal TSEs, but not in humans.

The human TSEs include several diseases: Creutzfeldt-Jakob disease (CJD), Gerstmann-Sträussler-Scheinker disease, fatal familial insomnia, kuru, and variant CJD (vCJD). Classic CJD can be sporadic (approximately 85% of cases), familial (approximately 15%), or iatrogenic (<1%). Iatrogenic CJD has been acquired through injection of cadaveric pituitary hormones (growth hormone and human gonadotropin), dura mater allografts, corneal transplantation, and instrumentation of the brain at neurosurgery or depth-electrode electroencephalographic recording. In 1996, an outbreak of vCJD linked to exposure to tissues from bovine spongiform encephalopathy (BSE)-infected cattle was reported in the United Kingdom. The best known TSEs affecting animals are scrapie of sheep, BSE, and a chronic wasting disease of North American deer and elk.

Creutzfeldt-Jakob disease manifests as a dementing syndrome with progressive defects in memory, personality, and other higher cortical functions in approximately two thirds of affected people. Approximately one third of patients have cerebellar dysfunction, including ataxia and dysarthria. Iatrogenic CJD may manifest as dementia (as in dural allograft transplants) or as cerebellar signs (as observed in virtually all peripherally inoculated disease). Myoclonus develops in at least 80% of affected people at some point in the course of disease. Death usually occurs in weeks to months; only approximately 10% of patients with sporadic CJD survive for more than a year.

The vCJD is distinguished from classic CJD by young age of onset, "psychiatric" manifestation, and other features, such as painful sensory symptoms, delayed onset of overt neurologic signs, absence of diagnostic electroencephalographic changes, and a more prolonged duration of illness. In vCJD, "florid" or "daisy" plaques and marked accumulation of PrP^{res} in the central nervous system and in lymphoid tissues are found.

ETIOLOGY: The infectious particle or prion responsible for the human and animal prion diseases is thought to be an abnormal glycoprotein, without a nucleic acid component, although some experts remain skeptical of the prion hypothesis. Proponents of the hypothesis postulate that sporadic CJD arises from a rare spontaneous structural change of the normal protease-sensitive host-encoded glycoprotein (PrP^{sen}) that normally is found on the surface of neurons in both humans and animals. Prion

---

* Whitley RJ, MacDonald N, Asher DM and the Committee on Infectious Diseases. Transmissible spongiform encephalopathies: a review for pediatricians. *Pediatrics.* 2000;106:1160–1165

protein (PrP) conformational changes are believed to be propagated by a "recruitment reaction" (the nature of which is unknown), in which abnormal PrP serves as a template or lattice for the conformational conversion of neighboring PrP^{sen} molecules.

EPIDEMIOLOGY: Classic CJD is rare, occurring at approximately 1 case per million people annually. The onset of disease peaks in the 60- to 69-year-old age group. Familial CJD occurs at approximately one tenth the frequency of sporadic CJD, with onset of disease approximately 10 years earlier than sporadic CJD.

Case-control studies of sporadic CJD have not identified any consistent environmental risk factor. No statistically significant increased risk has been observed for treatment with blood, blood components, or plasma derivatives, and the incidence of CJD is not increased in patients with several diseases associated with increased exposure to blood or blood products, specifically hemophilia A and B, thalassemia, and sickle cell disease.

As of March 2002, vCJD was reported in 117 patients in the United Kingdom, 6 patients in France, 1 patient in Hong Kong, 1 patient in Italy, and 1 patient in Ireland. The patients from Hong Kong and Ireland were long-term residents of the United Kingdom. Most patients with vCJD were younger than 30 years of age, and several were adolescents. All but one vCJD patient died before 55 years of age. On the basis of animal inoculation studies, strain typing, and epidemiologic investigations, cases of vCJD are believed to be associated with exposure to tissues from cattle infected with bovine spongiform encephalopathy.

The **incubation period** for iatrogenic CJD varies by route of exposure and ranges from 1.5 to more than 30 years.

DIAGNOSTIC TESTS: The diagnosis of human prion diseases can be obtained with certainty only by neuropathologic examination of affected brain tissue. In 75% to 85% of classic CJD patients, atypical 1-cycle to 2-cycles per second triphasic sharp-wave discharge on electroencephalographic tracing has been described. A newly developed 14-3-3 protein assay that detects the protein in the cerebrospinal fluid has been reported to be sensitive and specific as a marker for CJD. No blood test is available. A progressive neurologic syndrome in a person bearing a pathogenic mutation of the prion protein gene (PRNP) is presumed to be prion disease. The failure to identify a unique prion nucleic acid component precludes detection of the infective particle by genome amplification.

TREATMENT: No treatment has been shown in humans to slow or stop the progressive neurodegenerative syndromes of prion diseases. Experimental treatments are under study. Supportive therapy is necessary to manage dementia, spasticity, rigidity, and seizures arising during the course of the illness. Psychologic support may help families of affected people. Genetic counseling is indicated in familial disease.

ISOLATION OF THE HOSPITALIZED PATIENT: Standard precautions are recommended. The available evidence indicates that even prolonged intimate contact with CJD-infected people has not resulted in transmission of disease. Tissues associated with high levels of infectivity (eg, brain, eyes, and spinal cord of affected people) and instruments in contact with those tissues are considered biohazards; incineration, prolonged autoclaving at high temperature and pressure, and exposure to a solution of sodium hydroxide of 1N or greater or a solution of sodium hypochlorite of 5.25% or greater (undiluted household chlorine bleach) for 1 hour has been reported to decrease infectivity.* Cerebrospinal fluid should be regarded as infectious. Person-to-person transmission of CJD by blood, milk, saliva, urine, or feces has not been reported. These body fluids should be handled using standard infection control procedures.

CONTROL MEASURES: Immunization against prion diseases is not available, and no immune response to infection has been demonstrated. Iatrogenic transmission of CJD through cadaveric pituitary hormones has been obviated by use of recombinant products. Recognition that CJD can be spread by transplantation of infected dura and corneas has led to more stringent donor-selection criteria and improved collection protocols. The effect of vCJD on health care is unclear at present (see Blood Safety, p 106). Performing a brain autopsy in patients with suspected or clinically diagnosed CJD is encouraged to confirm the diagnosis and detect other emerging forms of CJD, such as vCJD. Free state-of-the-art diagnostic testing is available at the National Prion Disease Pathology Surveillance Center (telephone, 216-368-0587; Internet, www.cjdsurveillance.com). A suspected or confirmed diagnosis of CJD for which a special public health response may be needed (eg, suspected iatrogenic disease or vCJD) should be reported to the appropriate state or local health departments and to the CJD Surveillance Unit, Division of Viral and Rickettsial Diseases, Centers for Disease Control and Prevention, Atlanta, GA 30333; telephone, 404-639-3091). Current precautionary policies of the US Food and Drug Administration about risk of CJD and human blood or blood products are accessible on the Internet at www.fda.gov/cber/whatsnew.htm.

Q Fever

CLINICAL MANIFESTATIONS: Although up to 60% of initial infections are asymptomatic, disease attributable to Q fever occurs in 2 distinct forms: acute, which typically follows initial exposure; and chronic, which occurs years after acute infection. Acute Q fever usually is characterized by abrupt onset of fever, chills, weakness, headache, anorexia, and other nonspecific systemic symptoms. Weight loss and weakness can be pronounced. Cough and chest pain accompany pneumonia, which occurs in 20% to 40% of patients. Hepatitis is found in 40% to 60% of patients, and serum transaminase concentrations commonly are abnormal, but jaundice is rare. Rash is rare and nonspecific in character. The illness typically lasts 1 to 4 weeks and then resolves gradually. Life-threatening complications of acute infection, such as meningoencephalitis and myocarditis, occur rarely. Chronic Q fever occurs in approximately 1% of acutely infected patients and manifests as endocarditis in patients with underlying heart disease or prosthetic valves, vascular aneurysms, or vascular grafts. Hepatitis is another common manifestation. Q fever may manifest as

---

* *WHO Infection Control Guidelines for Transmissible Spongiform Encephalopathies.* Report of a WHO Consultation, Geneva, Switzerland, March 23–26, 1999. Available at: www.who.int/emc-documents/ tse/whocdscraph2003c.html.

fever of undetermined origin. Although acute Q fever rarely is fatal, chronic Q fever can be fatal if untreated; with appropriate long-term antimicrobial therapy, mortality among patients with endocarditis is decreased to approximately 10%. Q fever during pregnancy is associated with abortion, premature birth, and low birth weight.

ETIOLOGY: *Coxiella burnetii,* the cause of Q fever, is an intracellular rickettsial pathogen. The infectious form of *C burnetii* is highly resistant to heat, desiccation, and chemicals and can persist for long periods of time in the environment. *Coxiella burnetii* has been reclassified into the γ subgroup of Proteobacteria.

EPIDEMIOLOGY: Q fever is a zoonotic infection that has been reported worldwide. In animals, infection usually is asymptomatic. The most common reservoirs are domestic farm animals (especially sheep, goats, and cows), which most often are associated with human infection, but cats, dogs, rodents, marsupials, other mammalian species, and some wild and domestic bird species may transmit infection to humans. Tick vectors may be important for maintaining animal and bird reservoirs but are not thought to be important in transmission to humans. Human disease rarely is reported but is thought to be underrecognized. Humans typically acquire infection by inhalation of *C burnetii* in fine-particle aerosols generated from birthing fluids during animal parturition or through inhalation of dust contaminated by these materials. Infection can occur by direct exposure to infected animals or tissues on farms and ranches or in research facilities or by exposure to contaminated materials, such as wool, straw, fertilizer, or laundry. Airborne particles containing *Coxiella* species can be carried downwind a half-mile or more, contributing to sporadic cases for which no apparent animal contact can be demonstrated. Milk has not been proven to transmit the organism. Seasonal trends occur in farming areas with predictable frequency, and the disease coincides with the lambing season in the early spring. Evidence has been reported for human intrauterine infection and direct transmission by blood or marrow transfusion. The risk of chronic infection is increased by underlying cardiovascular disease, especially cardiac valve defects, immunodeficiency, and pregnancy.

The **incubation period** usually is 14 to 22 days but can vary from 9 to 39 days. Chronic Q fever can develop years to decades after initial infection.

DIAGNOSTIC TESTS: Isolation of *C burnetii* from blood usually is not attempted because of the hazard to laboratory workers. Cell culture systems, especially the shell vial method, have been the most successful in isolating *C burnetii* from humans but are most sensitive in chronic Q fever endocarditis in untreated patients. Confirmed Q fever requires one of the following: (1) a fourfold change in antibody titer to *C burnetii* antigen by immunofluorescence antibody assay or complement fixation antibody test; (2) positive polymerase chain reaction assay result; (3) culture of *C burnetii* from a clinical specimen; or (4) positive immunostaining of *C burnetii* in tissue, especially heart valve.

TREATMENT: Acute Q fever generally is a self-limited illness, and most patients recover without antimicrobial therapy. Doxycycline is the drug of choice, and treatment can hasten recovery by several days. A fluoroquinolone or chloramphenicol are alternatives. Tetracyclines should not be given to children younger than 8 years of age unless the benefit is greater than the potential risk of dental staining, and fluoro-quinolones are not approved for use in children younger than 18 years of age (see Antimicrobial Agents and Related Therapy, p 693). Therapy should be initiated promptly and continued until the patient is afebrile and clinically improved, usually for 10 to 14 days. In chronic Q fever, relapses can occur necessitating repeated courses of therapy. The organism can remain latent in tissues for years; treatment of chronic disease is extremely difficult. Treatment of chronic endocarditis is prolonged and requires doxycycline and hydroxychloroquine for a minimum of 18 months. Fluoro-quinolone treatment for at least 3 years has been recommended by some experts. Relapses can occur after discontinuation of treatment. Surgical replacement of the infected valve may be necessary in some patients.

ISOLATION OF THE HOSPITALIZED PATIENT: Standard precautions are recommended.

CONTROL MEASURES: Strict adherence to proper hygiene when handling parturient animals can help decrease the risk of infection in the farm setting. Improved biosecurity in research facilities using sheep may decrease the risk of infection. Special safety practices are recommended for nonpropagative laboratory procedures involving *C burnetii* and for all propagative procedures, necropsies of infected animals, and manipulation of infected human and animal tissues. No specific management is recommended for people who have been exposed. Experimental vaccines for domestic animals and laboratory and other high-risk workers have been developed but are not licensed or available in the United States. All human cases should be reported to the state health department. For additional information about Q fever, see www.cdc.gov/ncidod/dvrd/qfever/.

Rabies*

CLINICAL MANIFESTATIONS: Infection with rabies virus characteristically produces an acute illness with rapidly progressive central nervous system manifestations, including anxiety, dysphagia, and seizures. Some patients may have paralysis. Illness almost invariably progresses to death. The differential diagnosis of acute encephalitic illnesses of unknown cause with atypical focal neurologic signs or with paralysis should include rabies.

ETIOLOGY: Rabies virus is an RNA virus classified in the Rhabdoviridae family.

EPIDEMIOLOGY: Understanding the epidemiology of rabies has been aided by strain identification using monoclonal antibodies and nucleotide sequencing. In the United States, the number of cases of human rabies has decreased steadily since the 1950s, reflecting widespread rabies immunization of dogs and the availability

---

* For further information, see Centers for Disease Control and Prevention. Human rabies prevention: United States, 1999: recommendations of the Advisory Committee on Immunization Practices [published correction appears in *MMWR Morb Mortal Wkly Rep.* 1999;48:16]. *MMWR Recomm Rep.* 1999;48(RR-1):1–21

of effective immunoprophylaxis after exposure to a rabid animal. Between 1990 and 2001, a total of 26 (74%) of the 35 human rabies deaths in the United States have been associated with bat-variant rabies virus. Only 2 of these 26 human cases had known animal bites. Despite the large focus of rabies in raccoons in the eastern United States, no human deaths have been attributed to the raccoon rabies virus variant. Rarely, airborne transmission has been reported in the laboratory and in caves inhabited by bats. Transmission also has occurred by transplantation of corneas from patients dying of undiagnosed rabies. Person-to-person transmission by bite has not been documented in the United States, although the virus has been isolated from saliva of infected patients.

Wildlife rabies exists throughout the United States except for Hawaii, which remains rabies free. Wild animals, including raccoons, skunks, foxes, coyotes, bats, and other species, are the most important potential source of infection for humans and domestic animals in the United States. Rabies in small rodents (squirrels, hamsters, guinea pigs, gerbils, chipmunks, rats, and mice) and lagomorphs (rabbits and hares) is rare, but rabies may occur in woodchucks or other large rodents in areas where raccoon rabies is common. The virus is present in saliva and is transmitted by bites or, rarely, by contamination of mucosa or skin lesions by infectious material. Worldwide, most rabies cases in humans result from dog bites in areas where canine rabies is enzootic. Most dogs, cats, and ferrets become ill within 4 or 5 days of viral shedding, and no case of human rabies in the United States has been attributed to a dog, cat, or ferret that has remained healthy throughout the standard 10-day period of confinement.

The **incubation period** in humans averages 4 to 6 weeks but ranges from 5 days to more than 1 year. Incubation periods of up to 6 years have been confirmed by antigenic typing and nucleotide sequencing of strains.

DIAGNOSTIC TESTS: Infection in animals can be diagnosed by demonstration of virus-specific fluorescent antigen in brain tissue. Suspected rabid animals should be euthanatized in a manner that preserves brain tissue for appropriate examination. Virus can be isolated from saliva, brain, and other tissues in suckling mice or in tissue culture. The diagnosis in suspected human cases can be made postmortem by either immunofluorescence or immunohistochemical examination of brain. Antemortem diagnosis can be made by fluorescent microscopy of skin biopsy specimens from the nape of the neck, by isolation of the virus from saliva, by detection of antibody in the cerebrospinal fluid (CSF) or serum in unimmunized people, and by detection of viral nucleic acid in infected tissues. Laboratory personnel should be consulted before submission of specimens so that appropriate collection and transport of materials can be arranged.

TREATMENT: Once symptoms have developed, neither vaccine nor Rabies Immune Globulin improves the prognosis. There is no specific treatment. Only a few patients with human rabies have survived with intensive supportive care; all other patients have died despite treatment.

ISOLATION OF THE HOSPITALIZED PATIENT: Standard precautions are recommended for the duration of illness. If the patient has bitten another person or the patient's saliva has contaminated an open wound or mucous membrane, the involved area should be washed thoroughly and postexposure prophylaxis should be administered (see Care of Exposed People, p 518).

CONTROL MEASURES: Education of children to avoid contact with stray or wild animals is of primary importance. Children should be cautioned against provoking or attempting to capture stray or wild animals and against touching carcasses. Inadvertent contact of family members and pets with potentially rabid animals, such as raccoons, foxes, coyotes, and skunks, may be decreased by securing garbage and refuse to decrease attraction of domestic and wild animals. Similarly, chimneys and other potential entrances for wild animals, including bats, should be identified and covered. International travelers to areas of endemic canine rabies should be warned to avoid exposure to stray dogs, and, if traveling to an area where immediate access to medical care and biologicals is limited, preexposure prophylaxis is indicated.

Exposure Risk and Decisions to Give Immunoprophylaxis. Exposure to rabies results from a break in the skin caused by the teeth of a rabid animal or by contamination of scratches, abrasions, or mucous membranes with saliva from a rabid animal. The decision to immunize an exposed person should be made in consultation with the local health department, which can provide information on the risk of rabies in a particular area for each species of animal and in accordance with the guidelines in Table 3.50, p 517. In the United States, raccoons, skunks, foxes, and bats are more likely to be infected than other animals, but coyotes, cattle, dogs, cats, ferrets, and other species occasionally are infected. Bites of rodents (such as squirrels and rats) or lagomorphs (rabbits and hares) rarely require specific antirabies prophylaxis. Additional factors must be considered when deciding whether immunoprophylaxis is indicated. An unprovoked attack is more suggestive of a rabid animal than a bite that occurs during attempts to feed or handle an animal. Properly immunized dogs, cats, and ferrets have only a minimal chance of developing rabies. However, in rare instances, rabies has developed in properly immunized animals.

Postexposure prophylaxis for rabies is recommended for all people bitten by wild mammalian carnivores or bats or by domestic animals that may be infected. Exposures other than bites rarely have resulted in infection, but seemingly insignificant physical contact with bats may result in viral transmission even without a clear history of a bite. Postexposure prophylaxis is recommended for people who report an open wound, scratch, or mucous membrane that has been contaminated with saliva or other potentially infectious material (eg, brain tissue) from a rabid animal. Because the injury inflicted by a bat bite or scratch may be small and not evident or the circumstances of contact may preclude accurate recall (eg, a bat in a room of a sleeping person or previously unattended child), prophylaxis is indicated for situations in which a bat physically is present if a bite or mucous membrane exposure cannot reliably be excluded, unless prompt testing of the bat has excluded rabies virus infection. Prophylaxis always should be initiated as soon as possible after bites by known or suspected rabid animals.

Postexposure prophylaxis also is recommended for people who report a possibly infectious exposure (eg, bite, scratch, or open wound or mucous membrane contaminated with saliva or other infectious material) to a human with rabies. However, exposure to a human with rabies has not been documented in the United States as a means of rabies transmission, except after corneal transplantation from donors

Table 3.50. Rabies Postexposure Prophylaxis Guide

Animal Type	Evaluation and Disposition of Animal	Postexposure Prophylaxis Recommendations
Dogs, cats, and ferrets	Healthy and available for 10 days of observation	Prophylaxis only if animal develops signs of rabies[1]
	Rabid or suspected of being rabid[2]	Immediate immunization[3] and RIG
	Unknown (escaped)	Consult public health officials for advice
Bats, skunks, raccoons, foxes, and most other carnivores; woodchucks	Regarded as rabid unless geographic area is known to be free of rabies or until animal proven negative by laboratory tests[2]	Immediate immunization[3] and RIG
Livestock, rodents, and lagomorphs (rabbits and hares)	Consider individually	Consult public health officials. Bites of squirrels, hamsters, guinea pigs, gerbils, chipmunks, rats, mice, other rodents, rabbits, and hares almost never require antirabies treatment.

RIG indicates Rabies Immune Globulin.

[1] During the 10-day holding period, at the first sign of rabies in the biting dog, cat, or ferret, treatment with RIG (human) and vaccine should be initiated. The animal should be euthanatized immediately and tested.

[2] The animal should be euthanatized and tested as soon as possible. Holding for observation is not recommended. Immunization is discontinued if immunofluorescence test result for the animal is negative.

[3] See text.

who died of unsuspected rabies encephalitis. Casual contact with an infected person (eg, by touching a patient) or contact with noninfectious fluids or tissues (eg, urine or feces) alone does not constitute an exposure and is not an indication for prophylaxis (see Care of Hospital Contacts, p 518).

Handling of Animals Suspected of Having Rabies. A dog, cat, or ferret suspected of having rabies that has bitten a human should be captured, confined, and observed by a veterinarian for 10 days. Any illness in the animal should be reported immediately to the local health department. If signs of rabies develop, the animal should be euthanatized and its head should be removed and shipped under refrigeration (iced, not frozen) to a qualified laboratory for examination.

Other biting animals that may have exposed a person to rabies should be reported immediately to the local health department. Management of animals depends on the species, the circumstances of the bite, and the epidemiology of rabies in the area. Previous immunization of an animal may not preclude the necessity for euthanasia and testing if the period of viral shedding is unknown for that species. Because clinical manifestations of rabies in a wild animal cannot be interpreted reliably, a wild mammal suspected of having rabies should be euthanatized at once and its brain should be examined for evidence of rabies. The exposed person need not be treated if results of rapid examination of the brain by fluorescent antibody procedures are negative for rabies.

Care of Hospital Contacts. Immunization of hospital contacts of a patient with rabies should be reserved for people who were bitten or whose mucous membranes or open wounds have come in contact with saliva, CSF, or brain tissue of a patient with rabies (see Care of Exposed People). Other hospital contacts of a patient with rabies do not require immunization.

Care of Exposed People.

Local Wound Care. The immediate objective of postexposure prophylaxis is to prevent virus from entering neural tissue. Prompt and thorough local treatment of all lesions is essential, because virus may remain localized to the area of the bite for a variable time. All wounds should be flushed thoroughly and cleaned with soap and water. Quaternary ammonium compounds (such as benzalkonium chloride) no longer are considered superior to soap. The need for tetanus prophylaxis and measures to control bacterial infection also should be considered. The wound, if possible, should not be sutured.

Immunoprophylaxis. After wound care is completed, concurrent use of passive *and* active immunoprophylaxis is required for optimal therapy (see Table 3.50, p 517). Prophylaxis should begin as soon as possible after exposure, ideally within 24 hours. However, a delay of several days or more may not compromise effectiveness, and prophylaxis should be initiated if otherwise indicated, regardless of the interval between exposure and initiation of therapy. In the United States, only the human product Rabies Immune Globulin (RIG) is available for passive immunization. Licensed tissue culture rabies vaccine should be used for active immunization. Physicians can obtain expert counsel from their local or state health departments.

Active Immunization (Postexposure). Three rabies vaccines are approved commercially for prophylaxis in the United States (see Table 3.51, p 519). A 1.0-mL dose of any of the 3 vaccines is given intramuscularly in the deltoid area or anterolateral aspect of the thigh on the first day of postexposure prophylaxis, and repeated doses are given on days 3, 7, 14, and 28 after the first dose, for a total of 5 doses. Ideally, an immunization series should be initiated and completed with 1 vaccine product unless serious allergic reactions occur. Clinical studies evaluating efficacy or frequency of adverse reactions when the series is completed with a second product have not been conducted. The volume of the dose is not decreased for children. Serologic testing to document seroconversion after administration of any of the 3 rabies vaccine series is unnecessary but occasionally has been advised for recipients who may be immunocompromised.

Care should be taken to ensure that the vaccine is administered intramuscularly. Intradermal vaccine is not advised for postexposure prophylaxis in the United States, although for reasons of cost and availability, intradermal regimens are used in some countries. Because antibody responses in adults who received vaccine in the gluteal area sometimes have been less than in those who were injected in the deltoid muscle, the deltoid site always should be used except in infants and young children, in whom the anterolateral thigh is the appropriate site.

Table 3.51. US Food and Drug Administration-Licensed Rabies Vaccines and Rabies Immune Globulin

Category	Product	Manufacturer	Method of Administration
Human rabies vaccine	Human diploid cell vaccine (HDCV) (Imovax)	Aventis Pasteur	IM
	Rabies vaccine adsorbed (RVA)	Bio Port Corporation	IM
	Purified chicken embryo cell (PCEC) (RabAvert)	Chiron Corporation	IM
Rabies Immune Globulin	Imogam Rabies-HT	Aventis Pasteur	Infiltrate around wound[1]
	BayRab	Bayer	Infiltrate around wound[1]

IM indicates intramuscular.
[1] Any remaining volume should be administered IM.

- *Adverse reactions and precautions with human diploid cell vaccine (HDCV), rabies vaccine adsorbed (RVA), and purified chicken embryo cell (PCEC) vaccine.* Reactions after immunization, primarily reported in adults, are less common than those after immunization with previously used vaccines. Reactions are uncommon in children. In adults, local reactions, such as pain, erythema, and swelling or itching at the injection site are reported in 15% to 25%, and mild systemic reactions, such as headache, nausea, abdominal pain, muscle aches, and dizziness are reported in 10% to 20% of recipients. Several cases of neurologic illness resembling Guillain-Barré syndrome that resolved without sequelae in 12 weeks and an acute, generalized, transient neurologic syndrome temporally associated with HDCV have been reported but are not thought to be causally related.

  Immune complex-like reactions in people receiving booster doses of HDCV have been observed, possibly because of interaction between propiolactone and human albumin. The reaction, characterized by onset 2 to 21 days after inoculation, begins with generalized urticaria and can include arthralgia, arthritis, angioedema, nausea, vomiting, fever, and malaise. The reaction is not life threatening and occurs in as many as 6% of adults receiving booster doses as part of a preexposure immunization regimen. It is rare in people receiving primary immunization with HDCV. Similar allergic reactions with primary or booster doses have not been reported with PCEC or RVA.

  If the patient has a serious allergic reaction to HDCV, RVA or PCEC vaccine may be given according to the same schedule as HDCV. All suspected serious, systemic, neuroparalytic, or anaphylactic reactions to the rabies vaccine should be reported immediately (see Reporting of Adverse Events, p 40).

Although the safety of the use of rabies vaccine during pregnancy has not been studied specifically in the United States, pregnancy should not be considered a contraindication to the use of vaccine after exposure.

- **Nerve tissue vaccines.** Inactivated nerve tissue vaccines are not licensed in the United States but are available in many areas of the world. These preparations induce neuroparalytic reactions in between 1:2000 and 1:8000 recipients. Immunization with nerve tissue vaccine should be discontinued if meningeal or neuroparalytic reactions develop. Corticosteroids can be used for treatment of complications but should be used only for life-threatening reactions, because they increase the risk of rabies in experimentally inoculated animals.

Passive Immunization. Human RIG should be used concomitantly with the first dose of vaccine for postexposure prophylaxis to bridge the time between possible rabies exposure and active antibody production induced by the vaccine (see Table 3.51, p 519). If vaccine is not available immediately, RIG should be given alone and immunization started later. If RIG is not available immediately, vaccine should be given. Rabies Immune Globulin then is given subsequently if obtained within 7 days after initiating immunization. If administration of both vaccine and RIG is delayed, both should be used regardless of the interval between exposure and treatment.

The recommended dose of RIG is 20 IU/kg. As much of the dose as possible should be used to infiltrate the wound(s), if present. The remainder is given intramuscularly. In cases of multiple severe wounds in which RIG is insufficient for infiltration, dilution in saline solution to an adequate volume (twofold or threefold) has been recommended to ensure that all wound areas receive infiltrate. For children with a small muscle mass, it may be necessary to administer RIG at multiple sites. Human RIG is supplied in 2-mL (300 IU) and 10-mL (1500 IU) vials. Passive antibody can inhibit the response to rabies vaccines; therefore, the recommended dose should not be exceeded. Vaccine never should be administered in the same parts of the body or with the same syringe used to give RIG. Hypersensitivity reactions to RIG occur rarely, if ever.

Purified equine RIG containing rabies antibodies is available outside the United States and generally is accompanied by a low rate of serum sickness (<1%). It is administered at a dose of 40 IU/kg, and desensitization may be required.

Administration of RIG is not recommended for the following exposed people: (1) those who previously received postexposure prophylaxis with HDCV, RVA, or PCEC; (2) those who received a 3-dose, intramuscular, preexposure regimen of HDCV, RVA, or PCEC; (3) those who received a 3-dose, intradermal, preexposure regimen of HDCV with the product used in the United States; and (4) those who have a documented adequate rabies antibody titer after previous immunization with any other rabies vaccine. These people should receive two 1.0-mL doses of HDCV, RVA, or PCEC; doses are given on the day of exposure and 3 days later.

Preexposure Control Measures, Including Immunization. The relatively low frequency of reactions to HDCV, RVA, and PCEC has made the provision of preexposure immunization practical for people in high-risk groups, such as veterinarians, animal handlers, certain laboratory workers, and people moving to areas where canine rabies is common. Others, such as spelunkers, who have frequent exposures to bats and other wildlife, also should be considered for preexposure prophylaxis.

The HDCV, RVA, and PCEC vaccines are licensed for intramuscular administration. Previously, intradermal (0.1 mL) dosage formulations of HDCV were available for preexposure use. The preexposure immunization schedule is three 1-mL intramuscular injections each given on days 0, 7, and 21 **or** 28. This series of immunizations has resulted in development of antibodies in all people properly immunized. Therefore, routine serologic testing for rabies antibody is not indicated.

Serum antibodies usually persist for at least 2 years after the primary series given intramuscularly. Preexposure booster immunization with 1.0 mL of HDCV, RVA, or PCEC intramuscularly will produce an effective anamnestic response. Rabies serum antibody titers should be determined at 6-month intervals for people at continuous risk of infection (rabies research laboratory workers, rabies biologicals production workers). Titers should be determined approximately every 2 years for people with risk of frequent exposure (rabies diagnostic laboratory workers, spelunkers, veterinarians and staff, and animal-control and wildlife workers in rabies-enzootic areas). Booster doses of vaccine should be administered only as appropriate to maintain serum antibody concentrations. The Centers for Disease Control and Prevention currently specifies complete viral neutralization at a 1:5 or greater titer by the rapid fluorescent-focus inhibition test as acceptable; the World Health Organization specifies 0.5 IU/mL or more as acceptable.

Public Health. A variety of approved public health measures, including immunization of dogs, cats, and ferrets and elimination of stray dogs and selected wildlife, are used to control rabies in animals.* In regions where oral immunization of wildlife with recombinant rabies vaccine is undertaken, the incidence of rabies among foxes, coyotes, and raccoons may be decreased. Unimmunized dogs, cats, ferrets, or other pets bitten by a known rabid animal should be euthanatized immediately. If the owner is unwilling to allow the animal to be euthanatized, the animal should be placed in strict isolation for 6 months and immunized 1 month before release. If the animal has been immunized within 1 to 3 years, depending on the vaccine administered and local regulations, the animal should be reimmunized and observed for 45 days.

Case Reporting. All suspected cases of rabies should be reported promptly to public health authorities.

Rat-Bite Fever

CLINICAL MANIFESTATIONS: Rat-bite fever is caused by *Streptobacillus moniliformis* or *Spirillum minus*. *Streptobacillus moniliformis* infection (streptobacillary or Haverhill fever) is characterized by abrupt onset of fever, chills, a maculopapular or petechial rash predominantly on the extremities, muscle pain, vomiting, headache, and occasionally, adenopathy. The bite site usually heals promptly and exhibits no or minimal inflammation. Nonsuppurative migratory polyarthritis or arthralgia follows in approximately 50% of patients. Untreated infection usually has a relapsing course

---

* Centers for Disease Control and Prevention. Compendium of animal rabies prevention and control, 2001—National Association of State Public Health Veterinarians Inc. *MMWR Recomm Rep.* 2001;50(RR-8):1–9

for a mean of 3 weeks. Complications include soft tissue and solid-organ abscesses, pneumonia, endocarditis, myocarditis, and meningitis. With *S minus* infection, a period of initial apparent healing at the site of the bite usually is followed by fever and ulceration at the site, regional lymphangitis and lymphadenopathy, a distinctive rash of red or purple plaques, and rarely, arthritic symptoms. Infection with *S minus* is rare in the United States.

ETIOLOGY: The causes of rat-bite fever are *Streptobacillus moniliformis,* a micro-aerophilic, gram-negative, pleomorphic bacillus, and *Spirillum minus,* a small, gram-negative, spiral organism with bipolar flagellar tufts.

EPIDEMIOLOGY: Rat-bite fever is a zoonotic illness. The natural habitat of *S moniliformis* and *S minus* is the upper respiratory tract of rodents. *Streptobacillus moniliformis* is transmitted by bites of rats, squirrels, mice, cats, and weasels; by ingestion of contaminated food or milk products; and by contact with an infected animal. *Haverhill fever* refers to infection after ingestion of milk or water contaminated with *S moniliformis*. *Spirillum minus* is transmitted by bites of rats and mice. *Streptobacillus moniliformis* infection accounts for most cases of rat-bite fever in the United States; *S minus* infections occur primarily in Asia.

The **incubation period** for *S moniliformis* usually is 3 to 10 days but can be as long as 3 weeks; for *S minus,* it is 7 to 21 days.

DIAGNOSTIC TESTS: *Streptobacillus moniliformis* can be isolated from specimens of blood, synovial fluid, aspirates from abscesses, or material from the bite lesion by inoculation into bacteriologic media enriched with blood, serum, or ascitic fluid. Because it is a fastidious organism, laboratory personnel should be notified that *S moniliformis* is suspected. *Spirillum minus* has not been recovered on artificial media but can be visualized by darkfield microscopy in wet mounts of blood, exudate of a lesion, and lymph nodes. Blood specimens also should be viewed with Giemsa or Wright stain. *Spirillum minus* can be recovered from blood, lymph nodes, or local lesions by intraperitoneal inoculation of mice or guinea pigs.

TREATMENT: Penicillin G procaine should be administered intramuscularly for 7 to 10 days for rat-bite fever caused by either agent. Initial intravenous penicillin G therapy for 5 days followed by oral penicillin V also has been successful. Alternative drugs include ampicillin, cefuroxime, and cefotaxime sodium. Doxycycline, chloramphenicol, or streptomycin sulfate may be substituted when a patient is allergic to penicillin. Doxycycline should not be given to children younger than 8 years of age unless the benefits of therapy are greater than the risks of dental staining (see Antimicrobial Agents and Related Therapy, p 693). Patients with endocarditis should receive intravenous high-dose penicillin G for at least 4 weeks. The addition of streptomycin initially may be useful.

ISOLATION OF THE HOSPITALIZED PATIENT: Standard precautions are recommended.

CONTROL MEASURES: Exposed people should be observed for symptoms. Because the attack rate of *S moniliformis* after a rat bite is approximately 10%, some experts recommend postexposure administration of penicillin. Rat control is important in the control of disease.

Respiratory Syncytial Virus

CLINICAL MANIFESTATIONS: Respiratory syncytial virus (RSV) causes acute respiratory tract illness in patients of all ages. In infants and young children, RSV is the most important cause of bronchiolitis and pneumonia. During the first few weeks of life, particularly among preterm infants, infection with RSV may produce minimal respiratory tract signs. Lethargy, irritability, and poor feeding, sometimes accompanied by apneic episodes, may be the major manifestations. Most previously healthy infants infected with RSV do not require hospitalization, and many who are hospitalized improve with supportive care and are discharged in fewer than 5 days. Conditions that increase the risk of severe or fatal RSV infection are cyanotic or complicated congenital heart disease, especially conditions causing pulmonary hypertension; underlying pulmonary disease, especially bronchopulmonary dysplasia; prematurity; and immunodeficiency disease or therapy causing immunosuppression at any age. The association between RSV bronchiolitis early in life and subsequent reactive airway disease remains poorly understood. After RSV bronchiolitis, some children will develop long-term abnormalities in pulmonary function and experi ence recurrent wheezing. This association may reflect an underlying predisposition to reactive airway disease rather than a direct consequence of RSV infection.

Almost all children are infected at least once by 2 years of age, and reinfection throughout life is common. Older children and adults usually develop upper respiratory tract illness but also can develop more serious lower respiratory tract infection. Exacerbation of asthma or other chronic lung conditions may occur.

ETIOLOGY: Respiratory syncytial virus is an enveloped RNA paramyxovirus that lacks neuraminidase and hemagglutinin surface glycoproteins. Two major subtypes (A and B) have been identified and often circulate concurrently. The clinical and epidemiologic significance of strain variation has not been determined, but evidence suggests that antigenic differences may affect susceptibility to infection and that some strains may be more virulent than other strains.

EPIDEMIOLOGY: Humans are the only source of infection. Transmission usually is by direct or close contact with contaminated secretions, which may involve droplets or fomites. Respiratory syncytial virus can persist on environmental surfaces for many hours and for a half-hour or more on hands. Infection among hospital personnel and others can occur by self-inoculation with contaminated secretions. Enforcement of infection control policies is important to decrease the risk of health care-related transmission of RSV. Health care-related spread of RSV to organ transplant recipients or patients with cardiopulmonary abnormalities or immunocompromised conditions has been associated with severe and fatal disease in children and adults.

Respiratory syncytial virus usually occurs in annual epidemics during winter and early spring in temperate climates. However, sporadic infection may occur year round. Spread among household and child care contacts, including adults, is common. The period of viral shedding usually is 3 to 8 days, but it may last longer, especially in young infants, in whom shedding may continue for as long as 3 to 4 weeks.

The **incubation period** ranges from 2 to 8 days; 4 to 6 days is most common.

DIAGNOSTIC TESTS: Rapid diagnostic assays, including immunofluorescence and enzyme immunoassay techniques for detection of viral antigen in nasopharyngeal specimens, are available commercially and generally are reliable. The sensitivity of these assays in comparison with culture varies between 53% and 96%, with most in the 80% to 90% range. Viral isolation from nasopharyngeal secretions in cell cultures requires 3 to 5 days, but results and sensitivity vary among laboratories, because methods of isolation are exacting and RSV is a relatively labile virus. An experienced viral laboratory should be consulted for optimal methods of collection and transport of specimens. Serologic testing of acute and convalescent serum specimens can be used to confirm infection; however, the sensitivity of serologic diagnosis of infection is low among young infants. Polymerase chain reaction assay has been applied to detection of RSV in clinical specimens but is not available commercially.

TREATMENT: Primary treatment is supportive and should include hydration, careful clinical assessment of respiratory status, including measurement of oxygen saturation, use of supplemental oxygen, and if necessary, mechanical ventilation. Ribavirin has in vitro antiviral activity against RSV, but ribavirin aerosol treatment for RSV infection generally is not recommended. Placebo-controlled trials have failed to demonstrate a consistent decrease in need for mechanical ventilation, duration of stay in the pediatric intensive care unit, or duration of hospitalization among ribavirin recipients. The high cost, aerosol route of administration, concern about potential toxic effects among exposed health care professionals, and conflicting results of efficacy trials all contribute to this controversy. Decisions about ribavirin administration should be made on the basis of the particular clinical circumstances and physicians' experience.

Corticosteroids. In hospitalized infants with RSV bronchiolitis, corticosteroids are not effective and are not indicated.

Antimicrobial Agents. Antimicrobial agents rarely are indicated, because bacterial lung infection and bacteremia are uncommon in infants hospitalized with RSV bronchiolitis or pneumonia.

Prevention of RSV Infections. Two products are available to prevent RSV infection: Respiratory Syncytial Virus Immune Globulin Intravenous (RSV-IGIV)* prepared from donors selected for high serum titers of RSV neutralizing antibody, and palivizumab, a humanized mouse monoclonal antibody that is administered intramuscularly. Both products have been licensed for prevention of RSV disease in selected children younger than 24 months of age with chronic lung disease (CLD [formerly called bronchopulmonary dysplasia]) or with a history of preterm birth (<35 weeks' gestation). Both RSV-IGIV and palivizumab are administered approximately once per month (eg, every 30 days), beginning just before onset of the RSV

---

* RespiGam, Medimmune Inc, Gaithersburg, MD.

season, which typically occurs in November. In general, 4 subsequent monthly doses (total of 5 doses) are sufficient to provide protection during the entire RSV season. The dose of RSV-IGIV is 15 mL/kg (750 mg/kg), administered intravenously, and the dose of palivizumab is 15 mg/kg, administered intramuscularly. Because RSV-IGIV and palivizumab are not effective in the treatment of RSV disease, neither is approved for this indication.

Recommendations by the American Academy of Pediatrics for the use of palivizumab and RSV-IGIV are as follows:

- Palivizumab or RSV-IGIV prophylaxis should be considered for infants and children younger than 2 years of age with CLD who have required medical therapy (supplemental oxygen, bronchodilator, diuretic or corticosteroid therapy) for CLD within 6 months before the anticipated start of the RSV season. Palivizumab is preferred for most high-risk children because of its ease of administration, safety, and effectiveness. Patients with more severe CLD may benefit from prophylaxis during a second RSV season if they continue to require medical therapy for respiratory or cardiac dysfunction. Individual patients may benefit from decisions made in consultation with neonatologists, pediatric intensivists, pulmonologists, or infectious disease specialists. There are limited data regarding the effectiveness of palivizumab during the second year of life, although children with CLD who require ongoing medical therapy may experience severe RSV infections.

- Infants born at 32 weeks of gestation or earlier may benefit from RSV prophylaxis, even if they do not have CLD. For these infants, major risk factors to consider include their gestational age and chronologic age at the start of the RSV season. Infants born at 28 weeks of gestation or earlier may benefit from prophylaxis during their first RSV season, whenever that occurs during the first 12 months of life. Infants born at 29 to 32 weeks of gestation may benefit most from prophylaxis up to 6 months of age. For the purpose of this recommendation, 32 weeks' gestation refers to an infant born on or before the 32nd week of gestation (ie, 32 weeks, 0 days). Once a child qualifies for initiation of prophylaxis at the start of the RSV season, administration should continue throughout the season and not stop at the point an infant reaches either 6 months or 12 months of age.

- Although palivizumab and RSV-IGIV have been shown to decrease the likelihood of hospitalization in infants born between 32 and 35 weeks of gestation (ie, between 32 weeks, 1 day and 35 weeks, 0 days), the cost of administering prophylaxis to this large group of infants must be considered carefully. Therefore, most experts recommend that prophylaxis should be reserved for infants in this group who are at greatest risk of severe infection and who are younger than 6 months of age at the start of the RSV season. Epidemiologic data suggest that RSV infection is more likely to lead to hospitalization for these infants when the following risk factors are present: child care attendance, school-aged siblings, exposure to environmental air pollutants, congenital abnormalities of the airways, or severe neuromuscular disease. However, no single risk factor causes a very large increase in the rate of hospitalization, and the risk is additive as the number of risk factors for an individual infant increases. Therefore, prophylaxis should be considered for infants between

32 and 35 weeks of gestation only if 2 or more of these risk factors are present. Exposure to tobacco smoke is a risk factor that can be controlled by the family of an infant at increased risk of RSV disease, and preventive measures will be far less costly than palivizumab prophylaxis. High-risk infants never should be exposed to tobacco smoke. High-risk infants should be kept away from crowds and from situations in which exposure to infected individuals cannot be controlled. Participation in child care should be restricted during the RSV season for high-risk infants whenever feasible. Parents should be instructed on the importance of careful hand hygiene. In addition, all high-risk infants and their contacts should be immunized against influenza beginning at 6 months of age.

- Prophylaxis against RSV should be initiated just before onset of the RSV season and terminated at the end of the RSV season. In most seasons and in most regions of the Northern Hemisphere, the first dose of palivizumab should be administered at the beginning of November and the last dose should be administered at the beginning of March, which will provide protection into April. To understand the epidemiology of RSV in their area, physicians should consult with local health departments or diagnostic virology laboratories or the Centers for Disease Control and Prevention if such information is not available locally. Decisions about the specific duration of prophylaxis should be individualized according to the duration of the RSV season. Pediatricians may wish to use RSV rehospitalization data from their own region to assist in the decision-making process.

- Children who are 24 months of age or younger with hemodynamically significant cyanotic and acyanotic congenital heart disease will benefit from 5 monthly intramuscular injections of palivizumab (15 mg/kg). Decisions regarding prophylaxis with palivizumab in children with congenital heart disease should be made on the basis of the degree of physiologic cardiovascular compromise. Infants younger than 12 months of age with congenital heart disease who most likely are to benefit from immunoprophylaxis include:
  - Infants who are receiving medication to control congestive heart failure
  - Infants with moderate to severe pulmonary hypertension
  - Infants with cyanotic heart disease

    Because a mean decrease in palivizumab serum concentration of 58% was observed after surgical procedures that use cardiopulmonary bypass, for children who still require prophylaxis, a postoperative dose of palivizumab (15 mg/kg) should be considered as soon as the patient is medically stable.

    The following groups of infants are **not** at increased risk from RSV and generally should not receive immunoprophylaxis:
  - Infants and children with hemodynamically insignificant heart disease (eg, secundum atrial septal defect, small ventricular septal defect, pulmonic stenosis, uncomplicated aortic stenosis, mild coarctation of the aorta, and patent ductus arteriosus)

- Infants with lesions adequately corrected by surgery unless they continue to require medication for congestive heart failure
- Infants with mild cardiomyopathy who are not receiving medical therapy

Dates for initiation and termination of prophylaxis should be based on the same considerations as for high-risk preterm infants. As of April 2003, the US Food and Drug Administration had not licensed palivizumab for use in children with congenital heart disease, so recommendations may change (see www.aap.org). Unlike palivizumab, RSV-IGIV is contraindicated in children with cyanotic congenital heart disease.

- Palivizumab or RSV-IGIV prophylaxis has not been evaluated in randomized trials in immunocompromised children. Although specific recommendations for immunocompromised patients cannot be made, children with severe immunodeficiencies (eg, severe combined immunodeficiency or severe acquired immunodeficiency syndrome) may benefit from prophylaxis. If these infants and children are receiving standard IGIV monthly, physicians may consider substitution of RSV-IGIV during the RSV season.
- Because RSV-IGIV and palivizumab are not effective in the treatment of RSV disease, neither is licensed for this indication.
- Limited studies suggest that some patients with cystic fibrosis may be at increased risk of RSV infection. However, there are insufficient data to determine the effectiveness of palivizumab use in this patient population.
- If an infant or child who is receiving immunoprophylaxis experiences a break-through RSV infection, prophylaxis should continue through the RSV season. This recommendation is based on the observation that high-risk infants may be hospitalized more than once in the same season with RSV lower respiratory tract disease and the fact that more than one RSV strain often cocirculates in a community.
- Physicians should arrange for drug administration within 6 hours after opening a vial because this biologic product does not contain a preservative.
- Respiratory syncytial virus is known to be transmitted in the hospital setting and to cause serious disease in high-risk infants. In high-risk hospitalized infants, the major means to prevent RSV disease is strict observance of infection control practices, including the use of rapid means to identify and isolate RSV-infected infants. If an RSV outbreak is documented in a high-risk unit (eg, pediatric intensive care unit), primary emphasis should be placed on proper infection control practices, especially hand hygiene. Recommendations cannot be made regarding the use of palivizumab as a means of prevention of nosocomial RSV disease.
- Palivizumab does not interfere with response to vaccines. Infants and children receiving prophylaxis with RSV-IGIV should have immunization with measles-mumps-rubella and varicella vaccines deferred for 9 months after the last dose of RSV-IGIV. The use of RSV-IGIV should not alter the primary immuniza-

tion schedule for other recommended immunizations. Available data at this time do not support the need for supplemental doses of any of these routinely administered vaccines.

ISOLATION OF THE HOSPITALIZED PATIENT: In addition to standard precautions, contact precautions are recommended for the duration of RSV-associated illness among infants and young children, including patients treated with ribavirin. The effectiveness of these precautions depends on compliance and necessitates scrupulous adherence to appropriate hand hygiene practices. Patients with RSV infection should be cared for in single rooms or placed in a cohort.

CONTROL MEASURES: The control of nosocomial RSV transmission is complicated by the continuing chance of introduction through infected patients, staff, and visitors. During the peak of the RSV season, many infants and children hospitalized with respiratory tract symptoms will be infected with RSV and should be cared for with contact precautions (see Isolation of the Hospitalized Patient, above). Early identification of RSV-infected patients (see Diagnostic Tests, p 524) is important so that appropriate precautions can be instituted promptly. During large outbreaks, a variety of measures have been demonstrated to be effective, including the following: (1) laboratory screening of patients for RSV infection; (2) cohorting infected patients and staff; (3) excluding visitors with respiratory tract infections; (4) excluding staff with respiratory tract illness or RSV infection from caring for susceptible infants; and (5) use of gowns, gloves, goggles, and perhaps masks.

A critical aspect of RSV prevention among high-risk infants is education of parents and other caregivers about the importance of decreasing exposure to and transmission of RSV. Preventive measures include limiting, where feasible, exposure to contagious settings (eg, child care centers) and emphasis on hand hygiene in all settings, including the home, especially during periods when the contacts of high-risk children have respiratory infections. In addition, high-risk infants never should be exposed to tobacco smoke.

Rhinovirus Infections

CLINICAL MANIFESTATIONS: Rhinoviruses are the most frequent causes of the common cold or rhinosinusitis. Rhinoviruses also can be associated with pharyngitis, otitis media, less commonly bronchiolitis and pneumonia, and exacerbations of bronchitis and reactive airway disease. Nasal discharge usually is watery and clear at the onset but often becomes mucopurulent and viscus after a few days and may persist for 10 to 14 days. Malaise, headache, myalgias, and low-grade fever also may occur.

ETIOLOGY: Rhinoviruses are RNA viruses classified as picornaviruses. At least 100 antigenic serotypes have been identified by neutralizing antibodies. Infection with one type confers some type-specific immunity, but immunity is of variable degree and brief duration and offers little protection against other serotypes.

EPIDEMIOLOGY: Only humans and chimpanzees are infected with human rhino-viruses. Transmission occurs predominantly by person-to-person contact with self-inoculation by contaminated secretions on hands. Less commonly, transmission may occur by aerosol spread. Infections occur throughout the year, but peak activity is during autumn and spring. Several serotypes usually circulate simultaneously, but the prevalent serotypes circulating in a given population tend to change over time. By adulthood, antibodies to many serotypes have developed. Household spread is common. Viral shedding from nasopharyngeal secretions is most abundant during the first 2 to 3 days of infection and usually ceases by 7 to 10 days. However, shedding may continue for as long as 3 weeks.

The **incubation period** usually is 2 to 3 days but occasionally is up to 7 days.

DIAGNOSTIC TESTS: Inoculation of nasal secretions in appropriate cell cultures for viral isolation is the best means of establishing a specific diagnosis. The large number of antigenic types make serologic diagnosis of infection impractical.

TREATMENT: Placebo-controlled studies have indicated that over-the-counter antihistamine-decongestant cold medications are no more effective than placebo in children younger than 5 years of age. Antimicrobial agents do not prevent secondary bacterial infection and complicate later therapy by promoting the emergence of resistant bacteria (see Appropriate Use of Antimicrobial Agents, p 695).

ISOLATION OF THE HOSPITALIZED PATIENT: In addition to standard precautions, contact precautions are recommended for hospitalized infants and children for the duration of illness.

CONTROL MEASURES: Frequent hand hygiene and hygienic measures in schools, households, and other settings where transmission is common may help decrease the spread of rhinoviruses. Use of disinfectant sprays in the environment is of no proven benefit.

Rickettsial Diseases

Rickettsiae are small, coccobacillary bacteria, most of which have arthropod vectors, including ticks, fleas, and lice. Humans are incidental hosts, except for epidemic (louseborne) typhus, when humans are the principal reservoir and the human body louse is the vector. Rickettsiae are obligate intracellular pathogens and cannot be grown in cell-free media. They have typical bacterial cell walls and cytoplasmic membranes and divide by binary fission. Their natural life cycles typically involve mammalian reservoirs, and animal-to-human or vector-to-human transmission occurs as a result of environmental or occupational exposure.

Ticks are vectors for many rickettsial diseases. Thus, control measures involve prevention of tick transmission of rickettsial agents to humans (see Prevention of Tickborne Infections, p 186).

Rickettsial infections have many features in common, including the following:
- Multiplication of the organism occurs in an arthropod host.

- Intracellular replication.
- Geographic and seasonal occurrence is related to arthropod vector life cycles, activity, and distribution.
- They are zoonotic diseases.
- Humans are incidental hosts (except for louseborne typhus).
- Local primary eschars occur with some rickettsial diseases, particularly spotted fever group rickettsiae.
- Fever, rash (especially in spotted fever and typhus group rickettsiae), headache, myalgias, and respiratory tract symptoms are prominent features.
- Systemic capillary and small-vessel endothelial damage is the primary pathologic feature of spotted fever and typhus group rickettsial infections.
- Group-specific antibodies are detectable in the serum of most patients 7 to 14 days after onset of illness.
- Various serologic tests exist for detecting these antibodies. The indirect immunofluorescence antibody (IFA) assay is recommended in most cases because of its relative sensitivity and specificity.
- Polymerase chain reaction assays can detect rickettsiae in blood or tissue, although these tests are limited in their availability to research laboratories.
- In laboratories with experienced personnel, immunochemical staining or polymerase chain reaction testing of skin biopsy specimens from patients with rash can help to diagnose rickettsial infections.
- Treatment early in the course of illness can blunt or delay serologic responses.
- Rickettsial diseases can be rapidly life threatening, so prompt and specific therapy is important for optional patient outcome. Antimicrobial treatment is most effective for patients who are treated during the first week of illness. If the disease remains untreated during the second week, even optimal therapy is less effective in preventing complications of illness. Because confirmatory laboratory tests primarily are retrospective, treatment decisions should not be delayed until test results are known.
- Immunity against reinfection by the same agent after natural infection usually is of long duration, except in the case of scrub typhus caused by *Orientia tsutsugamushi*. Among the 4 groups of rickettsial diseases, partial or complete cross-immunity usually is conferred by infections within groups but not among groups. Reinfection with *Ehrlichia* and *Anaplasma* species has been described.
- Many rickettsial diseases, including Rocky Mountain spotted fever, ehrlichiosis, and Q fever are nationally notifiable diseases and should be reportable to state and local health departments.

For details, including treatment, the following chapters on rickettsial diseases should be consulted:
- *Ehrlichia* Infections (Human Ehrlichioses), p 266
- Q Fever, p 512
- Rickettsialpox, p 531
- Rocky Mountain Spotted Fever, p 532
- Endemic Typhus (Fleaborne Typhus or Murine Typhus), p 668
- Epidemic Typhus (Louseborne Typhus), p 669

A number of other epidemiologically distinct but clinically similar tickborne spotted fever infections caused by rickettsiae have been recognized. The causative agents of some of these infections share the same group antigen as *Rickettsia rickettsii;* these include *Rickettsia africae,* the causative agent of tick bite fever that is endemic to sub-Saharan Africa; *Rickettsia conorii,* the causative agent of boutonneuse fever (Mediterranean spotted fever, India tick typhus, and Marseilles fever) that is endemic in southern Europe, Africa, and the Middle East; *R sibirica,* the causative agent of Siberian tick typhus, endemic in central Asia; *R australis,* the causative agent of North Queensland tick typhus, endemic in eastern Australia; and *R japonica,* the causative agent of Japanese spotted fever, endemic in Japan. Each of these infections has clinical, pathologic, and epidemiologic features similar to those of Rocky Mountain spotted fever, and doxycycline is the drug of choice for therapy. The specific diagnosis is confirmed using indirect immunofluorescence antibody assay. These conditions are of importance among people traveling to or returning from areas where these agents are endemic.

Rickettsialpox

CLINICAL MANIFESTATIONS: Rickettsialpox is characterized by generalized erythematous papulovesicular eruptions on the trunk, face, extremities (including palms and soles), and mucous membranes after the appearance of an eschar at the site of the bite of a mouse mite vector. Regional lymph nodes in the area of the primary eschar typically become enlarged. Systemic disease lasts approximately 1 week; manifestations can include fever, chills, headache, drenching sweats, myalgias, anorexia, and photophobia. The disease is self-limited and rarely associated with complications.

ETIOLOGY: Rickettsialpox is caused by *Rickettsia akari,* which is classified with the spotted fever group rickettsiae and related antigenically to *Rickettsia rickettsii.*

EPIDEMIOLOGY: The natural host for *R akari* in the United States is *Mus musculus,* the common house mouse. The disease is transmitted by a mouse mite *(Liponyssoides sanguineus).* Disease risk is heightened in areas infested with mice. The disease is found in large urban settings and has been recognized in the northeastern United States, Ohio, Utah, Croatia, Ukraine, Russia, Korea, and South Africa. All age groups can be affected. No seasonal pattern of disease occurs. The disease is not communicable and currently is reported rarely in the United States.

The **incubation period** is 9 to 14 days.

DIAGNOSTIC TESTS: *Rickettsia akari* can be isolated from blood during the acute stage of disease, but culture is not attempted routinely and is available only in specialized laboratories. An indirect immunofluorescence antibody assay or complement fixation test for *R rickettsii* (the cause of Rocky Mountain spotted fever) will demonstrate a fourfold change in antibody titers between acute and convalescent serum specimens, because antibodies to *R akari* have extensive cross-reactivity with those against *R rickettsii.* Absorption of serum specimens before indirect immunofluorescence antibody assay can distinguish between antibody responses to *R rickettsii* and *R akari*. Direct fluorescent antibody testing of paraffin-embedded eschars and histopathologic examination of papulovesicles for distinctive features are useful diagnostic techniques.

TREATMENT: Doxycycline or chloramphenicol will shorten the course of disease; symptoms resolve within 48 hours after initiation of therapy. Tetracyclines should not be given to children younger than 8 years of age unless the benefits of therapy are greater than the risks of dental staining (see Antimicrobial Agents and Related Therapy, p 693). Treatment is effective when given for 3 to 5 days; relapse is rare.

ISOLATION OF THE HOSPITALIZED PATIENT: Standard precautions are recommended.

CONTROL MEASURES: Disinfestation with residual insecticides and rodent control measures limit or eliminate the vector. No specific management of exposed people is necessary.

Rocky Mountain Spotted Fever

CLINICAL MANIFESTATIONS: Rocky Mountain spotted fever (RMSF) is a systemic, small-vessel vasculitis with a characteristic rash that usually occurs before the sixth day of illness. Fever, myalgia, severe headache, nausea, vomiting, and anorexia are major clinical features. Abdominal pain and diarrhea often are present and can obscure the diagnosis. The rash initially is erythematous and macular and later can become maculopapular and, often, petechial. Rash usually appears first on the wrists and ankles, often spreading within hours proximally to the trunk. The palms and soles typically are involved. Although early development of a rash is a useful diagnostic sign, in up to 20% of cases, rash fails to develop. Thrombocytopenia of varying severity and hyponatremia develop in many cases, and anemia can occur. The white blood cell count typically is normal, but leukopenia can occur. The illness can last as long as 3 weeks and can be severe, with prominent central nervous system, cardiac, pulmonary, gastrointestinal tract, and renal involvement; disseminated intravascular coagulation; and shock leading to death. Significant long-term sequelae are common in patients with severe RMSF, including neurologic (paraparesis; hearing loss; peripheral neuropathy; bladder and bowel incontinence; and cerebellar, vestibular, and motor dysfunction) and nonneurologic (disability from limb amputation) effects.

ETIOLOGY: *Rickettsia rickettsii* is an obligate intracellular pathogen and a member of the spotted fever group of rickettsiae. The primary targets of infection in mammalian hosts are endothelial cells lining the small vessels of all major tissues and organs.

EPIDEMIOLOGY: The disease is transmitted to humans by the bite of a tick. Many small wild animals and dogs have antibodies to *R rickettsii,* but their role as natural hosts is not clear, because ticks are reservoirs and vectors of *R rickettsii.* In ticks, the agent is transmitted transovarially and between stages. People with occupational or recreational exposure to the tick vector (eg, pet owners, animal handlers, and people who spend time outdoors) are at increased risk of acquiring the organism. People of all ages can be infected, but most cases occur in people younger than 15 years of age. April through September are the months of highest incidence. Laboratory-acquired infection has resulted from accidental inoculation and aerosol contamination. Transmission has occurred on rare occasions by blood transfusion. Mortality is highest in males, people older than 50 years of age, and people with no known tick bite or attachment. Lack of known recent tick bite does not exclude the diagnosis. Delay in disease recognition and initiation of antirickettsial therapy increase the risk of death. Factors contributing to delayed diagnosis include absence of rash, initial presentation before the fourth day of illness, and onset of illness during months other than May through August.

The disease is widespread in the United States. Most cases are reported in the south Atlantic, southeastern, and south central states. The dog tick *(Dermacentor variabilis)* primarily is responsible for transmission in these geographic areas and some areas of western United States. In the western United States, the northern Rocky Mountain states have the highest incidence, where the vector usually is the wood tick *(Dermacentor andersoni)*. Transmission parallels the tick season in a given geographic area. The disease also occurs in Canada, Mexico, and Central and South America.

The **incubation period** usually is approximately 1 week but ranges from 2 to 14 days.

DIAGNOSTIC TESTS: The diagnosis can be established by one of the multiple rickettsial group-specific serologic tests. A fourfold or greater change in titer between acute- and convalescent-phase serum specimens is diagnostic when determined by indirect immunofluorescence antibody (IFA) assay, enzyme immunoassay, or complement fixation, latex agglutination, indirect hemagglutination, or microagglutination tests. The IFA assay is the most widely available confirmatory test. Antibodies generally are detected by IFA assay 7 to 10 days after onset of illness. A probable diagnosis can be established by a single serum titer of 1:64 or greater by IFA assay. The nonspecific and insensitive Weil-Felix serologic test (*Proteus vulgaris* OX-19 and OX-2 agglutinins) is not recommended.

Culture of *R rickettsii* usually is not attempted because of the danger of transmission to laboratory personnel; only laboratories with adequate biohazard containment equipment should attempt isolation of rickettsiae. *Rickettsia rickettsii* can be identified by immunohistochemical staining of tissue specimens (biopsy or autopsy) obtained from the site of the rash. This method is highly specific, but not sensitive. Ideally, a specimen should be obtained before antimicrobial therapy is initiated, because sensitivity diminishes within 24 to 48 hours of initiation of therapy. Polymerase chain reaction assay for detection of *R rickettsii* in blood and biopsy specimens during the acute phase of illness confirms the diagnosis, but this test is available only in reference laboratories.

TREATMENT: Doxycycline is the drug of choice; chloramphenicol is an alternative. Although tetracyclines generally are not given to children younger than 8 years of age because of the risk of dental staining (see Antimicrobial Agents and Related Therapy, p 693), most experts consider doxycycline to be the drug of choice for children of any age. Reasons for this preference include the following: (1) tetracycline staining of teeth is dose related; (2) doxycycline is less likely than other tetracyclines to stain developing teeth; (3) doxycycline is effective against ehrlichiosis, which may mimic RMSF, but chloramphenicol may not be (see *Ehrlichia* Infections, p 266); and (4) use of chloramphenicol is problematic because of serious adverse effects, the need to monitor serum concentrations, and lack of an oral preparation in the United States. Also, a retrospective study indicated that chloramphenicol may be less effective than doxycycline for the treatment of RMSF. Therapy is continued until the patient has been afebrile for at least 3 days and has demonstrated clinical improvement; the usual duration of therapy is 7 to 10 days. Treatment is initiated on the basis of clinical features and epidemiologic considerations. Treatment before day 5 of illness in children with compatible clinical manifestations affords the highest likelihood of good outcome.

ISOLATION OF THE HOSPITALIZED PATIENT: Standard precautions are recommended.

CONTROL MEASURES: Control of ticks in their natural habitat is not practical. Avoidance of tick-infested areas (ie, areas that border wooded regions) is the best preventive measure. If a tick-infested area is entered, people should wear protective clothing and apply tick or insect repellents to clothes and exposed body parts for added protection. Adults should be taught to thoroughly inspect themselves, their children (bodies and clothing), and pets for ticks after spending time outdoors during the tick season and to remove ticks promptly and properly (see Prevention of Tickborne Infections, p 186).

There is no role for antimicrobial agents in preventing RMSF. No licensed *R rickettsii* vaccine is available in the United States.

Rotavirus Infections

CLINICAL MANIFESTATIONS: Infection can result in nonbloody diarrhea, usually preceded or accompanied by emesis and fever. Symptoms generally persist for 3 to 8 days. In severe cases, dehydration, electrolyte abnormalities, and acidosis may occur. In immunocompromised children, including children with human immunodeficiency virus infection, persistent infection can develop. The risk of intussusception after wild-type rotavirus infection is unclear, but most information suggests that rotavirus is not a major cause of intussusception.

ETIOLOGY: Rotaviruses (Rvs) are segmented, double-stranded RNA viruses belonging to the family Reoviridae, with at least 7 distinct antigenic groups (A through G). Group A viruses are the major causes of Rv diarrhea worldwide. Group B and C viruses also have been identified as causes of gastroenteritis in humans. Serotyping is based on the VP7 glycoprotein (G) and VP4 protease-cleaved hemagglutinin (P); G types 1 through 4 and 9 and P types 1A and 1B are most common.

EPIDEMIOLOGY: Most human infections result from contact with infected people. Infections attributable to Rv occur in many animal species, but transmission from animals to humans has not been documented conclusively. However, because of the segmented nature of the genome, reassortment among Rvs, whether human or animal, can occur and generate new strains. Rotavirus is present in high titer in stools of infected patients with diarrhea, which is the only body specimen consistently positive for the virus. Rotavirus is present in stool before the onset of diarrhea and can persist for as long as 21 days after the onset of symptoms in immunocompetent hosts. Transmission is presumed to be by the fecal-oral route. Rotavirus can be found on toys and hard surfaces in child care centers, indicating that fomites may serve as a mechanism of transmission. Respiratory transmission also may have a role in disease transmission. Spread within families and institutions is common. Rotavirus is the most common cause of nosocomially acquired diarrhea in children and is an important cause of acute gastroenteritis in children attending child care. Rarely, common-source outbreaks from contaminated water or food have been reported.

Human Rv infections occur worldwide and may occur earlier in life and may be more common in lower socioeconomic areas. Rotaviruses are the single most common agent of severe diarrhea in children younger than 2 years of age. In developing countries, rotavirus infections are a major cause of dehydration and death.

In temperate climate, disease is most prevalent during the cooler months. In North America, the annual epidemic peak characteristically starts during autumn in Mexico and the southwest United States, moving sequentially to reach the northeast United States and maritime Canada by spring. Specific seasonal patterns in tropical climates are less pronounced, but disease is more common during the drier, cooler months.

Virtually all children are infected by 3 years of age. Rotavirus gastroenteritis most commonly occurs in infants and children between 4 and 24 months of age, and infections during the first 3 months of life and reinfections among older children are more likely to be asymptomatic. The rate of hospitalization from Rv diarrhea in infected children can be as high as 2.5%. From 30% to 50% of adult contacts of infected infants become infected, although only a minority manifest symptoms. Breastfeeding has not been proven to prevent infection but may be associated with milder disease and should be encouraged.

The **incubation period** ranges from 2 to 4 days.

DIAGNOSTIC TESTS: It is not possible to diagnose rotavirus infection by clinical presentation or nonspecific laboratory tests. Enzyme immunoassay and latex agglutination assays for group A Rv antigen detection in stool are available commercially. Both assays have high specificity, but false-positive and nonspecific reactions can occur in neonates and in people with underlying intestinal disease. Nonspecific reactions can be distinguished from true positive reactions by the performance of confirmatory assays. Virus also can be identified in stool by electron microscopy and by specific nucleic acid amplification techniques.

TREATMENT: No specific antiviral therapy is available. Oral or parenteral fluids are given to prevent and correct dehydration. Orally administered Human Immune Globulin given as an investigational therapy in immunocompromised patients with prolonged infections has decreased viral shedding and shortened the duration of diarrhea.

ISOLATION OF THE HOSPITALIZED PATIENT: In addition to standard precautions, contact precautions are indicated for the duration of illness. In view of the prolonged fecal shedding of low concentration of virus after recovery, continuation of contact precautions for the duration of hospitalization is justified, particularly if transmission can occur to immunocompromised and preterm infants.

CONTROL MEASURES:

Child Care. General measures for interrupting enteric transmission in child care centers are available (see Children in Out-of-Home Child Care, p 123). Surfaces should be washed with soap and water. A 70% ethanol solution or other disinfectants will inactivate Rv and may help prevent disease transmission resulting from contact with environmental surfaces.

Vaccines. A vaccine to prevent Rv infection and disease is not available commercially. The rhesus rotavirus tetravalent vaccine (Rotashield, previously manufactured by Wyeth-Ayerst Laboratories, Philadelphia, PA) licensed by the US Food and Drug Administration in August 1998 and incorporated into the 1999 routine immunization schedule no longer is recommended for use because of the association of this vaccine with intussusception. This product was withdrawn voluntarily from the market in October 1999. Children who received Rv vaccine during the period of approval are not at increased risk of developing intussusception in the future. Evaluation of other oral live-attenuated vaccines continues.

Rubella

CLINICAL MANIFESTATIONS:

Postnatal Rubella. Rubella usually is a mild disease characterized by a generalized erythematous maculopapular rash, generalized lymphadenopathy (commonly suboccipital, postauricular, and cervical), and slight fever. Transient polyarthralgia and polyarthritis rarely occur in children but are common in adolescents and adults, especially females. Encephalitis and thrombocytopenia are rare complications. Maternal rubella during pregnancy can result in miscarriage, fetal death, or a constellation of congenital anomalies (congenital rubella syndrome).

Congenital Rubella. The most commonly described anomalies associated with congenital rubella syndrome are ophthalmologic (cataracts, retinopathy, and congenital glaucoma), cardiac (patent ductus arteriosus, peripheral pulmonary artery stenosis), auditory (sensorineural hearing impairment), and neurologic (behavioral disorders, meningoencephalitis, and mental retardation). In addition, infants with congenital rubella syndrome often are growth retarded and may have radiolucent bone disease, hepatosplenomegaly, thrombocytopenia, and purpuric skin lesions (giving a "blueberry muffin" appearance). Mild forms of the disease can be associated with few or no obvious clinical manifestations at birth. The occurrence of congenital defects is as high as 85% if infection occurs during the first 4 weeks of gestation, 20% to 30% during the second month, and 5% during the third or fourth month.

ETIOLOGY: Rubella virus is an enveloped, positive-stranded RNA virus classified as a Rubivirus in the Togaviridae family.

EPIDEMIOLOGY: Humans are the only source of infection. Postnatal rubella is transmitted primarily through direct or droplet contact from nasopharyngeal secretions. The peak incidence of infection is during late winter and early spring. Approximately 25% to 50% of infections are asymptomatic. Immunity from wild-type or vaccine virus usually is prolonged, but reinfection on rare occasions has been demonstrated and rarely has resulted in congenital rubella. The period of maximal communicability extends from a few days before to 7 days after the onset of rash. Volunteer studies have demonstrated the presence of rubella virus in nasopharyngeal secretions from 7 days before to 14 days after the onset of the rash. A small number of infants with congenital rubella continue to shed virus in nasopharyngeal secretions and urine for 1 year or more and can transmit infection to susceptible contacts.

Before widespread use of rubella vaccine, rubella was an epidemic disease, occurring in 6- to 9-year cycles, with most cases occurring in children. The incidence of rubella in the United States has decreased by approximately 99% from the prevaccine era. The risk of acquiring rubella has decreased in all age groups, including adolescents and young adults. In the vaccine era, most cases have occurred in young, unimmunized adults in outbreaks on college campuses and in occupational settings. Although the number of susceptible people has decreased since introduction and widespread use of rubella vaccine, recent serologic surveys indicate that approximately 10% of young adults are susceptible to rubella. The percentage of susceptible people in certain immigrant population groups, especially adolescent and adult males from Latin America, may be higher.

The **incubation period** for postnatally acquired rubella ranges from 14 to 23 days, usually 16 to 18 days.

DIAGNOSTIC TESTS: Detection of rubella-specific immunoglobulin (Ig) M antibody usually indicates recent postnatal infection or congenital infection in a newborn infant, but false-positive results occur. Congenital infection also can be confirmed by stable or increasing serum concentrations of rubella-specific IgG over several months. Rubella virus can be isolated most consistently from nasal specimens by inoculation of appropriate cell culture. Laboratory personnel should be notified that rubella is suspected, because additional testing is required to detect the virus. Blood, urine, cerebrospinal fluid, and throat swab specimens also can yield virus, particularly in congenitally infected infants. A fourfold or greater increase in antibody titer or seroconversion between acute and convalescent serum titers indicates infection. Every effort should be made to establish a laboratory diagnosis when rubella infection is suspected in pregnant women or newborn infants. The diagnosis of congenital rubella infection in children older than 1 year of age is difficult; serologic testing usually is not diagnostic, and viral isolation, although confirmatory, is possible in only a small proportion of congenitally infected children of this age. The hemagglutination inhibition rubella antibody test, which previously was the most commonly used method of serologic screening, generally has been supplanted by a number of equally or more sensitive assays for determining rubella immunity, including enzyme immunoassay tests, latex agglutination, and immunofluorescence assay.

Some people in whom antibody has been absent by hemagglutination inhibition testing have been found to be immune when their serum specimens were tested by more sensitive assays.

TREATMENT: Supportive.

ISOLATION OF THE HOSPITALIZED PATIENT: In addition to standard precautions, for postnatal rubella, droplet precautions are recommended for 7 days after the onset of the rash. Contact isolation is indicated for children with proven or suspected congenital rubella until they are at least 1 year of age, unless nasopharyngeal and urine culture results after 3 months of age repeatedly are negative for rubella virus.

CONTROL MEASURES:

School and Child Care. Children with postnatal rubella should be excluded from school or child care for 7 days after onset of the rash. Children with congenital rubella should be considered contagious until they are at least 1 year of age, unless nasopharyngeal and urine culture results repeatedly are negative for rubella virus. Caregivers of these infants should be made aware of the potential hazard of the infants to susceptible pregnant contacts.

Care of Exposed People. When a pregnant woman is exposed to rubella, a blood specimen should be obtained as soon as possible and tested for rubella antibody. An aliquot of frozen serum should be stored for possible repeated testing at a later time. The presence of rubella-specific IgG antibody in a properly performed test at the time of exposure indicates that the person most likely is immune. If antibody is not detectable, a second blood specimen should be obtained 2 to 3 weeks later and tested concurrently with the first specimen. If the second test result is negative, another blood specimen should be obtained 6 weeks after the exposure and also tested concurrently with the first specimen; a negative test result in both specimens indicates that infection has not occurred, and a positive test result in the second or third specimen but not the first (seroconversion) indicates recent infection.

Immune Globulin. The routine use of Immune Globulin (IG) for postexposure prophylaxis of rubella-susceptible women exposed to rubella early in pregnancy is not recommended. Administration of IG should be considered only if termination of the pregnancy is not an option. Limited data indicate that intramuscular IG in a dose of 0.55 mL/kg may decrease clinically apparent infection in an exposed susceptible person from 87% to 18%, compared with placebo. However, the absence of clinical signs in a woman who has received intramuscular IG does not guarantee that fetal infection has been prevented. Infants with congenital rubella have been born to mothers who were given IG shortly after exposure.

Vaccine. Although live-virus rubella vaccine given after exposure has not been demonstrated to prevent illness, vaccine theoretically could prevent illness if administered within 3 days of exposure. Immunization of exposed nonpregnant people may be indicated, because if the exposure did not result in infection, immunization will protect these people in the future. Immunization of a person who is incubating natural rubella or who already is immune is not associated with an increased risk of adverse effects.

Rubella Vaccine. The live-virus rubella vaccine distributed in the United States is the RA 27/3 strain grown in human diploid cell cultures. Vaccine is administered by subcutaneous injection of 0.5 mL, alone or, preferably, as a combined vaccine containing measles-mumps-rubella (MMR). Vaccine can be given simultaneously with other vaccines (see Simultaneous Administration of Multiple Vaccines, p 33). Serum antibody to rubella is induced in 95% or more of the recipients after a single dose at 12 months of age or older. Clinical efficacy and challenge studies have demonstrated that 1 dose confers long-term, probably lifelong, immunity against clinical and asymptomatic infection in more than 90% of immunized people. Asymptomatic reinfection has occurred.

Because of the 2-dose recommendation for measles vaccine as MMR, 2 doses of rubella vaccine now are given routinely. This provides an added safeguard against primary vaccine failures.

Vaccine Recommendations. Rubella vaccine is recommended to be administered in combination with measles and mumps vaccines (MMR) when a child is 12 to 15 months of age, with a second dose at school entry at 4 to 6 years, according to recommendations for routine measles immunization. People who have not received the dose at school entry should receive their second dose as soon as possible but no later than 11 to 12 years of age (see Measles, p 419).

Special emphasis must continue to be placed on the immunization of at-risk postpubertal males and females, especially college students, military recruits, recent immigrants, and health care professionals. People who were born in 1957 or after and have not received at least 1 dose of vaccine or who have no serologic evidence of immunity to rubella are considered susceptible and should be immunized with MMR vaccine. Clinical diagnosis of infection usually is unreliable and should not be accepted as evidence of immunity. Women should be informed of the theoretic risk to the fetus if they are pregnant or become pregnant within 28 days of immunization (see Precautions and Contraindications, p 540, for further discussion). Specific recommendations are as follows:

- Postpubertal females without documentation of presumptive evidence of rubella immunity should be immunized unless they are known to be pregnant. Postpubertal females should be advised not to become pregnant for 28 days after receiving rubella containing vaccine.
- During annual health care examinations, premarital and family planning visits, and visits to sexually transmitted disease clinics, postpubertal females should be assessed for rubella susceptibility and, if deemed susceptible, should be immunized with MMR vaccine. Serologic prescreening is indicated only if follow-up of susceptible individuals is ensured.
- Routine prenatal screening for rubella immunity should be undertaken. If a woman is found to be susceptible, rubella vaccine should be administered during the immediate postpartum period before discharge. Physicians can help ensure immunization of susceptible women by inquiring about the immune status of the mothers of their patients during medical visits for well-child care of newborn infants.
- Previous or simultaneous administration of IG (Human) or blood products may require reimmunization (see Precautions and Contraindications, p 540).

- Breastfeeding is not a contraindication to postpartum immunization of the mother (for additional information, see Human Milk, p 117). Although the vaccine virus has been transmitted to breastfed infants, the infants remained asymptomatic.
- Special efforts should be made to be certain that all people who plan to attend or work in educational institutions, child care centers, or other places where there is a likelihood of exposure to or spread of rubella are immune to rubella.
- All susceptible health care professionals who may be exposed to patients with rubella should be immunized for the prevention or transmission of rubella to pregnant patients as well as for their own health.

Adverse Reactions.

- Of susceptible children who receive MMR vaccine, fever develops in 5% to 15% from 5 to 12 days after immunization. Rash occurs in approximately 5% of immunized people. Mild lymphadenopathy occurs commonly.
- Joint pain, usually in small peripheral joints, has been reported in approximately 0.5% of young children. Arthralgia and transient arthritis tend to be more common in susceptible postpubertal females, occurring in approximately 25% and 10%, respectively, of vaccine recipients. Joint involvement usually begins 7 to 21 days after immunization and generally is transient. Persistent or recurrent joint symptoms have been reported in adult women by 1 group of investigators from Canada, but subsequent studies in the United States and Israel have not noted this relationship.
- The incidence of joint manifestations after immunization is lower than that after natural infection at the corresponding age.
- Transient paresthesia and pain in the arms and legs also have been reported, although rarely.
- Central nervous system manifestations have been reported, but no causal relationship with rubella vaccine has been established.
- Thrombocytopenia can occur after rubella immunization with MMR vaccine (see Measles, p 419).

Precautions and Contraindications.

- *Pregnancy.* Rubella vaccine should not be given to pregnant women. If vaccine is given inadvertently or if pregnancy occurs within 28 days of immunization, the patient should be counseled on the theoretic risks to the fetus. Of offspring in such cases, 2% had asymptomatic infection, but none had congenital defects. In view of these observations, receipt of rubella vaccine during pregnancy is not an indication for termination of pregnancy.

   Routine serologic testing of postpubertal women before immunization is unnecessary. Serologic testing is a potential impediment to protection against rubella, because it requires 2 visits, 1 to identify susceptible people and 1 to administer vaccine. However, a specimen of blood may be obtained before immunization and stored for at least 28 days. If a woman becomes pregnant in the month after immunization, the preimmunization specimen can be tested. Demonstration of rubella antibody in the prevaccine specimen indicates immunity and eliminates anxiety about fetal injury from rubella vaccine virus. Immunizing susceptible children whose mothers or other household contacts are pregnant does not cause a risk. Most immunized people intermittently shed small amounts of virus from the pharynx 7 to 28 days after immunization, but no evidence of transmission of the vaccine virus from immunized children has been found in studies of more than 1200 susceptible household contacts.

- *Febrile illness.* Children with minor illnesses, such as upper respiratory tract infection, may be immunized (see Vaccine Safety and Contraindications, p 37). Fever is not a contraindication to immunization. However, if other manifestations suggest a more serious illness, the child should not be immunized until recovery has occurred.

- *Recent administration of IG.* Immune Globulin preparations may interfere with the serologic response to rubella vaccine (see p 35). Rubella vaccine may be given to postpartum women at the same time as anti-Rh$_o$ (D) IG (Human; RhoGAM [Ortho-Clinical Diagnostics, Raritan, NJ]) or after blood products are given, but these women should be tested 8 or more weeks later to determine whether they have developed an antibody response.

- *Altered immunity.* Immunocompromised patients with disorders associated with increased severity of viral infections should not receive live-virus rubella vaccine (see Immunocompromised Children, p 69). The exceptions are patients with human immunodeficiency virus infection who are not severely immunocompromised; these patients may be immunized against rubella with MMR (see Human Immunodeficiency Virus Infection, p 360). The risk of rubella exposure for patients with altered immunity can be decreased by immunizing their close susceptible contacts.

Corticosteroids. For patients who have received high doses of corticosteroids for 14 days or more and who are not otherwise immunocompromised, the recommended interval before immunization is at least 1 month (see Immunocompromised Children, p 69) after steroids have been discontinued.

Surveillance for Congenital Infections. Accurate diagnosis and reporting of the congenital rubella syndrome are extremely important in assessing control of rubella. All birth defects in which rubella infection is suspected etiologically should be investigated thoroughly and reported to the Centers for Disease Control and Prevention through local or state health departments.

Salmonella Infections

CLINICAL MANIFESTATIONS: Nontyphoidal *Salmonella* organisms cause asymptomatic carriage, gastroenteritis, bacteremia, and focal infections (such as meningitis and osteomyelitis). These disease categories are not mutually exclusive but represent a spectrum of illness. The most common illness associated with nontyphoidal *Salmonella* is gastroenteritis, in which diarrhea, abdominal cramps and tenderness, and fever are common manifestations. The site of infection usually is the small intestine, but colitis can occur. Sustained or intermittent bacteremia can occur, and focal infections are recognized in as many as 10% of patients with bacteremia resulting from *Salmonella* infection.

Salmonella serotype Typhi and several other *Salmonella* serotypes may cause a protracted bacteremic illness referred to as enteric or typhoid fever. The onset of illness typically is gradual, with manifestations such as fever, constitutional symptoms (eg, headache, malaise, anorexia, and lethargy), abdominal pain and tenderness, hepatomegaly, splenomegaly, rose spots, and changes in mental status. Enteric fever may manifest as a mild, nondescript febrile illness in young children in whom sustained or intermittent bacteremia can occur. Constipation may be an early feature. Diarrhea occurs commonly in children. Recurrent *Salmonella* bacteremia is an acquired immunodeficiency syndrome (AIDS)-defining condition for adolescents and adults infected with the human immunodeficiency virus (HIV).

ETIOLOGY: *Salmonella* organisms are gram-negative bacilli that belong to the Enterobacteriaceae family. Currently, there are more than 2460 *Salmonella* serotypes; most that cause human disease are divided among O-antigen groups A through E. *Salmonella* serotype Typhi is classified in serogroup D. In 2000, the most commonly reported human isolates in the United States were *Salmonella* serotype Typhimurium (serogroup B), *Salmonella* serotype Enteritidis (D), *Salmonella* serotype Newport (C2), *Salmonella* serotype Heidelberg (B), *Salmonella* serotype Javiana (D), *Salmonella* serotype Montevideo (C1), *Salmonella* serotype Muenchen (D), and *Salmonella* serotype Infantis (C1). The *Salmonella* nomenclature recently changed (see Table 3.52, p 543).

EPIDEMIOLOGY: The principal reservoirs for nontyphoidal *Salmonella* organisms are animals, including poultry, livestock, reptiles, and pets. The major vehicles of transmission are foods of animal origin, including poultry, beef, fish, eggs, and dairy products. Many other foods, including fruits, vegetables, and bakery products, have been implicated in outbreaks. These foods usually are contaminated by contact with an animal product or, occasionally, an infected human. Other modes of transmission include ingestion of contaminated water; contact with infected reptiles (eg, pet turtles, iguanas, lizards, snakes); and contact with contaminated medications, dyes, and medical instruments. Unlike nontyphoidal *Salmonella* serotypes, *S* serotype Typhi is found only in humans, and infection implies direct contact with an infected person or with an item contaminated by a carrier. Although uncommon in the United States (approximately 400 cases per year), typhoid fever is endemic in many countries. Consequently, typhoid fever infections in the United States usually are acquired during international travel.

Age-specific attack rates for *Salmonella* infection are highest in people younger than 4 years of age, with a peak during the first months of life. Rates of invasive infections and mortality are higher in infants, elderly people, and people with immunosuppressive conditions, hemoglobinopathies (including sickle cell disease), malignant neoplasms, and AIDS. Most reported cases are sporadic, but widespread outbreaks, including nosocomial, institutional, and nursery outbreaks, have been reported. From 1996 through 2000, *Salmonella* organisms were second to *Campylobacter* organisms as the cause of laboratory-confirmed cases of enteric disease as reported by the Foodborne Diseases Active Surveillance Network (FoodNet). In 3

Table 3.52. **Nomenclature for *Salmonella* Organisms**

Complete Name	CDC Designation	Commonly Used Name
S enterica[1] subspecies *enterica* serotype Typhi	*S* ser. Typhi	*S typhi*
S enterica subspecies *enterica* serotype Typhimurium	*S* ser. Typhimurium	*S typhimurium*
S enterica subspecies *enterica* serotype Newport	*S* ser. Newport	*S newport*
S enterica subspecies *enterica* serotype Choleraesuis	*S* ser. Choleraesuis	*S choleraesuis*
S enterica subspecies *arizona* serotype 18:z$_4$,z$_{23}$:−	*S* ser. 18:z$_4$,z$_{23}$:−	*Arizona hinshawii*
S enterica subspecies *houtenae* serotype Marina	*S* ser. Marina	*S marina*

CDC indicates Centers for Disease Control and Prevention.
[1] Some also use *choleraesuis* and *enteritidis* as species names.

of 8 state sites, *Salmonella* species were noted to be the most common enteric pathogens reported.

The risk of transmission exists throughout the variable duration of fecal excretion of organisms. Twelve weeks after infection, 45% of children younger than 5 years of age excrete *Salmonella* organisms, compared with 5% of older children and adults; antimicrobial therapy can prolong excretion. Approximately 1% of patients continue to excrete *Salmonella* organisms for more than 1 year (chronic carriers).

The **incubation period** for gastroenteritis is 6 to 48 hours. For enteric fever, the incubation period is 3 to 60 days (usually 7–14 days).

DIAGNOSTIC TESTS: Isolation of *Salmonella* organisms from cultures of stool, blood, urine, and material from foci of infection is diagnostic. Gastroenteritis is diagnosed by stool culture. Rapid tests using enzyme immunoassay, latex agglutination, DNA probes and monoclonal antibodies have been developed and are in use in some laboratories. Serologic tests for *Salmonella* agglutinins ("febrile agglutinins" [the Widal test]) are not recommended.

TREATMENT:
- Antimicrobial therapy usually is not indicated for patients with uncomplicated (noninvasive) gastroenteritis caused by nontyphoidal *Salmonella* species, because therapy does not shorten the duration of disease and may prolong the duration of carriage. Although of unproven benefit, antimicrobial therapy is recommended for gastroenteritis caused by *Salmonella* species in patients with an increased risk of invasive disease, including infants younger than 3 months of age and patients with chronic gastrointestinal tract disease, malignant neoplasms, hemoglobinopathies, HIV infection or other immunosuppressive illnesses or therapies, or severe colitis.

- Ampicillin, amoxicillin, trimethoprim-sulfamethoxazole, cefotaxime sodium, or ceftriaxone sodium are recommended for susceptible strains in patients for whom therapy is indicated. Strains acquired in developing countries often exhibit resistance to many antimicrobial agents but usually are susceptible to ceftriaxone or cefotaxime and to fluoroquinolones (eg, ciprofloxacin or ofloxacin). However, fluoroquinolones are not recommended for use in patients younger than 18 years of age unless the benefits of therapy outweigh the potential risks with use of the drug (see Antimicrobial Agents and Related Therapy, p 693). Domestically acquired *S* serotype Typhimurium and *S* serotype Newport infections increasingly are drug-resistant, with approximately one third of *S* serotype Typhimurium isolates resistant to ampicillin, chloramphenicol, streptomycin sulfate, sulfonamides, and tetracycline and approximately 11% of *S* serotype Newport isolates resistant to ceftriaxone.
- In invasive disease attributable to *Salmonella* species (such as typhoid, non-*S* serotype Typhi bacteremia, or osteomyelitis), appropriate drugs are ampicillin, amoxicillin, cefotaxime, ceftriaxone, chloramphenicol, trimethoprim-sulfamethoxazole, or a fluoroquinolone (see Antimicrobial Agents and Related Therapy, p 693). Drug of choice, route of administration, and duration of therapy are based on susceptibility of the organism, site of infection, host, and clinical response. For susceptible *S* serotype Typhi, administration of a 14-day course of ampicillin, chloramphenicol, or trimethoprim-sulfamethoxazole is adequate. For severely ill patients, parenteral therapy is indicated. For typhoid fever attributable to strains that are resistant to multiple antimicrobial agents (ampicillin, chloramphenicol, trimethoprim-sulfamethoxazole), such as are acquired routinely in India, Pakistan, and Egypt, therapeutic options include a 7- to 10-day course of ceftriaxone or a 5- to 7-day course of ofloxacin or ciprofloxacin. Some patients require more prolonged courses of treatment. Relapse is common after completion of therapy; retreatment is indicated. Strain susceptibility should be interpreted with caution; clinical failure has been reported in patients with typhoid fever treated with cephalexin, aminoglycosides, furazolidone, and second-generation cephalosporins despite in vitro susceptibility. For invasive, nonlocalized infections, such as bacteremia or enteric fever caused by nontyphoidal *Salmonella* species in immunocompetent hosts without localization, patients also should be treated for 14 days; patients with localized infection, such as osteomyelitis or abscess, and patients with concomitant bacteremia and HIV infection should receive 4 to 6 weeks of therapy to prevent relapse. For meningitis attributable to *Salmonella* species, ceftriaxone or cefotaxime is recommended for at least 4 weeks.
- Chronic (1 year or more) *S* serotype Typhi carriage may be eradicated in some children by high-dose parenteral ampicillin or high-dose oral amoxicillin combined with probenecid (see Antimicrobial Agents and Related Therapy, p 693). Ciprofloxacin is the drug of choice for elimination of organisms from adult carriers of *S* serotype Typhi. Cholecystectomy may be indicated in some instances in which gallstones provide a nidus for resistance to medical therapy.

- Corticosteroids may be beneficial in patients with severe enteric fever, which is characterized by delirium, obtundation, stupor, coma, or shock. These drugs, however, should be reserved for critically ill patients in whom relief of the manifestations of toxemia may be life saving. The usual regimen is high-dose dexamethasone given intravenously at an initial dose of 3 mg/kg, followed by 1 mg/kg, every 6 hours, for a total course of 48 hours.

ISOLATION OF THE HOSPITALIZED PATIENT: In addition to standard precautions, contact precautions should be used for diapered and incontinent children for the duration of illness. In children with typhoid fever, precautions should be continued until culture results for 3 consecutive stool specimens obtained at least 48 hours after cessation of antimicrobial therapy are negative.

CONTROL MEASURES: Important measures include proper sanitation methods for food processing and preparation, sanitary water supplies, proper hand hygiene, sanitary sewage disposal, exclusion of infected people from handling food or providing health care, prohibiting the sale of pet turtles and restricting the sale of other reptiles for pets, reporting cases to appropriate health authorities, and investigating outbreaks. Eggs and other foods of animal origin should be cooked thoroughly. Raw eggs and food containing raw eggs should not be eaten. Notification of public health authorities and determination of serotype are of primary importance in detection and investigation of outbreaks.

Child Care. Outbreaks of *Salmonella* infection are rare but have occurred in child care programs. Specific strategies for controlling infection in out-of-home child care include adherence to hygiene practices, including meticulous hand hygiene (see Children in Out-of-Home Child Care, p 123).

When *S* serotype Typhi infection is identified in a symptomatic child care attendee or staff member, stool cultures should be performed for other attendees and staff members, and all infected people should be excluded. The length of exclusion recommended varies with patient age; for those younger than 5 years of age, 3 negative stool specimens are recommended for return. For those 5 years of age and older, 24 hours without a diarrheal stool is recommended before return to a group setting.

When serotypes other than *S* serotype Typhi are identified in a symptomatic child care attendee or staff member with enterocolitis, older children and staff do not need to be excluded unless they are symptomatic. Stool cultures are not required for asymptomatic contacts. Antimicrobial therapy is not recommended for people with asymptomatic infection or uncomplicated diarrhea or for people who are contacts of an infected person.

Typhoid Vaccine. Resistance to infection with *S* serotype Typhi is enhanced by typhoid immunization, but the degree of protection with currently available vaccines is limited. Two typhoid vaccines are licensed for use in the United States (see Table 3.53, p 546).

The demonstrated efficacy of the 2 licensed vaccines ranges from 50% to 80%. Vaccine is selected on the basis of the age of the child, need for booster doses, and possible contraindications (see Precautions and Contraindications, p 547) and reactions (see Adverse Events, p 546).

Table 3.53. Commercially Available Typhoid Vaccines in the United States

Typhoid Vaccine	Type	Route	Minimum Age of Receipt, y	No. of Doses[1]	Booster Frequency, y	Adverse Effects (Incidence, %)
Ty21a	Live-attenuated	Oral	6	4	5	<5
Vi CPS	Polysaccharide	Intramuscular	2	1	2	<7

ViCPS indicates Vi capsular polysaccharide vaccine.

[1] Primary immunization. For further information on dosage, schedules, and adverse events, see text.

Indications. In the United States, immunization is recommended only for the following people:

- ***Travelers to areas where risk of exposure to S serotype Typhi is recognized.*** Risk is greatest for travelers to the Indian subcontinent, Latin America, Asia, and Africa who may have prolonged exposure to contaminated food and drink. Such travelers need to be cautioned that typhoid vaccine is not a substitute for careful selection of food and drink.
- ***People with intimate exposure to a documented typhoid fever carrier,*** such as occurs with continued household contact.
- ***Laboratory workers with frequent contact with S serotype Typhi and people living in typhoid-endemic areas outside the United States.***

Dosages. For primary immunization, the following dosage is recommended for each vaccine:

- ***Oral Ty21a vaccine.*** Children (6 years of age and older) and adults should take 1 enteric-coated capsule every 2 days for a total of 4 capsules. Each capsule should be taken with cool liquid, no warmer than 37°C (98°F), approximately 1 hour before a meal. The capsules must be kept refrigerated, and all 4 doses must be taken to achieve maximal efficacy.
- ***Vi capsular polysaccharide vaccine.*** Primary immunization of people 2 years of age and older with Vi capsular polysaccharide (ViCPS) vaccine consists of one 0.5-mL (25-µg) dose administered intramuscularly.

Booster Doses. In circumstances of continued or repeated exposure to S serotype Typhi, booster doses are recommended to maintain immunity after primary immunization.

Continued efficacy for 5 years after immunization with the oral Ty21a vaccine has been demonstrated; however, the manufacturer of Ty21a vaccine recommends reimmunization, completing the entire 4-dose series every 5 years if continued or renewed exposure to S serotype Typhi is expected.

The manufacturer of ViCPS vaccine recommends a booster dose every 2 years after the primary dose if continued or renewed exposure is expected.

No data have been reported concerning the use of one vaccine as a booster after primary immunization with the other.

Adverse Events. The Ty21a vaccine produces minimal adverse reactions that may include abdominal discomfort, nausea, vomiting, fever, headache, and rash or urticaria. Reported adverse reactions to ViCPS vaccine also are minimal and include fever (0%–1%), headache (1.5%–3%), and local reaction of erythema or induration of 1 cm or greater (7%).

Precautions and Contraindications. No data are available regarding the efficacy of typhoid vaccines in children younger than 2 years of age. However, there is evidence that breastfeeding and meticulous preparation of formula might prevent typhoid infection in endemic areas. A contraindication to administration of the parenteral typhoid (ViCPS) vaccine is a history of severe local or systemic reactions after a previous dose. No safety data have been reported for typhoid vaccines in pregnant women. The Ty21a vaccine is a live-attenuated vaccine and should not be administered to immunocompromised people, including those known to be infected with HIV; the parenteral ViCPS vaccine may be an alternative. The oral Ty21a vaccine requires replication in the gut for effectiveness; it should not be administered during gastrointestinal tract illness. Because the growth of Ty21a strain in vitro may be inhibited by antimalarial agents, previous recommendations have advised against the simultaneous administration of Ty21a with these agents. Subsequent studies have demonstrated that simultaneous administration of mefloquine hydrochloride and chloroquine hydrochloride with Ty21a results in an adequate in vivo response. However, the antimalarial proguanil hydrochloride should not be administered simultaneously with Ty21a vaccine but rather should be administered 10 or more days after the fourth dose of Ty21a vaccine. Antimicrobial agents also should be avoided for 7 days before the first dose of Ty21a vaccine and 7 days after the fourth dose of Ty21a vaccine.

Scabies

CLINICAL MANIFESTATIONS: Scabies is characterized by an intensely pruritic, erythematous, papular eruption caused by burrowing of adult female mites in upper layers of the epidermis, creating serpiginous burrows. Itching is most intense at night. In older children and adults, the sites of predilection are interdigital folds, flexor aspects of wrists, extensor surfaces of elbows, anterior axillary folds, waistline, thighs, navel, genitalia, areolae, abdomen, intergluteal cleft, and buttocks. In children younger than 2 years of age, the eruption generally is vesicular and often occurs in areas usually spared in older children and adults, such as the head, neck, palms, and soles. The eruption is caused by a hypersensitivity reaction to the proteins of the parasite.

The characteristic scabietic burrows appear as gray or white, tortuous, thread-like lines. Excoriations are common, and most burrows are obliterated by scratching before a patient is seen by a physician. Occasionally, 2- to 5-mm red-brown nodules are present, particularly on covered parts of the body, such as the genitalia, groin, and axilla. These scabies nodules are a granulomatous response to dead mite antigens and feces; the nodules can persist for weeks and even months after effective treatment. Cutaneous secondary bacterial infection can occur and usually is caused by *Streptococcus pyogenes* or *Staphylococcus aureus*.

Norwegian scabies is an uncommon clinical syndrome characterized by a large number of mites and widespread, crusted, hyperkeratotic lesions. Norwegian scabies usually occurs in debilitated, developmentally disabled, or immunologically compromised people.

ETIOLOGY: The mite, *Sarcoptes scabiei* subspecies *hominis,* is the cause of scabies. *Sarcoptes scabiei* subspecies *canis,* acquired from dogs (with clinical mange), can cause a self-limited and mild infestation usually involving the area in direct contact with the infested animal that will resolve without specific treatment.

EPIDEMIOLOGY: Humans are the source of infestation. Transmission usually occurs through prolonged, close, personal contact. Because of the large number of mites in exfoliating scales, even minimal contact with a patient with crusted (Norwegian) scabies may result in transmission. Infestation acquired from dogs and other animals is uncommon, and these mites do not replicate in humans. Scabies of human origin can be transmitted as long as the patient remains infested and untreated, including the interval before symptoms develop. Scabies is endemic in many countries and occurs worldwide in cycles thought to be 15 to 30 years long. Scabies affects people from all socioeconomic levels without regard to age, sex, or standards of personal hygiene. Scabies in adults often is acquired sexually.

The **incubation period** in people without previous exposure usually is 4 to 6 weeks. People who previously were infested are sensitized and develop symptoms 1 to 4 days after repeated exposure to the mite; however, these reinfestations usually are milder than the original episode.

DIAGNOSTIC TESTS: Diagnosis is confirmed by identification of the mite or mite eggs or scybala (feces) from scrapings of papules or intact burrows, preferably from the terminal portion where the mite generally is found. Mineral oil, microscope immersion oil, or water applied to skin facilitates the collection of scrapings. A number 15 scalpel is used to scrape the burrow. Scrapings and oil can be placed on a slide under a glass coverslip and examined microscopically under low power. Adult female mites average 330 to 450 µm in length.

TREATMENT: Infested children and adults should apply lotion or cream containing a scabicide over their entire body below the head. Because scabies can affect the head, scalp, and neck in infants and young children, treatment of the entire head, neck, and body in this age group is required. The drug of choice, particularly for infants, young children, and pregnant or nursing women, is 5% permethrin cream, a synthetic pyrethroid. Alternative drugs are 1% lindane cream or lotion and 10% crotamiton. Permethrin should be removed by bathing after 8 to 14 hours, and lindane should be removed by bathing after 8 to 12 hours. Crotamiton is applied once a day for 2 days followed by a cleansing bath 48 hours after the last application, but crotamiton is associated with frequent treatment failures. Ivermectin in a single dose administered orally is effective for treatment of severe or crusted (Norwegian) scabies and should be considered for patients whose infestation is refractory or who cannot tolerate topical therapy. This drug is not licensed for this indication by the US Food and Drug Administration.

Lindane should not be used for patients with crusted scabies, premature infants, people with known seizure disorders, people with hypersensitivity to the product, young infants, women who are pregnant or breastfeeding, and patients who have extensive dermatitis. The frequency of lindane applications should not exceed that recommended by the manufacturer to decrease the risk of possible neurologic toxic effects from absorption through skin. Lindane should not be used immediately after a bath or shower.

Because scabietic lesions are the result of a hypersensitivity reaction to the mite, itching may not subside for several weeks despite successful treatment. The use of oral antihistamines and topical corticosteroids can help relieve this itching. Topical or systemic antimicrobial therapy is indicated for secondary bacterial infections of the excoriated lesions.

ISOLATION OF THE HOSPITALIZED PATIENT: In addition to standard precautions, contact precautions are recommended until the patient has been treated with an appropriate scabicide.

CONTROL MEASURES:
- Prophylactic therapy is recommended for household members, particularly for those members who have had prolonged direct skin-to-skin contact. Manifestations of scabies infestation can appear as late as 2 months after exposure, during which time patients can transmit scabies. All household members should be treated at the same time to prevent reinfestation. Bedding and clothing worn next to the skin during the 4 days before initiation of therapy should be laundered in a washer with hot water and dried using a hot cycle. Mites do not survive more than 3 to 4 days without skin contact. Clothing that cannot be laundered should be removed from the patient and stored for several days to a week to avoid reinfestation.
- Children should be allowed to return to child care or school after treatment has been completed.
- Epidemics and localized outbreaks may require stringent and consistent measures to treat contacts. Caregivers who have had prolonged skin-to-skin contact with infested patients may benefit from prophylactic treatment.
- Environmental disinfestation is unnecessary and unwarranted. Thorough vacuuming of environmental surfaces is recommended after use of a room by a patient with crusted (Norwegian) scabies.
- People with crusted (Norwegian) scabies and their close contacts must be treated promptly and aggressively to avoid outbreaks.

Schistosomiasis

CLINICAL MANIFESTATIONS: Initial entry of the infecting larvae (cercariae) through the skin commonly is accompanied by a transient, pruritic, papular rash (cercarial dermatitis). After penetration, the organism enters the bloodstream and migrates through the lungs. Each of the 3 major human schistosome parasites lives in some part of the venous plexus that drains the intestines or the bladder. Four to 8 weeks after exposure to *Schistosoma mansoni* or *Schistosoma japonicum,* an acute illness that manifests as fever, malaise, cough, rash, abdominal pain, diarrhea, nausea, lymphadenopathy, and eosinophilia (Katayama fever) can develop. Heavy infestation can result in mucoid bloody diarrhea accompanied by tender hepatomegaly. The severity of symptoms associated with chronic disease is related to the worm burden. People with low to moderate worm burdens can be asymptomatic; heavily infected people can have a range of symptoms caused primarily by inflammation and fibrosis triggered by eggs produced by adult worms. Portal hypertension can develop and cause hepatosplenomegaly, ascites, and esophageal varices. Long-term involvement of the colon produces abdominal pain and bloody diarrhea. In *Schistosoma haematobium* infections, the bladder becomes inflamed and fibrotic. Symptoms and signs include dysuria, urgency, terminal microscopic and gross hematuria, secondary urinary tract infections, and nonspecific pelvic pain. Other organ systems can be involved from embolized eggs, for example, to the lungs, causing pulmonary hypertension; or to the central nervous system, notably the spinal cord in *S mansoni* or *S haematobium* infections and the brain in *S japonicum* infection.

Swimmer's itch (cercarial dermatitis or schistosome dermatitis) is caused by the larvae of other avian and mammalian schistosome species that penetrate human skin but do not complete the life cycle and do not cause chronic fibrotic disease. Manifestations include mild to moderate pruritus at the penetration site a few hours after exposure, followed in 5 to 14 days by an intermittent pruritic, sometimes papular, eruption. In previously sensitized people, more intense papular eruptions may occur for 7 to 10 days after exposure.

ETIOLOGY: The trematodes (flukes) *S mansoni, S japonicum, S haematobium,* and rarely, *Schistosoma mekongi* and *Schistosoma intercalatum* cause disease. All species have similar life cycles. Swimmer's itch is caused by multiple avian and mammalian species of *Schistosoma.*

EPIDEMIOLOGY: Humans are the principal hosts for the major species. Persistence of schistosomiasis depends on the presence of an appropriate snail as an intermediate host. Eggs excreted in stool (*S mansoni* and *S japonicum*) or urine *(S haematobium)* into fresh water hatch into motile miracidia, which infect snails. After development in snails, cercariae emerge and penetrate the skin of humans encountered in the water. Children commonly are infected after infancy when they begin to explore the environment. Children commonly are involved in transmission because of habits of uncontrolled defecation, urination, and frequent wading in infected waters. Communicability lasts as long as live eggs are excreted in the urine and feces.

Schistosoma mansoni occurs throughout tropical Africa, in several Caribbean islands, and in Venezuela, Brazil, Suriname, and the Arabian peninsula. *Schistosoma japonicum* is found in China, the Philippines, and Indonesia. *Schistosoma haematobium* occurs in Africa and the eastern Mediterranean region. *Schistosoma mekongi* is limited to a small area of the Mekong delta in Southeast Asia (Kampuchea and Laos). *Schistosoma intercalatum* is found in West and Central Africa. Adult worms of the *S mansoni* species have been documented to live as long as 26 years in the human host. Thus, schistosomiasis can be diagnosed in patients many years after they have left an endemic area. Swimmer's itch occurs in all regions of the world after exposure to fresh, brackish, or saltwater-containing larvae that do not complete their life cycle in humans.

The **incubation period** is variable but is approximately 8 weeks for *S haematobium* and 4 weeks for *S mansoni* and *S japonicum.*

DIAGNOSTIC TESTS: Infection with *S mansoni* and other species (except *S haematobium*) is determined by microscopic examination of concentrated stool specimens to detect characteristic eggs. In light infections, several specimens may need to be examined before eggs are found, and a biopsy of the rectal mucosa may be necessary. The fresh tissue obtained should be compressed between 2 glass slides and examined under low power (unstained) for eggs. *Schistosoma haematobium* is diagnosed by examining filtered urine for eggs. Egg excretion often peaks between noon and 3 PM. Biopsy of the bladder mucosa may be necessary. Serologic tests, available through the Centers for Disease Control and Prevention and some commercial laboratories, may be particularly helpful for detecting light infections or before eggs appear in the stool or urine.

Swimmer's itch can be difficult to differentiate from other causes of dermatitis. A skin biopsy may demonstrate larvae, but their absence does not exclude the diagnosis.

TREATMENT: The drug of choice for schistosomiasis caused by any species is praziquantel; the alternative drug for *S mansoni* is oxamniquine (see Drugs for Parasitic Infections, p 744). Swimmer's itch is a self-limited disease that requires only symptomatic treatment of the urticarial rash.

ISOLATION OF THE HOSPITALIZED PATIENT: Standard precautions are recommended.

CONTROL MEASURES: Elimination of the intermediate snail host is difficult to achieve in most areas. Thus, treatment of infected populations, sanitary disposal of human waste, and education about the source of infection are the key elements of current control measures. Travelers to endemic areas should be advised to avoid contact with freshwater streams and lakes.

Shigella Infections

CLINICAL MANIFESTATIONS: *Shigella* species primarily infect the large intestine, causing clinical manifestations that range from watery or loose stools with minimal or no constitutional symptoms to more severe symptoms, including fever, abdominal cramps or tenderness, tenesmus, and mucoid stools with or without blood. Clinical presentations vary with *Shigella* species; patients with *Shigella sonnei* infection usually exhibit watery diarrhea; people with *Shigella flexneri, Shigella boydii,* and *Shigella dysenteriae* infection typically have bloody diarrhea and severe systemic symptoms. Rare complications include bacteremia, Reiter syndrome (after *S flexneri* infection), hemolytic-uremic syndrome (after *S dysenteriae* type 1 infection), toxic megacolon and perforation, and toxic encephalopathy (ekiri syndrome).

ETIOLOGY: *Shigella* species are gram-negative bacilli in the family Enterobacteriaceae. Four species (with more than 40 serotypes) have been identified. Among *Shigella* isolates reported in the United States from 1989 to 2000, 78% were *S sonnei*, 19% were *S flexneri*, 2% were *S boydii*, and 1% were *S dysenteriae*. *Shigella dysenteriae* is rare in the United States but is widespread in rural Africa and the Indian subcontinent.

EPIDEMIOLOGY: Humans are the natural host for *Shigella*, although other primates may be infected. The primary mode of transmission is the fecal-oral route. Children 5 years of age or younger in child care settings, their caregivers, and other people living in crowded conditions are at increased risk of infection. Travel to resource-poor countries with inadequate sanitation may place the traveler at risk of infection. Transmission requires as few as 10 to 200 organisms for infection to occur. Other modes of transmission include ingestion of contaminated food or water, contact with a contaminated inanimate object, and sexual contact. Houseflies also may be vectors through physical transport of infected feces. *Shigella flexneri, S boydii,* and *S dysenteriae* infections are more common in older children and adults, and these infections often are associated with sources outside the United States. Transmission can occur while the organism is present in feces. Even without antimicrobial therapy, a carrier state usually ceases within 4 weeks of the onset of illness; a chronic carrier state (>1 year) is rare.

The **incubation period** varies from 1 to 7 days but typically is 2 to 4 days.

DIAGNOSTIC TESTS: Cultures of feces or rectal swab specimens containing feces yield the organism. The presence of fecal leukocytes on a methylene-blue stained stool smear is sensitive for a bacterial cause of diarrhea but is not specific for *Shigella* species. An enzyme immunoassay for Shiga toxin may be useful for detection of *S dysenteriae* type 1 in stool. Although bacteremia is rare, blood should be cultured in severely ill, immunocompromised, or malnourished patients. Other testing modalities, including the fluorescent antibody test, polymerase chain reaction assay, and enzyme-linked DNA probes, are being developed and may be available in research laboratories.

TREATMENT:
- Most clinical infections with *Shigella sonnei* are self-limited (48–72 hours) and may not require antimicrobial therapy. However, antimicrobial therapy is effective in shortening the duration of diarrhea and eradicating organisms from feces. Treatment is recommended for patients with severe disease, dysentery, or underlying immunosuppressive conditions. In mild disease, the primary indication for treatment is to prevent spread of the organism.
- Antimicrobial susceptibility testing of clinical isolates is indicated, because resistance to antimicrobial agents is common. Plasmid-mediated resistance has been identified in all *Shigella* species. In the United States, sentinel surveillance data from 1999 to 2000 indicated that 54% of *S sonnei* and 47% of *S flexneri* organisms were resistant to ampicillin and trimethoprim-sulfamethoxazole.

- For susceptible strains, ampicillin and trimethoprim-sulfamethoxazole are effective; amoxicillin is less effective because of its rapid absorption from the gastrointestinal tract. The oral route of therapy is recommended except for seriously ill patients. For cases in which susceptibility is unknown or an ampicillin and trimethoprim-sulfamethoxazole-resistant strain is isolated, parenteral ceftriaxone sodium, a fluoroquinolone (such as ciprofloxacin or ofloxacin), or azithromycin dihydrate may be given. Fluoroquinolones are not recommended for use for people younger than 18 years of age except in circumstances in which potential risks are less than potential benefits (see Antimicrobial Agents and Related Therapy, p 693).
- Antimicrobial therapy typically is administered for 5 days.
- Antidiarrheal compounds that inhibit intestinal peristalsis are contraindicated, because they may prolong the clinical and bacteriologic course of disease.
- Nutritional supplementation, including vitamin A (200 000 IU), can be given to hasten clinical resolution in geographic areas where children are at risk of malnutrition.

ISOLATION OF THE HOSPITALIZED PATIENT: In addition to standard precautions, contact precautions are indicated for the duration of illness.

CONTROL MEASURES:

Child Care. General measures for interrupting enteric transmission in child care centers are recommended (see Children in Out-of-Home Child Care, p 123). Meticulous hand hygiene is the single most important measure to decrease transmission. Eliminating access to shared water-play areas and contaminated diapers also can decrease infection rates.

When *Shigella* infection is identified in a child care attendee or staff member, stool specimens from other symptomatic attendees and staff members should be cultured. Stool specimens from household contacts who have diarrhea also should be cultured. All symptomatic people whose stool specimens test positive for *Shigella* organisms should receive appropriate antimicrobial therapy (see Treatment, p 552) and should not be permitted to reenter the child care facility until the diarrhea has ceased and stool cultures test negative for *Shigella* species. If several people are infected, a cohort system should be considered until stool cultures no longer yield *Shigella* organisms; this system should be combined with hand hygiene and antimicrobial therapy.

General Control Measures. Strict attention to hand hygiene is essential to limit spread. Other important control measures include improved sanitation, a safe water supply through chlorination, proper cooking and storage of food, the exclusion of infected people as food handlers, and measures to decrease contamination of food by house flies. Case reporting to appropriate health authorities (eg, hospital infection control personnel and public health department) is essential.

Immunization. No licensed vaccine is available.

Smallpox (Variola)

In 1980, the World Health Organization declared that smallpox (variola) had been eradicated successfully worldwide. The last naturally occurring case of smallpox occurred in Somalia in 1977, followed by 2 cases attributable to laboratory exposure in 1978. The United States discontinued routine childhood immunization against smallpox in 1971 and routine immunization of health care workers in 1976. The US military continued to immunize military personnel until 1990. Since 1980, the vaccine has been recommended only for people working with nonvariola orthopoxviruses. Two World Health Organization reference laboratories were authorized to maintain stocks of variola virus. There is increasing concern that the virus and the expertise to use it as a weapon of bioterrorism may have been misappropriated. Smallpox is included in this edition of the *Red Book* for the first time since 1977 because of this concern.

CLINICAL MANIFESTATIONS: An individual infected with variola major develops a severe prodromal illness characterized by high fever (102°F–104°F [38.9°C–40.0°C]) and constitutional symptoms, including malaise, severe headache, backache, abdominal pain, and prostration, lasting for 2 to 5 days. Infected children may suffer from vomiting and seizures during this prodromal period. Most patients with smallpox tend to be severely ill and bedridden during the febrile prodrome. The prodromal period is followed by enanthemas (lesions on the mucosa of the mouth or pharynx), which may not be noticed by the patient. This stage occurs less than 24 hours before the onset of rash, which usually is the first recognized manifestation of infectiousness. With the onset of enanthemas, the patient becomes infectious and remains so until all skin crust lesions have separated. The exanthem, or rash, typically begins on the face and rapidly progresses to involve the forearms, trunk, and legs in a centrifugal distribution (greatest concentration of lesions on the face and distal extremities). Many patients will have lesions on the palms and soles. With rash onset, fever decreases, but the patient does not defervesce fully. Lesions begin as maculae that progress to papules, then firm vesicles, and then deep-seated, hard pustules described as "pearls of pus," with each stage lasting 1 to 2 days. By the sixth or seventh day of rash, lesions may begin to umbilicate or become confluent. Lesions increase in size for approximately 8 to 10 days, after which they begin to crust. Once all the lesions have separated, 3 to 4 weeks after the onset of rash, the patient no longer is infectious. Infected people sustain significant scarring after separation of the crusts. Because of the relatively slow and steady evolution of the rash lesions, all lesions on any one part of the body are in the same stage of development.

Varicella (chickenpox) is the condition most likely to be mistaken for smallpox. Generally, children with varicella do not have a febrile prodrome; adults may have a brief, mild prodrome. Although the 2 diseases are confused easily in the first few days of the rash, smallpox lesions develop into pustules that are firm and deeply embedded in the dermis, whereas varicella lesions develop into superficial vesicles. Because varicella erupts in crops of lesions that evolve quickly, lesions on any one part of the body will be in different stages of evolution (papules, vesicles, and crusts). The rash distribution of the 2 diseases differ. Varicella most commonly affects the face and trunk with relative sparing of the extremities, and lesions on the palms or soles are rare.

In addition to the typical presentation of smallpox (≥90% of cases), there are 2 uncommon forms of variola major: hemorrhagic (characterized by hemorrhage into skin lesions and disseminated intravascular coagulation) and malignant or flat type (in which the skin lesions do not progress to the pustular stage but remain flat and soft). Each variant occurred in approximately 5% of cases and was associated with a 95% to 100% mortality rate. Hemorrhagic smallpox rash commonly was confused with meningococcemia. Flat-type (velvety) smallpox occurred more commonly in children. By contrast, variola minor, or alastrim, was associated with fewer lesions, more rapid progression of rash, and a much lower mortality rate (approximately 1%) than variola major, or typical smallpox.

Variola major in unimmunized people was associated with case fatality rates of approximately 30% during epidemics of smallpox. The mortality rate was highest in children younger than 1 year of age and adults older than 30 years of age. The potential for modern supportive therapy in improving outcome is not known. Death was most likely to occur during the second week of illness and was attributed to overwhelming viremia. Secondary bacterial infections occurred but were a less significant cause of mortality.

ETIOLOGY: Variola is a member of the Poxviridae family (genus *Orthopoxvirus*). These DNA viruses are among the largest and most complex viruses known and differ from most other DNA viruses by multiplying in the cytoplasm. Monkeypox, vaccinia, and cowpox are other members of the genus and can cause zoonotic infection of humans, but usually do not spread from person to person. Humans are the only natural reservoir for variola virus (smallpox). Although the original vaccine used by Edward Jenner contained cowpox virus, the current vaccine contains vaccinia virus.

EPIDEMIOLOGY: Smallpox is spread most commonly in droplets from the oropharynx of infected individuals, although infrequent transmission from aerosol and direct contact with infected lesions, clothing, or bedding has been reported. Patients are not infectious during the incubation period or febrile prodrome but become infectious with the onset of mucosal lesions (enanthemas), which occur within hours of the rash. The first week of rash illness is regarded as the most infectious period, although patients remain infectious until all scabs have separated. Because most smallpox patients are extremely ill and bedridden, spread generally is limited to household contacts, hospital workers, and other health care professionals. Secondary household attack rates for smallpox were considerably lower than for measles and similar to or lower than rates for varicella.

The **incubation period** is 7 to 17 days (mean, 12 days).

DIAGNOSTIC TESTS: Variola virus can be detected in vesicular or pustular fluid by culture or by polymerase chain reaction assay. Electron microscopy is able to detect orthopoxvirus infection but cannot distinguish between viruses. Variola diagnostic testing is conducted only at the Centers for Disease Control and Prevention (CDC) but may be expanded in the future. If a patient is suspected of having smallpox, standard, contact, and airborne precautions should be implemented immediately, and the state (and/or local) health department should be alerted at once. Reports of patients classified by the CDC as at high risk of having smallpox will trigger a rapid response with a team deployed to obtain specimens and advise on clinical management.

TREATMENT: There is no known effective antiviral therapy available to treat smallpox. Infected patients should receive supportive care. Cidofovir, currently licensed for cytomegalovirus retinitis, has been suggested as having a role in smallpox therapy, but data to support its use in smallpox are not available. The drug must be given intravenously and is associated with significant renal toxicity. Vaccinia Immune Globulin (VIG) is reserved for certain complications of immunization and has no role in treatment of smallpox.

ISOLATION OF THE HOSPITALIZED PATIENT: Standard, contact, and airborne precautions are essential for any patient suspected of having smallpox. On admission, hospital infection control personnel should be notified, and the patient should be placed in a private, airborne infection isolation room equipped with negative pressure ventilation with high-efficiency particulate air filtration. Anyone entering the room must wear an N95 or higher quality respirator, gloves, and gown, even if there is a history of recent successful immunization. If the patient leaves the room, he or she should wear a mask and be covered with sheets or gowns to decrease the risk of fomite transmission. Rooms vacated by patients should be decontaminated using standard hospital disinfectants, such as sodium hypochlorite or quaternary ammonia solutions. Laundry and waste should be discarded into biohazard bags and autoclaved, and bedding and clothing should be laundered in hot water with laundry detergent followed by hot air drying or incinerated.

CONTROL MEASURES

Care of Exposed People

Cases of febrile rash illness, for which smallpox is considered in the differential diagnosis, should be reported immediately to local or state health departments. After evaluation by the state or local health department, if smallpox laboratory diagnostics are considered necessary, the CDC Rash Illness Evaluation Team should be consulted at 770-488-7100. Laboratory confirmation of smallpox is available only at CDC.

Use of vaccine. Postexposure immunization (within 3–4 days of exposure) provides some protection against disease and significant protection against a fatal outcome. Any person with a significant exposure to a patient with proven smallpox during the infectious stage of illness requires immunization as soon after exposure as possible, but within 4 days of first exposure. Because infected individuals are not contagious until the rash (and/or enanthema) appears, individuals exposed only during the prodromal period are not at risk.

Vaccinia Immune Globulin. Vaccinia Immune Globulin prepared from plasma of immunized individuals was used in the past to prevent or modify smallpox when administered within 24 hours of a known exposure. Current supplies of VIG are used in the treatment of complications of smallpox immunization. The CDC is the only source of VIG in the United States. Supplies may be obtained by calling the CDC Smallpox Vaccine Adverse Events Clinical Information Line at 877-554-4625 for physicians in civilian medical facilities.

Preexposure Immunization of Adults.

Smallpox vaccine.[*] The only smallpox vaccine licensed in the United States is a lyophilized, live vaccinia virus preparation. The vaccine does not contain variola virus but contains a related virus called vaccinia virus, distinct from the cowpox virus initially used for vaccination by Jenner. Vaccinia vaccine is highly effective in preventing smallpox, with protection waning after 5 to 10 years after 1 dose; protection after reimmunization has lasted longer. However, substantial protection against death from smallpox persisted in the past for more than 30 years after immunization during infancy on the basis of experience at a time of worldwide smallpox virus circulation and routine smallpox immunization practices. A smallpox immunization plan has been implemented in the United States (www.bt.cdc.gov). The plan does not include immunization of children.[†] However, children may be at risk of vaccine complications as contacts of vaccinees. The federal government has contracted for production and purchase of newly developed tissue cell culture vaccine. Blood donation should be deferred for 21 days after immunization or until the scab has separated. Tuberculin skin testing should be deferred for 1 month after immunization.

Administration. Vaccine is administered using a bifurcated needle to deliver vaccine into the epidermis. Vaccine is held by capillarity between the 2 tines of the needle. Vaccine "take" is determined by the cutaneous reaction to the immunization: a papule should be evident at the immunization site at 3 to 5 days, progressing to a vesicle at 5 to 8 days then a pustule reaching maximum size in 8 to 10 days. The lesion scabs and heals after 14 to 21 days, leaving a scar. There may be associated swelling and tenderness of regional lymph nodes. Satellite lesions at the perimeter of the immunization site may occur. People occupationally exposed to vaccinia virus (the virus in the vaccine), recombinant vaccinia viruses, or other nonvariola orthopoxviruses should be immunized every 10 years.

Adverse events. Fever is common after immunization (as many as 70% of children) and less common after reimmunization (35%). Inadvertent inoculation of vaccinia virus by contact from the site of immunization to the face, eyes, or other sites is the most common serious complication of immunization. Other serious complications include erythema multiforme, postvaccinal encephalitis and encephalopathy, progressive vaccinia (vaccinia gangrenosa), eczema vaccinatum, generalized vaccinia, and fatal vaccinia. These complications are rare, but infants are at higher risk of complication from immunization than older children and adults. For this reason, smallpox immunization was delayed until after 1 year of age in the United States. Vaccinia Immune Globulin is recommended to treat patients with some of these complications. Cidofovir (available for use through an investigational new drug [IND] application from the CDC) also may be considered. Transmission of vaccinia virus from a recently immunized individual to a susceptible contact, including children, can occur. Vaccinia virus can be contained by keeping the immunization site covered with a semipermeable dressing over an absorbent material (eg, gauze) and changing the dressing frequently.

---

[*] Centers for Disease Control and Prevention. Recommendations for using smallpox vaccine in a pre-event vaccination program. *MMWR Dispatch.* 2003;52(Dispatch):1–16

[†] American Academy of Pediatrics, Committee on Infectious Diseases. Policy statement: smallpox vaccine. *Pediatrics.* 2002;110:841–845. Available at: http://aappolicy.aapjournals.org/cgi/content/full/pediatrics;110/4/841

Smallpox vaccine is not recommended for people younger than 18 years of age. In the event of a hostile release of smallpox virus, recommendations will be forthcoming from public health authorities.

Precautions and Contraindications*: In the absence of intentional release of smallpox virus, smallpox vaccine should not be administered to (1) people who have a history of or currently have atopic dermatitis (eczema); (2) people who have other active acute, chronic, or exfoliative skin conditions that disrupt the dermis; (3) pregnant women or women who desire to become pregnant in the 28 days after immunization; and (4) people who are immunocompromised as a result of human immunodeficiency virus, autoimmune conditions, cancer, radiation treatment, immunosuppressive medications, primary immunodeficiencies, or other immunodeficiencies. Other contraindications that apply only to immunization candidates but do not include close contacts of people who are immunized are people with vaccine component allergies, women who are breastfeeding, people using topical ocular steroids, people with moderate-to-severe illness, and people younger than 18 years of age. Current information for clinicians on all aspects of smallpox and smallpox vaccine is available at www.bt.cdc.gov. In the event of an outbreak of smallpox, outbreak-specific guidelines will be disseminated by the CDC.

Sporotrichosis

CLINICAL MANIFESTATIONS: Sporotrichosis manifests most commonly as cutaneous infection, although pulmonary and disseminated forms occur. Inoculation occurs at a site of minor trauma, causing an ulcerative subcutaneous nodule that is firm and slightly tender but often painless. Secondary lesions can spread along lymphatic channels to form multiple nodules that ulcerate and suppurate. The extremities and face are the most common sites of infection in children.

Extracutaneous sporotrichosis commonly affects bones and joints, particularly those of the hands, elbows, ankles, or knees, but any organ can be affected. Disseminated disease generally occurs after hematogenous spread from primary skin or lung infection. Disseminated sporotrichosis may involve multiple foci (eg, eyes, genitourinary system, or central nervous system) and occurs predominantly in immunocompromised patients. Pulmonary sporotrichosis clinically resembles tuberculosis and occurs after inhalation or aspiration of aerosolized spores. Pulmonary and disseminated sporotrichosis are uncommon in children.

ETIOLOGY: *Sporothrix schenckii* is a dimorphic fungus that grows as an oval or cigar-shaped yeast at 37°C (98°F).

EPIDEMIOLOGY: *Sporothrix schenckii* is a ubiquitous organism that has worldwide distribution but is most common in tropical and subtropical regions of Central and South America and parts of North America. The fungus is isolated from soil and plants, including hay, straw, thorny plants (especially roses), sphagnum moss, and decaying vegetation. Cutaneous disease occurs from inoculation of debris con-

---

* Centers for Disease Control and Prevention. Smallpox vaccination and adverse events. *MMWR Dispatch.* 2003;52:1–29.

taining the organism. People engaging in gardening or farming are at risk of infection. Inhalation of spores can lead to pulmonary disease. Rarely, transmission from infected cats has led to cutaneous disease.

The **incubation period** is 7 to 30 days after cutaneous inoculation but may be as long as 3 months.

DIAGNOSTIC TESTS: Culture of *S schenckii* from a tissue, wound drainage, or sputum specimen is diagnostic of infection. Culture of *S schenckii* from a blood specimen suggests the multifocal form of infection associated with immunodeficiency. Histopathologic examination of tissue can be helpful but requires special fungal stains to visualize the organism. Although reference laboratories (eg, Centers for Disease Control and Prevention) offer a latex agglutination assay, no standardized serologic test is available.

TREATMENT: Lymphocutaneous sporotrichosis usually does not resolve without treatment. Itraconazole is the drug of choice for cutaneous and lymphocutaneous disease in adults. Although there are no controlled trials to document the efficacy of itraconazole in pediatric patients, most experts now consider itraconazole the preferred treatment for children (see Recommended Doses of Parenteral and Oral Antifungal Drugs, p 722). The duration of therapy is 3 to 6 months. Oral fluconazole is less effective. The time-honored treatment for sporotrichosis, a saturated solution of potassium iodide, is much less costly and still is recommended as an alternative treatment. Saturated solution of potassium iodide is given orally until several weeks after all lesions are healed. Itraconazole is the treatment of choice for osteoarticular infection, because this form of sporotrichosis rarely is accompanied by systemic illness. Amphotericin B and itraconazole are treatment options for pulmonary infections, depending on severity. Amphotericin B is the drug of choice for disseminated sporotrichosis and infection in children with immunodeficiency, including human immunodeficiency virus (HIV) infection. Itraconazole may be required for lifelong maintenance therapy after initial treatment with amphotericin B in children with HIV infection. Pulmonary and disseminated infection respond less well than cutaneous infection, despite prolonged therapy. Surgical débridement or excision may be necessary to achieve resolution of cavitary pulmonary disease.

ISOLATION OF HOSPITALIZED PATIENTS: Standard precautions are indicated.

CONTROL MEASURES: Use of protective gloves and clothing in occupational and avocational activities associated with infection can decrease risk of disease.

Staphylococcal Food Poisoning

CLINICAL MANIFESTATIONS: Staphylococcal food poisoning is characterized by the abrupt and sometimes violent onset of severe nausea, abdominal cramps, vomiting, and prostration, often accompanied by diarrhea. Low-grade fever or subnormal temperature can occur. The duration of illness typically is 1 to 2 days, but the intensity of symptoms may require hospitalization. The short incubation period, brevity of illness, and usual lack of fever help distinguish staphylococcal from other types of food poisoning except that caused by *Bacillus cereus*. Chemical food poisoning usually has an even shorter incubation period. *Clostridium perfringens* food poisoning usually has a longer incubation period and rarely is accompanied by vomiting. Patients with foodborne *Salmonella* or *Shigella* infection usually have fever and a longer incubation period (see Appendix VI, Clinical Syndromes Associated With Foodborne Diseases, p 810).

ETIOLOGY: Enterotoxins produced by strains of *Staphylococcus aureus* and, rarely, *Staphylococcus epidermidis*, elicit the symptoms of staphylococcal food poisoning. Of the 8 immunologically distinct heat-stable enterotoxins (A, B, C1–3, D, E, and F), enterotoxin A is the most commonly identified cause of staphylococcal food poisoning outbreaks in the United States.

EPIDEMIOLOGY: Illness is caused by ingestion of food containing staphylococcal enterotoxins. Foods usually involved are those that come in contact with food handlers' hands without subsequent cooking or with inadequate heating or refrigeration, such as pastries, custards, salad dressings, sandwiches, poultry, sliced meats, and meat products. When these foods remain at room temperature for several hours before being eaten, toxin-producing staphylococci multiply and elaborate heat-stable toxin. The organisms may be of human origin from purulent discharges of an infected finger or eye, abscesses, acneiform facial eruptions, nasopharyngeal secretions, or apparently normal skin or, less commonly, of bovine origin, such as contaminated milk or milk products, especially cheese.

The **incubation period** ranges from 30 minutes to 8 hours, usually 2 to 4 hours.

DIAGNOSTIC TESTS: Recovery of large numbers of staphylococci or enterotoxin from stool or vomitus supports the diagnosis. In an outbreak setting, demonstration of enterotoxin or a large number of staphylococci ($>10^5$ colony-forming units/g of specimen) in epidemiologically implicated food confirms the diagnosis. Identification (by pulsed-field gel electrophoresis or phage type) of the same types of *S aureus* from stool or vomitus of 2 or more ill people or from stool or vomitus of an ill person and an implicated food or a person who handled the food also confirms the diagnosis. Local health authorities should be notified to help determine the source of the outbreak.

TREATMENT: Antimicrobial agents are not indicated. Treatment is supportive.

ISOLATION OF THE HOSPITALIZED PATIENT: Standard precautions are recommended.

CONTROL MEASURES: Prompt consumption or immediate cooling or refrigeration of cooked or baked foods will help to prevent the disease. Cooked foods should be refrigerated at temperatures less than 5°C (41°F). People with boils, abscesses, and other purulent lesions of the hands, face, or nose should be excluded temporarily from handling food. Hand hygiene before food handling should be enforced.

Staphylococcal Infections

CLINICAL MANIFESTATIONS: *Staphylococcus aureus* causes a variety of localized or invasive suppurative infections and 3 toxin-mediated syndromes: toxic shock syndrome (see Toxic Shock Syndrome, p 624), scalded skin syndrome, and food poisoning (see Staphylococcal Food Poisoning, p 559). Localized infections include hordeola, furuncles, carbuncles, impetigo (bullous and nonbullous), paronychia, ecthyma, cellulitis, parotitis, lymphadenitis, and wound infections. *Staphylococcus aureus* also causes foreign body infections, including infections associated with intravascular catheters or grafts, pacemakers, peritoneal catheters, cerebrospinal fluid shunts, and prosthetic joints, which may be associated with bacteremia. Bacteremia can be complicated by septicemia, endocarditis, pericarditis, pneumonia, pleural empyema, muscle or visceral abscesses, arthritis, osteomyelitis, septic thrombophlebitis of large vessels, and other foci of infection. Meningitis is rare. *Staphylococcus aureus* infections can be fulminant and commonly are associated with metastatic foci, abscess formation, and foreign bodies. These infections often require prolonged antimicrobial therapy, abscess drainage, and foreign body removal to achieve cure. Risk factors for severe staphylococcal infections include chronic diseases, such as diabetes mellitus, cirrhosis of the liver, and nutritional disorders; surgery; transplantation; disorders of neutrophil function; and acquired immunodeficiency syndrome.

Staphylococcal scalded skin syndrome (SSSS) is an *S aureus* toxin-mediated disease caused by circulation of exfoliative toxins A and B. The manifestations of SSSS are age-related and include Ritter disease (generalized exfoliation) in the neonate, a tender scarlatiniform eruption and localized bullous impetigo in older children, and a combination of these with thick white/brown flaky desquamation of the entire skin, especially on the face and neck, in older infants and toddlers. The hallmark of SSSS is the toxin-mediated cleavage of the stratum granulosum layer of the epidermis. Healing is without scarring. Bacteremia is rare, but dehydration and superinfections may occur with extensive exfoliation.

Coagulase-Negative Staphylococci: Most coagulase-negative staphylococci (CoNS) isolates represent contamination of culture material (see Diagnostic Tests, p 565). Of the isolates that do not represent contamination, most come from infections that are nosocomial, and most patients with CoNS infections have obvious disruptions of host defenses caused by surgery, catheter or prosthesis insertion, or immunosuppression. Coagulase-negative staphylococci are the most common cause of late-onset septicemia among premature infants, especially infants weighing less than 1500 g at birth and of episodes of nosocomial bacteremia in all age groups. Coagulase-negative staphylococci are responsible for bacteremia in children undergoing treatment for leukemia, lymphoma, or solid tumors as well as in bone marrow transplant recipients. Infections often are associated with intravascular catheters, cerebrospinal fluid shunts, peritoneal or urinary catheters, vascular grafts or intracardiac patches, prosthetic cardiac valves, pacemaker wires, or prosthetic joints. Mediastinitis after open-heart surgery, endophthalmitis after intraocular trauma, and omphalitis and scalp abscesses in neonates have been described. Coagulase-negative staphylococci also may enter the bloodstream from the respiratory tract of mechanically ventilated premature infants or from the gastrointestinal tract of infants with necrotizing enterocolitis. Some species of CoNS are associated with urinary tract infection, including *Staphylococcus saprophyticus* in adolescent girls and young adult women, often after sexual intercourse, and *Staphylococcus epidermidis* and *Staphylococcus haemolyticus* in hospitalized patients with urinary catheters. In general, CoNS infections have an indolent clinical manifestation.

ETIOLOGY: Staphylococci are catalase-positive, gram-positive cocci that appear microscopically as grape-like clusters. There are 32 species that are related closely on the basis of DNA base composition but only 17 species are indigenous to humans. *Staphylococcus aureus* is the only species that produces coagulase. Of the 16 coagulase-negative species, *S epidermidis, S haemolyticus, S saprophyticus, Staphylococcus schleiferi*, and *Staphylococcus lugdunensis* most often are associated with infections. Staphylococci are ubiquitous and can survive extreme conditions of drying, heat, and low-oxygen and high-salt environments. *Staphylococcus aureus* has many surface proteins, including the MSCRAMM (microbial surface components recognizing adhesive matrix molecule) receptors that allow the organism to bind to tissues and foreign bodies coated with fibronectin, fibrinogen, and collagen, permitting a low inoculum of organisms to adhere to sutures, catheters, prosthetic valves, and other devices. Coagulase-negative staphylococci produce an exopolysaccharide slime biofilm that makes these organisms, as they bind to medical devices (eg, catheters), relatively inaccessible to host defenses and to antimicrobial agents.

EPIDEMIOLOGY:

Staphylococcus aureus. *Staphylococcus aureus,* which is second only to coagulase-negative staphylococci as a cause of nosocomial bacteremia, is equal to *Pseudomonas aeruginosa* as the most common cause of nosocomial pneumonia and is responsible for most nosocomial surgical site infections. *Staphylococcus aureus* colonizes the skin and mucous membranes of 30% to 50% of healthy adults and children. The anterior nares, throat (infants and young children), axilla, perineum, vagina, or rectum are the usual sites of colonization. The anterior nares are colonized most densely, and colonization may persist for years in 10% to 20% of affected people. From 25% to 50% of nasal carriers transiently carry the organism on their hands and other skin areas. Rates of carriage of more than 50% occur in children with desquamating skin disorders or burns and in people with frequent needle use (eg, diabetes mellitus, hemodialysis, recreational drug use, allergy shots).

Transmission of S aureus *in Hospitals. Staphylococcus aureus* is transmitted most often by direct contact. Health care professionals can have colonization of *S aureus* in the nares or on the skin and can serve as an important reservoir for transmission of *S aureus* to patients. Health care professionals also can acquire transient hand colonization while caring for one patient and then transmit the organism to another patient. Infants colonized shortly after birth can serve as a reservoir for transmission to other infants. The role of clothing, gowns, environmental surfaces, and other fomites in the transmission of *S aureus* is unclear. Transmission by droplets may occur when patients have draining wounds, burns, or areas of dermatitis that are colonized or infected. Changing dressings or linens can cause these organisms to become droplet nuclei (ie, leading to airborne transmission). Dissemination of *S aureus* from people, including infants, with nasal carriage is related to density of colonization, and increased dissemination occurs during viral upper respiratory tract infections. Additional risk factors for nosocomial acquisition of *S aureus* include location on a high-risk ward, such as a newborn nursery or intensive care or burn unit; surgical procedures; prolonged hospitalization; an epidemic strain of *S aureus* in the hospital; and the presence of indwelling vascular catheters or prosthetic devices. Previous antimicrobial therapy increases the risk of acquiring an antimicrobial-resistant strain.

Staphylococcus aureus *Colonization and Disease*. Nasal and skin carriage are the primary reservoirs for *S aureus*. Adults who carry *S aureus* in the nose preoperatively are more likely to develop surgical site infections after general, cardiac, orthopedic, or solid organ transplant surgery than patients who are not carriers. Heavy cutaneous colonization at the insertion site is the single most important predictor of catheter-related infections for short-term percutaneously inserted catheters. For patients with *S aureus* skin colonization who receive hemodialysis, the incidence of vascular-access bacteremia is sixfold higher than for patients without skin colonization. After head trauma, adult nasal carriers of *S aureus* are more likely to develop *S aureus* pneumonia than are noncolonized patients.

Nosocomial Methicillin-Resistant S aureus. Methicillin-resistant *S aureus* (MRSA) accounts for 40% of nosocomial *S aureus* infections in hospitals with 500 or more beds. Methicillin-resistant *S aureus* strains of nosocomial origin usually are resistant to all β-lactamase resistant (BLR) β-lactam and cephalosporin antimicrobial agents as well as to antimicrobial agents of several other classes (multidrug resistance). Methicillin-susceptible *S aureus* (MSSA) strains can be heterogeneous for methicillin resistance (see Diagnostic Tests, p 565). These heterogeneous or heterotypic strains appear susceptible by disk testing. However, when a parent strain is cultured on methicillin-containing media, resistant subpopulations are apparent. When these resistant subpopulations are cultured on methicillin-free media, they may continue as stable resistant mutants or revert to susceptible strains *(heterogeneous resistance)*. When β-lactamase-resistant antimicrobial agents are used to treat infections caused by these heterotypic strains, the MSSA organisms are killed; MRSA organisms are selected and continue to grow.

Risk factors for nasal carriage of nosocomial MRSA include hospitalization within the previous year, recent (within the previous 60 days) antimicrobial use, prolonged hospital stay, frequent contact with a health care environment, presence of an intravascular catheter or tracheal tube, increased number of surgical procedures, or frequent contact with an individual with one or more of the preceding risk factors. After discharge from a hospital, a patient known to have had colonization of MRSA should be assumed to have continued colonization when rehospitalized, because carriage can persist for years.

Epidemic Strains of MRSA. Most nosocomial MRSA infections result from the patient's own organism or from endemic strains transmitted to the patient by the hands of health care professionals. On occasion, an epidemic strain of MRSA will be introduced into a community or a hospital environment where it spreads rapidly despite measures that contain the spread of nonepidemic strains. Identification of these epidemic MRSA strains using pulsed-field gel electrophoresis is important, because containment of epidemic MRSA strains requires strict adherence to and enhancement of infection control policies.

Methicillin-resistant *S aureus* and methicillin-resistant coagulase-negative staphylococci are responsible for a large portion of nosocomial infections. These strains are particularly difficult to treat, because they usually are multidrug resistant and predictably susceptible only to vancomycin hydrochloride.

Community-Acquired MRSA. Unique clones of MRSA increasingly are responsible for community-acquired infections in healthy children and adults without typical risk factors for health care-associated strains of MRSA. The antimicrobial susceptibility patterns of these strains are unique, because they are resistant to methicillin sodium and oxacillin sodium but are not multidrug resistant (uniform susceptibility to trimethoprim-sulfamethoxazole and gentamicin sulfate). These community-acquired MRSA strains have been isolated from people without risk factors from several cities, from child care centers, and from people in other countries.

Vancomycin-Intermediately Susceptible S aureus. Strains of MRSA with intermediate susceptibility to vancomycin (minimum inhibitory concentration [MIC], >4 µg/mL and ≤16 µg/mL) were isolated from 48 adults in the United States from 1996 to 2001. Each person had received multiple courses of vancomycin for a MRSA infection. Strains of MRSA can be heterogeneous for vancomycin resistance similar to MRSA and methicillin resistance (see Diagnostic Tests, p 565). Extensive vancomycin use allows the vancomycin-intermediately susceptible *S aureus* (VISA) strains to grow. Rapid and aggressive control measures have focused on containing VISA strains to prevent spread. Recommended measures from the Centers for Disease Control and Prevention (CDC) have included rapid diagnostic tests to detect VISA, confirmatory testing of isolated strains, measures to restrict vancomycin use, and strict infection control measures for the infected patient and the institution. Although rare, outbreaks of MRSA with decreased susceptibility to vancomycin and heteroresistance have been reported in France, Spain, and Japan. Communicability persists as long as lesions or the carrier state are present.

Vancomycin-Resistant S aureus. In 2002, 2 isolates of vancomycin-resistant *S aureus* (VRSA; minimum inhibitory concentration, ≥32 µg/mL) were identified in adults, 1 from each of 2 states. The guidelines for detecting these organisms and preventing spread are similar to those recommended for VISA. Guidelines from the CDC for preventing spread of VRSA are available at www.cdc.gov/ncidod/hip/10_20.pdf.

Coagulase-Negative Staphylococci. Coagulase-negative staphylococci are common inhabitants of the skin and mucous membranes. Virtually all infants have colonization at multiple sites by 2 to 4 days of age. Different species colonize specific areas of the body. *Staphylococcus epidermidis* is found most often, and *S haemolyticus* is found on areas of skin with numerous apocrine glands. The frequency of nosocomial CoNS infections has increased steadily during the past 2 decades. Infants and children in intensive care units, including intensive care nurseries, have the highest incidence of CoNS bloodstream infections. Coagulase-negative staphylococci colonizing the skin can be introduced at the time of medical device placement, through mucous membrane or skin breaks, or during catheter manipulation. Less often, health care professionals with environmental CoNS colonization on the hands transmit the organism. The roles of the environment or fomites in CoNS transmission are not known.

Methicillin-Resistant CoNS. Methicillin-resistant CoNS account for most nosocomial CoNS infections. Most methicillin-susceptible strains have heterogeneous resistance to methicillin, as described previously for MSSA. Methicillin-resistant strains are resistant to all β-lactam drugs, including cephalosporins, and usually several other drug classes. As for MRSA, once these strains become endemic in a hospital, eradication is difficult if not impossible, even when strict infection control techniques are followed.

Vancomycin-Intermediately Susceptible CoNS. Methicillin-resistant CoNS may be heterogeneous for vancomycin resistance, as described previously for MRSA. Use of vancomycin to treat methicillin-resistant CoNS infections selects for the emergence of strains with intermediate susceptibility to vancomycin. Although uncommon, infections caused by these strains are becoming more common. Among these, infections caused by *S hemolyticus* are most resistant. To prevent or delay development of resistance, the CDC has published recommendations for the prudent use of vancomycin (see Appropriate Use of Antimicrobial Agents, p 695).

For toxin-mediated scalded skin syndrome, the **incubation period** usually is 1 to 10 days. For other staphylococcal infections, the incubation period is variable. A long delay can occur between acquisition of the organism and onset of disease.

DIAGNOSTIC TESTS: Gram-stained smears of material from lesions can provide presumptive evidence of infection. Isolation of organisms from culture of an otherwise sterile body fluid is definitive. *Staphylococcus aureus* almost never is a contaminant when isolated from a blood culture. Isolation of CoNS from a blood culture commonly is dismissed as "a contaminant." In a neonate, an immunocompromised person, or a patient with a prosthetic implant, repeated isolation of the same phenotypic strain of CoNS (on the basis of antimicrobial susceptibility testing) from blood cultures suggests true infection, and genotyping more strongly supports an infection. For catheter-related bacteremia, quantitative cultures from the catheter will have 5 to 10 times more organisms than cultures from a peripheral blood vessel. Criteria that may suggest CoNS is a pathogen rather than a contaminant include the following: (1) growth within 24 hours; (2) multiple positive blood cultures; (3) identical antimicrobial susceptibility patterns for all isolates; (4) clinical findings of infection in the patient; (5) an intravascular catheter that has been in place for 3 days or more; and (6) multidrug resistance of the CoNS strain or similar or identical genotypes among isolates.

Quantitative antimicrobial susceptibility testing should be performed for all staphylococci, including CoNS, isolated from normally sterile sites. Some community-acquired *S aureus* strains will be methicillin resistant, and most hospital-acquired *S aureus* and more than 90% of hospital-acquired CoNS will be methicillin and multidrug resistant. All *S aureus* strains with an MIC to vancomycin of ≥4 g/mL should be confirmed and further characterized. Detection of VISA is critical (see Table 3.54, p 566).

Staphylococci have several mechanisms mediating resistance to the β-lactam antimicrobial agents. β-Lactamase enzymes break down the nonsemisynthetic penicillins. Resistance to the β-lactamase–resistant (BLR) semisynthetic penicillins is mediated by a novel cell wall penicillin-binding protein called PBP2a or PBP2′, which has decreased affinity for BLR β-lactam antimicrobial agents and is coded

Table 3.54. **Recommendations for Detecting and Preventing the Spread of** *Staphylococcus aureus* **With Decreased Susceptibility to Vancomycin**[1]

Strategies for selection of strains for additional testing:
- Select isolates with vancomycin MICs of ≥4 µg/mL. This is based on the apparent heterogeneity of strains, because organisms with MICs of ≥4 µg/mL have subpopulations with higher MICs. Clinical treatment failures have occurred with vancomycin in infections with these isolates.
- Select isolates with vancomycin MICs of ≥8 µg/mL (based on National Committee for Clinical Laboratory Standards breakpoints[2]).
- Select all methicillin-resistant *Staphylococcus aureus* (MRSA). All identified isolates of *S aureus* with decreased susceptibility to vancomycin have been MRSA.
- Select all *S aureus* isolates. Because little is known about the extent of this resistance, any *S aureus* potentially could have decreased susceptibility to vancomycin.

Testing and confirmation:
- Primary testing of *S aureus* against vancomycin requires 24 hours of incubation time.
- Disk diffusion is not an acceptable method for vancomycin susceptibility testing of *S aureus*. None of the known VISA strains have been or would be detected by this method.
- An MIC susceptibility testing method should be used to confirm vancomycin test results.

Infection control:
To minimize spread and prevent development of an endemic strain:
- Isolate patient in a private room and begin one-on-one care by specified personnel using contact precautions including masks.
- Initiate epidemiologic and laboratory investigations with assistance of state health departments and CDC.
- Educate health care professionals about epidemiologic implications and necessary infection control procedures.
- Monitor and strictly enforce compliance with contact precautions and other measures.
- Perform baseline cultures of hands and nares of:
  - Those with recent direct contact with patients with VISA
  - Health care professionals for patients with VISA
  - Roommates of patients with VISA
- Assess efficacy of precautions by monitoring personnel for acquisition of VISA.
- Consult with state health department and CDC before discharging and/or transferring the patient, and notify receiving institution or unit of presence of VISA and of appropriate precautions.[3]

MIC indicates minimum inhibitory concentration; VISA, vancomycin-intermediately susceptible *S aureus*; CDC, Centers for Disease Control and Prevention.

[1] Centers for Disease Control and Prevention. Laboratory capacity to detect antimicrobial resistance, 1998. *MMWR Morb Mortal Wkly Rep.* 2000;48:1167–1171.

[2] MIC breakpoints for vancomycin are as follows: susceptible, ≤4 µg/mL; intermediate, 8–16 µg/mL; and resistant, ≥32 µg/mL.

[3] For information regarding control of spread of VISA and vancomycin-resistant *S aureus*, e-mail SEARCH@cdc.gov or visit www.cdc.gov/ncidod/hip/default.htm.

for by the gene *mecA*. Clinical isolates of CoNS and of *S aureus* carrying the *mecA* gene vary widely in their resistance to methicillin (methicillin MICs of ≤4 µg/mL to ≥1000 µg/mL) in regard to the number of organisms of different susceptibilities and on the basis of culture conditions. This phenomenon is known as heterogeneous resistance. Strains of CoNS and *S aureus* with heterogeneous resistance are stable in the absence of selective pressure by certain antimicrobial agents. These strains may constitute 10% to 15% of CoNS or *S aureus* isolates.

The MIC breakpoints for CoNS or *S aureus* for methicillin are based on the presence of the *mecA* gene and, therefore, the potential for the organism to develop methicillin resistance. The presence of the gene, however, does not predict an accurate measure of gene expression (ie, susceptibility or resistance).

The mechanism for intermediate resistance of *S aureus* or CoNS to vancomycin is unknown. *Staphylococcus aureus* and CoNS strains with intermediate resistance to vancomycin have thickened and irregular cell walls, slow growth rates, and altered autolysis. Vancomycin resistance may be related to an increased number of cell wall vancomycin-binding sites, which prevent access to the cytoplasmic membrane.

Staphylococcus aureus and CoNS strain genotyping has become a necessary adjunct for determining whether several isolates from one patient or from different patients are the same. Typing may facilitate identification of the source, extent, and mechanism of transmission of an outbreak. Antimicrobial susceptibility testing is the most readily available method for typing by a phenotypic characteristic. Multilocus enzyme electrophoresis is another phenotypic tool for use, but pulsed-field gel electrophoresis typing by genotype has proven to be more discriminatory for identifying related isolates.

TREATMENT: Serious staphylococcal infections require intravenous therapy with a BLR β-lactam antimicrobial agent, such as nafcillin or oxacillin, because most *S aureus* strains in the community or in hospitals produce β-lactamase enzymes and are resistant to penicillin and ampicillin (see Table 3.55, p 568). The β-lactam/β-lactamase inhibitor combination ampicillin-sulbactam sodium is considered by some experts to be useful for treatment once antimicrobial susceptibility results are available. First- or second-generation cephalosporins (eg, cefazolin sodium or cefuroxime), vancomycin, and clindamycin are effective but less so than BLR β-lactam penicillins. The expanded-spectrum cephalosporins are not as active in vitro against MSSA or CoNS, and some may be ineffective in vivo. A parenteral formulation of nafcillin or oxacillin rather than vancomycin is recommended for treatment of MSSA infections to minimize the emergence of vancomycin-resistant strains. Patients who are allergic to penicillin can be treated with a first- or second-generation cephalosporin (if the patient is not also allergic to cephalosporins), clindamycin, or vancomycin.

For nosocomially acquired staphylococcal strains resistant to BLR β-lactam antimicrobial agents (eg, MRSA and methicillin-resistant CoNS), intravenous vancomycin is recommended for treatment of serious infections. For empiric therapy of serious or life-threatening suspected community-acquired MRSA infections, initial therapy should include vancomycin and a BLR β-lactam antimicrobial (eg, nafcillin or oxacillin). Subsequent therapy should be determined by antimicrobial susceptibility results. Clindamycin penetrates all tissues well except cerebrospinal

Table 3.55. **Parenteral Antimicrobial(s) for Treatment of Bacteremia and Other Serious *Staphylococcus aureus* Infections**

Susceptibility	Antimicrobial Agent	Comments
I. Initial empiric therapy (organism of unknown susceptibility) Drugs of choice:	• Vancomycin + nafcillin or oxacillin ± gentamicin	For life-threatening infections (ie, septicemia, endocarditis, osteomyelitis, pyarthrosis, pneumonia, meningitis); ampicillin-sulbactam could be added if the patient has received several recent courses of vancomycin
	• Nafcillin or oxacillin[1]	For non–life-threatening infection without signs of sepsis (eg, skin infection, cellulitis, osteomyelitis, pyarthrosis) when rates of MRSA colonization and infection in the community are low
	• Clindamycin	For non–life-threatening infection without signs of sepsis when rates of MRSA colonization and infection in the community are substantial
	• Vancomycin	For non–life-threatening, hospital-acquired infections
II. Methicillin-susceptible, penicillin-resistant *S aureus* (MSSA) Drugs of choice:	• Nafcillin or oxacillin[1,2]	…
	• Cefazolin[1]	…
Alternatives:	• Clindamycin	…
	• Vancomycin	Only for penicillin- and cephalosporin-allergic patients
	• Ampicillin + sulbactam	…
III. Methicillin-resistant *S aureus* (MRSA) (oxacillin MIC ≥4 µg/mL) A. Nosocomial (multidrug-resistant) Drugs of choice:	• Vancomycin ± gentamicin (or) ± rifampin[2]	…

Alternatives: susceptibility testing results available before alternative drugs are used

- Trimethoprim-sulfamethoxazole[3] ...
- Linezolid[3] ...
- Quinupristin-dalfopristin[3] ...
- Fluoroquinolones — Not recommended for people younger than 18 years of age or as monotherapy

B. Community (not multidrug-resistant)
Drugs of choice:

- Trimethoprim-sulfamethoxazole or clindamycin (if strain susceptible) ...

Alternatives:

- Vancomycin[2] ...

IV. Vancomycin-intermediate *S aureus* (minimum inhibitory concentration >4 µg/mL and ≤16 µg/mL)[2]
Drugs of choice:

- Optimal therapy is not known ...
- Linezolid[3] ...
- Quinupristin-dalfopristin[3] ...
- Vancomycin + ampicillin-sulbactam ± gentamicin ...

Alternatives:

- Vancomycin + trimethoprim-sulfamethoxazole[2] ...

---

[1] Penicillin and cephalosporin-allergic patients always should receive vancomycin as initial therapy for serious infections.

[2] One of the adjunctive agents, gentamicin or rifampin, should be added to the therapeutic regimen for life-threatening infections such as endocarditis or meningitis or infections with a vancomycin-intermediate *S aureus* strain. Consultation with an infectious diseases specialist should be considered to determine which agent to use and the duration of use.

[3] Linezolid and quinupristin-dalfopristin are 2 agents with activity in vitro and efficacy in adults with multidrug-resistant, gram-positive organisms, including *S aureus*. Because experience with these agents in children is limited, consultation with an infectious diseases specialist should be considered before use.

fluid and probably is comparable to vancomycin in efficacy for susceptible isolates from children who have infections other than endocarditis, meningitis, or ventriculitis (eg, ventriculoperitoneal shunt-associated infection).

Vancomycin-intermediately susceptible *S aureus* or vancomycin-intermediately susceptible CoNS strains rarely have been isolated. For seriously ill patients with a history of recurrent MRSA infections or for patients failing vancomycin therapy for whom VISA strains are a consideration, initial therapy could include vancomycin and ampicillin-sulbactam or trimethoprim-sulfamethoxazole, with or without gentamicin sulfate. For the penicillin-allergic patient, vancomycin plus gentamicin and trimethoprim-sulfamethoxazole could be considered. If antimicrobial susceptibility results document multidrug resistance, alternative agents, such as linezolid or quinupristin-dalfopristin, could be considered. Potential therapeutic options for these organisms on the basis of in vitro and limited clinical studies are outlined in Table 3.55 (p 568).

Gentamicin or rifampin could be added to an antimicrobial regimen depending on the severity and site of infection (eg, endocarditis or meningitis). Resistance rapidly emerges if rifampin is administered as a single agent. When gentamicin or rifampin is combined with BLR β-lactam antimicrobial agents, in vitro synergy commonly is demonstrated. The addition of gentamicin or rifampin to a regimen should be considered for serious infections and in consultation with an infectious diseases specialist.

For VISA strains, vancomycin plus nafcillin or oxacillin or vancomycin plus ampicillin-sulbactam have demonstrated synergy in vitro and efficacy in the rabbit endocarditis model. In all settings, vancomycin use should be minimized to discourage emergence of VISA from heteroresistant strains of MRSA.

Duration of therapy for serious *S aureus* infections depends on the site and severity of infection but usually is 4 weeks or more. After initial parenteral therapy and clinical improvement is noted, completion of the recommended antimicrobial course with an oral drug can be considered if compliance can be ensured and endocarditis is excluded. Monitoring blood concentrations of the antimicrobial agent also could be considered. For endocarditis, parenteral therapy is recommended for the entire treatment. Drainage of abscesses and removal of foreign bodies is desirable and almost always required.

Staphylococcal scalded skin syndrome in infants should be treated with a parenteral BLR β-lactam antimicrobial agent. In older children, depending on severity, oral agents can be considered. Skin and soft tissue infections, such as impetigo or cellulitis attributable to *S aureus*, usually can be treated with oral penicillinase-resistant β-lactam drugs, such as cloxacillin, dicloxacillin, or a first- or second-generation cephalosporin. For the penicillin-allergic patient, trimethoprim-sulfamethoxazole or clindamycin can be used. For localized superficial skin lesions, topical antimicrobial therapy with mupirocin or bacitracin zinc and local hygienic measures may be sufficient.

The duration of therapy for central venous catheter infections is controversial and depends on consideration of a number of factors, including the organism (*S aureus* vs CoNS), the type and location of the catheter, the site of infection (exit site vs tunnel vs bacteremia), the feasibility of using an alternative vessel at a later date, and the presence or absence of a catheter-related thrombus. Infections are more difficult to treat when associated with a thrombus, thrombophlebitis, or intra-atrial thrombus. If a catheter can be removed, there is no demonstrable thrombus, and bacteremia resolves promptly, a 3- to 5-day course of therapy seems appropriate for CoNS infections. A longer course of 2 or more weeks is suggested when the organism is *S aureus;* experts differ on optimal duration. If the patient needs a new catheter, waiting several days after bacteremia has resolved before insertion is optimal. If a tunneled catheter is needed for ongoing care, in situ treatment of the infection can be attempted. If the patient responds to antimicrobial therapy with immediate resolution of the *S aureus* bacteremia, the treatment can be continued for 10 to 14 days parenterally. If blood cultures remain positive for staphylococci for more than 3 to 5 days, the catheter should be removed, parenteral therapy should be continued, and the patient should be evaluated for metastatic foci of infection. If the patient develops hypotension at any time during therapy for a catheter-related infection, the catheter should be removed immediately. Vegetations or a thrombus in the heart or great vessels always should be considered when an intravascular catheter becomes infected. Transesophageal echocardiography is the most sensitive technique for identifying vegetations. Metastatic spread always should be evaluated in patients with *S aureus* bacteremia.

ISOLATION OF THE HOSPITALIZED PATIENT: Standard precautions are recommended for all patients. For patients with exposed lesions (eg, draining wounds, scalded skin syndrome, burns, bullous impetigo, or abscesses caused by MSSA), contact precautions are recommended for the duration of illness. For MSSA pneumonia, droplet precautions are recommended for the first 24 hours of antimicrobial therapy. Droplet precautions should be maintained throughout the illness for MSSA or MRSA tracheitis with a tracheostomy tube in place.

Patients infected or colonized with MRSA should be managed with contact precautions for multidrug-resistant organisms for the duration of illness, because MRSA carriage can persist for years. To prevent transmission of VISA and VRSA, the CDC has issued specific infection control recommendations that should be followed (see Table 3.54, p 566). For methicillin-resistant CoNS, standard precautions are recommended. For vancomycin-intermediately susceptible CoNS and known epidemic MRSA strains, contact precautions should be used.

CONTROL MEASURES:

Coagulase-Negative Staphylococci. Prevention and control of CoNS infections have focused on prevention of intraoperative contamination by skin flora and sterile insertion of intravascular and intraperitoneal catheters and other prosthetic devices. Prophylactic administration of an antimicrobial agent intraoperatively lowers the incidence of infection after cardiac surgery and the implantation of synthetic vascular grafts and prosthetic devices. There is no consensus about the role of intraoperative prophylaxis at the time of cerebrospinal fluid shunt placement.

Staphylococcus aureus. Measures to prevent and control *S aureus* infections can be considered separately for the individual patient and for the institution.

Individual Patient.

Community-acquired *S aureus* infections in immunocompetent hosts cannot be prevented, because the organism is ubiquitous and there is no vaccine. Frequently exercising hand hygiene, receiving appropriate treatment when indicated, and maintaining cleanliness of skin abrasions may prevent bacteremia. For patients with disorders of neutrophil function or with chronic skin conditions who are predisposed to *S aureus* infections, a variety of techniques have been used to prevent infection. These include scrupulous attention to skin hygiene and to the types of clothing and bed linen used to minimize sweating. Eradication of nasal carriage, if present, prompt use of antimicrobial agents for suspected infections, and in some instances, prolonged administration of trimethoprim-sulfamethoxazole also may be helpful.

Nosocomial *S aureus* infections may be prevented or controlled in an individual patient by general measures, intraoperative antimicrobial prophylaxis, and eradication of nasal carriage.

General Measures. The published recommendations of the CDC Hospital Infection Control Practices Advisory Committee (HICPAC)* for prevention of nosocomial pneumonia should be effective for decreasing the incidence of *S aureus* pneumonia. Careful preparation of the skin before surgery and before placement of intravascular catheters using barrier methods will decrease the incidence of *S aureus* wound and catheter infections. Meticulous surgical technique with minimal trauma to tissues, maintenance of good oxygenation, and minimal hematoma and dead space formation will minimize infection of the wound. Good hand hygiene, including before and after use of gloves, by health care professionals and strict adherence to contact precautions are of paramount importance.

Intraoperative Antimicrobial Prophylaxis. Bacteria are inoculated into wounds between the start and closure of the surgical incision. Antimicrobial agents can be given to achieve and maintain concentrations of antimicrobial agents during this critical period above the MICs of *S aureus* and CoNS in the blood and tissues. This pharmacologic defense can kill some inoculated bacteria directly and facilitate neutrophil killing of bacteria. The efficacy of prophylaxis for clean surgery is established. The antimicrobial agent is administered 15 to 30 minutes before the operation, and high serum concentrations are maintained throughout the procedure. A total duration of therapy of less than 24 hours is recommended. Staphylococci are the most common pathogens for several surgical procedures, and cefazolin is the most commonly recommended drug for most cardiac, general thoracic, vascular, orthopedic, and neurosurgical procedures. Vancomycin use for prophylaxis should be rare (see Principles of Appropriate Use of Vancomycin, p 697).

Eradication of Nasal Carriage. Detection and eradication of nasal carriage using mupirocin twice a day for 1 to 5 days has been shown to decrease the incidence of *S aureus* infections in some colonized adult patients after cardiothoracic, general, or neurosurgical procedures. The use of intermittent or continuous intranasal mupirocin for eradication of nasal carriage also has been shown to decrease the incidence of invasive *S aureus* infections in adult patients undergoing long-

---

* Centers for Disease Control and Prevention. Guidelines for prevention of nosocomial pneumonia. *MMWR*. In press

term hemodialysis or ambulatory peritoneal dialysis. Eradication of nasal carriage of *S aureus* is difficult, and mupirocin-resistant strains emerge with repeated or widespread use.

Institutions.

Measures to control the spread of *S aureus* within hospitals or hospital units involve use and careful monitoring of Hospital Infection Control Practices Advisory Committee guidelines published in 1996.* Strategies for controlling nosocomial transmission of MRSA vary widely among hospitals, and the guidelines recommend that hospitals individualize their recommendations. When a patient or health care professional is found to be a chronic carrier of *S aureus*, including MRSA, topical mupirocin therapy may eradicate carriage. Although an increasing number of MRSA strains are resistant in vitro to mupirocin, concentrations used topically (2% or 20 000 µg/mL) are high enough to be effective for many strains. Other topical preparations to be considered if mupirocin fails are ointments containing bacitracin and polymyxin B sulfate or a povidone-iodine cream. These preparations have not been studied in children. Decreasing the overuse of antimicrobial agents will decrease the emergence of VISA. Restriction and cycling of antimicrobial agents should be considered. Recommendations for containment of recently identified strains of VISA have been published by the CDC (Table 3.54, p 566). Ongoing review and restriction of vancomycin use is critical to attempting to control the emergence of VISA and VRSA (see Appropriate Use of Antimicrobial Agents, p 695). To date, the use of catheters impregnated with various antibacterial agents to prevent nosocomial infections has not been evaluated adequately in children.

Nurseries. Outbreaks of *S aureus* infections in newborn nurseries require unique measures of control. Application of triple dye, iodophor ointment, or hexachlorophene powder to the umbilical stump has been used to delay or prevent colonization. For full-term infants only, 3% hexachlorophene can be used for bathing followed by thorough rinsing. Other measures recommended during outbreaks include cohorting of ill infants and staff, alleviating overcrowding and understaffing, and emphasis on hand hygiene. Soaps containing antimicrobial agents are preferred during an outbreak. Culturing the umbilicus and nares of infants and nares and skin lesions of personnel for *S aureus* may help identify colonized infants. Pulsed-field gel electrophoresis should be used to determine strain identity. Epidemiologically implicated personnel can be treated for nasal carriage with mupirocin.

Group A Streptococcal Infections

CLINICAL MANIFESTATIONS: The most common clinical illness produced by group A streptococcal (GAS) infection is acute pharyngotonsillitis. In some patients who usually are untreated, purulent complications, including otitis media, sinusitis, peritonsillar and retropharyngeal abscesses, and suppurative cervical adenitis, develop.

---

* Centers for Disease Control and Prevention. Interim guidelines for the prevention and control of staphylococcal infection associated with reduced susceptibility to vancomycin. *MMWR Morb Mortal Wkly Rep.* 1997;46:626–628

The significance of streptococcal upper respiratory tract disease is related to acute morbidity and nonsuppurative sequelae (ie, acute rheumatic fever and acute glomerulonephritis). Scarlet fever occurs most commonly in association with pharyngitis and, rarely, with pyoderma or an infected wound. Scarlet fever has a characteristic confluent erythematous sandpaper-like rash, which is caused by one or more of several erythrogenic exotoxins produced by GAS strains. Severe scarlet fever with systemic toxic effects occurs rarely. Other than the occurrence of rash, the epidemiologic features, symptoms, sequelae, and treatment of scarlet fever are the same as those of streptococcal pharyngitis.

Toddlers (1–3 years of age) with GAS respiratory tract infection initially may have serous rhinitis and develop a protracted illness with moderate fever, irritability, and anorexia (streptococcal fever). The classic clinical presentation of streptococcal upper respiratory tract infection as acute pharyngitis is uncommon in children younger than 3 years of age. Rheumatic fever also is uncommon in children younger than 3 years of age.

The second most common site of GAS infection is the skin. Streptococcal skin infections (ie, pyoderma or impetigo) can result in acute glomerulonephritis, which occasionally occurs in epidemics, but acute rheumatic fever is not a sequela of streptococcal skin infection.

Other GAS infections include erysipelas, perianal cellulitis, vaginitis, bacteremia (with or without identified focus), pneumonia, endocarditis, pericarditis, septic arthritis, cellulitis, necrotizing fasciitis, osteomyelitis, myositis, puerperal sepsis, surgical wound infection, and neonatal omphalitis. Necrotizing fasciitis and other invasive GAS infections in children often occur as complications of varicella. Invasive GAS infections can be severe, with or without an identified focus of local infection, and can be associated with streptococcal toxic shock syndrome. The portal of entry of invasive infections often is the skin or soft tissue, and infection may follow minor or unrecognized trauma. An association between streptococcal infection and a condition referred to as PANDAS (pediatric autoimmune neuropsychiatric disorders associated with streptococcal infection) has been made. This condition manifests as a sudden onset or episodic course of obsessive-compulsive and/or tic disorders associated with streptococcal infection.

The toxic shock syndrome caused by GAS infection is reviewed in the chapter on Toxic Shock Syndrome (p 624).

ETIOLOGY: More than 100 distinct M-protein types of group A β-hemolytic streptococci *(Streptococcus pyogenes)* have been identified. Typing using emm types also is performed and may be more discriminating than M serotyping. Epidemiologic studies suggest an association between certain serotypes (eg, types 1, 3, 5, 6, 18, 19, and 24) and rheumatic fever, but a specific rheumatogenic factor has not been identified. Several serotypes (eg, types 49, 55, 57, and 59) are associated with pyoderma and acute glomerulonephritis. Other serotypes (eg, types 1, 6, and 12) are associated with pharyngitis and acute glomerulonephritis. Groups C and G streptococci have been associated with pharyngitis and, occasionally, acute nephritis but do not cause rheumatic fever.

EPIDEMIOLOGY: Pharyngitis usually results from contact with a person who has streptococcal pharyngitis. Fomites and household pets, such as dogs, are not vectors of GAS infection. Transmission of GAS infection, including school outbreaks of pharyngitis, almost always follows contact with respiratory tract secretions. Pharyngitis and impetigo (and their nonsuppurative complications) may be associated with crowding, which often is present in socioeconomically disadvantaged populations. The close contact that occurs in schools, child care centers, and military installations facilitates transmission. Foodborne outbreaks have occurred and are a consequence of human contamination of food in conjunction with improper preparation or refrigeration procedures.

Streptococcal pharyngitis occurs at all ages but it is most common among school-aged children and adolescents. Group A streptococcal pharyngitis and pyoderma are less common in adults than in children.

Geographically, streptococcal pharyngitis and pyoderma are ubiquitous. Pyoderma is more common in tropical climates and warm seasons, presumably because of antecedent insect bites and other minor skin trauma. Streptococcal pharyngitis is more common during late autumn, winter, and spring in temperate climates, presumably because of close person-to-person contact in schools. Communicability of patients with streptococcal pharyngitis is highest during the acute infection and, in untreated people, gradually diminishes over a period of weeks. Patients no longer are contagious within 24 hours after initiation of appropriate antimicrobial therapy.

Throat culture surveys of asymptomatic children during school outbreaks of pharyngitis have yielded GAS prevalence rates as high as 15% to 50%. These include children with asymptomatic infections and pharyngeal carriers with no subsequent immune response to GAS cellular or extracellular antigens. Carriage of GAS may persist for many months, but the risk of transmission to others is minimal.

The incidence of acute rheumatic fever in the United States has decreased sharply over several decades, but focal outbreaks of rheumatic fever in the 1990s in school-aged children in various geographic areas demonstrated that acute rheumatic fever remains a risk. Although the reason(s) for these local outbreaks is not clear, their occurrence reemphasizes the importance of diagnosing GAS pharyngitis and of compliance with recommended duration of antimicrobial therapy.

In streptococcal impetigo, the organism usually is acquired from another person with impetigo by direct physical contact. Colonization of healthy skin by GAS usually precedes development of skin infection. Impetiginous lesions occur at the site of breaks in skin (insect bites, burns, traumatic wounds), because GAS organisms do not penetrate intact skin. After development of impetiginous lesions, the upper respiratory tract often becomes colonized. Infection of surgical wounds and postpartum (puerperal) sepsis usually result from contact transmission via hand carriage. Anal or vaginal carriers and people with pyoderma or local suppurative infections can transmit GAS to surgical and obstetrical patients, resulting in nosocomial outbreaks. Infections in neonates can result from intrapartum or contact transmission; in the latter situation, infection often begins with omphalitis.

In recent years, the incidence of severe invasive GAS infections, including bacteremia, streptococcal toxic shock syndrome, and necrotizing fasciitis, appears to have increased. The incidence seems to be highest in infants and in older people.

Varicella is the most commonly identified risk factor in children. Other risk factors include intravenous drug use, human immunodeficiency virus infection, diabetes mellitus, and chronic cardiac or pulmonary disease. The portal of entry is unknown in almost 50% of invasive GAS infections; in most cases, it is believed to be the skin or mucous membrane. Such infections rarely follow GAS pharyngitis. Although numerous case reports have described a temporal association between use of non-steroidal anti-inflammatory drugs and invasive GAS infections in children with varicella, a causal relationship has not been established.

The **incubation period** for streptococcal pharyngitis is 2 to 5 days. For impetigo, a 7- to 10-day period between the acquisition of GAS on healthy skin and development of lesions has been demonstrated.

DIAGNOSTIC TESTS: Laboratory confirmation of GAS is recommended for children with pharyngitis, because accurate clinical differentiation of viral and GAS pharyngitis is not possible. A specimen should be obtained by vigorous swabbing of the tonsils and posterior pharynx. Culture on sheep blood agar can confirm GAS infection, and latex agglutination, fluorescent antibody, coagglutination, or precipitation techniques performed on colonies growing on the agar plate can differentiate group A from other β-hemolytic streptococci. Appropriate use of bacitracin-susceptibility disks (containing 0.04 units) allows presumptive identification of GAS but is a less accurate method of diagnosis. False-negative culture results occur for fewer than 10% of symptomatic patients when an adequate throat swab specimen is obtained and cultured properly by trained personnel using appropriate media and technique. Recovery of GAS from the pharynx does not distinguish patients with true streptococcal infection (defined by a serologic antibody response) from streptococcal carriers who have an intercurrent viral pharyngitis. The number of colonies of GAS on the agar culture plate does not accurately differentiate true infection from carriage. Cultures that are negative for GAS after 24 hours should be incubated for a second day to optimize recovery of GAS.

Several rapid diagnostic tests for GAS pharyngitis are available. Most are based on nitrous acid extraction of group A carbohydrate antigen from organisms obtained by throat swab. The specificities of these tests generally are high, but the reported sensitivities vary considerably. As with throat cultures, the accuracy of these tests is highly dependent on the quality of the throat swab specimen, which must contain pharyngeal and/or tonsillar secretions, on the experience of the person performing the test, and the rigor of the culture standard used for comparison. Therefore, when a patient suspected on clinical grounds of having GAS pharyngitis has a negative rapid streptococcal test, a throat culture should be obtained to ensure that the patient does not have GAS infection. Because of the very high specificity of these rapid tests, a positive test result generally does not require throat culture confirmation. Rapid diagnostic tests using techniques, such as optical immunoassay and chemiluminescent DNA probes, have been developed. Published data suggest that these tests may be as sensitive as standard throat cultures on sheep blood agar. Some experts believe that the optical immunoassay is sufficiently sensitive to be used without throat culture backup. Physicians who use any of these rapid tests without culture backup may wish to compare their results with those of culture to validate adequate sensitivity in their practice.

Indications for GAS Testing. Factors to be considered in the decision to obtain a throat swab specimen for testing in children with pharyngitis are the patient's age; clinical signs and symptoms; the season; and family and community epidemiology, including contact with a case of GAS infection or presence in the family of a person with acute rheumatic fever or history thereof or with poststreptococcal glomerulonephritis. Group A streptococcal infection is less common in children younger than 3 years of age, but outbreaks of streptococcal pharyngitis have been reported in young children in child care settings. The risk of acute rheumatic fever is so remote in developed countries in such young children that diagnostic studies for streptococcal pharyngitis are not recommended routinely for children younger than 3 years of age. Children with manifestations highly suggestive of viral infection, such as coryza, conjunctivitis, hoarseness, cough, anterior stomatitis, discrete ulcerative lesions, or diarrhea are unlikely to have GAS as the cause of their pharyngitis and generally should not be tested for GAS. Children with acute onset of sore throat, fever, headache, pain on swallowing, abdominal pain, nausea, vomiting, and enlarged tender anterior cervical lymph nodes are more likely to have GAS as the cause of their pharyngitis and should have a rapid antigen test or throat culture performed.

Indications for testing contacts for GAS vary according to circumstances. Testing asymptomatic household contacts for GAS usually is not recommended except during outbreaks or when contacts are at increased risk of developing sequelae of GAS infection. Throat swab specimens should be obtained from siblings and all other household contacts of a child who has acute rheumatic fever or post-streptococcal glomerulonephritis, and if test results are positive, contacts should be treated regardless of whether they are currently or were recently symptomatic. Household contacts of an index case with streptococcal pharyngitis who have recent or current symptoms suggestive of streptococcal infection also should be tested. Pyoderma lesions should be cultured in families with one or more cases of acute nephritis or streptococcal toxic shock syndrome so that antimicrobial therapy can be administered to eradicate GAS.

Post-treatment throat swab cultures are indicated only for patients at particularly high risk of rheumatic fever or who remain symptomatic at that time. Repeated courses of antimicrobial therapy are not indicated for asymptomatic patients who remain GAS positive after appropriate antimicrobial therapy; the exceptions are people who have had, or whose family members have had, rheumatic fever or rheumatic heart disease or in other uncommon epidemiologic circumstances, such as outbreaks of rheumatic fever or acute poststreptococcal glomerulonephritis.

Patients in whom repeated episodes of pharyngitis occur at short intervals with GAS documented by culture or antigen detection test present a special problem. Often, these people are long-term GAS carriers who are experiencing frequent viral illnesses. In assessing such patients, inadequate compliance with oral treatment also should be considered. Although uncommon, in some areas erythromycin resistance may occur, resulting in treatment failures. Such strains also are resistant to other macrolides, such as clarithromycin and azithromycin dihydrate. Testing asymptomatic household contacts usually is not helpful. However, if multiple household members have symptomatic pharyngitis or other GAS infection, such as pyoderma, simultaneous cultures of all household members and treatment of all people with positive cultures or rapid antigen tests may be of value.

In schools, child care centers, or other environments in which a large number of people are in close contact, the prevalence of GAS pharyngeal carriage in healthy children can be as high as 15% in the absence of an outbreak of streptococcal disease. Therefore, classroom or more widespread culture surveys are not indicated routinely and should be considered only if multiple cases of rheumatic fever, glomerulonephritis, or severe invasive GAS disease have occurred.

Cultures of impetiginous lesions are not indicated routinely, because lesions often yield both streptococci and staphylococci, and determination of the primary pathogen may not be possible.

In suspected invasive GAS infections, cultures of blood and focal sites of possible infection are indicated. In necrotizing fasciitis, magnetic resonance imaging can be helpful for confirming the anatomic diagnosis.

TREATMENT:

Pharyngitis.

- Penicillin V is the drug of choice for treatment of GAS pharyngitis, except in people who are allergic to penicillin. A clinical isolate of group A streptococci resistant to penicillin never has been documented. Ampicillin or amoxicillin often is used in place of penicillin V, but these drugs have no microbiologic advantage over penicillin. However, preliminary data suggest that orally administered amoxicillin given as a single daily dose for 10 days is as effective as orally administered penicillin V given 3 times per day for 10 days. Penicillin therapy prevents acute rheumatic fever even when therapy is started as long as 9 days after the onset of the acute illness, shortens the clinical course, decreases the risk of transmission, and decreases the risk of suppurative sequelae. For all patients with acute rheumatic fever, a complete course of penicillin or other appropriate antimicrobial agent for GAS pharyngitis should be given to eradicate GAS from the throat, even though the organism may not be recovered in the initial throat culture.

  The dose of orally administered penicillin V is 400 000 U (250 mg), 2 to 3 times per day for 10 days for children weighing less than 27 kg and 800 000 U (500 mg), 2 to 3 times per day, for heavier children, adolescents, and adults. To prevent acute rheumatic fever, oral treatment with penicillin should be given for the full 10 days, regardless of the promptness of clinical recovery. Although different preparations of oral penicillin vary in absorption, their clinical efficacy is similar. Treatment failures may occur more often with oral penicillin than with intramuscularly administered benzathine penicillin G as a result of inadequate compliance with oral therapy.

- Intramuscular penicillin G benzathine is appropriate therapy. It ensures adequate blood concentrations and avoids the problem of compliance, but administration is painful. For children who weigh less than 60 lb (27 kg), penicillin G benzathine is given in a single dose of 600 000 U; for larger children and adults, the dose is 1.2 million U. Discomfort is less if the preparation of penicillin G benzathine is brought to room temperature before intramuscular injection. Mixtures containing shorter-acting penicillins (eg, penicillin G procaine) in addition to penicillin G benzathine have not been demonstrated to be more effective than penicillin G benzathine alone but are less painful when administered. Although supporting data are limited, the combination of 900 000 U of penicillin G benzathine and 300 000 U of penicillin G procaine is satisfactory therapy for most children; however, the efficacy of this combination for heavier patients, such as adolescents and adults, has not been demonstrated.

- Orally administered erythromycin is indicated for patients who are allergic to penicillin. Treatment should be given for 10 days. Erythromycin estolate (20 to 40 mg/kg per day in 2–4 divided doses) or erythromycin ethylsuccinate (40 mg/kg per day in 2–4 divided doses) is effective for treating streptococcal pharyngitis; the maximum dose is 1 g/day. Other macrolides, such as clarithromycin for 10 days or azithromycin for 5 days (regimens licensed by the US Food and Drug Administration) also are effective. Although GAS strains resistant to erythromycin and other macrolides have been prevalent in some areas of the world (eg, Japan and Finland) and have resulted in treatment failures, they remain uncommon in most areas of the United States.

- A 10-day course of a narrow-spectrum (first-generation) oral cephalosporin is an acceptable alternative, particularly for people who are allergic to penicillin. However, as many as 15% of penicillin-allergic people also are allergic to cephalosporins. Patients with immediate, anaphylactic-type hypersensitivity to penicillin should not be treated with a cephalosporin. A number of reports have suggested that a 5-day course of certain oral cephalosporins is similar to a 10-day course of oral penicillin in eradicating GAS from the upper respiratory tract. However, additional studies are warranted to expand and confirm these observations before these regimens can be recommended. The additional cost of most cephalosporins and their wider range of antibacterial activity compared with penicillin preclude recommending them for routine use in either conventional or short-course regimens in people with GAS pharyngitis who are not allergic to penicillin.

- Tetracyclines and sulfonamides should not be used for treating GAS pharyngitis. Many strains are resistant to tetracycline, and sulfonamides do not eradicate GAS, even though they are effective for continuous prophylaxis for recurrent rheumatic fever (see Secondary Prophylaxis for Rheumatic Fever, p 582).

Children who have a recurrence of GAS pharyngitis shortly after completing a 10-day course of a recommended oral antimicrobial agent can be retreated with the same antimicrobial agent, given an alternative oral drug, or given an intramuscular dose of penicillin G benzathine, especially if inadequate compliance with oral therapy is likely. Alternative drugs include a narrow-spectrum cephalosporin, amoxicillin-clavulanate potassium, clindamycin, erythromycin, or another macrolide. Expert opinions differ about the most appropriate therapy in this circumstance.

Management of a patient who has repeated and frequent episodes of acute pharyngitis associated with a positive laboratory test for GAS is problematic. To determine whether the patient is a long-term streptococcal pharyngeal carrier who is experiencing repeated episodes of intercurrent viral pharyngitis (which is the situation in most cases), the following should be determined: (1) whether the clinical findings are more suggestive of a GAS or a viral cause; (2) whether epidemiologic factors in the community are more suggestive of a GAS or a viral cause; (3) the nature of the clinical response to the antimicrobial therapy (in true GAS, response to therapy usually is rapid); (4) whether laboratory tests are positive for GAS between episodes of acute pharyngitis; and (5) whether a serologic response to GAS extracellular antigens (eg, antistreptolysin O) has occurred. Serotyping of GAS isolates generally is available only in research laboratories, but if performed, repeated isolation of the same serotype suggests carriage, and isolation of differing serotypes indicates repeated infections.

Pharyngeal Carriers. Antimicrobial therapy is not indicated for most GAS pharyngeal carriers. Exceptions (ie, specific situations in which eradication of carriage may be indicated) include the following: (1) an outbreak of acute rheumatic fever or poststreptococcal glomerulonephritis occurs; (2) an outbreak of GAS pharyngitis in a closed or semiclosed community occurs; (3) a family history of rheumatic fever exists; (4) multiple episodes of documented symptomatic GAS pharyngitis continue to occur within a family during a period of many weeks despite appropriate therapy; (5) a family has excessive anxiety about GAS infections; or (6) tonsillectomy is considered only because of chronic GAS carriage.

Streptococcal carriage can be difficult to eradicate with conventional antimicrobial therapy. A number of antimicrobial agents, including clindamycin, amoxicillin-clavulanate, and a combination of rifampin for the last 4 days of treatment with either penicillin V or penicillin G benzathine, have been demonstrated to be more effective than penicillin in eliminating chronic streptococcal carriage. Of these drugs, oral clindamycin, given as 20 mg/kg per day in 3 doses (maximum 1.8 g/day) for 10 days, has been reported to be the most effective. Data also suggest that orally administered azithromycin is an effective short-course regimen for eradication of oropharyngeal GAS; however, widespread use may contribute to emergence of macrolide-resistant bacteria. Documented eradication of the carrier state is helpful in the evaluation of subsequent episodes of acute pharyngitis; however, long-term carriage may recur after reacquisition of GAS.

Streptococcal Impetigo.

- Local mupirocin ointment may be useful for limiting person-to-person spread of GAS impetigo and for eradicating localized disease. With multiple lesions or with impetigo in multiple family members, child care groups, or athletic teams, impetigo should be treated with antimicrobial regimens administered systemically. Because episodes of impetigo may be caused by *Staphylococcus aureus* or *Streptococcus pyogenes,* children with impetigo usually should be treated with an antimicrobial active against both GAS and *S aureus.*

Other Infections.

- High-dose parenteral antimicrobial therapy is required for severe infections, such as endocarditis, pneumonia, septicemia, meningitis, arthritis, osteomyelitis, necrotizing fasciitis, neonatal omphalitis, and streptococcal toxic shock syndrome. Treatment often is prolonged (2–6 weeks).
- For treatment of patients with severe invasive GAS infection, including toxic shock syndrome, see Toxic Shock Syndrome (p 624).

Prevention of Sequelae. Acute rheumatic fever and acute glomerulonephritis are serious nonsuppurative sequelae of GAS infections. During epidemics of GAS infections on military bases in the 1950s, rheumatic fever developed in 3% of untreated patients with acute streptococcal pharyngitis. The current attack rate after endemic infections is not known but is believed to be substantially lower. The risk of rheumatic fever virtually can be eliminated by adequate treatment of the antecedent GAS infection; however, rare cases of rheumatic fever have occurred even after apparently appropriate therapy. The effectiveness of antimicrobial therapy for preventing acute poststreptococcal glomerulonephritis after pyoderma has not been established. Suppurative sequelae, such as peritonsillar abscesses and cervical adenitis, usually are prevented by treatment of the primary infection.

ISOLATION OF THE HOSPITALIZED PATIENT: In addition to standard precautions, droplet precautions are recommended for children with pharyngitis or pneumonia until 24 hours after initiation of appropriate therapy. For burns with secondary GAS infection and extensive or draining cutaneous infections that cannot be covered or contained adequately by dressings, contact precautions should be used for at least 24 hours after the start of appropriate therapy.

CONTROL MEASURES: The most important means of controlling GAS disease and its sequelae is prompt identification and treatment of infections.

School and Child Care. Children with streptococcal pharyngitis or skin infections should not return to school or child care until at least 24 hours after beginning appropriate antimicrobial therapy. Close contact with other children during this time should be avoided, if possible.

Care of Exposed People. People who are contacts of documented cases of streptococcal infection and who have recent or current clinical evidence of a GAS infection should undergo appropriate laboratory tests and should be treated if test results are positive. Rates of GAS carriage are higher among sibling contacts than among parent contacts in nonepidemic settings; rates as high as 50% for sibling contacts and 20% for parent contacts have been reported during epidemics. More than half of the contacts who acquire the organism will become ill. Asymptomatic acquisition of GAS may pose some risk of nonsuppurative complications; studies indicate that as many as one third of patients with rheumatic fever had no history of recent streptococcal infection and another third had minor respiratory tract symptoms that were not brought to medical attention. However, laboratory evaluation of asymptomatic household contacts usually is not indicated except during outbreaks or when the contacts are at increased risk of developing sequelae of infection (see Indications for GAS Testing, p 577). Short courses (<10 days) of an antimicrobial agent for contacts are inappropriate. In rare circumstances, such as a large family with documented, repeated, intrafamilial transmission resulting in frequent episodes of GAS pharyngitis during a prolonged period, physicians may elect to treat all family members identified by laboratory tests as harboring GAS.

Some experts recommend oral penicillin prophylaxis during the period of the year of greatest risk for children with repeated episodes of GAS pharyngitis. However, this approach should be limited because of concerns about selecting resistant pathogens, such as *Streptococcus pneumoniae,* but not GAS.

Household contacts of patients with severe invasive GAS disease, including streptococcal toxic shock syndrome, are at increased risk of developing severe invasive GAS disease compared with the general population, but the risk is not sufficiently high to warrant routine testing for GAS colonization or routine chemoprophylaxis of all household contacts of people with invasive GAS disease. However, because of the increased risk of sporadic, invasive GAS disease among certain populations and because of the risk of death in people 65 years of age and older who develop invasive GAS disease, health care professionals should consider targeted chemoprophylaxis in household contacts who are 65 years of age and older or who are members of other high-risk populations (eg, people with human immunodeficiency virus infection, chickenpox, diabetes mellitus). Because of the rarity of subsequent cases and the low risk of invasive GAS infections in children in general, chemoprophylaxis is not recommended in schools or child care facilities.

Secondary Prophylaxis for Rheumatic Fever. Patients who have a well-documented history of acute rheumatic fever (including cases manifested solely as Sydenham chorea) and patients who have documented evidence of rheumatic heart disease should be given continuous antimicrobial prophylaxis to prevent recurrent attacks (secondary prophylaxis), because asymptomatic and symptomatic GAS infections can result in a rheumatic recurrence. Continuous prophylaxis should be initiated as soon as the diagnosis of acute rheumatic fever or rheumatic heart disease is made.

Duration. Secondary prophylaxis should be long-term, perhaps for life, for patients with rheumatic heart disease (even after prosthetic valve replacement, because these patients remain at risk of recurrence of rheumatic fever). The risk of recurrence decreases as the interval from the most recent episode increases, and patients without rheumatic heart disease are at a lower risk of recurrence than are patients with cardiac involvement. These considerations influence the duration of secondary prophylaxis in adults but should not alter the practice of secondary prophylaxis for children and adolescents. Secondary prophylaxis for all patients who have had rheumatic fever should be continued for at least 5 years or until the person is 21 years of age, whichever is longer (see Table 3.56, p 583). Prophylaxis also should be continued if the risk of contact with people with GAS infection is high, such as for parents with school-aged children and teachers.

When streptococcal infections occur in household contacts of patients with a history of rheumatic fever, infected people should be treated promptly with an appropriate antimicrobial (see Indications for GAS Testing, p 577, and Treatment, p 578).

The drug regimens in Table 3.57 (p 584) are effective for secondary prophylaxis. The intramuscular regimen has been shown to be the most reliable, because the success of oral prophylaxis depends primarily on patient compliance; however, inconvenience and the pain of injection may cause some patients to discontinue intramuscular prophylaxis. In some countries and in situations in which the risk of GAS infection is particularly high, penicillin G benzathine is given every 3 weeks because of greater effectiveness. In the United States, administration every 4 weeks seems adequate in most circumstances. Oral sulfadiazine is as effective as oral penicillin for secondary prophylaxis but may not be readily available in the United States. By

Table 3.56. Duration of Prophylaxis for People Who Have Had Rheumatic Fever: Recommendations of the American Heart Association[1]

Category	Duration
Rheumatic fever without carditis	5 y or until 21 y of age, whichever is longer
Rheumatic fever with carditis but without residual heart disease (no valvular disease[2])	10 y or well into adulthood, whichever is longer
Rheumatic fever with carditis and residual heart disease (persistent valvular disease[2])	At least 10 y since last episode and at least until 40 y of age; sometimes lifelong prophylaxis

[1] Modified from Dajani A, Taubert K, Ferrieri P, Peter G, Shulman S. Treatment of acute streptococcal pharyngitis and prevention of rheumatic fever: a statement for health professionals: Committee on Rheumatic Fever, Endocarditis, and Kawasaki Disease of the Council on Cardiovascular Disease in the Young, The American Heart Association. *Pediatrics.* 1995;96:758–764.
[2] Clinical or echocardiographic evidence.

extrapolating from data demonstrating effectiveness of sulfadiazine, sulfisoxazole acetyl has been deemed an appropriate alternative.

Allergic reactions to oral penicillin are similar to those with intramuscular penicillin, but they usually are less severe and occur less commonly. These reactions also occur less commonly in children than in adults. Anaphylaxis is rare in patients receiving oral penicillin. Severe allergic reactions in patients receiving continuous penicillin G benzathine prophylaxis also are rare. The rare reports of anaphylaxis and death generally have involved patients older than 12 years of age with severe rheumatic heart disease. Most of these severe reactions seem to represent vasovagal responses rather than anaphylaxis. Reactions also include a serum sickness-like reaction characterized by fever and joint pains, which can be mistaken for recurrence of acute rheumatic fever.

Reactions to continuous sulfadiazine or sulfisoxazole prophylaxis are rare and usually minor; evaluation of blood cell counts may be advisable after 2 weeks of prophylaxis, because leukopenia has been reported. Prophylaxis with a sulfonamide during late pregnancy is contraindicated because of interference with fetal bilirubin metabolism. Febrile mucocutaneous syndromes (erythema multiforme, Stevens-Johnson syndrome, or toxic epidermal necrolysis) have been associated with penicillin and with sulfonamides. When an adverse event occurs with any of these therapeutic regimens, the drug should be stopped immediately and an alternative drug should be selected. For the rare patient allergic to both penicillins and sulfonamides, erythromycin is recommended. Newer macrolides, such as azithromycin or clarithromycin, also should be acceptable; they have less risk of gastrointestinal intolerance but increased costs.

Poststreptococcal Reactive Arthritis. After an episode of acute GAS pharyngitis, reactive arthritis may develop in the absence of sufficient clinical manifestations and laboratory findings to fulfill the Jones criteria for the diagnosis of acute rheumatic fever. This syndrome has been termed poststreptococcal reactive arthritis (PSRA). The precise relationship of PSRA to acute rheumatic fever is unclear. In

Table 3.57. **Chemoprophylaxis for Recurrences of Rheumatic Fever[1]**

Drug	Dose	Route
Penicillin G benzathine	1.2 million U, every 4 wk[2]	Intramuscular
OR		
Penicillin V	250 mg, twice a day	Oral
OR		
Sulfadiazine or sulfisoxazole	0.5 g, once a day for patients ≤27 kg (≤60 lb) 1.0 g, once a day for patients >27 kg (>60 lb)	Oral
For people who are allergic to penicillin and sulfonamide drugs		
Erythromycin	250 mg, twice a day	Oral

[1] Modified from Dajani A, Taubert K, Ferrieri P, Peter G, Shulman S. Treatment of acute streptococcal pharyngitis and prevention of rheumatic fever: a statement for health professionals: Committee on Rheumatic Fever, Endocarditis, and Kawasaki Disease of the Council on Cardiovascular Disease in the Young, The American Heart Association. *Pediatrics.* 1995;96:758–764

[2] In high-risk situations, administration every 3 weeks is recommended.

contrast with the arthritis of acute rheumatic fever, the arthritis of PSRA does not respond dramatically to nonsteroidal anti-inflammatory agents. Because some patients with PSRA apparently may have silent or delayed-onset carditis, patients should be observed carefully for several months for the subsequent development of carditis. Some experts recommend prophylaxis for these patients for several months to a year if carditis does not develop; if carditis occurs, the patient should be considered to have had rheumatic fever, and prophylaxis should be continued (see Secondary Prophylaxis for Rheumatic Fever, p 582).

Bacterial Endocarditis Prophylaxis. Patients with rheumatic valvular heart disease also require additional short-term antimicrobial prophylaxis at the time of certain procedures (including dental and surgical procedures) to prevent the possible development of bacterial endocarditis (see Prevention of Bacterial Endocarditis, p 778). Patients who have had rheumatic fever without evidence of valvular heart disease do not need prophylaxis for prevention of endocarditis. Penicillin, ampicillin, and amoxicillin should not be used for endocarditis prophylaxis for patients who are receiving oral penicillin for secondary rheumatic fever prophylaxis because of relative penicillin and aminopenicillin resistance among viridans streptococci in the oral cavity in such patients. Clindamycin, azithromycin, and clarithromycin are the alternative antimicrobial agents recommended for such patients.

Group B Streptococcal Infections

CLINICAL MANIFESTATIONS: Group B streptococci are a major cause of perinatal bacterial infections, including bacteremia, endometritis, chorioamnionitis, and urinary tract infections in parturient women and systemic and focal infections in infants from birth until 3 months of age or older. Invasive disease in young infants is categorized into 2 entities on the basis of chronologic age at onset. Early-onset disease usually occurs within the first 24 hours of life (range, 0–6 days) and is characterized by signs of systemic infection, respiratory distress, apnea, shock, pneumonia, and less often, meningitis (5%–10% of cases). Late-onset disease, which typically occurs at 3 to 4 weeks of age (range, 7 days–3 months), commonly manifests as occult bacteremia or meningitis; other focal infections, such as osteomyelitis, septic arthritis, adenitis, and cellulitis, can occur. Group B streptococci also cause systemic infections in nonpregnant adults with underlying medical conditions, such as diabetes mellitus, chronic liver or renal disease, malignancy, or other immunocompromising conditions, and adults 65 years of age and older.

ETIOLOGY: Group B streptococci *(Streptococcus agalactiae)* are gram-positive, aerobic diplococci that typically produce beta hemolysis and are divided into 9 serotypes on the basis of capsular polysaccharides (Ia, Ib, II, and III through VIII). Serotypes Ia, Ib, II, III, and V account for approximately 95% of cases in the United States. Serotype III is the predominant cause of early-onset meningitis and most late-onset infections.

EPIDEMIOLOGY: Group B streptococci are common inhabitants of the gastrointestinal and genitourinary tracts. Less commonly, they colonize the pharynx. The colonization rate in pregnant women and newborn infants ranges from 15% to 40%. Colonization during pregnancy can be constant or intermittent. Before recommendations for prevention of early-onset group B streptococcal (GBS) disease by maternal intrapartum antimicrobial prophylaxis (see Control Measures, p 586) were made, the incidence was 1 to 4 cases per 1000 live births; early-onset disease accounted for approximately 75% of infant cases and occurred in approximately 1 infant per 100 to 200 colonized women. Associated with widespread maternal intrapartum antimicrobial prophylaxis, the incidence of early-onset disease has decreased by approximately 70% to approximately 0.5 cases per 1000 live births. Case-fatality ratios range from 5% to 8% but are higher in preterm neonates. Transmission from mother to infant occurs shortly before or during delivery. After delivery, person-to-person transmission can occur. Although uncommon, GBS can be acquired in the nursery from hospital personnel (probably via hand contamination) or more commonly in the community from healthy colonized people. The risk of early-onset disease is increased in preterm infants born at less than 37 weeks of gestation, in infants born after the amniotic membranes have been ruptured 18 hours or more, and in infants born to women with high genital GBS inoculum, intrapartum fever (temperature ≥38°C [≥100.4°F]), chorioamnionitis, or GBS bacteriuria during the pregnancy. A low or an absent concentration of serotype-specific serum antibody also is a predisposing factor. Other risk factors are maternal age younger than 20 years and black race or Hispanic ethnicity. The period of communicability is unknown but may extend throughout the duration of colonization or of disease. Infants can remain colonized for several months after birth and after treatment for systemic infection. Recurrent GBS disease affects an estimated 1% to 3% of appropriately treated infants.

The **incubation period** of early-onset disease is fewer than 7 days. In late-onset disease, the incubation period from GBS acquisition to disease is unknown. Late-onset disease usually occurs from 7 days to 3 months of age, but up to 10% of pediatric cases occur beyond early infancy, and many but not all of these are in infants who were born prematurely.

DIAGNOSTIC TESTS: Gram-positive cocci in body fluids that typically are sterile (such as cerebrospinal [CSF], pleural, or joint fluid) provide presumptive evidence of infection. Cultures of blood, other typically sterile body fluids, or a suppurative focus are necessary to establish the diagnosis. Serotype identification is available in reference laboratories. Rapid tests that identify group B streptococcal antigen in body fluids other than CSF are not recommended.

TREATMENT:
- Ampicillin plus an aminoglycoside is the initial treatment of choice for a newborn infant with presumptive invasive GBS infection.
- Penicillin G alone can be given when GBS has been identified as the cause of the infection and when clinical and microbiologic responses have been documented.
- For infants with meningitis attributable to GBS, the recommended dosage of penicillin G for infants 7 days of age or younger is 250 000 to 450 000 U/kg per day, intravenously, in 3 divided doses; for infants older than 7 days of age, 450 000 to 500 000 U/kg per day, intravenously, in 4 to 6 divided doses is recommended. For ampicillin, the recommended dosage for infants with meningitis 7 days of age or younger is 200 to 300 mg/kg per day, intravenously, in 3 divided doses; for infants older than 7 days of age, 300 mg/kg per day, intravenously, in 4 to 6 divided doses is recommended.
- For meningitis, some experts believe that a second lumbar puncture approximately 24 to 48 hours after initiation of therapy assists in management and prognosis. Additional lumbar punctures and diagnostic imaging studies are indicated if response to therapy is in doubt or neurologic abnormalities persist. Consultation with a specialist in pediatric infectious diseases is useful.
- For infants with bacteremia without a defined focus, treatment should be continued for 10 days. For infants with uncomplicated meningitis, 14 days of treatment is satisfactory, but longer periods of treatment may be necessary for infants with prolonged or complicated courses. Osteomyelitis or ventriculitis requires treatment for 4 weeks.
- Because of the reported risk of coinfection, the twin or any multiples of an index case with early- or late-onset disease should be observed carefully and evaluated and treated empirically for suspected systemic infection if any manifestations of illness occur.

ISOLATION OF THE HOSPITALIZED PATIENT: Only standard precautions are recommended except during a nursery outbreak of disease attributable to GBS (see Control Measures, Nursery Outbreak, p 591).

CONTROL MEASURES:

Chemoprophylaxis. Recommendations for prevention of early-onset neonatal GBS infection are based on data comparing a culture screening method to a risk-based method to identify women who should receive intrapartum antimicrobial prophylaxis that demonstrated significantly better efficacy for the culture screening method.

Recommendations from the Centers for Disease Control and Prevention (CDC)* indicate the following:

- All pregnant women should be screened at 35 to 37 weeks' gestation for vaginal and rectal colonization (see Fig 3.1, p 588). The only exceptions to this recommendation for universal culture screening are women with GBS bacteriuria during the current pregnancy or women who have had a previous infant with invasive GBS disease; these women always should receive intrapartum chemoprophylaxis. At the onset of labor or rupture of membranes, intrapartum chemoprophylaxis should be given to all pregnant women identified as GBS carriers. Colonization during a previous pregnancy is not an indication for intrapartum chemoprophylaxis unless screening results are positive in the current pregnancy.
- Women with GBS isolated from the urine in any concentration (eg, 10^3) during their current pregnancy should receive intrapartum chemoprophylaxis, because such women usually are heavily colonized with GBS and are at increased risk of delivering an infant with early-onset GBS disease; prenatal culture screening is not necessary.
- Women who previously have given birth to an infant with invasive GBS disease should receive intrapartum chemoprophylaxis; prenatal culture screening is not necessary.
- If GBS status is not known at onset of labor or rupture of membranes, intrapartum chemoprophylaxis should be administered to women with any of the following risk factors: gestation less than 37 weeks, duration of membrane rupture 18 hours or longer, or intrapartum temperature of ≥38.0°C (≥100.4°F).
- Culture techniques that maximize the likelihood of GBS recovery are required for prenatal screening. The optimal method for GBS screening cultures is collection of swabs of the lower vagina and rectum; placement of swabs in a nonnutrient transport medium, removal of swabs and inoculation into selective broth medium, such as Trans-Vag Broth supplemented with 5% defibrinated sheep blood or Lim broth; overnight incubation; and subculture onto solid blood agar medium.
- Oral antimicrobial agents should *not* be used to treat women who are found to have GBS colonization during prenatal screening unless there is GBS bacteriuria. Such treatment is *not* effective in eliminating GBS carriage or preventing neonatal disease and may cause adverse consequences.
- Women who have GBS colonization and have a planned cesarean delivery performed before rupture of membranes and onset of labor should *not* receive intrapartum chemoprophylaxis routinely.

The following recommendations are summarized in Fig 3.1 (p 588):

- For intrapartum chemoprophylaxis, intravenous penicillin G (5 million U initially, then 2.5 million U every 4 hours until delivery) is the preferred agent because of its effectiveness and narrow spectrum of antimicrobial activity. An alternative regimen is intravenous ampicillin (2 g initially, then 1 g every 4 hours until delivery).

---

* Centers for Disease Control and Prevention. Prevention of perinatal group B streptococcal disease. Revised guidelines from CDC. *MMWR Recomm Rep.* 2002;51(RR-11):1–22

Fig 3.1. Indications for intrapartum antimicrobial prophylaxis (IAP) to prevent early-onset group B streptococcal (GBS) disease using a universal prenatal culture screening strategy at 35 to 37 weeks' gestation for all women.

Vaginal and Rectal GBS Cultures at 35–37 Weeks' Gestation for ALL Pregnant Women[1]

IAP INDICATED

- Previous infant with invasive GBS disease
- GBS bacteriuria during *current* pregnancy
- Positive GBS screening culture during current pregnancy (*unless* a planned cesarean delivery is performed in the absence of labor or membrane rupture)
- Unknown GBS status AND any of the following:
  - Delivery at <37 weeks' gestation
  - Membranes ruptured for ≥18 hours
  - Intrapartum fever (temperature ≥38.0°C [≥100.4°F])[2]

IAP *NOT* INDICATED

- Previous pregnancy with a positive GBS screening culture (unless a culture also was positive during the current pregnancy or previous infant with invasive GBS disease)
- Planned cesarean delivery performed in the absence of labor or membrane rupture (regardless of GBS culture status)
- Negative vaginal and rectal GBS screening culture in late gestation, regardless of intrapartum risk factors

---

[1] Exceptions: women with GBS bacteriuria during the current pregnancy or women with a previous infant with invasive GBS disease.

[2] If chorioamnionitis is suspected, broad-spectrum antimicrobial therapy that includes an agent known to be active against GBS should replace GBS IAP.

- Because of the increasing prevalence of GBS resistance to erythromycin and clindamycin, cefazolin sodium, 2 g initially, then 1 g every 8 hours, is recommended for women who are allergic to penicillin but at low risk of anaphylaxis because of its narrow spectrum of activity and ability to achieve high amniotic fluid concentrations. Women whose GBS isolates are tested and found to be clindamycin susceptible and who are at high risk of anaphylaxis with penicillin can receive this drug at a dose of 900 mg every 8 hours. Vancomycin hydrochloride should be reserved for penicillin-allergic women who are at high risk of anaphylaxis and for whom GBS isolate susceptibility testing has not been performed; vancomycin should be administered intravenously, 1 g every 12 hours until delivery.
- Routine use of antimicrobial agents as chemoprophylaxis for neonates born to mothers who have received adequate intrapartum chemoprophylaxis for GBS disease is *not* recommended. However, therapeutic use of these agents is appropriate for infants with clinically suspected systemic infection.

An approach for empiric management of newborn infants born to women who receive intrapartum chemoprophylaxis to prevent early-onset GBS disease or to treat suspected chorioamnionitis is provided in Fig 3.2, p 590. These guidelines are based on recently published information as well as expert opinion and are as follows:

- If a woman receives intrapartum antimicrobial agents for treatment of suspected chorioamnionitis, her newborn infant should have a full diagnostic evaluation and empiric therapy pending culture results, regardless of clinical condition at birth, duration of maternal therapy before delivery, or weeks of gestation at delivery. Empiric therapy for the infant should include antimicrobial agents active against GBS as well as other organisms that might cause early-onset neonatal sepsis (eg, ampicillin and gentamicin sulfate).
- When clinical signs in the infant suggest sepsis, a full diagnostic evaluation should include a lumbar puncture, if feasible. Blood cultures can be sterile in as many as 15% of newborns with meningitis, and the clinical management of an infant with abnormal cerebrospinal fluid (CSF) differs from that of an infant with normal CSF. If a lumbar puncture has been deferred for a neonate receiving empiric antimicrobial therapy and therapy is continued beyond 48 hours because of ongoing clinical findings suggesting infection, CSF should be obtained for measurement of white blood cell count and differential, glucose, and protein and for culture.
- In addition to penicillin or ampicillin, initiation of intrapartum antimicrobial prophylaxis with cefazolin at least 4 hours before delivery can be considered adequate on the basis of achievable amniotic fluid concentrations of cefazolin. Although other agents may be substituted for penicillin if the woman has a history of penicillin allergy, the effectiveness of these agents (eg, clindamycin or vancomycin hydrochloride) in preventing early-onset GBS disease has not been studied, and no data are available to suggest the duration before delivery of these regimens that can be considered adequate.
- On the basis of the demonstrated effectiveness of intrapartum antimicrobial prophylaxis in preventing early-onset GBS disease and data indicating that clinical onset occurs within the first 24 hours of life in more than 90% of infants, hospital discharge as early as 24 hours after birth may be reasonable

Fig 3.2. Empiric management of a neonate whose mother received intrapartum antimicrobial prophylaxis (IAP) for prevention of early-onset group B streptococcal (GBS) disease[1] or suspected chorioamnionitis. This algorithm is not an exclusive course of management. Variations that incorporate individual circumstances or institutional preferences may be appropriate.

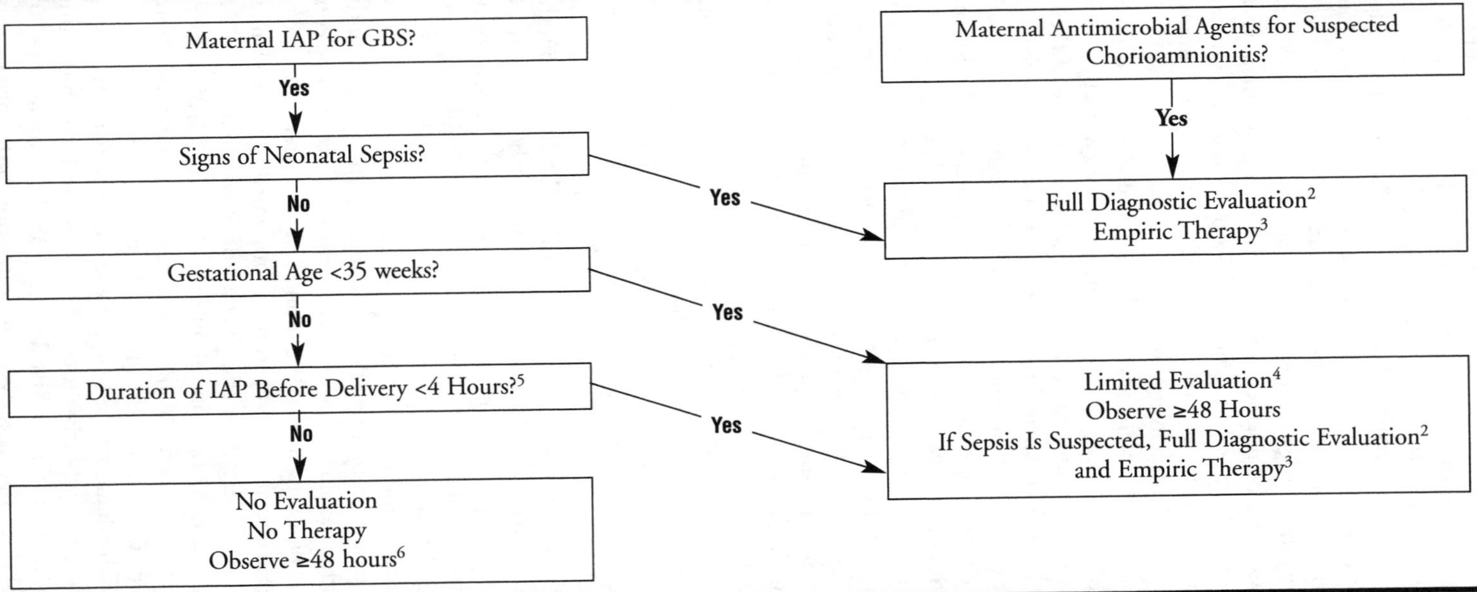

1 If no maternal IAP for GBS was administered despite an indication being present, data are insufficient on which to recommend a single management strategy.
2 Includes complete blood cell (CBC) count with differential, blood culture, and chest radiograph if respiratory abnormalities are present. When signs of sepsis are present, a lumbar puncture, if feasible, should be performed.
3 Duration of therapy varies depending on results of blood culture, cerebrospinal fluid findings (if obtained), and the clinical course of the infant. If laboratory results and clinical course do not indicate bacterial infection, duration may be as short as 48 hours.
4 CBC including WBC count with differential and blood culture.
5 Applies only to penicillin, ampicillin, or cefazolin and assumes recommended dosing regimens.
6 A healthy-appearing infant who was ≥38 weeks' gestation at delivery and whose mother received ≥4 hours of IAP before delivery may be discharged home after 24 hours if other discharge criteria have been met and a person able to comply fully with instructions for home observation will be present. If any one of these conditions is not met, the infant should be observed in the hospital for at least 48 hours and until criteria for discharge are achieved.

under certain circumstances. Specifically, a healthy-appearing infant who is at least 38 weeks' gestation at delivery and whose mother received 4 or more hours of intrapartum penicillin, ampicillin, or cefazolin before delivery may be discharged home as early as 24 hours after delivery if other discharge criteria have been met and a person able to comply fully with instructions for home observation will be present. A key component of following instructions is the ability of the person observing the infant to communicate with health care professionals by telephone and to transport the infant promptly to an appropriate health care facility if clinical signs of systemic infection develop. If these conditions are not met, the infant should remain in the hospital for at least 48 hours of observation.

Neonatal Infection Control. Routine cultures to determine whether infants have colonization with GBS are not recommended. Epidemiologic evaluation of late-onset cases in a special care nursery may be required to exclude a nosocomial source.

Nursery Outbreak. Cohorting of ill and colonized infants and use of contact precautions during an outbreak are recommended. Other methods of control (eg, treatment of asymptomatic carriers with penicillin) are impractical or ineffective. Routine hand hygiene by health care professionals caring for infants colonized or infected with GBS is the best way to prevent spread to other infants.

Non-Group A or B Streptococcal and Enterococcal Infections

CLINICAL MANIFESTATIONS: Streptococci of groups other than A or B can be associated with invasive disease in infants, children, adolescents, and adults. Urinary tract infection, endocarditis, upper and lower respiratory tract infections, and meningitis are the principal clinical syndromes. Viridans streptococci are associated with a variety of infections, perhaps the most significant being endocarditis and bacteremia in neutropenic patients with cancer. Enterococci are associated with bacteremia in neonates and bacteremia, intra-abdominal abscesses, and urinary tract infections in older children and adults.

ETIOLOGY: Changes in taxonomy and nomenclature of the *Streptococcus* genus have evolved as a result of the application of molecular technology.* Among gram-positive organisms that are catalase negative and that display chains in Gram stains, the 2 genera associated most often with human disease are *Streptococcus* and *Enterococcus*. The *Streptococcus* genus contains organisms that are (a) hemolytic on blood agar plates (*Streptococcus pyogenes* [see Group A Streptococcal Infections, p 573], *Streptococcus agalactiae* [see Group B Streptococcal Infections, p 584], and groups C, G, and F streptococci); (b) nonhemolytic on blood agar plates (*Streptococcus pneumoniae* [see Pneumococcal Infections, p 490], *Streptococcus bovis* group, and other group D streptococci); (c) 26 species of viridans streptococci, which are divided into 6 groups by phenotypic characteristics; (d) nutritionally variant strep-

---

* Facklam R. What happened to the streptococci: overview of taxonomic and nomenclature changes. *Clin Microbiol Rev.* 2002;15:613

tococci (now referred to as *Abiotrophia* and *Granulicatella*); and (e) unusual streptococcal species that do not fit into any of the other *Streptococcus* species groups.

The genus *Enterococcus* (previously included with group D streptococci) contains more than 20 species, with *Enterococcus faecalis* and *Enterococcus faecium* accounting for most cases of human enterococcal infection.

EPIDEMIOLOGY: The habitats that streptococci occupy in humans include skin (groups C, F, and G), oropharynx (groups C, F, and G), gastrointestinal tract (groups D, F, and G and *Enterococcus* species), and vagina (groups C, D, F, and G and *Enterococcus* species). The typical human habitats of different species of viridans streptococci include the oropharynx, dental surfaces, skin, and genitourinary tract. Intrapartum transmission probably is responsible for most cases of early-onset neonatal infection. Environmental contamination or transmission via hands of health care professionals can lead to colonization of patients.

The **incubation period** and the period of communicability are unknown.

DIAGNOSTIC TESTS: Microscopic examination of fluids that ordinarily are sterile can yield presumptive evidence of infections by streptococci and enterococci. Diagnosis is established by culture and serogrouping of the isolate, using group-specific antisera. Identification of the *Enterococcus* species may be useful to predict antimicrobial susceptibility. In some circumstances, biochemical testing may be necessary to accurately identify the organism. Antimicrobial susceptibility testing of enterococci isolated from sterile sites is important to determine ampicillin and vancomycin hydrochloride susceptibility as well as gentamicin sulfate susceptibility to assess potential of gentamicin for synergy with ampicillin. Some automated methods may not detect vancomycin resistance. Disk diffusion methods are not always reliable for determination of vancomycin susceptibility.

TREATMENT: For most streptococcal infections, treatment with penicillin G alone is adequate. However, for penicillin-resistant isolates, options include penicillin and gentamicin, other β-lactam agents, and vancomycin. Enterococci and some streptococcal strains (especially viridans streptococci and nutritionally variant streptococci requiring growth media additives) are resistant to penicillin. Enterococci uniformly are resistant to cephalosporins and may be resistant to ampicillin and vancomycin as well, making treatment challenging. In invasive enterococcal infections, including endocarditis and meningitis, ampicillin or vancomycin in combination with an aminoglycoside (usually gentamicin), for synergy and for bactericidal activity, should be administered until in vitro susceptibility is established and appropriate combination therapy can be selected. Quinupristin-dalfopristin has been licensed for adults for treatment of infections attributable to vancomycin-resistant *E faecium*. Quinupristin-dalfopristin is not effective against *E faecalis*. Linezolid is licensed for use in adults for treatment of vancomycin-resistant enterococcal infections, including *E faecium* and *E fecalis*.

Endocarditis. Guidelines for antimicrobial therapy in adults have been formulated by the American Heart Association and should be consulted for regimens that may be appropriate for children and adolescents.*

---

* Wilson WR, Karchmer AW, Dajani AS, et al. Antibiotic treatment of adults with infective endocarditis due to streptococci, enterococci, staphylococci, and HACEK microorganisms. *JAMA.* 1995;274:1706–1713

ISOLATION OF THE HOSPITALIZED PATIENT: Standard precautions are recommended. For patients with infection or colonization attributable to vancomycin-resistant enterococci (VRE), standard and contact precautions are indicated. The duration of isolation may vary by institution. Common practice is to maintain precautions until the patient no longer harbors the organism. Negative culture results from body fluid or tissue specimens from multiple sites (may include stool or rectal swab, perineal area, axilla or umbilicus, wound, and indwelling urinary catheter or colostomy sites, if present) on at least 3 separate occasions (more than 1 week apart) define resolution of VRE colonization.

CONTROL MEASURES: Patients with valvular or congenital heart disease should receive antimicrobial prophylaxis to prevent endocarditis at the time of dental and other selected surgical procedures (see Prevention of Bacterial Endocarditis, p 778). Use of vancomycin and treatment with broad-spectrum antimicrobial agents are risk factors for colonization and infection with VRE. Hospitals should develop institution-specific guidelines for the proper use of vancomycin.*

Strongyloidiasis
(Strongyloides stercoralis)

CLINICAL MANIFESTATIONS: Asymptomatic infection accompanied by peripheral blood eosinophilia may be the only manifestation of infection. Hence, strongyloidiasis warrants consideration whenever eosinophilia (blood eosinophil concentration >500/μL) without an obvious cause occurs in a patient who has resided in an endemic area. Infective larvae entering the body produce transient pruritic papules at the site of penetration of the skin, usually on the feet. Larval migration through lungs can cause pneumonitis with a cough productive of blood-streaked sputum. The intestinal phase of infection can be accompanied by vague abdominal pain, distention, vomiting, and diarrhea that may be mucoid and voluminous. Malabsorption has been reported. Larval migration from defecated stool can result in pruritic skin lesions in the perianal area, buttocks, and upper thighs. Lesions may present as migrating, pruritic, serpiginous, erythematous tracks called *larva currens*. In immunocompromised patients, particularly patients receiving corticosteroids, and less commonly in people who are malnourished, alcoholic, or infected with human T-lymphotropic virus type I, complications include disseminated strongyloidiasis (caused by hyperinfection), diffuse pulmonary infiltrates, and septicemia or meningitis from enteric gram-negative bacilli.

ETIOLOGY: *Strongyloides stercoralis* is a nematode (roundworm).

EPIDEMIOLOGY: Strongyloidiasis is endemic in the tropics and subtropics, including the southern and southwestern United States, wherever suitable moist soil and improper disposal of human waste coexist. Humans are the principal hosts. Dogs,

---

* Centers for Disease Control and Prevention. Recommendations for preventing the spread of vancomycin resistance: recommendations of the Hospital Infection Control Practices Advisory Committee (HICPAC). *MMWR Recomm Rep.* 1995;44(RR-12):1–13

cats, and other animals also can be reservoirs. Transmission involves penetration of the skin by infective (filariform) larvae from contact with infected soil or auto-infection. Infections rarely can be acquired from intimate skin contact or from inadvertent coprophagy, such as from ingestion of contaminated food scavenged from garbage. Because some larvae mature into infective forms in the colon, autoinfection can occur. Larvae are transported to lungs, from which they migrate to the trachea and eventually are swallowed. Adult females lodge in the lamina propria of the duodenum and proximal jejunum, where they lay eggs that become free-living rhabditiform larvae that generally pass into the external environment in feces. Because of internal autoinfection, patients may remain infected for decades. In immunocompromised patients, autoinfection is more common, resulting in disseminated strongyloidiasis, wherein organs and tissues are hyperinfected with larvae, and the number of adult worms in the small intestine is high.

The **incubation period** in humans is unknown.

DIAGNOSTIC TESTS: Stool examination may disclose characteristic larvae, but several fresh stool specimens may need to be examined. Stool concentration procedures may be required. Examination of duodenal contents obtained by a commercially available string test (Entero-Test [HDC Corporation, San Jose, CA]) or a direct aspirate through a flexible endoscope may demonstrate larvae. Serodiagnosis can be helpful but is available only in a few reference laboratories, and false-negative results occur. The enzyme immunoassay for antibodies is positive in approximately 85% of infected people; however, serologic cross-reactions with filarial infections limits specificity of serodiagnosis. Eosinophilia (blood eosinophil count >500/μL) is common. In disseminated strongyloidiasis, larvae can be found in the sputum.

TREATMENT: Treatment with ivermectin or thiabendazole is curative in most patients, but these drugs are not recommended for use during pregnancy (see Drugs for Parasitic Infections, p 744). Common adverse effects of thiabendazole are nausea, vomiting, and malaise. If treatment is required for heavy infection during pregnancy, ivermectin would be the drug of choice. Treatment with ivermectin is associated with exceedingly low risks of adverse effects. Treatment may need to be repeated or prolonged in the hyperinfection syndrome or in immunocompromised patients. Relapses occur and should be treated with the same drugs.

ISOLATION OF THE HOSPITALIZED PATIENT: Standard precautions are recommended.

CONTROL MEASURES: Sanitary disposal measures for human waste should be followed. Education about the risk of infection through bare skin is important.

For a patient who has an immunologic defect or who requires immunosuppressive therapy and is from an endemic region, examination of stool and, possibly, duodenal fluid and respiratory tract secretions for *S stercoralis* should be considered before immunosuppressive therapy is started. Serologic tests seem to be most sensitive for diagnosis but do not distinguish between past and current infection, and results from a reference laboratory may not be available immediately. If a patient's status requires initiation of immunosuppressive therapy before results of diagnostic tests can be obtained, the risks of empiric antiparasitic therapy for strongyloidiasis must be weighed against the risks of a disseminated infection.

Syphilis

CLINICAL MANIFESTATIONS:

Congenital Syphilis. Intrauterine infection can result in stillbirth, hydrops fetalis, or prematurity. Infants may have hepatosplenomegaly, snuffles, lymphadenopathy, mucocutaneous lesions, osteochondritis and pseudoparalysis, edema, rash, hemolytic anemia, or thrombocytopenia at birth or within the first months of life. Untreated infants, regardless of whether they have manifestations in early infancy, may develop late manifestations, which usually appear after 2 years of age and involve the central nervous system (CNS), bones and joints, teeth, eyes, and skin. Some consequences of intrauterine infection may not become apparent until many years after birth, such as interstitial keratitis (5–20 years of age), eighth cranial nerve deafness (10–40 years of age), Hutchinson teeth (peg-shaped, notched central incisors), anterior bowing of the shins, frontal bossing, mulberry molars, saddle nose, rhagades, and Clutton joints (symmetric, painless swelling of the knees). The first 3 manifestations are referred to as the Hutchinson triad.

Acquired Syphilis. Infection can be divided into 3 stages. The **primary stage** appears as one or more painless indurated ulcers (chancres) of the skin or mucous membranes at the site of inoculation. These lesions most commonly appear on the genitalia. The **secondary stage,** beginning 1 to 2 months later, is characterized by rash, mucocutaneous lesions, and lymphadenopathy. The polymorphic maculopapular rash is generalized and typically includes the palms and soles. In moist areas around the vulva or anus, hypertrophic papular lesions (condylomata lata) can occur. Generalized lymphadenopathy, fever, malaise, splenomegaly, sore throat, headache, and arthralgia can be present. A variable latent period follows but sometimes is interrupted during the first few years by recurrences of symptoms of secondary syphilis. **Latent** syphilis is defined as the period after infection when patients are seroreactive but demonstrate no clinical manifestations of disease. Latent syphilis acquired within the preceding year is referred to as *early latent syphilis;* all other cases of latent syphilis are *late latent syphilis* or *syphilis of unknown duration.* The tertiary stage of infection refers to gumma formation and cardiovascular involvement but not neurosyphilis. The tertiary stage can be marked by aortitis or gummatous changes of the skin, bone, or viscera, occurring from years to decades after the primary infection. Neurosyphilis is defined as infection of the central nervous system with *Treponema pallidum.* Manifestations of neurosyphilis can occur at any stage of infection, especially in people infected with human immunodeficiency virus (HIV).

ETIOLOGY: *Treponema pallidum* is a thin, motile spirochete that is extremely fastidious, surviving only briefly outside the host. The organism has not been cultivated successfully on artificial media.

EPIDEMIOLOGY: Syphilis, which is rare in much of the industrialized world, persists in the United States and in developing countries. The incidence of acquired and congenital syphilis increased dramatically in the United States during the late 1980s and early 1990s but subsequently decreased. Rates of infection remain disproportionately high in large urban areas and the rural South of the United States. In adults, syphilis is more common among people with HIV infection.

Congenital syphilis is contracted from an infected mother via transplacental transmission of *T pallidum* at any time during pregnancy or at birth. Among women with untreated early syphilis, 40% of pregnancies result in spontaneous abortion, stillbirth, or perinatal death. Infection can be transmitted to the fetus at any stage of disease; the rate of transmission is 60% to 100% during secondary syphilis and slowly decreases with time. The moist secretions of congenital syphilis are highly infectious. However, organisms rarely are found in lesions more than 24 hours after treatment has begun.

Acquired syphilis almost always is contracted through direct sexual contact with ulcerative lesions of the skin or mucous membranes of infected people. Sexual abuse must be suspected in any young child with acquired syphilis. Open, moist lesions of the primary or secondary stages are highly infectious. Relapses of secondary syphilis with infectious mucocutaneous lesions can occur up to 4 years after primary infection.

The **incubation period** for acquired primary syphilis typically is 3 weeks but ranges from 10 to 90 days.

DIAGNOSTIC TESTS: Definitive diagnosis is made when spirochetes are identified by microscopic darkfield examination or direct fluorescent antibody tests of lesion exudate or tissue, such as placenta or umbilical cord. Specimens should be scraped from moist mucocutaneous lesions or aspirated from a regional lymph node. Specimens from mouth lesions require direct fluorescent antibody techniques to distinguish *T pallidum* from nonpathogenic treponemes. Because false-negative microscopic results are common, serologic testing often is necessary. Polymerase chain reaction tests and immunoglobulin (Ig) M immunoblotting have been developed but are not yet available commercially.

Presumptive diagnosis is possible using nontreponemal and treponemal tests. The use of only 1 type of test is insufficient for diagnosis, because false-positive nontreponemal test results occur with various medical conditions, and false-positive treponemal test results occur with other spirochetal diseases.

The standard nontreponemal tests for syphilis include the Venereal Disease Research Laboratory (VDRL) slide test, the rapid plasma reagin (RPR) test, and the automated reagin test (ART). These tests measure antibody directed against lipoidal antigen from *T pallidum,* antibody interaction with host tissues, or both. These tests are inexpensive and rapidly performed and provide quantitative results. Quantitative results help define disease activity and monitor response to therapy. Nontreponemal test results may be falsely negative (ie, nonreactive) with early primary syphilis, latent acquired syphilis of long duration, and late congenital syphilis. Occasionally, a nontreponemal test performed on serum samples containing high concentrations of antibody against *T pallidum* will be weakly reactive or falsely negative, a reaction termed the *prozone* phenomenon. This reaction usually can be detected by experienced laboratory technicians; diluting serum results in a positive test result. When nontreponemal tests are used to monitor treatment response, the same specific test (eg, VDRL, RPR, or ART) must be used throughout the follow-up period, preferably by the same laboratory. This helps to ensure comparability of results.

A reactive nontreponemal test from a patient with typical lesions indicates the need for treatment. However, any reactive nontreponemal test must be confirmed by one of the specific treponemal tests to exclude a false-positive test result. False-positive results can be caused by certain viral infections (eg, infectious mononucleosis, hepatitis, varicella, and measles), lymphoma, tuberculosis, malaria, endocarditis, connective tissue disease, pregnancy, abuse of injection drugs, laboratory or technical error, or Wharton jelly contamination when cord blood specimens are used. Treatment should not be delayed while awaiting the results of the treponemal test results if the patient is symptomatic or at high risk of infection. A sustained fourfold decrease in titer of the nontreponemal test result after treatment demonstrates adequate therapy; a fourfold increase in titer after treatment suggests reinfection or relapse. The quantitative nontreponemal test result usually becomes nonreactive within 1 year after successful therapy if the initial titer was low (≤1:8) and the infection (primary or secondary syphilis) was treated early. The patient usually becomes seronegative within 2 years even if the initial titer was high or the infection was congenital. Some people will continue to have low nontreponemal antibody titers despite effective therapy. The serofast state is more common in patients treated for latent or tertiary syphilis.

Treponemal tests currently in use are fluorescent treponemal antibody absorption (FTA-ABS) and *T pallidum* particle agglutination (TP-PA) tests. People who have positive FTA-ABS and TP-PA test results usually remain reactive for life, even after successful therapy. Treponemal test antibody titers correlate poorly with disease activity and should not be used to assess response to therapy.

Treponemal tests also are not 100% specific for syphilis; positive reactions variably occur in patients with other spirochetal diseases, such as yaws, pinta, leptospirosis, rat-bite fever, relapsing fever, and Lyme disease. Nontreponemal tests can be used to differentiate Lyme disease from syphilis, because the VDRL is nonreactive in Lyme disease.

Usually, a serum nontreponemal test is obtained initially, and if it is reactive, a treponemal test is performed. The probability of syphilis is high in a sexually active person whose serum is reactive on both nontreponemal and treponemal tests. Differentiating syphilis treated in the past from reinfection often is difficult unless the nontreponemal titer is increasing.

In summary, nontreponemal antibody tests (VDRL, RPR, and ART) are used for screening, and treponemal tests (FTA-ABS and TP-PA) are used to establish a presumptive diagnosis. Quantitative nontreponemal antibody tests are useful in assessing the adequacy of therapy and in detecting reinfection and relapse. All patients who have syphilis should be tested for HIV infection.

Cerebrospinal Fluid Tests. For evaluation of possible neurosyphilis, the VDRL test should be performed on cerebrospinal fluid (CSF). In addition to VDRL testing of CSF, evaluation of CSF protein and white blood cell count is used to assess the likelihood of CNS involvement. Some experts also use the FTA-ABS test, believing it to be more sensitive although less specific than the VDRL test of CSF. Results from the VDRL test should be interpreted cautiously, because a negative result on a VDRL test of CSF does not exclude a diagnosis of neurosyphilis. Fewer data exist for the TP-PA test for CSF, and none exist for the RPR test; these tests should not be used for CSF evaluation.

Testing During Pregnancy. All women should be screened serologically for syphilis early in pregnancy with a nontreponemal test (eg, VDRL or RPR) and preferably again at delivery. In areas of high prevalence and in patients considered at high risk of syphilis, a nontreponemal serum test at the beginning of the third trimester (28 weeks' gestation) is indicated. For women treated during pregnancy, follow-up serologic testing is necessary to assess the efficacy of therapy. Low-titer false-positive nontreponemal antibody test results occasionally occur in pregnancy. The result of a positive nontreponemal antibody test should be confirmed with a treponemal antibody test (eg, FTA-ABS). When a pregnant woman has a reactive nontreponemal test result and a persistently negative treponemal test result, a false-positive test result is confirmed.

Evaluation of Newborn Infants for Congenital Infection. No newborn infant should be discharged from the hospital without determination of the mother's serologic status for syphilis. Testing of cord blood or an infant serum sample is inadequate for screening, because these test results can be nonreactive even when the mother is seropositive. All infants born to seropositive mothers require a careful examination and a quantitative nontreponemal syphilis test. The test performed on the infant should be the same as that performed on the mother to enable comparison of titer results.

An infant should be evaluated further for congenital syphilis if the maternal titer has increased fourfold, if the infant titer is fourfold greater than the mother's titer, or if the infant is symptomatic. In addition, an infant should be evaluated further if born to a mother with positive nontreponemal and treponemal test results if the mother has one or more of the following conditions:
- Syphilis untreated or inadequately treated or treatment not documented (see Treatment, p 599)
- Syphilis during pregnancy treated with a nonpenicillin regimen, such as erythromycin
- Syphilis during pregnancy treated with an appropriate penicillin regimen, but without the expected decrease in nontreponemal antibody titer after therapy
- Syphilis treated less than 1 month before delivery (because treatment failures occur and the efficacy of treatment cannot be assumed)
- Syphilis treated before pregnancy but with insufficient serologic follow-up to assess the response to treatment and current infection status

Evaluation for syphilis in an infant should include the following:
- Physical examination
- Quantitative nontreponemal serologic test of serum from the infant for syphilis (not cord blood, because false-positive and false-negative results can occur)
- A VDRL test of CSF and analysis for cells and protein concentration (see Cerebrospinal Fluid Testing, p 599, for indications)
- Long-bone radiographs (unless the diagnosis has been established otherwise)

- Complete blood cell and platelet count
- Other clinically indicated tests (eg, chest radiograph and liver function tests)

Pathologic examination of the placenta or umbilical cord using specific fluorescent antitreponemal antibody staining, if available, also is recommended.

A guide for interpretation of the results of nontreponemal and treponemal serologic tests is given in Table 3.58 (p 600). An infected infant's test may be reactive or nonreactive, depending on the timing of maternal and fetal infection, thus the emphasis on screening maternal blood. Conversely, transplacental transmission of nontreponemal and treponemal antibodies to the fetus can occur in a mother who has been treated appropriately for syphilis during pregnancy, resulting in positive test results in the uninfected newborn infant. The neonate's nontreponemal test titer in these circumstances usually reverts to negative in 4 to 6 months, whereas a positive FTA-ABS or TP-PA test result from passively acquired antibody may not become negative for 1 year or longer.

In an infant with clinical or tissue findings suggestive of congenital syphilis, a positive serum nontreponemal test result strongly supports the diagnosis regardless of the therapy the mother received during the pregnancy.

Cerebrospinal Fluid Testing. Cerebrospinal fluid should be examined in all infants who are evaluated for congenital syphilis if the infant has any of the following: (1) abnormal physical examination findings consistent with congenital syphilis; (2) a serum quantitative nontreponemal titer that is fourfold greater than the mother's titer; or (3) a positive darkfield or fluorescent antibody test result on body fluid(s). Testing of CSF also may be indicated in other situations to help determine appropriate treatment (see Evaluation of Newborn Infants for Congenital Infection, p 598, and Treatment, below). Cerebrospinal fluid also should be examined in all patients with suspected neurosyphilis or with acquired untreated syphilis of more than 1 year's duration. Abnormalities in CSF in patients with neurosyphilis include increased protein concentration and white blood cell count and a reactive VDRL test result. Some experts also recommend performing the FTA-ABS test on CSF, believing it to be more sensitive but less specific than VDRL testing of CSF for neurosyphilis. Because of the wide range of normal values for CSF white blood cell counts and protein concentrations in the newborn infant, interpretation may be difficult. Although a white blood cell count as high as 25/µL and a protein concentration greater than 150 mg/dL might be normal, some experts recommend that a white blood cell count of 5/µL and a protein concentration of 40 mg/dL be considered the upper limits of normal. A negative result on VDRL or FTA-ABS testing of CSF does not exclude congenital neurosyphilis, and that is one of the reasons why infants with proven or probable congenital syphilis require 10 days of parenteral treatment with penicillin G regardless of CSF test results.

TREATMENT*: Parenteral penicillin G remains the preferred drug for treatment of syphilis at any stage. Recommendations for penicillin G and duration of therapy vary, depending on the stage of disease and clinical manifestations. Parenteral penicillin G is the only documented effective therapy for patients who have neurosyphilis, congenital syphilis, or syphilis during pregnancy and is recommended

---

* Centers for Disease Control and Prevention. Sexually transmitted diseases treatment guidelines—United States, 2002. *MMWR Recomm Rep.* 2002;51(RR-6):1–80

Table 3.58. **Guide for Interpretation Syphilis Serologic Test Results of Mothers and Their Infants**

Nontreponemal Test Result (eg, VDRL, RPR, ART)		Treponemal Test Result (eg, MHA-TP, FTA-ABS)		Interpretation[1]
Mother	Infant	Mother	Infant	
−	−	−	−	No syphilis or incubating syphilis in the mother or infant or prozone phenomenon
+	+	−	−	No syphilis in mother (false-positive result of nontreponemal test with passive transfer to infant)
+	+ or −	+	+	Maternal syphilis with possible infant infection; mother treated for syphilis during pregnancy; or mother with latent syphilis and possible infant infection[2]
+	+	+	+	Recent or previous syphilis in the mother; possible infant infection
−	−	+	+	Mother successfully treated for syphilis before or early in pregnancy; or mother with Lyme disease, yaws, or pinta (ie, false-positive serologic test result)

VDRL indicates Venereal Disease Research Laboratory; RPR, rapid plasma reagin; ART, automated reagin test; MHA-TP, microhemagglutination test for *Treponema pallidum;* FTA-ABS, fluorescent treponemal antibody absorption; +, reactive; −, nonreactive.

[1] Table presents a guide and not a definitive interpretation of serologic test results for syphilis in mothers and their newborn infants. Maternal history is the most important aspect for interpretation of test results. Factors that should be considered include timing of maternal infection, nature and timing of maternal treatment, quantitative maternal and infant titers, and serial determination of nontreponemal test titers in both mother and infant.

[2] Mothers with latent syphilis may have nonreactive nontreponemal test results.

strongly for HIV-infected patients. Such patients always should be treated with penicillin, even if desensitization for penicillin allergy is necessary. If penicillin G cannot be given, alternate treatment recommendations can be found online (www.cdc.gov/nchstp/dstd/penicillinG.htm).

Penicillin Allergy. Skin testing for penicillin hypersensitivity with the major and minor determinants can reliably identify people at high risk of reacting to penicillin; currently, only the major determinant (benzylpenicilloyl poly-L-lysine) and penicillin G skin tests are available commercially. Testing with the major determinant of penicillin G is estimated to miss 3% to 6% of penicillin-allergic patients who are at risk of serious or fatal reactions. Thus, a cautious approach to penicillin therapy is advised when the patient cannot be tested with all of the penicillin skin test reagents. An oral or intravenous desensitization protocol for patients with a positive skin test result is available and should be performed in a hospital setting.* Oral desensitization is regarded as safer and easier to perform. Desensitization usually can be completed in approximately 4 hours, after which the first dose of penicillin can be given.

Congenital Syphilis: Newborn Infants (see Table 3.59, p 602). Infants should be treated for congenital syphilis if they have proven or probable disease demonstrated by one or more of the following: (1) physical, laboratory, or radiographic evidence of active disease; (2) positive placenta or umbilical cord test results for treponemes using DFA-TP staining or darkfield test; (3) a reactive result on VDRL testing of CSF; or (4) a serum quantitative nontreponemal titer that is at least fourfold higher than the mother's titer using the same test and preferably the same laboratory. If the mother's titer is 4 times higher than that of the infant, congenital syphilis still can be present. When an infant warrants evaluation for congenital syphilis (see Evaluation of Newborn Infants for Congenital Infection, p 598), the infant should be treated if test results cannot exclude infection, if the infant cannot be evaluated fully, or if adequate follow-up cannot be ensured.

In infants with proven or probable disease, aqueous crystalline penicillin G is preferred. The dosage should be based on chronologic, not gestational, age (see Table 3.59, p 602). Alternatively, some experts recommend penicillin G procaine for treatment of congenital syphilis; however, adequate CSF concentrations may not be achieved by this regimen. If more than 1 day of therapy is missed, the entire course should be restarted. Data supporting the use of ampicillin for the treatment of congenital syphilis are not available.

Asymptomatic infants are at minimal risk of syphilis if (1) they are born to mothers who received appropriate penicillin treatment for syphilis more than 4 weeks before delivery; (2) the mother had an appropriate serologic response to treatment (in early or high-titer syphilis, a documented fourfold or greater decrease in VDRL, RPR, or ART titer or in latent low-titer syphilis, titers remained stable and low); (3) infants have a serum quantitative nontreponemal serologic titer the same as or less than fourfold the maternal titer; and (4) the mother had no evidence of reinfection or relapse. Although a full workup may be unnecessary, these infants should be examined carefully, preferably monthly, until their nontreponemal serologic test results are negative. If this is not possible, many experts would treat such infants with a single injection of penicillin G benzathine.

Infants whose mothers received no treatment or inadequate treatment for syphilis require special consideration. Maternal treatment for syphilis is deemed inadequate if: (1) the mother's penicillin dose is unknown, undocumented, or inadequate; (2) the mother received erythromycin or any other nonpenicillin regimen during pregnancy for syphilis; (3) treatment was given within 30 days of the infant's birth; or (4) the mother's response to treatment of early or high-titer syphilis has not been established by demonstrating a fourfold decrease in titer by nontreponemal serologic testing for syphilis.

Asymptomatic infants whose quantitative nontreponemal serologic titer is the same or less than fourfold their mother's titer and born to women who received no treatment or inadequate treatment (as defined by one or more of these criteria) should be evaluated fully, including CSF examination (see Evaluation of Newborn

---

* Centers for Disease Control and Prevention. Sexually transmitted diseases treatment guidelines— United States, 2002. *MMWR Recomm Rep.* 2002;51(RR-6):1–80

Table 3.59. Recommended Treatment of Neonates (≤4 Weeks of Age) With Proven or Possible Congenital Syphilis

Clinical Status	Antimicrobial Therapy[1]
Proven or highly probable disease[2]	Aqueous crystalline penicillin G, 100 000–150 000 U/kg per day, administered as 50 000 U/kg per dose, IV, every 12 h during the first 7 days of life and every 8 h thereafter for a total of 10 days OR Penicillin G procaine,[3] 50 000 U/kg per day, IM, in a single dose for 10 days
Asymptomatic: normal CSF examination results, CBC and platelet count, and radiographic examination; and follow-up is certain with the following maternal treatment history: • (a) No penicillin treatment or inadequate or no documentation of penicillin treatment[4]; (b) mother was treated with erythromycin or other nonpenicillin regimen; (c) mother received treatment ≤4 weeks before delivery; (d) sequential serologic tests on the mother do not demonstrate a fourfold or greater decrease in a nontreponemal antibody titer	Aqueous crystalline penicillin G, IV, for 10–14 days[2] OR Penicillin G procaine,[3] 50 000 U/kg per day, IM, in a single dose for 10 days OR Clinical, serologic follow-up, and penicillin G benzathine,[3] 50 000 U/kg, IM, in a single dose
• (a) Adequate therapy given >1 mo before delivery; (b) mother's nontreponemal titers decreased fourfold after appropriate therapy for early syphilis and remained stable and low for late syphilis; (c) mother has no evidence of reinfection or relapse	Clinical, serologic follow-up, and penicillin G benzathine, 50 000 U/kg, IM, in a single dose[5]

IV indicates intravenously; IM, intramuscularly; CSF, cerebrospinal fluid; and CBC, complete blood cell.

[1] See text for details.

[2] If more than 1 day of therapy is missed, the entire course should be restarted.

[3] Penicillin G benzathine and penicillin G procaine are approved for IM administration *only*.

[4] See text for definition (includes infants in whom a serum quantitative nontreponemal serologic titer is the same or less than fourfold the maternal titer). If any part of the infant's evaluation is abnormal or not performed or if the CSF analysis is uninterpretable, the 10-day course of penicillin is required.

[5] Some experts would not treat the infant but would provide close serologic follow-up.

Infants for Congenital Infection, p 598). Some experts would treat all such infants with aqueous crystalline penicillin G (or aqueous penicillin G procaine) for 10 days, because physical examination and laboratory test results cannot reliably exclude the diagnosis in all cases. However, if the infant's physical examination, including ophthalmologic examination, CSF findings, radiographs of long bones and chest, and complete blood cell and platelet counts all are normal, some experts would treat infants in the specific circumstances given in Table 3.59 (p 602) with a single dose of penicillin G benzathine (50 000 U/kg intramuscularly). In the case in which maternal response to treatment has not been demonstrated but the mother received an appropriate regimen of penicillin therapy more than 1 month before delivery, the infant's evaluation is normal, and clinical and serologic follow-up can be ensured, some experts would give a single dose of penicillin G benzathine and continue to observe the infant.

Congenital Syphilis: Older Infants and Children. Because establishing the diagnosis of neurosyphilis is difficult, infants older than 4 weeks of age who possibly have congenital syphilis or who have neurologic involvement should be treated with aqueous crystalline penicillin, 200 000 to 300 000 U/kg per day, intravenously (administered every 6 hours), for 10 days. This regimen also should be used to treat children older than 1 year of age who have late and previously untreated congenital syphilis. Some experts also suggest giving such patients penicillin G benzathine, 50 000 U/kg, intramuscularly, in 3 weekly doses after the 10-day course of intravenous aqueous crystalline penicillin. If the patient has minimal clinical manifestations of disease, the CSF examination is normal, and the result of the VDRL test of CSF is negative, some experts would treat with 3 weekly doses of penicillin G benzathine (50 000 U/kg, intramuscularly).

Syphilis in Pregnancy. Regardless of the stage of pregnancy, patients should be treated with penicillin according to the dosage schedules appropriate for the stage of syphilis as recommended for nonpregnant patients. For women with early acquired syphilis, some experts recommend 2 doses of penicillin G benzathine (2.4 million U each, intramuscularly) given 1 week apart, rather than 1 dose. For penicillin-allergic patients, no proven alternative therapy has been established. A pregnant woman with a history of penicillin allergy should be treated with penicillin after desensitization. In some patients, skin testing may be helpful. Desensitization should be performed in consultation with a specialist and only in facilities in which emergency assistance is available (see Penicillin Allergy, p 600).

Erythromycin or any other nonpenicillin treatment of syphilis during pregnancy cannot be considered reliable to cure infection in the fetus. Tetracycline is not recommended for pregnant women because of potential adverse effects on the fetus.

Early Acquired Syphilis (Primary, Secondary, Early Latent Syphilis). A single intramuscular dose of penicillin G benzathine is the preferred treatment for children and adults (see Table 3.60, p 604). All children should have a CSF examination before treatment to exclude a diagnosis of neurosyphilis. Evaluation of CSF in adolescents and adults is necessary only if clinical signs or symptoms of neurologic or ophthalmic involvement are present. Neurosyphilis should be considered in the differential diagnosis of neurologic disease in HIV-infected people.

For nonpregnant patients who are allergic to penicillin, doxycycline or tetracycline should be given for 14 days. Children younger than 8 years of age should not

Table 3.60. Recommended Treatment for Syphilis

	Children	Adults
Primary, secondary, and early latent syphilis[1]	Penicillin G benzathine,[2] 50 000 U/kg, IM, up to the adult dose of 2.4 million U in a single dose	Penicillin G benzathine, 2.4 million U, IM, in a single dose **OR** *If allergic to penicillin and not pregnant,* Doxycycline, 100 mg, orally, twice a day for 14 days **OR** Tetracycline, 500 mg, orally, 4 times/day for 14 days
Late latent syphilis or latent syphilis of unknown duration	Penicillin G benzathine, 50 000 U/kg, IM, up to the adult dose of 2.4 million U, administered as 3 single doses at 1-wk intervals (total 150 000 U/kg, up to the adult dose of 7.2 million U)	Penicillin G benzathine, 7.2 million U total, administered as 3 doses of 2.4 million U, IM, each at 1-wk intervals **OR** *If allergic to penicillin and not pregnant,* Doxycycline, 100 mg, orally, twice a day for 4 wk **OR** Tetracycline, 500 mg, orally, 4 times/day for 4 wk
Tertiary	…	Penicillin G benzathine, 7.2 million U total, administered as 3 doses of 2.4 million U, IM, at 1-wk intervals
Neurosyphilis[3]	Aqueous crystalline penicillin G, 200 000 to 300 000 U/kg per day, given every 4–6 h for 10–14 days in doses not to exceed the adult dose	Aqueous crystalline penicillin G, 18–24 million U per day, administered as 3–4 million U, IV, every 4 h for 10–14 days **OR** Penicillin G procaine,[2] 2.4 million U, IM, once daily **PLUS** probenecid, 500 mg, orally, 4 times/day, both for 10–14 days

IM indicates intramuscularly; IV, intravenously.

[1] Early latent syphilis is defined as being acquired within the preceding year.
[2] Penicillin G benzathine and penicillin G procaine are approved for IM administration *only*.
[3] Patients who are allergic to penicillin should be desensitized.

be given tetracycline or doxycycline unless the benefits of therapy are greater than the risks of dental staining (see Antimicrobial Agents and Related Therapy, p 693). Drugs other than penicillin and tetracycline do not have proven efficacy in the treatment of syphilis. Limited clinical studies, along with biologic and pharmacologic considerations, suggest ceftriaxone should be effective for early syphilis. The optimal dose and duration of ceftriaxone therapy are undefined. However, some experts recommend 1 g daily via either the intramuscular or intravenous route for 8 to 10 days (for adolescents and adults). Single-dose therapy with ceftriaxone sodium is not effective. Preliminary data suggest that azithromycin dihydrate may be effective in a single oral dose of 2 g. Because the efficacy of these therapies is not well documented, close follow-up is essential. When follow-up cannot be ensured, especially for children younger than 8 years of age, consideration must be given to hospitalization and desensitization followed by administration of penicillin G (see Penicillin Allergy, p 600).

Syphilis of More Than 1 Year's Duration (Except Neurosyphilis). Penicillin G benzathine should be given intramuscularly weekly for 3 successive weeks (see Table 3.60, p 604). In patients who are allergic to penicillin, doxycycline or tetracycline for 4 weeks should be given only if a CSF examination has excluded neurosyphilis. Children younger than 8 years of age should not be given tetracycline or doxycycline unless the benefits of therapy are greater than the risks of dental staining (see Antimicrobial Agents and Related Therapy, p 693). Performing a VDRL test of CSF, protein concentration test, and leukocyte cell count is mandatory for people with suspected neurosyphilis, people who have concurrent HIV infection, people who have failed treatment, and people receiving antimicrobial agents other than penicillin.

Neurosyphilis. The recommended regimen for adults is aqueous crystalline penicillin G, intravenously, for 10 to 14 days (see Table 3.60, p 604). If compliance with therapy can be ensured, patients may be treated with an alternative regimen of penicillin G procaine plus probenecid for 10 to 14 days. Some experts recommend following this regimen with penicillin G benzathine, 2.4 million U, intramuscularly, weekly for 1 to 3 doses. For children, aqueous crystalline penicillin G for 10 to 14 days is recommended, and some experts recommend additional therapy with penicillin G benzathine, 50 000 U/kg per dose (not to exceed 2.4 million U) in 3 single weekly doses.

If the patient has a history of allergy to penicillin, consideration should be given to desensitization, and the patient should be managed in consultation with a specialist (see Penicillin Allergy, p 600).

Other Considerations.

- Mothers of infants with congenital syphilis should be tested for other sexually transmitted diseases (STDs), including gonorrhea and *Chlamydia trachomatis,* HIV, and hepatitis B virus infection. Because of lifestyle, the mother also may be at risk of hepatitis C virus infection.
- All recent sexual contacts of people with acquired syphilis should be evaluated for other STDs as well as syphilis (see Control Measures, p 607).

- All patients with syphilis should be tested for other STDs, including HIV. Patients who have primary syphilis should be retested for HIV after 3 months if the first HIV test result is negative.
- For HIV-infected patients with syphilis, careful follow-up is essential. Patients infected with HIV who have early syphilis may be at increased risk of neurologic complications and higher rates of treatment failure with currently recommended regimens.

Follow-up and Management.

Congenital syphilis. Treated infants should have careful follow-up evaluations at 1, 2, 3, 6, and 12 months of age. Serologic nontreponemal tests should be performed 3, 6, and 12 months after conclusion of treatment or until results become nonreactive or the titer has decreased fourfold. Nontreponemal antibody titers should decrease by 3 months of age and should be nonreactive by 6 months of age if the infant was infected and adequately treated or was not infected and initially seropositive because of transplacentally acquired maternal antibody. Patients with increasing titers or with persistent stable titers, including infants with low titers at 6 to 12 months of age should be evaluated, including a CSF examination, and treated with a 10-day course of parenteral penicillin G, even if they were treated previously.

Treated infants with congenital neurosyphilis and initially positive results of VDRL tests of CSF or abnormal or uninterpretable CSF cell counts and/or protein concentrations should undergo repeated clinical evaluation and CSF examination at 6-month intervals until their CSF examination is normal. A reactive result of VDRL testing of CSF at the 6-month interval is an indication for retreatment. If white blood cell counts still are abnormal at 2 years or are not decreasing at each examination, retreatment is indicated.

Acquired syphilis. Treated pregnant women with syphilis should have quantitative nontreponemal serologic tests performed monthly for the remainder of their pregnancy. Other patients with early acquired syphilis should return for repeated quantitative nontreponemal tests at 3, 6, and 12 months after the conclusion of treatment. Patients with syphilis for more than 1 year also should undergo serologic testing 24 months after treatment. Careful follow-up serologic testing particularly is important for patients treated with antimicrobial agents other than penicillin.

Indications for Retreatment.

Primary/secondary syphilis:
- If clinical signs or symptoms persist or recur or if a fourfold increase in titer of a nontreponemal test occurs, evaluate CSF and HIV status and retreat.
- If nontreponemal titer fails to decrease fourfold within 6 months after therapy, evaluate for HIV; retreat unless follow-up for continued clinical and serologic assessment can be ensured. Some experts recommend CSF evaluation.

Latent syphilis: In the following situations, CSF examination should be performed and retreatment should be provided:
- Titers increase fourfold
- An initially high titer (>1:32) fails to decrease at least fourfold within 12 to 24 months

- Signs or symptoms attributable to syphilis develop

In all these instances, retreatment, when indicated, should be performed with 3 weekly injections of penicillin G benzathine, 2.4 U, intramuscularly, unless CSF examination indicates that neurosyphilis is present, at which time treatment for neurosyphilis should be initiated. Retreated patients should be treated with the schedules recommended for patients with syphilis for more than 1 year. In general, only 1 retreatment course is indicated. The possibility of reinfection or concurrent HIV infection always should be considered when retreating patients with early syphilis.

Patients with neurosyphilis must have periodic serologic testing, clinical evaluation at 6-month intervals, and repeated CSF examinations. If the CSF cell count has not decreased after 6 months or CSF is not entirely normal after 2 years, retreatment should be considered.

ISOLATION OF THE HOSPITALIZED PATIENT: Standard precautions are recommended for all patients, including infants with suspected or proven congenital syphilis. In addition, for infants with suspected or proven congenital syphilis, parents, visitors, hospital personnel, and medical staff should use gloves when handling the infant until 24 hours of treatment has been completed. Because moist open lesions and possibly blood are contagious in all patients with syphilis, gloves should be worn when caring for patients with primary and secondary syphilis with skin and mucous membrane lesions until 24 hours of treatment has been completed.

CONTROL MEASURES:
- All women should be screened for syphilis early in pregnancy and preferably at delivery. Women at high risk of syphilis also should be screened at 28 weeks of gestation.
- Education of patients and populations about STDs, treatment of sexual contacts, reporting of each case to local public health authorities for contact investigation and appropriate follow-up, and serologic screening of high-risk populations are indicated.
- All recent sexual contacts of a person with acquired syphilis should be identified, examined, serologically tested, and treated appropriately. Sexual contacts within the last 3 months are at high risk of early syphilis and should be treated for early acquired syphilis whether or not they are seropositive. Every effort, including physical examination and serologic testing, should be made to establish a diagnosis in these patients.
- All people, including hospital personnel, who have had close unprotected contact with a patient with early congenital syphilis before identification of the disease or during the first 24 hours of therapy should be examined clinically for the presence of lesions 2 to 3 weeks after contact. Serologic testing should be performed and repeated 3 months after contact or sooner if symptoms occur. If the degree of exposure is considered substantial, immediate treatment should be considered.

Tapeworm Diseases
(Taeniasis and Cysticercosis)

CLINICAL MANIFESTATIONS:

Taeniasis. Infection often is asymptomatic; however, mild gastrointestinal tract symptoms, such as nausea, diarrhea, and pain, can occur. Tapeworm segments can be seen migrating from the anus or feces.

Cysticercosis. Manifestations depend on the location and numbers of pork tapeworm cysts (cysticerci) and the host response. Cysts may be found anywhere in the body. The most common and serious manifestations are caused by those in the central nervous system. Cysts of *Taenia solium* in the brain (neurocysticercosis) can cause seizures, behavioral disturbances, obstructive hydrocephalus, and other neurologic signs and symptoms. Neurocysticercosis can be a leading cause of epilepsy, depending on epidemiologic circumstances. The host reaction to degenerating cysts can produce signs and symptoms of meningitis. Cysts in the spinal column can cause gait disturbance, pain, or transverse myelitis. Subcutaneous cysts produce palpable nodules, and ocular involvement can cause visual impairment.

ETIOLOGY: Taeniasis is caused by intestinal infection by the adult tapeworm, *Taenia saginata* (beef tapeworm) or *T solium* (pork tapeworm). Usually, only 1 adult worm is present in the intestine. Human cysticercosis is caused only by the larvae of *T solium (Cysticercus cellulosae).*

EPIDEMIOLOGY: These tapeworm diseases have worldwide distribution. Prevalence rates are high in areas with poor sanitation and human fecal contamination in areas where cattle graze or swine are fed. Most cases of *T solium* infection in the United States are imported from Latin America or Asia. High rates of *T saginata* infection also occur in Mexico, Argentina, Africa (especially Ethiopia), and central Europe. Taeniasis is acquired by eating undercooked beef *(T saginata)* or pork *(T solium)* that contains encysted larvae. Infection often is asymptomatic.

Cysticercosis is acquired by ingesting eggs of the pork tapeworm by hetero-infection from a contact harboring the adult tapeworm or by autoinfection. The eggs are found in human feces only, because humans are the only definitive host. The eggs liberate oncospheres in the intestine that migrate through the blood and lymphatics to tissues throughout the body, including the central nervous system, where cysts form. Although most cases of cysticercosis in the United States have been imported, cysticercosis can be acquired in the United States from tapeworm carrier cases who recently immigrated from an endemic area and still have *T solium* intestinal stage infection.

The **incubation period** for taeniasis, the time from ingestion of the larvae until segments are passed in the feces, is 2 to 3 months. For cysticercosis, the time between infection and onset of symptoms may be several years.

DIAGNOSIS: Diagnosis of taeniasis (adult tapeworm infection) is based on demonstration of the proglottids or ova in feces or the perianal region. Species identification of the parasite is based on the different structures of the terminal gravid segments.

Diagnosis of neurocysticercosis is made primarily on the basis of computed tomography (CT) scanning or magnetic resonance imaging (MRI) of the brain or spinal cord. The enzyme immunotransfer blot assay that detects antibody to *T solium* in serum and cerebrospinal fluid (CSF) is the antibody test of choice. This test is available through the Centers for Disease Control and Prevention and several commercial laboratories. The test is more sensitive with serum specimens than with CSF specimens. Serum antibody assay results often are negative in children with solitary parenchymal lesions but usually are positive in patients with multiple lesions.

TREATMENT:

Taeniasis. Praziquantel is highly effective for eradicating infection with the adult tapeworm, and niclosamide is an alternative (see Drugs for Parasitic Infections, p 744).

Cysticercosis. Neurocysticercosis treatment should be individualized on the basis of the number and viability of cysticerci as assessed by neuroimaging studies (MRI or CT scan) and where they are located. For patients with only nonviable cysts (eg, only calcifications on CT scan), management should be aimed at symptoms and should include anticonvulsants for patients with seizures and insertion of shunts for patients with hydrocephalus. Two antiparasitic drugs, albendazole and praziquantel, are available. Although both drugs are cysticercidal and hasten radiologic resolution of cysts, most symptoms result from the host inflammatory response and may be exacerbated by treatment. In some clinical trials, patients treated with albendazole had better radiologic and clinical responses than patients treated with low doses of praziquantel. However, neither drug has been proven better than placebo in controlled trials. Several studies have indicated that patients with single inflamed cysts within the brain parenchyma do well without antiparasitic therapy, and most experts do not recommend antiparasitic therapy. However, many experts recommend therapy for patients with nonenhancing or multiple cysticerci. Coadministration of corticosteroids for the first 2 to 3 days of therapy may decrease adverse effects and is recommended for patients with multiple cysts and associated cerebral edema (cysticercal encephalitis). Antiparasitic therapy should be deferred at least until cerebral edema is controlled.

Seizures may recur for months. Anticonvulsant therapy is recommended until there is neuroradiologic evidence of resolution and seizures have not occurred for 1 to 2 years. Calcification of cysts may require indefinite use of anticonvulsants. Intraventricular cysts and hydrocephalus usually require surgical therapy with placement of intraventricular shunts. Adjunctive chemotherapy with antiparasitic agents and corticosteroids may decrease the rate of subsequent shunt failure. Ocular cysticercosis is treated by surgical excision of the cysts. Ocular and spinal cysts generally are not treated with antihelmintic drugs, which can exacerbate inflammation. An ophthalmic examination should be performed before treatment to rule out intraocular cysts.

ISOLATION OF THE HOSPITALIZED PATIENT: Standard precautions are recommended.

CONTROL MEASURES: Eating raw or undercooked beef or pork should be avoided. People known to harbor the adult tapeworm of *T solium* should be treated immediately. Careful attention to hand hygiene and appropriate disposal of fecal material is important.

Examination of stool specimens obtained from food handlers who recently have emigrated from endemic countries for detection of eggs and proglottids is advisable. People traveling to developing countries with high endemic rates of cysticercosis should avoid eating uncooked vegetables and fruits that cannot be peeled.

Other Tapeworm Infections
(Including Hydatid Disease)

Ingestion of certain cestode (tapeworm) eggs or accidental contact with certain larval forms can lead to tissue infection. Most infections are asymptomatic, but nausea, abdominal pain, and diarrhea have been observed in people who are heavily infected.

Hymenolepis nana. This tapeworm, also called dwarf tapeworm because it is the smallest of the adult tapeworms, has its entire cycle within humans. Therefore, direct person-to-person transmission is possible. More problematic is autoinfection, which tends to perpetuate the infection in the host, because the eggs can hatch within the intestine and reinitiate the cycle, leading to development of new worms and a large worm burden. This cycle makes eradicating the infection with praziquantel difficult. If infection persists after treatment, retreatment with praziquantel is indicated.

Dipylidium caninum. This tapeworm is the most common and widespread adult tapeworm of dogs and cats. *Dipylidium caninum* infects children when they inadvertently swallow a dog or cat flea, which serves as the intermediate host. Diagnosis is made by finding the characteristic eggs or motile tapeworm segments in stool. Tapeworm segments resemble rice kernels. Therapy with praziquantel is effective. Niclosamide is an alternative therapeutic option.

Diphyllobothrium latum *(and related species).* This tapeworm, also called fish tapeworm, has fish as one of its intermediate hosts. Consumption of infected, raw freshwater fish (including salmon) leads to infection. Three to 5 weeks are needed for the adult tapeworm to mature and begin to lay eggs. The worm sometimes causes mechanical obstruction of the bowel or diarrhea, abdominal pain, or rarely, megaloblastic anemia secondary to vitamin B_{12} deficiency. The diagnosis is made by recognition of the characteristic eggs or proglottids passed in stool. Therapy with praziquantel is effective, and niclosamide is an alternative.

Echinococcus granulosus *and* Echinococcus multilocularis. The larval forms of these tapeworms are the causes of hydatid disease. The distribution of *Echinococcus granulosus* is related to sheep or cattle herding. Countries with the highest prevalence include Argentina, China, Greece, Italy, Lebanon, Romania, South Africa, Spain, Syria, Turkey, and the countries in the former Soviet Union. In the United States, small endemic foci exist in Arizona, California, New Mexico, and Utah, and a strain adapted to wolves, moose, and caribou occurs in Alaska and Canada. Dogs, coyotes, wolves, dingoes, and jackals can become infected by swallowing protoscolices of the parasite within hydatid cysts in the organs of sheep or other intermediate hosts.

Dogs pass embryonated eggs in their stools, and sheep become infected by swallowing the eggs. If humans swallow *Echinococcus* eggs, they can become inadvertent intermediate hosts, and cysts can develop in various organs, such as the liver, lungs, kidney, and spleen. These cysts usually grow slowly (1 cm in diameter per year) and eventually can contain several liters of fluid. If a cyst ruptures, anaphylaxis and multiple secondary cysts from seeding of protoscolices can result. Clinical diagnosis often is difficult. A history of contact with dogs in an endemic area is helpful. Space-occupying lesions can be demonstrated by radiographs, ultrasonography, or computed tomography of various organs. Serologic tests, available at the Centers for Disease Control and Prevention, are helpful, but false-negative results occur. Surgical treatment is indicated for some patients and requires meticulous care to prevent spillage of cyst contents. Injection of scolecidal solutions into the cyst before attempted removal can minimize the risk of dissemination if spillage occurs. Treatment with albendazole for several months is of benefit in many cases.

Echinococcus multilocularis, a species for which the life cycle involves foxes, dogs, and rodents, causes the alveolar form of hydatid disease, which is characterized by invasive growth of the larvae in the liver with occasional metastatic spread. The alveolar form of hydatid disease is limited to the northern hemisphere and usually is diagnosed in people 50 years of age or older. The preferred treatment is surgical extirpation of the entire larval mass. In nonresectable cases, continuous treatment with albendazole has been associated with clinical improvement.

ISOLATION OF THE HOSPITALIZED PATIENT: Standard precautions are recommended.

CONTROL MEASURES: Preventive measures for *H nana* include educating the public about personal hygiene and sanitary disposal of feces.

Infection with *D caninum* is prevented by keeping dogs and cats free of fleas and worms.

Thorough cooking (56°C [133°F] for 5 minutes), freezing (−18°C [0°F] for 24 hours), or irradiation of freshwater fish ensures protection against *D latum.*

Control measures for prevention of *E granulosus* and *E multilocularis* include educating the public about good hand hygiene and avoiding exposure to dog feces. Prevention and control of the infection in dogs decreases the risk.

Tetanus
(Lockjaw)

CLINICAL MANIFESTATIONS: Generalized tetanus (lockjaw) is a neurologic disease that manifests as trismus and severe muscular spasms. Tetanus is caused by neurotoxin produced by the anaerobic bacterium *Clostridium tetani* in a contaminated wound. Onset is gradual, occurring over 1 to 7 days, and symptoms progress to severe generalized muscle spasms, which often are aggravated by any external stimulus. Severe spasms persist for 1 week or more and subside in a period of weeks in people who recover.

Localized tetanus manifests as local muscle spasms in areas contiguous to a wound. Cephalic tetanus is a dysfunction of cranial nerves associated with infected wounds on the head and neck. Both conditions may precede generalized tetanus.

ETIOLOGY: *Clostridium tetani,* the tetanus bacillus, is a spore-forming, anaerobic, gram-positive bacillus. This organism is a wound contaminant that causes neither tissue destruction nor an inflammatory response. The vegetative form of *C tetani* produces a potent plasmid-encoded exotoxin (tetanospasmin), which binds to gangliosides at the myoneural junction of skeletal muscle and on neuronal membranes in the spinal cord, blocking inhibitory pulses to motor neurons. The action of tetanus toxin on the brain and sympathetic nervous system is less well documented.

EPIDEMIOLOGY: Tetanus occurs worldwide and is more common in warmer climates and during warmer months, in part because of the higher frequency of contaminated wounds associated with those locations and seasons. The organism, a normal inhabitant of soil and animal and human intestines, is ubiquitous in the environment, especially where contamination by excreta is common. Wounds, recognized or unrecognized, are the sites at which the organism multiplies and elaborates toxin. Contaminated wounds, especially those with devitalized tissue and deep-puncture trauma, are at greatest risk. Neonatal tetanus is common in many developing countries where women are not immunized appropriately against tetanus and nonsterile umbilical cord-care practices are followed. Widespread active immunization against tetanus has modified the epidemiology of the disease in the United States, where fewer than 50 cases have been reported annually since 1995. Tetanus is not transmissible from person to person.

The **incubation period** ranges from 2 days to months, with most cases occurring within 14 days. In neonates, the incubation period usually is 5 to 14 days. Shorter incubation periods have been associated with more heavily contaminated wounds, more severe disease, and a worse prognosis.

DIAGNOSTIC TESTS: The diagnosis of tetanus is made clinically by excluding other causes of tetanic spasms, such as hypocalcemic tetany, phenothiazine reaction, strychnine poisoning, and hysteria. Attempts to culture *C tetani* could be made; however, the yield is poor and a negative culture does not rule out disease. A protective serum antitoxin concentration should not be used to exclude the diagnosis of tetanus.

TREATMENT:
- Human Tetanus Immune Globulin (TIG) is recommended for treatment in a single total dose of 3000 to 6000 U for children and adults. The optimum therapeutic dose has not been established, and doses as small as 500 U have been effective and cause less discomfort to the patient. Available preparations must be given intramuscularly. Some authorities recommend infiltration of part of the dose locally around the wound, although the efficacy of this approach has not been proven. Results of studies on the benefit from intrathecal TIG are conflicting. The TIG preparation in use in the United States is not licensed or formulated for intrathecal or intravenous use.

- In countries where TIG is not available, equine tetanus antitoxin may be available. This product no longer is available in the United States. Equine antitoxin is administered after appropriate testing for sensitivity and desensitization if necessary (see Sensitivity Tests for Reactions to Animal Sera, p 60, and Desensitization to Animal Sera, p 61).
- Immune Globulin Intravenous contains antibodies to tetanus and can be considered for treatment if TIG is not available. The US Food and Drug Administration has not licensed TIG for this use, and the dosage has not been determined.
- All wounds should be properly cleaned and débrided, especially if extensive necrosis is present. In neonatal tetanus, wide excision of the umbilical stump is not indicated.
- Supportive care and pharmacotherapy to control tetanic spasms are of major importance.
- Oral (or intravenous) metronidazole (30 mg/kg per day, given at 6-hour intervals; maximum 4 g/day) is effective in decreasing the number of vegetative forms of *C tetani* and is the antimicrobial agent of choice. Parenteral penicillin G (100 000 U/kg per day, given at 4- to 6-hour intervals; maximum 12 million U/day) is an alternative treatment. Therapy for 10 to 14 days is recommended.

ISOLATION OF THE HOSPITALIZED PATIENT: Standard precautions are recommended.

CONTROL MEASURES:

Care of Exposed People (see Table 3.61, p 614). After primary immunization with tetanus toxoid, antitoxin persists at protective concentrations in most people for at least 10 years and for a longer time after a booster immunization.

- The use of tetanus toxoid and TIG or antitoxin in the management of wounds depends on the nature of the wound and the history of immunization with tetanus toxoid as described in Table 3.61.
- Although any open wound is a potential source of tetanus, wounds contaminated with dirt, feces, soil, or saliva are at increased risk of contamination. Wounds containing devitalized tissue, including necrotic or gangrenous wounds, frostbite, crush and avulsion injuries, and burns particularly are prone to contamination with *C tetani*.
- If tetanus immunization is incomplete at the time of wound treatment, a dose of vaccine should be given, and the immunization series should be completed according to the primary immunization schedule. Tetanus Immune Globulin should be administered for tetanus-prone wounds in patients infected with human immunodeficiency virus, regardless of the history of tetanus immunizations.
- In usual practice, when tetanus toxoid is required for wound prophylaxis in a child 7 years of age or older, the use of adult-type diphtheria and tetanus toxoids (Td) instead of tetanus toxoid alone is advisable so that diphtheria immunity also is maintained. When a booster injection is indicated for wound

Table 3.61. Guide to Tetanus Prophylaxis in Routine Wound Management

History of Absorbed Tetanus Toxoid (Doses)	Clean, Minor Wounds		All Other Wounds[1]	
	Td[2]	TIG[3]	Td[2]	TIG[3]
<3 or unknown	Yes	No	Yes	Yes
≥3[4]	No[5]	No	No[6]	No

Td indicates adult-type diphtheria and tetanus toxoids vaccine; TIG, Tetanus Immune Globulin (human).

[1] Such as, but not limited to, wounds contaminated with dirt, feces, soil, and saliva; puncture wounds; avulsions; and wounds resulting from missiles, crushing, burns, and frostbite.

[2] For children younger than 7 years of age, diphtheria and tetanus toxoids and acellular pertussis (DTaP) vaccine is recommended; if pertussis vaccine is contraindicated, diphtheria and tetanus toxoids (DT) vaccine is given. For people 7 years of age or older, Td vaccine is recommended.

[3] Equine tetanus antitoxin should be used, if available, when TIG is not available.

[4] If only 3 doses of fluid toxoid have been received, a fourth dose of toxoid, preferably an adsorbed toxoid, should be given. Although licensed, fluid tetanus toxoid rarely is used.

[5] Yes, if more than 10 years since last dose.

[6] Yes, if more than 5 years since last dose. More frequent boosters are not needed and can accentuate adverse effects.

prophylaxis in a child younger than 7 years of age, diphtheria and tetanus toxoids and acellular pertussis vaccine (DTaP) should be used unless pertussis vaccine is contraindicated (see Pertussis, p 472), in which case immunization with diphtheria and tetanus toxoids (DT) is recommended.

- When TIG is required for wound prophylaxis, it is given intramuscularly in a dose of 250 U. Equine tetanus antitoxin is recommended if TIG is unavailable after appropriate testing of the patient for sensitivity (see Sensitivity Tests for Reactions to Animal Sera, p 60). Equine antitoxin is not available in the United States. If tetanus toxoid and TIG or equine tetanus antitoxin are given concurrently, separate syringes and sites should be used. Administration of TIG or equine tetanus antitoxin does not preclude initiation of active immunization with tetanus toxoid. Efforts should be made to initiate immunization and arrange for its completion. Administration of tetanus toxoid simultaneously or at an interval after receipt of Immune Globulin should not substantially impair development of protective antibody.

- Regardless of immunization status, dirty wounds should be properly cleaned and débrided if dirt or necrotic tissue is present. Wounds should receive prompt surgical treatment to remove all devitalized tissue and foreign material as an essential part of tetanus prophylaxis. It is not necessary or appropriate to extensively débride puncture wounds.

Immunization. Active immunization with tetanus toxoid is indicated for all people. For all indications, tetanus immunization is administered with diphtheria toxoid-containing vaccines. Vaccine is given intramuscularly and may be given concurrently with other vaccines (see Simultaneous Administration of Multiple Vaccines, p 33). *Haemophilus influenzae* type b conjugate vaccines containing tetanus toxoid (PRP-T) are not substitutes for tetanus toxoid immunization. Recommendations for use of tetanus and diphtheria toxoid-containing vaccines summarized in Fig 1.1 (p 24) and Table 1.6 (p 26) are as follows:

- Immunization for children from 2 months of age to the seventh birthday (see Fig 1.1, p 24, and Table 1.6, p 26) should consist of 5 doses of tetanus and diphtheria toxoid-containing vaccine. The initial 3 doses are given as DTaP administered at 2-month intervals beginning at approximately 2 months of age. A fourth dose is recommended 6 to 12 months after the third dose, usually at 15 to 18 months of age (see Pertussis, p 472). An additional dose of DTaP is recommended before school entry (kindergarten or elementary school) at 4 to 6 years of age, unless the fourth dose was given after the fourth birthday. The DTaP vaccine can be given concurrently with other vaccines (see Simultaneous Administration of Multiple Vaccines, p 33).

Immunization against tetanus and diphtheria for children younger than 7 years of age in whom pertussis immunization is contraindicated (see Pertussis, p 472) should be accomplished with DT instead of DTaP, as follows:

- For children younger than 1 year of age, 3 doses of DT are given at 2-month intervals; a fourth dose should be given 6 to 12 months after the third dose, and the fifth dose should be given before school entry at 4 to 6 years of age.
- For children 1 through 6 years of age who have not received previous doses of DT, DTaP, or diphtheria and tetanus toxoids and pertussis vaccine (DTP), 2 doses of DT approximately 2 months apart should be given, followed by a third dose 6 to 12 months later to complete the initial series. The DT vaccine can be given concurrently with other vaccines. An additional dose is recommended before school entry at 4 to 6 years of age unless the preceding dose was given after the fourth birthday.
- For children 1 through 6 years of age who have received 1 or 2 doses of DTaP, DTP, or DT during the first year of life and for whom further pertussis immunization is contraindicated, additional doses of DT should be given until a total of 5 doses of diphtheria and tetanus toxoids are received by the time of school entry. The fourth dose is administered 6 to 12 months after the third dose. The preschool (fifth) dose is omitted if the fourth dose was given after the fourth birthday.
- For children who have received fewer than the recommended number of doses of pertussis vaccine but who have received the recommended number of DT doses for their age (ie, those in whom immunization was started with DT and who were then given DTaP [or DTP]), dose(s) of DTaP should be given to complete the recommended pertussis immunization schedule (see Pertussis, p 472). However the total number of doses of diphtheria and tetanus toxoids (as DT, DTaP, or DTP) should not exceed 6 before the seventh birthday.

Other recommendations for tetanus and diphtheria immunization, including those for older children, are as follows:

- For children after their seventh birthday (see Table 1.6, p 26), tetanus immunization should be accomplished with Td (ie, adult-type diphtheria and tetanus toxoids). The Td preparation contains not more than 2 Lf (flocculation units) of diphtheria toxoid per dose, compared with 6.7 to 25.0 Lf per dose in the DTaP and DT preparations for use in infants and younger children. Because of the lower dose of diphtheria toxoid, the Td vaccine is less likely than DTaP or DT to produce adverse reactions in older children and adults.

Two doses are given 1 to 2 months apart; a third dose should be given 6 to 12 months after the second.

- After the initial immunization series is completed at 4 to 6 years of age, a booster dose of diphtheria and tetanus toxoids (given as Td) is recommended at 11 to 12 years of age, and should be given no later than by 16 years of age, and every 10 years thereafter. This 10-year period is determined from the time that the last dose was administered, regardless of whether it was given earlier as a routine childhood immunization or as part of wound management. Because the immunity conferred by adsorbed preparations of tetanus toxoid has proved to be of long duration, routine boosters more often than every 10 years are not indicated and may be associated with an increased incidence and severity of adverse reactions.
- If more than 5 years have elapsed since the last dose, a booster of Td should be considered for people who are going on wilderness expeditions where tetanus boosters may not be readily available.
- Prevention of neonatal tetanus can be accomplished by prenatal immunization of the previously unimmunized mother. Pregnant women who have not completed their primary series should do so before delivery if time permits. If there is insufficient time, 2 doses of Td should be administered at least 4 weeks apart, and the second dose should be given at least 2 weeks before delivery. Immunization with tetanus toxoid or Td is not contraindicated during pregnancy.
- Active immunization against tetanus always should be undertaken during convalescence from tetanus, because this exotoxin-mediated disease usually does not confer immunity.

Adverse Events, Precautions, and Contraindications. Severe anaphylactic reactions, Guillain-Barré syndrome, and brachial neuritis attributable to tetanus toxoid have been reported but are rare. No increased risk of Guillain-Barré syndrome has been observed with use of DTaP vaccine in children, and therefore, no special precautions are recommended when immunizing children with a history of Guillain-Barré syndrome.

An immediate anaphylactic reaction to tetanus and diphtheria toxoid-containing vaccine (ie, DTaP, DT, or Td) is a contraindication to further doses unless the patient can be desensitized to these toxoids (see Pertussis, p 472). Because of uncertainty about which vaccine component (ie, diphtheria, tetanus, or pertussis) might be responsible and the importance of tetanus immunization, people who experience anaphylactic reactions may be referred to an allergist for evaluation and possible desensitization.

Other Control Measures. Sterilization of hospital supplies will prevent the rare instances of tetanus that may occur in a hospital from contaminated sutures, instruments, or plaster casts.

For prevention of neonatal tetanus, preventive measures (in addition to maternal immunization) include community immunization programs for adolescent girls and women of childbearing age and appropriate training of midwives in recommendations for immunization and sterile technique.

Tinea Capitis
(Ringworm of the Scalp)

CLINICAL MANIFESTATIONS: Fungal infection of the scalp may manifest as one of the following distinct clinical syndromes:
- Patchy areas of dandruff-like scaling, with subtle or extensive hair loss, which easily is confused with dandruff, seborrheic dermatitis, or atopic dermatitis
- Discrete areas of hair loss studded by stubs of broken hairs, which is referred to as *black-dot ringworm*
- Numerous discrete pustules or excoriations with little hair loss or scaling
- Kerion, a boggy inflammatory mass surrounded by follicular pustules, is a hypersensitivity reaction to the fungal infection. Kerion may be accompanied by fever and local lymphadenopathy and commonly is misdiagnosed as impetigo, cellulitis, or an abscess of the scalp.

A pruritic, fine, papulovesicular eruption (dermatophytid or id reaction) involving the trunk, hands, or face caused by a hypersensitivity response to the infecting fungus, may accompany scalp lesions.

Tinea capitis may be confused with many other diseases, including seborrheic dermatitis, atopic dermatitis, psoriasis, alopecia areata, trichotillomania, folliculitis, impetigo, and lupus erythematosus.

ETIOLOGY: *Trichophyton tonsurans* is the cause of tinea capitis in more than 90% of cases in North and Central America. *Microsporum canis, Microsporum audouinii,* and *Trichophyton mentagrophytes* are less common. The causative agents may vary in different geographic areas.

EPIDEMIOLOGY: Infection of the scalp with *T tonsurans* results from person-to-person transmission. Although the organism remains viable on combs, hairbrushes, and other fomites for long periods of time, the role of fomites in transmission has not been defined. Occasionally, *T tonsurans* is cultured from the scalp of asymptomatic children and is cultured readily from asymptomatic family members of infected people. Asymptomatic people who harbor the organism are thought to have a significant role as reservoirs for infection and reinfection within families, schools, and communities. Tinea capitis attributable to *T tonsurans* occurs most commonly in children between the ages of 3 and 9 years and seems to be more common in black children.

Microsporum canis infection results from animal-to-human transmission. Infection often is the result of contact with household pets.

The **incubation period** is unknown.

DIAGNOSTIC TESTS: Hairs may be obtained by gentle scraping of a moistened area of the scalp with a blunt scalpel, toothbrush, or tweezers for potassium hydroxide wet mount examination and culture. In black-dot ringworm, broken hairs should be obtained for diagnosis. In cases of *T tonsurans* infection, microscopic examination of a potassium hydroxide wet mount preparation will disclose numerous arthroconidia within the hair shaft. In *Microsporum* infection, spores surround the hair shaft. Use of dermatophyte test medium also is a reliable, simple, and inexpensive method of diagnosing tinea capitis. Skin scrapings, brushings, or hairs from lesions are inoculated directly onto culture medium and incubated at room temperature. After 1 to 2 weeks, a phenol red indicator in the agar will turn from yellow to red in the area surrounding a dermatophyte colony. When necessary, the diagnosis also may be confirmed by culture on Sabouraud dextrose agar by direct plating technique or by moistened cotton-tipped applicators or by Culturettes (Becton Dickinson and Co, Franklin Lakes, NJ) transported to reference laboratories.

Examination of hair of patients with *Microsporum* infection using Wood light results in brilliant green fluorescence. However, because *T tonsurans* does not fluoresce under Wood light, this diagnostic test is not helpful for most patients with tinea capitis.

TREATMENT: Topical antifungal medications are not effective for treatment of tinea capitis. Tinea capitis requires systemic antifungal therapy. Microsize griseofulvin is given orally, 15 to 20 mg/kg per day (maximum 1 g), once daily. The dose of ultramicrosize griseofulvin is 5 to 10 mg/kg per day (maximum 750 mg), once daily. Optimally, griseofulvin is given after a meal containing fat (eg, peanut butter or ice cream). Treatment for 4 to 6 weeks usually is required and should be continued 2 weeks beyond clinical resolution. Some children may require higher doses of microsize griseofulvin (20–25 mg/kg per day) or the ultramicrosize drug formulation to achieve clinical cure. Treatment with oral itraconazole, oral terbinafine hydrochloride, or oral fluconazole also is effective for tinea capitis, but these products have not been licensed by the US Food and Drug Administration for this indication. Selenium sulfide shampoo, either 1% or 2.5%, used twice a week, decreases fungal shedding and may help curb the spread of infection.

Kerion is treated with griseofulvin. Corticosteroid therapy consisting of prednisone or prednisolone given orally in dosages of 1.5 to 2 mg/kg per day (maximum 20 mg/day) may be used in addition. Treatment with corticosteroids should be continued for approximately 2 weeks, with tapering doses toward the end of therapy. Antimicrobial agents generally are not needed, except if there is suspected secondary infection, and surgery is not indicated.

ISOLATION OF THE HOSPITALIZED PATIENT: Standard precautions are recommended.

CONTROL MEASURES: Early treatment of infected people is indicated, as is examination of siblings and other household contacts for evidence of tinea capitis. Ribbons, combs, and hairbrushes should not be shared by family members.

Children receiving treatment for tinea capitis may attend school if they are using a topical treatment, such as selenium sulfide shampoo, to decrease shedding. Hair cuts, shaving of the head, or wearing a cap during treatment are unnecessary.

Tinea Corporis
(Ringworm of the Body)

CLINICAL MANIFESTATIONS: Superficial tinea infections of the nonhairy (glabrous) skin may involve the face, trunk, or limbs but not the scalp, beard, groin, hands, or feet. The lesion generally is circular (hence, the term "ringworm"), slightly erythematous, and well demarcated with a scaly, vesicular, or pustular border. Pruritus is common. Lesions often are mistaken for atopic, seborrheic, or contact dermatitis. A frequent source of confusion is an alteration in the appearance of lesions resulting from application of a topical corticosteroid preparation, termed *tinea incognita.* In patients with diminished T-lymphocyte function (eg, human immunodeficiency virus infection), the rash may appear as grouped papules or pustules unaccompanied by scaling or erythema.

A pruritic, fine, papulovesicular eruption (dermatophytic or id reaction) involving the trunk, hands, or face, caused by a hypersensitivity response to infecting fungus, may accompany the rash.

ETIOLOGY: The prime causes of the disease are fungi of the genus *Trichophyton,* especially *Trichophyton rubrum, Trichophyton mentagrophytes,* and *Trichophyton tonsurans;* the genus *Microsporum,* especially *Microsporum canis;* and *Epidermophyton floccosum.*

EPIDEMIOLOGY: These causative fungi occur worldwide and are transmissible by direct contact with infected humans, animals, or fomites. Fungi in lesions are communicable.

The **incubation period** is unknown.

DIAGNOSIS: The fungi responsible for tinea corporis can be detected by microscopic examination of a potassium hydroxide wet mount of skin scrapings. Use of dermatophyte test medium also is a reliable, simple, and inexpensive method of diagnosis. Skin scrapings from lesions are inoculated directly onto culture medium and incubated at room temperature. After 1 to 2 weeks, a phenol red indicator in the agar will turn from yellow to red in the area surrounding a dermatophyte colony. When necessary, the diagnosis also can be confirmed by culture on Sabouraud dextrose agar.

TREATMENT: Topical application of a miconazole nitrate, clotrimazole, terbinafine, tolnaftate, naftifine hydrochloride, or ciclopirox olamine preparation twice a day or of a ketoconazole, econazole nitrate, oxiconazole nitrate, butenafine hydrochloride, or sulconazole nitrate preparation once a day is recommended (see Topical Drugs for Superficial Fungal Infections, p 726). Although clinical resolution may be evident within 2 weeks of therapy, a minimum duration of 4 weeks generally is indicated. Topical preparations of antifungal medication mixed with high-potency corticosteroids should not be used, because corticosteroids can cause striae and atrophy of the skin.

If lesions are extensive or unresponsive to topical therapy, griseofulvin is administered orally for 4 weeks (see Tinea Capitis, p 617). Oral itraconazole, fluconazole, and terbinafine may be effective alternative therapies for tinea corporis, but these products are not licensed by the US Food and Drug Administration for this indication.

ISOLATION OF THE HOSPITALIZED PATIENT: Standard precautions are recommended.

CONTROL MEASURES: Direct contact with known or suspected sources of infection should be avoided. Periodic inspections of contacts for early lesions and prompt therapy are recommended.

Tinea Cruris
(Jock Itch)

CLINICAL MANIFESTATIONS: Tinea cruris is a common superficial fungal disorder of the groin and upper thighs. The eruption is marginated sharply and usually is bilaterally symmetric. Involved skin is erythematous and scaly and varies from red to brown; occasionally, the eruption is accompanied by central clearing and a vesiculopapular border. In chronic infections, the margin may be subtle, and lichenification may be present. Tinea cruris skin lesions may be extremely pruritic. These lesions should be differentiated from intertrigo, seborrheic dermatitis, psoriasis, primary irritant dermatitis, allergic contact dermatitis (generally caused by the therapeutic agents applied to the area), or erythrasma, which is a superficial bacterial infection of the skin caused by *Corynebacterium minutissimum.*

ETIOLOGY: The fungi *Epidermophyton floccosum, Trichophyton rubrum,* and *Trichophyton mentagrophytes* are the most common causes.

EPIDEMIOLOGY: Tinea cruris occurs predominantly in adolescent and adult males, mainly via indirect contact from desquamated epithelium or hair. Moisture, close-fitting garments, friction, and obesity are predisposing factors. Direct or indirect person-to-person transmission may occur. This infection commonly occurs in association with tinea pedis.

The **incubation period** is unknown.

DIAGNOSTIC TESTS: The fungi responsible for tinea cruris may be detected by microscopic examination of a potassium hydroxide wet mount of scales. Use of dermatophyte test medium also is a reliable, simple, and inexpensive method of diagnosing tinea cruris. Skin scrapings from lesions are inoculated directly onto culture medium and incubated at room temperature. After 1 to 2 weeks, a phenol red indicator in the agar will turn from yellow to red in the area surrounding a dermatophyte colony. When necessary, the diagnosis also can be confirmed by culture on Sabouraud dextrose agar. A characteristic coral-red fluorescence under Wood light can identify the presence of erythrasma and, thus, exclude tinea cruris.

TREATMENT: Topical application for 4 to 6 weeks of a clotrimazole, haloprogin, miconazole nitrate, terbinafine, tolnaftate, or ciclopirox olamine preparation gently rubbed into the affected areas and surrounding skin twice daily or a topical econazole nitrate, ketoconazole, naftifine hydrochloride, oxiconazole nitrate, butenafine, or sulconazole nitrate preparation once daily is effective (see Topical Drugs for Superficial Fungal Infections, p 726). Tinea pedis, if present, should be treated concurrently (see Tinea Pedis, p 621).

Topical preparations of antifungal medication mixed with high-potency corticosteroids should not be used, because corticosteroids can cause striae and atrophy of the skin. Loose-fitting, washed, cotton underclothes to decrease chafing as well as the use of a bland absorbent powder can be helpful adjuvants to therapy. Griseofulvin, given orally for 2 to 6 weeks, may be effective in unresponsive cases (see Tinea Capitis, p 617). Oral itraconazole, fluconazole, or terbinafine are effective alternative therapies, but these products are not licensed by the US Food and Drug Administration for treatment of tinea cruris and usually are unnecessary. Because many conditions mimic tinea cruris, a differential diagnosis should be considered if primary treatments fail.

ISOLATION OF THE HOSPITALIZED PATIENT: Standard precautions are recommended.

CONTROL MEASURES: Infections should be treated promptly. Potentially involved areas should be kept dry, and loose undergarments should be recommended. Patients should be advised to dry the groin area before drying their feet to avoid inoculating dermatophytes of tinea pedis into the groin area.

Tinea Pedis
(Athlete's Foot, Ringworm of the Feet)

CLINICAL MANIFESTATIONS: Tinea pedis manifests as fine vesiculopustular or scaly lesions that commonly are pruritic. The lesions can involve all areas of the foot, but usually they are patchy in distribution, with a predisposition to fissures and scaling between toes, particularly in the third and fourth interdigital spaces. Toenails may be infected and can be dystrophic (tinea unguium). Tinea pedis must be differentiated from dyshidrotic eczema, atopic dermatitis, contact dermatitis, juvenile plantar dermatosis, and erythrasma (a superficial bacterial infection caused by *Corynebacterium minutissimum*). Tinea pedis commonly occurs in association with tinea cruris.

Tinea pedis and many other fungal infections can be accompanied by a hypersensitivity reaction to the fungi (the dermatophytid or id reaction), with resulting vesicular eruptions on the palms and the sides of fingers and, occasionally, by an erythematous vesicular eruption on the extremities and trunk.

ETIOLOGY: The fungi *Trichophyton rubrum, Trichophyton mentagrophytes,* and *Epidermophyton floccosum* are the most common causes.

EPIDEMIOLOGY: Tinea pedis is a common infection worldwide in adolescents and adults but is relatively uncommon in young children. The fungi are acquired by contact with skin scales containing fungi or with fungi in damp areas, such as swimming pools, locker rooms, and shower rooms. Tinea pedis tends to spread throughout the household among family members. It is communicable for as long as the infection is present.

The **incubation period** is unknown.

DIAGNOSIS: Tinea pedis usually is diagnosed by clinical manifestations and may be confirmed by microscopic examination of a potassium hydroxide wet mount of the cutaneous scrapings. Use of dermatophyte test medium is a reliable, simple, and inexpensive method of diagnosis in complicated or unresponsive cases. Skin scrapings are inoculated directly onto the culture medium and incubated at room temperature. After 1 to 2 weeks, a phenol red indicator in the agar will turn from yellow to red in the area surrounding a dermatophyte colony. When necessary, the diagnosis also can be confirmed by culture on Sabouraud dextrose agar. Infection of the nail can be verified by direct microscopic examination and fungal culture of desquamated subungual material.

TREATMENT: Topical application of a miconazole nitrate, haloprogin, clotrimazole, ciclopirox olamine, terbinafine, butenafine, or tolnaftate preparation twice a day or of a ketoconazole, econazole nitrate, naftifine hydrochloride, oxiconazole nitrate, or sulconazole nitrate preparation once a day for 2 to 3 weeks, can be used for active infections (see Topical Drugs for Superficial Fungal Infections, p 726). Acute vesicular lesions may be treated with intermittent use of open wet compresses (eg, with Burrow solution, 1:80). Tinea cruris, if present, should be treated concurrently (see Tinea Cruris, p 620).

Griseofulvin, administered orally for 6 to 8 weeks, may be necessary for treatment of severe, chronic, or recalcitrant tinea pedis. Oral itraconazole or terbinafine also are effective alternative therapies for tinea pedis unresponsive to topical therapy, but these products have not been licensed by the US Food and Drug Administration for this indication. Id (hypersensitivity response) reactions are treated by wet compresses, topical corticosteroids, occasionally systemic corticosteroids, and eradication of the primary source of infection.

Recurrence is prevented by proper foot hygiene, which includes keeping the feet dry and cool, gentle cleaning, drying between the toes, the use of absorbent antifungal foot powder, frequent airing of affected areas, and avoidance of occlusive footwear and nylon socks or other fabrics that interfere with dissipation of moisture.

In the past, most nail infections, particularly toenail infections, have been highly resistant to oral griseofulvin therapy. Studies in adult patients have demonstrated a modest cure rate after therapy with oral itraconazole, terbinafine, or fluconazole. Further studies on the safety and efficacy of these drugs in children are necessary before these drugs can be recommended. Recurrences are common. Removal of the nail plate followed by use of oral therapy during the period of regrowth can help to effect a cure in resistant cases.

ISOLATION OF THE HOSPITALIZED PATIENT: Standard precautions are recommended.

CONTROL MEASURES: Treatment of patients with active infections should decrease transmission. Public areas conducive to transmission (eg, swimming pools) should not be used by those with active infection. Chemical foot baths are of no value and can facilitate spread of infection. Because recurrence after treatment is common, proper foot hygiene is important (as described in Treatment, p 622). Patients should be advised to dry the groin area before drying their feet to avoid inoculating tinea pedis dermatophytes into the groin area.

Tinea Versicolor
(Pityriasis Versicolor)

CLINICAL MANIFESTATIONS: Pityriasis versicolor (formerly tinea versicolor) is a common superficial yeast infection of the skin characterized by multiple, scaling, oval, and patchy macular lesions usually distributed over upper portions of the trunk, proximal areas of the arms, and neck. Facial involvement particularly is common in children. Lesions may be hypopigmented or hyperpigmented (fawn colored or brown). Lesions fail to tan during the summer and during the winter are relatively darker, hence the term *versicolor*. Common conditions confused with this disorder include pityriasis alba, postinflammatory hypopigmentation, vitiligo, melasma, seborrheic dermatitis, pityriasis rosea, and secondary syphilis.

ETIOLOGY: The cause of pityriasis versicolor is *Malassezia furfur,* a dimorphic lipid-dependent yeast that exists on healthy skin in yeast phase and causes clinical lesions only when substantial growth of hyphae occurs. Moist heat and lipid-containing sebaceous secretions encourage rapid overgrowth.

EPIDEMIOLOGY: Pityriasis versicolor occurs worldwide but is more prevalent in tropical and subtropical areas. Although primarily a disorder of adolescents and young adults, tinea versicolor also may occur in prepubertal children and infants. The yeast is transmitted by personal contact during periods of scaling.

The **incubation period** is unknown.

DIAGNOSIS: The clinical appearance usually is diagnostic. Involved areas are fluorescent yellow under examination by Wood light. Skin scrapings examined microscopically in a potassium hydroxide wet mount preparation or stained with methylene blue or May-Grünwald-Giemsa stain disclose the pathognomonic clusters of yeast cells and hyphae ("spaghetti and meatball" appearance). Growth of this yeast on culture requires a source of long-chain fatty acids, which may be provided by overlaying Sabouraud dextrose agar medium with sterile olive oil.

TREATMENT: Topical treatment with selenium sulfide as 2.5% lotion or 1% shampoo has been the traditional treatment of choice. These preparations are applied in a thin layer covering the body surface from the face to the knees daily for 30 minutes for a week, followed by monthly applications for 3 months to help prevent recurrences. Topical ketoconazole 2% shampoo used as a single application daily for 1 to 3 days is an effective alternative. Other topical preparations with therapeutic efficacy include sodium hyposulfite or thiosulfate in 15% to 25% concentrations (eg, Tinver lotion) applied twice a day for 2 to 4 weeks. Small focal infections may be treated with topical antifungal agents, such as ciclopirox olamine, clotrimazole, econazole nitrate, haloprogin, ketoconazole, miconazole nitrate, or naftifine hydrochloride (see Topical Drugs for Superficial Fungal Infections, p 726). Because *M furfur* is part of normal flora, relapses are common. Multiple topical treatments may be necessary.

Oral antifungal therapy has advantages over topical therapy, including ease of administration and shorter duration of treatment, but oral therapy is more expensive and associated with a greater risk of adverse reactions. A single dose of ketoconazole (400 mg orally) or fluconazole (400 mg orally) or a 5-day course of itraconazole (200 mg orally once a day) has been effective in adults. Some experts recommend that children receive 3 days of ketoconazole therapy rather than the single dose given to adults. For pediatric dosage recommendations for ketoconazole, fluconazole, and itraconazole, see Recommended Doses of Parenteral and Oral Antifungal Drugs, p 722. These drugs have not been studied extensively in children for this disorder and are not yet licensed by the US Food and Drug Administration for this indication. Exercise to increase sweating and skin concentrations of medication may enhance the effectiveness of systemic therapy. Patients should be advised that repigmentation may not occur for several months after successful treatment.

ISOLATION OF THE HOSPITALIZED PATIENT: Standard precautions are recommended.

CONTROL MEASURES: Infected people should be treated.

Toxic Shock Syndrome

CLINICAL MANIFESTATIONS: Toxic shock syndrome (TSS) may be caused by toxin-producing *Staphylococcus aureus* or *Streptococcus pyogenes* (group A streptococci). Both organisms cause an acute illness characterized by fever, rapid-onset hypotension, rapidly accelerated renal failure, and multisystem organ involvement (see Tables 3.62, p 625, and 3.63, p 626). Profuse watery diarrhea, vomiting, generalized erythroderma, conjunctival injection, and severe myalgias commonly are present with *S aureus*-mediated TSS but are less common with *S pyogenes*-mediated TSS. Evidence of local soft tissue infection (eg, cellulitis, abscess, myositis, or necrotizing fasciitis) associated with severe increasing pain is common with *S pyogenes*-mediated TSS but not with *S aureus*-mediated TSS. The presence of a foreign body at the site of infection is common with *S aureus*-mediated TSS, but not with *S pyogenes*-mediated TSS. Both forms of TSS may occur without a readily identifiable focus of infection. Both forms of TSS also may be associated with invasive infections, such as pneumonia, osteomyelitis, bacteremia, pyarthrosis, or endocarditis. Patients with *S aureus*-mediated TSS, especially menses associated, are at risk of a recurrent episode of TSS. Recurrent episodes have not been reported for *S pyogenes*-mediated TSS. Toxic shock can be confused with many infectious and noninfectious causes of fever with mucocutaneous manifestations.

ETIOLOGY: *Staphylococcus aureus*-mediated TSS usually is caused by strains producing toxic-shock syndrome toxin-1 (TSST-1). Most of these strains also produce at least one of the staphylococcal enterotoxins. Some TSST-1 negative strains of

Table 3.62. Staphylococcal Toxic Shock Syndrome: Clinical Case Definition[1]

- Fever: temperature ≥38.9°C (≥102.0°F)
- Rash: diffuse macular erythroderma
- Desquamation: 1–2 wk after onset, particularly on palms, soles, fingers, and toes
- Hypotension: systolic pressure ≤90 mm Hg for adults; lower than fifth percentile for age for children younger than 16 years of age; orthostatic drop in diastolic pressure of ≥15 mm Hg from lying to sitting; orthostatic syncope or orthostatic dizziness
- Multisystem organ involvement: 3 or more of the following:
  - Gastrointestinal: vomiting or diarrhea at onset of illness
  - Muscular: severe myalgia or creatinine phosphokinase concentration greater than twice the upper limit of normal
  - Mucous membrane: vaginal, oropharyngeal, or conjunctival hyperemia
  - Renal: serum urea nitrogen or serum creatinine concentration greater than twice the upper limit of normal or urinary sediment with ≥5 white blood cells per high-power field in the absence of urinary tract infection
  - Hepatic: total bilirubin, aspartate transaminase, or alanine transaminase concentration greater than twice the upper limit of normal
  - Hematologic: platelet count, ≤100 × 10^9/L (≤100 × 10^3/µL)
  - Central nervous system: disorientation or alterations in consciousness without focal neurologic signs when fever and hypotension are absent
- Negative results on the following tests, if obtained:
  - Blood, throat, or cerebrospinal fluid cultures; blood culture may be positive for *Staphylococcus aureus*
  - Serologic tests for Rocky Mountain spotted fever, leptospirosis, or measles

Case Classification

Probable: a case with 5 of the 6 aforementioned clinical findings

Confirmed: a case with all 6 of the clinical findings, including desquamation. If the patient dies before desquamation could have occurred, the other 5 criteria constitute a definitive case.

---

[1] Adapted from Wharton M, Chorba TL, Vogt RL, Morse DL, Buehler JW. Case definitions for public health surveillance. *MMWR Recomm Rep.* 1990;39(RR-13):1–43

S aureus have been implicated in nonmenstrual cases of TSS. Most cases of *S pyogenes*-mediated TSS are caused by strains producing at least 1 of several different protein superantigenic exotoxins: streptococcal pyrogenic exotoxins A, B, or C; mitogenic factor; or streptococcal superantigen.

EPIDEMIOLOGY:

Staphylococcus aureus-*Mediated TSS*. This syndrome was first recognized in 1978, occuring in children and adults both male and female; many early cases frequently were associated with tampon use in menstruating women, with a predilection for adolescents and young women with no circulating antibody to TSST-1. Changes in tampon composition and a decrease in absorbency during the past 2 decades were coincident with a significant decrease in the proportion of cases associated with men-

Table 3.63. Streptococcal Toxic Shock Syndrome: Clinical Case Definition[1]

I. Isolation of group A β-hemolytic streptococci *(Streptococcus pyogenes)*
   A. From a normally sterile site (eg, blood, cerebrospinal fluid, peritoneal fluid, or tissue biopsy specimen)
   B. From a nonsterile site (eg, throat, sputum, vagina, surgical wound, or superficial skin lesion)

II. Clinical signs of severity
   A. Hypotension: systolic pressure ≤90 mm Hg in adults or lower than the fifth percentile for age in children

AND

   B. Two or more of the following signs:
   • Renal impairment: creatinine concentration ≥177 μmol/L (≥2 mg/dL) for adults or 2 times or more the upper limit of normal for age
   • Coagulopathy: platelet count, ≤100 × 10⁹/L (≤100 × 10³/μL) or disseminated intravascular coagulation
   • Hepatic involvement: alanine transaminase, aspartate transaminase, or total bilirubin concentrations 2 times or more the upper limit of normal for age
   • Adult respiratory distress syndrome
   • A generalized erythematous macular rash that may desquamate
   • Soft tissue necrosis, including necrotizing fasciitis or myositis, or gangrene

---

[1] An illness fulfilling criteria IA and IIA and IIB can be defined as a *definite* case. An illness fulfilling criteria IB and IIA and IIB can be defined as a *probable* case if no other cause for the illness is identified.

Adapted from The Working Group on Severe Streptococcal Infections. Defining the group A streptococcal toxic shock syndrome: rationale and consensus definition. *JAMA.* 1993;269:390–391

struation, which accounted for fewer than 50% of reported cases in 1996. Risk factors for nonmenstrual TSS are outlined in Table 3.64, p 627.

In adults, TSST-1–producing strains of *S aureus* may be part of the normal flora of the anterior nares and the vagina. Colonization is believed to produce protective antibody, and more than 90% of adults have antibodies to TSST-1. People in whom *S aureus*-mediated TSS with TSST-1–producing strains develops usually do not have antibodies to TSST-1. Person-to-person transmission of TSS is rare. Nosocomial cases are uncommon and most often have followed surgical procedures. In postoperative cases, the organism generally originates from the patient's own flora.

The **incubation period** for postoperative TSS can be as short as 12 hours. Menses-related cases generally develop on the third or fourth day of menses. The mortality rate is less than 5% overall and is highest in men and women older than 45 years of age.

Streptococcus pyogenes-*Mediated TSS.* The incidence of *S pyogenes*-mediated TSS seems to be highest among young children, particularly children with concomitant varicella, and the elderly, although it may occur in people of any age. Of all cases of severe invasive streptococcal infections in children, fewer than 10% are associated with TSS, compared with as many as one third of such infections in people older than 75 years of age. Other people at increased risk include people with diabetes mellitus, chronic cardiac or pulmonary disease, and human immun-

Table 3.64. Risk Factors for Nonmenstrual Staphylococcal Toxic Shock Syndrome

I. Colonization with or introduction of toxin-producing *Staphylococcus aureus*

II. Absence of protective antitoxin antibody

III. Infected site

- Primary *S aureus* infection

Carbuncle	Endocarditis	Peritonitis	Pyomyositis
Cellulitis	Folliculitis	Peritonsillar abscess	Sinusitis
Dental abscess	Mastitis	Pneumonia	Tracheitis
Empyema	Osteomyelitis	Pyarthrosis	

- Postoperative wound infection

Abdominal	Ear, nose, and throat	Cesarean section	Neurosurgical
Breast	Genitourinary	Dermatologic	Orthopedic

- Skin or mucous membrane disruption

Burns (eg, chemical, scald)	Superficial or penetrating trauma
Dermatitis	(eg, insect bite, needlestick)
Postpartum (vaginal delivery)	

- Surgical or nonsurgical foreign body placement

Augmentation mammoplasty	Surgical prostheses, stents, packing
Catheters	material, or sutures
Diaphragm	Tampons
Sponge (contraceptive)	

- No obvious focus of infection (often sinusitis, occult abscess, or bacteremia)

odeficiency virus infection and intravenous drug and alcohol users. In 2 studies, the risk of severe invasive infection in contacts has been estimated to be at least 15-fold greater than for the general population but still is rare. Most contacts will have asymptomatic colonization.

Mortality rates are higher for adults than for children and depend on whether the *S pyogenes*-mediated TSS is associated only with bacteremia or with a specific focal infection (eg, necrotizing fasciitis, myositis, or pneumonia).

The **incubation period** is not defined clearly and may depend on the route of inoculation. The incubation period has been as short as 14 hours in cases associated with the accidental subcutaneous inoculation of organisms, such as during childbirth or after penetrating trauma.

DIAGNOSTIC TESTS:

Staphylococcus aureus-*Mediated TSS*. *Staphylococcus aureus*-mediated TSS remains a clinical diagnosis. Blood culture results are positive for *S aureus* in fewer than 5% of patients with *S aureus*-mediated TSS. Culture results usually are positive from the site of infection and should be obtained as soon as the site is identified. Specialized serologic testing, such as enzyme immunoassay for TSST-1, may be available from the Centers for Disease Control and Prevention or other reference laboratories. If

S aureus is isolated in the laboratory, it is important to obtain antimicrobial susceptibilities, because methicillin-resistant *S aureus* strains have caused TSS, although
rarely. Because approximately one third of isolates of *S aureus* from nonmenstrual
cases produce toxins other than TSST-1, and TSST-1 producing organisms can be
present as part of the normal flora of the anterior nares and vagina, production of
TSST-1 by an isolate of *S aureus* is not helpful diagnostically.

Streptococcus pyogenes-*Mediated TSS.* Blood culture results are positive for
S pyogenes in more than 50% of patients with *S pyogenes*-mediated TSS. Culture
results from the site of infection usually are positive and may remain positive for
several days after appropriate antimicrobial agents have been initiated. *Streptococcus
pyogenes* uniformly is susceptible to β-lactam antimicrobial agents. Antimicrobial
susceptibility should be determined only for non–β-lactam antimicrobial agents,
such as clindamycin and erythromycin, to which *S pyogenes* may be resistant. A significant increase in antibody titers to antistreptolysin O, antideoxyribonuclease B,
or other streptococcal extracellular products 4 to 6 weeks after infection may help
confirm the diagnosis if culture results were negative.

For both forms of TSS, laboratory studies may reflect multisystem organ
involvement and disseminated intravascular coagulation.

TREATMENT: As outlined in Tables 3.65 (below) and 3.66 (p 629), most aspects
of management are the same for TSS caused by *S aureus* and *S pyogenes*. The first
priority is aggressive fluid replacement as well as management of respiratory or cardiac failure or arrhythmias if present. Because distinguishing between the 2 forms
of TSS may not be possible, initial empiric antimicrobial therapy should include a
β-lactamase–resistant antistaphylococcal antimicrobial agent and a protein synthesis-
inhibiting antimicrobial drug, such as clindamycin. Both should be given parenterally at maximal doses for age. In mice, clindamycin is more effective than penicillin
for treating well-established *S pyogenes* infections, because the antimicrobial activity
of clindamycin is not affected by inoculum size, has a long postantimicrobial effect,
and acts on bacteria by inhibiting protein synthesis. Inhibition of protein synthesis

Table 3.65. **Management of Staphylococcal or Streptococcal Toxic Shock Syndrome *Without* Necrotizing Fasciitis**

- Fluid management to maintain adequate venous return and cardiac filling pressures to prevent end-organ damage
- Anticipatory management of multisystem organ failure
- Parenteral antimicrobial therapy at maximum doses for age
  - Kill organism with bactericidal cell wall inhibitor (eg, β-lactamase–resistant antistaphylococcal antimicrobial agent)
  - Stop enzyme, toxin, or cytokine production with protein synthesis inhibitor (eg, clindamycin)
- Immune Globulin Intravenous may be considered for infection refractory to several hours of aggressive therapy, presence of an undrainable focus, or persistent oliguria with pulmonary edema

Table 3.66. **Management of Streptococcal Toxic Shock Syndrome *With* Necrotizing Fasciitis**

- Principles outlined in Table 3.65 (p 628)
- Immediate surgical evaluation
  - Exploration or incisional biopsy for diagnosis and culture
  - Resection of all necrotic tissue
- Repeated resection of tissue may be needed if infection persists or progresses

results in suppression of synthesis of the *S pyogenes* antiphagocytic M protein and bacterial toxins. Clindamycin should not be used alone as initial empiric therapy, because in the United States, 1% to 2% of *S pyogenes* strains are resistant to clindamycin. Methicillin-resistant *S aureus* has caused fewer than 1% of cases of TSS, and vancomycin hydrochloride should not be used routinely as initial empiric therapy.

Once the organism has been identified, antimicrobial therapy can be changed to penicillin and clindamycin for *S pyogenes*-mediated TSS. For *S aureus*-mediated TSS, the most appropriate parenteral β-lactam antimicrobial agent on the basis of susceptibility testing should be given with clindamycin.

For *S aureus*-mediated TSS, antimicrobial therapy should be continued for a minimum of 10 to 14 days to eradicate the organism, thus preventing recurrent disease. The antimicrobial agent(s) may be changed to high-dose oral therapy once the patient's condition is stable hemodynamically and clearly improved and the patient is receiving oral alimentation. The total duration of therapy should be based on the usual duration established for the underlying focus, such as osteomyelitis or pneumonia.

For *S pyogenes*-mediated TSS, intravenous therapy should be continued until the patient is afebrile and is in hemodynamically stable condition and negative blood culture results have been documented. The total duration of therapy should be based on the duration established for infection of the underlying focus.

Aggressive drainage and irrigation of accessible sites of infection should be performed as soon as possible. Concerted efforts should be made to identify a foreign body at the site of infection, and all foreign bodies, including those recently inserted during surgery, should be removed if possible. If necrotizing fasciitis is suspected, immediate surgical exploration or biopsy is crucial to identify a deep soft tissue infection that should be débrided immediately.

The use of Immune Globulin Intravenous (IGIV) may be considered in treatment of either form of TSS. The mechanism of action of IGIV is unclear but may be neutralization of circulating bacterial toxins. For *S pyogenes*-mediated TSS, in vitro data, case reports, and a comparative observational study from Canada support a potential role for IGIV, but further studies are needed. For *S aureus*-mediated TSS, IGIV may be considered for patients who remain unresponsive to all other therapeutic measures and for patients with infection in an area that cannot be drained. Various regimens of IGIV, including 150 to 400 mg/kg per day for 5 days and a single dose of 1 to 2 g/kg, have been used, but the optimal regimen is unknown.

The clearance of IGIV may be as short as 4 to 6 days in TSS patients, and some experts have suggested additional doses.

ISOLATION OF THE HOSPITALIZED PATIENT: Standard precautions, as well as droplet and contact precautions, are recommended for all patients with TSS attributable to *S pyogenes*. Because person-to-person transmission of *S aureus*-mediated TSS is uncommon, only standard precautions are needed.

CONTROL MEASURES: Control measures for *S pyogenes*-mediated TSS are the same as those for other forms of severe, invasive group A streptococcal infections (see p 573).

For *S aureus*-mediated TSS, the control measures are the same as those for other forms of severe staphylococcal diseases (see p 561).

Toxocariasis
(Visceral Larva Migrans, Ocular Larva Migrans)

CLINICAL MANIFESTATIONS: The severity of symptoms depends on the number of larvae ingested and the degree of allergic response. Most people who are infected lightly are asymptomatic. Visceral larva migrans typically occurs in children 1 to 4 years of age with a history of pica but can occur in older children and adults. Characteristic manifestations include fever, leukocytosis, eosinophilia, hypergammaglobulinemia, and hepatomegaly. Other manifestations include malaise, anemia, cough, and in rare instances, pneumonia, myocarditis, and encephalitis. When ocular invasion (endophthalmitis or retinal granulomas) occurs, other evidence of infection usually is lacking, suggesting that the visceral and ocular manifestations are distinct syndromes. Atypical manifestations include hemorrhagic rash and seizures. In some cases, so-called covert toxocariasis may manifest only as asymptomatic eosinophilia or pulmonary wheezing.

ETIOLOGY: Toxocariasis is caused by *Toxocara* species, which are common roundworms of dogs and cats (especially puppies or kittens), specifically *Toxocara canis* and *Toxocara cati* in the United States; most cases are caused by *T canis*. Other nematodes of animals also can cause this syndrome, although rarely.

EPIDEMIOLOGY: Humans are infected by ingestion of soil containing infective eggs of the parasite. A history of pica, particularly eating soil, is common. Direct contact with dogs is of secondary importance, because eggs are not infective immediately when shed in the feces. Most reported cases involve children. Toxocariasis is endemic in Puerto Rico and the contiguous United States. The infection is endemic in many underserved urban areas. Eggs may be found wherever dogs and cats defecate.

The **incubation period** is unknown.

DIAGNOSTIC TESTS: Hypereosinophilia and hypergammaglobulinemia associated with increased titers of isohemagglutinin to the A and B blood group antigens are presumptive evidence of infection. Microscopic identification of larvae in a liver biopsy specimen is diagnostic, but this finding is rare. A liver biopsy negative for larvae, therefore, does not exclude the diagnosis. An enzyme immunoassay for *Toxocara* antibodies in serum, available at the Centers for Disease Control and Prevention and some commercial laboratories, can provide presumptive evidence of toxocariasis. This assay is specific and sensitive for the diagnosis of visceral larva migrans but is less sensitive for the diagnosis of ocular larva migrans.

TREATMENT: Albendazole or mebendazole are the recommended drugs for treatment of toxocariasis. Both drugs have been licensed by the US Food and Drug Administration, but not for this indication. In severe cases with myocarditis or involvement of the central nervous system, corticosteroid therapy is indicated. Correcting the underlying causes of pica helps prevent reinfection.

Treatment of ocular larva migrans may not be effective. Inflammation may be decreased by injection of corticosteroids, and secondary damage may be aided by surgery.

ISOLATION OF THE HOSPITALIZED PATIENT: Standard precautions are recommended.

CONTROL MEASURES: Proper disposal of cat and dog feces is essential. Treatment of puppies and kittens with anthelmintics at 2, 4, 6, and 8 weeks of age prevents excretion of eggs by worms acquired transplacentally or through mother's milk. Covering sandboxes when not in use is helpful. No specific management of exposed people is recommended.

Toxoplasma gondii Infections
(Toxoplasmosis)

CLINICAL MANIFESTATIONS: Infants with congenital infection are asymptomatic at birth in 70% to 90% of cases, although visual impairment, learning disabilities, or mental retardation will become apparent in a large proportion of children several months to years later. Signs of congenital toxoplasmosis at birth can include a maculopapular rash, generalized lymphadenopathy, hepatomegaly, splenomegaly, jaundice, and thrombocytopenia. As a consequence of intrauterine meningoencephalitis, cerebrospinal fluid (CSF) abnormalities, hydrocephalus, microcephaly, chorioretinitis, seizures, and deafness can develop. Some of the severely affected infants die in utero or within a few days of birth. Cerebral calcifications may be demonstrated by radiography, ultrasonography, or computed tomography of the head.

Toxoplasma gondii infection acquired after birth usually is asymptomatic. When symptoms develop, they are nonspecific and include malaise, fever, sore throat, and myalgia. Lymphadenopathy, frequently cervical, is the most common sign. Occasionally, patients may have a mononucleosis-like illness associated with a macular rash and hepatosplenomegaly. The clinical course usually is benign and self-limited. Myocarditis, pericarditis, and pneumonitis are rare complications.

Isolated ocular toxoplasmosis most commonly results from congenital infection but also occurs in a small percentage of people with acquired infection. Acute ocular involvement manifests as blurred vision, and characteristic retinal infiltrates develop in up to 85% of young adults after congenital infection. Ocular disease can become reactivated years after the initial infection in healthy and immunocompromised people.

In chronically infected immunodeficient patients, including people with human immunodeficiency virus (HIV) infection, reactivated infection can result in encephalitis, pneumonitis, or less commonly, systemic toxoplasmosis. Rarely, infants who are born to HIV-infected mothers or mothers who are immunocompromised for other reasons who have chronic infection with *T gondii* may have acquired congenital toxoplasmosis in utero as a result of reactivated maternal parasitemia.

ETIOLOGY: *Toxoplasma gondii,* a protozoan parasite, is the only known species of *Toxoplasma.*

EPIDEMIOLOGY: *Toxoplasma gondii* is worldwide in distribution and infects most species of warm-blooded animals. Members of the cat family are definitive hosts. Cats generally acquire the infection by feeding on infected animals, such as mice or uncooked household meats. The parasite replicates sexually in the feline small intestine. Cats may begin to excrete oocysts in their stools 3 to 30 days after primary infection and may shed oocysts for 7 to 14 days. After excretion, oocysts require a maturation phase (sporulation) of 24 to 48 hours in temperate climates before they are infective by the oral route. Intermediate hosts (including sheep, pigs, and cattle) can have tissue cysts in the brain, myocardium, skeletal muscle, and other organs. These cysts remain viable for the lifetime of the host. Humans usually become infected by consumption of raw or undercooked meat that contains cysts or by accidental ingestion of sporulated oocysts from soil or in contaminated food. A large outbreak epidemiologically linked to contamination of a municipal water supply also has been reported. Transmission of *T gondii* has been documented to result from blood or blood product transfusion and organ (eg, heart) or bone marrow transplantation from a seropositive donor with latent infection. Rarely, infection has occurred as a result of a laboratory accident. In most cases, congenital transmission occurs as a result of primary maternal infection during gestation. The incidence of congenital toxoplasmosis in the United States has been estimated to be 1 in 1000 to 1 in 10 000 live births.

The **incubation period** of acquired infection, on the basis of a well-studied outbreak, is estimated to be approximately 7 days, with a range of 4 to 21 days.

DIAGNOSTIC TESTS: Serologic tests are the primary means of diagnosis, but results must be interpreted carefully. Laboratories with special expertise in toxoplasma serologic assays and their interpretation particularly are useful to the practitioner. Immunoglobulin (Ig) G-specific antibodies (eg, measured by indirect immunofluorescence or enzyme immunoassay) achieve a peak concentration 1 to 2 months after infection and remain positive indefinitely. For patients with seroconversion or a fourfold increase in IgG antibody titer, specific IgM antibody determinations should be performed by a reference laboratory to confirm acute infection. The presence of *T gondii*-specific IgM antibodies may indicate acute or recent infection. Enzyme immunoassay tests are the more sensitive assays for IgM, and indirect fluorescent antibody tests are the least sensitive in detecting IgM. Immunoglobulin M-specific antibodies can be detected 2 weeks after infection, achieve peak concentrations in 1 month, decrease thereafter, and usually become undetectable within 6 to 9 months but uncommonly persist for as long as 2 years, confounding the differentiation of acute and remote infection. Tests to detect IgA and IgE antibodies, which decrease to undetectable concentrations sooner than IgM antibodies, are useful for the diagnosis of congenital infections and infections in other patients, such as pregnant women, for whom more precise information about the duration of infection is needed. *Toxoplasma gondii*-specific IgA and IgE antibody tests are available commercially but are not used commonly in routine laboratories.

Special Situations.

Prenatal. A definitive diagnosis of congenital toxoplasmosis can be made prenatally by detecting the parasite in fetal blood or amniotic fluid or documenting the presence of *T gondii* IgM or IgA antibodies in fetal blood. The parasite rarely can be isolated by mouse inoculation. Detection of *T gondii* DNA in amniotic fluid by polymerase chain reaction assay in a reference laboratory has been shown to be a safe and accurate method of diagnosis. Serial fetal ultrasonographic examinations should be performed in cases of suspected congenital infection to detect any increase in size of the lateral ventricles of the central nervous system or other signs of fetal infection.

Postnatal. Infants who are born to women who have evidence of primary *T gondii* infection during gestation or women who are infected with HIV *and* have serologic evidence of past infection with *T gondii* should be assessed for congenital toxoplasmosis.

If the diagnosis for an infant is unclear at the time of delivery, evaluation of the infant should include ophthalmologic, auditory, and neurologic examinations; lumbar puncture; and computed tomography of the head. An attempt should be made to isolate *T gondii* from the placenta, umbilical cord, or blood specimen from the infant by mouse inoculation. Alternatively, peripheral blood white blood cells, CSF, and amniotic fluid specimens should be assayed for *T gondii* by polymerase chain reaction assay in a reference laboratory.

Congenital infection is serologically confirmed on the basis of a positive IgM or IgA assay within the first 6 months of life or persistently positive IgG titers beyond the first 12 months of life. The sensitivity of *T gondii*-specific IgM by the double-sandwich enzyme immunoassay or an immunosorbent assay is 75% to 80%. The indirect fluorescent assay for IgM should not be relied on to diagnose congenital infection. In an uninfected infant, a continuous decrease in IgG titer without IgM or IgA will occur. Transplacentally transmitted IgG antibody usually will become undetectable by 6 to 12 months of age.

HIV Infection. Patients with HIV infection who are infected latently with *T gondii* have variable titers of IgG antibody to *T gondii* but rarely have IgM antibody. Although seroconversion and fourfold increases in IgG antibody titers may occur, the ability to diagnose active disease in patients with acquired immunodeficiency syndrome commonly is impaired by immunosuppression. In HIV-infected patients who are seropositive for *T gondii* IgG, *T gondii* encephalitis is diagnosed presumptively on the basis of the presence of characteristic clinical and radiographic findings. If the infection does not respond to an empiric trial of anti-*T gondii* therapy, demonstration of *T gondii* organisms, antigen, or DNA in biopsied tissue, blood, or cerebrospinal fluid may be necessary to confirm the diagnosis.

Infants born to women who are infected simultaneously with HIV and *T gondii* should be evaluated for congenital toxoplasmosis because of an increased likelihood of maternal reactivation and congenital transmission in this setting.

Ocular toxoplasmosis is diagnosed on the basis of observation of characteristic retinal lesions in conjunction with serum *T gondii*-specific IgG or IgM antibodies.

TREATMENT: Most cases of acquired infection in an immunocompetent host do not require specific antimicrobial therapy. When indicated (eg, chorioretinitis or significant organ damage), the combination of pyrimethamine and sulfadiazine,* which is synergistic against *T gondii*, is the most widely accepted regimen for children and adults with acute symptomatic disease (see Drugs for Parasitic Infections, p 744). Alternatively, pyrimethamine can be used in combination with clindamycin if the patient does not tolerate sulfadiazine. Corticosteroids appear to be useful in the management of ocular complications and central nervous system disease in certain patients.

Patients infected with HIV who have had toxoplasmic encephalitis should receive lifelong suppressive therapy to prevent recurrence. Regimens for primary treatment also are effective for suppressive therapy.

For HIV-infected adults, primary chemoprophylaxis with trimethoprim-sulfamethoxazole against toxoplasmosis has been recommended by the US Public Health Services and Infectious Diseases Society of America Prevention of Opportunistic Infections Working Group[†] for people who are *T gondii*-seropositive and have CD4+ T-lymphocyte counts less than 100×10^6/L (<100/µL). Current data are insufficient for formulation of specific guidelines for children; chemoprophylaxis should be considered and is recommended by some experts. Trimethoprim-sulfamethoxazole administered for *Pneumocystis* pneumonia prophylaxis will provide prophylaxis against toxoplasmosis. Severely immunosuppressed children who are not receiving trimethoprim-sulfamethoxazole or atovaquone who are found to be seropositive for *Toxoplasma* species should be given prophylaxis for both *Pneumocystis* pneumonia and toxoplasmosis (ie, dapsone plus pyrimethamine).

For symptomatic and asymptomatic congenital infection, pyrimethamine combined with sulfadiazine (supplemented with folinic acid) is recommended as initial therapy. Duration of therapy is prolonged and often is 1 year. However, the optimal dosage and duration are not established definitively and should be determined in consultation with appropriate specialists.

Treatment of primary *T gondii* infection in pregnant women, including women with HIV infection, is recommended. Appropriate specialists should be consulted for management. Spiramycin treatment of primary infection during gestation is used in an attempt to decrease transmission of *T gondii* from the mother to the fetus. Maternal therapy may decrease the severity of sequelae in the fetus once congenital toxoplasmosis has occurred. Spiramycin is available only as an investi-

---

* Available from Eon Labs, Laurelton, NY (800-526-0225).
† Centers for Disease Control and Prevention. Guidelines for preventing opportunistic infections among HIV-infected persons—2002. Recommendations of the US Public Health Service and the Infectious Diseases Society of America. *MMWR Recomm Rep.* 2002;51(RR-8):1–46. Available at: www.cdc.gov/mmwr/preview/mmwrhtml/rr5108a1.htm

gational drug in the United States. Spiramycin may be obtained from the manufacturer with authorization from the US Food and Drug Administration.* If fetal infection is confirmed after 17 weeks of gestation or if the mother acquires infection during the third trimester, consideration should be given to starting therapy with pyrimethamine and sulfadiazine.

ISOLATION OF THE HOSPITALIZED PATIENT: Standard precautions are recommended.

CONTROL MEASURES: Pregnant women whose serostatus for *T gondii* is negative or unknown should avoid activities that potentially expose them to cat feces (such as changing litter boxes, gardening, and landscaping), or they should wear gloves and wash their hands if such activities are unavoidable. Daily changing of cat litter will decrease the chance of infection, because oocysts are not infective during the first 1 to 2 days after passage. Domestic cats can be protected from infection by feeding them commercially prepared cat food and preventing them from eating undercooked kitchen meat scraps and hunting wild rodents.

Oral ingestion of *T gondii* can be avoided by the following measures: (1) cooking meat, particularly pork, lamb, and venison, to an internal temperature of 65.5°C to 76.6°C (150°F–170°F [no longer pink]) before consumption (smoked meat and meat cured in brine are considered safe); (2) washing fruits and vegetables; (3) washing hands and cleaning kitchen surfaces after handling fruits, vegetables, and raw meat; (4) washing hands after gardening or other contact with soil; and (5) preventing contamination of food with raw or undercooked meat or soil. All HIV-infected people and pregnant women should be counseled about the various sources of toxoplasmic infection.

Trichinosis
(Trichinella spiralis)

CLINICAL MANIFESTATIONS: The clinical spectrum of infection ranges from inapparent to fulminant and fatal illness, but most infections are inapparent. The severity of the disease is proportional to the infective dose. During the first week after ingesting infected meat, a person may be asymptomatic or experience abdominal discomfort, nausea, vomiting, and/or diarrhea. Two to 8 weeks later, as larvae migrate into tissues, fever, myalgia, periorbital edema, urticarial rash, and conjunctival and subungual hemorrhages may develop. Larvae may remain viable in tissues for years; calcification of some larvae in skeletal muscle usually occurs within 6 to 24 months and may be detected on radiographs. In severe infections, myocarditis, neurologic involvement, and pneumonitis can follow in 1 or 2 months.

ETIOLOGY: Infection is caused by nematodes (roundworms) of the genus *Trichinella*. At least 5 species capable of infecting only warm-blooded animals

---

* US Food and Drug Administration, Division of Special Pathogen and Immunologic Drug Products. Telephone, 301-827-2127; fax, 301-927-2475.

have been identified. Worldwide, *Trichinella spiralis* is the most common cause
of human infection.

EPIDEMIOLOGY: The infection is enzootic worldwide in many carnivores, especially scavengers. Infection occurs as a result of ingestion of raw or insufficiently cooked meat containing encysted larvae of *T spiralis*. The usual source of human infections is pork, but horse meat and wild carnivorous game, such as bear, seal, and walrus meat in North America, can be sources. Feeding pigs uncooked garbage perpetuates the cycle of infection. In the United States, the incidence of infection in humans has decreased considerably, but infection occurs sporadically, often within a family or among friends who have prepared uncooked sausage from fresh pork. The disease is not transmitted from person to person.

The **incubation period** usually is 1 to 2 weeks.

DIAGNOSTIC TESTS: Eosinophilia approaching 70%, in conjunction with compatible symptoms and dietary history, suggests the diagnosis. Increases in concentrations of muscle enzymes, such as creatinine phosphokinase and lactic dehydrogenase, also occur. Encapsulated larvae in a skeletal muscle biopsy specimen (particularly deltoid and gastrocnemius) can be visualized microscopically beginning 2 weeks after infection. Fresh tissue, compressed between 2 microscope slides, should be examined. Digestion of muscle tissue in artificial gastric juice followed by examination of the sediment for larvae is more sensitive. Identification of larvae in suspect meat can be the most rapid source of diagnostic information. Serologic tests are available through some private and state laboratories and the Centers for Disease Control and Prevention. Serum antibody titers rarely become positive before the second week of illness. Testing paired acute and convalescent serum specimens usually is diagnostic.

TREATMENT: Mebendazole and albendazole have comparable efficacy for treatment of trichinosis (see Drugs for Parasitic Infections, p 744). Neither drug is very effective for *Trichinella* larvae already in the muscles. Coadministration of corticosteroids with mebendazole or albendazole often is recommended when symptoms are severe. Corticosteroids alleviate symptoms of the inflammatory reaction and can be lifesaving when the central nervous system or heart is involved.

ISOLATION OF THE HOSPITALIZED PATIENT: Standard precautions are recommended.

CONTROL MEASURES: Transmission to pigs can be decreased by not feeding pigs garbage and by effective rat control. The public should be educated about the necessity of cooking pork thoroughly (until the meat is no longer pink). Freezing pork at −23°C (−10°F) for 10 days kills larvae. However, *Trichinella* organisms in Arctic wild animals can survive this procedure. People known to have ingested contaminated meat recently should be treated with mebendazole (or albendazole).

Trichomonas vaginalis Infections
(Trichomoniasis)

CLINICAL MANIFESTATIONS: Infection with *Trichomonas vaginalis* commonly is asymptomatic. The usual clinical manifestations in symptomatic postmenarcheal female patients consist of a frothy vaginal discharge and mild vulvovaginal itching. Dysuria and, rarely, lower abdominal pain can occur. The vaginal discharge usually is pale yellow to gray-green and has a musty odor. Symptoms commonly are more severe just before or after menstruation. The vaginal mucosa often is deeply erythematous, and the cervix is friable and diffusely inflamed, sometimes covered with numerous petechiae ("strawberry cervix"). Urethritis and, more rarely, epididymitis or prostatitis can develop in infected males, but most are asymptomatic. Reinfection is common.

ETIOLOGY: *Trichomonas vaginalis* is a flagellated protozoan that is slightly larger than a granulocyte.

EPIDEMIOLOGY: *Trichomonas vaginalis* infection primarily is transmitted sexually and commonly coexists with other conditions, particularly infection with *Neisseria gonorrhoeae* and bacterial vaginitis. The presence of *T vaginalis* in a prepubertal child should raise suspicion of sexual abuse. *Trichomonas vaginalis* acquired during birth by newborn infants can cause a vaginal discharge during the first weeks of life.

The **incubation period** averages 1 week but ranges from 4 to 28 days.

DIAGNOSTIC TESTS: Diagnosis usually is established by examination of a wet-mount preparation of the vaginal discharge. Lashing of the flagella and jerky motility of the organism are distinctive. Positive preparation results, found more commonly in women who have symptoms, are related directly to the number of organisms but are identified in only 60% to 70% of cases. Culture of the organism and tests using enzyme immunoassay and immunofluorescence techniques for demonstration of the organism are more sensitive than wet-mount preparations but generally are not required for diagnosis. Culture for *T vaginalis* is positive in more than 80% of cases. No FDA-licensed polymerase chain reaction assay for *T vaginalis* is available in the United States but may be available as a research diagnostic test or from commercial laboratories.

TREATMENT: Metronidazole is the treatment of choice, resulting in cure rates of approximately 95%. The sexual partner should be treated concurrently, even if asymptomatic. Patients should abstain from alcohol for 48 hours after treatment because of the disulfiram-like effects of the drug. During pregnancy, patients can be treated with a 2-g single dose of metronidazole or with the 7-day regimen.

Patients whose infections do not respond to treatment should be retreated with metronidazole (1 g in 2 divided doses for adolescents and adults) for 7 days. Patients who repeatedly fail to respond should be treated with metronidazole, 2 g, once a day for 3 to 5 days. *Trichomonas* strains with decreased susceptibility to metronidazole have been reported. In the event of continued treatment failure, consultation with an expert is advised. Consultation is available from the Centers for Disease Control and Prevention at www.cdc.gov/std or 770-488-4115.

People infected with *T vaginalis* should be evaluated for the presence of other sexually transmitted diseases, including syphilis, *N gonorrhoeae, Chlamydia trachomatis,* hepatitis B virus, and human immunodeficiency virus infection.

ISOLATION OF THE HOSPITALIZED PATIENT: Standard precautions are recommended.

CONTROL MEASURES: Measures to prevent sexually transmitted diseases, particularly the consistent use of condoms, are indicated. Patients should be instructed to avoid sexual activity until they and their sexual partners are cured.

Trichuriasis
(Whipworm Infection)

CLINICAL MANIFESTATIONS: Most infected children harbor only small numbers of the organism and are asymptomatic. Children with heavy infestations can develop a *Trichuris trichiura* dysentery syndrome consisting of abdominal pain, tenesmus, and bloody diarrhea with mucus or a chronic *T trichiura* colitis. *Trichuris trichiura* colitis can mimic other forms of inflammatory bowel disease and lead to physical growth retardation. Chronic illness associated with heavy infestation also can be associated with rectal prolapse.

ETIOLOGY: *Trichuris trichiura,* the whipworm, is the causative agent. Adult worms are 30- to 50-mm long with a large, thread-like anterior end that is embedded in the mucosa of the large intestine.

EPIDEMIOLOGY: The parasite has a worldwide distribution but is more common in the tropics and in areas of poor sanitation. In some areas of Asia, the prevalence of infestation is 50%. In the United States, trichuriasis generally has been limited to rural areas of the southeast and no longer is a serious public health problem. Migrants from tropical areas also may be infected. Eggs require a minimum of 10 days of incubation in the soil before they are infectious. The disease is not communicable from person to person.

The **incubation period** is unknown. However, the time required for mature worms to begin laying eggs that are passed in feces is approximately 90 days after ingestion of the eggs.

DIAGNOSTIC TESTS: Eggs may be found on direct examination of stool or by using concentration techniques.

TREATMENT: Mebendazole or albendazole given for 3 days usually is effective in eradicating most of the worms.

ISOLATION OF THE HOSPITALIZED PATIENT: Standard precautions are recommended.

CONTROL MEASURES: Proper disposal of fecal material is indicated.

African Trypanosomiasis
(African Sleeping Sickness)

CLINICAL MANIFESTATIONS: The rapidity and severity of clinical manifestations vary with the infecting subspecies. With *Trypanosoma brucei gambiense* (West African) infection, a cutaneous nodule or chancre may appear at the site of parasite inoculation within a few days of a bite by an infected tsetse fly. Systemic illness is chronic, occurring months to years later, and is characterized by intermittent fever, posterior cervical lymphadenopathy (Winterbottom sign), and multiple nonspecific complaints, including malaise, weight loss, arthralgia, rash, pruritus, and edema. If the central nervous system (CNS) is involved, chronic meningoencephalitis with behavioral changes, cachexia, headache, hallucinations, delusions, and somnolence can occur. In contrast, *Trypanosoma brucei rhodesiense* (East African) infection is an acute, generalized illness that develops days to weeks after parasite inoculation, with manifestations including high fever, cutaneous chancre, myocarditis, hepatitis, anemia, thrombocytopenia, and laboratory evidence of disseminated intravascular coagulation. Clinical meningoencephalitis can develop as early as 3 weeks after onset of the untreated systemic illness. *Trypanosoma brucei rhodesiense* infection has a high fatality rate; without treatment, infected patients usually die within days to months after clinical onset of disease.

ETIOLOGY: The West African (Gambian) form of sleeping sickness is caused by *T brucei gambiense,* whereas the East African (Rhodesian) form is caused by *T brucei rhodesiense*. Both are extracellular protozoan hemoflagellates that live in the blood and tissue of the human host.

EPIDEMIOLOGY: Approximately 50 000 human cases are reported annually worldwide, although only a few cases, acquired in Africa, are reported every year in the United States. There has been a recent increase of trypanosomiasis in travelers after short visits to game parks in Tanzania. Transmission is confined to an area in Africa between the latitudes of 15° north and 20° south, corresponding precisely with the distribution of the tsetse fly vector (*Glossina* species). In East Africa, wild animals, such as antelope, bushbuck, and hartebeest, constitute the major reservoirs for of *T brucei rhodesiense*, although cattle serve as reservoir hosts in local outbreaks. Domestic pigs and dogs have been found as incidental reservoirs of *T brucei gambiense;* however, humans are the only important reservoir in West and Central Africa.

The **incubation period** for *T brucei rhodesiense* infection is 3 to 21 days and usually is 5 to 14 days; for *T brucei gambiense* infection, the incubation period is usually longer and variable, ranging from several months to years.

DIAGNOSTIC TESTS: Diagnosis is made by identification of trypomastigotes in specimens of blood, cerebrospinal fluid (CSF), or fluid aspirated from a chancre or lymph node or by inoculation of susceptible laboratory animals (mice) with heparinized blood. Examination of the CSF is critical to management and should be performed using the double-centrifugation technique. Concentration and Giemsa staining of the buffy coat layer of peripheral blood also can be helpful. *Trypanosoma brucei gambiense* is more likely to be found in lymph node aspirates. Although an increased concentration of immunoglobulin M in serum or CSF is considered characteristic of African trypanosomiasis, polyclonal hyperglobulinemia is common.

TREATMENT: When no evidence of CNS involvement is present (including absence of trypanosomes and CSF pleocytosis), the drug of choice for the acute hemolymphatic stage of infection is pentamidine for *T brucei gambiense* infection and suramin sodium for *T brucei rhodesiense* infection. For treatment of hemolymphatic and CNS disease, see Drugs for Parasitic Infections, p 744. Because of the risk of relapse, patients who have had CNS involvement should undergo repeated CSF examinations every 6 months for 2 years.

ISOLATION OF THE HOSPITALIZED PATIENT: Standard precautions are recommended.

CONTROL MEASURES: Travelers to endemic areas should avoid known foci of sleeping sickness and tsetse fly infestation and minimize fly bites by the use of protective clothing, insecticide-impregnated bed netting, and insect repellents. Infected patients should not breastfeed or donate blood.

American Trypanosomiasis
(Chagas Disease)

CLINICAL MANIFESTATIONS: Patients can have acute or chronic disease. The early phase of this disease commonly is asymptomatic. However, children are more likely to exhibit symptoms than are adults. In some patients, a red nodule known as a *chagoma* develops at the site of the original inoculation, usually on the face or arms. The surrounding skin becomes indurated and, later, hypopigmented. Unilateral firm edema of the eyelids, known as Romaña sign, is the earliest indication of the infection but is not always present. The edematous skin is violaceous and associated with conjunctivitis and enlargement of the ipsilateral preauricular lymph node. A few days after the appearance of Romaña sign, fever, generalized lymphadenopathy, and malaise can develop. Acute myocarditis, hepatosplenomegaly, edema, and meningoencephalitis can follow. In nearly all cases, acute Chagas disease resolves after 1 to 3 months, and an asymptomatic period follows. In 20% to 30% of cases, serious sequelae, consisting of cardiomyopathy and heart failure (the major cause of death), megaesophagus, and/or megacolon, develop many years after the initial infection. Congenital disease is characterized by low birth weight, hepatomegaly, and meningoencephalitis with seizures and tremors.

ETIOLOGY: *Trypanosoma cruzi,* a protozoan hemoflagellate, is the cause.

EPIDEMIOLOGY: Parasites are transmitted through feces of the insects of the triatomine family, usually an infected reduviid (cone-nose or kissing) bug. These insects defecate during or after taking blood. The bitten person is inoculated by inadvertently rubbing the insect feces containing the parasite into the site of the bite or mucous membranes of the eye or the mouth. The parasite also can be transmitted congenitally, during organ transplantation, through blood transfusion, and by consumption of the vector or the vector's excretion. Accidental laboratory infections can result from handling blood from infected people or laboratory animals. The disease is limited to the Western hemisphere, predominantly Mexico and Central and South America. Although some small mammals in the southern and southwestern United States harbor *T cruzi,* vectorborne transmission to humans is rare in the United States. Several transfusion- and transplantation-associated cases have been documented in the United States. Infection is common in immigrants from Central and South America. The disease is an important cause of death in South America, where between 7 and 15 million people are infected.

The **incubation period** for the acute phase of disease is 1 to 2 weeks or longer. Chronic manifestations do not appear for years to decades.

DIAGNOSTIC TESTS: During the acute phase of disease, the parasite is demonstrable in blood specimens by Giemsa staining or by direct wet-mount preparation. In chronic infections, which are characterized by low-level parasitemia, recovery of the parasite requires culture on special media or xenodiagnosis. Serologic tests include indirect hemagglutination, indirect immunofluorescence, and enzyme immunoassay.

TREATMENT: The acute phase of Chagas disease is treated with benznidazole or nifurtimox (see Drugs for Parasitic Infections, p 744). Although treatment of children during the latent and chronic phases of infection is routine in some Latin American countries, the effectiveness of this approach has not been established.

ISOLATION OF THE HOSPITALIZED PATIENT: Standard precautions should be followed.

CONTROL MEASURES: Travelers to endemic areas should avoid contact with reduviid insects by avoiding habitation in buildings that do not have control measures for these insects, particularly buildings constructed of mud, palm thatch, or adobe brick, and especially those with cracks in the walls or roof. The use of insecticide-impregnated bed nets also may be beneficial. Camping or sleeping outdoors in highly endemic areas is not recommended. Blood and serologic examinations should be performed on members of households with an infected patient if they have had exposure to the vector similar to that of the patient. Serologic testing before and after travel should be considered if exposure to the vector through residence in reduviid bug-infested houses in highly endemic areas is unavoidable.

Education about the mode of spread and the methods of prevention is warranted in endemic areas. Homes should be examined for the presence of the vectors, and if found, measures to eliminate the vector should be taken.

Blood donors in endemic areas should be screened by serologic tests (see Blood Safety, p 106). Infected patients should not donate blood. Blood recipients can be protected in endemic areas by treatment of the donated blood with gentian violet at a dilution of 1:4000.

Tuberculosis

CLINICAL MANIFESTATIONS: Most tuberculosis infections in children and adolescents are asymptomatic. When disease does occur, clinical manifestations most often appear 1 to 6 months after infection and include fever, growth delay or weight loss, cough, night sweats, and chills. Pulmonary radiographic findings range from normal to diverse abnormalities, such as lymphadenopathy of the hilar, subcarinal, or mediastinal nodes; atelectasis or infiltrate of a segment or lobe; pleural effusion; cavitary lesions; or miliary disease. Extrapulmonary manifestations are meningitis and disease of the middle ear and mastoid, lymph nodes, bones, joints, and skin. Renal tuberculosis and reactivation or adult-type pulmonary tuberculosis are rare in young children but can occur in adolescents. Clinical findings in patients with drug-resistant tuberculosis are indistinguishable from manifestations in patients with drug-susceptible disease.

ETIOLOGY: The agent is *Mycobacterium tuberculosis,* an acid-fast bacillus (AFB). Human disease caused by *Mycobacterium bovis,* the cause of bovine tuberculosis, occurs in the United States in children who have ingested unpasteurized milk or milk products.

DEFINITIONS:
- **Positive tuberculin skin test (TST).** A positive TST result (see Table 3.67, p 643) indicates likely infection with *M tuberculosis.* Tuberculin reactivity appears 2 to 12 weeks after initial infection; the median interval is 3 to 4 weeks (see Tuberculin Testing, p 645).
- **Exposed person** refers to a patient who has had recent contact with a person with suspected or confirmed contagious pulmonary tuberculosis and who has a negative TST result, normal physical examination findings, and chest radiographic findings that are not compatible with tuberculosis. Some exposed people have infection (and subsequently develop a positive TST result) and some do not; the 2 groups cannot be distinguished initially.
- **Source case** is defined as the person who has transmitted *M tuberculosis* to a child with tuberculosis infection or disease.
- **Latent tuberculosis infection (LTBI)** is defined as *M tuberculosis* infection in a person who has a positive TST result, no physical findings of disease, and chest radiograph findings that are normal or reveal evidence of healed infection (eg, granulomas or calcification in the lung, hilar lymph nodes, or both).
- **Tuberculosis disease** is defined as disease in a person with infection in whom symptoms, signs, or radiographic manifestations caused by *M tuberculosis* are apparent; disease may be pulmonary, extrapulmonary, or both.
- **Directly observed therapy (DOT)** is defined as an intervention by which medication is provided directly to the patient by a health care professional or trained third party (not a relative or friend), who observes and documents that the patient ingests each dose of medication.

EPIDEMIOLOGY: Case rates of tuberculosis disease for all ages are higher in urban, low-income areas and in nonwhite racial and ethnic groups; two thirds of reported cases in the United States occur in nonwhite individuals. In recent years, foreign-

Table 3.67. Definitions of Positive Tuberculin Skin Test (TST) Results in Infants, Children, and Adolescents[1]

Induration ≥5 mm

Children in close contact with known or suspected contagious cases of tuberculosis disease

Children suspected to have tuberculosis disease:
- Findings on chest radiograph consistent with active or previously active tuberculosis
- Clinical evidence of tuberculosis disease[2]

Children receiving immunosuppressive therapy[3] or with immunosuppressive conditions, including HIV infection

Induration ≥10 mm

Children at increased risk of disseminated disease:
- Those younger than 4 years of age
- Those with other medical conditions, including Hodgkin disease, lymphoma, diabetes mellitus, chronic renal failure, or malnutrition (see Table 3.68, p 646)

Children with increased exposure to tuberculosis disease:
- Those born, or whose parents were born, in high-prevalence regions of the world
- Those frequently exposed to adults who are HIV infected, homeless, users of illicit drugs, residents of nursing homes, incarcerated or institutionalized, or migrant farm workers
- Those who travel to high-prevalence regions of the world

Induration ≥15 mm

Children 4 years of age or older without any risk factors

HIV indicates human immunodeficiency virus.

[1] These definitions apply regardless of previous bacille Calmette-Guérin (BCG) immunization (see also Interpretation of TST Results in Previous Recipients of BCG Vaccine, p 647); erythema at TST site does not indicate a positive test result. TSTs should be read at 48 to 72 hours after placement.

[2] Evidence by physical examination or laboratory assessment that would include tuberculosis in the working differential diagnosis (eg, meningitis).

[3] Including immunosuppressive doses of corticosteroids (see Corticosteroids, p 654).

born children have accounted for more than one third of newly diagnosed cases in children 14 years of age or younger. Specific groups with high LTBI and disease rates include first-generation immigrants from high prevalence regions (eg, Asia, Africa, and Latin America), homeless people, and residents of corrections facilities.

Infants and postpubertal adolescents are at increased risk of progression of LTBI to tuberculosis disease. Other predictive factors for development of disease include recent infection (within the past 2 years); immunodeficiency, including human immunodeficiency virus (HIV) infection; use of immunosuppressive drugs, such as prolonged or high-dose corticosteroid therapy or chemotherapy; intravenous drug use; and certain diseases or medical conditions, including Hodgkin disease, lymphoma, diabetes mellitus, chronic renal failure, and malnutrition.

A diagnosis of LTBI or tuberculosis disease in a child is a sentinel event usually representing recent transmission of *M tuberculosis*. Transmission of *M tuberculosis* is airborne, with inhalation of droplet nuclei produced by an adult or adolescent with contagious, cavitary, pulmonary tuberculosis. The duration of contagiousness of an adult receiving effective treatment depends on drug susceptibilities of the organism, the number of organisms in sputum, and frequency of cough. Although contagiousness usually lasts only a few days to weeks after initiation of effective drug therapy, it may last longer, especially when the adult patient does not adhere to medical therapy or is infected with a drug-resistant strain. If the sputum smear is negative for AFB organisms on 3 separate days and coughing has ceased, the treated person can be considered noncontagious. Children younger than 12 years of age with primary pulmonary tuberculosis rarely are contagious, because their pulmonary lesions are small, cough is not productive, and there is little or no expulsion of bacilli.

The **incubation period** from infection to development of a positive TST result is 2 to 12 weeks. The risk of developing tuberculosis disease is highest during the 6 months after infection and remains high for 2 years; however, many years can elapse between initial infection and disease.

DIAGNOSTIC TESTS: Isolation of *M tuberculosis* by culture from specimens of gastric aspirates, sputum, bronchial washings, pleural fluid, cerebrospinal fluid (CSF), urine, or other body fluids or a biopsy specimen establishes the diagnosis. The best specimen for diagnosis of pulmonary tuberculosis in any young child or adolescent in whom the cough is nonproductive or absent is an early morning gastric aspirate. Gastric aspirate specimens should be obtained with a nasogastric tube on awakening the child and before ambulation or feeding. Aspirates collected on 3 separate days should be submitted. Results of AFB smears of gastric aspirates usually are negative, and false-positive results caused by the presence of other mycobacteria can occur. Attempts should be made to demonstrate AFB in sputum, body fluids, or both by the Ziehl-Neelsen method or by auramine-rhodamine staining with fluorescent microscopy. Fluorescent methods are more sensitive and, if available, preferred. Histologic examination for and demonstration of AFB in biopsy specimens from lymph node, pleura, liver, bone marrow, or other tissues can be useful, but *M tuberculosis* cannot reliably be distinguished from other mycobacteria in stained specimens. Regardless of results of the AFB smears, each specimen should be cultured.

Because *M tuberculosis* is slow growing, detection of this organism may take as long as 10 weeks using solid media; liquid media allows detection within 1 to 6 weeks. Even with optimal culture techniques, organisms are isolated from fewer than 50% of children and 75% of infants with pulmonary tuberculosis diagnosed by other criteria. Species identification of isolates by culture can be more rapid if a DNA probe or high-pressure liquid chromatography is used.

Nucleic acid amplification tests for rapid diagnosis are licensed by the US Food and Drug Administration (FDA) only for acid-fast stain positive respiratory tract specimens. Polymerase chain reaction assay has comparable sensitivity to culture for gastric aspirate specimens, but false-negative and false-positive results can occur with these specimens as well as with sputum, CSF, and tissue specimens.

Identification of the source case supports the child's presumptive diagnosis and defines the likely drug susceptibility of the child's organism.

Culture material should be obtained from children with evidence of tuberculosis disease, especially when (1) an isolate from a source case is not available; (2) the source case has drug-resistant tuberculosis; (3) the child is immunocompromised, including children with HIV infection; or (4) the child has extrapulmonary disease.

Tuberculin Testing. The TST is the only practical tool for diagnosing LTBI in asymptomatic people. The test containing 5 tuberculin units of purified protein derivative, which is administered using a 27-gauge needle and a 1.0-mL syringe intradermally into the volar aspect of the forearm, is recommended. Creation of a visible wheal is crucial to accurate testing. Other strengths of TSTs (1 or 250 tuberculin units) should not be used. Multiple puncture tests are not recommended, because they lack adequate sensitivity and specificity.

The American Academy of Pediatrics recommends a TST for children who are at increased risk of acquiring LTBI and tuberculosis disease (see Table 3.68, p 646). Routine TST administration, including school-based programs that include populations at low risk, will result in either a low yield of positive results or a large proportion of false-positive results, leading to an inefficient use of health care resources. Simple questionnaires can identify children with risk factors for LTBI who should have a TST. Factors that have correlated consistently with increased risk of LTBI in several published studies include recent contact with a case of tuberculosis, family history of tuberculosis, positive TST reactions in other current household members, and foreign birth or prolonged travel to a country with high tuberculosis rates.

A TST can be administered during the same visit that immunizations, including live-virus vaccines, are given. Because measles vaccine temporarily can suppress tuberculin reactivity, if tuberculin testing is indicated and cannot be performed at the same time as measles immunization, tuberculin testing should be deferred for 4 to 6 weeks. Previous immunization with bacille Calmette-Guérin (BCG) vaccine is not a contraindication to TST.

Administration of TSTs and interpretation of results should be performed by experienced health care professionals who have been trained in the proper methods, because administration and interpretation by unskilled people (eg, family members) is unreliable. The recommended time for assessing the TST result (eg, measurement of the size of induration by the ballpoint pen technique) is 48 to 72 hours after administration. However, a reaction that develops at the site of administration more than 72 hours later should be measured and considered the result. The diameter of induration in millimeters is measured transversely to the long axis of the forearm. Positive test results, as defined in Table 3.67 (p 643), can persist for several weeks.

A negative TST result cannot exclude LTBI or tuberculosis disease. Approximately 10% of immunocompetent children with culture-documented disease do not react initially to a TST. Host factors, such as young age, poor nutrition, immunosuppression, other viral infections (especially measles, varicella, and influenza), and disseminated tuberculosis can decrease TST reactivity. Many children and adults coinfected with HIV and *M tuberculosis* do not react to a TST. Control skin tests to assess cutaneous anergy are not recommended.

Interpretation of TST Results (see Table 3.67, p 643). The classification of TST results is based on epidemiologic and clinical factors. The size of induration (mm) for a positive result varies with the person's risks of LTBI and progression to tuberculosis disease.

Table 3.68. Tuberculin Skin Test (TST) Recommendations for Infants, Children, and Adolescents[1]

Children for whom immediate TST is indicated:
- Contacts of people with confirmed or suspected contagious tuberculosis (contact investigation)
- Children with radiographic or clinical findings suggesting tuberculosis disease
- Children immigrating from endemic countries (eg, Asia, Middle East, Africa, Latin America)
- Children with travel histories to endemic countries and/or significant contact with indigenous people from such countries

Children who should have annual TST[2]:
- Children infected with HIV
- Incarcerated adolescents

Some experts recommend that children should be tested every 2–3 years[2]:
- Children with ongoing exposure to the following people: HIV infected people, homeless people, residents of nursing homes, institutionalized adolescents or adults, users of illicit drugs, incarcerated adolescents or adults, and migrant farm workers; foster children with exposure to adults in the preceding high-risk groups are included

Some experts recommend that children should be considered for TST at 4–6 and 11–16 years of age:
- Children whose parents immigrated (with unknown TST status) from regions of the world with high prevalence of tuberculosis; continued potential exposure by travel to the endemic areas and/or household contact with people from the endemic areas (with unknown TST status) should be an indication for a repeated TST

Children at increased risk of progression of infection to disease: Children with other medical conditions, including diabetes mellitus, chronic renal failure, malnutrition, and congenital or acquired immunodeficiencies deserve special consideration. Without recent exposure, these people are not at increased risk of acquiring tuberculosis infection. Underlying immune deficiencies associated with these conditions theoretically would enhance the possibility for progression to severe disease. Initial histories of potential exposure to tuberculosis should be included for all of these patients. If these histories or local epidemiologic factors suggest a possibility of exposure, immediate and periodic TST should be considered. **An initial TST should be performed before initiation of immunosuppressive therapy, including prolonged steroid administration, for any child with an underlying condition that necessitates immunosuppressive therapy.**

HIV indicates human immunodeficiency virus.
[1] Bacille Calmette-Guérin immunization is not a contraindication to TST.
[2] Initial TST is at the time of diagnosis or circumstance, beginning at 3 months of age.

Current guidelines from the Centers for Disease Control and Prevention (CDC), American Thoracic Society, and the American Academy of Pediatrics accept 15 mm or greater of induration as a positive TST result for any person. Interpretation of 5 mm or more or 10 mm or more induration is summarized in Table 3.67 (p 643). Interpretation is aided by knowledge of the child's risk factors for tuberculosis infection and disease. Prompt radiographic evaluation of all children with a positive TST reaction is recommended.

Interpretation of TST Results in Previous Recipients of BCG Vaccine. Generally, interpretation of TST results in BCG recipients is the same as for people who have not received BCG vaccine. After BCG immunization, distinguishing between a positive TST result caused by *M tuberculosis* infection and that caused by BCG can be difficult. Reactivity of the TST after receipt of BCG vaccine does not occur in some patients. The size of the TST reaction (ie, induration) attributable to BCG immunization depends on many factors, including age at BCG immunization, quality and strain of BCG vaccine used, number of doses of BCG received, nutritional and immunologic status of the vaccine recipient, and frequency of TST administration.

Disease caused by *M tuberculosis* should be suspected strongly in any symptomatic person with a positive TST result, regardless of history of BCG immunization. When evaluating an asymptomatic child who has a positive TST result but who possibly received BCG, verification of previous BCG immunization by written documentation or identification of the typical BCG immunization scar should be undertaken. Although a positive TST result never can be proven to be attributable to BCG vaccine, certain factors, such as documented receipt of multiple BCG immunizations (as evidenced by multiple BCG scars), decrease the likelihood that the positive TST result is attributable to LTBI. Evidence that increases the probability that a positive TST result is attributable to LTBI includes known contact with a person with contagious tuberculosis, a family history of tuberculosis, immigration from a country with a high prevalence of tuberculosis, a long interval (>5 years) since the last BCG immunization, and a TST reaction ≥15 mm.

Prompt radiographic evaluation of all children with a positive TST reaction is recommended, regardless of the child's BCG immunization status. Chest radiographic findings of a granuloma, calcification, or adenopathy can be caused by *M tuberculosis* but not by BCG immunization. In most situations, an asymptomatic BCG-immunized child with a positive TST result will have normal chest radiograph findings. In such children, LTBI should be assumed and antituberculosis therapy should be initiated to prevent progression to *M tuberculosis* disease. For some children, such as children recently immunized with BCG, children with documented multiple BCG immunizations, or children who immigrated from a country with a low prevalence of tuberculosis, treatment may not be indicated. In such cases, follow-up should include patient education and awareness of the signs and symptoms of tuberculosis disease.

Recommendations for TST Usage. The most reliable strategies for preventing LTBI and tuberculosis disease in children are based on aggressive, expedient contact investigations rather than nonselective TST screening of large populations. Specific recommendations for TST use are found in Table 3.68 (p 646). All children need routine health care evaluations that include an assessment of their risk of exposure to tuberculosis. Only children deemed to have increased risk of contact with people with contagious tuberculosis or children with suspected tuberculosis disease should be considered for a TST. Household investigation is indicated whenever a TST result of a household member converts from negative to positive (indicating recent infection). In many locales, the health department does not have enough resources to perform this investigation in the absence of a case of suspected tuberculosis disease.

HIV Testing. People with tuberculosis disease should be tested for HIV infection, because the risk of tuberculosis disease is increased in HIV infected people.

TREATMENT (SEE TABLE 3.69, P 649):

Specific Drugs. Antituberculosis drugs kill *M tuberculosis* or inhibit multiplication of the organism, thereby arresting progression of tuberculosis and preventing most complications of early primary disease. Chemotherapy does not cause rapid disappearance of already caseous or granulomatous lesions (eg, mediastinal lymphadenitis with endobronchial breakthrough). Dosage recommendations and the more commonly reported adverse reactions of major antituberculosis drugs are summarized in Tables 3.70 and 3.71, (p 650 and p 651). For treatment of tuberculosis disease, these drugs must always be used in combination to hinder emergence of drug-resistant strains.

Isoniazid is bactericidal, rapidly absorbed, and well tolerated and penetrates into body fluids, including CSF. Isoniazid is metabolized in the liver and excreted primarily through the kidneys. Hepatotoxic effects are rare in children but can be life threatening. In children and adolescents given recommended doses, peripheral neuritis or seizures caused by inhibition of pyridoxine metabolism are rare, and most do not need pyridoxine supplements. Pyridoxine is recommended for children and adolescents on meat- and milk-deficient diets; children with nutritional deficiencies, including all symptomatic HIV-infected children; and pregnant adolescents and women. For infants and young children, isoniazid tablets can be pulverized.

Rifampin is a bactericidal agent that is absorbed rapidly and penetrates into body fluids, including CSF. Rifampin is metabolized by the liver and can alter the pharmacokinetics and serum concentrations of many other drugs. Hepatotoxic effects occur rarely. Rifampin is excreted in bile and urine and can cause orange urine, sweat, and tears and discoloration of soft contact lenses. Rifampin can make oral contraceptives ineffective, so other birth control methods should be adopted when rifampin is administered to sexually active women. For infants and young children, the contents of the capsules can be suspended in wild cherry-flavored syrup or sprinkled on applesauce. *Mycobacterium tuberculosis* resistant to rifampin is uncommon in the United States. Other rifamycins (rifabutin and rifapentine) used in adults are not licensed by the FDA for use in children.

Pyrazinamide attains therapeutic CSF concentrations, is detectable in macrophages, is administered orally, and is metabolized by the liver. Administration of pyrazinamide with isoniazid and rifampin allows for 6-month regimens. In doses of 30 mg/kg per day or less, pyrazinamide seldom has hepatotoxic effects and is well tolerated by children. Some adolescents and many adults develop arthralgia because of inhibition of uric acid excretion. Pyrazinamide is not recommended for people with underlying liver disease or who have had isoniazid-associated liver injury.

Streptomycin sulfate is administered by the intramuscular route but is available only on a limited basis. When streptomycin is not available, kanamycin, capreomycin, or amikacin are alternatives that are prescribed for the initial 4 to 8 weeks of therapy.

Ethambutol hydrochloride is well absorbed after oral administration, diffuses well into tissues, and is excreted in urine. At 15 mg/kg per day, ethambutol is bacteriostatic only, and its primary therapeutic role is to prevent emergence of drug

Table 3.69. Recommended Treatment Regimens for Drug-Susceptible Tuberculosis in Infants, Children, and Adolescents

Infection or Disease Category	Regimen	Remarks
Latent tuberculosis infection (positive TST result, no disease)		
• Isoniazid-susceptible	9 mo of isoniazid, once a day	If daily therapy is not possible, DOT twice a week can be used for 9 mo.
• Isoniazid-resistant	6 mo of rifampin, once a day	
• Isoniazid-rifampin-resistant[1]	Consult a tuberculosis specialist	
Pulmonary and extrapulmonary (except meningitis)	2 mo of isoniazid, rifampin, and pyrazinamide daily, followed by 4 mo of isoniazid and rifampin[2]	If possible drug resistance is a concern (see text), another drug (ethambutol or an aminoglycoside) is added to the initial 3-drug therapy until drug susceptibilities are determined. DOT is highly desirable. If hilar adenopathy only, a 6-mo course of isoniazid and rifampin is sufficient. Drugs can be given 2 or 3 times/wk under DOT in the initial phase if nonadherence is likely
Meningitis	2 mo of isoniazid, rifampin, pyrazinamide, and an aminoglycoside or ethionamide, once a day, followed by 7–10 mo of isoniazid and rifampin, once a day or twice a week (9–12 mo total)	A fourth drug, usually an aminoglycoside, is given with initial therapy until drug susceptibility is known. For patients who may have acquired tuberculosis in geographic areas where resistance to streptomycin is common, capreomycin, kanamycin, or amikacin may be used instead of streptomycin.

TST indicates tuberculin skin test; DOT, directly observed therapy.

[1] Duration of therapy is longer for human immunodeficiency virus (HIV)-infected people, and additional drugs may be indicated (see Tuberculosis Disease and HIV Infection, p 654).

[2] Medications should be administered daily for the first 2 weeks to 2 months of treatment and then can be administered 2–3 times per week by DOT.

Table 3.70. Commonly Used Drugs for the Treatment of Tuberculosis in Infants, Children, and Adolescents

Drugs	Dosage Forms	Daily Dosage, mg/kg	Twice a Week Dosage, mg/kg per Dose	Maximum Dose	Adverse Reactions
Ethambutol	Tablets 100 mg 400 mg	15–25	50	2.5 g	Optic neuritis (usually reversible), decreased red-green color discrimination, gastrointestinal tract disturbances, hypersensitivity
Isoniazid[1]	Scored tablets 100 mg 300 mg Syrup 10 mg/mL	10–15[2]	20–30	Daily, 300 mg Twice a week, 900 mg	Mild hepatic enzyme elevation, hepatitis,[2] peripheral neuritis, hypersensitivity
Pyrazinamide[1]	Scored tablets 500 mg	20–40	50	2 g	Hepatotoxic effects, hyperuricemia
Rifampin[1]	Capsules 150 mg 300 mg Syrup formulated in syrup from capsules	10–20	10–20	600 mg	Orange discoloration of secretions or urine, staining of contact lenses, vomiting, hepatitis, influenza-like reaction, thrombocytopenia; oral contraceptives may be ineffective

[1] Rifamate (Aventis Pharmaceuticals, Bridgewater, NJ) is a capsule containing 150 mg of isoniazid and 300 mg of rifampin. Two capsules provide the usual adult (>50 kg) daily doses of each drug. Rifater is a capsule containing 50 mg of isoniazid, 120 mg of rifampin, and 300 mg of pyrazinamide. Isoniazid and rifampin also are available for parenteral administration.

[2] When isoniazid in a dosage exceeding 10 mg/kg per day is used in combination with rifampin, the incidence of hepatotoxic effects may be increased.

Table 3.71. Less Commonly Used Drugs for Treatment of Drug-Resistant Tuberculosis in Infants, Children, and Adolescents[1]

Drugs	Dosage Forms	Daily Dosage, mg/kg	Maximum Dose	Adverse Reactions
Capreomycin	Vials, 1g	15–30 (intramuscular administration)	1 g	Ototoxic and nephrotoxic effects
Ciprofloxacin[2]	Tablets 250 mg 500 mg 750 mg	Adults 500–1500 mg total per day (twice a day)	1.5 g	Theoretic effect on growing cartilage, gastro-intestinal tract disturbances, rash, headache
Cycloserine	Capsules, 250 mg	10–20	1 g	Psychosis, personality changes, seizures, rash
Ethionamide	Tablets, 250 mg	15–20, given in 2–3 divided doses	1 g	Gastrointestinal tract disturbances, hepatotoxic effects, hypersensitivity reactions
Kanamycin	Vials 75 mg/2 mL 500 mg/2 mL 1 g/3 mL	15–30 (intramuscular administration)	1 g	Auditory and vestibular toxic effects, nephro-toxic effects
Levofloxacin[2]	Tablets 250 mg 500 mg Vials 25 mg/mL	Adults 500–1000 mg (once daily)	1 g	Theoretic effect on growing cartilage, gastro-intestinal tract disturbances, rash, headache
Para-aminosalicylic acid (PAS)	Packets, 3g	200–300 (2 to 4 times a day)	10 g	Gastrointestinal tract disturbances, hyper-sensitivity, hepatotoxic effects
Streptomycin (intramuscular administration)	Vials 1 g 4 g	20–40	1 g	Auditory and vestibular toxic effects, nephrotoxic effects, rash

[1] These drugs should be used in consultation with a specialist in tuberculosis.
[2] Fluoroquinolones currently are not licensed for use in people younger than 18 years of age; their use in younger patients necessitates assessment of the potential risks and benefits (see Antimicrobial Agents and Related Therapy, p 693).

resistance. A dose of 25 mg/kg per day is necessary for bactericidal activity. Because ethambutol may cause reversible or irreversible optic neuritis, recipients should be monitored monthly for visual acuity and red-green color discrimination. Use of ethambutol in young children whose visual acuity cannot be monitored requires consideration of risks and benefits. However, ethambutol-associated optic neuritis is exceedingly rare in children with normal renal function.

The less commonly used (eg, "second-line") antituberculosis drugs, their doses, and adverse effects are listed in Table 3.71 (p 651). These drugs have limited usefulness because of lesser effectiveness and greater toxicity and should be used only in consultation with a specialist. Ethionamide is an orally administered antituberculosis drug that is well tolerated by children, achieves therapeutic CSF concentrations, and may be useful for treatment of people with meningitis or drug-resistant tuberculosis. Fluoroquinolones have antituberculosis activity and can be used in special circumstances. Because these drugs are licensed by the FDA for use only in people 18 years of age and older, their use in younger patients necessitates careful assessment of the potential risks and benefits (see Antimicrobial Agents and Related Therapy, p 693). In cases of multidrug-resistant LTBI or tuberculosis disease, these drugs should be considered for therapy.

Occasionally, a patient cannot tolerate oral medications. Isoniazid, rifampin, streptomycin and related drugs, and fluoroquinolones can be administered parenterally. Some pharmacies have formulated suppository preparations for isoniazid and rifampin, but there is no standard formulation; serum drug concentrations should be monitored if rectal medication is administered.

Therapy for LTBI. Isoniazid given to adults who have LTBI (eg, no clinical or radiographic abnormalities suggesting tuberculosis disease) provides substantial protection (54%–88%) against development of tuberculosis disease for at least 20 years. Among children, efficacy approaches 100% with appropriate adherence to therapy. All infants, children, and adolescents who have a positive TST result but no evidence of tuberculosis disease and who never have received antituberculosis therapy should receive isoniazid unless resistance to isoniazid is suspected or a specific contraindication exists. Isoniazid in this circumstance is therapeutic and prevents development of disease. A chest radiograph should be obtained at the time therapy is initiated to exclude active disease; if radiographic findings are normal, the child remains asymptomatic, and treatment is completed, radiography need not be repeated.

Duration of Therapy for LTBI. For infants, children, and adolescents, the recommended duration of isoniazid therapy is 9 months. Isoniazid is given daily in a single dose. When adherence with daily therapy with isoniazid cannot be ensured, twice-a-week DOT can be considered.

Therapy for Contacts of Patients With Isoniazid-Resistant M tuberculosis. The incidence of isoniazid resistance among *M tuberculosis* isolates from US patients is approximately 9%. Risk factors for drug resistance are listed in Table 3.72, p 653. However, most experts recommend that isoniazid be used to treat LTBI in children unless the child has had contact with a person known to have isoniazid-resistant tuberculosis. If the source case is found to have isoniazid-resistant organisms, isoniazid should be discontinued and rifampin should be given for a total course of at least 6 months. The effectiveness and safety of a 2-month course of rifampin

Table 3.72. **People at Increased Risk of Drug-Resistant Tuberculosis Infection or Disease**

- People with a history of treatment for active tuberculosis (or whose source case for the contact received such treatment)
- Contacts of a patient with drug-resistant contagious tuberculosis disease
- People born in countries with high prevalence of drug-resistant tuberculosis
- Residents of areas where the prevalence of drug-resistant *Mycobacterium tuberculosis* is documented to be high (defined by most experts as isoniazid resistance rates ≥4%)
- Infected people whose source case has positive smears for acid-fast bacilli or cultures after 2 months of appropriate antituberculosis therapy

and pyrazinamide in children to treat LTBI is unknown and cannot be recommended. Optimal therapy for children with LTBI caused by organisms with resistance to isoniazid and rifampin is unknown. In these circumstances, multidrug regimens have been used. Drugs to consider include pyrazinamide, a fluoroquinolone, and ethambutol, depending on susceptibility of the isolate. Consultation with a tuberculosis specialist is indicated.

Treatment of Tuberculosis Disease. The goal of treatment is to achieve sterilization of the tuberculous lesion in the shortest possible time. Achievement of this goal minimizes the possibility of development of resistant organisms. The major problem limiting successful treatment is poor adherence to prescribed treatment regimens. The use of DOT decreases the rates of relapse, treatment failures, and drug resistance and, therefore, DOT is recommended for treatment of children and adolescents with tuberculosis disease in the United States.

A 6-month regimen consisting of isoniazid, rifampin, and pyrazinamide for the first 2 months and isoniazid and rifampin for the remaining 4 months is recommended for treatment of **drug-susceptible** *M tuberculosis* disease, including pulmonary, pulmonary with hilar adenopathy, and hilar adenopathy disease in infants, children, and adolescents. For children with hilar adenopathy in whom drug resistance is not a consideration, a 6-month regimen of only isoniazid and rifampin is adequate.

When **drug resistance** is suspected (see Table 3.72, above), initial therapy should include a fourth drug, either ethambutol or an aminoglycoside, until drug susceptibility results are available. If an isolate from the pediatric case under treatment is not available, drug susceptibilities can be inferred by the drug susceptibility pattern of isolates from the adult source case. If this information is not available, local endemic rates of single and multiple drug resistance can be helpful. Data may not be available for foreign-born children or in circumstances of foreign travel. If this information is not available, a 4-drug initial regimen is recommended.

In the 6-month regimen with triple-drug therapy, isoniazid, rifampin, and pyrazinamide are given once a day for the first 2 weeks. Between 2 weeks and 2 months of treatment, isoniazid, rifampin, and pyrazinamide can be given daily or twice a week by DOT. After the initial 2 month period, a DOT regimen of isoniazid and rifampin given twice a week is acceptable (see Table 3.69, p 649, for doses). Several alternative regimens with differing durations of daily therapy and total therapy have been used successfully in adults and children. These alternative regimens should be prescribed and managed by a specialist in tuberculosis.

Therapy for Drug-Resistant Tuberculosis Disease. In some areas of North America, the incidence of drug resistance in previously untreated patients has increased in recent years. Drug resistance is most common in the following: (1) people born in areas such as Russia and the former Soviet Union, Asia, Africa, and Latin America; (2) people previously treated for tuberculosis disease; and (3) contacts, especially children, with tuberculosis disease whose source case is a person from one of these groups (see also Table 3.72, p 653). Most cases of pulmonary tuberculosis in children that are caused by an isoniazid-resistant but rifampin-susceptible strain of *M tuberculosis* can be treated with a 9-month regimen of rifampin, pyrazinamide, and ethambutol. For cases of suspected drug-resistant tuberculosis disease, an initial treatment regimen should include at least 4 antituberculosis drugs. Treatment should include at least 2 bactericidal drugs, such as isoniazid and rifampin, pyrazinamide, and an aminoglycoside (also bactericidal) or ethambutol at 25 mg/kg per day. In cases of tuberculosis with isoniazid- or rifampin-resistant strains, 6-month drug regimens are not recommended. Twelve to 18 months of therapy usually is necessary for cure. Twice-a-week regimens also are not recommended for drug-resistant disease; DOT is critical to cure children with drug-resistant tuberculosis disease and to prevent emergence of further resistance.

Extrapulmonary Tuberculosis. In general, extrapulmonary tuberculosis—with the exception of meningitis—can be treated with the same regimens as used for pulmonary tuberculosis. For drug-susceptible tuberculous meningitis, daily treatment with isoniazid; rifampin; pyrazinamide; and ethambutol, streptomycin, or another aminoglycoside or ethionamide for the first 1 or 2 months, followed by isoniazid and rifampin once a day or twice a week by DOT is recommended for a total of 9 to 12 months. For life-threatening tuberculosis, 4 drugs are given initially because of the possibility of drug resistance and the severe consequences of treatment failure (see Therapy for Drug-Resistant Tuberculosis Disease, above).

Corticosteroids. The evidence supporting adjuvant treatment with corticosteroids for children with tuberculosis disease is incomplete. Corticosteroids are indicated for children with tuberculous meningitis, because they decrease rates of mortality and long-term neurologic impairment. Corticosteroids may be considered for children with pleural and pericardial effusions (to hasten reabsorption of fluid), severe miliary disease (to mitigate alveolocapillary block), and endobronchial disease (to relieve obstruction and atelectasis). Corticosteroids should be given only when accompanied by appropriate antituberculosis therapy. Most experts consider 1 to 2 mg/kg per day of prednisone (maximum 60 mg/day) or its equivalent for 6 to 8 weeks to be appropriate.

Tuberculosis Disease and HIV Infection. Adults and children with HIV infection have an increased incidence of tuberculosis disease. Hence, testing for HIV is indicated for all people with tuberculosis disease. The clinical manifestations and radiographic appearance of tuberculosis disease in children with HIV infection tend to be similar to those in immunocompetent children, but manifestations in these children can be more severe and unusual and can include extrapulmonary involvement of multiple organs. In HIV-infected patients, a TST result of 5-mm induration or more is considered positive (see Table 3.67, p 643); however, a negative TST result attributable to HIV-related immunosuppression also can occur. Specimens for culture should be obtained from all HIV-infected children with suspected tuberculosis.

Most HIV-infected adults with drug-susceptible tuberculosis respond well to antituberculosis drugs when appropriate therapy is given early. However, optimal therapy for tuberculosis in children with HIV infection has not been established. Therapy always should include at least 3 drugs initially and be continued for at least 9 months. Isoniazid, rifampin, and pyrazinamide, usually with ethambutol or an aminoglycoside, should be given for at least the first 2 months. A 3-drug regimen can be used once drug-resistant disease is excluded. Consultation with a specialist who has experience in managing HIV-infected patients with tuberculosis is advised.

Evaluation and Monitoring of Therapy in Children and Adolescents. Careful monthly monitoring of the clinical and bacteriologic responses to therapy is important. With DOT, clinical evaluation is an integral component of each visit for drug administration. For patients with pulmonary tuberculosis, chest radiographs should be obtained after 2 to 3 months of therapy to evaluate response. Even with successful 6-month regimens, hilar adenopathy may persist for 2 to 3 years; normal radiographic findings are not necessary to discontinue therapy. Follow-up chest radiographs beyond the termination of successful therapy usually are not necessary unless clinical deterioration occurs.

If therapy has been interrupted, the date of completion should be extended. Although guidelines cannot be provided for every situation, factors to consider when establishing the date of completion include the following: (1) length of interruption of therapy; (2) time during therapy (early or late) when interruption occurred; and (3) the patient's clinical, radiographic, and bacteriologic status before, during, and after interruption of therapy. Consultation with a specialist in tuberculosis is advised.

Untoward effects of isoniazid therapy, including severe hepatitis in otherwise healthy infants, children, and adolescents, are rare. Routine determination of serum transaminase concentrations is not recommended. However, for children with severe tuberculosis, especially children with meningitis or disseminated disease, transaminase concentrations should be monitored approximately monthly during the first several months of treatment. Other indications for testing include the following: (1) having concurrent or recent liver or biliary disease; (2) being pregnant or in the first 6 weeks postpartum; (3) having clinical evidence of hepatotoxic effects; or (4) concurrently using other hepatotoxic drugs (especially anticonvulsant agents). In most other circumstances, monthly clinical evaluations to observe for signs or symptoms of hepatitis and other adverse effects of drug therapy without routine monitoring of transaminase concentrations is appropriate follow-up. In all cases, regular physician-patient contact to assess drug adherence, efficacy, and toxic effects is an important aspect of management.

Immunizations. Patients who are receiving treatment for tuberculosis can be given measles and other age appropriate live-virus vaccines unless they are receiving high-dose corticosteroids, are severely ill, or have other specific contraindications to immunization.

Tuberculosis During Pregnancy and Breastfeeding. Tuberculosis treatment
during pregnancy varies because of the complexity of management decisions. During
pregnancy, if tuberculosis disease is diagnosed, a regimen of isoniazid, rifampin,
and ethambutol is recommended. Pyrazinamide commonly is used in a 3- or 4-drug
regimen, but safety during pregnancy has not been established. At least 6 months of
therapy is indicated for drug-susceptible tuberculosis disease if pyrazinamide is used;
at least 9 months of therapy is indicated if pyrazinamide is not used. Prompt initiation of therapy is mandatory to protect mother and fetus.

Asymptomatic pregnant women with a positive TST result, normal chest radiographic findings, and contact with a contagious person should receive isoniazid
therapy. The recommended duration of therapy is 9 months. Therapy in these
circumstances should begin after the first trimester. Pyridoxine is indicated for all
pregnant and breastfeeding women receiving isoniazid.

Isoniazid, ethambutol, and rifampin are relatively safe for the fetus. The benefit
of ethambutol and rifampin for therapy of tuberculosis disease in the mother outweighs the risk to the infant. Because streptomycin can cause ototoxic effects in the
fetus, it should not be used unless administration is essential for effective treatment.

Although isoniazid is secreted in human milk, no adverse effects of isoniazid on
nursing infants have been demonstrated (see Human Milk, p 117). Breastfed infants
do not require pyridoxine unless they are receiving isoniazid.

Congenital Tuberculosis. Women who have only pulmonary tuberculosis
are not likely to infect the fetus but may infect their infant after delivery. Congenital tuberculosis is rare, but in utero infections can occur after maternal
M tuberculosis bacillemia.

If a newborn is suspected of having congenital tuberculosis, a TST, chest radiograph, lumbar puncture, and appropriate cultures should be performed promptly.
The TST result usually is negative in newborn infants with congenital or perinatally
acquired infection. Hence, regardless of the TST results, treatment of the infant
should be initiated promptly with isoniazid, rifampin, pyrazinamide, and streptomycin or kanamycin. The placenta should be examined histologically and cultured
for *M tuberculosis*. The mother should be evaluated for the presence of pulmonary
or extrapulmonary, including uterine, tuberculosis. If the maternal physical examination or chest radiographic findings support the diagnosis of tuberculosis disease,
the newborn infant should be treated with regimens recommended for tuberculosis
disease. If meningitis is confirmed, corticosteroids should be added (see Corticosteroids, p 654). Drug susceptibility testing of the organism recovered from the
mother, infant, or both should be performed.

***Management of the Newborn Infant Whose Mother (or Other Household Contact)
Has LTBI or Disease.*** Management of the newborn infant is based on categorization
of the maternal (or household contact) infection. Although protection of the infant
from tuberculosis disease is of paramount importance, separation of the infant from
the mother (or household contact) should be avoided when possible. Differing circumstances and resulting recommendations are as follows:

- ***Mother (or household contact) has a positive TST result and normal chest
  radiographic findings.*** If the mother (or household contact) is asymptomatic,
  no separation is required. The mother usually is a candidate for treatment of
  LTBI. The newborn infant needs no special evaluation or therapy. Because the

positive TST result could be a marker of an unrecognized case of contagious tuberculosis within the household, other household members should have a TST and further evaluation, but this should not delay the child's discharge from the hospital.

- **Mother (or household contact) has a positive TST result and abnormal findings on chest radiography consistent with tuberculosis disease.** If the radiograph appears abnormal, the mother (or household contact) and infant should be separated until the mother (or household contact) has been evaluated and, if tuberculosis disease is found, until the mother or contact has been receiving appropriate antituberculosis therapy for at least 2 weeks. Some experts permit immediate contact if the mother and infant are on appropriate medication, the mother wears a mask, and infection control measures are discussed with the mother. If the mother has a risk factor for or known disease attributable to a multidrug-resistant strain, the mother and infant should be separated and an expert in tuberculosis should be consulted. Other household members should have a TST and further evaluation.

- **Mother (or household contact) has a positive TST result and abnormal findings on chest radiography but no evidence of tuberculosis disease.** If the chest radiograph of the mother (or household contact) appears abnormal but is not characteristic of tuberculosis and the history, physical examination, and sputum smear indicate no evidence of tuberculosis disease, the infant can be assumed to be at low risk of *M tuberculosis* infection and need not be separated from the mother (or household contact). The mother and her infant should receive follow-up care and the mother should be treated. Other household members should have a TST and further evaluation.

- **Mother (or household contact) has a positive TST result and clinical or radiographic evidence of possibly contagious tuberculosis.** Cases in mothers (or household contacts) should be reported immediately to the local health department, and investigation of all household members should be performed within several days. All contacts should have a TST, chest radiograph, and physical examination. The infant should be evaluated for congenital tuberculosis (see Congenital Tuberculosis, p 656), the mother should be treated, and the mother and infant should be tested for HIV infection. If the infant is receiving isoniazid, separation is not necessary unless the mother has a risk factor for a multidrug-resistant strain. If the mother (or household contact) has tuberculosis disease attributable to multidrug-resistant *M tuberculosis* or has poor adherence to treatment and DOT is not possible, the infant should be separated from the ill mother or household member, and BCG immunization should be considered for the infant. Because the response to BCG in infants may be delayed and inadequate for prevention of tuberculosis, DOT for the mother (or household contact) and infant is preferred. Other household members should have a TST and further evaluation.

  If congenital tuberculosis is excluded, isoniazid is given until the infant is 3 or 4 months of age, when a TST should be performed. If the TST result is positive, the infant should be reassessed for tuberculosis disease. If disease is not present, isoniazid should be continued for 9 months. If the TST result is negative and the mother or other household contacts with tuberculosis have good adherence and response to treatment and no longer are contagious, isoniazid is discontinued. The infant should be evaluated at monthly intervals during treatment.

ISOLATION OF THE HOSPITALIZED PATIENT: Most children with tuberculosis disease are not contagious and require only standard precautions. Exceptions are children with the following: (1) cavitary pulmonary tuberculosis; (2) positive sputum AFB smears; (3) laryngeal involvement; (4) extensive pulmonary infection; or (5) suspected congenital tuberculosis. Precautions for tuberculosis or AFB are indicated until effective therapy has been initiated, sputum smears demonstrate a diminishing number of organisms, and cough is abating. Children with no cough and negative sputum AFB smears can be hospitalized in an open ward. Infection control measures for hospital personnel in contagious cases should include the use of personally "fitted" and "sealed" particulate respirators for all patient contacts (see Infection Control for Hospitalized Children, p 146). The contagious patient should be placed in a negative-pressure room in the hospital.

The major concern in infection control relates to adult household members and contacts who may be the source case. These people should have a chest radiograph to exclude contagious tuberculosis and a TST. Household members and contacts should be managed with tuberculosis or AFB precautions when visiting until they are demonstrated not to have contagious tuberculosis. Nonadherent household contacts should be excluded from hospital visitation until evaluation is complete and tuberculosis disease is excluded or treatment has rendered source cases noncontagious.

CONTROL MEASURES:

The control of tuberculosis in the United States requires collaboration between health care professionals and health department personnel, obtaining a thorough history of exposure(s) to people with contagious tuberculosis, timely and effective contact investigations, proper interpretation of TST results, and appropriate anti-tuberculosis therapy, including DOT services.

Management of Contacts, Including Epidemiologic Investigation. Children with a positive TST result or tuberculosis disease should be the starting point for epidemiologic investigation by the local health department. Close contacts of a TST-positive child should have a TST, and people with a positive TST result or symptoms consistent with tuberculosis disease should be investigated further. Because children with primary tuberculosis usually are not contagious, their contacts are not likely to be infected unless they also have been in contact with the same adult source case. After the presumptive adult source of the child's tuberculosis is identified, other contacts of that adult should be evaluated.

Therapy for Contacts. People exposed within the previous 3 months to a contagious case of tuberculosis disease should have a TST and a chest radiograph. For exposed contacts with impaired immunity (eg, HIV infection) and all household contacts younger than 4 years of age, isoniazid therapy should be initiated, even if the TST result is negative, once tuberculosis disease is excluded (see Therapy for LTBI, p 652). Infected people can have a negative TST result because cellular reactivity has not yet developed or because of cutaneous anergy. People with a negative TST result should be retested 12 weeks after the last contact. If the TST result still is negative in a immunocompetent person, isoniazid is discontinued. If the contact is immunocompromised, LTBI cannot be excluded, and treatment should be continued for 9 months. If a contact's TST result becomes positive, isoniazid should be continued for 9 months.

Child Care and Schools. Children with tuberculosis disease can attend school or child care if they are receiving therapy (see Children in Out-of-Home Child Care, p 123). They can return to regular activities as soon as effective therapy has been instituted, adherence to therapy has been documented, and clinical symptoms have diminished substantially. Children with LTBI can participate in all activities whether they are receiving treatment or not.

BCG Vaccine. The BCG vaccine is a live-virus vaccine prepared from attenuated strains of *M bovis*. Use of BCG vaccine is recommended by the Expanded Programme on Immunization of the World Health Organization for administration at birth (see Table 1.3, p 8) and currently is used in more than 100 countries. Bacille Calmette-Guérin vaccine is used to prevent disseminated and other life-threatening manifestations of *M tuberculosis* infection in infants and young children. However, BCG immunization does not prevent infection with *M tuberculosis*. The various BCG vaccines used throughout the world differ in composition and efficacy.

Two meta-analyses of published clinical trials and case-control studies concerning the efficacy of BCG vaccines concluded that BCG vaccine has relatively high protective efficacy (approximately 80%) against meningeal and miliary tuberculosis in children. The protective efficacy against pulmonary tuberculosis differed significantly among the studies, precluding a specific conclusion. Protection afforded by BCG vaccine in one meta-analysis was estimated to be 50%. Two BCG vaccines, one manufactured by Organon Teknika Corporation (Durham, NC) and the other by Connaught Laboratories (Willowdale, Ontario), are licensed in the United States. Comparative evaluations of these and other BCG vaccines have not been performed.

Indications. In the United States, administration of BCG vaccine should be considered only in limited and select circumstances, such as unavoidable risk of exposure to *M tuberculosis* and failure or unfeasibility of other methods of control of tuberculosis. Recommendations for use of BCG vaccine for control of tuberculosis among children and health care professionals have been published by the Advisory Committee on Immunization Practices and the Advisory Council for the Elimination of Tuberculosis of the CDC.* For infants and children, BCG immunization should be considered only for people with a negative TST result who are not infected with HIV in the following circumstances:

- The child is exposed continually to a person or people with contagious pulmonary tuberculosis resistant to isoniazid and rifampin and the child cannot be removed from this exposure.
- The child is exposed continually to a person or people with untreated or ineffectively treated contagious pulmonary tuberculosis and the child cannot be removed from such exposure or given antituberculosis therapy.

---

* Centers for Disease Control and Prevention. The role of BCG vaccine in the prevention and control of tuberculosis in the United States: a joint statement by the Advisory Committee for the Elimination of Tuberculosis and the Advisory Committee on Immunization Practices. *MMWR Recomm Rep.* 1996;45(RR-4):1–18

Careful assessment of the potential risks and benefits of BCG vaccine and consultation with personnel in local tuberculosis control programs strongly are recommended before use of BCG vaccine.

When BCG vaccine is given, care should be taken to observe precautions and directions for administration in the product label. Healthy infants from birth to 2 months of age may be given BCG vaccine without a TST unless congenital infection is suspected; thereafter, BCG vaccine should be given only to children with a negative TST result.

Adverse Reactions. Uncommonly (1%–2% of immunizations), BCG vaccine can result in local adverse reactions, such as subcutaneous abscess and regional lymphadenopathy, which generally are not serious. One rare complication, osteitis affecting the epiphysis of long bones, may occur as long as several years after BCG immunization. Disseminated fatal infection occurs rarely (approximately 2 per 1 million people), primarily in people with severe immunocompromise. Antituberculosis therapy is recommended to treat osteitis and disseminated disease caused by BCG vaccine. Pyrazinamide is not believed to be effective against BCG and should not be included in treatment regimens. Most experts do not recommend treatment of draining skin lesions or chronic suppurative lymphadenitis caused by BCG vaccine, because spontaneous resolution occurs in the majority of cases. People with complications caused by BCG vaccine should be referred for management, if possible, to a tuberculosis expert.

Contraindications. People with burns, skin infections, and primary or secondary immunodeficiencies, including HIV infection, should not receive BCG vaccine. In populations of the world in which the risk of LTBI and tuberculosis disease is high, the World Health Organization recommends BCG immunization for asymptomatic HIV-infected children. Use of BCG vaccine is contraindicated for people receiving immunosuppressive medications, including high-dose corticosteroids (see Corticosteroids, p 654). Although no untoward effects of BCG vaccine on the fetus have been observed, immunization during pregnancy is not recommended.

Reporting of Cases. Reporting of suspected and confirmed cases of tuberculosis disease is mandated by laws in all states. A diagnosis of tuberculosis infection or disease in a child is a sentinel event representing recent transmission of *M tuberculosis* in the community. Physicians should assist in the search for a source case and others infected by the source case. Members of the household, such as relatives, baby-sitters, au pairs, boarders, domestic workers, and frequent visitors or other adults, such as child care providers and teachers with whom the child has frequent contact, potentially are source cases.

Diseases Caused by Nontuberculous Mycobacteria
(Atypical Mycobacteria, Mycobacteria Other Than *Mycobacterium tuberculosis*)

CLINICAL MANIFESTATIONS: Several syndromes are caused by nontuberculous mycobacteria (NTM). In children, the most common of these syndromes is cervical lymphadenitis. Less common infections include cutaneous infection, osteomyelitis, otitis media, central catheter infections, and pulmonary disease. Disseminated infections almost always are associated with impaired cell-mediated immunity, as found in congenital immune defects or human immunodeficiency virus (HIV) infection. Manifestations of disseminated NTM infections depend on the species and route of infection but include fever, night sweats, weight loss, abdominal pain, fatigue, diarrhea, and anemia. Nontuberculous mycobacteria, especially *M avium* complex (MAC [including *Mycobacterium avium* and *Mycobacterium intracellulare*]) and *M abscessus*, can be recovered from 10% to 20% of adolescents and young adults with cystic fibrosis and may be associated with fever and declining clinical status despite aggressive antipseudomonal therapy.

ETIOLOGY: Of the many species of NTM that have been identified, only a small number account for most human infections. The species most commonly encountered in infected children are MAC, *Mycobacterium fortuitum*, *Mycobacterium kansasii*, and *Mycobacterium marinum* (see Table 3.73, p 662). Several new species that can be detected by nucleic acid amplification but cannot be grown by routine culture methods have been identified in lymph nodes of children with cervical adenitis. Nontuberculous mycobacteria disease in patients with HIV infection usually is caused by MAC. *Mycobacterium fortuitum*, *Mycobacterium chelonae*, and *M abscessus* commonly are referred to as "rapidly growing" mycobacteria, because sufficient growth and identification can be achieved in the laboratory within 3 to 7 days, whereas other NTM and *Mycobacterium tuberculosis* often require weeks before sufficient growth occurs. Rapidly growing mycobacteria occasionally have been implicated in wound, soft tissue, bone, pulmonary, central catheter, and middle-ear infections. Other mycobacterial species that usually are not pathogenic have caused infections in immunocompromised hosts or have been associated with the presence of a foreign body.

EPIDEMIOLOGY: Many NTM species are ubiquitous in nature and are found in soil, food, water, and animals. The major reservoir for *M kansasii*, *M simiae*, and health care-associated infections attributable to the rapidly growing mycobacteria is tap water. For *M marinum*, water in a fish tank or aquarium is the major source of infection. Although many people are exposed to NTM, only a few of these exposures result in chronic infection or disease. The usual portals of entry for NTM infection are believed to be abrasions in the skin (eg, cutaneous lesions caused by *M marinum*), surgical incisions (especially central catheters), oropharyngeal mucosa (the presumed portal of entry for cervical lymphadenitis), gastrointestinal or respiratory tract for disseminated MAC, and respiratory tract (including tympanostomy tubes) for otitis media, pulmonary disease, and rare cases of mediastinal adenitis and endobronchial disease. Most infections remain localized at the portal of entry or in

Table 3.73. **Diseases Caused by Nontuberculous Mycobacterial Species**

Clinical Disease	Common Species	Less Common Species
Cutaneous infection	*M chelonae, M fortuitum, M abscessus, M marinum*	*M ulcerans*[1]
Lymphadenitis	MAC	*M kansasii, M fortuitum, M malmoense*[2]
Otologic infection	*M abscessus*	*M fortuitum*
Pulmonary infection	MAC, *M kansasii, M abscessus*	*M xenopi, M malmoense,*[2] *M szulgai, M fortuitum, M simiae*
Catheter-associated infection	*M chelonae, M fortuitum*	*M abscessus*
Skeletal infection	MAC, *M kansasii, M fortuitum*	*M chelonae, M marinum, M abscessus*
Disseminated	MAC	*M kansasii, M genavense, M haemophilum, M chelonae*

MAC indicates *Mycobacterium avium* complex.
1 Not endemic in the United States.
2 Found primarily in Northern Europe.

regional lymph nodes. Dissemination to distal sites primarily occurs in immunocompromised hosts, especially in people with acquired immunodeficiency syndrome (AIDS). No definitive evidence of person-to-person transmission of NTM exists. Outbreaks of otitis media caused by *M abscessus* have been associated with polyethylene ear tubes and use of contaminated equipment or water. A waterborne route of transmission has been implicated for MAC infection in immunodeficient hosts.

The **incubation period** is variable.

DIAGNOSTIC TESTS: Definitive diagnosis of NTM disease requires isolation of the organism. However, because these organisms commonly are found in the environment, contamination of cultures or transient colonization can occur. Therefore, caution must be exercised in the interpretation of cultures obtained from nonsterile sites, such as gastric washing specimens, a single acid-fast bacillus smear-negative sputum specimen, or a urine specimen and if the species cultured usually is nonpathogenic (eg, *Mycobacterium gordonae*). Repeated isolation of numerous colonies of a single species is more likely to indicate disease than culture contamination or transient colonization. Unlike bacteria, isolates from draining sinus tracts almost always are significant clinically. Recovery of NTM from sites that usually are sterile, such as cerebrospinal fluid, pleural fluid, bone marrow, blood, lymph node aspirates, middle ear or mastoid aspirates, or surgically excised tissue, is the most reliable diagnostic test. With the radiometric broth or lysis-centrifugation techniques, blood cultures are highly sensitive in recovery of MAC and other bloodborne NTM species. Disseminated MAC disease should prompt a search for underlying immunodeficiency, usually HIV infection.

Patients with NTM infection can have a positive tuberculin skin test (TST), because the purified protein derivative preparation, derived from *M tuberculosis,* shares a number of antigens with NTM species. These TST reactions usually measure less than 10 mm of induration but can measure more than 15 mm (see Tuberculosis, p 642).

TREATMENT: Many NTM are relatively resistant in vitro to antituberculosis drugs. In vitro resistance, however, does not necessarily correlate with clinical response. Only limited controlled trials have been performed in patients with NTM infections. The approach to therapy should be dictated by the following: (1) the species causing the infection; (2) the results of drug-susceptibility testing; (3) the site(s) of infection; (4) the patient's underlying disease (if any); and (5) the need to treat a patient presumptively for tuberculosis while awaiting culture reports that subsequently reveal NTM.

For NTM lymphadenitis in otherwise healthy children, especially when the disease is caused by MAC, complete surgical excision almost always is curative. Antituberculosis chemotherapy offers no benefit. Therapy with clarithromycin combined with ethambutol or rifabutin may be beneficial for children in whom surgical excision is incomplete or for children with recurrent disease but has not been studied in a clinical trial (see Table 3.74, p 664).

Isolates of rapidly growing mycobacteria (*M fortuitum, M abscessus,* and *M chelonae*) should be tested in vitro against drugs (such as amikacin sulfate, imipenem, sulfamethoxazole or trimethoprim-sulfamethoxazole, cefoxitin sodium, ciprofloxacin, gatifloxacin, clarithromycin, linezolid, and doxycycline), to which they commonly are susceptible and which have been used with some therapeutic success. Clarithromycin and at least one other agent commonly is the treatment of choice for cutaneous (disseminated) infections attributable to *M chelonae.* Details about choice of drugs, dosages, and duration should be reviewed with a consultant experienced in the management of NTM infections.

In patients with AIDS and in other immunocompromised people with disseminated MAC infection, multidrug therapy is recommended. Single-drug therapy with a macrolide antimicrobial agent commonly results in development of antimicrobial resistance. Clinical isolates of MAC usually are resistant to many of the approved antituberculosis drugs, including isoniazid, but often are susceptible to clarithromycin, azithromycin dihydrate, ethambutol hydrochloride, rifabutin, rifampin, amikacin, streptomycin, and fluoroquinolones, which are not licensed for use in people younger than 17 years of age. The optimal regimen has yet to be determined. Treatment of disseminated MAC infection should be done in consultation with an expert. In addition, the following treatment guidelines should be considered:

- Susceptibility testing to drugs other than the macrolides is not predictive of in vivo response and should not be used to guide therapy.
- Unless there is clinical or laboratory evidence of macrolide resistance, treatment regimens should contain clarithromycin or azithromycin combined with ethambutol.
- Many clinicians have added a third agent (rifampin, rifabutin), and in some situations, a fourth agent (amikacin or streptomycin).

Table 3.74. Treatment of Nontuberculous Mycobacteria Infections in Children

Organism	Disease	Treatment
Mycobacterium avium complex (MAC)	Lymphadenitis	Excision of major nodes; if excision incomplete or disease recurs, clarithromycin or azithromycin plus ethambutol with rifampin.
	Pulmonary infection	Clarithromycin or azithromycin plus ethambutol with rifampin or rifabutin (pulmonary resection in some patients). For severe disease, an initial course of amikacin or streptomycin often is included.
	Disseminated	See text.
Mycobacterium fortuitum complex	Cutaneous infection	Excision of tissue; initial therapy is amikacin plus cefoxitin, IV, followed by erythromycin, clarithromycin, doxycycline,[1] or ciprofloxacin orally.
	Catheter infection	Catheter removal and amikacin plus cefoxitin, IV; clarithromycin, trimethoprim-sulfamethoxazole, or ciprofloxacin orally based on in vitro susceptibility testing.
Mycobacterium kansasii	Pulmonary infection	Rifampin plus ethambutol with isoniazid.
	Osteomyelitis	Surgical débridement and prolonged antimicrobial therapy using rifampin plus ethambutol with isoniazid.
Mycobacterium marinum	Cutaneous infection	None, if minor; rifampin, trimethoprim- sulfamethoxazole, clarithromycin, or doxycycline[1] for moderate disease; extensive lesions may require surgical débridement.
Mycobacterium abscessus	Otitis media	Clarithromycin plus initial course of amikacin plus cefoxitin; may require surgical débridement.
	Pulmonary infection (in cystic fibrosis)	Serious disease, clarithromycin, amikacin, and cefoxitin based on susceptibility testing; may require surgical resection; seek expert advice.

IV indicates intravenously.

[1] Doxycycline should not be given to children younger than 8 years of age unless the benefits of therapy are greater than the risks of dental staining (see Antimicrobial Agents and Related Therapy, p 693).

- Patients receiving protease inhibitor antiretroviral therapy generally should not be treated with rifabutin. However, if coadministration of rifabutin and a protease inhibitor is necessary, indinavir sulfate and nelfinavir mesylate are the preferred protease inhibitors, and the dose of rifabutin should be decreased by 50%.
- Clofazimine is ineffective for treatment of MAC disease and should not be used.
- Patients receiving therapy should be monitored. Considerations are as follows:
  - Clinical manifestations of disseminated MAC infection, such as fever, weight loss, and night sweats, should be monitored several times during the initial weeks of therapy. Microbiologic response, as assessed by blood culture every 4 weeks during initial therapy, also can be helpful for interpreting the efficacy of a therapeutic regimen.
  - Most patients who ultimately respond show substantial clinical improvement in the first 4 to 6 weeks of therapy. Elimination of the organisms from blood cultures may take somewhat longer, often requiring up to 12 weeks.
  - Patients receiving clarithromycin plus rifabutin or high-dose rifabutin (with another drug) should be observed for the rifabutin-related development of leukopenia, uveitis, polyarthralgias, and pseudojaundice.

Chemoprophylaxis. According to the 2002 US Public Health Service and Infectious Diseases Society of America guidelines* for preventing the first MAC episode, prophylaxis with azithromycin or clarithromycin should be considered for HIV-infected children 6 years of age and older, adolescents, and adults with CD4+ T-lymphocyte counts of less than 50 cells × 10^6/L (50 cells/μL). Rifabutin is an alternative agent but should not be used until active tuberculosis has been excluded. Disseminated MAC should be excluded by a negative blood culture result before prophylaxis is initiated.

Prophylaxis for preventing the first MAC infection should be offered to HIV-infected children younger than 13 years of age with the following CD4+ T-lymphocyte counts: children 6 years of age or older, less than 50 cells × 10^6/L (<50/μL); children 2 to 6 years of age, less than 75 cells × 10^6/L (<75/μL); children 1 to 2 years of age, less than 500 cells × 10^6/L (<500/μL); and children younger than 12 months of age, less than 750 cells × 10^6/L (<750/μL).

Oral suspensions of clarithromycin and azithromycin are available in the United States. No pediatric formulation of rifabutin is available, but a dosage of 5 mg/kg per day seems appropriate. Rifabutin should be used only for children older than 6 years of age. Children with a history of disseminated MAC should receive lifelong prophylaxis to prevent recurrence.

ISOLATION OF THE HOSPITALIZED PATIENT: Standard precautions are recommended.

CONTROL MEASURES: Control measures include chemoprophylaxis for certain patients with HIV infection (see Treatment, p 663) and use of sterile equipment for middle-ear instrumentation, including otoscopic equipment, for prevention of

---

* Centers for Disease Control and Prevention. Guidelines for preventing opportunistic infections among HIV-infected persons—2002. Recommendations of the US Public Health Service and the Infectious Diseases Society of America. *MMWR Recomm Rep.* 2002;51(RR-8):1–46

M abscessus otitis media. Because MAC organisms are common in environmental sources, such as food and water, current information does not support specific recommendations about avoidance of exposure for HIV-infected people.

Tularemia

CLINICAL MANIFESTATIONS: Most patients with tularemia experience an abrupt onset of fever, chills, myalgia, and headache. Illness usually conforms to one of the several tularemic syndromes. Most common is the ulceroglandular syndrome, characterized by a painful, maculopapular lesion at the portal of bacterial entry, with subsequent ulceration and slow healing associated with painful, acutely inflamed regional lymph nodes, which may drain spontaneously. The glandular syndrome (regional lymphadenopathy with no ulcer) also is common. Less common disease syndromes are: oculoglandular (severe conjunctivitis and preauricular lymphadenopathy), oropharyngeal (severe exudative stomatitis, pharyngitis, or tonsillitis and cervical lymphadenopathy), typhoidal (high fever, hepatomegaly, and splenomegaly), intestinal (intestinal pain, vomiting, and diarrhea), and pneumonic (primary pleuropulmonary disease).

ETIOLOGY: *Francisella tularensis,* the causative agent, is a gram-negative pleomorphic coccobacillus.

EPIDEMIOLOGY: Sources of the organism include approximately 100 species of wild mammals (eg, rabbits, hares, muskrats, and voles); at least 9 species of domestic animals (eg, sheep, cattle, and cats); blood-sucking arthropods that bite these animals (eg, ticks, deerflies, and mosquitoes); and water and soil contaminated by infected animals. In the United States, ticks and rabbits are major sources of human infection. Infected animals and arthropods, especially ticks, are infective for prolonged periods; frozen rabbits can remain infective for more than 3 years. People at risk are those with occupational or recreational exposure to infected animals or their habitats, such as rabbit hunters and trappers, people exposed to certain ticks or biting insects, and laboratory technicians working with *F tularensis,* which is highly infectious, especially when aerosolized. In the United States, ticks are the most important arthropod vectors, and most cases occur during summer months. Infection also may be acquired by direct contact with infected animals, ingestion of contaminated water or inadequately cooked meat, or inhalation of aerosolized organisms or contaminated particles. Person-to-person transmission does not occur. Organisms can be present in blood during the first 2 weeks of disease and in cutaneous lesions for as long as 1 month if untreated.

The **incubation period** usually is 3 to 5 days, with a range of 1 to 21 days.

DIAGNOSTIC TESTS: Diagnosis is established most often by serologic testing. A single serum antibody titer of ≥1:128 determined by microagglutination (MA) or of ≥1:160 determined by tube agglutination (TA) is consistent with recent or past infection and constitutes a presumptive diagnosis. Confirmation by serologic testing requires a fourfold or greater titer change between 2 sera obtained at least 2 weeks apart, with one of the specimens having a minimum titer of ≥1:128 (MA) or ≥1:160 (TA). Slide agglutination tests are less reliable than TA tests. Nonspecific cross-reactions can occur with specimens containing heterophil antibodies or antibodies to *Brucella* species, *Legionella* species, or other gram-negative bacteria. However, cross-reactions rarely result in MA or TA titers that are diagnostic. Most clinical laboratories can identify presumptively *F tularensis* in ulcer exudate or aspirate material by direct fluorescent antibody or polymerase chain reaction assays. Suspect growth on culture may be identified presumptively by direct fluorescent antibody, polymerase chain reaction, or rapid slide agglutination tests. Isolation of *F tularensis* from specimens of blood, skin, ulcers, lymph node drainage, gastric washings, or respiratory tract secretions is best achieved by inoculation of cysteine-enriched media. Immunohistochemical staining is specific for detection of *F tularensis* in fixed tissues; however, it is not available in most clinical laboratories. Because of its propensity for causing laboratory-acquired infections, laboratory personnel should be alerted to the suspicion of *F tularensis*.

TREATMENT: Streptomycin sulfate, gentamicin sulfate, or amikacin sulfate are recommended for treatment of tularemia. Duration of therapy usually is 10 days. A longer course is required for more severe illness. Alternative drugs include imipenem-cilastatin, doxycycline (which should not be given to children younger than 8 years of age unless the benefits of therapy are greater than the risks [see Antimicrobial Agents and Related Therapy, p 693]), ciprofloxacin (which is not approved for patients younger than 18 years of age), and chloramphenicol. These drugs are associated with prompt clinical response, but relapses have been reported after treatment with tetracyclines.

ISOLATION OF THE HOSPITALIZED PATIENT: Standard precautions are recommended.

CONTROL MEASURES:
- People should protect themselves against arthropod bites by wearing protective clothing, by frequent inspection for and removal of ticks from the skin and scalp, and by using insect repellents (see Prevention of Tickborne Infections, p 186).
- Children should be instructed not to handle sick or dead animals.
- Rubber gloves should be worn by hunters, trappers, and food preparers when handling the carcasses of wild rabbits and other potentially infected animals.
- Game meats should be cooked thoroughly.
- Face masks and rubber gloves should be worn by people working with cultures or infective material in the laboratory, and the work should be performed in a biologic safety cabinet.
- Standard precautions should be used for handling clinical materials.

Endemic Typhus
(Fleaborne Typhus or Murine Typhus)

CLINICAL MANIFESTATIONS: Fleaborne typhus resembles epidemic (louseborne) typhus but usually is milder and can have a less abrupt onset with less severe systemic symptoms. In young children, the disease is mild. Fever can be accompanied by persistent headache and myalgias. A rash typically appears on day 4 to 7 of illness, is macular or maculopapular, lasts 4 to 8 days, and tends to remain discrete, with sparse lesions and no hemorrhage. The illness seldom lasts longer than 2 weeks; visceral involvement is uncommon.

ETIOLOGY: Fleaborne typhus is caused by *Rickettsia typhi* (formerly *Rickettsia mooseri*) and *Rickettsia felis*.

EPIDEMIOLOGY: Rats, in which infection is inapparent, are the natural reservoirs. Opossums and domestic cats and dogs also can be infected and can serve as hosts. The vector for transmission among rats and to humans is the rat flea (usually *Xenopsylla cheopis*). Infected flea feces are rubbed into broken skin or mucous membranes or inhaled as an aerosol. The disease is worldwide in distribution, tends to occur more commonly in adults and in males, is most common from April to October, and is rare in the United States, with most cases occurring in southern California, southern Texas, the southeastern Gulf Coast, and Hawaii. Exposure to rats and their fleas is the major risk factor for infection, although a history of such exposure commonly is absent. In some regions, the classic rat-flea-rat cycle has been replaced by a peridomestic cycle involving cats, dogs, and opossums and their fleas.

The **incubation period** is 6 to 14 days.

DIAGNOSTIC TESTS: Antibody titers determined by an indirect fluorescent antibody test, enzyme immunoassay, latex agglutination test, or complement fixation test peak around 4 weeks after infection. A fourfold titer change between acute and convalescent serum specimens is diagnostic, and an enzyme immunoassay specific for immunoglobulin M antibody may aid in confirmation of clinical diagnoses. However, serologic tests cannot differentiate murine typhus from epidemic (louseborne) typhus without antibody cross-absorption tests, which are not available routinely. Isolation of the organism in culture is possible but is hazardous and requires specialized laboratories.

TREATMENT: Doxycycline administered intravenously or orally is the treatment of choice (2.2 mg/kg every 12 hours; maximum 300 mg/24 hours). Treatment should be administered for at least 3 days after defervescence and evidence of clinical improvement is documented, usually for 5 to 10 days. Despite concerns regarding dental staining after the use of tetracycline-class antimicrobial agents in young children (see Antimicrobial Agents and Related Therapy, p 693), doxycycline provides superior therapy for this potentially severe or life-threatening disease. Furthermore, available data suggest that one course of doxycycline does not cause discoloration of permanent teeth. Chloramphenicol can be considered in patients for whom life-threatening reactions to doxycycline have been documented.

ISOLATION OF THE HOSPITALIZED PATIENT: Standard precautions are recommended.

CONTROL MEASURES: Rat fleas should be controlled by appropriate insecticides before the use of rodenticides, because the flea will seek alternative hosts. Rat populations should be controlled by appropriate means. Vaccine no longer is available in the United States. No treatment is recommended for exposed people. The disease should be reported to local or state public health departments.

Epidemic Typhus
(Louseborne Typhus)

CLINICAL MANIFESTATIONS: Epidemic louseborne typhus is characterized by the abrupt onset of high fever, chills, and myalgias accompanied by severe headache and malaise. Influenza illness commonly is suspected. A rash appears 4 to 7 days after illness onset, beginning on the trunk and spreading to the limbs. A concentrated eruption is present in the axillae. The rash is maculopapular, becomes petechial or hemorrhagic, then develops into brownish pigmented areas. The face, palms, and soles usually are not affected. Changes in mental status are common, and delirium or coma often occur. Myocardial and renal failure can occur when the disease is severe. Illness varies from moderately severe to fatal. The fatality rate in untreated people is as high as 30%. Untreated patients who recover typically have an illness lasting 2 weeks. Mortality is less common in children, and the rate increases with advancing age. Brill-Zinsser disease is a relapse of epidemic louseborne typhus that occurs years after the initial episode. Factors that reactivate the rickettsiae are unknown. The recrudescent illness is similar to the primary infection but generally is milder and of shorter duration.

ETIOLOGY: Epidemic typhus is caused by *Rickettsia prowazekii*.

EPIDEMIOLOGY: Humans are the usual source of the organism, which is transmitted from person to person by the body louse, *Pediculus humanus* subspecies *corporis*. Infected louse feces are rubbed into broken skin or mucous membranes or inhaled as an aerosol. All ages are affected. Poverty, crowding, poor sanitary conditions, and poor personal hygiene contribute to the spread of lice and, hence, the disease. Currently, cases of typhus are rare but have occurred throughout the world, including Asia, Africa, some parts of Europe, and Central and South America. Typhus is most common during winter, when conditions favor person-to-person transmission of the vector, the body louse. Rickettsiae are present in the blood and tissues of patients during the early febrile phase but are not found in secretions. Direct person-to-person spread of the disease does not occur in the absence of the louse vector. Occasional cases in humans have been reported in the United States that appear to be associated with contact with infected flying squirrels, their nests, or their ectoparasites. Flying squirrel-related disease typically presents as a milder illness.

The **incubation period** is 1 to 2 weeks.

DIAGNOSTIC TESTS: *Rickettsia prowazekii* can be isolated from blood specimens by inoculation into guinea pigs and mice or the yolk sac of embryonated hens eggs or through tissue culture but isolation is hazardous and rarely is attempted. Definitive diagnosis requires visualization of rickettsiae in tissues, isolation of the organism, detecting rickettsiae by polymerase chain reaction assay, or testing of serum specimens obtained during the acute and convalescent phases of disease. The indirect fluorescent antibody test is the preferred serologic assay, but enzyme immunoassay, microagglutination, and latex agglutination also are available. A fourfold change in antibody titer between acute and convalescent serum specimens is diagnostic of epidemic louseborne typhus or endemic fleaborne typhus. An antibody absorption test can differentiate the 2 diseases but is not available routinely. An immunohistochemical assay for *R prowazekii* in formalin-fixed tissue specimens is available at the Centers for Disease Control and Prevention.

TREATMENT: Doxycycline given intravenously or orally, 2.2 mg/kg every 12 hours (maximum 300 mg/24 hours), is the treatment of choice for epidemic louseborne typhus. Therapy should be administered until the patient is afebrile for at least 3 days and clinical improvement is documented; the usual duration of therapy is 7 to 10 days. Severe disease can require a longer course of treatment. Despite concerns regarding dental staining after use of a tetracycline-class antimicrobial agent in children 8 years of age or younger (see Antimicrobial Agents and Related Therapy, p 693), doxycycline provides superior therapy for this potentially life-threatening disease. In people who are intolerant of tetracyclines, intravenous chloramphenicol or fluoroquinolones can be considered. Fluoroquinolones are not recommended for people younger than 18 years of age. To halt the spread of disease to other people, louse-infested patients should be treated with cream or gel pediculicides containing pyrethrins (0.16%–0.33%), piperonyl butoxide (2%–4%), crotamiton (10%), or lindane (1%). In epidemic situations in which antimicrobial agents may be limited (eg, refugee camps), a single dose of doxycycline may provide effective treatment (4.4 mg/kg for children weighing less than 45 kg, or 200 mg for heavier children).

ISOLATION OF THE HOSPITALIZED PATIENT: Standard precautions are recommended. Precautions should be taken to delouse hospitalized patients.

CONTROL MEASURES: Thorough delousing in epidemic situations, particularly among exposed contacts of cases, is recommended. Several applications may be needed, because lice eggs are resistant to most insecticides. Washing clothes in hot water kills lice and eggs. During epidemics, insecticides dusted onto clothes of louse-infested populations are effective. Prevention and control of flying squirrel-associated typhus requires precautions to prevent animals from living in human dwellings, such as sealing access routes. Vaccine no longer is available in the United States. Cases should be reported to local or state public health departments.

Ureaplasma urealyticum Infections

CLINICAL MANIFESTATIONS: The most common syndrome associated with *Ureaplasma urealyticum* infections is nongonococcal urethritis (NGU). Although 15%–55% of cases of NGU are caused by *Chlamydia trachomatis, U urealyticum* may be responsible for up to 20% to 30% of the remaining cases in some studies, with the etiology of most of the other cases unknown. Without treatment, the disease usually resolves within 1 to 6 months, although asymptomatic infection may persist thereafter. Prostatitis and epididymitis also have been associated with *U urealyticum* infection in men. In women, salpingitis, endometritis, and chorioamnionitis can occur.

Ureaplasma urealyticum has been isolated from the lower respiratory tract and from lung biopsy specimens of preterm infants and may contribute to pneumonia and chronic lung disease of prematurity. Although the organism also has been recovered from respiratory tract secretions of infants 3 months of age or younger with pneumonia, its role in development of lower respiratory tract disease in otherwise healthy young infants is controversial. *Ureaplasma urealyticum* has been isolated from cerebrospinal fluid of newborn infants with meningitis, intraventricular hemorrhage, and hydrocephalus. The contribution of *U urealyticum* to the outcome of these newborn infants is unclear given the confounding effects of prematurity and intraventricular hemorrhage.

Isolated cases of *U urealyticum* arthritis, osteomyelitis, pericarditis, and progressive sinopulmonary disease in immunocompromised patients have been reported.

ETIOLOGY: The genera *Ureaplasma* and *Mycoplasma* comprise the Mycoplasmataceae family. *Ureaplasma* organisms are small pleomorphic bacteria that characteristically lack a cell wall. The genus *Ureaplasma* contains a single species, *U urealyticum*, which includes at least 16 serotypes.

EPIDEMIOLOGY: The principal reservoir of human *U urealyticum* is the genital tract of sexually active adults. Colonization occurs in approximately half of sexually active women; the incidence in sexually active men is lower. Colonization is uncommon in prepubertal children and adolescents who are not sexually active, but a positive genital culture is not in itself an indication of sexual abuse. Transmission during delivery is likely from an asymptomatic colonized mother to her newborn. *Ureaplasma urealyticum* may colonize the throat, eyes, umbilicus, and perineum of newborn infants and may persist for several months after birth.

Because *U urealyticum* commonly is isolated from the female lower genital tract and neonatal respiratory tract in the absence of disease, a positive culture does not establish its causative role in acute infection.

The **incubation period** for NGU after sexual transmission is 10 to 20 days.

DIAGNOSTIC TESTS: Specimens for culture require specific *Ureaplasma* species transport media with refrigeration at 4°C (39°F). The use of cotton swabs should be avoided. Several rapid, sensitive polymerase chain reaction assays for detection of *U urealyticum* have been developed but are not available routinely. *Ureaplasma urealyticum* can be cultured in urea-containing broth in 1 to 2 days. Serologic testing for *U urealyticum* antibodies is of limited value and should not be used for routine diagnosis.

TREATMENT: A positive culture does not indicate need for therapy if the patient is asymptomatic. For symptomatic older children, adolescents, and adults, doxycycline is the drug of choice. Recurrences are common. Erythromycin is the preferred antimicrobial agent for people who are allergic to tetracycline and for people with infections caused by tetracycline-resistant strains. Studies in adult men with NGU indicate that single-dose azithromycin dihydrate (1 g orally) also is effective. Results of trials of antimicrobial therapy in pregnant women to prevent preterm delivery and in preterm infants to prevent pulmonary disease generally have not demonstrated efficacy. Thus, antimicrobial therapy cannot be recommended for these indications. Similarly, definitive evidence of efficacy of antimicrobial agents in the treatment of central nervous system (CNS) infections in infants and children is lacking.

ISOLATION OF THE HOSPITALIZED PATIENT: Standard precautions are recommended.

CONTROL MEASURES: Partners of infected sexually active people should be notified so they can be offered treatment if symptomatic.

Varicella-Zoster Infections

CLINICAL MANIFESTATIONS: Primary infection results in varicella (chickenpox), manifesting as a generalized, pruritic, vesicular rash typically consisting of 250 to 500 lesions, mild fever, and other systemic symptoms. Complications include bacterial superinfection of skin lesions, thrombocytopenia, arthritis, hepatitis, cerebellar ataxia, encephalitis, meningitis, and glomerulonephritis. Varicella tends to be more severe in adolescents and adults than in young children. Reye syndrome can follow some cases of chickenpox, although the incidence of Reye syndrome has decreased dramatically with decreased use of salicylates during varicella or influenza-like illnesses. In immunocompromised children, progressive severe varicella characterized by continuing eruption of lesions and high fever persisting into the second week of illness, as well as encephalitis, hepatitis, and pneumonia, can develop. Hemorrhagic varicella also is more common among immunocompromised patients than immunocompetent hosts. Pneumonia is relatively less common among immunocompetent children but is the most common complication in adults. In children with human immunodeficiency virus (HIV) infection, chronic or recurrent varicella (disseminated herpes zoster) can develop, with new lesions appearing for months. Severe and even fatal varicella has been reported in otherwise healthy children receiving intermittent courses of corticosteroids for treatment of asthma and other illnesses. The risk is especially high when corticosteroids are given during the incubation period for chickenpox.

The virus establishes latency in the dorsal root ganglia during primary infection. Reactivation results in herpes zoster ("shingles"). Grouped vesicular lesions appear in the distribution of 1 to 3 sensory dermatomes, sometimes accompanied by pain localized to the area. *Postherpetic neuralgia* is defined as pain that persists after resolution of the rash. Systemic symptoms are few. Zoster occasionally can become disseminated in immunocompromised patients, with lesions appearing outside the primary dermatomes and with visceral complications.

Fetal infection after maternal varicella during the first or early second trimester of pregnancy occasionally results in varicella embryopathy, which is characterized by limb atrophy and scarring of the skin of the extremities (the congenital varicella syndrome). Central nervous system and eye manifestations also can occur. The incidence of congenital varicella syndrome among infants born to mothers with varicella is approximately 2% when infection occurs before 20 weeks of gestation. Children exposed to varicella-zoster virus in utero during the second 20 weeks of pregnancy can develop inapparent varicella and subsequent zoster early in life without having had extrauterine varicella. Varicella infection can be fatal for an infant if the mother develops varicella from 5 days before to 2 days after delivery. When varicella develops in a mother more than 5 days before delivery and gestational age is 28 weeks or more, the severity of disease in the newborn is modified by transplacental transfer of varicella-zoster virus (VZV)-specific maternal immunoglobulin (Ig) G antibody.

ETIOLOGY: Varicella-zoster virus is a member of the herpesvirus family.

EPIDEMIOLOGY: Humans are the only source of infection for this highly contagious virus. Humans are infected when the virus comes in contact with the mucosa of the upper respiratory tract or the conjunctiva. Person-to-person transmission occurs primarily by direct contact with patients with varicella or zoster and occasionally occurs by airborne spread from respiratory tract secretions and, rarely, from zoster lesions. In utero infection also can occur as a result of transplacental passage of virus during maternal varicella infection. Varicella-zoster virus infection in a household member usually results in infection of almost all susceptible people in that household. Children who acquire their infection at home (secondary family cases) may have more severe disease than that in the index case. Nosocomial transmission is well documented in pediatric units, but transmission is rare in newborn nurseries.

In temperate climates, varicella is a childhood disease with a marked seasonal distribution with peak incidence during late winter and early spring. In tropical climates, the epidemiology of varicella is different; acquisition of disease occurs at later ages, resulting in a higher proportion of adults being susceptible to varicella compared with adults in temperate climates. In the prevaccine era, most cases of varicella in the United States occurred in children younger than 10 years of age; however, with implementation of universal immunization, a higher proportion of cases is expected to occur among adolescents and adults. Immunity generally is lifelong. Cellular immunity is more important than humoral immunity for limiting the extent of primary infection with VZV and for preventing reactivation of virus with herpes zoster. Symptomatic reinfection is uncommon in immunocompetent people, although asymptomatic reinfection occurs. Asymptomatic primary infection is unusual, but because some cases are mild, they may not be recognized.

As vaccine coverage increases and the incidence of wild-type varicella decreases, a higher proportion of varicella cases will occur in immunized people as breakthrough disease. In sites where active surveillance is being conducted, cases of breakthrough disease have increased as a percentage of all cases from 4% in 1995 to approximately 25% in 2000. This should not be confused as an increasing rate of breakthrough disease or as evidence of increasing vaccine failure.

Immunocompromised people with primary (varicella) or recurrent (zoster) infection are at increased risk of severe disease. Disseminated varicella and zoster are more likely to develop in children with congenital T-cell defects or acquired immunodeficiency syndrome than in people with B-cell abnormalities. Other groups of pediatric patients who may experience more severe or complicated disease include infants, adolescents, patients with chronic cutaneous or pulmonary disorders, and patients receiving systemic corticosteroids or long-term salicylate therapy.

Patients are most contagious from 1 to 2 days before to shortly after onset of the rash. Contagiousness persists until crusting of lesions. Immunocompromised patients with progressive varicella remain contagious throughout the period of eruption of new lesions.

The **incubation period** usually is 14 to 16 days, occasionally as short as 10 or as long as 21 days after contact. It may be prolonged for as long as 28 days after use of Varicella-Zoster Immune Globulin (VZIG) and shortened in immunocompromised patients. Varicella can develop between 1 and 16 days of life in infants born to mothers with active varicella around the time of delivery; the usual interval from onset of rash in a mother to onset in her neonate is 9 to 15 days.

DIAGNOSTIC TESTS: Diagnostic tests for VZV are summarized in Table 3.75, p 675. Varicella zoster virus can be isolated from scrapings of a vesicle base during the first 3 to 4 days of the eruption but rarely from other sites, including respiratory tract secretions. A significant increase in serum varicella IgG antibody by any standard serologic assay can retrospectively confirm a diagnosis. These antibody tests are reliable for determining immune status in healthy hosts after natural infection but may not be reliable in immunocompromised people (see Care of Exposed People, p 677). Most commercially available tests are not sufficiently sensitive to demonstrate a vaccine-induced antibody response.

TREATMENT: The decision to use antiviral therapy and the route and duration of therapy should be determined by specific host factors, extent of infection, and initial response to therapy. Antiviral drugs have a limited window of opportunity to affect the outcome of varicella-zoster infection. In immunocompetent hosts, most virus replication has stopped by 72 hours after onset of rash; the duration is extended in immunocompromised hosts. Oral acyclovir is not recommended for routine use in otherwise healthy children with varicella. Administration within 24 hours of the onset of rash results in only a modest decrease in symptoms. Oral acyclovir should be considered for otherwise healthy people at increased risk of moderate to severe varicella, such as people older than 12 years of age, people with chronic cutaneous or pulmonary disorders, people receiving long-term salicylate therapy, and people receiving short, intermittent, or aerosolized courses of corticosteroids. Some experts also recommend use of oral acyclovir for secondary household cases in which the disease usually is more severe than in the primary case. For recommendations on dosage and duration of therapy, see Antiviral Drugs for Non-Human Immunodeficiency Virus Infections (p 729).

Table 3.75. Diagnostic Tests for Varicella-Zoster Virus (VZV) Infection

Test	Specimen	Comments
Tissue cultures	Vesicular fluid	Distinguish VZV from HSV. Cost, limited availability.
DFA	Vesicle scraping	Distinguish VZV from HSV. More rapid and sensitive than culture.
Tzanck smear	Vesicle scraping	See multinucleated giant cells with inclusion. Not specific for VZV. Less sensitive and accurate than DFA.
EIA	Acute and convalescent serum specimens for IgG	Requires special equipment. May not be sensitive enough to identify vaccine-induced immunity.
LA	Acute and convalescent serum specimens for IgG	Rapid (15 min), special equipment not needed. More sensitive but less specific than EIA.
IFA	Acute and convalescent serum specimens for IgG	Requires special equipment. Good sensitivity, specificity
FAMA	Acute and convalescent serum specimens for IgG	Very sensitive and specific but not available widely.
CF	Acute and convalescent serum specimens for IgG	Poor sensitivity.
PCR	Body fluid or tissue	Can distinguish wild type strains from vaccine virus. Very sensitive.

HSV indicates herpes simplex virus; DFA, direct fluorescent antibody test; EIA, enzyme immunoassay; IgG, immunoglobulin G; LA, latex agglutination test; IFA, indirect immunofluorescence antibody test; FAMA, fluorescent antibody to membrane assay; CF, complement fixation test; PCR, polymerase chain reaction assay.

Oral acyclovir is not recommended routinely for pregnant women with uncomplicated varicella, because the risks and benefits to the fetus and mother are unknown. Some experts, however, recommend oral acyclovir for pregnant women with varicella, especially during the second and third trimesters. Intravenous acyclovir is recommended for the pregnant patient with serious complications of varicella.

Intravenous antiviral therapy is recommended for immunocompromised patients. Therapy initiated early in the course of the illness, especially within 24 hours of rash onset, maximizes efficacy. Oral acyclovir should not be used to treat immunocompromised children with varicella because of poor oral bioavailability. However, some experts have used oral high-dose acyclovir in selected immunocompromised patients perceived to be at lower risk of developing severe varicella, such as HIV-infected patients with relatively normal concentrations of CD4+ T-lymphocytes and children with leukemia in whom careful follow-up is ensured. Although VZIG given shortly after exposure can prevent or modify the course of disease, it is not effective once disease is established (see Care of Exposed People, p 677).

Famciclovir and valacyclovir have been licensed for treatment of zoster in adults. Famciclovir is converted to penciclovir, which has an extended half-life in infected cells. Valacyclovir hydrochloride is converted to acyclovir and produces fourfold greater serum concentrations than those produced by acyclovir. No pediatric formulation is available for either medication, and insufficient data exist on the use or dose of these drugs in children to support therapeutic recommendations. Infections caused by acyclovir-resistant VZV strains should be treated with parenteral foscarnet sodium.

Children with varicella should not receive salicylates, because administration of salicylates to such children increases the risk of Reye syndrome. Acetaminophen may be used for control of fever.

ISOLATION OF THE HOSPITALIZED PATIENT: In addition to standard precautions, airborne and contact precautions are recommended for patients with varicella for a minimum of 5 days after onset of the rash and as long as vesicular lesions are present, which in immunocompromised patients can be a week or longer. For exposed susceptible patients, airborne and contact precautions from 8 until 21 days after onset of the rash in the index patient also are indicated; these precautions should be maintained until 28 days after exposure for those who received VZIG.

Airborne and contact precautions are recommended for neonates born to mothers with varicella and, if still hospitalized, should be continued until 21 days of age or 28 days of age if they received VZIG. Infants with varicella embryopathy do not require isolation.

Immunocompromised patients who have zoster (localized or disseminated) and immunocompetent patients with disseminated zoster require airborne and contact precautions for the duration of illness. For immunocompetent patients with localized zoster, contact precautions are indicated until all lesions are crusted.

CONTROL MEASURES:

Child Care and School. Children with uncomplicated chickenpox who have been excluded from school or child care may return when the rash has crusted, which may be several days in mild cases and several weeks in severe cases or in immunocompromised children.

Exclusion of children with zoster whose lesions cannot be covered is based on similar criteria. Children who are excluded may return after the lesions have crusted. Lesions that are covered seem to pose little risk to susceptible people. Older children and staff members with zoster should be instructed to wash their hands if they touch potentially infectious lesions.

CARE OF EXPOSED PEOPLE:

Potential interventions for susceptible people exposed to a person with varicella include either VZIG (1 dose up to 96 hours after exposure) or varicella vaccine (1 dose up to 72 hours after exposure).

Hospital Exposure. If an inadvertent exposure in the hospital to an infected patient, health care professional, or visitor occurs, the following control measures are recommended:

- Personnel and patients who have been exposed (see Table 3.76, p 678) and are susceptible to varicella should be identified.
- Varicella-Zoster Immune Globulin should be administered to appropriate candidates (see Table 3.77, p 679).
- All exposed susceptible patients should be discharged as soon as possible.
- All exposed susceptible patients who cannot be discharged should be placed in isolation from day 8 to day 21 after exposure to the index patient. For people who have received VZIG, isolation should be continued until day 28.
- All susceptible exposed personnel should be furloughed or excused from patient contact from day 8 to day 21 after exposure to an infectious patient. The interval should be extended to 28 days for people who have received VZIG (see p 35).
- Serologic testing for immunity is not necessary for personnel who have been immunized, because 99% of adults are seropositive after the second vaccine dose. For more information, see the recommendations of the Advisory Committee on Immunization Practices (ACIP) of the Centers for Disease Control and Prevention (CDC).*
- Varicella immunization is recommended for susceptible personnel if varicella does not develop from the exposure.

Postexposure Immunization. Administration of varicella vaccine to susceptible children within 72 hours and possibly up to 120 hours after varicella exposure may prevent or significantly modify disease and should be considered in these circumstances. Physicians should advise parents and their children that the vaccine may not protect against disease in all cases, because some children may have been exposed at the same time as the index case. However, if exposure to varicella does not cause

---

* Centers for Disease Control and Prevention. Prevention of varicella update: recommendations of the Advisory Committee on Immunization Practices (ACIP). *MMWR Recomm Rep.* 1999;48(RR-6):1–5

Table 3.76. **Types of Exposure to Varicella or Zoster for Which VZIG Is Indicated for Susceptible People¹**

- Household: residing in the same household
- Playmate: face-to-face² indoor play
- Hospital:

    Varicella: In same 2- to 4-bed room or adjacent beds in a large ward, face-to-face² contact with an infectious staff member or patient, or visit by a person deemed contagious

    Zoster: Intimate contact (eg, touching or hugging) with a person deemed contagious.

- Newborn infant: onset of varicella in the mother 5 days or less before delivery or within 48 h after delivery; VZIG is not indicated if the mother has zoster

---

VZIG indicates Varicella-Zoster Immune Globulin.
¹ Patients should meet criteria of both significant exposure and candidacy for receiving VZIG, as given in Table 3.77, (p 679). Varicella-Zoster Immune Globulin should be administered as soon as possible and no later than 96 hours after exposure.
² Experts differ in opinion about the duration of face-to-face contact that warrants administration of VZIG. However, the contact should be nontransient. Some experts suggest a contact of 5 or more minutes as constituting significant exposure for this purpose; others define close contact as more than 1 hour.

infection, postexposure immunization with varicella vaccine will result in protection against subsequent exposure. There is no evidence that administration of varicella vaccine during the presymptomatic or prodromal stage of illness increases the risk of vaccine-associated adverse events or more severe natural disease.

Chemoprophylaxis. Oral acyclovir is not recommended.

Passive Immunoprophylaxis. Susceptible people at high risk of developing severe varicella should be given VZIG within 96 hours; for maximum effectiveness, it should be given as soon as possible after exposure. Varicella-Zoster Immune Globulin can be obtained by contacting the local American Red Cross Blood Services or FFF Enterprises (41093 County Center, Temecula, CA 92591; telephone, 800-843-7477). The Red Cross has contracted with FFF Enterprises to handle distribution of VZIG in all states except Massachusetts (where VZIG is distributed by Massachusetts Biologic Laboratories, Boston, MA), New Hampshire, New York, and Maine.

The decision to administer VZIG depends on 3 factors: (1) the likelihood that the exposed person is susceptible to varicella; (2) the probability that a given exposure to varicella or zoster will result in infection; and (3) the likelihood that complications of varicella will develop if the person is infected.

Household exposure to varicella poses an almost certain risk of infection; exposure to an immunocompetent contact with varicella whose rash has been present for more than 5 days is low risk. People with a history of varicella usually are considered immune. However, people without such a history also may be immune. In deciding whether an adolescent or young adult with no history of varicella infection is likely

Table 3.77. Candidates for VZIG, Provided Significant Exposure Has Occurred[1]

- Immunocompromised children[2] without history of varicella or varicella immunization[3]
- Susceptible pregnant women
- Newborn infant whose mother had onset of chickenpox within 5 days before delivery or within 48 h after delivery
- Hospitalized premature infant (≥28 wk of gestation) whose mother lacks a reliable history of chickenpox or serologic evidence of protection against varicella
- Hospitalized premature infants (<28 wk of gestation or ≤1000 g birth weight), regardless of maternal history of varicella or varicella-zoster virus serostatus

VZIG indicates Varicella-Zoster Immune Globulin.
[1] See text and Table 3.76 (p 678) for additional discussion.
[2] Including children who are infected with human immunodeficiency virus.
[3] Immunocompromised adolescents and adults known to be susceptible also should receive VZIG.

to be immune, careful questioning about the following can be helpful: (1) history of varicella in other siblings (particularly younger siblings); (2) whether the patient attended an urban school; (3) previous exposure to people with chickenpox or zoster; (4) childhood in temperate climates; and (5) other clues, such as clinical description of disease.

Although serologic testing of immunocompetent people to determine immune status is reliable, it may not be reliable in immunocompromised patients. A carefully obtained history of varicella should be the primary determinant of immunity in immunocompromised patients. Administration of VZIG to exposed immunocompromised children with no history of varicella, regardless of serologic test results, usually is advised. Some experts, however, do not recommend administration of VZIG when the child is seropositive if determined by a sensitive assay (eg, latex agglutination test or enzyme immunoassay) and has not received a blood product that could have provided the passive antibody.

Patients receiving monthly high-dose Immune Globulin Intravenous (IGIV) (400 mg/kg or greater) are likely to be protected and probably do not require VZIG if the last dose of IGIV was given 3 weeks or less before exposure.

Administration and Dose. Varicella-Zoster Immune Globulin is given by intramuscular (IM) injection and contains between 10% and 18% Globulin and does not contain thimerosal. One vial (approximate volume, 1.25 mL) containing 125 U is given for each 10 kg of body weight and is the minimal dose. The suggested maximal dose of VZIG is 625 U (ie, 5 vials).

Use of VZIG for patients with a bleeding diathesis should be avoided, if possible. Immune Globulin Intravenous would be an acceptable alternative in this situation. Varicella-Zoster Immune Globulin never should be given intravenously.

Indications for VZIG. Tables 3.76 (p 678) and 3.77 (above) indicate susceptible people who should receive VZIG if exposed, including immunocompromised people, susceptible pregnant women, and certain newborn infants.

For healthy term infants exposed postnatally to varicella, including infants whose mother's rash developed more than 48 hours after delivery, VZIG is not indicated. However, some experts advise use of VZIG for any exposed susceptible newborn who has severe skin disease.

- **Healthy adults.** Varicella-Zoster Immune Globulin can be given to healthy susceptible adults after exposure to varicella, but VZIG is not recommended routinely. A 7-day course of acyclovir may be given to susceptible adults beginning 7 to 9 days after varicella exposure if vaccine is contraindicated or more than 72 hours has elapsed from the time of exposure. Most adults with no history or an uncertain history of chickenpox are nonetheless immune.

- **Subsequent exposures and follow-up of VZIG recipients.** Because administration of VZIG can cause varicella infection to be asymptomatic, testing of recipients 2 months or later after administration of VZIG to ascertain their immune status may be helpful in the event of subsequent exposure. Some experts, however, would advise VZIG administration after subsequent exposures, regardless of serologic results because of the unreliability of serologic test results in immunocompromised people and the uncertainty about whether asymptomatic infection after VZIG administration confers lasting protection.

The duration for which VZIG recipients are protected against varicella is unknown. If a second exposure occurs more than 3 weeks after administration of VZIG in a recipient in whom varicella did not develop, another dose of VZIG should be given.

Active Immunization. *

Vaccine. Varicella vaccine is a live-attenuated preparation of the serially propagated and attenuated wild Oka strain. The product contains trace amounts of neomycin and gelatin. The vaccine was licensed in March 1995 by the US Food and Drug Administration for use in healthy people 12 months of age or older who have not had varicella illness.

Dose and Administration. The recommended dose of the vaccine is 0.5 mL, which provides at least 1350 plaque-forming units of VZV. One dose is recommended for children 12 years of age or younger, and 2 doses separated by an interval of at least 4 to 8 weeks are recommended for individuals older than 12 years of age. Subcutaneous administration is recommended, although IM administration has been demonstrated to result in similar rates of seroconversion.

Immunogenicity. More than 95% of immunized healthy children between 12 months and 12 years of age develop humoral and cell-mediated immune response to VZV after a single dose of varicella vaccine. In people 13 years of age and older, seroconversion rates are 78% to 82% after 1 dose and 99% after 2 doses.

Effectiveness. The currently licensed product is more than 95% effective in preventing moderate or severe disease. Effectiveness in preventing mild infection is less uniform, generally ranging from 70% to 85%. After varicella immunization, a mild varicella-like syndrome develops in 1% to 4% of immunized children per year; these rates depend on exposure and are likely to decrease as coverage increases. Neither the

---

* American Academy of Pediatrics, Committee on Infectious Diseases. Recommendations for the use of live attenuated varicella vaccine. *Pediatrics.* 1995;95:791–796 and American Academy of Pediatrics, Committee on Infectious Diseases. Varicella vaccine update. *Pediatrics.* 2000,105:136–141

rate nor the severity of breakthrough varicella increases with time after immunization. Varicella in vaccine recipients is milder than that occurring in unimmunized children, with a median of 15 to 32 vesicles, lower rate of fever (10% with temperature ≥39°C [≥102°F]), and rapid recovery. At times, the disease is so mild that it is not easily recognizable as varicella because the skin lesions may resemble insect bites. In contrast, the median number of lesions in unimmunized children with varicella is more than 250. Varicella transmission from vaccine recipients with mild breakthrough disease has been documented but is rare.

Duration of Immunity. Although there has been concern about waning immunity, follow-up evaluations of children immunized during prelicensure clinical trials in the United States indicate protection for at least 11 years. Studies in Japan indicate protection for at least 20 years. However, these studies were conducted during a period when a substantial amount of wild-type VZV was present in the community, with many opportunities for boosting of immunity by subclinical infection in immunized people. Experience with other live-virus vaccines (eg, measles, rubella) suggests that immunity remains high throughout life; the primary reason for second doses of measles vaccine is to induce protection in children without an adequate response to the first dose, not because of waning immunity. Follow-up studies of clinical trials in children and postlicensure studies are being performed to determine the need, if any, for additional doses of varicella vaccine.

Simultaneous Administration With Other Vaccines. Varicella vaccine may be given simultaneously with other recommended childhood immunizations (see Recommended Childhood and Adolescent Immunization Schedule, p 24), but separate syringes and injection sites must be used. Although further immunogenicity studies are needed on the use of varicella vaccine administered simultaneously with inactivated poliovirus vaccine, there is no reason to suspect that varicella vaccine will affect the immune response to this vaccine. If not given simultaneously, the interval between administration of varicella vaccine and MMR vaccine should be at least 28 days.

Adverse Events. Varicella vaccine is safe; reactions generally are mild and occur with an overall frequency of approximately 5% to 35%. Approximately 20% of immunized people will experience minor injection site reactions (eg, pain, redness, swelling). In approximately 3% to 5% of immunized children, a localized rash develops, and in an additional 3% to 5%, a generalized varicella-like rash develops. These rashes typically consist of 2 to 5 lesions and may be maculopapular rather than vesicular; lesions usually appear 5 to 26 days after immunization. Most generalized varicelliform rashes that occur within the first 2 weeks after varicella immunization are attributable to wild-type VZV infection and are not an adverse effect of the vaccine. Although a temperature higher than 39°C (102°F) has been observed from 1 to 42 days after immunization in 15% of healthy immunized children, fever also occurs in a similar percentage of children receiving placebo and is not considered to be a common adverse reaction to varicella immunization. A temperature higher than 38°C (100°F) has been reported in 10% of adolescents and adults who are immunized with the vaccine. Serious adverse events, such as anaphylaxis, encephalitis, ataxia, erythema multiforme, Stevens-Johnson syndrome, pneumonia, thrombocytopenia, seizures, neuropathy, Guillian-Barré syndrome, secondary bacterial infections, and death have been reported rarely in temporal association with varicella vaccine. In rare instances, a causal relationship between the varicella vaccine and some of these serious adverse events has been established, although the frequency is much lower than after natural infection. In most cases, data are insufficient to determine a causal association.

Herpes Zoster After Immunization. The varicella vaccine virus has been associated with development of herpes zoster in immunocompetent and immunocompromised people within 25 to 722 days after immunization. Data from postlicensure surveillance indicate that the age-specific risk of herpes zoster seems to be lower among immunocompetent children immunized with varicella vaccine than among children who have had natural varicella infection. A population-based study indicated that the annual incidence of herpes zoster after natural varicella infection among immunocompetent children younger than 20 years of age was 68 per 100 000 people, and the reported annual rate of herpes zoster after varicella immunization among immunocompetent people was approximately 2.6 per 100 000 vaccine doses distributed (CDC, unpublished data). However, comparison of these rates should be made cautiously, because the rates of zoster after natural infection are based on populations monitored actively for longer periods of time than the duration of passive surveillance after immunization. Wild-type VZV has been isolated from vesicles in people with herpes zoster after immunization, indicating that herpes zoster in immunized people also may result from antecedent natural varicella infection.

Transmission of Vaccine-Associated Virus. Experience since 1995 with more than 30 million doses of varicella vaccine distributed in the United States indicates that vaccine-associated virus transmission to contacts is rare (only 3 well-documented cases) and the risk of transmission exists only if a rash develops on the immunized person (Merck & Co Inc, unpublished data).

The role of VZIG or acyclovir as prophylaxis for high-risk people exposed to immunized people with lesions will be difficult to evaluate given the rarity of transmission. If contact inadvertently occurs, the routine use of VZIG is not recommended, because transmission is rare and disease, if it were to develop, would be expected to be mild. However, some experts believe that immunocompromised people in whom skin lesions develop, possibly related to vaccine virus, should receive acyclovir treatment.

Storage. The lyophilized vaccine should be stored in a frost-free freezer at an average temperature of −15°C (+5°F) or colder. Vaccine may be stored at refrigerator temperature of 2°C to 8°C (36°F–46°F) for up to 72 continuous hours before administration. The diluent used for reconstitution should be stored separately in a refrigerator or at room temperature. Once the vaccine has been reconstituted, it should be injected as soon as possible and discarded if not used within 30 minutes.

Recommendations for Immunization. Universal immunization of infants and immunization of susceptible older children and adolescents without a contraindication is recommended on the basis of the frequency of serious complications and deaths after natural infection, the excessive cost to the family and society resulting from varicella infection, and the efficacy and safety of the live-attenuated varicella vaccine. Susceptibility is defined by lack of proof of varicella immunization, lack of a reliable history of varicella, or absence of serologic evidence of varicella. Age-specific recommendations are as follows:

- **Age 12 months to the 13th birthday:**

  Age 12 to 18 months. One dose of varicella vaccine is recommended for universal immunization for all immunocompetent children who lack a reliable history or serologic evidence of varicella.

  Age 19 months to the 13th birthday. Immunization of susceptible children is recommended, and immunization may be given any time during childhood but before the 13th birthday because of the potential increased severity of natural varicella after this age.

- **Healthy adolescents and young adults.** Healthy adolescents past their 13th birthday who are susceptible should be immunized against varicella by administration of 2 doses of vaccine 4 to 8 weeks apart. Longer intervals between doses do not necessitate a third dose but may leave the person unprotected during the intervening months.

- **Adults.** Recommendations for the use of varicella vaccine in adults have been issued by the ACIP.* Immunization is recommended by the ACIP for the following high-risk groups; however, varicella immunization of all susceptible adults is encouraged:

  - Close contacts of people at high risk of serious complications, including family contacts of immunocompromised people
  - Health care professionals
  - People who live or work in environments where transmission of VZV is likely (eg, teachers of young children, child care employees, and residents and staff members in institutional settings)
  - People who live and work in environments where transmission can occur (eg, college students, inmates and staff members of correctional institutions, and military personnel)
  - Nonpregnant women of childbearing age
  - Adolescents and adults living in households with children
  - International travelers

Serologic Testing Before and After Immunization

An adult, adolescent, or child with a reliable history of varicella can be assumed to be immune, and immunization is unnecessary. Because approximately 70% to 90% of people 18 years of age or older without a reliable history of varicella also will be immune, it may be cost-effective to perform serologic tests on people 13 years of age or older and immunize only those who are seronegative. If serologic testing is performed, a tracking system for seronegative people should be developed to ensure that susceptible people are immunized. However, serologic testing is not required, because varicella vaccine is well tolerated by people immune from earlier disease. In some situations, universal immunization may be easier to implement than serologic testing and tracking. Most children younger than 13 years of age without a reliable history of varicella should be considered susceptible and immunized without serologic testing. However, data from some populations indicate that a large proportion of 9- to 12-year old children with an uncertain history of varicella are immune and that

---

* Centers for Disease Control and Prevention. Prevention of varicella update: recommendations of the Advisory Committee on Immunization Practices (ACIP). *MMWR Morb Mortal Wkly Rep.* 1999;45(RR-6):1–5

serologic testing before deciding about immunization may be cost-effective. Seroconversion rates after 1 dose of varicella vaccine in children younger than 13 years of age and after 2 doses in adolescents and adults are so high that serologic testing after immunization is unnecessary.

Whole-cell enzyme immunoassay is the most commonly used commercially available serologic test for VZV. The sensitivity of this test is sufficient to determine immunity after natural varicella, but it may not be sensitive enough to determine vaccine-induced immunity. Tests such as the fluorescent antibody to membrane antigen and latex agglutination tests are more sensitive, but the fluorescent antibody to membrane antigen test assay is not commercially available, and the latex agglutination assay is not convenient for mass testing.

Booster Immunization. Reimmunization is not recommended currently, but the need for recommendations for reimmunization will be reassessed with time.

Contraindications and Precautions.

Intercurrent Illness. As with other vaccines, varicella vaccine should not be administered to people who have moderate or severe illnesses, with or without fever (see Vaccine Safety and Contraindications, p 37).

Immunocompromised Patients.

General recommendations. Varicella vaccine should not be administered routinely to children who have T-lymphocyte immunodeficiency, including people with leukemia, lymphoma, other malignant neoplasms affecting the bone marrow or lymphatic systems, and congenital T-cell abnormalities (see Immunocompromised Children, p 69). Exceptions include children with acute lymphocytic leukemia, to whom vaccine may be administered under a study with protocol (see Acute lymphocytic leukemia, below) and certain asymptomatic children infected with HIV (see Human Immunodeficiency Virus Infection, p 360). Children with impaired humoral immunity may be immunized.

Immunodeficiency should be excluded before immunization in children with a family history of hereditary immunodeficiency. The presence of an immunodeficient or HIV-seropositive family member does not contraindicate vaccine use in other family members.

Acute lymphocytic leukemia. Although the current vaccine is not licensed for routine use in children with malignant neoplasms, immunization should be considered when a susceptible child with acute lymphocytic leukemia has been in continuous remission for at least 1 year and has a lymphocyte count greater than 700/μL (0.7 × 10^9/L) and a platelet count greater than 100 × 10^3/μL (100 × 10^9/L). Immunization has been demonstrated to be safe, immunogenic, and effective in these children, and the vaccine may be obtained free for use in a research protocol. This protocol requires approval by the appropriate institutional review board as well as monitoring for safety.*

Human immunodeficiency virus infection. Routine screening for HIV infection is not indicated before routine varicella immunization. Children known to be infected with HIV may be at increased risk of morbidity from varicella and herpes

---

* To immunize a child with acute lymphocytic leukemia, contact The Varivax Coordinating Center, Omnicare Clinical Research, 630 Allendale Rd, King of Prussia, PA 19406; telephone, 484-679-2856.

zoster compared with healthy children. Limited data on immunization of HIV-infected children in CDC Class 1 with a CD4+ T-lymphocyte percentage of 25% or greater indicate that the vaccine is safe, immunogenic, and effective. Therefore, after weighing potential risks and benefits, varicella vaccine should be considered for HIV-infected children in CDC Class 1 with a CD4+ T-lymphocyte percentage of 25% or greater. Eligible children should receive 2 doses of varicella vaccine with a 3-month interval between doses and return for evaluation if they experience a postimmunization varicella-like rash. With increased use of varicella vaccine and the resulting decrease in incidence of varicella in the community, exposure of immunocompromised hosts to VZV will decrease. As the risk of exposure decreases and more data are generated on the use of varicella vaccine in high-risk populations, the risk versus benefit of varicella immunization in HIV-infected children will need to be reassessed.

Children receiving corticosteroids. Varicella vaccine should not be administered to people who are receiving high doses of systemic corticosteroids (2 mg/kg per day or more of prednisone or its equivalent or 20 mg/day of prednisone or its equivalent if weight >10 kg) for 14 days or more. The recommended interval between discontinuation of corticosteroid therapy and immunization with varicella vaccine is at least 1 month. Other recommendations about varicella vaccine use in children receiving corticosteroids can be found in Immunocompromised Children, p 69.

Households with potential contact with immunocompromised people. Transmission of vaccine-type VZV from healthy people has been documented, albeit rarely (see Adverse Events, p 681). Even in families with immunocompromised people, including people with HIV infection, no precautions are needed after immunization of healthy children in whom a rash does not develop. Immunized people in whom a rash develops should avoid direct contact with immunocompromised susceptible hosts for the duration of the rash.

Pregnancy and Lactation. Varicella vaccine should not be administered to pregnant women, because the possible effects on fetal development are unknown.* When postpubertal females are immunized, pregnancy should be avoided for at least 1 month after immunization. A pregnant mother or other household member is not a contraindication for immunization of a child in the household. This recommendation is based on the following: transmission of vaccine virus is rare; more than 95% of adults are immune, and immunization of the child likely will protect the susceptible mother from exposure to wild-type VZV.

A study of nursing mothers and their infants showed no evidence of excretion of vaccine strain in human milk or of transmission to infants who are breastfeeding. Varicella vaccine should be administered to susceptible nursing mothers.

Immune Globulin. Whether Immune Globulin (IG) can interfere with varicella vaccine-induced immunity is unknown, although IG can interfere with immunity induction by measles vaccine. Pending additional data, varicella vaccine should be withheld for the same intervals after receipt of any form of IG or other blood product as measles vaccine (see Measles, p 419). Conversely, IG should be withheld for at least 2 weeks after receipt of varicella vaccine. Transplacental antibodies to VZV

---

* The manufacturer, in collaboration with the CDC, has established the Varivax Pregnancy Registry to monitor the maternal and fetal outcomes of women who inadvertently are given varicella vaccine 3 months before or at any time during pregnancy. Reporting cases is encouraged and may be done by telephone (800-986-8999).

do not interfere with the immunogenicity of varicella vaccine administered at 12 months of age or older.

Salicylates. Whether Reye syndrome results from administration of salicylates after immunization for varicella in children is unknown. No cases have been reported. However, because of the association between Reye syndrome, natural varicella infection, and salicylates, the vaccine manufacturer recommends that salicylates be avoided for 6 weeks after administration of varicella vaccine. Physicians need to weigh the theoretic risks associated with varicella vaccine against the known risks of wild-type virus in children receiving long-term salicylate therapy.

Allergy to Vaccine Components. Varicella vaccine should not be administered to people who have had an anaphylactic-type reaction to any component of the vaccine, including gelatin and neomycin. Most people with allergy to neomycin have resulting contact dermatitis, a reaction that is not a contraindication to immunization. The vaccine does not contain preservatives or egg protein.

VIBRIO INFECTIONS

Cholera
(Vibrio cholerae)

CLINICAL MANIFESTATIONS: Cholera is characterized by painless voluminous diarrhea without abdominal cramps or fever. Dehydration, hypokalemia, metabolic acidosis, and occasionally, hypovolemic shock can occur in 4 to 12 hours if fluid losses are not replaced. Coma, seizures, and hypoglycemia also can occur, particularly in children. Stools are colorless, with small flecks of mucus ("rice-water"), and contain high concentrations of sodium, potassium, chloride, and bicarbonate. Most infected people with toxigenic *Vibrio cholerae* O1 have no symptoms, and some have only mild to moderate diarrhea; fewer than 5% have severe watery diarrhea, vomiting, and dehydration *(cholera gravis)*.

ETIOLOGY: *Vibrio cholerae* is a gram-negative, curved, motile bacillus with many serogroups. Until recently, only enterotoxin-producing organisms of serogroup O1 have caused epidemics. *Vibrio cholerae* O1 is divided into 2 serotypes, Inaba and Ogawa, and 2 biotypes, classical and El Tor. The predominant biotype is El Tor. In 1992, a cholera epidemic attributable to toxigenic *V cholerae* serogroup O139 Bengal (a non-O1 toxigenic strain) caused epidemic cholera in the Indian subcontinent and southeast Asia; cases of cholera caused by this serogroup have been confined to Southeast Asia since 1993. Serogroups of *V cholerae* other than O1 and O139 Bengal and nontoxigenic strains of *V cholerae* O1 can cause sporadic diarrheal illness, but they do not cause epidemics.

EPIDEMIOLOGY: During the last 4 decades, *V cholerae* O1, biotype El Tor, has spread from India and Southeast Asia to Africa, the Middle East, Southern Europe, and the Western Pacific Islands (Oceania). In 1991, epidemic cholera caused by toxigenic *V cholerae* O1, serotype Inaba, biotype El Tor, appeared in Peru and spread to most countries in South and North America. In the United States, cases resulting from travel to Latin America or Asia and attributable to ingestion of contaminated food transported from Latin America or Asia were reported. In addition, the Gulf Coast of Louisiana and Texas has an endemic focus of a unique strain of toxigenic *V cholerae* O1. Most cases of disease from this strain have resulted from consumption of raw or undercooked shellfish. Humans are the only documented natural host, but free-living *V cholerae* organisms can exist in the aquatic environment. The usual mode of infection is ingestion of contaminated water or less commonly, food (particularly raw or undercooked shellfish, moist grains held at ambient temperature, and raw or partially dried fish). Boiling or treating water with chlorine or iodine and adequately cooking food kills the organism. Direct person-to-person spread has not been documented. People with low gastric acidity are at increased risk of cholera infection.

The **incubation period** usually is 1 to 3 days, with a range of a few hours to 5 days.

DIAGNOSTIC TESTS: *Vibrio cholerae* can be cultured from fecal specimens or vomitus plated on thiosulfate citrate bile salts sucrose agar. Because most laboratories in the United States do not routinely culture for *V cholerae* or other *Vibrio* organisms, clinicians should request appropriate cultures for clinically suspected cases. Isolates of *V cholerae* should be sent to a state health department laboratory for serogrouping; those of serogroup O1 or O139 Bengal then are sent to the Centers for Disease Control and Prevention for testing for production of cholera toxin. A fourfold increase in vibriocidal antibody titers between acute and convalescent serum specimens or a fourfold decrease in vibriocidal titers between early and late convalescent (more than a 2-month interval) serum specimens can confirm the diagnosis.

TREATMENT: Oral or parenteral rehydration therapy to correct dehydration and electrolyte abnormalities is the most important modality of therapy and should be initiated as soon as the diagnosis is suspected.* Oral rehydration is preferred unless the patient is in shock, is obtunded, or has intestinal ileus. The World Health Organization's Oral Rehydration Solution (ORS) has been the standard, but recent data suggest that rice-based ORS or amylase-resistant starch ORS is more effective.

Antimicrobial therapy results in prompt eradication of vibrios, decreases the duration of diarrhea, and decreases requirements for fluid replacement. It should be considered for people who are moderately to severely ill. Oral doxycycline as a single dose or tetracycline for 3 days are the drugs of choice for cholera attributable to *V cholerae* O1 and O139 Bengal. The use of tetracyclines generally is not recommended for children younger than 8 years of age, but in cases of severe cholera, the benefits may offset the small risk of staining of developing teeth (see Antimicrobial Agents and Related Therapy, p 693). If strains are resistant to tetracyclines, trimethoprim-sulfamethoxazole, erythromycin, or furazolidone may be used. *Vibrio cholerae* O139 Bengal strains typically are not susceptible to trimethoprim-sulfamethoxazole or furazolidone. Ciprofloxacin or ofloxacin usually are effective therapeutic agents for infection attributable to *V cholerae* O1 and O139 Bengal but generally should

---

* American Academy of Pediatrics, Committee on Quality Improvement, Subcommittee on Acute Gastroenteritis. The management of acute gastroenteritis in young children. *Pediatrics.* 1996;97:424-435

be used only for people at least 18 years of age (see Antimicrobial Agents and Related Therapy, p 693). Antimicrobial susceptibility testing of newly isolated organisms should be determined.

ISOLATION OF THE HOSPITALIZED PATIENT: In addition to standard precautions, contact precautions are indicated for diapered or incontinent children for the duration of illness.

CONTROL MEASURES:

Hygiene. Because cholera spreads by contaminated food or water and infection commonly requires ingestion of large numbers of organisms, disinfection or boiling of water prevents transmission. Thoroughly cooking crabs, oysters, and other shellfish from the Gulf Coast before eating is recommended to decrease the likelihood of transmission. Foods such as fish, rice, or grain gruels should be refrigerated promptly after meals and thoroughly reheated before eating. Appropriate hand hygiene after defecating and before preparing or eating food is important for preventing transmission.

Treatment of Contacts. The administration of doxycycline, tetracycline, or trimethoprim-sulfamethoxazole within 24 hours of identification of the index case may effectively prevent coprimary cases of cholera among household contacts. However, antimicrobial prophylaxis plays a limited role in cholera control. The use of tetracyclines generally is not recommended for children younger than 8 years of age (see Antimicrobial Agents and Related Therapy, p 693). Chemoprophylaxis is not recommended in the United States, because secondary spread is rare, unless unusual sanitary and hygienic conditions indicate that the rate of secondary transmission could be high.

Vaccine. No cholera vaccines are available in the United States. Two oral vaccines are available outside of the United States (WC/r BS and CDV 103 Hgr). Neither vaccine provides established protection in children younger than 2 years of age, and they are not effective against *V cholerae* 0139 Bengal. Furthermore, travelers using appropriate precautions in countries with cholera are at a low risk of infection. Cholera immunization is not required for travelers entering the United States from cholera-affected areas, and the World Health Organization no longer recommends immunization for travel to or from cholera-infected areas. No country requires cholera vaccine for entry.

Reporting. Confirmed cases of cholera must be reported to health authorities in any country in which they occur or were contracted. State health departments should be notified immediately of presumed or known cases of cholera attributable to *V cholerae* O1 or O139 Bengal.

Other *Vibrio* Infections

CLINICAL MANIFESTATIONS: Noncholera *Vibrio* species are associated with 3 major syndromes: diarrhea, septicemia, and wound infection. Diarrhea is the most common and is characterized by acute onset of watery stools and crampy abdominal pain. Approximately half of those afflicted will have low-grade fever, headache, and chills; approximately 30% will have vomiting. Spontaneous recovery follows in 2 to 5 days. Bacteremia rarely accompanies gastroenteritis. Infection can develop in contaminated wounds. Skin infections in immunocompromised people can cause extensive and rapid tissue necrosis. Patients with immunodeficiency or liver disease are susceptible to septicemia from bowel or skin infections, often resulting in shock, bullous or necrotic skin lesions, and death. Primary septicemia can develop in immunocompromised people with a preceding gastroenteritis or wound infection.

ETIOLOGY: *Vibrio* organisms are facultatively anaerobic, motile, gram-negative bacilli that are tolerant of salt. The most important noncholera *Vibrio* species associated with diarrhea are *Vibrio parahaemolyticus, V cholerae* non-O1, *Vibrio mimicus, Vibrio hollisae, Vibrio fluvialis,* and *Vibrio furnissii. Vibrio vulnificus* causes primary septicemia and wound infections in immunocompromised patients, especially people with liver disease. *Vibrio parahaemolyticus, Vibrio damsela,* and *Vibrio alginolyticus* also are associated with wound infections. *Vibrio alginolyticus* has been associated with otitis externa.

EPIDEMIOLOGY: Noncholera *Vibrio* species commonly are found in seawater, increasing quantitatively during summer. Most infections occur during summer and fall. Enteritis usually is acquired from seafood that is eaten raw or undercooked, especially oysters, crabs, and shrimp. The disease probably is not communicable person to person. Wound infections commonly result from exposure of abrasions to contaminated seawater or from punctures resulting from handling of contaminated shellfish. People with increased susceptibility to infection with *Vibrio* species include people with liver disease, low gastric acidity, and immunodeficiency, including people with human immunodeficiency virus infection.

The median **incubation period** of enteritis is 23 hours, with a range of 5 to 92 hours.

DIAGNOSTIC TESTS: *Vibrio* organisms can be isolated from stool or vomitus of patients with diarrhea, from blood specimens, and from wound exudates. Because identification of the organism requires special techniques, laboratory personnel should be notified when infection with *Vibrio* species is suspected.

TREATMENT: Most episodes of diarrhea are mild and self-limited and do not require treatment other than oral rehydration. Antimicrobial therapy may benefit those with severe diarrhea, wound infection, or septicemia. Most organisms are susceptible to doxycycline or tetracycline, cefotaxime sodium, gentamicin sulfate, and chloramphenicol. Doxycycline should not be given to children younger than 8 years of age unless the benefits of therapy are greater than the risks of dental staining (see Antimicrobial Agents and Related Therapy, p 693).

ISOLATION OF THE HOSPITALIZED PATIENT: In addition to standard precautions, contact precautions are recommended for diapered or incontinent children.

CONTROL MEASURES: Seafood should be cooked adequately, and if not ingested immediately, it should be refrigerated. Uncooked mollusks and crustaceans should be handled with care. Abrasions suffered by ocean bathers should be rinsed with clean fresh water. All children and immunocompromised people should be warned to avoid eating raw oysters or clams.

Yersinia enterocolitica and *Yersinia pseudotuberculosis* Infections
(Enteritis and Other Illnesses)

CLINICAL MANIFESTATIONS: *Yersinia enterocolitica* and *Yersinia pseudotuberculosis* cause several age-specific syndromes and a variety of other uncommon presentations. The most common manifestation of infection with *Y enterocolitica* is enterocolitis with fever and diarrhea; stool often contains leukocytes, blood, and mucus. This syndrome occurs most often in young children, and relapsing disease and, rarely, necrotizing enterocolitis have been described. A pseudoappendicitis syndrome (fever, abdominal pain, tenderness in the right lower quadrant of the abdomen, and leukocytosis) occurs primarily in older children and young adults. Bacteremia with *Y enterocolitica* most often occurs in children younger than 1 year of age and in older children with predisposing conditions, such as excessive iron storage (eg, desferrioxamine use, sickle cell disease, β-thalassemia) and immunosuppressive states. Focal manifestations of *Y enterocolitica* are uncommon and include pharyngitis, meningitis, osteomyelitis, pyomyositis, conjunctivitis, pneumonia, empyema, endocarditis, acute peritonitis, abscesses of the liver and spleen, and primary cutaneous infection. Postinfectious sequelae observed with *Y enterocolitica* infection include erythema nodosum, proliferative glomerulonephritis, and reactive arthritis; these sequelae occur most often in older children and adults, particularly those with HLAB27 antigen.

The major manifestations of *Y pseudotuberculosis* infection are fever, rash, and abdominal symptoms. The rash usually is scarlatiniform. Acute pseudoappendiceal abdominal pain is most common, resulting from ileocecal mesenteric adenitis, appendicitis, or terminal ileitis. Other findings include diarrhea, erythema nodosum, septicemia, and sterile pleural and joint effusions. Clinical features can mimic those of Kawasaki syndrome.

ETIOLOGY: *Yersinia enterocolitica* and *Y pseudotuberculosis* are gram-negative bacilli that, along with *Y pestis,* represent the 3 most commonly encountered human pathogenic species of the 11 in the genus *Yersinia.* Fifteen pathogenic O groups of *Y enterocolitica* are recognized. Differences in virulence exist among various O groups of *Y enterocolitica;* O:3 and O:9 now predominate as the most common causes of diarrhea in the United States.

EPIDEMIOLOGY: *Yersinia enterocolitica* infections are uncommon in the United States; the annual incidence, according to the Foodborne Disease Active Surveillance Network (FoodNet), is 0.4 per 100 000 people. *Yersinia pseudotuberculosis* infections are rare. The principal reservoir of *Y enterocolitica* is swine; feral *Y pseudotuberculosis* has been isolated from ungulates (deer, elk, goats, sheep, cattle), rodents (rats, rabbits, squirrels, beaver), and many bird species. Infection is believed to be transmitted by ingestion of contaminated food (raw or incompletely cooked pork products and unpasteurized milk), by contaminated surface or well water, by direct or indirect contact with animals, by transfusion with packed Red Blood Cells, and possibly although rarely by fecal-oral, person-to-person transmission. Bottle-fed infants can be infected if their caregivers simultaneously are handling raw pork intestines (chitterlings). *Yersinia enterocolitica* is isolated more often in cooler climates, with a predominance in November through January in the northern United States. The period of communicability is unknown; organisms are excreted for an average of 6 weeks after diagnosis.

The **incubation period** typically is 4 to 6 days, varying from 1 to 14 days.

DIAGNOSTIC TESTS: *Yersinia enterocolitica* and *Y pseudotuberculosis* can be recovered from throat swabs, mesenteric lymph nodes, peritoneal fluid, and blood. Stool cultures generally are positive during the first 2 weeks of illness, regardless of the nature of gastrointestinal tract manifestations. *Yersinia enterocolitica* also has been isolated from synovial fluid, bile, urine, cerebrospinal fluid, sputum, and wounds. Because of the relatively low incidence of *Yersinia* infection in the United States, it is not routinely sought in stool specimens by most laboratories. Consequently, laboratory personnel should be notified when *Yersinia* infection is suspected. Biotyping and serotyping for further identification of pathogenic strains is available through public health reference laboratories. Infection can be confirmed by demonstrating increases in serum antibody titer after infection, but these tests generally are available only in reference or research laboratories. Cross-reactions of these antibodies with *Brucella, Vibrio, Salmonella,* and *Rickettsia* species and *Escherichia coli* lead to false-positive *Y enterocolitica* and *Y pseudotuberculosis* titers. In patients with thyroid disease, persistently increased *Y enterocolitica* antibody titers can result from antigenic similarity of the organism with antigens of the thyroid epithelial cell membrane. Characteristic ultrasonographic features demonstrating edema of the wall of the terminal ileum and cecum help to distinguish pseudoappendicitis from appendicitis and may help avoid exploratory surgery.

TREATMENT: *Yersinia enterocolitica* and *Y pseudotuberculosis* usually are susceptible to trimethoprim-sulfamethoxazole, aminoglycosides, cefotaxime sodium, fluoroquinolones (for patients 18 years of age and older), tetracycline or doxycycline (for children 8 years of age and older), and chloramphenicol. *Yersinia enterocolitica* isolates usually are resistant to first-generation cephalosporins and most penicillins. Patients with septicemia or sites of infection other than the gastrointestinal tract and immunocompromised hosts with enterocolitis should receive antimicrobial therapy. Other than decreasing the duration of fecal excretion of *Y enterocolitica* and *Y pseudotuberculosis,* a clinical benefit of antimicrobial therapy for patients with enterocolitis, pseudoappendicitis syndrome, or mesenteric adenitis has not been established.

ISOLATION OF THE HOSPITALIZED PATIENT: Standard precautions are recommended.

CONTROL MEASURES: Ingestion of uncooked meat, unpasteurized milk, or contaminated water should be avoided. People handling pork intestines should wash their hands after contact and should not care for a young infant at the same time.

Antimicrobial Agents and Related Therapy

....

INTRODUCTION

In some instances, antimicrobial agents are recommended for specific indications other than indications in the product label (package insert) approved by the US Food and Drug Administration (FDA). An FDA-licensed indication means that adequate and well-controlled studies were conducted and then reviewed by the FDA. However, accepted medical practice often includes drug use that is not reflected in approved drug labeling. Lack of licensing for an indication does not necessarily mean lack of effectiveness but indicates that the appropriate studies have not been performed or data have not been submitted to the FDA for a license for that indication. Unlicensed use does not imply improper use, provided that reasonable medical evidence justifies such use and that use of the drug is deemed in the best interest of the patient. The decision to prescribe a drug resides with the physician, who must weigh risks and benefits of using the drug, regardless of whether the drug has received FDA licensure for the specific indication and age of the patient.

Some antimicrobial agents with proven therapeutic benefit in humans are not licensed by the FDA for use in pediatric patients or are considered contraindicated in children because of possible toxicity. Some of these drugs, however, such as fluoroquinolones (in people younger than 18 years of age) and tetracyclines (in children younger than 8 years of age), may be used in special circumstances after careful assessment of the risks and benefits. Obtaining informed consent before use is prudent. The following information delineates general principles for use of these classes of drugs.

Fluoroquinolones

Use of fluoroquinolones (for example, ciprofloxacin, enoxacin, gatifloxacin, levofloxacin, lomefloxacin, moxifloxacin, norfloxacin, ofloxacin, sparfloxacin, and trovafloxacin) generally is contraindicated, according to FDA-approved product labeling, in children and adolescents younger than 18 years of age, because fluoroquinolones have been shown to cause cartilage damage in every juvenile animal model tested at doses that approximate those needed to be therapeutic. The mechanism for this damage is unknown. Pefloxacin, a fluoroquinolone that had been used extensively in France, causes arthropathy in children and adults. Furthermore, data suggest that alatrofloxacin mesylate and trovafloxacin can cause acute liver failure that has resulted in a number of deaths.

To date, ciprofloxacin is the fluoroquinolone that has been used most extensively in children (mostly in adolescents). On the basis of relatively limited experience, this drug appears to be well tolerated, does not appear to cause arthropathy, and is effective as an oral agent for treating a number of diseases in children that otherwise would require parenteral therapy. Accordingly, in special circumstances after careful assessment of the risks and benefits for the individual patient, use of a fluoroquinolone can be justified. Circumstances in which fluoroquinolones may be useful include those in which (1) no other oral agent is available, necessitating an alternative drug given parenterally; and (2) infection is caused by multidrug-resistant, gram-negative, enteric, and other pathogens, such as certain *Pseudomonas* and *Mycobacterium* strains. Possible uses, accordingly, include the following:

- To decrease the incidence or progression of disease after exposure to aerosolized *Bacillus anthracis* (see Anthrax, p 196)
- Urinary tract infection caused by *Pseudomonas aeruginosa* or other multidrug-resistant, gram-negative bacteria
- Chronic suppurative otitis media or malignant otitis externa
- Chronic osteomyelitis
- Exacerbation of cystic fibrosis
- Mycobacterial infections
- Other gram-negative bacterial infections in immunocompromised hosts in which prolonged oral therapy is desired

Licensure by the FDA of one or more fluoroquinolones for use in children, and with limited indications, may occur. Until then, if use of a fluoroquinolone is recommended for a patient younger than 18 years of age, the risks and benefits should be explained to the patients and parents.

Tetracyclines

Use of tetracyclines in pediatric patients has been limited, because these drugs can cause permanent dental discoloration in children younger than 8 years of age. Studies have documented that tetracyclines and their colored degradation products that are bound to teeth are observed in the dentin and incorporated diffusely in the enamel. The period of odontogenesis to completion of the formation of enamel in permanent teeth appears to be the critical time for the effects of these drugs and is virtually complete by 8 years of age, at which time the drug can be given without concern for dental staining. The degree of staining appears to depend on dosage and duration of therapy, with the total dosage received being the most important factor. In addition to dental discoloration, tetracyclines also may cause enamel hypoplasia and reversible delay in rate of bone growth.

These possible adverse events have resulted in use of alternative, equally effective antimicrobial agents in most circumstances in young children in which tetracyclines are likely to be effective. However, in some cases, the benefits of therapy with a tetracycline can exceed the risks, particularly if alternative drugs are associated with significant adverse effects or may be less effective. In these cases, the use of tetracyclines in young children is justified. Examples include life-threatening rickettsial infections such as Rocky Mountain spotted fever (see p 532) and ehrlichiosis (see p 266), cholera (see p 686), and anthrax (see p 196). Doxycycline usually is the agent of choice in children with these infections, because the risk of dental staining is less with this product than that with other tetracyclines. In addition, the drug is given only twice a day, in contrast to the more frequent dosing regimens of other tetracyclines.

....

APPROPRIATE USE OF
ANTIMICROBIAL AGENTS

The increasing prevalence of antimicrobial resistance is an issue of major concern to patients as well as health care professionals. Rarely, highly resistant pathogens, such as *Burkholderia cepacia, Staphylococcus aureus,* or *Enterococcus faecium* are not treatable with available agents. More commonly, the presence of resistant pathogens complicates therapy, increases expense, and makes treatment failure more likely. Resistant foodborne pathogens, such as fluoroquinolone-resistant *Campylobacter jejuni;* community-acquired pathogens, such as drug-resistant *Streptococcus pneumoniae;* and hospital-acquired pathogens, such as vancomycin-resistant enterococci, have unique epidemiologic features and require specific control measures. Control of antimicrobial resistance among foodborne pathogens has focused on measures such as irradiating food products before consumption and decreasing addition of antimicrobial agents to animal feed. Among community-acquired and hospital-acquired pathogens, the overuse of antimicrobial agents in humans largely is responsible for the increase in resistance. The following principles for appropriate use of antimicrobial agents have become a central focus of public health measures to combat the spread of resistant organisms.

Principles of Appropriate Use for Upper Respiratory Tract Infections

Approximately three fourths of all outpatient prescriptions for children are given for 5 conditions: otitis media, sinusitis, cough illness/bronchitis, pharyngitis, and nonspecific upper respiratory tract infection (the common cold). Physicians report that many patients and parents try to persuade them to dispense unnecessary antimicrobial agents. Children treated with an antimicrobial agent are at increased risk of becoming carriers of resistant bacteria, including *S pneumoniae* and *Haemophilus influenzae.* Carriers of a resistant strain who develop illness from that strain are more likely to have antimicrobial therapy failure. In some conditions, such as otitis media with effusion, observation without antimicrobial therapy is recommended, and in other conditions such as the common cold or cough, antimicrobial therapy is not indicated. The following principles, with detailed supporting evidence, were published by the American Academy of Pediatrics, American Academy of Family Physicians, and Centers for Disease Control and Prevention (CDC) to identify clinical conditions for which antimicrobial therapy could be curtailed without compromising patient care.*

---

* Dowell SF, Marcy SM, Phillips WR, Gerber MA, Schwartz B. Principles of judicious use of antimicrobial agents for pediatric upper respiratory tract infections. *Pediatrics.* 1998;101:S163–S165; and Dowell SF, Schwartz B, Phillips WR. Appropriate use of antibiotics for URIs in children: part II. Cough, pharyngitis and the common cold. The Pediatric URI Consensus Team. *Am Fam Phys.* 1998;58:1335–1342, 1345

OTITIS MEDIA

- Episodes of otitis media should be classified as acute otitis media (AOM) or otitis media with effusion (OME).
- Antimicrobial agents are indicated for treatment of AOM; however, diagnosis requires documented middle ear effusion *and* signs or symptoms of acute local or systemic illness.
- Acute otitis media can be treated with a 5- to 7-day course of antimicrobial agents in most children 2 years of age or older. Younger children and children with underlying medical conditions, craniofacial abnormalities, chronic or recurrent otitis media, or perforation of the tympanic membrane, should be treated with a standard 10-day course. A narrow-spectrum antimicrobial agent (eg, amoxicillin) should be used for initial episodes of acute otitis media.
- Persistent middle ear effusion (OME) for 2 to 3 months after therapy for AOM is expected and does not require retreatment.
- Antimicrobial agents are not indicated for initial treatment of OME; treatment may be indicated if effusions persist for 3 months or more.
- Antimicrobial prophylaxis should be reserved for control of recurrent AOM, defined as 3 or more distinct and well-documented episodes in 6 months or 4 or more episodes in 12 months.

ACUTE SINUSITIS

- Clinical diagnosis of bacterial sinusitis requires the following: nasal discharge and daytime cough without improvement for 10 to 14 days, or more severe signs and symptoms of acute sinusitis (ie, temperature of ≥39°C [≥102°F], facial swelling, facial pain).
- The common cold is a rhinosinusitis that often includes radiologic evidence of sinus involvement; radiographs, therefore, should be used only in selected circumstances and should be interpreted with caution. Radiographs may be indicated when episodes of sinusitis are recurrent or when complications are suspected.
- Initial antimicrobial treatment of acute sinusitis should be with an agent with the narrowest spectrum that is active against the likely pathogens.

COUGH ILLNESS/BRONCHITIS

- Nonspecific cough illness/bronchitis in children, regardless of duration, does not warrant antimicrobial treatment.
- Antimicrobial treatment for prolonged cough (>10–14 days) may be indicated in certain conditions, including *Bordetella pertussis* and *Mycoplasma pneumoniae* infections, and appropriate diagnostic studies for these infections should be obtained. Pertussis should be treated according to established recommendations (see Pertussis, p 472). *Mycoplasma pneumoniae* can cause bronchitis or pneumonia and prolonged cough, usually in children older than 5 years of age; a macrolide agent (or a tetracycline for children 8 years of age or older) can be used for treatment (see *Mycoplasma pneumoniae*, p 443). Children with underlying chronic pulmonary disease other than asthma (eg, cystic fibrosis) may benefit from antimicrobial therapy for acute exacerbations.

PHARYNGITIS

(See Group A Streptococcal Infections, p 573)

- Diagnosis of group A streptococcal pharyngitis should be made on the basis of results of appropriate laboratory tests in conjunction with clinical and epidemiologic findings.
- Antimicrobial therapy should not be given to a child with pharyngitis in the absence of identified group A streptococci. Rarely, other bacteria may cause pharyngitis (eg, *Corynebacterium diphtheriae, Francisella tularensis,* groups G and C hemolytic streptococci, *Neisseria gonorrhoeae, Arcanobacterium haemolyticum*), and treatment should be provided according to recommendations in disease-specific chapters in Section 3.
- Penicillin remains the drug of choice for treating group A streptococcal pharyngitis.

THE COMMON COLD

- Antimicrobial agents should not be given for the common cold.
- Mucopurulent rhinitis (thick, opaque, or discolored nasal discharge) commonly accompanies the common cold and is not an indication for antimicrobial treatment unless it persists without signs of improvement for 10 to 14 days, suggesting possible sinusitis.

Principles of Appropriate Use of Vancomycin*

During the past decade, vancomycin-resistant enterococci have emerged rapidly as nosocomial pathogens in hospitals throughout the United States. Strains of *S aureus* with intermediate and high-level resistance to vancomycin and other glycopeptides have been reported. The major risk factor for emergence of vancomycin-resistant enterococci and *S aureus* with intermediate and high-level resistance to vancomycin has been increased use of vancomycin, particularly among patients receiving hematology-oncology, neonatology, cardiac surgery, and neurosurgery services. Prevention of further emergence of vancomycin resistance will depend on more appropriate use of vancomycin.

Situations in which the use of vancomycin is appropriate include the following:

- For treatment of serious infections attributable to β-lactam–resistant gram-positive organisms
- For treatment of infections attributable to gram-positive microorganisms in patients with serious allergy to β-lactam agents
- When antimicrobial-associated colitis fails to respond to metronidazole therapy or if it is severe and potentially life threatening (see *Clostridium difficile,* p 246)
- For prophylaxis, as recommended by the American Heart Association, for endocarditis after certain procedures in patients at high risk of endocarditis (see Prevention of Bacterial Endocarditis, p 778)

---

* Recommendations for preventing the spread of vancomycin resistance. Recommendations of the Hospital Infection Control Practices Advisory Committee. *MMWR Recomm Rep.* 1995; 44(RR-12):1–13

- For prophylaxis for major surgical procedures involving implantation of prosthetic materials or devices at institutions with a high rate of infections attributable to methicillin-resistant *S aureus* or methicillin-resistant coagulase-negative staphylococci.

  Situations in which the use of vancomycin should be discouraged:
- Routine prophylaxis for:
  - Surgical patients other than patients with a life-threatening allergy to β-lactam antimicrobial agents
  - Very low birth weight infants
  - Patients receiving continuous ambulatory peritoneal dialysis or hemodialysis
  - Preventing infection or colonization of indwelling central or peripheral intravascular catheters (either systemic or antibiotic lock)
- Empiric antimicrobial therapy for a febrile neutropenic patient, unless strong evidence indicates an infection attributable to gram-positive microorganisms and the prevalence of infections attributable to methicillin-resistant *S aureus* in the hospital is substantial
- Treatment in response to a single positive result of a blood culture for coagulase-negative staphylococcus, if other blood culture results obtained in the same period are negative
- Continued empiric use for presumed infections in patients whose culture results are negative for β-lactam–resistant, gram-positive microorganisms
- Selective decontamination of the digestive tract
- Attempted eradication of methicillin-resistant *S aureus* colonization
- Primary treatment of antimicrobial-associated colitis (see *Clostridium difficile,* p 246)
- Treatment of infections attributable to β-lactam–susceptible gram-positive microorganisms, including vancomycin given for dosing convenience in patients with renal failure
- Topical application or irrigation

Prevention of Antimicrobial Resistance in Health Care Settings

The CDC has initiated a campaign designed to highlight the importance of antimicrobial resistance and to engage clinicians, health care facilities, and patients in efforts to prevent resistance and promote safer care. The Campaign to Prevent Antimicrobial Resistance focuses on 4 integrated strategies: preventing infection, diagnosing and treating infection effectively, using antimicrobial agents wisely, and preventing transmission. Additional information about the campaign is available at www.cdc.gov/drugresistance/healthcare/.

TABLES OF ANTIBACTERIAL DRUG DOSAGES

Recommended dosages for antimicrobial agents commonly used for newborn infants (see Table 4.1, p 700) and for older infants and children (see Table 4.2, p 702) are given separately because of the physiologic immaturity of the newborn infant and resulting different pharmacokinetics. The table for newborn infants is divided by postnatal age and birth weight because of age-related differences in pharmacokinetics.

Recommended dosages are not absolute and are intended only as a guide. Clinical judgment about the disease, alterations in renal or hepatic function, coadministration of other drugs, and other factors affecting pharmacokinetics, patient response, and laboratory results may dictate modifications of these recommendations in an individual patient. In some cases, monitoring of serum drug concentrations is recommended to avoid toxicity and to ensure therapeutic efficacy.

Product label information should be consulted for details, such as the diluent for reconstitution of injectable preparations, measures to be taken to avoid incompatibilities, drug interactions, and other precautions.

Table 4.1. Antibacterial Drugs for Newborn Infants: Dose[1] (mg/kg or U/kg) and Frequency of Administration

Drug	Route	Infants 0–4 wk of age BW <1200 g	Infants <1 wk of age BW ≤1200–2000 g	Infants <1 wk of age BW >2000 g	Infants ≥1 wk of age BW ≤1200–2000 g	Infants ≥1 wk of age BW >2000 g
Aminoglycosides[2,3]						
Amikacin	IV, IM	7.5 every 18–24 h	7.5 every 12 h	7.5–10 every 12 h	7.5–10 every 8 or 12 h	10 every 8 h
Gentamicin	IV, IM	2.5 every 18–24 h	2.5 every 12 h	2.5 every 12 h	2.5 every 8 or 12 h	2.5 every 8 h
Neomycin	PO only	…	25 every 6 h	25 every 6 h	25 every 6 h	25 every 6 h
Tobramycin	IV, IM	2.5 every 18–24 h	2.5 every 12 h	2.5 every 12 h	2.5 every 8 or 12 h	2.5 every 8 h
Antistaphylococcal penicillins[4]						
Methicillin	IV, IM	25 every 12 h	25–50 every 12 h	25–50 every 8 h	25–50 every 8 h	25–50 every 6 h
Nafcillin	IV, IM	25 every 12 h	25 every 12 h	25 every 8 h	25 every 8 h	25–35 every 6 h
Oxacillin	IV, IM	25 every 12 h	25–50 every 12 h	25–50 every 8 h	25–50 every 8 h	25–50 every 6 h
Aztreonam	IV, IM	30 every 12 h	30 every 12 h	30 every 8 h	30 every 8 h	30 every 6 h
Carbapenems[5]						
Imipenem/cilastatin	IV	25 every 12 h	25 every 12 h	25 every 12 h	25 every 8 h	25 every 8 h
Cephalosporins						
Cefotaxime	IV, IM	50 every 12 h	50 every 12 h	50 every 8 or 12 h	50 every 8 h	50 every 6 or 8 h
Ceftazidime	IV, IM	50 every 12 h	50 every 12 h	50 every 8 or 12 h	50 every 8 h	50 every 8 h
Ceftriaxone[6]	IV, IM	50 every 24 h	50 every 24–36 h	50 every 24 h	50 every 24 h	50–75 every 24 h
Clindamycin	IV, IM, PO	5 every 12 h	5 every 12 h	5 every 8 h	5 every 8 h	5–7.5 every 6 h
Erythromycin	PO	10 every 12 h	10 every 12 h	10 every 12 h	10 every 8 h	10 every 8 h
Metronidazole[5]	IV, PO	7.5 every 24–48 h	7.5 every 24 h	7.5 every 12 h	7.5 every 12 h	15 every 12 h

Table 4.1. Antibacterial Drugs for Newborn Infants: Dose[1] (mg/kg or U/kg) and Frequency of Administration, continued

Drug	Route	Infants 0–4 wk of age BW <1200 g	Infants <1 wk of age BW ≤1200–2000 g	Infants <1 wk of age BW >2000 g	Infants ≥1 wk of age BW ≤1200–2000 g	Infants ≥1 wk of age BW >2000 g
Penicillins						
Ampicillin[4]	IV, IM	25–50 every 12 h	25–50 every 12 h	25–50 every 8 h	25–50 every 8 h	25–50 every 6 h
Penicillin G,[4] aqueous	IV, IM	25 000–50 000 U every 12 h	25 000–50 000 U every 12 h	25 000–50 000 U every 8 h	25 000–50 000 U every 8 h	25 000–50 000 U every 6 h
Penicillin G procaine	IM	…	50 000 U every 24 h	50 000 U every 24 h	50 000 U every 24 h	50 000 U every 24 h
Ticarcillin[7]	IV, IM	75 every 12 h	75 every 12 h	75 every 8 h	75 every 8 h	75 every 6 h
Vancomycin[2]	IV	15 every 24 h	10–15 every 12–18 h	10–15 every 8–12 h	10–15 every 8–12 h	10–15 every 6 or 8 h

BW indicates birth weight; IV, intravenous; IM, intramuscular; PO, oral.

1 Unless otherwise listed, dosages are given as mg/kg.
2 Optimal dosage should be based on determination of serum concentrations, especially in low birth weight (<1500 g) infants. In very low birth weight infants (<1200 g), dosing every 18 to 24 hours may be appropriate in the first week of life.
3 Dosages for aminoglycosides may differ from those recommended by the manufacturer in the package insert.
4 For meningitis, the larger dosage is recommended. Some experts recommend even larger dosages for group B streptococcal meningitis.
5 Safety in infants and children has not been established. Meropenem is preferred if a carbapenem is to be used in newborn infants.
6 Drug should not be administered to hyperbilirubinemic neonates, especially infants born prematurely.
7 Same dosage for ticarcillin and clavulanate potassium.

Table 4.2. Antibacterial Drugs for Pediatric Patients Beyond the Newborn Period

Drug, Generic (Trade Name)	Route	Dosage per kg per Day		Comments
		Mild to Moderate Infections	Severe Infections	
Aminoglycosides[1]				
Amikacin (Amikin)	IV, IM	Inappropriate	15–22.5 mg in 3 doses (daily adult dose, 15 mg/kg; maximum, 1.5 g)	30 mg in 3 doses is recommended by some consultants.
Gentamicin (Garamycin)	IV, IM	Inappropriate	3–7.5 mg in 3 doses (daily adult dose is the same)	Once daily dosing (5–6 mg/kg every 24 h) is investigational in children.
Kanamycin (Kantrex)	IV, IM	Inappropriate	15–22.5 mg in 3 doses (daily adult dose, 1–1.5 g)	30 mg in 3 doses is recommended by some consultants.
Neomycin (numerous types)	PO only	100 mg in 4 doses	100 mg in 4 doses	For some enteric infections.
Paromomycin (Humatin)	PO	30 mg in 3 doses (maximum daily adult dose, 4 g)	Inappropriate	...
Tobramycin (Nebcin)	IV, IM	Inappropriate	3–7.5 mg in 3 doses (daily adult dose, 3–5 mg in 3 doses)	Once daily dosing (5–6 mg/kg every 24 h) is investigational in children.
Aztreonam[2] (Azactam)	IV, IM	90 mg in 3 doses (daily adult dose, 3 g)	120 mg in 4 doses (maximum daily adult dose, 8 g)	...
Cephalosporins[2]				
Cefaclor (Ceclor)	PO	20–40 mg in 2 or 3 doses (daily adult dose, 750 mg–1.5 g)	Inappropriate	A twice daily regimen has been demonstrated to be effective for treatment of acute otitis media.
Cefadroxil (Duricef, Ultracef)	PO	30 mg in 2 doses (maximum daily adult dose, 2 g)	Inappropriate	...

Table 4.2. **Antibacterial Drugs for Pediatric Patients Beyond the Newborn Period, continued**

Drug, Generic (Trade Name)	Route	Dosage per kg per Day		Comments
		Mild to Moderate Infections	Severe Infections	
Cefdinir (Omnicef)	PO	14 mg in 1 or 2 doses (maximum 600 mg/day)	Inappropriate	Inadequate activity against resistant pneumococcus.
Cefditoren (Spectracef)	PO	800 mg in 2 doses	No data available	Not licensed for children younger than 12 years of age.
Cefepime (Maxipime)	IV, IM	100–150 mg in 3 doses (daily adult dose, 1–2 g)	150 mg in 3 doses (daily adult dose, 2–4 g)	Not licensed for treatment of meningitis.
Cefonicid (Monocid)	IV, IM	20–40 mg in 1 dose (maximum daily adult dose, 2 g)	No data available	Not licensed for use in children.
Cefoperazone (Cefobid)	IV, IM	100–150 mg in 2 or 3 doses (maximum daily adult dose, 4 g)	No data available	Not licensed for use in children.
Cefotaxime (Claforan)	IV, IM	75–100 mg in 3 or 4 doses (daily adult dose, 4–6 g)	150–200 mg in 3 or 4 doses (daily adult dose, 8–10 g)	A regimen of 300 mg in 3 or 4 doses can be used for treatment of meningitis.
Cefotetan (Cefotan)	IV, IM	Inappropriate	40–80 mg in 2 doses (maximum daily adult dose, 6 g)	Not licensed for use in children.
Cefoxitin (Mefoxin)	IV, IM	80–100 mg in 3–4 doses (daily adult dose, 3–4 g)	80–160 mg in 4–6 doses (daily adult dose, 6–12 g)	...
Cefpodoxime proxetil (Vantin)	PO	10 mg in 2 doses (maximum daily adult dose, 800 mg)	Inappropriate	...

Table 4.2. Antibacterial Drugs for Pediatric Patients Beyond the Newborn Period, *continued*

Drug, Generic (Trade Name)	Route	Dosage per kg per Day		Comments
		Mild to Moderate Infections	Severe Infections	
Cefprozil (Cefzil)	PO	15–30 mg in 2 doses (maximum daily adult dose, 1 g)	Inappropriate	30-mg dosage recommended for treatment of acute otitis media.
Ceftazidime (Fortaz, Tazicef, Tazidime)	IV, IM	75–100 mg in 3 doses (daily adult dose, 3 g)	125–150 mg in 3 doses (daily adult dose, 6 g)	Only cephalosporin with anti-*Pseudomonas* activity that has been licensed for use in children.
Ceftibuten (Cedax)	PO	9 mg in 1 dose (maximum daily adult dose: see package insert)	Inappropriate	Inadequate activity against intermediate and resistant pneumococci.
Cefizoxime (Cefizox)	IV, IM	100–150 mg in 3 doses (daily adult dose, 3–4 g)	150–200 mg in 3 or 4 doses (daily adult dose, 4–6 g)	⋯
Ceftriaxone (Rocephin)	IV, IM	50–75 mg in 1 or 2 doses (daily adult dose, 2 g)	80–100 mg in 1 or 2 doses (daily adult dose, 4 g)	Larger dosage appropriate for penicillin-resistant pneumococcal meningitis.
Cefuroxime (Zinacef)	IV, IM	75–100 mg in 3 doses (daily adult dose, 2–4 g)	100–150 mg in 3 doses (daily adult dose, 4–6 g)	⋯
Cefuroxime axetil (Ceftin)	PO	20–30 mg in 2 doses (daily adult dose, 1–2 g)	Inappropriate	The higher dosage recommended for treatment of otitis media. Limited activity against penicillin-resistant *Streptococcus pneumoniae.*
Cephalexin (Keflex)	PO	25–50 mg in 3–4 doses (daily adult dose, 1–4 g)	Inappropriate	⋯
Cephalothin (Keflin)	IV, IM	80–100 mg in 4 doses (daily adult dose, 2–4 g)	100–150 mg in 4–6 doses (daily adult dose, 8–12 g)	⋯
Cephradine (Anspor)	PO	25–50 mg in 2–4 doses (daily adult dose, 1–4 g)	Inappropriate	⋯

Table 4.2. **Antibacterial Drugs for Pediatric Patients Beyond the Newborn Period, continued**

Drug, Generic (Trade Name)	Route	Dosage per kg per Day		Comments
		Mild to Moderate Infections	Severe Infections	
Cephradine, continued (Velosef)	IV, IM	50–100 mg in 4 doses (daily adult dose, 2–8 g)	100 mg in 4 doses (daily adult dose, 6–8 g)	…
Loracarbef (Lorabid)	PO	30 mg for otitis media and 15 mg for other indications in 2 doses (maximum daily adult dose, 800 mg)	Inappropriate	…
Chloramphenicol (Chloromycetin)				
Chloramphenicol succinate	IV	Inappropriate	50–100 mg in 4 doses (daily adult dose, 2–4 g)	Optimal dosage is determined by measurement of serum concentrations with resulting modifications to achieve therapeutic concentrations. Use only for serious infections because of the rare occurrence of aplastic anemia after administration. Oral formulation (palmitate) not available in US.
Clindamycin (Cleocin)	IM, IV	15–25 mg in 3–4 doses (daily adult dose, 600 mg–3.6 g)	25–40 mg in 3–4 doses (daily adult dose, 1.2–2.7 g)	Active against anaerobes, especially *Bacteroides* species. Active against many multidrug-resistant pneumococci. Effective for otitis media caused by many multidrug-resistant pneumococci.
	PO	10–20 mg in 3–4 doses (daily adult dose, 600 mg–1.8 g)	Inappropriate	

Table 4.2. **Antibacterial Drugs for Pediatric Patients Beyond the Newborn Period, continued**

| Drug, Generic (Trade Name) | Route | Dosage per kg per Day | | Comments |
		Mild to Moderate Infections	Severe Infections	
Fluoroquinolones[3]				
Ciprofloxacin (Cipro)	PO	20–30 mg in 2 doses (daily adult dose, 0.5–1.5 g)	30 mg in 2 doses (daily adult dose, 1.0–1.5 g)	Not licensed for use in people younger than 18 years of age[3]; however, drug has selective indications in children and adolescents (see p 693).
	IV	Inappropriate	20–30 mg in 2 doses (daily adult dose, 400–800 mg in 2 doses)	…
Carbapenems				
Imipenem[2,4] (Primaxin)	IV, IM	40–60 mg in 4 doses (daily adult dose, 1–2 g)	60 mg in 4 doses (daily adult dose, 2–4 g)	Caution in use for treatment of meningitis because of possible seizures.
Meropenem[2,4] (Merrem)	IV	60 mg in 3 doses (daily adult dose, 4 g)	60–120 mg in 3 doses (daily adult dose, 4–6 g)	Larger dosage is used for treatment of meningitis.
Ertapenem (Invanz)	IV	Inappropriate	1 g, every 24 hours	Not licensed for people younger than 18 years of age. Not active against *Pseudomonas* species and *Actinobacter* species.
Macrolides/ streptogramins				
Erythromycins (numerous types)	PO	30–50 mg in 2–4 doses (daily adult dose, 1–2 g)	Inappropriate	Available in base, stearate, ethylsuccinate, and estolate preparations.
	IV	Inappropriate	15–50 mg in 4 doses (daily adult dose, 1–4 g)	Administer in a continuous drip or by slow infusion over 60 min or longer. May cause cardiac arrhythmia.

Table 4.2. **Antibacterial Drugs for Pediatric Patients Beyond the Newborn Period, continued**

Drug, Generic (Trade Name)	Route	Mild to Moderate Infections	Severe Infections	Comments
		Dosage per kg per Day		
Azithromycin (Zithromax)	PO	5–12 mg once daily (maximum daily adult dose, 600 mg)	Inappropriate	Otitis media: 10 mg/kg on first day, 5 mg/kg per day for additional 4 days. Pharyngitis: 12 mg/kg per day for 5 days.
Clarithromycin (Biaxin)	PO	15 mg in 2 doses (maximum daily adult dose, 1 g)	Inappropriate	…
Quinupristin/ dalfopristin (Synercid)	IV	15 mg in 2 doses (daily adult dose, same)	22.5 mg in 3 doses (daily adult dose, same)	Modestly effective for vancomycin-resistant *Enterococcus faecium*. Limited use in children.
Methenamine mandelate (Mandelamine)	PO	50–75 mg in 3–4 doses (daily adult dose, 2–4 g)	Inappropriate	Should not be used for infants; urine pH must be adjusted to 5–5.5.
Metronidazole (Flagyl)	PO	15–35 mg in 3 doses (maximum daily adult dose, 1–2 g)	Inappropriate	Safety in infants and children has not been established.
Nitrofurantoin (Furadantin)	PO	5–7 mg in 4 doses (daily adult dose, 200–400 mg)	Inappropriate	Should not be used for young infants; prophylactic dose is 1–2 mg/kg per day in 1 dose.
Oxazolidinones Linezolid (Zyvox)	PO, IV	20–30 mg in 3 doses (daily adult dose, 800 mg)	20–30 mg in 3 doses (daily adult dose, 1200 mg)	Myelosuppression may occur.

Table 4.2. **Antibacterial Drugs for Pediatric Patients Beyond the Newborn Period, continued**

Drug, Generic (Trade Name)	Route	Dosage per kg per Day		Comments
		Mild to Moderate Infections	Severe Infections	
PENICILLINS[2]				
Broad-spectrum penicillins				
Ampicillin (numerous types)	IV, IM	100–150 mg in 4 doses (daily adult dose, 2–4 g)	200–400 mg in 4 doses (daily adult dose, 6–12 g)	Larger dosage recommended for treatment of meningitis.
	PO	50–100 mg in 4 doses (daily adult dose, 2–4 g)	Inappropriate	Diarrhea occurs in approximately 20% of recipients.
Ampicillin-sulbactam (Unasyn)	IV	100–150 mg of ampicillin in 4 doses	200–400 mg of ampicillin in 4 doses (daily adult dose, 6–12 g)	Not licensed for use in infants and children.
Amoxicillin (numerous types)	PO	25–50 mg in 3 doses (daily adult dose, 750 mg–1.5 g)	Inappropriate	Larger dosage (80–90 mg in 2 doses) for otitis media caused by penicillin-resistant pneumococci.
Amoxicillin-clavulanic acid				
(Augmentin, 7:1 ratio)	PO	45 mg of amoxicillin in 2 doses	Inappropriate	…
(Augmentin ES-600; 14:1 ratio)	PO	90 mg of amoxicillin in 2 doses	Inappropriate	For multidrug-resistant pneumococcal otitis media and β-lactamase-positive *H influenzae*.
(Augmentin XR)	PO	2 g, twice a day (total 4000 mg)	Inappropriate	Oral extended-release formulation licensed for adults.
Mezlocillin (Mezlin)	IV, IM	100–150 mg in 4 doses (daily adult dose, 6–8 g)	200–300 mg in 4–6 doses (daily adult dose, 12–18 g)	…
Piperacillin[5] (Pipracil)	IV, IM	100–150 mg in 4 doses (daily adult dose, 6–8 g)	200–300 mg in 4–6 doses daily adult dose, 12–18 g)	…

Table 4.2. **Antibacterial Drugs for Pediatric Patients Beyond the Newborn Period, continued**

Drug, Generic (Trade Name)	Route	Dosage per kg per Day		Comments
		Mild to Moderate Infections	Severe Infections	
Piperacillin-tazobactam[5] (Zosyn)	IV	Inappropriate	240 mg of piperacillin in 3 doses	Not licensed for use in children.
Ticarcillin (Ticar)	IV, IM	100–200 mg in 4 doses (daily adult dose, 4–6 g)	200–300 mg in 4 doses (daily adult dose, 12–24 g)	Contains 5.2 mEq of sodium per gram.
Ticarcillin-clavulanate (Timentin)	IV, IM	100–200 mg of ticarcillin in 4 doses (4–6 g)	200–300 mg of ticarcillin in 4 doses (12–24 g)	...
Penicillin G and V[2,5]				
Penicillin G, crystalline potassium or sodium (numerous types)	IV, IM	25 000–50 000 U in 4 doses	250 000–400 000 U in 4–6 doses. Maximum adult dose 24 million U/24 h.	Larger dosage appropriate for central nervous system infections.
Penicillin G procaine (numerous types)	IM	25 000–50 000 U in 1–2 doses. Maximum adult dose 4.8 million U/24 h.	Inappropriate	Contraindicated in procaine allergy.
Penicillin G benzathine (Bicillin, Permapen)	IM	<27.3 kg (60 lb) in body weight: 600 000 U ≥27.3 kg (60 lb): 1.2 million U	Inappropriate	Major use is prevention of rheumatic fever by treatment and prophylaxis of streptococcal infections.
Penicillin V (numerous types)	PO	25 000–50 000 U in 3 or 4 doses. Maximum adult dose 500 mg/dose, every 6–8 h (2 g/24 h).	Inappropriate	Optimal to administer on an empty stomach.

Table 4.2. **Antibacterial Drugs for Pediatric Patients Beyond the Newborn Period, continued**

| Drug, Generic (Trade Name) | Route | Dosage per kg per Day | | Comments |
		Mild to Moderate Infections	Severe Infections	
Penicillinase-resistant penicillins[2]				Methicillin (oxacillin)-resistant staphylococci usually are resistant to all other semi-synthetic antistaphylococcal cephalosporins.
Methicillin (Staphcillin)	IV, IM	100–150 mg in 4 doses (daily adult dose, 4–8 g)	150–200 mg in 4–6 doses (daily adult dose, 4–12 g)	Interstitial nephritis (ie, hematuria) occurs in 0%–4% of patients.
Oxacillin (Prostaphlin, Bactocill)	IV, IM	100–150 mg in 4 doses (daily adult dose, 2–4 g)	150–200 mg in 4–6 doses (daily adult dose, 4–12 g)	...
Nafcillin (Unipen, Nafcil)	IV, IM, PO	50–100 mg in 4 doses (daily adult dose, 2–4 g)	100–150 mg in 4 doses (daily adult dose, 4–12 g)	Oral formulation not used because of poor absorption.
Cloxacillin (Tegopen, Cloxapen)	PO	50–100 mg in 4 doses (daily adult dose, 2–4 g)	Inappropriate	...
Dicloxacillin (Dynapen, Pathocil)	PO	25–50 mg in 4 doses (daily adult dose, 1–2 g)	Inappropriate	Excellent serum concentrations after oral administration.
Rifampin (numerous types)	PO	10–20 mg in 1–2 doses (daily adult dose, 600 mg)	20 mg in 2 doses. Maximum adult dose 600 mg/24 h.	Should not be used as monotherapy except when given for prophylaxis.
	IV	10–20 mg in 1–2 doses (daily adult dose, 600 mg)	20 mg in 2 doses. Maximum adult dose 600 mg/24 h.	...
Sulfonamides				
Sulfadiazine	PO	100–150 mg in 4 doses	120–150 mg in 4–6 doses	...
Sulfisoxazole (Gantrisin)	PO	120–150 mg in 4–6 doses	120–150 mg in 4–6 doses	...
Triple sulfonamides (numerous types)	PO	120–150 mg in 4 doses	120–150 mg in 4 doses	...

Table 4.2. Antibacterial Drugs for Pediatric Patients Beyond the Newborn Period, continued

Drug, Generic (Trade Name)	Route	Dosage per kg per Day			Comments
		Mild to Moderate Infections	Severe Infections		
Trimethoprim–sulfamethoxazole (Bactrim, Septra)	PO	8–12 mg of trimethoprim, 40–60 mg of sulfamethoxazole in 2 doses (daily adult dose, 320 mg of trimethoprim, 1.6 g of sulfamethoxazole)	20 mg of trimethoprim, 100 mg of sulfamethoxazole in 4 doses (for use only in *Pneumocystis* pneumonia)		For prophylaxis in immunocompromised patients, recommended dose is 5 mg of trimethoprim, 25 mg of sulfamethoxazole per kg per day in 2 doses.
	IV	Inappropriate	8–12 mg of trimethoprim, 40–60 mg of sulfamethoxazole in 4 doses OR 20 mg of trimethoprim, 100 mg of sulfamethoxazole in 4 doses		Use intravenous formulation when PO formulation cannot be administered. Treatment of *Pneumocystis* infection.
Tetracyclines (numerous types)	IV	Inappropriate	10–25 mg in 2–4 doses (daily adult dose, 1–2 g)		Responsible for staining of developing teeth; use only in children 8 years of age or older except in circumstances in which the benefits of therapy exceed the risks and alternative drugs are less effective or more toxic (see p 694).
	PO	20–50 mg in 4 doses (daily adult dose, 1–2 g)	Inappropriate		Responsible for staining of developing teeth; use only in children 8 years of age or older except in circumstances in which the benefits of therapy exceed the risks and alternative drugs are less effective or more toxic (see p 694).

Table 4.2. Antibacterial Drugs for Pediatric Patients Beyond the Newborn Period, continued

Drug, Generic (Trade Name)	Route	Dosage per kg per Day		Comments
		Mild to Moderate Infections	Severe Infections	
Doxycycline (numerous types)	PO, IV	2–4 mg in 1–2 doses (daily adult dose, 100–200 mg)	Inappropriate	Adverse effects similar to those of other tetracycline products except that risk of dental staining in children younger than 8 years of age is less.
Vancomycin (Vancocin, Vancoled, Vancor)	IV	40 mg in 3–4 doses (daily adult dose,[6] 1–2 g)	40–60 mg in 4 doses (daily adult dose,[6] 2–4 g)	In meningitis, 60 mg/kg dose should be given over a period of at least 60 min; routine monitoring of serum concentrations is unnecessary.

IV, indicates intravenous; IM, intramuscular; PO, oral.

1 Dosages for aminoglycosides may differ from those recommended by the manufacturers (see package insert).

2 In patients with history of allergy to penicillin or one of its many congeners, alternative drugs are recommended. In some circumstances, a cephalosporin or other β-lactam–class drug may be acceptable. However, these drugs should not be used in patients with an immediate hypersensitivity (anaphylaxis) to penicillin, because approximately 5% to 15% of penicillin-allergic patients also will be allergic to cephalosporins.

3 Not licensed for use in patients younger than 18 years of age. Some fluoroquinolones currently are being studied in selected children and adolescents (see Fluoroquinolones, p 693).

4 Not licensed for use in patients younger than 12 years of age.

5 Patients with a history of allergy to penicillin G or penicillin V should be considered for subsequent skin testing. Many such patients can be treated safely with penicillin, because only 10% of children with such history are proven allergic when skin tested.

6 In adults, daily dose is given in 2 to 4 divided doses.

For more information on individual drugs, see *Physicians' Desk Reference* (Greenwood Village, CO: Thomson Micromedex) or http://pdrel.thomsonhc.com/pdrel/librarian/action/command.Command.

SEXUALLY TRANSMITTED DISEASES

Table 4.3. Guidelines for Treatment of Sexually Transmitted Diseases in Children and Adolescents According to Syndrome
Preferred regimens are listed. For further information concerning other acceptable regimens and diseases not included, see specific recommendations in disease-specific chapters in Section 3. In addition, revised recommendations on the treatment of sexually transmitted diseases have been issued by the Centers for Disease Control and Prevention in 2002.[1]

Syndrome	Organisms/Diagnoses	Treatment of Adolescent	Treatment of Infant/Child
Urethritis and cervicitis	*Neisseria gonorrhoeae*, *Chlamydia trachomatis*	Ceftriaxone, 125 mg, IM, in a single dose **OR**	***Children <45 kg:*** Ceftriaxone, 125 mg, IM, in a single dose **OR**
Urethritis: Inflammation of urethra with mucoid, mucopurulent, or purulent discharge	Other causes of urethritis and cervicitis include *Ureaplasma urealyticum*, possibly *Mycoplasma genitalium*, and sometimes	Ciprofloxacin, 500 mg, orally, in a single dose[2,3] **OR**	Spectinomycin, 40 mg/kg (maximum 2 g) IM in a single dose **If chlamydial infection not ruled out, PLUS**
Cervicitis: Inflammation of cervix with mucopurulent or purulent cervical discharge. Cervicitis occurs rarely in prepubertal girls (see Prepubertal vaginitis)	*Trichomonas vaginalis* and herpes simplex virus (HSV)	Ofloxacin, 400 mg, orally, in a single dose[2,3] **OR** Levofloxacin, 250 mg, orally, in single dose[2,3] **If chlamydial infection not ruled out, PLUS EITHER** Azithromycin, 1 g, orally, in a single dose **OR** Doxycycline, 100 mg, orally, twice a day for 7 days	Erythromycin base or ethylsuccinate, 50 mg/kg per day, orally, in 4 divided doses (maximum 2 g/day) for 14 days ***Children ≥45 kg but younger than 8 years of age:*** Azithromycin, 1 g, orally, in a single dose ***Children 8 years of age or older:*** Azithromycin, 1 g, orally, in a single dose **OR** Doxycycline, 100 mg, orally, twice a day for 7 days
Prepubertal vaginitis (STD related):	*N gonorrhoeae*[1]	…	***Children <45 kg:*** Ceftriaxone, 125 mg, in a single dose
	C trachomatis[1]	…	***Children <45 kg:*** Erythromycin base or ethylsuccinate, 50 mg/kg per day, orally, in 4 divided doses (maximum 2 g/day) for 14 days

Table 4.3. **Guidelines for Treatment of Sexually Transmitted Diseases in Children and Adolescents According to Syndrome, continued**

Syndrome	Organisms/Diagnoses	Treatment of Adolescent	Treatment of Infant/Child
Prepubertal vaginitis (STD related, continued):	*C trachomatis,*[1] continued		***Children ≥45 kg but younger than 8 years of age:*** Azithromycin, 1 g, orally, in a single dose ***Children 8 years of age or older:*** Azithromycin, 1 g, orally, in a single dose **OR** Doxycycline, 100 mg, orally, twice a day for 7 days
	T vaginalis	...	***Children <45 kg:*** Metronidazole, 15 mg/kg per day, orally, in 3 divided doses (maximum 2 g/day) for 7 days
	Bacterial vaginosis	...	***Children <45 kg:*** Metronidazole, 15 mg/kg per day, orally, in 2 divided doses (maximum 1 g/day) for 7 days
	HSV—primary infection	Acyclovir, 400 mg, orally, 3 times/day for 7–10 days **OR** Acyclovir, 200 mg, orally, 5 times/day for 7–10 days **OR** Famciclovir (250 mg, orally, 3 times/day) for 7–10 days **OR** Valacyclovir (1 g, orally, twice daily) for 7–10 days	***Children <45 kg:*** Acyclovir, 80 mg/kg per day, orally, in 3–4 divided doses (maximum 1.2 g/day) for 7–10 days

Table 4.3. Guidelines for Treatment of Sexually Transmitted Diseases in Children and Adolescents According to Syndrome, continued

Syndrome	Organisms/Diagnoses	Treatment of Adolescent	Treatment of Infant/Child
Adolescent vulvo-vaginitis	T vaginalis	Metronidazole, 2 g, orally, in a single dose **OR** Metronidazole, 500 mg, twice daily for 7 days	...
	Bacterial vaginosis	Metronidazole, 500 mg, orally, twice daily for 7 days **OR** Metronidazole gel 0.75%, 1 full applicator (5 g), intravaginally, once a day for 5 days **OR** Clindamycin cream 2%, 1 full applicator (5 g), intravaginally at bedtime, for 7 days **OR** Metronidazole, 2 g, orally, in a single dose **OR** Clindamycin, 300 mg, orally, twice a day for 7 days **OR** Clindamycin ovules, 100 g, intravaginally, once at bedtime for 3 days	...
	Candida species	See Table 4.4, Recommended Regimens for Vulvovaginal Candidiasis (p 718)	...
	HSV—primary infection	Acyclovir, 1000–1200 mg/day, orally, in 3–5 divided doses for 7–10 days	...

Table 4.3. Guidelines for Treatment of Sexually Transmitted Diseases in Children and Adolescents According to Syndrome, continued

Syndrome	Organisms/Diagnoses	Treatment of Adolescent	Treatment of Infant/Child
Pelvic inflammatory disease (PID)	*N gonorrhoeae*, *C trachomatis*, anaerobes, coliform bacteria, and *Streptococcus* species	See Pelvic Inflammatory Disease (Table 3.41, p 471)	PID occurs rarely, if at all, in prepubertal girls
Syphilis	*Treponema pallidum*	See Syphilis, p 595	***Children <45 kg:*** Same as for congenital syphilis (see p 601 and Table 3.59, p 602)
Genital ulcer disease	*T pallidum*	Same as for syphilis	***Children <45 kg:*** Same as for congenital syphilis (see p 601 and Table 3.59, p 602)
	HSV—primary infection	See prepubertal vaginitis.	***Children <45 kg:*** See prepubertal vaginitis.
	Haemophilus ducreyi (chancroid)	Azithromycin, 1 g, orally, in a single dose **OR** Ceftriaxone, 250 mg, IM, in a single dose **OR** Ciprofloxacin, 500 mg, orally, twice daily for 3 days[3] **OR** Erythromycin base, 500 mg, orally, 4 times/day for 7 days	***Children <45 kg:*** Ceftriaxone, 50 mg/kg, IM, in a single dose **OR** ***Children <45 kg:*** Azithromycin, 20 mg/kg, orally, in a single dose (maximum 1 g)
Sexually acquired epididymitis	*C trachomatis*, *N gonorrhoeae*	Ceftriaxone, 250 mg, IM, in a single dose **PLUS** Doxycycline, 100 mg, orally, twice daily for 10 days	…
	Enteric organisms (for patients allergic to cephalosporins and/or tetracycline or for patients >35 years of age)	Ofloxacin, 300 mg, orally, twice a day for 10 days **OR** Levofloxacin, 500 mg, orally, once daily for 10 days	…

Table 4.3. Guidelines for Treatment of Sexually Transmitted Diseases in Children and Adolescents According to Syndrome, continued

Syndrome	Organisms/Diagnoses	Treatment of Adolescent	Treatment of Infant/Child
Anogenital warts	Human papillomavirus	*Patient-applied:* Podofilox 0.5% solution or gel[4] **OR** Imiquimod 5% cream *Provider-administered:* Cryotherapy **OR** Podophyllin resin 10%–25%[4] **OR** Trichloroacetic acid **OR** Bichloroacetic acid **OR** Surgical removal	*Children <45 kg:* Same as for adolescents

IM indicates intramuscularly; STD, sexually transmitted disease.

1 For additional information and recommendations, see Centers for Disease Control and Prevention. Sexually transmitted diseases treatment guidelines—2002. *MMWR Recomm Rep.* 2002;51(RR-6):1–80. Some regimens are not indicated for pregnant adolescents.

2 Quinolones should not be used for infections acquired in Asia or the Pacific, including Hawaii. Use of quinolones is inadvisable for treating infections acquired in California.

3 Ciprofloxacin, ofloxacin, and levofloxacin are contraindicated for pregnant and lactating women and for people younger than 18 years of age.

4 Not tested for safety in children and contraindicated in pregnancy.

Table 4.4. Recommended Regimens for Vulvovaginal Candidiasis

Intravaginal agents:

Butoconazole, 2% cream, 5 g, intravaginally, for 3 days[1,2]

OR

Butoconazole, 2% cream (sustained release), 5 g, single intravaginal application

OR

Clotrimazole, 1% cream, 5 g, intravaginally, for 7–14 days[1,2]

OR

Clotrimazole, 100-mg vaginal tablet for 7 days[1]

OR

Clotrimazole, 100-mg vaginal tablet, 2 tablets for 3 days[1]

OR

Clotrimazole, 500-mg vaginal tablet, 1 tablet in a single application[1]

OR

Miconazole, 2% cream, 5 g, intravaginally, for 7 days[1,2]

OR

Miconazole, 200-mg vaginal suppository, 1 suppository for 3 days[1,2]

OR

Miconazole, 100-mg vaginal suppository, 1 suppository for 7 days[1,2]

OR

Nystatin, 100 000-U vaginal tablet, 1 tablet for 14 days

OR

Tioconazole, 6.5% ointment, 5 g, intravaginally, in a single application[1,2]

OR

Terconazole, 0.4% cream, 5 g, intravaginally, for 7 days[1]

OR

Terconazole, 0.8% cream, 5 g, intravaginally, for 3 days[1]

OR

Terconazole, 80-mg vaginal suppository, 1 suppository for 3 days[1]

Oral agent:

Fluconazole 150-mg oral tablet, 1 tablet in single dose

---

[1] These creams and suppositories are oil-based and might weaken latex condoms and diaphragms. Refer to condom or diaphragm product labeling for additional information.

[2] Over-the-counter preparations.

....

ANTIFUNGAL DRUGS FOR SYSTEMIC FUNGAL INFECTIONS

Polyenes

Amphotericin B deoxycholate (conventional amphotericin B) is the drug of choice for most disseminated, potentially life-threatening fungal infections. Amphotericin B is fungicidal against a broad array of fungal species, excluding *Fusarium* species and *Pseudallescheria boydii*. Amphotericin B may cause adverse reactions, particularly renal toxicity, that limit its use in certain patients. Lipid formulations of amphotericin B also are available.

Amphotericin B is given intravenously in a single daily dose of 0.5 to 1.5 mg/kg (maximum 1.5 mg/kg per day). Amphotericin B is administered in 5% dextrose in water at a concentration of 0.1 mg/mL and delivered through a central or peripheral venous catheter (see Table 4.5, p 722). Infusion over 4 to 8 hours previously was recommended to avoid toxicity. More recently, infusion times of 1 to 2 hours have been shown to be well tolerated in adults and older children and theoretically increase the blood-to-tissue gradient, thereby improving drug delivery. After completing 1 week of daily therapy, adequate serum concentrations of the drug usually can be maintained by administering double the daily dose (maximum, 1.5 mg/kg) on alternate days. The duration of therapy depends on the type and extent of the specific fungal infection.

Amphotericin B is eliminated by a renal mechanism for weeks after therapy is discontinued. No adjustment in dose is required for neonates or for children with impaired renal function, because serum concentrations are not significantly increased in these patients. Neither hemodialysis nor peritoneal dialysis significantly decreases serum concentrations of the drug.

Infusion-related reactions to amphotericin B include fever, chills, and sometimes nausea, vomiting, headache, generalized malaise, hypotension, and arrhythmias. Onset usually is within 1 to 3 hours after starting the infusion; duration typically is less than an hour. Hypotension and arrhythmias are idiosyncratic reactions that are unlikely to occur if not observed after the initial dose but also can occur in association with rapid infusion. Multiple regimens have been used to attempt to prevent infusion-related reactions, but few have been studied in controlled clinical trials. Pretreatment with acetaminophen, alone or combined with diphenhydramine, may alleviate febrile reactions, although these reactions appear to be less common in children than in adults. Hydrocortisone (25–50 mg in adults and older children) also can be added to the infusion to decrease febrile and other systemic reactions. Tolerance to febrile reactions develops with time, allowing tapering and eventual discontinuation of the hydrocortisone and often diphenhydramine and antipyretics.

Meperidine hydrochloride and ibuprofen have been effective in preventing or treating fever and chills in some patients who are refractory to the conventional premedication regimen. Toxicity from amphotericin B may include nephrotoxicity, hepatotoxicity, thrombophlebitis, anemia, or neurotoxicity. Nephrotoxicity is caused by decreased renal blood flow and can be prevented or ameliorated by hydration, saline solution loading (0.9% saline solution over 30 minutes) before infusion of amphotericin B, and avoiding diuretic drugs. Hypokalemia is common and can be exacerbated by sodium loading. Renal tubular acidosis can occur but usually is mild. Permanent nephrotoxicity is related to cumulative dose. Nephrotoxicity can be enhanced by concomitant administration of amphotericin B and aminoglycosides, cyclosporine, tacrolimus, cisplatin, nitrogen mustard compounds, and acetazolamide. Anemia is secondary to inhibition of erythropoietin production. Neurotoxicity occurs rarely and can manifest as confusion, delirium, obtundation, psychotic behavior, seizures, blurred vision, or hearing loss.

Lipid formulations of amphotericin B have a role in some children who are intolerant of or refractory to amphotericin B deoxycholate (see Table 4.5, p 722). In adults, none of these formulations have been demonstrated to be more efficacious than has conventional amphotericin B. Amphotericin B lipid complex (Abelcet [The Liposome Co, Princeton, NJ]) is licensed by the US Food and Drug Administration (FDA) for treatment of invasive fungal infections in children and adults who are refractory to or intolerant of conventional amphotericin B therapy, defined as (1) renal dysfunction with a serum creatinine concentration of 1.5 mg/dL or greater that develops during therapy; or (2) disease progression after a total dose of amphotericin B of at least 10 mg/kg. Amphotericin B cholesteryl sulfate complex (Amphotec [manufactured by BenVenue Laboratories, Bedford, OH; distributed by Intermune Inc, Brisbane, CA]) is a colloidal complex that is licensed by the Food and Drug Administration for treatment of invasive aspergillosis in adults who cannot tolerate or fail to respond to amphotericin B deoxycholate. The liposomal formulation of amphotericin B (AmBisome [manufactured by Gilead Sciences Inc, San Dimas, CA for Fujisawa Healthcare Inc, Deerfield, IL]) is licensed for use in adults who cannot tolerate or fail to respond to conventional amphotericin B therapy for aspergillosis, candidiasis, cryptococcosis, or febrile neutropenia. In recommended doses, these lipid formulations cost 10 to 65 times more per day than does amphotericin B deoxycholate. These lipid formulations are being evaluated for treatment of other fungal infections and for use in children.

Pyrimidines

Among pyrimidine antifungal agents, only flucytosine (5-fluorocytosine) is licensed for use in children. Flucytosine has a limited spectrum of activity against fungi and potential for toxicity (see Table 4.5, p 722), and when used as a single agent, resistance often emerges. Flucytosine is used in combination with amphotericin B for cryptococcal meningitis and some life-threatening *Candida* infections, such as meningitis.

Azoles

Four oral azoles, which include ketoconazole and especially fluconazole, itraconazole, and voriconazole, have a relatively broad spectrum of activity against common fungi and can be alternatives to amphotericin B therapy in certain patients (see Table 4.5, p 722). Limited data are available regarding the safety and efficacy of azoles in pediatric patients, and trials comparing these agents to amphotericin B have not been conducted. Azoles are easy to administer and have little toxicity, but their use can be limited by the frequency of their interactions with coadministered drugs. These drug interactions may result in decreased serum concentrations of the azole (ie, poor therapeutic activity) or unexpected toxicity from the coadministered drug (ie, increased serum concentrations of the coadministered drug resulting from alteration of the cytochrome P-450 system). When considering the use of azoles, the physician should review carefully the patient's concurrent medications to avoid potential adverse clinical outcomes. Another potential limitation of azoles is the emergence of resistant fungi, especially *Candida* species resistant to fluconazole. Use of fluconazole for therapy or prophylaxis has resulted in an increased frequency of non-*albicans Candida* species as a cause of bloodstream infections. A triazole derivative of fluconazole with activity similar to itraconazole is voriconazole, which has been licensed by the FDA for primary treatment of invasive *Aspergillus* species and for refractory infection with *Scedosporium apiospermum* (the asexual form of *P boydii*) or *Fusarium* species. This new agent also is active against other opportunistic molds. Limited data are available regarding the use of voriconazole in children.

Echinocandins

Caspofungin acetate is a water-soluble lipopeptide that is licensed by the FDA for treatment of invasive aspergillosis in patients who are refractory to or intolerant of other antifungal drugs. Clinical trials assessing safety or efficacy in pediatric patients have not been conducted. Caspofungin, like azoles, has important drug interactions. Table 4.6 (p 725) provides recommendations for treatment of serious fungal infections with amphotericin B, flucytosine, azoles, caspofungin, and other antifungal agents.

RECOMMENDED DOSES OF PARENTERAL AND ORAL ANTIFUNGAL DRUGS

Table 4.5. **Recommended Doses of Parenteral and Oral Antifungal Drugs**

Drug	Route[1]	Dose (per day)	Adverse Reactions[2,3]
Amphotericin B (see Antifungal Drugs for Systemic Fungal Infections, p 719, for detailed information)	IV	0.25–0.5 mg/kg initially, increase as tolerated to 0.5–1.5 mg/kg; infuse as single dose over 2 h; 0.5–1.0 mg/kg weekly for suppressive therapy	Fever, chills, gastrointestinal tract symptoms, headache, hypotension, renal dysfunction, hypokalemia, anemia, cardiac arrhythmias, neurotoxicity, anaphylaxis
	IT	0.025 mg, increase to 0.5 mg, twice a week	Headache, gastrointestinal tract symptoms, arachnoiditis/radiculitis
Amphotericin B lipid complex (Abelcet)[4,5]	IV	5 mg/kg, infused over 2 h	Fever, chills, other reactions associated with amphotericin B, but less nephrotoxicity; hepatotoxicity
Amphotericin B cholesteryl sulfate complex (Amphotec)[4,5]	IV	3–6 mg/kg, infused at a rate of 1 mg/kg per hour	Fever, chills, other reactions associated with amphotericin B, but less nephrotoxicity; hepatotoxicity
Liposomal Amphotericin B (AmBisome)[4,5]	IV	3–5 mg/kg, infused over 1–2 h	Fever, chills, other reactions associated with amphotericin B, but less nephrotoxicity; hepatotoxicity
Caspofungin[4,5]	IV	Adults: 70 mg, loading dose, then 50 mg once daily	Fever, rash, pruritus, phlebitis, headache, gastrointestinal tract symptoms, anemia. Concomitant use with cyclosporine is not recommended unless potential benefits outweigh potential risks.
Clotrimazole	PO	10-mg tablet 5 times per day (dissolved slowly in mouth)	Gastrointestinal tract symptoms, hepatotoxicity
Fluconazole[3,5]	IV	Children: 3–6 mg/kg per day, single dose	Rash, gastrointestinal tract symptoms, hepatotoxicity, Stevens-Johnson syndrome, anaphylaxis

Table 4.5. Recommended Doses of Parenteral and Oral Antifungal Drugs, continued

Drug	Route[1]	Dose (per day)	Adverse Reactions[2,3]
Fluconazole,[3,5] continued	PO	Children: 6 mg/kg per day once, then 3 mg/kg per day for oropharyngeal or esophageal candidiasis; 6–12 mg/kg per day for invasive fungal infections; 6 mg/kg per day for suppressive therapy in HIV-infected children with cryptococcal meningitis Adults: 200 mg once, followed by 100 mg/day for oropharyngeal or esophageal candidiasis; 400–800 mg/day for other invasive fungal infections; 200 mg/day for suppressive therapy in HIV-infected patients with cryptococcal meningitis	
Flucytosine	PO	50–150 mg/kg per day in 4 doses at 6-h intervals (adjust dose if renal dysfunction)	Bone marrow suppression, renal dysfunction, gastrointestinal tract symptoms, rash, neuropathy, hepatotoxicity, confusion, hallucinations
Griseofulvin	PO	Ultramicrosize: 5–10 mg/kg, single dose; maximum dose, 750 mg Microsize: 10–20 mg/kg per day divided in 2 doses; maximum dose, 1000 mg	Rash, paresthesias, leukopenia, gastrointestinal tract symptoms, proteinuria, hepatotoxicity, mental confusion, headache
Itraconazole[3,5]	IV, PO	Children: 5–10 mg/kg per day as a single dose or divided into 2 doses Adults: 200 mg/day once or twice a day; 200 mg once a day for suppressive therapy in HIV-infected patients with histoplasmosis	Gastrointestinal tract symptoms, rash, edema, headache, hypokalemia, hepatotoxicity, thrombocytopenia, leukopenia; cardiac toxicity is possible in patients also taking terfenadine or astemizole

Table 4.5. Recommended Doses of Parenteral and Oral Antifungal Drugs, continued

Drug	Route[1]	Dose (per day)	Adverse Reactions[2,3]
Ketoconazole[3,5]	PO	Children[6]: 3.3–6.6 mg/kg per day, single dose Adults: 200 mg, twice a day for 4 doses, then 200 mg, once a day	Hepatotoxicity, gastrointestinal tract symptoms, rash, anaphylaxis, thrombocytopenia, hemolytic anemia, gynecomastia, adrenal insufficiency; cardiac toxicity is possible in patients also taking terfenadine or astemizole
Nystatin	PO	Infants: 200 000 U, 4 times a day, after meals Children and adults: 400 000–600 000 U, 3 times a day, after meals	Gastrointestinal tract symptoms, rash
Terbinafine[4]	PO	Adults: 250 mg, once a day	Gastrointestinal tract symptoms, rash, taste abnormalities, cholestatic hepatitis
Voriconazole	IV, PO	Adults: 200 mg, IV or PO, every 12 h	Visual disturbance, rash, increased liver function tests

[1] IV indicates intravenous; IT, intrathecal; PO, oral; HIV, human immunodeficiency virus.

[2] See package insert or listing in current edition of the *Physicians' Desk Reference* (Greenwood Village, CO: Thomson Micromedex) or http://pdrel.thomsonhc.com/pdrel/librarian/action/command.Command.

[3] Interactions with other drugs are common. Consult the *Physicians' Desk Reference*, a drug interaction reference or database, or a pharmacist before prescribing these medications.

[4] Experience with drug in children is limited.

[5] Limited or no information about use in newborn infants is available.

[6] For children 2 years of age and younger, the daily dose has not been established.

DRUGS FOR INVASIVE AND OTHER SERIOUS FUNGAL INFECTIONS IN CHILDREN

Table 4.6. Drugs for Invasive and Other Serious Fungal Infections[1]

Disease	Intravenous	Oral, Absorbable			Intravenous or Oral		
	Amphotericin B	Caspofungin[2]	Flucytosine	Ketoconazole[2]	Itraconazole	Fluconazole	Voriconazole
Aspergillosis	P	A	...	...	A, M	...	A
Blastomycosis	P	...	...	A, M	M, (P)	A, M	...
Candidiasis:							
Chronic, mucocutaneous	A	...	...	A	A	P	...
Oropharyngeal, esophageal	A	...	...	A	A	P	...
Systemic	P, S (severe cases)	...	S	...	...	(P), A, M	...
Coccidioidomycosis	P	...	...	A, M	A, M	(P), A, M	...
Cryptococcosis	P, S	...	P, S	...	A	A, M	...
Histoplasmosis	P	...	...	A, M	(P), A	A, M	...
Mucormycosis (zygomycosis)	P	...	...	...	...	...	...
Paracoccidioidomycosis	(P3)	...	...	M	P, M	...	...
Pseudallescheriasis	...	...	...	A	P	...	A
Sporotrichosis	(P)	...	...	...	P	A, M	...

[1] P indicates preferred treatment in most cases (parentheses indicate drug is considered preferred treatment by some experts); A, efficacy less well established or alternative drug; M, for mild and moderately severe cases; S, combination recommended if infection is severe or central nervous system is involved.

[2] Efficacy and safety have not been established for children.

[3] Usually in combination with itraconazole or a sulfonamide.

TOPICAL DRUGS FOR SUPERFICIAL FUNGAL INFECTIONS

Table 4.7. Topical Drugs for Superficial Fungal Infections

Drug	Strength	Formulation	Trade Name Examples	Application(s) per Day	Adverse Reactions/Notes
Amphotericin B (Rx)	3%	C, L, O	Fungizone	2–4	Discoloration of the skin, clothes, nails
Basic fuchsin, phenol, resorcinol, and acetone (Rx)		S	Castellani Paint Modified	1	Excellent for intertriginous areas in all age groups. Stains everything. Also available as a colorless solution with alcohol and without basic fuchsin. This is an alternative if the patient cannot tolerate other topical antifungals.
Butenafine (Rx)	1%	C	Mentax	1	Safety and efficacy in patients <12 years of age have not been established.
Ciclopirox (Rx)	1%; 8%	C, L, S	Loprox; Penlac	2	Irritant dermatitis; shake lotion vigorously before application; safety and efficacy in children <10 years of age have not been established.
Clotrimazole (Rx and OTC)	1%	C, L, S, Com	Topical solution >10 preparations; check with pharmacist[1]	1 (Rx) 2 (OTC)	Irritant dermatitis; safety and efficacy in children have not been established. Beware of topical steroid combinations.[2]
Clotrimazole and betamethasone dipropionate (Rx)		C, L	Lotrisone[3]	2[2]	Irritant dermatitis: safety and efficacy in children have been established. Beware of topical steroid combinations,[2] especially when applied to the diaper area, because high systemic steroid exposure can occur.
Econazole (Rx)	1%	C	Spectazole	1 (dermatophyte) 2 (candidiasis)	Irritant dermatitis.
Haloprogin (Rx)	1%	C, S	Halotex	2	Irritant dermatitis.

Table 4.7. Topical Drugs for Superficial Fungal Infections, continued

Drug	Strength	Formulation	Trade Name Examples	Application(s) per Day	Adverse Reactions/Notes
Hydrocortisone-iodoquinol (Rx)	1%	C	Vytone Dermazene	3–4	Do not use in children <2 years of age.[2] May stain clothes and skin and interfere with thyroid function and phenylketonuria tests.
Ketoconazole (Rx)	2%	C, Sh	Nizoral	1 (candidiasis), tinea dermatophyte	Potential sulfite reaction with anaphylactic or asthmatic reaction; shampoo can cause dry or oily hair and increase hair loss.
Miconazole (Rx and OTC)	2%	O, C, P, S, SpP, SpL	>10 preparations; check with pharmacist[1]	2 (seborrhea), apply 2 times/ wk for 4 wk 2 (C, L) 2 (P, L)	Irritant and allergic contact dermatitis.
Naftifine (Rx)	1%	C, Gel	Naftin	1 (C) 2 (Gel)	Irritant dermatitis.
Nystatin (Rx and OTC)	100 000 U/mL or 100 000 U/g	C, P, O, Com	Nystatin, Nystop powder, Pedi-Dri powder	2 (C) 2–3 (P)	Nontoxic except with topical steroid combinations.[4]
Nystatin and triamcinolone acetonide (Rx)		C, O	Mytrex cream, Mytrex ointment	2[3]	
Oxiconazole (Rx)	1%	C, L	Oxistat	1–2 (tinea dermatophyte)	Irritant dermatitis.
Sulconazole (Rx)	1%	C, S	Exelderm	1–2 (tinea vesicular)	Irritant dermatitis.

Table 4.7. Topical Drugs for Superficial Fungal Infections, continued

Drug	Strength	Formulation	Trade Name Examples	Application(s) per Day	Adverse Reactions/Notes
Terbinafine (OTC)	1%	C, Gel	Lamisil	2	Irritant dermatitis; avoid use of occlusive clothing or dressings.
Tolnaftate (OTC)	1%	C, P, S, Gel, SpP, SpL	>10 preparations; check with pharmacist	2	Irritant and allergic contact dermatitis.
Triacetin (Rx)	% varies	S, C, Sp	Fungoid tincture, fungoid cream only-clean nail	3(C, S)	Irritant dermatitis.
Undecylenic acid and derivatives (OTC)	8%–25%	C, O, S, F, SpP, P, soap	See pharmacist for formulations and applications[1]	2 (tincture) Spray 1–2 sec	Irritant dermatitis.
Other Remedies					
Gentian violet (OTC)	2%	S	…	2	Staining.
Selenium sulfide (OTC)	2.5%	L, Sh	Exsel	1	For tinea capitis, to decrease spore formation and to decrease the potential spread of the dermatophyte.
	1%	Sh	Head & Shoulders, Selsun Blue	1	For tinea capitis, to decrease spore formation and to decrease the potential spread of the dermatophyte.

Rx indicates prescription; C, cream; L, lotion; O, ointment; S, solution; OTC, over the counter; Com, combinations; Sh, shampoo; P, powder; Sp, spray; F, foam.

[1] The pharmacist is your best resource to check formulations that are available and new. They use *Facts and Comparisons* reference products (*Facts and Comparisons*, St Louis, MO [Division of Lippincott Williams & Wilkins]).

[2] Topical steroids must be used with caution in young children and in areas of thin skin (eg, diaper area). In these circumstances, high systemic exposure may occur, resulting in endogenous synthesis suppression with the potential for serious adverse effects. Potential adverse effects include irritant dermatitis, folliculitis, hypertrichosis, acneform eruptions, hypopigmentation, perioral dermatitis, allergic contact dermatitis, maceration, secondary infection, skin atrophy, striae, and miliaria.

[3] Lotrisone cream no longer is available; lotion is available.

[4] Any topical preparation has the potential to irritate the skin and cause itching, burning, stinging, erythema, edema, vesicles, and blister formation.

For more information on individual drugs, see *Physician's Desk Reference* (Greenwood Village, CO: Thomson Micromedex) or http://pdrel.thomsonhc.com/pdrel/librarian/action/command.Command.

ANTIVIRAL DRUGS FOR NON-HUMAN IMMUNODEFICIENCY VIRUS INFECTIONS

Table 4.8. Antiviral Drugs for Non-Human Immunodeficiency Virus Infections

Generic (Trade Name)	Indication	Route	Usually Recommended Dosage
Acyclovir[1,2] (Zovirax)	Genital herpes simplex virus (HSV) infection; first episode	Oral	1000–1200 mg/day in 3–5 divided doses for 5–10 days. Oral pediatric dose: 40–80 mg/kg per day divided in 3–4 doses for 5–10 days (maximum 1.0 g/day).
		IV	15 mg/kg per day in 3 divided doses for 5–7 days.
	Genital HSV infection: recurrence	Oral	1000–1200 mg/day in 3–5 divided doses for 5 days.
	Recurrent genital and cutaneous (ocular) HSV episodes in a patient with frequent recurrences, chronic suppressive therapy	Oral	400–1200 mg/day in 2–3 divided doses for as long as 12 continuous months.
	HSV in immunocompromised host (localized, progressive, or disseminated)	IV	15–30 mg/kg per day in 3 divided doses for 7–14 days.
		Oral	1000 mg/day in 3–5 divided doses for 7–14 days.
	Prophylaxis of HSV in immunocompromised host	Oral	600–1000 mg/day in 3–5 divided doses during period of risk.
	HSV-seropositive patients	IV	15 mg/kg in 3 divided doses during period of risk.
	HSV encephalitis	IV	30 mg/kg per day in 3 divided doses for a minimum of 14–21 days.
	Neonatal HSV	IV	60 mg/kg per day in 3 divided doses for 14–21 days.
	Varicella in immunocompromised host	IV	For children <1 year of age: 30 mg/kg per day in 3 divided doses for 7–10 days; some experts also recommend this dose for children ≥1 year of age. For children ≥1 year of age: 1500 mg/m² of body surface area per day in 3 divided doses for 7–10 days.
	Zoster in immunocompetent host	IV	Same as for varicella in immunocompromised host.
		Oral	4000 mg/day in 5 divided doses for 5–7 days for patients ≥12 years of age.

Table 4.8. Antiviral Drugs for Non–Human Immunodeficiency Virus Infections, continued

Generic (Trade Name)	Indication	Route	Usually Recommended Dosage
	Varicella in immunocompetent host[3]	Oral	80 mg/kg per day in 4 divided doses for 5 days; maximum dose, 3200 mg/day.
Amantadine (Symmetrel)	Influenza A: treatment and prophylaxis	Oral	Treatment: 1–9 y of age: 5 mg/kg per day, maximum 150 mg/day, in 2 divided doses ≥10 y of age, <40 kg: 5 mg/kg per day, in 2 divided doses; ≥40 kg: 200 mg/day in 2 divided doses Prophylaxis: Same as for treatment. An alternative and equally acceptable dosage is 100 mg/day for children weighing >20 kg and adults. See Influenza (p 382).
Cidofovir (Vistide)	Cytomegalovirus (CMV) retinitis	IV	Induction: 5 mg/kg once with probenecid with hydration. Weekly maintenance: 3 mg/kg once with probenecid and hydration.
Famciclovir (Famvir)	Genital HSV infection	Oral	For adolescents, 750 mg/day in 3 divided doses for 7–10 days.
	Episodic recurrent genital HSV infection	Oral	For adolescents, 250 mg/day in 2 divided doses for 5 days.
	Daily suppressive therapy	Oral	For adolescents, 250–500 mg/day in 2 divided doses for 1 y, then reassess for recurrence of HSV infection.
Fomivirsen (Vitravene)	CMV retinitis	IO	1 vial (330 µg) injected into the vitreous, then repeated every 2–4 wk.
Foscarnet[1] (Foscavir)	CMV retinitis in patients with acquired immunodeficiency syndrome	IV	180 mg/kg per day in 3 divided doses for 14–21 days, then 90–120 mg/kg once a day as maintenance dose.
	HSV infection resistant to acyclovir in immunocompromised host	IV	80–120 mg/kg per day in 2–3 divided doses until infection resolves.
Ganciclovir[1] (Cytovene)	Acquired CMV retinitis in immuno-compromised host[4]	IV	10 mg/kg per day in 2 divided doses for 14–21 days; for long-term suppression, 5 mg/kg per day for 5–7 days/wk.
	Prophylaxis of CMV in high-risk host	IV	10 mg/kg per day in 2 divided doses for 1 wk, then 5 mg/kg per day in 1 dose for 100 days.
		Oral	1 g, orally, 3 times/day.

Table 4.8. Antiviral Drugs for Non–Human Immunodeficiency Virus Infections, continued

Generic (Trade Name)	Indication	Route	Usually Recommended Dosage
Lamivudine (Epivir-HBV)	Treatment of chronic hepatitis B	Oral	For people ≥2 years of age, 3 mg/kg per day (maximum 100 mg/day).
Oseltamivir (Tamiflu)	Influenza A and B: treatment	Oral[5]	Treatment for people 1–12 years of age: ≤15 kg: 30 mg, twice daily; >15 kg to 23 kg: 45 mg, twice daily; >23 kg to 40 kg: 60 mg, twice daily; >40 kg: 75 mg, twice daily. Prophylaxis ≥13 years of age: 75 mg, twice daily. See Influenza (p 382).
	Influenza A and B: prophylaxis	Oral[5]	For adolescents (≥13 years of age): 75 mg, daily.
Ribavirin (Virazole)	Treatment of respiratory syncytial virus infection	Aerosol	Given by a small-particle generator, in a solution of 6 g in 300 mL sterile water (20 mg/mL), delivered for 18 h per day for 3–7 days or 6 g in 100 mL of sterile water for 2 h, 3 times/day; longer treatment may be necessary in some patients.
Ribavirin (Rebetol)	Treatment of hepatitis C in combination with interferon	Oral	Fixed dose by weight is suggested: 25–36 kg: 200 mg AM and PM; >36–49 kg: 200 mg AM and 400 mg PM; >49–61 kg: 400 mg AM and PM; >61–75 kg: 400 mg AM and 600 mg PM; >75 kg: 600 mg AM and PM.
Rimantadine (Flumadine)	Influenza A: treatment and prophylaxis	Oral	Treatment: ≥13 years of age, 200 mg/day in 2 divided doses Prophylaxis: 1–9 y of age: 5 mg/kg per day, maximum 150 mg/day, in 2 divided doses ≥10 y of age, <40 kg: 5 mg/kg per day, in 2 divided doses; ≥40 kg: 200 mg/day in 2 divided doses See Influenza (p 382).

Table 4.8. Antiviral Drugs for Non–Human Immunodeficiency Virus Infections, continued

Generic (Trade Name)	Indication	Route	Usually Recommended Dosage
Valacyclovir (Valtrex)	Genital HSV infection	Oral	For adolescents, 2 g/day in 2 divided doses for 7–10 days.
	Episodic recurrent genital HSV infection	Oral	For adolescents, 1 g/day in 2 divided doses for 5 days.
	Daily suppressive therapy for HSV infection	Oral	For adolescents, 500–1000 mg, once daily for 1 year, then reassess for recurrences.
Zanamivir (Relenza)	Influenza A and B: treatment	Inhalation	Treatment for children 7 y of age or older and adults, 10 mg, twice daily. See Influenza (p 382). Not licensed for prophylaxis.

IV indicates intravenous; IO, intraocular.

1 Dose should be decreased in patients with impaired renal function.
2 Oral dosage of acyclovir in children should not exceed 80 mg/kg per day.
3 Selective indications; see Varicella-Zoster Infections (p 672).
4 Some experts use ganciclovir in immunocompromised host with CMV gastrointestinal tract disease and CMV pneumonitis (with or without CMV Immune Globulin Intravenous).
5 Oseltamivir oral suspension is packaged with a dispensing syringe calibrated with graduations of 30, 45, and 60 mg; 75 mg may be dispensed using a combination of 30- and 45-mg graduations.

For more information on individual drugs, see *Physician's Desk Reference* (Greenwood Village, CO: Thomson Micromedex) or http://pdrel.thomsonhc.com/pdrel/librarian/action/command.Command.

ANTIRETROVIRAL THERAPY

Table 4.9. Characteristics of Antiretroviral Drugs:
Nucleoside/Nucleotide Reverse Transcriptase Inhibitors

Drug (Abbreviation)/ Trade Name	Dosage[1]	Special Instructions
Abacavir (ABC)/Ziagen Component of Combivir	*Neonatal:* 1 to 3 mo of age: 8 mg/kg, twice daily, is under study. *Pediatric and adolescent:* 8 mg/kg, twice daily; maximum dosage 300 mg, twice daily *Adult:* 300 mg, twice daily	An abacavir warning card, which lists signs and symptoms of abacavir hypersensitivity, should be provided with each prescription of abacavir.
Didanosine (ddI)/Videx	*Usual pediatric range:* 90–120 mg/m^2, every 12 h *Neonatal (<90 days of age):* 100 mg/m^2 age 14 days to 6 wk *Adolescent and adult:* Weight >60 kg: 200 mg, twice daily Weight <60 kg: 125 mg, twice daily *Videx EC, adolescent and adult:* Weight >60 kg: 400 mg, once daily Weight <60 kg: 250 mg, once daily	All formulations except Videx EC contain buffering agents or antacids. Food decreases absorption; administer ddI on an empty stomach (1 h before or 2 h after meal). Concomitant therapy with quinolones: ddI should be given 2 h after or 6 h before the quinolone dose. For oral solution: shake well and keep refrigerated; admixture stable for 30 days.
Lamivudine (3TC)/Epivir Component of Combivir, Trizivir.	*Pediatric:* 4 mg/kg, every 12 h *Neonatal (<30 days of age):* under study in clinical trials: 2 mg/kg, every 12 h *Adolescent and adult:* 150 mg, twice daily	Can be administered with or without food. For oral solution: store at room temperature. Decrease dosage for patients with impaired renal function.
Stavudine (d4T)/Zerit	*Pediatric:* 1 mg/kg, every 12 h (up to weight of 30 kg) *Neonatal:* birth to 13 days: 0.5 mg/kg, every 12 h; >13 days of age: 1 mg/kg, every 12 h *Adolescent and adult:* Weight >60 kg: 40 mg, twice daily Weight 30–60 kg: 30 mg, twice daily	Can be administered with food. For oral solution: shake well and keep refrigerated; solution stable for 30 days.

Table 4.9. Characteristics of Antiretroviral Drugs: Nucleoside/Nucleotide Reverse Transcriptase Inhibitors, continued

Drug (Abbreviation)/ Trade Name	Dosage[1]	Special Instructions
Tenofovir (DF)/Viread	*Pediatric:* Unknown *Neonatal:* Unknown *Adolescent and adult:* 300 mg/day	Tenofovir should be taken with food to enhance bioavailability. When used in combination with ddI, tenofovir should be taken 2 h before or 1 h after ddI. Should not be administered to patients with renal insufficiency (creatinine clearance <60 mL/min).
Zalcitabine (ddC)/HIVID	*Usual pediatric:* 0.01 mg/kg, every 8 h *Pediatric range:* 0.005 to 0.01 mg/kg, every 8 h *Neonatal:* Unknown *Adolescent and adult:* 0.75 mg, 3 times/day	Administer on an empty stomach (1 h before or 2 h after a meal). Decrease dosage in patients with impaired renal function.
Zidovudine (AZT, ZDV)/Retrovir Component of Combivir, Trizivir	*Usual pediatric: (>6 wk of age)* Oral: 160 mg/m², every 8 h *Pediatric range:* 90–180 mg/m², every 6–8 h Some experts use a dosage of 180 mg/m², every 12 h in combinations with other antiretroviral compounds. *Neonatal prophylaxis (birth–6 wk of age)* Oral: 2 mg/kg, every 6 h IV: 1.5 mg/kg, every 6 h Dose may need to be decreased for premature infants. *Adolescent and adult:* 200 mg, 3 times/day or 300 mg, twice daily	Can be administered with food.
Combivir (fixed dose combination of zidovudine, lamivudine)	**See individual drugs for information.**	

Table 4.9. Characteristics of Antiretroviral Drugs: Nucleoside/Nucleotide Reverse Transcriptase Inhibitors, continued

Drug (Abbreviation)/ Trade Name	Dosage[1]	Special Instructions
Trizivir: (fixed dose combination of abacavir, zidovudine, lamivudine)	**See individual drugs for information.**	An abacavir warning card, which lists signs and symptoms of abacavir hypersensitivity, should be provided with each prescription of abacavir.

AUC, area under the curve; TMP-SMX, trimethoprim-sulfamethoxazole; IV, intravenous.

[1] Adolescent dosing by Tanner Stage: adolescents in early puberty (Tanner stages I-II) should be dosed using pediatric schedules, and those in late puberty (Tanner stage V) should be dosed using adult schedules. Youth who are in the midst of their growth spurt (Tanner stage III females and Tanner stage IV males) should be closely monitored for medication efficacy and toxic effects when choosing adult or pediatric dosing guidelines.

For more information on individual drugs, see *Physician's Desk Reference* (Greenwood Village, CO: Thomson Micromedex) or http://pdrel.thomsonhc.com/pdrel/librarian/action/command.Command or www.aidsinfo.nih.gov/.

Table 4.10. Characteristics of Antiretroviral Drugs: Nonnucleoside Reverse Transcriptase Inhibitors

Drug (Abbreviation)/ Trade Name	Dosage	Special Instructions
Delavirdine (DLV)/ Rescriptor	*Pediatric:* Unknown *Neonatal:* Unknown *Adolescent and adult:* 400 mg, 3 times/day	Can be administered with food. Should be taken 1 h before or 1 h after ddI (other than extended-release formulation) or antacids. 100-mg tablets can be dissolved in water and the resulting dispersion can be taken promptly. Dispersion cannot be achieved with 200-mg tablets.
Efavirenz (EFV)/Sustiva	*Pediatric (>3 y of age):* administered once daily. Body weight 10–<15 kg; 200 mg; 15–<20 kg; 250 mg; 20–<25 kg; 300 mg; 25–<32.5 kg; 350 mg; 32.5–<40 kg; 400 mg; ≥40 kg; 600 mg. No data are available on the appropriate dosage for children <3 y of age. *Adolescent and adult:* 600 mg, once daily	Efavirenz should be taken on an empty stomach. Capsules may be opened and added to liquids or foods, but efavirenz has a peppery taste; grape jelly has been used to disguise the taste. Bedtime dosing is recommended; particularly during the first 2–4 wk of therapy, to improve tolerability of CNS adverse effects. Use in pregnancy should be avoided, and women of child-bearing potential should undergo pregnancy testing before initiating therapy.
Nevirapine (NVP)/Viramune	*Pediatric:* 120–200 mg/m², every 12 h. Note: initiate therapy with 120 mg/m², once daily for 14 days. Increase to full dose administered every 12 h if no rash or other untoward effects. OR	Can be administered with food. May be administered concurrently with ddI. Suspension must be shaken well; store at room temperature. Increased incidence of hepatotoxicity in patients with increased alanine transaminase or aspartate transaminase concentrations before starting therapy and in patients coinfected with hepatitis B or hepatitis C.

Table 4.10. Characteristics of Antiretroviral Drugs:
Nonnucleoside Reverse Transcriptase Inhibitors, continued

Drug (Abbreviation)/ Trade Name	Dosage	Special Instructions
Nevirapine (NVP)/Viramune, continued	2 mo–8 y of age: 4 mg/kg, once daily for 14 days, then increase to 7 mg/kg, twice daily. Older than 8 years: 4 mg/kg, once daily for 14 days, then 4 mg/kg, twice daily. Maximum 400 mg/day. *Neonatal: unknown* *Adolescent and adult:* 200 mg, every 12 h. Note: initiate therapy at half dose for the first 14 days. Increase to full dose if no rash or other untoward effects.	

ddI indicates didanosine; CNS, central nervous system; AUC, area under the curve.

1 Note: drugs metabolized by the hepatic cytochrome P-450 3A (CYP 3A) enzyme system have the potential for significant interactions with multiple drugs, some of which may be life threatening. These interactions are outlined in detail in Centers for Disease Control and Prevention. Guidelines for using antiretroviral agents among HIV-infected adults and adolescents. Recommendations of the Panel on Clinical Practice for Treatment of HIV. *MMWR Recomm Rep.* 2002;51 (RR-7):1–56 and at www.aidsinfo.nih.gov and in prescribing information available from drug companies. These interactions will not be reiterated in this document, and the health care professional should review those documents for detailed information. Before therapy with these drugs is initiated, the patient's medication profile should be reviewed carefully for potential drug interactions.

For more information on individual drugs, see *Physician's Desk Reference* (Greenwood Village, CO: Thomson Micromedex) or http://pdrel.thomsonhc.com/pdrel/librarian/action/command.Command or www.aidsinfo.nih.gov/.

Table 4.11. Characteristics of Antiretroviral Drugs: Protease Inhibitors[1]

Drug (Trade Name)	Dosage	Special Instructions
Amprenavir (Agenerase)	Neonatal dose: Not recommended in children <4 years of age. Pediatric/adolescent (<50 kg in body weight): 4–16 y of age Oral solution: 22.5 mg/kg, twice daily or 17 mg/kg, 3 times/day (maximum daily dose 2800 mg). Capsules: 20 mg/kg, twice daily or 15 mg/kg, 3 times/day (maximum daily dose 2400 mg). Adult dose: 1200 mg (eight 150-mg capsules), twice daily	Amprenavir should not be used in children <4 y of age because of the uncertain effect of extremely high doses of vitamin E and the propylene glycol content of the oral liquid solution. The oral solution and capsule formulation are not interchangeable on a mg/mg basis. Amprenavir may be taken with or without food but should not be given with a high-fat content meal. Patients taking antacids (or buffered formulations of ddI) should take amprenavir at least 1 h before or after antacid (or buffered ddI) use.
Indinavir (Crixivan)	*Pediatric:* Under study in clinical trials: 350–500 mg/m² of body surface area, every 6–8 h *Neonatal:* Unknown. Because of adverse effect of hyperbilirubinemia, should not be given to neonates *Adolescent and adult:* 800 mg, every 8 h	Administer on an empty stomach 1 h before or 2 h after a meal (or can take with a light meal). Aggressive hydration required to minimize risk of nephrolithiasis. If coadministered with ddI, give at least 1 h apart on an empty stomach. Decrease dosage for patients with hepatic insufficiency or cirrhosis. Capsules are sensitive to moisture and should be stored in original container with desiccant.
Lopinavir + ritonavir (Kaletra) (lopinavir + ritonavir is a coformulation of the 2 individual PIs in a fixed drug combination)	*Pediatric (>6 mo of age):* 7–15 kg: 12 mg/kg, twice daily 15–40 kg: 10 mg/kg, twice daily >40 kg: 400 mg, then 100 mg, daily *Neonatal:* unknown *Adolescent and adult:* 400 mg, then 100 mg, daily	

Table 4.11. Characteristics of Antiretroviral Drugs: Protease Inhibitors,[1] continued

Drug (Trade Name)	Dosage	Special Instructions
Nelfinavir (Viracept)	*Pediatric:* 30 mg/kg, 3 times/day *Neonatal:* unknown *Adolescent and adult:* 750 mg, 3 times/day OR 1250 mg, twice daily	Administer with meal or light snack. Powder may be mixed with water, milk, pudding, ice cream, or formula (for up to 6 h). Do not mix with acidic food or juice because of resulting poor taste. Do not add water to bottles of oral powder; a special scoop is provided with oral powder for measuring. Tablets readily dissolve in water and produce a dispersion that can be mixed with milk, chocolate milk; tablets also can be crushed and administered with pudding.
Ritonavir (Norvir)	*Pediatric:* 400 mg/m^2, every 12 h To minimize nausea and vomiting, initiate therapy starting at 250 mg/m^2, every 12 h, and increase stepwise to full dose over 5 days as tolerated. *Pediatric range:* 350–400 mg/m^2, every 12 h *Neonatal:* unknown *Adolescent and adult:* 600 mg, every 12 h	Administration with food increases absorption. If administered with ddI (other than ddI EC), should be administered 2.5 h apart. Oral capsules and solution must be kept refrigerated. Techniques to increase tolerance by children may include preceding dose with foods that coat or cool the tongue, mixing with better-tasting ingredients, or following dose with strongly flavored foods. Ritonavir oral solution is 43% ethanol (vol/vol). Accidental ingestion could result in ethanol toxicity. When used in low doses as a pharmacologic enhancer, ritonavir does not have antiviral activity and should not be considered a second therapeutic PI.

Table 4.11. Characteristics of Antiretroviral Drugs: Protease Inhibitors,[1] continued

Drug (Trade Name)	Dosage	Special Instructions
Saquinavir (Fortovase, Invirase)	*Pediatric:* 50 mg/kg, 3 times/day under study *Neonatal:* Unknown *Adolescent and adult:* Soft gel capsules (Fortovase): 1200 mg, 3 times/day OR Soft or hard gel capsules, 400 mg, in combination with ritonavir 400 mg **Inverase** and **Fortovase** are not bioequivalent and cannot be used interchangeably. **Invirase** should not be used as a single PI in a HAART regimen but should be used in combination with ritonavir as noted above.	Administer within 2 h of a full meal to increase absorption. Concurrent administration of grapefruit juice increases saquinavir concentration. Sun exposure can cause photosensitivity reactions; sunscreen or protective clothing is recommended.

PI indicates protease inhibitor; WHO, World Health Organization; ddI, didanosine; HAART, highly active antiretroviral therapy.

1 Data for children are limited, and doses may change as more information is obtained about the pharmacokinetics of these drugs in children.

2 Note: drugs metabolized by the hepatic cytochrome P-450 3A (CYP 3A) enzyme system have the potential for significant interactions with multiple drugs, some of which may be life threatening. These interactions are outlined in detail in Centers for Disease Control and Prevention. Report of the NIH Panel to Define Principles of Therapy of HIV Infection and guidelines for the use of antiretroviral agents in HIV-infected adults and adolescents. *MMWR Morb Mortal Wkly Rep.* 1998;47(RR-5):1–82 and at www.aidsinfo.nih.gov and in prescribing information available from the drug companies. These interactions will not be reiterated in this document, and the health care professional should review those documents for detailed information. Before therapy with these drugs is initiated, the patient's medication profile should be reviewed carefully for potential drug interactions.

For more information on individual drugs, see *Physician's Desk Reference* (Greenwood Village, CO: Thomson Micromedex) or http://pdrel.thomsonhc.com/pdrel/librarian/action/command.Command.

Table 4.12. Common Class Adverse Events and Drug Interactions

Drug Class	Drug Name	Common Class Adverse Events	Common Class Drug Interactions
Nucleoside/nucleotide reverse transcriptase inhibitors (NRTIs)	Abacavir Didanosine (ddI) Lamivudine (3TC) Stavudine (d4T) Tenofovir Zalcitabine (ddc) Zidovudine (ZDV, AZT) ZDV plus lamivudine ZDV plus lamivudine and abacavir	• Lactic acidosis • Increased liver function tests, hepatitis, hepatic steatosis	See www.aidsinfo.nih.gov for individual drug interactions.
Nonnucleoside reverse transcriptase inhibitors (NNRTIs)	Delavirdine (DLV) Efavirenz (EFV) Nevirapine (NVP)	• Rash, possibly severe, including Stevens-Johnson syndrome and toxic epidermal necrolysis	Mixed inducers/inhibitors of cytochrome P450; doses of concomitant drugs metabolized by P450 may require adjustment. Protease inhibitors (PIs): saquinavir and indinavir concentrations decreased; ritonavir concentrations may increase or decrease. Antifungals: ketoconazole concentrations decreased. Rifampin nevirapine concentrations significantly decreased. Rifabutin has less of an effect on nevirapine concentrations. Methadone: decreased methadone concentrations when used concomitantly with efavirenz and nevirapine; patients should be monitored for withdrawal symptoms. Anticonvulsants and psychotropics: these are metabolized via similar pathways. Anticonvulsant (phenobarbital, phenytoin, and carbamazepine) serum concentrations should be monitored.

Table 4.12. Common Class Adverse Events and Drug Interactions, continued

Drug Class	Drug Name	Common Class Adverse Events	Common Class Drug Interactions
Nonnucleoside reverse transcriptase inhibitors (NNRTIs), continued			Psychotropic agents: patients should be monitored carefully when these medications are used concomitantly with NNRTIs. Oral contraceptives: NNRTIs may decrease plasma concentrations of oral contraceptives and other hormonal contraceptives. Oral contraceptives should not be the only means of birth control when used by patients treated with NNRTIs.
Protease inhibitors (PIs)	Amprenavir Indinavir Nelfinavir Ritonavir Saquinavir Lopinavir + ritonavir	• Hyperglycemia/diabetes mellitus including new onset diabetes mellitus • Body fat redistribution • Hyperlipidemia/hypercholesterolemia • Nausea, vomiting, diarrhea • Increased hepatic transaminases	Extensively metabolized by hepatic cytochrome P450 3A(CYP3A). Potential for multiple drug interactions. Before administration, the patient's medication profile should be reviewed carefully for potential drug interactions. PIs are not recommended for concurrent use with the following: antihistamines astemizole or terfenadine; cisapride; ergot alkaloid derivatives; certain cardiac drugs (quinidine, amiodarone); lipid-lowering agents (simvastatin and lovastatin); St John's Wort; or sedative-hypnotics (midazolam and triazolam). PI concentrations are greatly decreased with concurrent use of rifampin. Concurrent use is not recommended. Rifabutin causes less decrease in PI concentrations; if coadministered with PI, rifabutin should be decreased to one half the usual dose.

Table 4.12. Common Class Adverse Events and Drug Interactions, continued

Drug Class	Drug Name	Common Class Adverse Events	Common Class Drug Interactions
Protease inhibitors (PIs), continued			Grapefruit juice may substantially increase or decrease serum concentrations of PIs. Clarithromycin concentrations may be increased when given concomitantly with PIs. Sildenafil concentrations are increased when used in patients also receiving PIs. The coadministration of ketoconazole and PIs may result in increased PI concentrations or increased ketoconazole concentrations. Estradiol concentrations are decreased by PIs, and alternative or additional methods of birth control should be used if coadministering with hormonal methods of birth control. Coadministration with efavirenz decreases concentrations of saquinavir, amprenavir, and indinavir and increases the concentrations of ritonavir and nelfinavir. The coadministration of nevirapine results in decreased concentrations of PIs. The concentrations of NNRTIs may be decreased when used with PIs. The coadministration of delavirdine and PIs increases PI concentrations.

DRUGS FOR PARASITIC INFECTIONS

The following tables (4.13 and 4.14) are reproduced from *The Medical Letter.**
These tables provide recommendations that are likely to be consistent in many cases
with those of the Committee on Infectious Diseases, as given in the disease-specific
chapters in Section 3. However, because *The Medical Letter* recommendations are
developed independently, these recommendations occasionally may differ from recommendations of the committee. Accordingly, both should be consulted. The committee thanks *The Medical Letter* for their courtesy in allowing this information to
be reprinted.

In Table 4.13 (p 745), first-choice and alternative drugs with recommended
adult and pediatric dosages for most parasitic infections are given. In each case,
the need for treatment must be weighed against the toxic effects of the drug. A
decision to withhold therapy often may be correct, particularly when the drugs
can cause severe adverse effects. When the first-choice drug initially is ineffective
and the alternative is more hazardous, a second course of treatment with the first
drug before giving the alternative may be prudent.

Several drugs recommended in Table 4.13 (p 745) have not been licensed by
the US Food and Drug Administration and, thus, are investigational (see footnotes).
When prescribing an unlicensed drug, the physician should inform the patient of
the investigational status and adverse effects of the drug.

These recommendations periodically (usually every other year) are updated
by *The Medical Letter* and, thus, likely are to be superseded by new ones before
the next edition of the *Red Book* is published (www.medletter.com).

---

* Reprinted with permission from *The Medical Letter.*

Table 4.13. Drugs for Parasitic Infections

Parasitic infections are found throughout the world. With increasing travel, immigration, use of immunosuppressive drugs and the spread of AIDS, physicians anywhere may see infections caused by previously unfamiliar parasites. The table below lists first-choice and alternative drugs for most parasitic infections. The manufacturers of the drugs are listed on page 770.

Infection	Drug	Adult Dosage	Pediatric Dosage
Acanthamoeba keratitis			
Drug of choice:	See footnote 1		
AMEBIASIS (*Entamoeba histolytica*)			
asymptomatic			
Drug of choice:	Iodoquinol	650 mg tid × 20d	30–40 mg/kg/d (max. 2g) in 3 doses × 20d
OR	Paromomycin	25–35 mg/kg/d in 3 doses × 7d	25–35 mg/kg/d in 3 doses × 7d
Alternative:	Diloxanide furoate[2]	500 mg tid × 10d	20 mg/kg/d in 3 doses × 10d
mild to moderate intestinal disease[3]			
Drug of choice:[4]	Metronidazole	500–750 mg tid × 7–10d	35–50 mg/kg/d in 3 doses × 7–10d
OR	Tinidazole[5]	2 grams/d divided tid × 3d	50 mg/kg (max. 2g) qd × 3d
severe intestinal and extraintestinal disease[3]			
Drug of choice:	Metronidazole	750 mg tid × 7–10d	35–50 mg/kg/d in 3 doses × 7–10d
OR	Tinidazole[5]	800 mg tid × 5d	60 mg/kg/d (max. 2 g) × 5d

* Availability problems. See table on page 770.

1. For treatment of keratitis caused by *Acanthamoeba*, concurrent topical use of 0.1% propamidine isethionate (*Brolene*) plus neomycin-polymyxin B-gramicidin ophthalmic solution has been successful (SL Hargrave et al, Ophthalmology 1999; 106:952). In addition, 0.02% topical polyhexamethylene biguanide (PHMB) and/or chlorhexadine has been used successfully in a large number of patients (G Tabin et al, Cornea 2001; 20:757; YS Wysenbeek et al, Cornea 2000; 19:464). PHMB is available from Leiters Park Avenue Pharmacy, San Jose, CA (800-292-6773).

2. The drug is not available commercially, but as a service can be compounded by Medical Center Pharmacy, New Haven, CT (203-688-6816) or Panorama Compounding Pharmacy 6744 Balboa Blvd, Van Nuys, CA 91406 (800-247-9767).

3. Treatment should be followed by a course of iodoquinol or paromomycin in the dosage used to treat asymptomatic amebiasis.

4. Nitazoxanide (an investigational drug in the US manufactured by Romark Laboratories, Tampa, Florida, 813-282-8544, www.romarklabs.com) 500 mg bid × 3d is also effective for treatment of amebiasis (JF Rossignol et al, *J Infect Dis* 2001; 184:381).

5. A nitro-imidazole similar to metronidazole, but not marketed in the US, tinidazole appears to be at least as effective as metronidazole and better tolerated. Ornidazole, a similar drug, is also used outside the US.

Table 4.13. Drugs for Parasitic Infections, continued

Infection	Drug	Adult Dosage	Pediatric Dosage
AMEBIC MENINGOENCEPHALITIS, PRIMARY			
Naegleria			
Drug of choice:	Amphotericin B[6,7]	1 mg/kg/d IV, uncertain duration	1 mg/kg/d IV, uncertain duration
Acanthamoeba			
Drug of choice:	See footnote 8		
Balamuthia mandrillaris			
Drug of choice:	See footnote 9		
Sappinia diploidea			
Drug of choice:	See footnote 10		
ANCYLOSTOMA caninum (Eosinophilic enterocolitis)			
Drug of choice:	Albendazole[7]	400 mg once	400 mg once
OR	Mebendazole	100 mg bid × 3d	100 mg bid × 3d
OR	Pyrantel pamoate[7]	11 mg/kg (max. 1g) × 3d	11 mg/kg (max. 1g) × 3d
OR	Endoscopic removal		

Ancylostoma duodenale, see HOOKWORM

* Availability problems. See table on page 770.

6. A *Naegleria* infection was treated successfully with intravenous and intrathecal use of both amphotericin B and miconazole, plus rifampin (J Seidel et al, *N Engl J Med* 1982; 306:346). Other reports of successful therapy are questionable.

7. An approved drug, but considered investigational for this condition by the U.S. Food and Drug Administration.

8. Strains of *Acanthamoeba* isolated from fatal granulomatous amebic encephalitis are usually susceptible *in vitro* to pentamidine, ketoconazole (*Nizoral*), flucytosine (*Ancobon*) and (less so) to amphotericin B. Chronic *Acanthamoeba* meningitis has been successfully treated in 2 children with a combination of oral trimethoprim/sulfamethoxazole, rifampin and ketoconazole (T Singhal et al, *Pediatr Infect Dis J* 2001; 20:623), and in an AIDS patient with fluconazole and sulfadiazine combined with surgical resection of the CNS lesion (M Seijo Martinez et al, *J Clin Microbiol* 2000; 38:3892). Disseminated cutaneous infection in an immunocompromised patient has been treated successfully with IV pentamidine isethionate, topical chlorhexidine, and 2% ketoconazole cream, followed by oral itraconazole (*Sporanox*) (CA Slater et al, *N Engl J Med* 1994; 331:85).

9. A free-living leptomyxid ameba that causes subacute to chronic granulomatous CNS disease. *In vitro* pentamidine isethionate 10 µg/ml is amebastatic (CF Denney et al, *Clin Infect Dis* 1997; 25:1354). One patient, according to Medical Letter consultants, was successfully treated with clarithromycin (*Biaxin*) 500 mg t.i.d., fluconazole (*Diflucan*) 400 mg once daily, sulfadiazine 1.5 g q6h and flucytosine (*Ancobon*) 1.5 g q6h.

10. A recently described free-living ameba not previously known to be pathogenic to humans. It was successfully treated with azithromycin, IV pentamidine, itraconazole and flucytosine (BB Gelman et al, *JAMA* 2001; 285:2450).

Table 4.13. Drugs for Parasitic Infections, continued

Infection	Drug	Adult Dosage	Pediatric Dosage
ANGIOSTRONGYLIASIS			
Angiostrongylus cantonensis			
Drug of choice:	See footnote 11		
Angiostrongylus costaricensis			
Drug of choice:	See footnote 12		
ANISAKIASIS (*Anisakis*)			
Treatment of choice:	Surgical or endoscopic removal		
ASCARIASIS (*Ascaris lumbricoides*, roundworm)			
Drug of choice:	Albendazole[7]	400 mg once	400 mg once
OR	Mebendazole	100 mg bid × 3d or 500 mg once	100 mg bid × 3d or 500 mg once
OR	Pyrantel pamoate[7]	11 mg/kg once (max. 1 gram)	11 mg/kg once (max. 1 gram)
BABESIOSIS (*Babesia microti*)			
Drugs of choice:[13]	Clindamycin[7]	1.2 grams bid IV or 600 mg tid PO × 7–10d	20–40 mg/kg/d PO in 3 doses × 7d
	plus quinine	650 mg tid PO × 7d	25 mg/kg/d PO in 3 doses × 7d
OR	Atovaquone[7]	750 mg bid × 7–10d	20 mg/kg bid × 7–10d
	plus azithromycin[7]	600 mg PO daily × 7–10d	12 mg/kg daily × 7–10d

Balamuthia mandrillaris, see AMEBIC MENINGOENCEPHALITIS, PRIMARY

---

* Availability problems. See table on page 770.

11. Most patients have a self-limited course and recover completely. Analgesics, corticosteroids, and careful removal of CSF at frequent intervals can relieve symptoms (FD Pien and BC Pien, *Int J Infect Dis* 1999; 3:161; V Lo Re and SJ Gluckman, *Clin Infect Dis* 2001; 33:e112). In a recent report, mebendazole and a glucocorticosteroid appeared to shorten the course of infection (H-C Tsai et al, *Am J Med* 2001; 111:109). No drug is proven to be effective and some patients have worsened when given thiabendazole, albendazole, mebendazole or ivermectin.

12. Mebendazole has been used in experimental animals.

13. Exchange transfusion has been used in severely ill patients and those with high (>10%) parasitemia (JC Hatcher et al, *Clin Infect Dis* 2001; 32:1117). Combination therapy with atovaquone and azithromycin is as effective as clindamycin/quinine and may be better tolerated (PJ Krause et al, *N Engl J Med* 2000;343:1454). Concurrent use of pentamidine and trimethoprim-sulfamethoxazole has been reported to cure an infection with *B. divergens*, the most common *Babesia* species in Europe (D Raoult et al, *Ann Intern Med* 1987; 107:944).

Table 4.13. **Drugs for Parasitic Infections, continued**

Infection	Drug	Adult Dosage	Pediatric Dosage
BALANTIDIASIS (*Balantidium coli*)			
Drug of choice:	Tetracycline[7,14]	500 mg qid × 10d	40 mg/kg/d (max. 2 g) in 4 doses × 10d
Alternatives:	Metronidazole[7]	750 mg tid × 5d	35–50 mg/kg/d in 3 doses × 5d
	Iodoquinol[7]	650 mg tid × 20d	40 mg/kg/d in 3 doses × 20d
BAYLISASCARIASIS (*Baylisascaris procyonis*)			
Drug of choice:	See footnote 15		
BLASTOCYSTIS hominis infection			
Drug of choice:	See footnote 16		
CAPILLARIASIS (*Capillaria philippinensis*)			
Drug of choice:	Mebendazole[7]	200 mg bid × 20d	200 mg bid × 20d
Alternatives:	Albendazole[7]	400 mg daily × 10d	400 mg daily × 10d
Chagas' disease, see TRYPANOSOMIASIS			
Clonorchis sinensis, see FLUKE infection			
CRYPTOSPORIDIOSIS (*Cryptosporidium*)			
Drug of choice:	See footnote 17		

*   Availability problems. See table on page 770.
14. Use of tetracyclines is contraindicated in pregnancy and in children less than 8 years old.
15. No drugs have been demonstrated to be effective. Albendazole 25 mg/kg/d × 10d started up to 3d after possible infection might prevent clinical disease and is recommended for children with known exposure (ingestion of racoon stool or contaminated soil) (*MMWR Morb Mortal Wkly Rep* 2002; 50:1153). Mebendazole, thiabendazole, levamisole (*Ergamisol*) and ivermectin could also be tried. Steroid therapy may be helpful, especially in eye and CNS infections. Ocular baylisascariasis has been treated successfully using laser photocoagulation therapy to destroy the intraretinal larvae.
16. Clinical significance of these organisms is controversial, but metronidazole 750 mg tid × 10d or iodoquinol 650 mg tid × 20d has been reported to be effective (DJ Stenzel and PFL Borenam, *Clin Microbiol Rev* 1996; 9:563). Metronidazole resistance may be common (K Haresh et al, *Trop Med Int Health* 1999; 4:274). Trimethoprim-sulfamethoxazole is an alternative regimen (UZ Ok et al, *Am J Gastroenterol* 1999; 94:3245).
17. Three days of treatment with nitazoxanide (see footnote 4) may be useful for treating cryptosporidial diarrhea in immunocompetent patients. The recommended dose in adults is 500 mg bid, in children 4–11 years old, 200 mg bid, and in children 1–3 years old, 100 mg bid (JA Rossignol et al, *J Infect Dis* 2001; 184:103). A small randomized, double-blind trial in symptomatic HIV-infected patients found paromomycin similar to placebo (RG Hewitt et al, *Clin Infect Dis* 2000;3:1084).

Table 4.13. Drugs for Parasitic Infections, continued

Infection	Drug	Adult Dosage	Pediatric Dosage
CUTANEOUS LARVA MIGRANS (creeping eruption, dog and cat hookworm)			
Drug of choice:[18]	Albendazole[7]	400 mg daily × 3d	400 mg daily × 3d
OR	Ivermectin[7]	200 µg/kg daily × 1–2d	200 µg/kg daily × 1–2d
OR	Thiabendazole	Topically	Topically
CYCLOSPORA infection			
Drug of choice:[19]	Trimethoprimsulfamethoxazole[7]	TMP 160 mg, SMX 800 mg bid × 7–10d	TMP 5 mg/kg, SMX 25 mg/kg bid × 7–10d
CYSTICERCOSIS, see TAPEWORM infection			
DIENTAMOEBA *fragilis* infection			
Drug of choice:	Iodoquinol	650 mg tid × 20d	30–40 mg/kg/d (max. 2g) in 3 doses × 20d
OR	Paromomycin[7]	25–35 mg/kg/d in 3 doses × 7d	25–35 mg/kg/d in 3 doses × 7d
OR	Tetracycline[7,14]	500 mg qid × 10d	40 mg/kg/d (max. 2g) in 4 doses × 10d
OR	Metronidazole	500–750 mg tid × 10d	20–40 mg/kg/d in 3 doses × 10d
Diphyllobothrium latum, see TAPEWORM infection			
DRACUNCULUS *medinensis* (guinea worm) infection			
Drug of choice:	Metronidazole[7,20]	250 mg tid × 10d	25 mg/kg/d (max. 750 mg) in 3 doses × 10d
Echinococcus, see TAPEWORM infection			
Entamoeba *histolytica,* see AMEBIASIS			

* Availability problems. See table on page 770.
18. G Albanese et al, *Int J Dermatol* 2001; 40:67.
19. HIV infected patients may need higher dosage and long-term maintenance. In cases of cotrimoxazole intolerance, ciprofloxacin 500 mg bid × 7d has been effective (R-I Verdier et al, *Ann Intern Med* 2000; 132:885).
20. Not curative, but decreases inflammation and facilitates removing the worm. Mebendazole 400–800 mg/d for 6d has been reported to kill the worm directly.

Table 4.13. **Drugs for Parasitic Infections, continued**

Infection	Drug	Adult Dosage	Pediatric Dosage
***ENTAMOEBA** polecki* infection			
Drug of choice:	Metronidazole[7]	750 mg tid × 10d	35–50 mg/kg/d in 3 doses × 10d
***ENTEROBIUS** vermicularis* (pinworm) infection			
Drug of choice:[21]	Pyrantel pamoate	11 mg/kg base once (max. 1 gram); repeat in 2 weeks	11 mg/kg base once (max. 1 gram); repeat in 2 weeks
OR	Mebendazole	100 mg once; repeat in 2 weeks	100 mg once; repeat in 2 weeks
OR	Albendazole[7]	400 mg once; repeat in 2 weeks	400 mg once; repeat in 2 weeks
Fasciola hepatica, see FLUKE infection			
FILARIASIS[22]			
Wuchereria bancrofti, Brugia malayi, Brugia timori			
Drug of choice:[23,24]	Diethylcarbamazine[25]*	Day 1: 50 mg, p.c. Day 2: 50 mg tid Day 3: 100 mg tid Days 4 through 14: 6 mg/kg/d in 3 doses	Day 1: 1 mg/kg p.c. Day 2: 1 mg/kg tid Day 3: 1–2 mg/kg tid Days 4 through 14: 6 mg/kg/d in 3 doses

* Availability problems. See table on page 770.

21. Since all family members are usually affected, treatment of the entire household is recommended.

22. Endosymbiotic *Wolbachia* bacteria may have a role in filarial development and host response, and may represent a new target for therapy (HF Cross et al, *Lancet* 2001; 358:1873). Doxycycline 100 mg daily × 6 weeks has eradicated *Wolbachia* and led to sterility of adult worms in onchocerciasis (A Hoerauf et al, *Lancet* 2000; 355:1241).

23. Most symptoms caused by the adult worm. Single-dose combination of albendazole (400 mg) with either ivermectin (200 μg/kg) or diethylcarbamazine (6 mg/kg) is effective for reduction or suppression of *W. bancrofti* microfilaremia (MM Ismail et al, *Trans R Soc Trop Med Hyg* 2001; 95:332; TB Nutman, *Curr Opin Infect Dis* 2001; 14:539).

24. Antihistamines or corticosteroids may be required to decrease allergic reactions due to disintegration of microfilariae in treatment of filarial infections, especially those caused by *Loa loa.*

25. For patients with no microfilariae in the blood, full doses can be given from day one.

Table 4.13. Drugs for Parasitic Infections, continued

Infection	Drug	Adult Dosage	Pediatric Dosage
FILARIASIS (continued)			
Loa loa			
Drug of choice:[24,26]	Diethylcarbamazine[25]*	Day 1: 50 mg p.c. Day 2: 50 mg tid Day 3: 100 mg tid Days 4 through 21: 9 mg/kg/d in 3 doses	Day 1: 1 mg/kg p.c. Day 2: 1 mg/kg tid Day 3: 1–2 mg/kg tid Days 4 through 21: 9 mg/kg/d in 3 doses
Mansonella ozzardi			
Drug of choice:[24]	See footnote 27		
Mansonella perstans			
Drug of choice:[24]	Mebendazole[7]	100 mg bid × 30d	100 mg bid × 30d
OR	Albendazole[7]	400 mg bid × 10d	400 mg bid × 10d
Mansonella streptocerca			
Drug of choice:[24,28]	Diethylcarbamazine* Ivermectin[7]	6 mg/kg/d × 14d 150 µg/kg once	6 mg/kg/d × 14d 150 µg/kg once
Tropical Pulmonary Eosinophilia (TPE)			
Drug of choice:	Diethylcarbamazine*	6 mg/kg/d in 3 doses × 21d	6 mg/kg/d in 3 doses × 21d
Onchocerca volvulus (River blindness)			
Drug of choice:	Ivermectin[29]	150 µg/kg once, repeated every 6 to 12 months until asymptomatic	150 µg/kg once, repeated every 6 to 12 months until asymptomatic

* Availability problems. See table on page 770.

26. In heavy infections with *Loa loa*, rapid killing of microfilariae can provoke an encephalopathy. Apheresis has been reported to be effective in lowering microfilarial counts in patients heavily infected with *Loa loa* (EA Ottesen, *Infect Dis Clin North Am* 1993; 7:619). Albendazole or ivermectin have also been used to reduce microfilaremia; albendazole is preferred because of its slower onset of action (AD Klion et al, *J Infect Dis* 1993; 168:202; M Kombila et al, *Am J Trop Med Hyg* 1998; 58:458). Albendazole may be useful for treatment of loiasis when diethylcarbamazine is ineffective or cannot be used but repeated courses may be necessary (AD Klion et al, *Clin Infect Dis* 1999; 29:680). Diethylcarbamazine, 300 mg once weekly, has been recommended for prevention of loiasis (TB Nutman et al, *N Engl J Med* 1988; 319:752).

27. Diethylcarbamazine has no effect. Ivermectin, 200 µg/kg once, has been effective.

28. Diethylcarbamazine is potentially curative due to activity against both adult worms and microfilariae. Ivermectin is only active against microfilariae.

29. Annual treatment with ivermectin 150 µg/kg can prevent blindness due to ocular onchocerciasis (D Mabey et al, *Ophthalmology* 1996; 103:1001).

Table 4.13. Drugs for Parasitic Infections, continued

Infection	Drug	Adult Dosage	Pediatric Dosage
FLUKE, hermaphroditic, infection			
Clonorchis sinensis (Chinese liver fluke)			
Drug of choice:	Praziquantel	75 mg/kg/d in 3 doses × 1d	75 mg/kg/d in 3 doses × 1d
OR	Albendazole[7]	10 mg/kg × 7d	10 mg/kg × 7d
Fasciola hepatica (sheep liver fluke)			
Drug of choice:[30]	Triclabendazole*	10 mg/kg once	10 mg/kg once
Alternative:	Bithionol*	30–50 mg/kg × 10–15 doses	30–50 mg/kg on alternate days × 10–15 doses
Fasciolopsis buski, Heterophyes heterophyes, Metagonimus yokogawai (intestinal flukes)			
Drug of choice:	Praziquantel[7]	75 mg/kg/d in 3 doses × 1d	75 mg/kg/d in 3 doses × 1d
Metorchis conjunctus (North American liver fluke)[31]			
Drug of choice:	Praziquantel[7]	75 mg/kg/d in 3 doses × 1d	75 mg/kg/d in 3 doses × 1d
Nanophyetus salmincola			
Drug of choice:	Praziquantel[7]	60 mg/kg/d in 3 doses × 1d	60 mg/kg/d in 3 doses × 1d
Opisthorchis viverrini (Southeast Asian liver fluke)			
Drug of choice:	Praziquantel	75 mg/kg/d in 3 doses × 1d	75 mg/kg/d in 3 doses × 1d
Paragonimus westermani (lung fluke)			
Drug of choice:	Praziquantel[7]	75 mg/kg/d in 3 doses × 2d	75 mg/kg/d in 3 doses × 2d
Alternative:[32]	Bithionol*	30–50 mg/kg on alternate days × 10–15 doses	30–50 mg/kg on alternate days × 10–15 doses

*   Availability problems. See table on page 770.

30. Unlike infections with other flukes, *Fasciola hepatica* infections may not respond to praziquantel. Triclabendazole, a veterinary fasciolide, may be safe and effective but data are limited (CS Graham et al, *Clin Infect Dis* 2001; 33:1). It is available from Victoria Pharmacy, Zurich, Switzerland, 41-1-211-24-32. It should be given with food for better absorption.

31. JD MacLean et al, *Lancet* 1996; 347:154.

32. Triclabendazole may be effective in a dosage of 5 mg/kg once daily for 3 days or 10 mg/kg twice in one day (M Calvopiña et al, *Trans R Soc Trop Med Hyg* 1998;92:566). See footnote 30.

Table 4.13. Drugs for Parasitic Infections, continued

Infection	Drug	Adult Dosage	Pediatric Dosage
GIARDIASIS (*Giardia lamblia*)			
Drug of choice:	Metronidazole[7]	250 mg tid × 5d	15 mg/kg/d in 3 doses × 5d
Alternatives:[33]	Quinacrine[2]	100 mg tid × 5d (max. 300 mg/d)	2 mg/kg tid × 5d (max. 300 mg/d)
	Tinidazole[5]	2 grams once	50 mg/kg once (max. 2 g)
	Furazolidone	100 mg qid × 7–10d	6 mg/kg/d in 4 doses × 7–10d
	Paromomycin[7,34]	25–35 mg/kg/d in 3 doses × 7d	25–35 mg/kg/d in 3 doses × 7d
GNATHOSTOMIASIS (*Gnathostoma spinigerum*)			
Treatment of choice:[35]	Albendazole[7]	400 mg bid × 21d	400 mg bid × 21d
OR	Ivermectin[7]	200 µg/kg/d × 2d	200 µg/kg/d × 2d
OR	Surgical removal		
GONGYLONEMIASIS (*Gongylonema sp.*)			
Treatment of choice:	Surgical removal		
OR	Albendazole[7,36]	10 mg/kg/d × 3 d	10 mg/kg/d × 3 d
HOOKWORM infection (*Ancylostoma duodenale, Necator americanus*)			
Drug of choice:	Albendazole[7]	400 mg once	400 mg once
OR	Mebendazole	100 mg bid × 3d or 500 mg once	100 mg bid × 3d or 500 mg once
OR	Pyrantel pamoate[7]	11 mg/kg (max. 1g) × 3d	11 mg/kg (max. 1g) × 3d

Hydatid cyst, see TAPEWORM infection

* Availability problems. See table on page 770.

33. In one study, nitazoxanide (see footnote 4) was as effective as metronidazole and has been used successfully in high doses to treat a case of *Giardia* resistant to metronidazole and albendazole (JJ Ortiz et al, *Aliment Pharmacol Ther* 2001; 15:1409; P Abboud et al, *Clin Infect Dis* 2001; 32:1792). Albendazole 400 mg daily × 5d may be effective (A Hall and Q Nahar, *Trans R Soc Trop Med Hyg* 1993; 87:84; AK Dutta et al, Indian *J Pediatr* 1994; 61:689). Bacitracin zinc or bacitracin 120,000 U bid for 10 days may also be effective (BJ Andrews et al, *Am J Trop Med Hyg* 1995; 52:318). Combination treatment with standard doses of metronidazole and quinacrine given for 3 weeks has been effective for a small number of refractory infections (TE Nash et al, *Clin Infect Dis* 2001; 33:22).

34. Not absorbed; may be useful for treatment of giardiasis in pregnancy.

35. F Chappuis et al, *Clin Infect Dis* 2001; 33:e17; P Nontasut et al, Southeast Asian *J Trop Med Public Health* 2000; 31:374.

36. One patient has been successfully treated with albendazole (ML Eberhard and C Busillo, *Am J Trop Med Hyg* 1999; 61:51).

Table 4.13. Drugs for Parasitic Infections, continued

Infection	Drug	Adult Dosage	Pediatric Dosage
Hymenolepis nana, see TAPEWORM infection			
ISOSPORIASIS (*Isospora belli*)			
Drug of choice:[37]	Trimethoprimsulfa-methoxazole[7]	160 mg TMP, 800 mg SMX bid × 10d	TMP 5 mg/kg, SMX 25 mg/kg bid × 10d
LEISHMANIASIS[38]			
Drug of choice:[39]	Sodium stibogluconate*	20 mg Sb/kg/d IV or IM × 20–28d[40]	20 mg Sb/kg/d IV or IM × 20–28d[40]
OR	Meglumine antimonate*	20 mg Sb/kg/d IV or IM × 20–27d[40]	20 mg Sb/kg/d IV or IM × 20–28d[40]
OR	Amphotericin B[7]	0.5 to 1 mg/kg IV daily or every 2d for up to 8 wks	0.5 to 1 mg/kg IV daily or every 2d for up to 8 wks

* Availability problems. See table on page 770.

37. Immunosuppressed patients: TMP/SMX qid × 10d followed by bid × 3 weeks. In sulfonamide-sensitive patients, pyrimethamine 50–75 mg daily in divided doses has been effective. HIV-infected patients may need long-term maintenance. Ciprofloxacin 500 mg bid × 7d has also been effective (R-I Verdier et al, *Ann Intern Med* 2000; 132:885).

38. Treatment dosage and duration vary based on the disease symptoms, host immune status, species, and the area of the world where infection was acquired. Cutaneous infection is due to *L. mexicana, L. tropica, L. major, L. braziliensis*; mucocutaneous is mostly due to *L. braziliensis*, and visceral is due to *L. donovani* (Kala-azar). *L. infantum, L. chagasi.* Dosage range listed includes many, but not all possibilities.

39. For treatment of kala-azar, oral miltefosine 100 mg daily for 4 weeks was 97% effective after 6 months in one study. Gastrointestinal adverse effects are common and the drug is contraindicated in pregnancy (TK Jha et al, *N Engl J Med* 1999; 341:1795). In an uncontrolled trial, oral miltefosine was effective for the treatment of American cutaneous leishmaniasis at a dosage of about 2.25 mg/kg/day for 3–4 wks. "Motion sickness" was the most frequent adverse effect (J Soto et al, *Clin Infect Dis* 2001; 33:e57).

40. May be repeated or continued. A longer duration may be needed for some forms of visceral leishmaniasis (BL Herwaldt, *Lancet* 1999; 354:1191).

41. Three preparations of lipid-encapsulated amphotericin B have been used for treatment of visceral leishmaniasis. Largely based on clinical trials in patients infected with *L. infantum*, the FDA approved liposomal amphotericin B (*AmBisome*) for treatment of visceral leishmaniasis (A Meyerhoff, *Clin Infect Dis* 1999; 28:42; JD Berman, *Clin Infect Dis* 1999; 28:49). Amphotericin B lipid complex (*Abelcet*) and amphotericin B cholesteryl sulfate (*Amphotec*) have also been used with good results. Limited data in a few patients suggest that liposomal amphotericin B may also be effective for mucocutaneous disease (VS Amato et al, *J Antimicrob Chemother* 2000; 46:341; RNR Sampaio and PD Marsden, *Trans R Soc Trop Med Hyg* 1997; 91:77). Some studies indicate that *L. donovani* resistant to pentavalent antimonial agents may respond to lipid-encapsulated amphotericin B (S Sundar et al, *Ann Trop Med Parasitol* 1998; 92:755).

Table 4.13. Drugs for Parasitic Infections, continued

Infection	Drug	Adult Dosage	Pediatric Dosage
LEISHMANIASIS[38], continued			
OR	Liposomal Amphotericin B[41]	3 mg/kg/d (days 1-5) and 3 mg/kg/d days 14, 21[42]	3 mg/kg/d (days 1-5) and 3 mg/kg/d days 14, 21[42]
Alternatives:	Pentamidine	2–4 mg/kg daily or every 2d IV or IM for up to 15 doses[43]	2–4 mg/kg daily or every 2d IV or IM for up to 15 doses[43]
OR	Paromomycin[44]*	Topically 2x/d × 10–20d	
LICE infestation (*Pediculus humanus, P. capitis, Phthirus pubis*)[45]			
Drug of choice:	1% Permethrin[46]	Topically	Topically
OR	0.5% Malathion[47]	Topically	Topically
Alternative:	Pyrethrins with piperonyl butoxide[46]	Topically	Topically
OR	Ivermectin[7,48]	200 μg/kg once	200 μg/kg once
Loa loa, see FILARIASIS			

* Availability problems. See table on page 770.

42. The dose for immunocompromised patients with HIV is 4 mg/kg/d (days 1–5) and 4 mg/kg/d on days 10,17,24,31,38. The relapse rate is high, suggesting that maintenance therapy may be indicated.

43. For *L. donovani:* 4 mg/kg once/day × 15 doses; for cutaneous disease: 2 mg/kg once/day × 7 or 3 mg/kg once/day × 4 doses.

44. Topical paromomycin can only be used in geographic regions where cutaneous leishmaniasis species have low potential for mucosal spread. A formulation of 15% paromomycin and 12% methylbenzethonium chloride (*Leshcutan*) in soft white paraffin for topical use, has been reported to be effective in some patients against cutaneous leishmaniasis due to *L. major* (O Ozgoztasi and I Baydar, *Int J Dermatol* 1997; 36:61; BA Arana et al, *Am J Trop Med Hyg* 2001; 65:466).

45. For infestation of eyelashes with crab lice, use petrolatum. For pubic lice, treat with 5% permethrin or ivermectin as for scabies (see page 9).

46. A second application is recommended one week later to kill hatching progeny. Some lice are resistant to pyrethrins and permethrin (RJ Pollack, *Arch Pediatr Adolesc Med* 1999; 153:969).

47. RJ Roberts et al, *Lancet* 2000; 356:540.

48. Ivermectin is effective against adult lice but has no effect on nits (TA Bell, *Pediatr Infect Dis J* 1998; 17:923).

Table 4.13. **Drugs for Parasitic Infections, continued**

Infection	Drug	Adult Dosage	Pediatric Dosage
MALARIA, Treatment of (*Plasmodium falciparum, P. ovale, P. vivax, and P. malariae*)			
Chloroquine-resistant *P. falciparum* [49]			
ORAL			
Drugs of choice:	Quinine sulfate	650 mg q8h × 3–7d [50]	25mg/kg/d in 3 doses × 3–7d [50]
	plus		
	doxycycline [7,14]	100 mg bid × 7d	2 mg/kg/d × 7d
	or plus		
	tetracycline [7,14]	250 mg qid × 7d	6.25 mg/kg qid × 7d
	or plus		
	pyrimethamine-sulfadoxine [51]	3 tablets at once on last day of quinine	<1 yr: ¼ tablet 1–3 yrs: ½ tablet 4–8 yrs: 1 tablet 9–14 yrs: 2 tablets
	or plus		
	clindamycin [7,52]	900 mg tid × 5d	20–40 mg/kg/d in 3 doses × 5d
OR	Atovaquone/proguanil [53]	2 adult tablets bid × 3d	11–20 kg: 1 adult tablet/day × 3d 21–30 kg: 2 adult tablets/day × 3d 31–40 kg: 3 adult tablets/day × 3d >40 kg: 2 adult tablets bid × 3d

* Availability problems. See table on page 770.

49. Chloroquine-resistant *P. falciparum* occur in all malarious areas except Central America west of the Panama Canal Zone, Mexico, Haiti, the Dominican Republic, and most of the Middle East (chloroquine resistance has been reported in Yemen, Oman, Saudi Arabia and Iran).

50. In Southeast Asia, relative resistance to quinine has increased and the treatment should be continued for 7 days.

51. *Fansidar* tablets contain 25 mg of pyrimethamine and 500 mg of sulfadoxine. Resistance to pyrimethamine-sulfadoxine has been reported from Southeast Asia, the Amazon basin, sub-Saharan Africa, Bangladesh and Oceania.

52. For use in pregnancy.

53. Atovaquone plus proguanil is available as a fixed-dose combination tablet: adult tablets (250 mg atovaquone/100 mg proguanil, *Malarone*) and pediatric tablets (62.5 mg atovaquone/25 mg proguanil, *Malarone Pediatric*). To enhance absorption, it should be taken within 45 minutes after eating (S Looaresuwan et al, *Am J Trop Med Hyg* 1999; 60:533). Although approved for once daily dosing, to decrease nausea and vomiting the dose for treatment is usually divided in two.

Table 4.13. Drugs for Parasitic Infections, continued

Infection	Drug	Adult Dosage	Pediatric Dosage
MALARIA, Treatment of, continued			
Alternatives:[54]	Mefloquine[55, 56]	750 mg followed by 500 mg 12 hrs later	<45 kg: 15 mg/kg PO followed by 10 mg/kg PO 8–12 hours later
	Halofantrine[57]*	500 mg q6h × 3 doses; repeat in 1 week[58]	<40 kg: 8 mg/kg q6h × 3 doses; repeat in 1 week[58]
OR	Artesunate[59]* **plus**	4 mg/kg/d × 3d	
	mefloquine[55, 56]	750 mg followed by 500 mg 12 hrs later	15 mg/kg followed 8–12 hrs later by 10 mg/kg
Chloroquine-resistant P. vivax[60]			
Drug of choice:	Quinine sulfate **plus**	650 mg q8h × 3–7d[50]	25 mg/kg/d in 3 doses × 3–7d[50]
	doxycycline[7,14]	100 mg bid × 7d	2 mg/kg/d × 7d
OR	Mefloquine[55,56]	750 mg followed by 500 mg 12 hr later	15 mg/kg followed 8–12 hrs later by 10 mg/kg

* Availability problems. See table on page 770.

54. For treatment of multiple-drug-resistant *P. falciparum* in Southeast Asia, especially Thailand, where resistance to mefloquine and halofantrine is frequent, a 7-day course of quinine and tetracycline is recommended (G Watt et al, *Am J Trop Med Hyg* 1992; 47:108). Artesunate plus mefloquine (C Luxemburger et al, *Trans R Soc Trop Med Hyg* 1994; 88:213), artemether plus mefloquine (J Karbwang et al, *Trans R Soc Trop Med Hyg* 1995; 89:296), mefloquine plus doxycycline or atovaquone/proguanil may also be used to treat multiple-drug-resistant *P. falciparum*.

55. At this dosage, adverse effects including nausea, vomiting, diarrhea, dizziness, disturbed sense of balance, toxic psychosis and seizures can occur. Mefloquine is teratogenic in animals and should not be used for treatment of malaria in pregnancy. It should not be given together with quinine, quinidine or halofantrine, and caution is required in using quinine, quinidine or halofantrine to treat patients with malaria who have taken mefloquine for prophylaxis. The pediatric dosage has not been approved by the FDA. Resistance to mefloquine has been reported in some areas, such as the Thailand-Myanmar and -Cambodia borders and in the Amazon basin, where 25 mg/kg should be used.

56. In the US, a 250-mg tablet of mefloquine contains 228 mg mefloquine base. Outside the US, each 275-mg tablet contains 250 mg base.

Table 4.13. Drugs for Parasitic Infections, continued

Infection	Drug	Adult Dosage	Pediatric Dosage
MALARIA, Treatment of, continued			
Alternatives:	Halofantrine[57, 61]*	500 mg q6h × 3 doses	8 mg/kg q6h × 3 doses
	Chloroquine **plus**	25 mg base/kg in 3 doses over 48 hrs	
	primaquine[62]	2.5 mg base/kg in 3 doses over 48 hrs	
All *Plasmodium* except Chloroquine-resistant *P. falciparum*[49] and Chloroquine-resistant *P. vivax*[60]			
ORAL			
Drug of choice:	Chloroquine phosphate[63]	1 gram (600 mg base), then 500 mg (300 mg base) 6 hrs later, then 500 mg (300 mg base) at 24 and 48 hrs	10 mg base/kg (max. 600 mg base), then 5 mg base/kg 6 hrs later, then 5 mg base/kg at 24 and 48 hrs

* Availability problems. See table on page 770.

57. May be effective in multiple-drug-resistant *P. falciparum* malaria, but treatment failures and resistance have been reported, and the drug has caused lengthening of the PR and QTc intervals and fatal cardiac arrhythmias. It should not be used for patients with cardiac conduction defects or with other drugs that may affect the QT interval, such as quinine, quinidine and mefloquine. Cardiac monitoring is recommended. Variability in absorption is a problem; halofantrine should not be taken one hour before to two hours after meals because food increases its absorption. It should not be used in pregnancy.

58. A single 250-mg dose can be used for repeat treatment in mild to moderate infections (JE Touze et al, *Lancet* 1997; 349:255).

59. K Na-Bangchang, *Trop Med Int Health* 1999; 4:602.

60. *P. vivax* with decreased susceptibility to chloroquine is a significant problem in Papua-New Guinea and Indonesia. There are also a few reports of resistance from Myanmar, India, Thailand, the Solomon Islands, Vanuatu, Guyana, Brazil, Colombia and Peru.

61. JK Baird el al, *J Infect Dis* 1995; 171:1678.

62. Primaquine phosphate can cause hemolytic anemia, especially in patients whose red cells are deficient in glucose-6-phosphate dehydrogenase. This deficiency is most common in African, Asian and Mediterranean peoples. Patients should be screened for G-6-PD deficiency before treatment. Primaquine should not be used during pregnancy.

63. If chloroquine phosphate is not available, hydroxychloroquine sulfate is as effective; 400 mg of hydroxychloroquine sulfate is equivalent to 500 mg of chloroquine phosphate.

Table 4.13. **Drugs for Parasitic Infections, continued**

Infection	Drug	Adult Dosage	Pediatric Dosage
MALARIA, Treatment of, continued			
All *Plasmodium*			
PARENTERAL			
Drug of choice:[64]	Quinidine gluconate[65]	10 mg/kg loading dose (max. 600 mg) in normal saline slowly over 1 to 2 hrs, followed by continuous infusion of 0.02 mg/kg/min until oral therapy can be started	Same as adult dose
OR	Quinine dihydro-chloride[65]	20 mg/kg loading dose IV in 5% dextrose over 4 hrs, followed by 10 mg/kg over 2–4 hrs q8h (max. 1800 mg/d) until oral therapy can be started	Same as adult dose
Alternative:	Artemether[66]*	3.2 mg/kg IM, then 1.6 mg/kg daily × 5–7d	Same as adult dose
Prevention of relapses: *P. vivax* and *P. ovale* only			
Drug of choice:	Primaquine phosphate[62,67]	26.3 mg (15 mg base)/d × 14d or 79 mg (45 mg base)/wk × 8 wks	0.3 mg base/kg/d × 14d

* Availability problems. See table on page 770.

64. Exchange transfusion has been helpful for some patients with high-density (>10%) parasitemia, altered mental status, pulmonary edema or renal complications (KD Miller et al, *N Engl J Med* 1989; 321:65).

65. Continuous EKG, blood pressure and glucose monitoring are recommended, especially in pregnant women and young children. For problems with quinidine availability, call the manufacturer (Eli Lilly, 800-821-0538) or the CDC Malaria Hotline (770-488-7788). Quinidine may have greater antimalarial activity than quinine. The loading dose should be decreased or omitted in those patients who have received quinine or mefloquine. If more than 48 hours of parenteral treatment is required, the quinine or quinidine dose should be reduced by ⅓ to ½.

66. Artemether-Quinine Meta-Analysis Study Group, *Trans R Soc Trop Med Hyg* 2001; 95:637. Not available in the US.

67. Relapses have been reported with this regimen, and should be treated with a second 14-day course of 30 mg base/day. In Southeast Asia and Somalia the higher dose (30 mg base/day) should be used initially.

Table 4.13. Drugs for Parasitic Infections, continued

Infection	Drug	Adult Dosage	Pediatric Dosage
MALARIA, Prevention of[68]			
Chloroquine-sensitive areas[49]			
Drug of choice:	Chloroquine phosphate[69,70]	500 mg (300 mg base), once/week[71]	5 mg/kg base once/week, up to adult dose of 300 mg base[71]
Chloroquine-resistant areas[49]			
Drug of choice:	Mefloquine[56,70,72]	250 mg once/week[71]	<15 kg: 5 mg/kg[71] 15–19 kg: ¼ tablet[71] 20–30 kg: ½ tablet[71] 31–45 kg: ¾ tablet[71] >45 kg: 1 tablet[71]
OR	Doxycycline[7,70]	100 mg daily[73]	2 mg/kg/d, up to 100 mg/day[73]
OR	Atovaquone/ Proguanil[53,70]	250 mg/100 mg (1 adult tablet) daily[74]	11–20 kg: 62.5 mg/25 mg[53,74] 21–30 kg: 125 mg/50 mg[53,74] 31–40 kg: 187.5 mg/75 mg[53,74] >40 kg: 250 mg/100 mg[53,74]

*   Availability problems. See table on page 770.

68. No drug regimen guarantees protection against malaria. If fever develops within a year (particularly within the first two months) after travel to malarious areas, travelers should be advised to seek medical attention. Insect repellents, insecticide-impregnated bed nets and proper clothing are important adjuncts for malaria prophylaxis.

69. In pregnancy, chloroquine prophylaxis has been used extensively and safely.

70. For prevention of attack after departure from areas where *P. vivax* and *P. ovale* are endemic, which includes almost all areas where malaria is found (except Haiti), some experts prescribe in addition primaquine phosphate 26.3 mg (15 mg base)/d or, for children, 0.3 mg base/kg/d during the last two weeks of prophylaxis. Others prefer to avoid the toxicity of primaquine and rely on surveillance to detect cases when they occur, particularly when exposure was limited or doubtful. See also footnotes 62 and 67.

71. Beginning one to two weeks before travel and continuing weekly for the duration of stay and for four weeks after leaving.

72. The pediatric dosage has not been approved by the FDA, and the drug has not been approved for use during pregnancy. However, it has been reported to be safe for prophylactic use during the second or third trimester of pregnancy and possibly during early pregnancy as well (CDC Health Information for International Travel, 2001–2002, page 113; BL Smoak et al, J Infect Dis 1997; 176:831). Mefloquine is not recommended for patients with cardiac conduction abnormalities. Patients with a history of seizures or psychiatric disorders should avoid mefloquine (*Medical Letter* 1990; 32:13). Resistance to mefloquine has been reported in some areas, such as Thailand; in these areas, doxycycline should be used for prophylaxis. In children less than eight years old, proguanil plus sulfisoxazole has been used (KN Suh and JS Keystone, *Infect Dis Clin Pract* 1996; 5:541).

Table 4.13. Drugs for Parasitic Infections, continued

Infection	Drug	Adult Dosage	Pediatric Dosage
MALARIA, Prevention of (continued)			
Chloroquine-resistant areas[49], continued			
Alternatives:	Primaquine[7,62,75]	30 mg base daily	0.5 mg/kg base daily
	Chloroquine phosphate	500 mg (300 mg base) once/week[71]	5 mg/kg base once/week, up to adult dose of 300 mg base[71]
	plus proguanil[76]	200 mg once/day	<2 yrs: 50 mg once/day
			2–6 yrs: 100 mg once/day
			7–10 yrs: 150 mg once/day
			>10 yrs: 200 mg once/day
Presumptive treatment	Atovaquone/proguanil[53]	2 adult tablets bid × 3d[74]	11–20 kg: one adult tablet/day × 3d[74]
			21–30 kg: 2 adult tablets/day × 3d[74]
			31–40 kg: 3 adult tablets/day × 3d[74]
			>40 kg: 2 adult tablets bid × 3d[74]
OR	Pyrimethamine-sulfadoxine[51]	Carry a single dose (3 tablets) for self treatment of febrile illness when medical care is not immediately available	<1 yr: ¼ tablet
			1–3 yrs: ½ tablet
			4–8 yrs: 1 tablet
			9–14 yrs: 2 tablets

* Availability problems. See table on page 770.

73. Beginning 1–2 days before travel and continuing for the duration of stay and for 4 weeks after leaving. Use of tetracyclines is contraindicated in pregnancy and in children less than eight years old. Doxycycline can cause gastrointestinal disturbances, vaginal moniliasis and photosensitivity reactions.

74. GE Shanks et al, *Clin Infect Dis* 1998; 27:494; B Lell et al, *Lancet* 1998; 351:709. Beginning 1 to 2 days before travel and continuing for the duration of stay and for 1 week after leaving. In one study of malaria prophylaxis, atovaquone/proguanil was better tolerated than mefloquine in nonimmune travelers (D Overbosch et al, *Clin Infect Dis* 2001; 33:1015).

75. Several studies have shown that daily primaquine beginning one day before departure and continued until 7 days after leaving the malaria area provides effective prophylaxis against chloroquine-resistant *P. falciparum* (JK Baird et al, *Clin Infect Dis* 2001; 33:1990). Some studies have shown less efficacy against *P. vivax*. Nausea and abdominal pain can be diminished by taking with food.

76. Proguanil (*Paludrine*—Wyeth Ayerst, Canada; AstraZeneca, United Kingdom), which is not available alone in the US but is widely available in Canada and Europe, is recommended mainly for use in Africa south of the Sahara. Prophylaxis is recommended during exposure and for four weeks afterwards. Proguanil has been used in pregnancy without evidence of toxicity (PA Phillips-Howard and D Wood, *Drug Saf* 1996; 14:131).

Table 4.13. Drugs for Parasitic Infections, continued

Infection	Drug	Adult Dosage	Pediatric Dosage
MICROSPORIDIOSIS			
Ocular (*Encephalitozoon hellem, Encephalitozoon cuniculi, Vittaforma corneae [Nosema corneum]*)			
Drug of choice:	Albendazole[7]	400 mg bid	
	plus fumagillin[77]*		
Intestinal (*Enterocytozoon bieneusi, Encephalitozoon [Septata] intestinalis*)			
E. bieneusi[78]			
Drug of choice:	Fumagillin*	60 mg/d PO × 14d	
E. intestinalis			
Drug of choice:	Albendazole[7]	400 mg bid × 21d	
Disseminated (*E. hellem, E. cuniculi, E. intestinalis, Pleistophora sp., Trachipleistophora sp. and Brachiola vesicularum*)			
Drug of choice:[79]	Albendazole[7]	400 mg bid	
Mites, see SCABIES			
MONILIFORMIS moniliformis infection			
Drug of choice:	Pyrantel pamoate[7]	11 mg/kg once, repeat twice, 2 wks apart	11 mg/kg once, repeat twice, 2 wks apart
***Naegleria* species,** see AMEBIC MENINGOENCEPHALITIS, PRIMARY			
Necator americanus, see HOOKWORM infection			
OESOPHAGOSTOMUM* *bifurcum			
Drug of choice:	See footnote 80		

---

* Availability problems. See table on page 770.

77. Ocular lesions due to *E. hellem* in HIV-infected patients have responded to fumagillin eyedrops prepared from *Fumidil-B*, a commercial product (Mid-Continent Agrimarketing, Inc., Olathe, Kansas, 800-547-1392) used to control a microsporidial disease of honey bees (MC Diesenhouse, *Am J Ophthalmol* 1993; 115:293). For lesions due to *V. corneae*, topical therapy is generally not effective and keratoplasty may be required (RM Davis et al, *Ophthalmology* 1990; 97:953).

78. Oral fumagillin (see footnote 77, Sanofi Recherche, Gentilly, France) has been effective in treating *E. bieneusi* (J-M Molina et al, *AIDS* 2000; 14:1341), but has been associated with thrombocytopenia. Highly active antiretroviral therapy (HAART) may lead to microbiologic and clinical response in HIV-infected patients with microsporidial diarrhea (NA Foudraine et al, *AIDS* 1998; 12:35; A Carr et al, *Lancet* 1998; 351:256). Octreotide (*Sandostatin*) has provided symptomatic relief in some patients with large volume diarrhea.

79. J-M Molina et al, *J Infect Dis* 1995; 171:245. There is no established treatment for *Pleistophora.*

80. Albendazole or pyrantel pamoate may be effective (HP Krepel et al, *Trans R Soc Trop Med Hyg* 1993; 87:87).

Table 4.13. **Drugs for Parasitic Infections, continued**

Infection	Drug	Adult Dosage	Pediatric Dosage
Onchocerca volvulus, see FILARIASIS			
Opisthorchis viverrini, see FLUKE infection			
Paragonimus westermani, see FLUKE infection			
Pediculus capitis, humanus, Phthirus pubis, see LICE			
Pinworm, see ENTEROBIUS			
PNEUMOCYSTIS carinii pneumonia (PCP)[81]			
Drug of choice:	Trimethoprimsulfa-methoxazole	TMP 15 mg/kg/d, SMX 75 mg/kg/d, oral or IV in 3 or 4 doses × 14–21d	Same as adult dose
Alternatives:	Primaquine[7,62] **plus** clindamycin[7]	30 mg base PO daily × 21 days 600 mg IV q6h × 21 days, or 300–450 mg PO q6h × 21 days	
OR	Trimethoprim[7] **plus** dapsone[7]	5 mg/kg PO tid × 21 days 100 mg PO daily × 21 days	
	Pentamidine	3–4 mg/kg IV daily × 14–21 days	Same as adult dose
OR	Atovaquone	750 mg bid PO × 21d	
Primary and secondary prophylaxis[82]			
Drug of Choice:	Trimethoprimsulfa-methoxazole	1 tab (single or double strength) daily	TMP 150 mg/m², SMX 750 mg/m² in 2 doses on 3 consecutive days per week
Alternatives:[83]	Dapsone[7]	50 mg bid, or 100 mg daily	2 mg/kg (max. 100 mg) daily or 4 mg/kg (max. 200 mg each week)

* Availability problems. See table on page 770.
81. In severe disease with room air PO$_2$ ≤ 70 mmHg or Aa gradient ≥ 35 mmHg, prednisone should also be used (S Gagnon et al, *N Engl J Med* 1990; 323:1444; E Caumes et al, *Clin Infect Dis* 1994; 18:319).
82. Primary/secondary prophylaxis in patients with HIV can be discontinued after CD4 count increases to >200 × 10⁶/L for more than 3 months (HIV/AIDS Treatment Information Service, US Department of Health and Human Services 2001; www.hivatis.org).
83. An alternative trimethoprim/sulfamethoxazole regimen is one DS tab 3x/week. Weekly therapy with sulfadoxine 500 mg/pyrimethamine 25 mg/leucovorin 25 mg was effective PCP prophylaxis in liver transplant patients (J Torre-Cisneros et al, *Clin Infect Dis* 1999; 29:771).

Table 4.13. Drugs for Parasitic Infections, continued

Infection	Drug	Adult Dosage	Pediatric Dosage
PNEUMOCYSTIS carinii pneumonia (PCP)[81], continued			
OR	Dapsone[7]	50 mg daily or 200 mg each week	
	plus pyrimethamine[84]	50 mg or 75 mg each week	
OR	Pentamidine aerosol	300 mg inhaled monthly via *Respirgard II* nebulizer	≥5 yrs: same as adult dose
OR	Atovaquone[7]	1500 mg daily	
Roundworm, see ASCARIASIS			
Sappinia Diploidea, See AMEBIC MENINGOENCEPHALITIS, PRIMARY			
SCABIES (*Sarcoptes scabiei*)			
Drug of choice:	5% Permethrin	Topically	Topically
Alternatives:	Ivermectin[7,85]	200 μg/kg PO once	200 μg/kg PO once
	10% Crotamiton	Topically once/daily × 2	Topically once/daily × 2
SCHISTOSOMIASIS (*Bilharziasis*)			
S. haematobium			
Drug of choice:	Praziquantel	40 mg/kg/d in 2 doses × 1d	40 mg/kg/d in 2 doses × 1d
S. japonicum			
Drug of choice:	Praziquantel	60 mg/kg/d in 3 doses × 1d	60 mg/kg/d in 3 doses × 1d
S. mansoni			
Drug of choice:	Praziquantel	40 mg/kg/d in 2 doses × 1d	40 mg/kg/d in 2 doses × 1d
Alternative:	Oxamniquine[86]	15 mg/kg once[87]	20 mg/kg/d in 2 doses × 1d[87]
S. mekongi			
Drug of choice:	Praziquantel	60 mg/kg/d in 3 doses × 1d	60 mg/kg/d in 3 doses × 1d

*   Availability problems. See table on page 770.

84. Plus leucovorin 25 mg with each dose of pyrimethamine.

85. Effective for crusted scabies in immunocompromised patients (M Larralde et al, *Pediatr Dermatol* 1999; 16:69;
A Patel et al, *Australas J Dermatol* 1999; 40:37; O Chosidow, *Lancet* 2000; 355:819).

86. Oxamniquine has been effective in some areas in which praziquantel is less effective (FF Stelma et al, *J Infect Dis* 1997; 176:304).
Oxamniquine is contraindicated in pregnancy.

Table 4.13. Drugs for Parasitic Infections, continued

Infection	Drug	Adult Dosage	Pediatric Dosage
Sleeping sickness, see TRYPANOSOMIASIS			
STRONGYLOIDIASIS (*Strongyloides stercoralis*)			
Drug of choice:[88]	Ivermectin	200 µg/kg/d × 1–2d	200 µg/kg/d × 1–2d
Alternative:	Thiabendazole	50 mg/kg/d in 2 doses (max. 3 grams/d) × 2d[89]	50 mg/kg/d in 2 doses (max. 3 grams/d) × 2d[89]
TAPEWORM infection			
— Adult (intestinal stage)			
Diphyllobothrium latum (fish), *Taenia saginata* (beef), *Taenia solium* (pork), *Dipylidium caninum* (dog)			
Drug of choice:	Praziquantel[7]	5–10 mg/kg once	5–10 mg/kg once
Alternative:	Niclosamide	2 g once	50 mg/kg once
Hymenolepis nana (dwarf tapeworm)			
Drug of choice:	Praziquantel[7]	25 mg/kg once	25 mg/kg once
— Larval (tissue stage)			
Echinococcus granulosus (hydatid cyst)			
Drug of choice:[90]	Albendazole	400 mg bid × 1–6 months	15 mg/kg/d (max. 800 mg) × 1–6 months
Echinococcus multilocularis			
Treatment of choice:	See footnote 91		

* Availability problems. See table on page 770.

87. In East Africa, the dose should be increased to 30 mg/kg, and in Egypt and South Africa to 30 mg/kg/d × 2d. Some experts recommend 40–60 mg/kg over 2–3 days in all of Africa (KC Shekhar, *Drugs* 1991; 42:379).

88. In immunocompromised patients or disseminated disease, it may be necessary to prolong or repeat therapy or use other agents. A veterinary parenteral formulation of ivermectin was used in one patient (PL Chiodini et al, *Lancet* 2000; 355:43).

89. This dose is likely to be toxic and may have to be decreased.

90. Patients may benefit from or require surgical resection of cysts. Praziquantel is useful preoperatively or in case of spill during surgery. Percutaneous drainage with ultrasound guidance plus albendazole therapy has been effective for management of hepatic hydatid cyst disease (MS Khuroo et al, *N Engl J Med* 1997; 337:881; O Akhan and M Ozman, *Eur J Radiol* 1999; 32:76).

91. Surgical excision or the PAIR (Puncture, Aspirate, Inject, Re-aspirate) technique is the only reliable means of cure. Reports have suggested that in nonresectable cases use of albendazole or mebendazole can stabilize and sometimes cure infection (W Hao et al, *Trans R Soc Trop Med Hyg* 1994; 88:340; WHO Group, *Bull WHO* 1996; 74:231).

Table 4.13. Drugs for Parasitic Infections, continued

Infection	Drug	Adult Dosage	Pediatric Dosage
TAPEWORM infection, continued			
Cysticercus cellulosae (**cysticercosis**)			
Treatment of choice:	See footnote 92		
Alternative:	Albendazole	400 mg bid × 8–30d; can be repeated as necessary	15 mg/kg/d (max. 800 mg) in 2 doses × 8–30d; can be repeated as necessary
OR	Praziquantel[7]	50–100 mg/kg/d in 3 doses × 30d	50–100 mg/kg/d in 3 doses × 30d
Toxocariasis, see VISCERAL LARVA MIGRANS			
TOXOPLASMOSIS (*Toxoplasma gondii*)[93]			
Drugs of choice:[94]	Pyrimethamine[95]	25–100 mg/d × 3–4 wks	2 mg/kg/d × 3d, (max. 25 mg/d) × 4 wks[96]
	plus sulfadiazine	1–1.5 grams qid × 3–4 wks	100–200 mg/kg/d × 3–4 wks

* Availability problems. See table on page 770.

92. Initial therapy of parenchymal disease with seizures should focus on symptomatic treatment with anticonvulsant drugs. Treatment of parenchymal disease with albendazole and praziquantel is controversial and randomized trials have not been conclusive. Obstructive hydrocephalus is treated with surgical removal of the obstructing cyst or CSF diversion. Prednisone 40 mg daily may be given in conjunction with surgery. Arachnoiditis, vasculitis or cerebral edema is treated with prednisone 60 mg daily or dexamethasone 4–16 mg/d combined with albendazole or praziquantel (AC White, Jr, *Annu Rev Med* 2000; 51:187). Patients with subarachnoid cysts or giant cysts in the fissures should receive albendazole for at least 30 days (JV Proano et al, *N Engl J Med* 2001; 345:879). Any cysticercocidal drug may cause irreparable damage when used to treat ocular or spinal cysts, even when corticosteroids are used. An ophthalmic exam should always be done before treatment to rule out intraocular cysts.

93. In ocular toxoplasmosis with macular involvement, corticosteroids are recommended for an anti-inflammatory effect on the eyes.

94. To treat CNS toxoplasmosis in HIV-infected patients, some clinicians have used pyrimethamine 50 to 100 mg daily (after a loading dose of 200 mg) with sulfadiazine and, when sulfonamide sensitivity developed, have given clindamycin 1.8 to 2.4 g/d in divided doses instead of the sulfonamide (JS Remington et al, *Lancet* 1991; 338:1142; BJ Luft et al, *N Engl J Med* 1993; 329:995). Atovaquone plus pyrimethamine appears to be an effective alternative in sulfa-intolerant patients (JA Kovacs et al, *Lancet* 1992; 340:637). Treatment is followed by chronic suppression with lower dosage regimens of the same drugs. For primary prophylaxis in HIV patients with <100 CD4 cells, either trimethoprim-sulfamethoxazole, pyrimethamine with dapsone or atovaquone with or without pyrimethamine can be used. Primary/Secondary prophylaxis may be discontinued when the CD4 count increases to >200 × 10⁶/L for more than 3 months (HIV/AIDS Treatment Information Service US Department of Health and Human Services 2001; (www.hivatis.org). See also footnote 95.

95. Plus leucovorin 10 to 25 mg with each dose of pyrimethamine.

96. Congenitally infected newborns should be treated with pyrimethamine every two or three days and a sulfonamide daily for about one year (JS Remington and G Desmonts in JS Remington and JO Klein, eds, *Infectious Disease of the Fetus and Newborn Infant*, 5th ed, Philadelphia:Saunders, 2001, page 290).

Table 4.13. Drugs for Parasitic Infections, continued

Infection	Drug	Adult Dosage	Pediatric Dosage
TOXOPLASMOSIS (*Toxoplasma gondii*)[93], continued			
Alternative:[97]	Spiramycin*	3–4 grams/d × 3–4 wks	50–100 mg/kg/d × 3–4 wks
TRICHINOSIS (*Trichinella spiralis*)			
Drugs of choice:	Steroids for severe symptoms **plus**		
	mebendazole[7]	200–400 mg tid × 3d, then 400–500 mg tid × 10d	200–400 mg tid × 3d, then 400–500 mg tid × 10d
Alternative:	Albendazole[7]	400 mg bid × 8–14d	400 mg bid × 8–14d
TRICHOMONIASIS (*Trichomonas vaginalis*)			
Drug of choice:[98]	Metronidazole	2 grams once or 500 mg bid × 7d	15 mg/kg/d orally in 3 doses × 7d
OR	Tinidazole[5]	2 grams once or 500 mg bid	50 mg/kg once (max. 2 g)
TRICHOSTRONGYLUS infection			
Drug of choice:	Pyrantel pamoate[7]	11 mg/kg base once (max. 1 g)	11 mg/kg once (max. 1 gram)
Alternative:	Mebendazole[7]	100 mg bid × 3d	100 mg bid × 3d
OR	Albendazole[7]	400 mg once	400 mg once
TRICHURIASIS (*Trichuris trichiura*, whipworm)			
Drug of choice:	Mebendazole	100 mg bid × 3d or 500 mg once	100 mg bid × 3d or 500 mg once
Alternative:	Albendazole[7]	400 mg × 3d	400 mg × 3d

* Availability problems. See table on page 770.

97. For prophylactic use during pregnancy. If it is determined that transmission has occurred *in utero*, therapy with pyrimethamine and sulfadiazine should be started. Pyrimethamine is a potential teratogen and should be used only after the first trimester.

98. Sexual partners should be treated simultaneously. Metronidazole-resistant strains have been reported and should be treated with metronidazole 2–4 g/d × 7–14d. Desensitization has been recommended for patients allergic to metronidazole (MD Pearlman et al, *Am J Obstet Gynecol* 1996; 174:934). High dose tinidazole has also been used for the treatment of metronidazole-resistant trichomoniasis (JD Sobel et al, *Clin Infect Dis* 2001; 33:1341).

Table 4.13. Drugs for Parasitic Infections, continued

Infection	Drug	Adult Dosage	Pediatric Dosage
TRYPANOSOMIASIS			
***T. cruzi* (American trypanosomiasis, Chagas' disease)**			
Drug of choice:	Benznidazole*	5–7 mg/kg/d in 2 divided doses × 30–90d	Up to 12 yrs: 10 mg/kg/d in 2 doses × 30–90d
OR	Nifurtimox[99]*	8–10 mg/kg/d in 3–4 doses × 90–120d	1–10 yrs: 15–20 mg/kg/d in 4 doses × 90d; 11–16 yrs: 12.5–15 mg/kg/d in 4 doses × 90d
***T. brucei gambiense* (West African trypanosomiasis, sleeping sickness) hemolymphatic stage**			
Drug of choice:[100]	Pentamidine isethionate[7]	4 mg/kg/d IM × 10d	4 mg/kg/d IM × 10d
Alternative:	Suramin*	100–200 mg (test dose) IV, then 1 gram IV on days 1,3,7,14, and 21	20 mg/kg on days 1,3,7,14, and 21
OR	Eflornithine*	See footnote 101	
***T. b. rhodesiense* (East African trypanosomiasis, sleeping sickness) hemolymphatic stage**			
Drug of choice:	Suramin*	100–200 mg (test dose) IV, then 1 gram IV on days 1,3,7,14, and 21	20 mg/kg on days 1,3,7,14, and 21

*　Availability problems. See table on page 770.

99. Available from CDC. The addition of gamma interferon to nifurtimox for 20 days in a limited number of patients and in experimental animals appears to have shortened the acute phase of Chagas' disease (RE McCabe et al, *J Infect Dis* 1991; 163:912).

100. For treatment of *T.b. gambiense*, pentamidine and suramin have equal efficacy but pentamidine is better tolerated.

101. Eflornithine is highly effective in *T.b. gambiense* and variably effective in *T.b. rhodesiense* infections. It is available in limited supply only from the WHO, and is given 400 mg/kg/d IV in 4 divided doses for 14 days.

Table 4.13. Drugs for Parasitic Infections, continued

Infection	Drug	Adult Dosage	Pediatric Dosage
TRYPANOSOMIASIS, continued			
late disease with CNS involvement (*T.b. gambiense* or *T.b. rhodesiense*)			
Drug of choice:	Melarsoprol[102]*	2–3.6 mg/kg/d IV × 3d; after 1 wk 3.6 mg/kg per day IV × 3d; repeat again after 10–21 days	18–25 mg/kg total over 1 month; initial dose of 0.36 mg/kg IV, increasing gradually to max. 3.6 mg/kg at intervals of 1–5d for total of 9–10 doses
OR	Eflornithine	See footnote 101	
VISCERAL LARVA MIGRANS[103] (Toxocariasis)			
Drug of choice:	Albendazole[7]	400 mg bid × 5d	400 mg bid × 5d
	Mebendazole[7]	100–200 mg bid × 5d	100–200 mg bid × 5d
Whipworm, see TRICHURIASIS			
Wuchereria bancrofti, see FILARIASIS			

* Availability problems. See table on page 770.

102. In frail patients, begin with as little as 18 mg and increase the dose progressively. Pretreatment with suramin has been advocated for debilitated patients. Corticosteroids have been used to prevent arsenical encephalopathy (J Pepin et al, *Trans R Soc Trop Med Hyg* 1995; 89:92). Up to 20% of patients with *T. gambiense* fail to respond to melarsoprol (MP Barrett, *Lancet* 1999; 353:1113). A shortened course consisting of 10 daily injections of 2.2 mg/kg gave a similar outcome to the usual 26-treatment schedule (C Burri et al, *Lancet* 2000; 355:1419).

103. Optimum duration of therapy is not known; some *Medical Letter* consultants would treat for up to 20 days. For severe symptoms or eye involvement, corticosteroids can be used in addition.

Table 4.14. Manufacturers of Some Antiparasitic Drugs

albendazole—*Albenza* (GlaxoSmithKline)

§ artemether—*Artenam* (Arenco, Belgium)

§ artesunate—(Guilin No. 1 Factory, People's Republic of China)

§ atovaquone—*Mepron* (GlaxoSmithKline)

atovaquone/proguanil—*Malarone* (GlaxoSmithKline)

bacitracin—many manufacturers

§ bacitracin-zinc—(Apothekernes Laboratorium A.S., Oslo, Norway)

§ benznidazole—*Rochagan* (Roche, Brazil)

† bithionol—*Bitin* (Tanabe, Japan)

chloroquine HCl and chloroquine phosphate—*Aralen* (Sanofi), others

crotamiton—*Eurax* (Westwood-Squibb)

dapsone—(Jacobus)

† diethylcarbamazine citrate USP—(University of Iowa School of Pharmacy)

§ diloxanide furoate—*Furamide* (Boots, United Kingdom)

§ eflornithine (Difluoromethylornithine, DFMO)—*Ornidyl* (Aventis)

furazolidone—*Furoxone* (Roberts)

§ halofantrine—*Halfan* (GlaxoSmithKline)

iodoquinol—*Yodoxin* (Glenwood), others

ivermectin—*Stromectol* (Merck)

malathion—*Ovide* (Medicis)

mebendazole—*Vermox* (McNeil)

mefloquine—*Lariam* (Roche)

§ meglumine antimonate—*Glucantime* (Aventis, France)

† melarsoprol—*Mel-B* (Specia)

metronidazole—*Flagyl* (Searle), others

§ miltefosine—(Zentaris)

§ niclosamide—*Yomesan* (Bayer, Germany)

† nifurtimox—*Lampit* (Bayer, Germany)

* nitazoxanide—*Cryptaz* (Romark)

§ ornidazole—*Tiberal* (Roche, France)

oxamniquine—*Vansil* (Pfizer)

paromomycin—*Humatin* (Monarch); *Leshcutan* (Teva Pharmaceutical Industries, Ltd., Israel; (topical formulation not available in US)

pentamidine isethionate—*Pentam 300*, NebuPent (Fujisawa)

permethrin—*Nix* (GlaxoSmithKline), *Elimite* (Allergan)

praziquantel—*Biltricide* (Bayer)

primaquine phosphate USP

§ proguanil—*Paludrine* (Wyeth Ayerst, Canada; AstraZeneca, United Kingdom); in combination with atovaquone as *Malarone* (GlaxoSmithKline)

§ propamidine isethionate—*Brolene* (Aventis, Canada)

pyrantel pamoate—*Antiminth* (Pfizer)

pyrethrins and piperonyl butoxide—*RID* (Pfizer), others

§ pyrimethamine USP—*Daraprim* (GlaxoSmithKline)

quinine dihydrochloride

quinine sulfate—many manufacturers

† sodium stibogluconate—*Pentostam* (GlaxoSmithKline, United Kingdom)

* spiramycin—*Rovamycine* (Aventis)

† suramin sodium—(Bayer, Germany)

§ thiabendazole—*Mintezol* (Merck)

§ tinidazole—*Fasigyn* (Pfizer)

* triclabendazole—*Egaten* (Novartis, Switzerland)

trimetrexate—*Neutrexin* (US Bioscience)

* Available in the US only from the manufacturer.

§ Not available in the US.

† Available under an Investigational New Drug (IND) protocol from the CDC Drug Service, Centers for Disease Control and Prevention, Atlanta, Georgia 30333; 404-639-3670 (evenings, weekends, or holidays: 404-639-2888).

MEDWATCH—THE FDA SAFETY INFORMATION AND ADVERSE EVENT REPORTING PROGRAM

MEDWATCH, the Food and Drug Administration (FDA) Safety Information and Adverse Event Reporting Program, is an outreach program for the health care system, including doctors, nurses, pharmacists, and patients, to enhance the effectiveness of the FDA's risk management activities for all regulated clinical medical products. These products include drugs, biologics, medical devices, and dietary supplements.

The MEDWATCH program has 2 goals: (1) to provide clinically useful and timely safety information to health care professionals and their patients; and (2) to encourage and facilitate reporting of the serious adverse events. Reports are used by the FDA as a data source to identify and evaluate new safety concerns with drugs and devices after they are approved and more widely used in clinical practice. With this new information, the FDA can develop, with the manufacturer, a modified product, revised and strengthened professional labeling and patient instructions, and a modified use strategy that will lead to a safer product.

Health care professionals are in the best position to recognize serious, unexpected adverse drug reactions (ADRs), medication errors, and product quality problems arising from the use of medical products. In the interest of public health, the FDA and manufacturers depend on clinicians to recognize and voluntarily report these events when they suspect an association between a product and a serious harm or outcome.

Vaccine-related adverse events are not reported to MEDWATCH but should be reported to the Vaccine Adverse Events Reporting System (www.fda.gov/cber/vaers/report.htm; see Reporting of Adverse Events, p 40).

The MEDWATCH voluntary form is a simple, 1-page, postage-paid form (see Fig 4.1, p 772). The MEDWATCH Web site (www.fda.gov/medwatch) offers an online version that can be completed and submitted immediately to the FDA. The Web site also offers the form for downloading and printing. This form then can be returned by fax (800-FDA-0178) or mail. A toll-free number (800-FDA-1088) is available for health care professionals and consumers to report by phone or request blank forms with instructions.

Fig 4.1. **MedWatch reporting form.**

U.S. Department of Health and Human Service

MEDWATCH
The FDA Safety Information and
Adverse Event Reporting Program

For **VOLUNTARY** reporting of
adverse events and product problems

Page ____ of ____

Form Approved: OMB No. 0910-0230 Expires: 09/30/05
See OMB statement on reverse

FDA Use Only

Triage unit
sequence #

PLEASE TYPE OR USE BLACK INK

A. Patient information

1. Patient identifier

In confidence

2. Age at time
of event:

or

Date
of birth:

3. Sex

☐ female

☐ male

4. Weight

____ lbs

or

____ kgs

B. Adverse event or product problem

1. ☐ Adverse event   and/or   ☐ Product problem (e.g., defects/malfunctions)

2. Outcomes attributed to adverse event
(check all that apply)

☐ death _____ (mo/day/yr)

☐ life-threatening

☐ hospitalization - initial or prolonged

☐ disability

☐ congenital anomaly

☐ required intervention to prevent
permanent impairment/damage

☐ other: _____

3. Date of
event
(mo/day/yr)

4. Date of
this report
(mo/day/yr)

5. Describe event or problem

6. Relevant tests/laboratory data, including dates

7. Other relevant history, including preexisting medical conditions (e.g., allergies,
race, pregnancy, smoking and alcohol use, hepatic/renal dysfunction, etc.)

C. Suspect medication(s)

1. **Name** (give labeled strength & mfr/labeler, if known)

#1

#2

2. Dose, frequency & route used

#1

#2

3. Therapy dates (if unknown, give duration)
from/to (or best estimate)

#1

#2

4. Diagnosis for use (indication)

#1

#2

5. Event abated after use
stopped or dose reduced

#1 ☐ yes ☐ no ☐ doesn't apply

#2 ☐ yes ☐ no ☐ doesn't apply

6. Lot # (if known)

#1

#2

7. Exp. date (if known)

#1

#2

8. Event reappeared after
reintroduction

#1 ☐ yes ☐ no ☐ doesn't apply

#2 ☐ yes ☐ no ☐ doesn't apply

9. NDC # (for product problems only)

10. Concomitant medical products and therapy dates (exclude treatment of event)

D. Suspect medical device

1. Brand name

2. Type of device

3. Manufacturer name & address

4. Operator of device

☐ health professional

☐ lay user/patient

☐ other:

5. Expiration date
(mo/day/yr)

6.
model # _____
catalog # _____
serial # _____
lot # _____
other # _____

7. If implanted, give date
(mo/day/yr)

8. If explanted, give date
(mo/day/yr)

9. Device available for evaluation?   (Do not send to FDA)

☐ yes   ☐ no   ☐ returned to manufacturer on _____ (mo/day/yr)

10. Concomitant medical products and therapy dates (exclude treatment of event)

E. Reporter (see confidentiality section on back)

1. Name & address

phone #

2. Health professional?

☐ yes ☐ no

3. Occupation

4. Also reported to

☐ manufacturer

☐ user facility

☐ distributor

5. If you do NOT want your identity disclosed to
the manufacturer, place an " X " in this box. ☐

FDA

Mail to: **MEDWATCH**
5600 Fishers Lane
Rockville, MD 20852-9787

or FAX to:
1-800-FDA-0178

FDA Form 3500 (11/02)   Submission of a report does not constitute an admission that medical personnel or the product caused or contributed to the event.

NOTE: You also may download this and the mandatory reporting form (www.fda.gov/medwatch/getforms.htm).

Antimicrobial Prophylaxis

ANTIMICROBIAL PROPHYLAXIS

Antimicrobial agents commonly are prescribed to prevent infections in infants and children. The efficacy of prophylactic use of antimicrobial agents has been documented for some conditions but is unsubstantiated for most. *Prophylaxis* is defined as the use of antimicrobial drugs in the absence of suspected or documented infection to decrease the incidence of infection.

Chemoprophylaxis is directed at different but not mutually exclusive targets: specific pathogens, infection-prone body sites, and vulnerable hosts. Effective prophylaxis is achieved more readily with specific pathogens and certain body sites. In any situation in which prophylactic antimicrobial therapy is being considered, the risk of emergence of resistant organisms must be weighed against potential benefits. Prophylactic agents should have as narrow a spectrum of antimicrobial activity as possible and should be used for as brief a period of time as possible.

Specific Pathogens

Prophylaxis may be appropriate or indicated if there is increased risk of serious infection with a specific pathogen, and a specific antimicrobial agent may eliminate the pathogen from people at risk with minimal adverse effects. For some pathogens that colonize the upper respiratory tract, elimination of the carrier state can be difficult and may require use of an antimicrobial agent, such as rifampin, that achieves effective concentrations in nasopharyngeal secretions, a property often lacking among antimicrobial agents ordinarily used to treat infections caused by such pathogens. In instances in which prophylaxis is recommended, the regimen is described in the disease-specific chapter in Section 3.

Infection-Prone Body Sites

Prevention of infection of vulnerable body sites may be possible if (1) the period of risk is defined and brief; (2) the expected pathogens have predictable antimicrobial susceptibility; and (3) the site is accessible to antimicrobial agents. Prevention of surgical site infection and neonatal ophthalmia is discussed in this section.

Acute otitis media recurs less frequently in otitis-prone children treated prophylactically with antimicrobial agents. Studies have demonstrated that either amoxicillin or sulfisoxazole is effective. However, antimicrobial prophylaxis may alter the nasopharyngeal flora and foster colonization with resistant organisms, compromising long-term efficacy of the prophylactic drug. Antimicrobial prophylaxis should be reserved for control of recurrent acute otitis media, defined as 3 or more distinct and well-documented episodes during a period of 6 months or 4 or more episodes during a period of 12 months.

Protection afforded to the urinary tract by chemoprophylaxis depends on the rate of emergence of antimicrobial resistance in the gastrointestinal tract flora, the usual source of bacteria that invade the urinary tract. The long-term effectiveness of nitrofurantoin or trimethoprim-sulfamethoxazole is explained by the minimal effect of these drugs on development of resistant flora. Both drugs are concentrated in urine, and adequate inhibitory activity can be obtained with less than the usual therapeutic dose. Use of a single dose at bedtime has been successful. Chemoprophylaxis has proven to be of benefit only in urinary-continent children and has not been studied adequately in younger children and infants.

Chemoprophylaxis of human and animal bite wounds has become common practice even though dog bites, the most common wound, are infected infrequently (see Bite Wounds, p 182, for recommendations).

Vulnerable Hosts

Most attempts to prevent bacterial infections in vulnerable patients with antimicrobial prophylaxis have been unsuccessful because of the rapid emergence of bacteria resistant to the antimicrobial agents used. Recommendations for prevention of opportunistic infections in people infected with human immunodeficiency virus are available.*

....

ANTIMICROBIAL PROPHYLAXIS IN PEDIATRIC SURGICAL PATIENTS

A major use of antimicrobial agents in hospitalized children is for prevention of postoperative wound infections through perioperative prophylaxis. Because of this common use, consensus recommendations for prevention of surgical site infections in children have been developed.

Frequency of Antimicrobial Prophylaxis

Two studies have demonstrated that approximately 75% of antimicrobial use in pediatric surgical services is for prophylaxis. The efficacy of antimicrobial agents in decreasing the incidence of postoperative infection and infection after invasive nonsurgical procedures, such as cystoscopy or cardiac catheterization, has been demonstrated in controlled clinical trials. The principles for effective use of antimicrobial agents in prophylaxis of operative wound infections, including choice of drugs, optimal time of administration, and duration, have been delineated by experimental studies in animals and through clinical trials.

---

* Centers for Disease Control and Prevention. Guidelines for preventing opportunistic infections among HIV-infected persons—2002. Recommendations of the US Public Health Service and the Infectious Diseases Society of America. *MMWR Recomm Rep.* 2002;51(RR-8):1–46

Inappropriate Antimicrobial Prophylaxis

The consequences of inappropriate prophylactic use of antimicrobial agents include increased costs as a result of unnecessary drug use, potential emergence of resistant organisms, and adverse events. Prophylaxis has been associated with a high frequency of inappropriate use of antimicrobial agents. In a study of children younger than 6 years of age undergoing surgery, antimicrobial agents were administered for prophylaxis inappropriately to 42% of children preoperatively, 67% intraoperatively, and 55% postoperatively. Similarly, in another study, 66% of antimicrobial use in children hospitalized in surgical wards was considered inappropriate because of lack of indication or wrong drug, dose, time of initiation, or duration.

Guidelines for Appropriate Use

Studies documenting that systemic antimicrobial prophylaxis decreases the incidence of surgical site infections primarily have been performed in adults. Because the pathogenesis of these infections is the same in children, the principles that guide surgical prophylaxis in children should be similar. In the absence of specific studies in children, guidelines recommended in *The Medical Letter** and by the American College of Surgeons, the Surgical Infection Society,[†] and the Hospital Infections Program of the Centers for Disease Control and Prevention[‡] are available to direct use of systemic antimicrobial agents for prophylaxis in pediatric surgical patients. The following general principles are presented with the understanding that future studies in children or application to settings unique to infants and children, such as prematurity or certain immunodeficiencies, may justify modification of these recommendations.

Indications for Prophylaxis

Systemic prophylaxis is indicated when the probability or morbidity of postoperative infection is high and benefits of preventing wound infection outweigh potential risks from adverse drug reactions or emergence of antimicrobial-resistant organisms. The latter poses a potential risk not only to the recipient but also to other hospitalized patients in whom a health care-associated infection caused by antimicrobial-resistant organisms may develop. Procedures in which the benefits justify the risks incurred in antimicrobial prophylaxis are those associated with an increased incidence of postoperative infection and those in which the likelihood of infection may not be great but the adverse consequences of infection are extreme, such as with prosthetic materials.

A major determinant of the probability of surgical site infection is the number of microorganisms in the wound at completion of the procedure. The classification

---

* Antimicrobial prophylaxis in surgery. *Med Lett Drugs Ther.* 1999;41:75–79

† Page CP, Bohnen JM, Fletcher JR, McManus AT, Solomkin JS, Wittmann DH. Antimicrobial prophylaxis for surgical wounds. Guidelines for clinical care [published correction appears in *Arch Surg.* 1993;128:410]. *Arch Surg.* 1993;128:79–88

‡ Mangram AJ, Horan TC, Pearson ML, Silver LC, Jarvis WR. Guideline for prevention of surgical site infection, 1999. Hospital Infection Control Practices Advisory Committee. *Infect Control Hosp Epidemiol.* 1999;20:250–278

of surgical procedures is based on an estimation of bacterial contamination and, thus, risk of subsequent infection. The 4 classes are: (1) clean wounds; (2) clean-contaminated wounds; (3) contaminated wounds; and (4) dirty and infected wounds. As evidenced by the wide variation in infection rates within these classes, wound classification is not the only factor affecting risk of surgical site infection. Additional independent factors include site of operation, duration of the procedure, and patient's preoperative health status. A patient risk index, which incorporates the American Society of Anesthesiologists preoperative physical status assessment score and the duration of the operation in addition to the aforementioned wound classification, has been demonstrated to be a better predictor of postoperative surgical site infection.*

CLEAN WOUNDS

Clean wounds are uninfected operative wounds in which no inflammation is encountered and the respiratory, alimentary, and genitourinary tracts or oropharyngeal cavity are not entered. The operative procedures are elective, and wounds are closed primarily and, if necessary, drained with closed drainage. No break in aseptic technique occurs. Operative incisional wounds that follow nonpenetrating (blunt) abdominal trauma should be included in this category, provided that the surgical procedure does not entail entry into the gastrointestinal or genitourinary tracts. The benefits of systemic antimicrobial prophylaxis do not justify the potential risks associated with antimicrobial use in most clean wound procedures, because the risk of infection is low (1%–2%). Some exceptions exist in which either the risks or consequences of infection are high. Examples are implantation of intravascular prosthetic material (eg, insertion of a prosthetic heart valve) or a prosthetic joint, open-heart surgery for repair of structural defects, body cavity exploration in neonates, and most neurosurgical operations. Prophylaxis generally is given in these circumstances.

CLEAN-CONTAMINATED WOUNDS

In clean-contaminated operative wounds, the respiratory, alimentary, or genitourinary tract is entered under controlled conditions with no significant contamination. Operations involving the biliary tract, appendix, vagina, or oropharynx and urgent or emergency surgery in an otherwise clean procedure are included in this category, provided that no evidence of infection is encountered and no major break in aseptic technique occurs. Prophylaxis is limited to procedures in which a substantial amount of wound contamination has occurred. The overall risk of infection for the surgical site is 3% to 15%. On the basis of data from adults, procedures for which prophylaxis is indicated for pediatric patients include the following: (1) all gastrointestinal tract procedures in which there is obstruction or when the patient is receiving H_2 receptor antagonists or proton pump blockers or has a permanent foreign body; (2) selected biliary tract operations (eg, when there is obstruction from common bile duct stones); and (3) urinary tract surgery or instrumentation in the presence of bacteriuria or obstructive uropathy.

---

* Culver DH, Horan TC, Gaynes RP, et al. Surgical wound infection rates by wound class, operative procedure, and patient risk index. National Nosocomial Infections Surveillance System. *Am J Med.* 1991;91(suppl 3B):152S–157S

CONTAMINATED WOUNDS

Contaminated wounds include open, fresh, accidental wounds; operative wounds in the setting of major breaks in aseptic technique or gross spillage from the gastrointestinal tract; penetrating trauma of fewer than 4 hours' duration; and incisions in which acute nonpurulent inflammation is encountered. The estimated rate of infection for the surgical site is 15%. In contaminated wound procedures, antimicrobial prophylaxis is appropriate for some patients with acute nonpurulent inflammation isolated to and contained within an inflamed viscus (such as acute appendicitis or cholecystitis). In contaminated wounds resulting from other causes, antimicrobial therapy should be considered treatment rather than prophylaxis.

DIRTY AND INFECTED WOUNDS

Dirty and infected wounds include penetrating traumatic wounds of more than 4 hours' duration, wounds with retained devitalized tissue, and wounds involving existing clinical infection or perforated viscera. This definition suggests that the organisms causing postoperative infection were present in the operative field before surgery. The estimated rate of infection for the surgical site is 40%. In dirty and infected wound procedures, such as those for a perforated abdominal viscus, a compound fracture, or a laceration attributable to an animal or human bite, or if a major break in sterile technique has occurred, antimicrobial agents are given as treatment rather than prophylaxis.

Timing of Administration of Prophylactic Antimicrobial Agents

Effective prophylaxis occurs when adequate drug concentrations in tissues are present when bacterial contamination occurs intraoperatively. Administration of an antimicrobial agent within 2 hours before surgery has been demonstrated to decrease the risk of wound infection. Accordingly, administration is recommended at least 30 minutes before surgical incision to ensure adequate tissue concentrations at the start of the procedure.

Duration of Administration of Antimicrobial Agents

A single antimicrobial dose that provides adequate tissue concentrations throughout the surgical procedure is sufficient. When surgery is prolonged (more than 4 hours), major blood loss occurs, or an antimicrobial agent with a short half-life is used, it is advisable to follow the preincision dose with 1 or more doses during the procedure. Although published studies of antimicrobial prophylaxis commonly use 1 or 2 doses postoperatively in addition to 1 preoperative dose, there are no data to suggest that this practice improves outcome.

Recommended Antimicrobial Agents

An antimicrobial agent is chosen on the basis of bacterial pathogens most likely to cause infectious complications after the specific procedure, the antimicrobial susceptibility pattern of these pathogens, and the safety and efficacy of the drug. New, more costly antimicrobial agents generally are not recommended unless prophylactic efficacy has been proven to be superior to drugs of established benefit. Drugs do not have to be active against every potential organism. Routine use of vancomycin hydrochloride and extended-spectrum cephalosporins for surgical prophylaxis is not recommended. Doses and routes of administration are determined on the basis of the need to achieve therapeutic blood and tissue concentrations throughout the procedure. Antimicrobial prophylaxis for most surgical procedures (including gastric, biliary, thoracic [noncardiac], vascular, neurosurgical, and orthopedic operations) can be achieved effectively using an agent such as a first-generation cephalosporin (eg, cefazolin sodium). For colorectal surgery or appendectomy, effective prophylaxis requires antimicrobial agents that are active against intestinal flora. Table 5.1 (p 779) provides recommendations for drugs, including preoperative doses, to be used in children undergoing surgical manipulation or invasive procedures. Physicians should be aware of potential interactions and adverse effects associated with prophylactic antimicrobial agents and other medications the patient may be receiving.

PREVENTION OF BACTERIAL ENDOCARDITIS

The Committee on Rheumatic Fever, Endocarditis, and Kawasaki Disease of the American Heart Association issues detailed recommendations on the rationale, indications, and antimicrobial regimens for the prevention of bacterial endocarditis for people at increased risk. The most recent recommendations were published in 1997.* The cardiac conditions associated with endocarditis, procedures for which endocarditis prophylaxis is recommended for people with cardiac conditions that put them at risk, and specific prophylactic regimens are presented in Tables 5.2 through 5.6 (pp 782–786). Health care professionals should consult the published recommendations for further details.

PREVENTION OF NEONATAL OPHTHALMIA

Ophthalmia neonatorum is defined as conjunctivitis occurring within the first 4 weeks of life. The major causes of ophthalmia neonatorum are presented in Table 5.7, p 787. The prevalence of infection with *Chlamydia trachomatis* and *Neisseria gonorrhoeae* in newborn infants is related directly to the prevalence of infection among pregnant women and whether pregnant women are screened and treated and newborn infants are given ophthalmia prophylaxis. Screening of all pregnant women for chlamydia and gonorrhea infection followed by appropriate treatment and follow-up of all infected women and their partner(s) can minimize the risk of perinatal transmission (see Chlamydial Infections, p 235, and Gonococcal Infections, p 285).

Gonococcal Ophthalmia

For newborn infants, topical 1% silver nitrate aqueous solution, 0.5% erythromycin ointment, and 1% tetracycline ophthalmic ointment are considered equally effective

---

* Dajani AS, Taubert KA, Wilson W, et al. Prevention of bacterial endocarditis. Recommendations by the American Heart Association. *JAMA*. 1997;277:1794–1801

Table 5.1. Recommendations for Preoperative Antimicrobial Prophylaxis[1]

Operation	Likely Pathogens	Recommended Drugs	Preoperative Dose
Neonatal (<72 h of age)—all major procedures	Group B streptococci, enteric gram-negative bacilli, enterococci	Ampicillin PLUS gentamicin sulfate	50 mg/kg 2.5–3 mg/kg
Cardiac (prosthetic valve or pacemaker)	*Staphylococcus epidermidis, Staphylococcus aureus, Corynebacterium* species, enteric gram-negative bacilli	Cefazolin sodium OR, if MRSA is likely, vancomycin hydrochloride	25 mg/kg 10 mg/kg
Gastrointestinal			
Esophageal	Gram-positive cocci, enteric gram-negative bacilli	Cefazolin	25 mg/kg
Gastroduodenal	Gram-positive cocci, enteric gram-negative bacilli	Cefazolin	25 mg/kg
Biliary	Enteric gram-negative bacilli	Cefazolin	25 mg/kg
Colorectal or appendectomy	Enteric gram-negative bacilli, enterococci, anaerobes	Cefoxitin sodium OR cefotetan disodium[2]; if high risk, gentamicin PLUS clindamycin ± ampicillin	40 mg/kg 40 mg/kg 2 mg/kg 10 mg/kg 50 mg/kg
Genitourinary	Enteric gram-negative bacilli, enterococci	Ampicillin PLUS gentamicin	50 mg/kg 2 mg/kg
Head and neck surgery (incision through oral mucosa)	Anaerobes, enteric gram-negative bacilli, *S aureus*	Gentamicin PLUS clindamycin	2 mg/kg 10 mg/kg
Neurosurgery (craniotomy)	*S epidermidis, S aureus*	Cefazolin OR, if MRSA is likely, vancomycin	25 mg/kg 10 mg/kg

Table 5.1. Recommendations for Preoperative Antimicrobial Prophylaxis,[1] continued

Operation	Likely Pathogens	Recommended Drugs	Preoperative Dose
Ophthalmic (open globe procedures)	*S epidermidis*, *S aureus*, streptococci, enteric gram-negative bacilli, *Pseudomonas* species	Gentamicin, ciprofloxacin, ofloxacin, tobramycin, or neomycin-gramicidin-polymyxin B sulfate,	Multiple drops topically for 2–24 h before procedure
		OR cefazolin	100 mg, subconjunctivally
Orthopedic (internal fixation of fractures or prosthetic joints)	*S epidermidis*, *S aureus*	Cefazolin OR, if MRSA is likely, vancomycin	25 mg/kg 10 mg/kg
Thoracic (noncardiac)	*S epidermidis*, *S aureus*	Cefazolin OR, if MRSA is likely, vancomycin	25 mg/kg 10 mg/kg
Ruptured viscus	Enteric gram-negative bacilli, anaerobes, enterococci	Cefoxitin or cefotetan[2] ± gentamicin OR gentamicin PLUS clindamycin	40 mg/kg 2 mg/kg 2 mg/kg 10 mg/kg
Traumatic wound (nonbites)	*S aureus*, group A streptococci, *Clostridium* species	Cefazolin	25 mg/kg

MRSA indicates methicillin-resistant *Staphylococcus aureus*.
[1] Antimicrobial prophylaxis in surgery. *Med Lett Drugs Ther.* 1999;41:75–79
[2] Safety and effectiveness of cefotetan have not been established in children.

for prophylaxis of ocular gonorrheal infection. Each is available in single-dose forms. Povidone-iodine in a 2.5% solution also may be useful, but more studies are required, and a product for this purpose currently is not available in the United States. Silver nitrate causes more chemical conjunctivitis than other agents but is recommended in areas where the incidence of penicillinase-producing *N gonorrhoeae* (PPNG) is appreciable. The efficacy of erythromycin or povidone-iodine prophylaxis against PPNG is not known, but one study has demonstrated tetracycline to be effective. Infants born to women with untreated gonococcal infection should receive 1 dose of ceftriaxone sodium (25–50 mg/kg, intravenously [IV] or intramuscularly [IM], not to exceed 125 mg) or cefotaxime sodium (100 mg/kg, IV or IM). Topical antimicrobial therapy alone is inadequate and is not necessary if systemic therapy is administered. Infants who have gonococcal ophthalmia should be hospitalized, evaluated for signs of disseminated infection, and treated (see Gonococcal Infections, p 285).

Chlamydial Ophthalmia

Neonatal ophthalmia attributable to *C trachomatis,* although not as severe as gono-coccal conjunctivitis, is common in the United States and should be evaluated and treated (see Chlamydial Infections, p 235). Results of clinical efficacy studies of ery-thromycin and of tetracycline ointment for prophylaxis of chlamydial conjunctivitis have been conflicting, and they do not have proven efficacy in preventing nasopha-ryngeal colonization.

Nongonococcal Nonchlamydial Ophthalmia

Silver nitrate, povidone-iodine, and probably, erythromycin are effective for prevent-ing nongonococcal nonchlamydial conjunctivitis during the first 2 weeks of life.

Administration of Neonatal Ophthalmic Prophylaxis. Before administering local prophylaxis, each eyelid should be wiped gently with sterile cotton. Two drops of a 1% silver nitrate solution or a 1-cm ribbon of antimicrobial ointment (0.5% erythromycin or 1% tetracycline) are placed in each lower conjunctival sac. The eyelids then should be massaged gently to spread the solution or ointment. After 1 minute, excess solution or ointment may be wiped away with sterile cotton. None of the prophylactic agents should be flushed from the eyes after instillation, because flushing may decrease the efficacy of prophylaxis.

Infants born by cesarean delivery should receive prophylaxis against neonatal gonococcal ophthalmia. Although gonococcal and chlamydial infections usually are transmitted to the infant during passage through the birth canal, infection by the ascending route also occurs.

Prophylaxis should be given shortly after birth. Some experts suggest that prophylaxis may be administered more effectively in the nursery than in the delivery room. Delaying prophylaxis for as long as 1 hour after birth to facilitate parent-infant bonding is unlikely to influence efficacy. Longer delays have not been studied for efficacy. Hospitals should establish a system to ensure that all infants are given prophylaxis.

Table 5.2. Cardiac Conditions Associated With Endocarditis

Endocarditis Prophylaxis:	
Recommended	**Not Recommended**
HIGH RISK	*NEGLIGIBLE RISK[1]*
Prosthetic cardiac valves, including bioprosthetic and homograft valves	Isolated secundum atrial septal defect
Previous bacterial endocarditis	Surgical repair of atrial septal defect, ventricular septal defect, or patent ductus arteriosus (without residua and beyond 6 mo of age)
Complex cyanotic congenital heart disease (eg, single ventricle states, transposition of the great arteries, tetralogy of Fallot)	Previous coronary artery bypass graft surgery
Surgically constructed systemic pulmonary shunts or conduits	Mitral valve prolapse without valvular regurgitation[2]
	Physiologic, functional, or innocent heart murmurs[2]
MODERATE RISK	Previous Kawasaki syndrome without valvular dysfunction
Most other congenital cardiac malformations (other than those in the high-risk and negligible-risk categories)	Previous rheumatic fever without valvular dysfunction
Acquired valvular dysfunction (eg, rheumatic heart disease)	Cardiac pacemakers (intravascular and epicardial) and implanted defibrillators
Hypertrophic cardiomyopathy	
Mitral valve prolapse with valvular regurgitation and/or thickened leaflets[2]	

[1] No greater risk than the general population.

[2] For further details, see Dajani AS, Taubert KA, Wilson W, et al. Prevention of bacterial endocarditis. Recommendations by the American Heart Association. *JAMA.* 1997;277:1794–1801

Table 5.3. **Dental Procedures and Endocarditis Prophylaxis**

Endocarditis Prophylaxis	
Recommended[1]	**Not Recommended**
Dental extractions	Restorative dentistry[2] (operative and prosthodontic) with or without retraction cord[3]
Periodontal procedures, including surgery, scaling and root planing, probing, and routine maintenance	Local anesthetic injections (nonintraligamentary)
Dental implant placement and reimplantation of avulsed teeth	Intracanal endodontic treatment; postplacement and buildup
Endodontic (root canal) instrumentation or surgery only beyond the apex	Placement of rubber dams
Subgingival placement of antimicrobial fibers or strips	Postoperative suture removal
Initial placement of orthodontic bands but not brackets	Placement of removable prosthodontic or orthodontic appliances
Intraligamentary local anesthetic injections	Taking of oral impressions
Prophylactic cleaning of teeth or implants during which bleeding is anticipated	Fluoride treatments
	Taking of oral radiographs
	Orthodontic appliance adjustment
	Shedding of primary teeth

[1] Prophylaxis is recommended for patients with high- and moderate-risk cardiac conditions.

[2] This includes restoration of decayed teeth (filling cavities) and replacement of missing teeth.

[3] Clinical judgment may indicate antimicrobial use in some circumstances that may create significant bleeding.

Table 5.4. Other Procedures and Endocarditis Prophylaxis

	Endocarditis Prophylaxis	
	Recommended[1]	**Not Recommended**
Respiratory tract	Tonsillectomy, adenoidectomy, or both Surgical operations that involve respiratory mucosa Bronchoscopy with a rigid bronchoscope	Endotracheal intubation Bronchoscopy with a flexible bronchoscope, with or without biopsy[2] Tympanostomy tube insertion
Gastrointestinal tract[3]	Sclerotherapy for esophageal varices Esophageal stricture dilation Endoscopic retrograde cholangiography with biliary obstruction Biliary tract surgery Surgical operations that involve intestinal mucosa	Transesophageal echocardiography[2] Endoscopy with or without gastrointestinal biopsy[2]
Genitourinary tract	Prostatic surgery Cystoscopy Urethral dilation	Vaginal hysterectomy[2] Vaginal delivery[2] Cesarean delivery In uninfected tissue: Urethral catheterization Uterine dilatation and curetage Therapeutic abortion Sterilization procedures Insertion or removal of intrauterine devices
Other		Cardiac catheterization, including balloon angioplasty Implanted cardiac pacemakers, implanted defibrillators, and coronary stents Incision or biopsy of surgically scrubbed skin Circumcision

[1] Prophylaxis is recommended for high- and moderate-risk cardiac conditions.
[2] Prophylaxis is optional for high-risk patients.
[3] Prophylaxis is recommended for high-risk patients; optional for medium-risk patients.

Table 5.5. Prophylactic Regimens for Dental, Oral, Respiratory Tract, or Esophageal Procedures

Situation	Agent	Regimen[1]
Standard general prophylaxis	Amoxicillin	Adults: 2.0 g; children: 50 mg/kg of body weight, orally, 1 h before procedure
Unable to take oral medications	Ampicillin	Adults: 2.0 g, intramuscularly (IM) or intravenously (IV); children: 50 mg/kg, IM or IV, within 30 min before procedure
Allergic to penicillin	Clindamycin	Adults: 600 mg; children: 20 mg/kg, orally, 1 h before procedure
	OR	
	Cephalexin[2] or cefadroxil[2]	Adults: 2.0 g; children: 50 mg/kg, orally, 1 h before procedure
	OR	
	Azithromycin or clarithromycin	Adults: 500 mg; children: 15 mg/kg, orally, 1 h before procedure
Allergic to penicillin and unable to take oral medications	Clindamycin	Adults: 600 mg; children: 20 mg/kg, IV, within 30 min before procedure
	OR	
	Cefazolin[2]	Adults: 1.0 g; children: 25 mg/kg, IM or IV, within 30 min before procedure

[1] Total children's dose should not exceed adult dose.
[2] Cephalosporins should not be used for people with immediate-type hypersensitivity reaction (urticaria, angioedema, or anaphylaxis) to penicillins.

Table 5.6. Prophylactic Regimens for Genitourinary and Gastrointestinal Tract (Excluding Esophageal) Procedures

Situation	Agents[1]	Regimen[2]
High-risk patients	Ampicillin **PLUS** gentamicin sulfate	Adults: ampicillin, 2.0 g, intramuscularly (IM) or intravenously (IV), plus gentamicin, 1.5 mg/kg (maximum 120 mg), within 30 min of starting procedure; 6 h later: ampicillin, 1 g, IM or IV, or amoxicillin, 1 g, orally Children: ampicillin, 50 mg/kg, IM or IV (maximum 2.0 g), plus gentamicin, 1.5 mg/kg, within 30 min of starting procedure; 6 h later: ampicillin, 25 mg/kg, IM or IV, or amoxicillin, 25 mg/kg, orally.
High-risk patients allergic to ampicillin or amoxicillin	Vancomycin hydrochloride **PLUS** gentamicin	Adults: vancomycin, 1.0 g, IV, over 1–2 h plus gentamicin, 1.5 mg/kg, IV or IM (maximum 120 mg), complete injection/infusion within 30 min of starting procedure. Children: vancomycin, 20 mg/kg, IV, over 1–2 h plus gentamicin, 1.5 mg/kg, IV or IM, complete injection/infusion within 30 min of starting procedure.
Moderate-risk patients	Amoxicillin **OR** ampicillin	Adults: amoxicillin, 2.0 g, orally, 1 h before procedure, or ampicillin, 2.0 g, IM or IV, within 30 min of starting procedure. Children: amoxicillin, 50 mg/kg, orally, 1 h before procedure, or ampicillin, 50 mg/kg, IM or IV, within 30 min of starting procedure.
Moderate-risk patients allergic to ampicillin or amoxicillin	Vancomycin	Adults: vancomycin, 1.0 g, IV, over 1–2 h, complete infusion within 30 min of starting procedure. Children: vancomycin, 20 mg/kg, IV, over 1–2 h, complete infusion within 30 min of starting procedure.

[1] Total children's dose should not exceed adult dose.
[2] No second dose of vancomycin or gentamicin is recommended.

Table 5.7. **Major and Minor Pathogens in Ophthalmia Neonatorum**

Etiology of Ophthalmia Neonatorum	Percentage of Cases	Incubation Period (Days)	Severity of Conjunctivitis[1]	Associated Problems
Chlamydia trachomatis	2–40	5–14	+	Pneumonitis 3 wk to 3 mo (see Chlamydial Infections, p 235)
Neisseria gonorrhoeae	<1	2–7	+++	Disseminated infection (see Gonococcal Infections, p 285)
Other bacterial microbes[2]	30–50	5–14	+	Variable
Herpes simplex virus	<1	6–14	+	Disseminated infection (see Herpes Simplex, p 344); keratitis and ulceration also possible
Chemical	Varies with silver nitrate use	1	+	...

[1] + indicates mild; +++, severe.

[2] *Staphylococcus* species; *Streptococcus pneumoniae*; *Haemophilus influenzae*, nontypeable; *Streptococcus mitis*; group A and B streptococci; *Neisseria cinerea*; *Corynebacterium* species; *Moraxella catarrhalis*; *Escherichia coli*; *Klebsiella pneumoniae*; *Pseudomonas aeruginosa*.

....
APPENDIX I.

Directory of Resources[1]

Organization	Telephone/Fax Numbers	Web Site
AIDSinfo PO Box 6303 Rockville, MD 20849-6303 USA	1-800-HIV-0440 (1-800-448-0440, USA & Canada) 1-301-519-0459 (International) TTY: 1-888-480-3739 1-301-519-6616 (Fax)	www.aidsinfo.nih.gov

American Academy of Pediatrics (AAP)
141 Northwest Point Blvd
Elk Grove Village, IL 60007-1098
USA
	1-847-434-4000
	1-847-434-8000 (Fax)
	Publications/Customer Service:
	    1-866-THEAAP1
	        (1-866-843-2271)
		www.aap.org

Canadian Paediatric Society (CPS) 2204 Walkley Rd, Ste 100 Ottawa, Ontario K1G 4G8 Canada	1-613-526-9397 1-613-526-3332 (Fax)	www.cps.ca
Centers for Disease Control and Prevention (CDC) 1600 Clifton Rd Atlanta, GA 30333 USA	1-404-639-3311	www.cdc.gov
• 24-Hour Service	1-404-639-2888	
• Division of Bacterial and Mycotic Diseases	1-404-639-1603	www.cdc.gov/ncidod/dbmd
• Division of Parasitic Diseases	1-770-488-7775 OR 1-770-488-7760	www.cdc.gov/ncidod/dpd/default.htm
• Division of Tuberculosis Elimination	1-404-639-8120	www.cdc.gov/nchstp/tb/default.htm

[1] Internet addresses and telephone/fax numbers are current at the time of publication.

Directory of Resources[1], continued

Organization	Telephone/Fax Numbers	Web Site
CDC, continued		
• Division of Viral Hepatitis	1-888-4-HEP-CDC (1-888-443-7232)	www.cdc.gov/ncidod/diseases/hepatitis
• Division of Viral & Rickettsial Diseases	1-404-639-3574	www.cdc.gov/ncidod/dvrd/index.htm
• Drug Service (weekdays, 8 AM to 4:30 PM ET)	1-404-639-3670	www.cdc.gov/ncidod/srp/drugservice/index.htm
• Drug Service (weekends, nights, holidays)	1-404-639-2888	www.cdc.gov/ncidod/srp/drugservice/index.htm
• Immunization, Infectious Diseases, and Other Health Information— Voice Information System	1-800-232-SHOT (1-800-232-7468)	
• Malaria Hotline	1-770-488-7788	www.cdc.gov/ncidod
• National Center for Infectious Diseases	1-404-639-3401	www.ashastd.org/nah
• National HIV and AIDS Hotline	1-800-342-AIDS (1-800-342-2437)	www.cdc.gov/nip
• National Immunization Program	1-404-639-8200 English Hotline: 1-800-232-2522 Spanish Hotline: 1-800-232-0233 1-888-CDC-FAXX (Fax) (1-888-232-3299)	
• National Prevention Information Network	1-800-458-5231	www.cdc.gov/hiv/hivinfo/npin.htm
• National Vaccine Injury Compensation Program (for information on filing claims)	1-800-338-2382	www.cdc.gov/od/nvpo/vacsafe.htm

[1] Internet addresses and telephone/fax numbers are current at the time of publication.

Directory of Resources[1], continued

Organization	Telephone/Fax Numbers	Web Site
CDC, continued		
• Public Inquiries	1-404-639-3534	
• Publications	1-800-232-2522	www.cdc.gov/publications.htm#pubs
	1-404-639-8828 (Fax)	
• Rash Illness Evaluation Team	1-770-488-7100	
• Smallpox Adverse Events Clinical Information Line	1-877-554-4225	
• Software		www.cdc.gov/publications.htm#soft
• Traveler's Health Hotline and Fax	1-877-FYI-TRIP (877-394-8747)	www.cdc.gov/travel
	1-888-232-3299 (Fax toll free)	
• Vector-Borne Infectious Diseases	1-970-221-6400	www.cdc.gov/ncidod/dvbid/index.htm
• Voice/Fax Information Service (including international travel and immunization)	1-404-332-4555 (Voice)	www.cdc.gov/epo/mmwr/preview/mmwrhtml/00033199.htm
	1-404-332-4565 (Fax)	
Food and Drug Administration (FDA) 5600 Fishers Ln Rockville, MD 20857-0001 USA	1-888-463-6332	www.fda.gov
• Center for Biologics Evaluation and Research	1-301-827-2000 OR 1-800-835-4709	www.fda.gov/cber
• Center for Drug Evaluation and Research	1-301-594-6740	www.fda.gov/cder
• Division of Special Pathogen and Immunologic Drug Products	1-301-827-2127	
	1-301-827-2475 (Fax)	

[1] Internet addresses and telephone/fax numbers are current at the time of publication.

Directory of Resources[1], continued

Organization	Telephone/Fax Numbers	Web Site
FDA, continued		
• HIV/AIDS Office of Special Health Issues	1-301-827-4460	www.fda.gov/oashi/aids/hiv.html
• Kids' Vaccinations	1-800-FDA-1088 (1-800-332-1088)	www.fda.gov/fdac/reprints/vaccine.html
• MEDWATCH	1-800-FDA-0178 (Fax) (1-800-332-0178)	www.fda.gov/medwatch
• Vaccine Adverse Events Reporting System (VAERS)	1-800-822-7967	www.fda.gov/cber/vaers/vaers.htm
Immunization Action Coalition (IAC) 1573 Selby Ave, Ste 234 St Paul, MN 55104 USA	1-651-647-9009 1-651-647-9131 (Fax)	www.immunize.org
Infectious Diseases Society of America (IDSA) 66 Canal Center Plaza, Ste 600 Alexandria, VA 22314 USA	1-703-299-0200 1-703-299-0204 (Fax)	www.idsociety.org
Institute of Medicine (IOM) The National Academies 500 Fifth St, NW Washington, DC 20001 USA	1-202-334-3300	www.iom.edu

[1] Internet addresses and telephone/fax numbers are current at the time of publication.

Directory of Resources[1], continued

Organization	Telephone/Fax Numbers	Web Site
National Institutes of Health (NIH) 9000 Rockville Pike Bethesda, MD 20892 USA	1-301-496-4000	www.nih.gov
• National Institute of Allergy and Infectious Diseases (NIAID)	1-301-496-2263	www.niaid.nih.gov
• NIAID Collaborative Antiviral Study Group	1-205-934-5316	www.peds.uab.edu/casg
• National Library of Medicine 8600 Rockville Pike Bethesda, MD 20894 USA	1-888-346-3656	www.nlm.nih.gov
National Network for Immunization Information (NNii) 66 Canal Center Plaza, Ste 600 Alexandria, VA 20001 USA	1-877-341-6644 1-703-299-0204 (Fax)	www.immunizationinfo.org
National Pediatric & Family HIV Resource Center (NPHRC) University of Medicine & Dentistry of New Jersey 30 Bergen St, ADMC #4 Newark, NJ 07103 USA	1-800-362-0071 1-973-972-0399 (Fax)	www.pedhivaids.org

[1] Internet addresses and telephone/fax numbers are current at the time of publication.

Directory of Resources[1], continued

Organization	Telephone/Fax Numbers	Web Site
National Vaccine Program Office (NVPO)	1-770-488-2040	www.cdc.gov/od/nvpo
Pediatric AIDS Drug Trials—Information		
• Pediatric Branch, National Cancer Institute	1-301-496-4256	
• Pediatric Clinical Trials Group (NIAID-sponsored)	1-800-TRIALS-A (1-800-874-2572)	
Pediatric Infectious Diseases Society 66 Canal Center Plaza, Ste 600 Alexandria, VA 20001 USA	1-703-299-6764 1-703-299-0473 (Fax)	www.pids.org
World Health Organization (WHO) Avenue Appia 20 1211 Geneva 27 Switzerland	(+41 22) 791 21 11 (+41 22) 791 3111 (Fax)	www.who.int

[1] Internet addresses and telephone/fax numbers are current at the time of publication.

························

APPENDIX II.

Standards for Child and Adolescent Immunization Practices*

Recommended by the
National Vaccine Advisory Committee (2003)
Approved by the
United States Public Health Service
Endorsed by the
American Academy of Pediatrics

The Standards represent the consensus of the National Vaccine Advisory Committee (NVAC) and are endorsed by a variety of medical and public health organizations including the American Academy of Pediatrics. The Standards constitute the most essential and desirable immunization practices and represent an important element in our national strategy to protect America's children against vaccine-preventable diseases. The Standards can be useful in helping health care professionals identify needed changes in their office practices and obtain resources to implement the desirable immunization practices.

Since the Standards were published initially in 1992, vaccine delivery in the United States has changed in several important ways. First, immunization coverage rates among preschool children have increased substantially and now are monitored by the National Immunization Survey. Second, immunization of children has shifted markedly from the public to the private sector, with an emphasis on immunization in the context of primary care and the medical home. The Vaccines for Children Program has provided critical support to this shift by covering the cost of immunizations for the most economically disadvantaged children and adolescents. Third, the development and introduction of performance measures, such as the National Committee for Quality Assurance's HEDIS (Health Employer Data and Information Set), have focused national attention on the quality of preventive care, including immunization. Finally, high-quality research in health services has helped to refine strategies for raising and sustaining immunization coverage levels among children, adolescents, and adults.

Health care professionals who immunize children and adolescents continue to face important challenges. These challenges include a diminishing level of experience with the diseases that vaccines prevent among patients, parents, and physicians, the ready availability of vaccine-related information that may be inaccurate or misleading, the increasing complexity of the immunization schedule, the failure of many health plans to pay for the costs associated with immunization, and the focus on adolescent immunization.

---

* The National Vaccine Advisory Committee. Standards for Pediatric and Adolescent Immunization Practices. *Pediatrics.* In press

The Standards are directed toward *health care professionals,* an inclusive term for the many people in clinical settings who share in the responsibility for immunization of children and adolescents: physicians, nurses, mid-level practitioners (eg, nurse practitioners, physician assistants), medical assistants, and clerical staff. In addition to this primary audience, the Standards are intended to be useful to public health professionals, policy makers, health plan administrators, employers who purchase health care coverage, and others whose efforts shape and support the delivery of immunization services.

The use of the term *standards* should not be confused with a minimum standard of care. Rather, these Standards represent the most desirable immunization practices, which health care professionals should strive to achieve. Given current resource limitations, some health care professionals may find it difficult to implement all of the Standards, resulting from circumstances over which they have little control. The expectation is that, by summarizing the best immunization practices in a clear and concise format, the Standards will assist these health care professionals in securing the resources necessary to implement this set of recommendations.

By adopting these Standards, health care professionals can enhance their own policies and practices, making achievement of immunization objectives for children and adolescents as outlined in *Healthy People 2010* both feasible and likely. Achieving these objectives will improve the health and welfare of all children and adolescents as well as the communities in which they live. Provided here are the Standards and resource information. Supporting information for each Standard can be found at www.aap.org and in *Pediatrics.**

STANDARDS FOR CHILD AND ADOLESCENT IMMUNIZATION PRACTICES

Availability of vaccines
1. Immunization services are readily available.
2. Immunizations are coordinated with other health care services and provided within a medical home[†] when possible.
3. Barriers to immunization are identified and minimized.
4. Patient costs are minimized. For information about the Vaccines for Children Program, see www.cdc.gov/nip/vfc/.

Assessment of immunization status
5. Health care professionals review the immunization and health status of patients at every encounter to determine which vaccines are indicated (see Fig 1.1, p 24).
6. Health care professionals assess for and follow only medically accepted contraindications (see Precautions and Indications, p 45).

Effective communication about vaccine benefits and risks
7. Parents/guardians and patients are educated about the benefits and risks of immunization in a culturally appropriate manner and in easy-to-understand language (see Table 1.2, p 5; Risk Communication, p 6; and Risks and Adverse Events, p 37).

---

* The National Vaccine Advisory Committee. Standards for Child and Adolescent Immunization Practices. *Pediatrics.* In press
† American Academy of Pediatrics, Medical Home Initiatives for Children With Special Needs Project Advisory Committee. The medical home. *Pediatrics.* 2002;110:184–186

Proper storage, administration, and documentation of immunizations

8. Health care professionals follow appropriate procedures for vaccine storage and handling (see Vaccine Handling and Storage, p 10).

9. Up-to-date, written immunization protocols are accessible at all locations where vaccines are administered.

10. People who administer vaccines and staff members who manage or support vaccine administration are knowledgeable and receive ongoing education. Information about training programs is available at www.cdc.gov/nip/ed/.

11. Health care professionals simultaneously administer as many indicated vaccine doses as possible.

12. Immunization records for patients are accurate, complete, and easily accessible (see Record Keeping and Immunization Registries, p 36).

13. Health care professionals report adverse events after immunization promptly and accurately to the Vaccine Adverse Event Reporting System (VAERS) and are aware of a separate program, the National Vaccine Injury Compensation Program (VICP) (see Vaccine Safety and Contraindications, p 37).

14. All personnel who have contact with patients are appropriately immunized (see www.cdc.gov/nip/recs/adult-schedule.htm).

Implementation of strategies to improve immunization coverage

15. Systems are used to remind parents/guardians, patients, and health care professionals when immunizations are due and to recall those who are overdue.

16. Office- or clinic-based patient record reviews and immunization coverage assessments are performed annually.

17. Health care professionals practice community-based approaches.

APPENDIX III.

Guide to Contraindications and Precautions to Immunizations, 2003

This information is based on the recommendations of the Advisory Committee on Immunization Practices (ACIP) and the Committee on Infectious Diseases of the American Academy of Pediatrics (AAP). Sometimes, these recommendations vary from those in the manufacturers' package inserts. For more detailed information, health care professionals should consult the published recommendations of the ACIP, AAP, and the manufacturers' package inserts. These guidelines, originally issued in 1993, have been updated to give current recommendations as of 2003 (based on information available as of February 2003).

Vaccine	Contraindications	Precautions[1]	Not Contraindications (Vaccines May Be Given)
General for all vaccines (DTaP, IPV, MMR, Hib, pneumococcal, hepatitis B, varicella, hepatitis A, influenza)	Anaphylactic reaction to a vaccine contraindicates further doses of that vaccine Anaphylactic reaction to a vaccine constituent contraindicates the use of vaccines containing that substance	Moderate or severe illnesses with or without a fever Latex allergy[2]	Mild to moderate local reaction (soreness, redness, swelling) after a dose of an injectable antigen Low-grade or moderate fever after a previous vaccine dose Mild acute illness with or without low-grade fever Current antimicrobial therapy Convalescent phase of illnesses Prematurity (same dosage and indications as for healthy, full-term infants) Recent exposure to an infectious disease History of penicillin or other nonspecific allergies or fact that relatives have such allergies Pregnancy of mother or household contact Unimmunized household contact Immunodeficient household contact Breastfeeding (nursing infant OR lactating mother)

DTaP indicates diphtheria and tetanus toxoids and acellular pertussis; DTP, diphtheria and tetanus toxoids and pertussis; IPV, inactivated poliovirus; MMR, measles-mumps-rubella; Hib, *Haemophilus influenzae* type b; GBS, Guillain-Barré syndrome; HIV, human immunodeficiency virus; PPD, purified protein derivative (tuberculin).

[1] The events or conditions listed as precautions, although not contraindications, should be reviewed carefully. The benefits and risks of administering a specific vaccine to a person under the circumstances should be considered. If the risks are believed to outweigh the benefits, the immunization should be withheld; if the benefits are believed to outweigh the risks (for example, during an outbreak or foreign travel), the immunization should be given. Whether and when to administer DTaP to children with proven or suspected underlying neurologic disorders should be decided on an individual basis.

[2] If a person reports a severe (anaphylactic) allergy to latex, vaccines supplied in vials or syringes that contain natural rubber should not be administered unless the benefits of immunization outweigh the risks of an allergic reaction to the vaccine. For latex allergies other than anaphylactic allergies (eg, a history of contact allergy to latex gloves), vaccines supplied in vials or syringes that contain dry natural rubber or latex can be administered.

Guide to Contraindications and Precautions to Immunizations, 2003, continued

Vaccine	Contraindications	Precautions[1]	Not Contraindications (Vaccines May Be Given)
DTaP	Encephalopathy within 7 days of administration of previous dose of DTaP/DTP	Temperature of 40.5°C (104.8°F) within 48 h after immunization with a previous dose of DTaP/DTP Collapse or shock-like state hypotonic-(hyporesponsive episode) within 48 h of receiving a previous dose of DTaP/DTP Seizures within 3 days of receiving a previous dose of DTaP/DTP[3] Persistent inconsolable crying lasting 3 h, within 48 h of receiving a previous dose of DTaP/DTP GBS within 6 wk after a dose[4]	Family history of seizures[3] Family history of sudden infant death syndrome Family history of an adverse event after DTaP/DTP administration
IPV	Anaphylactic reactions to neomycin, streptomycin, or polymyxin B	Pregnancy	...

[3] Acetaminophen given before administering DTaP and thereafter every 4 hours for 24 hours should be considered for children with a personal or family (ie, siblings or parents) history of seizures.

[4] The decision to give additional doses of DTaP should be made on the basis of consideration of the benefit of further immunization versus the risk of recurrence of GBS. For example, completion of the primary series in children is justified.

Guide to Contraindications and Precautions to Immunizations, 2003, continued

Vaccine	Contraindications	Precautions[1]	Not Contraindications (Vaccines May Be Given)
MMR[5,6]	Pregnancy Anaphylactic reaction to neomycin or gelatin Known altered immunodeficiency (hematologic and solid tumors, congenital immunodeficiency, severe HIV infection, and long-term immunosuppressive therapy)	Recent (within 3 to 11 mo, depending on product and dose) Immune Globulin administration[7] (see Table 3.33, p 423) Thrombocytopenia or history of thrombocytopenic purpura[7] Tuberculosis or positive PPD[8]	Simultaneous tuberculin skin testing[9] Breastfeeding Pregnancy of mother of recipient Immunodeficient family member or household contact Infection with HIV Nonanaphylactic reactions to gelatin or neomycin

5 A theoretic risk exists that the administration of multiple live-virus vaccines within 30 days (4 weeks) of one another if not given on the same day will result in suboptimal immune response. No data substantiate this risk, however.

6 An anaphylactic reaction to egg ingestion previously was considered a contraindication unless skin testing and, if indicated, desensitization had been performed. However, skin testing no longer is recommended as of 1997.

7 The decision to immunize should be made on the basis of consideration of the benefits of immunity to measles, mumps, and rubella versus the risk of recurrence or exacerbation of thrombocytopenia after immunization or from natural infections of measles or rubella. In most instances, the benefits of immunization will be much greater than the potential risks and justify giving MMR, particularly in view of the even greater risk of thrombocytopenia after measles or rubella disease. However, if a previous episode of thrombocytopenia occurred in temporal proximity to immunization, not giving a subsequent dose may be prudent.

8 A theoretic basis exists for concern that measles vaccine might exacerbate tuberculosis. Consequently, before administering MMR to people with untreated active tuberculosis, initiating antituberculosis therapy is advisable.

9 Measles immunization may suppress tuberculin reactivity temporarily. MMR vaccine may be given after, or on the same day as, tuberculin testing. If MMR has been given recently, postpone the tuberculin skin test until 4 to 6 weeks after administration of MMR.

Guide to Contraindications and Precautions to Immunizations, 2003, continued

Vaccine	Contraindications	Precautions[1]	Not Contraindications (Vaccines May Be Given)
Hib	None	...	...
Hepatitis B	Anaphylactic reaction to baker's yeast	Prematurity[10]	Pregnancy
Pneumococcal	None	...	...
Varicella[5]	Pregnancy Anaphylactic reaction to neomycin or gelatin Infection with HIV[11] Known altered immunodeficiency (hematologic and solid tumors, congenital immunodeficiency, and long-term immunosuppressive therapy)[12]	Recent Immune Globulin administration (see Table 3.33, p 423) Family history of immunodeficiency[13]	Pregnancy of mother of recipient Immunodeficiency in a household contact Household contact with HIV
Hepatitis A	Anaphylactic reaction to 2-phenoxyethanol or alum	Pregnancy	...
Influenza	Anaphylactic reaction to eggs	GBS within 6 wk after a previous influenza immunization	Pregnancy

[10] For preterm infants weighing less than 2 kg at birth and born to hepatitis B surface antigen (HBsAg)-negative mothers, initiation of immunization should be delayed until just before hospital discharge if the infant weighs 2 kg or more, or until approximately 2 months of age, when other routine immunizations are given, to improve response. All preterm infants born to HBsAg-positive mothers should receive immunoprophylaxis (Hepatitis B Immune Globulin and vaccine) beginning as soon as possible after birth, followed by appropriate postimmunization testing.

[11] Varicella vaccine should be considered for asymptomatic or mildly symptomatic HIV-infected children, specifically children in Centers for Disease Control and Prevention class N1 or A1, with age-specific T-cell percentages of 25% or higher.

[12] Varicella vaccine should not be administered to people who have cellular immunodeficiencies, but people with impaired humoral immunity may be immunized.

[13] Varicella vaccine should not be administered to a person who has a family history of congenital or hereditary immunodeficiency in parents or siblings unless that person's immune competence has been substantiated clinically or verified by a laboratory.

APPENDIX IV.

National Childhood Vaccine Injury Act. Reporting and Compensation Table.

This table includes adverse events that are reportable to the Vaccine Adverse Event Reporting System (VAERS) (see Vaccine Safety and Contraindications, p 37) as well as vaccines covered by the National Vaccine Injury Compensation Program. The intervals from immunization to the onset of an event for reporting to VAERS and for possible compensation by the Vaccine Injury Compensation Program are provided.

National Childhood Vaccine Injury Act Reporting and Compensation Table[1]

Vaccine	Adverse Event	Interval from Vaccination to Onset of Event	
		For Reporting[2]	For Compensation[3]
I. Tetanus toxoid-containing vaccines (eg, DTaP, DTP; DTP-Hib; DT; Td, or TT)	A. Anaphylaxis or anaphylactic shock	0–7 days	0–4 h
	B. Brachial neuritis	0–28 days	2–28 days
	C. Any acute complication or sequela (including death) of above events	Not applicable	Not applicable
	D. Events described in manufacturer's package insert as contraindications to additional doses of vaccine	See package insert	Not applicable
II. Pertussis antigen-containing vaccines (eg, DTaP, DTP, P, DTP-Hib)	A. Anaphylaxis or anaphylactic shock	0–7 days	0–4 h
	B. Encephalopathy (or encephalitis)	0–7 days	0–72 h
	C. Any acute complication or sequela (including death) of above events	Not applicable	Not applicable
	D. Events described in manufacturer's package insert as contraindications to additional doses of vaccine	See package insert	Not applicable
III. Measles, mumps, and rubella virus-containing vaccines in any combination (eg, MMR, MR, M, R)	A. Anaphylaxis or anaphylactic shock	0–7 days	0–4 h
	B. Encephalopathy (or encephalitis)	0–15 days	5–15 days
	C. Any acute complication or sequela (including death) of above events	Not applicable	Not applicable
	D. Events described in manufacturer's package insert as contraindications to additional doses of vaccine	See package insert	Not applicable
IV. Rubella virus-containing vaccines (eg, MMR, MR, R)	A. Chronic arthritis	0–42 days	7–42 days
	B. Any acute complication or sequela (including death) of above event	Not applicable	Not applicable
	C. Events described in manufacturer's package insert as contraindications to additional doses of vaccine	See package insert	Not applicable
V. Measles virus-containing vaccines (eg, MMR, MR, M)	A. Thrombocytopenic purpura	0–30 days	7–30 days
	B. Vaccine-strain measles viral infection in an immunodeficient recipient	0–6 mo	0–6 mo
	C. Any acute complication or sequela (including death) of above events	Not applicable	Not applicable
	D. Events described in manufacturer's package insert as contraindications to additional doses of vaccine	See package insert	Not applicable

National Childhood Vaccine Injury Act Reporting and Compensation Table,[1] continued

Vaccine	Adverse Event	Interval from Vaccination to Onset of Event	
		For Reporting[2]	For Compensation[3]
VI. Live poliovirus-containing vaccines (OPV)	A. Paralytic polio		
	• in a nonimmunodeficient recipient	0–30 days	0–30 days
	• in an immunodeficient recipient	0–6 mo	0–6 mo
	• in a vaccine-associated community case	No limit	Not applicable
	B. Vaccine-strain polio viral infection		
	• in a nonimmunodeficient recipient	0–30 days	0–30 days
	• in an immunodeficient recipient	0–6 mo	0–6 mo
	• in a vaccine-associated community case	No limit	Not applicable
	C. Any acute complication or sequela (including death) of above events	Not applicable	Not applicable
	D. Events described in manufacturer's package insert as contraindications to additional doses of vaccine	See package insert	Not applicable
VII. Inactivated poliovirus-containing vaccines (eg, IPV)	A. Anaphylaxis or anaphylactic shock	0–7 days	0–4 h
	B. Any acute complication or sequela (including death) of above event	Not applicable	Not applicable
	C. Events described in manufacturer's package insert as contraindications to additional doses of vaccine	See package insert	Not applicable
VIII. Hepatitis B antigen–containing vaccines	A. Anaphylaxis or anaphylactic shock	0–7 days	0–4 h
	B. Any acute complication or sequela (including death) of above event	Not applicable	Not applicable
	C. Events described in manufacturer's package insert as contraindications to additional doses of vaccine	See package insert	Not applicable
IX. *Haemophilus influenzae* type b (polysaccharide conjugate vaccines)	A. No condition specified for compensation	Not applicable	Not applicable
	B. Events described in manufacturer's package insert as contraindications to additional doses of vaccine	See package insert	Not applicable
X. Varicella vaccine	A. No condition specified for compensation	Not applicable	Not applicable
	B. Events described in manufacturer's package insert as contraindications to additional doses of vaccine	See package insert	Not applicable

National Childhood Vaccine Injury Act Reporting and Compensation Table, [1] continued

Vaccine	Adverse Event	Interval from Vaccination to Onset of Event	
		For Reporting[2]	For Compensation[3]
XI. Rotavirus vaccine	A. No condition specified for compensation	Not applicable	Not applicable
	B. Events described in manufacturer's package insert as contraindications to additional doses of vaccine	See package insert	Not applicable
XII. Vaccines containing live, oral, rhesus-based rotavirus	A. Intussusception	0–30 days	0–30 days
	B. Events described in manufacturer's package insert as contraindications to additional doses of vaccine	See package insert	Not applicable
XII. Pneumococcal conjugate vaccines	A. No condition specified for compensation	Not applicable	Not applicable
	B. Events described in manufacturer's package insert as contraindications to additional doses of vaccine Not applicable	See package insert	Not applicable
XIV. Any new vaccine recommended by the Centers for Disease Control and Prevention for routine administration to children, after publication by Secretary, HHS of a notice of coverage	A. No condition specified for compensation	Not applicable	Not applicable
	B. Events described in manufacturer's package insert as contraindications to additional doses of vaccine	Not applicable	Not applicable

DTaP, diphtheria and tetanus toxoids and acellular pertussis; DTP, diphtheria and tetanus toxoids and pertussis; Hib, *Haemophilus influenzae* type b; DT, diphtheria and tetanus toxoids; Td, adult-type diphtheria and tetanus toxoids; TT, tetanus toxoid vaccine; OPV, oral poliovirus; PRP, polyribosylribitol phosphate polysaccharide; HHS, US Department of Health and Human Services.

[1] Effective date: August 26, 2002.

2 Taken from the Reportable Events Table (RET), which lists conditions reportable by law (42 USC §300aa-25) to the Vaccine Adverse Event Reporting System (VAERS), including conditions found in the manufacturer's package insert. In addition, physicians are encouraged to report any clinically significant or unexpected events (even if you are not certain the vaccine caused the event) for any vaccine, whether or not it is listed on the RET. Manufacturers also are required by regulation (21 CFR §600.80) to report to the VAERS program all adverse events made known to them for any vaccine. VAERS reporting forms and information can be obtained by calling 1-800-822-7967 or from the Web site (www.vaers.org).

3 Taken from the Vaccine Injury Table (VIT) used in adjudication of claims filed with the National Vaccine Injury Compensation Program (VICP). Claims also may be filed for a condition with onset outside the designated time intervals or a condition not included in the VIT. The Qualifications and Aids to Interpretation below define conditions or injuries listed on the VIT. Information on filing a claim can be obtained by calling 1-800-338-2382 or through the VICP Web site (www.hrsa.gov/osp/vicp).

Qualifications and Aids to Interpretation

(1) *Anaphylaxis and anaphylactic shock* mean an acute, severe, and potentially lethal systemic allergic reaction. Most cases resolve without sequelae. Signs and symptoms begin minutes to a few hours after exposure. Death, if it occurs, usually results from airway obstruction caused by laryngeal edema or bronchospasm and may be associated with cardiovascular collapse. Other significant clinical signs and symptoms include the following: cyanosis, hypotension, bradycardia, tachycardia, arrhythmia, edema of the pharynx and/or trachea and/or larynx with stridor, and dyspnea. Autopsy findings may include acute emphysema, which results from lower respiratory tract obstruction; edema of the hypopharynx, epiglottis, larynx, or trachea; and minimal findings of eosinophilia in the liver, spleen, and lungs. When death occurs within minutes of exposure and without signs of respiratory distress, there may not be significant pathologic findings.

(2) *Encephalopathy.* For purposes of the VIT, a vaccine recipient shall be considered to have suffered an encephalopathy only if such recipient manifests, within the applicable period, an injury meeting the following description of an acute encephalopathy, and then a chronic encephalopathy persists in such person for more than 6 months beyond the date of immunization.

    (i) An *acute encephalopathy* is one that is sufficiently severe so as to require hospitalization (whether or not hospitalization occurred).

        (A) *For children younger than 18 months of age* who present without an associated seizure event, an acute encephalopathy is indicated by a "significantly decreased level of consciousness" (see "D" below) lasting for at least 24 hours. Children younger than 18 months of age who present after a seizure shall be viewed as having an acute encephalopathy if their significantly decreased level of consciousness persists beyond 24 hours and cannot be attributed to a postictal state (seizure) or medication.

        (B) *For adults and children 18 months of age or older,* an acute encephalopathy is one that persists for at least 24 hours and is characterized by at least 2 of the following:

            (1) A significant change in mental status that is not medication-related, specifically a confusional state, a delirium, or a psychosis;

            (2) A significantly decreased level of consciousness, which is independent of a seizure and cannot be attributed to the effects of medication; and

            (3) A seizure associated with loss of consciousness.

        (C) Increased intracranial pressure may be a clinical feature of acute encephalopathy in any age group.

(D) A "significantly decreased level of consciousness" is indicated by the presence of at least one of the following clinical signs for at least 24 hours or greater (see paragraphs (2)(i)(A) and (2)(i)(B) of this section for applicable time frames):

(1) Decreased or absent response to environment (responds, if at all, only to loud voice or painful stimuli);

(2) Decreased or absent eye contact (does not fix gaze on family members or other persons); or

(3) Inconsistent or absent responses to external stimuli (does not recognize familiar people or things).

(E) The following clinical features alone or in combination do not demonstrate an acute encephalopathy or a significant change in either mental status or level of consciousness as described above: sleepiness, irritability (fussiness), high-pitched and unusual screaming, persistent inconsolable crying, and bulging fontanelle. Seizures in themselves are not sufficient to constitute a diagnosis of encephalopathy. In the absence of other evidence of an acute encephalopathy, seizures shall not be viewed as the first symptom or manifestation of the onset of an acute encephalopathy.

(ii) *Chronic encephalopathy* occurs when a change in mental or neurologic status, first manifested during the applicable time period, persists for a period of at least 6 months from the date of immunization. People who return to a normal neurologic state after the acute encephalopathy shall not be presumed to have suffered residual neurologic damage from that event; any subsequent chronic encephalopathy shall not be presumed to be a sequela of the acute encephalopathy. If a preponderance of the evidence indicates that a child's chronic encephalopathy is secondary to genetic, prenatal, or perinatal factors, that chronic encephalopathy shall not be considered to be a condition set forth in the VIT.

(iii) An encephalopathy shall not be considered to be a condition set forth in the VIT if, in a proceeding on a petition, it is shown by a preponderance of the evidence that the encephalopathy was caused by an infection, a toxin, a metabolic disturbance, a structural lesion, a genetic disorder, or trauma (without regard to whether the cause of the infection, toxin, trauma, metabolic disturbance, structural lesion, or genetic disorder is known). If at the time a decision is made on a petition filed under section 2111(b) of the Act for a vaccine-related injury or death it is not possible to determine the cause by a preponderance of the evidence of an encephalopathy, the encephalopathy shall be considered to be a condition set forth in the VIT.

(iv) In determining whether or not an encephalopathy is a condition set forth in the VIT, the Court shall consider the entire medical record.

(3) *Seizure and convulsion.* For purposes of paragraphs (2) and (3) of this section, the terms, "seizure" and "convulsion" include myoclonic, generalized tonic-clonic (grand mal), and simple and complex partial seizures. Absence (petit mal) seizures shall not be considered to be a condition set forth in the VIT. Jerking movements or staring episodes alone are not necessarily an indication of seizure activity.

(4) *Sequela.* The term sequela means a condition or event that actually was caused by a condition listed in the VIT.

(5) *Chronic arthritis.* For purposes of the VIT, chronic arthritis may be found in a person with no history in the 3 years before immunization of arthropathy (joint disease) on the basis of:

(A) Medical documentation, recorded within 30 days after the onset, of objective signs of acute arthritis (joint swelling) that occurred between 7 and 42 days after a rubella immunization;

(B) Medical documentation (recorded within 3 years after the onset of acute arthritis) of the persistence of objective signs of intermittent or continuous arthritis for more than 6 months after immunization;

(C) Medical documentation of an antibody response to the rubella virus

For purposes of the VIT, the following shall not be considered as chronic arthritis: musculoskeletal disorders such as diffuse connective tissue diseases (including but not limited to rheumatoid arthritis, juvenile rheumatoid arthritis, systemic lupus erythematosus, systemic sclerosis, mixed connective tissue disease, polymyositis/dermatomyositis, fibromyalgia, necrotizing vasculitis and vasculopathies, and Sjögren syndrome), degenerative joint disease, infectious agents other than rubella (whether by direct invasion or as an immune reaction), metabolic and endocrine diseases, trauma, neoplasms, neuropathic disorders, bone and cartilage disorders, and arthritis associated with ankylosing spondylitis, psoriasis, inflammatory bowel disease, Reiter syndrome, or blood disorders. Arthralgia (joint pain) or stiffness without joint swelling shall not be viewed as chronic arthritis for purposes of the VIT.

(6) *Brachial neuritis* is defined as dysfunction limited to the upper extremity nerve plexus (ie, its trunks, divisions, or cords) without involvement of other peripheral (eg, nerve roots or a single peripheral nerve) or central (eg, spinal cord) nervous system structures. A deep, steady, often severe aching pain in the shoulder and upper arm usually heralds onset of the condition. The pain is followed in days or weeks by weakness and atrophy in upper extremity muscle groups. Sensory loss may accompany the motor deficits but is generally a less notable clinical feature. The neuritis, or plexopathy, may be present on the same side as or the opposite side of the injection; it is sometimes bilateral, affecting both upper extremities. Weakness is required before the diagnosis can be made. Motor, sensory, and reflex findings on physical examination and the results of nerve conduction and electromyographic studies must be consistent in confirming that dysfunction is attributable to the brachial plexus. The condition should thereby be distinguishable from conditions that may give rise to dysfunction of nerve roots (ie, radiculopathies) and peripheral nerves (ie, including multiple mononeuropathies) as well as other peripheral and central nervous system structures (eg, cranial neuropathies and myelopathies).

(7) *Thrombocytopenic purpura* is defined by a serum platelet count less than 50 000/mm³. Thrombocytopenic purpura does not include cases of thrombocytopenia associated with other causes such as hypersplenism, autoimmune disorders (including alloantibodies from previous transfusions), myelodysplasias, lymphoproliferative disorders, congenital thrombocytopenia, or hemolytic-uremic syndrome. This does not include cases of immune (formerly called idiopathic) thrombocytopenic purpura (ITP) that are mediated, for example, by viral or fungal infections, toxins, or drugs. Thrombocytopenic purpura does not include cases of thrombocytopenia associated with disseminated intravascular coagulation, as observed with bacterial and viral infections. Viral infections include, for example, those infections secondary to Epstein-Barr virus, cytomegalovirus, hepatitis A and hepatitis B, rhinovirus, human immunodeficiency virus (HIV), adenovirus, and dengue virus. An antecedent viral infection may be demonstrated by clinical signs and symptoms and need not be confirmed by culture or serologic testing. Bone marrow examination, if performed, must reveal a normal or an increased number of megakaryocytes in an otherwise normal marrow.

(8) *Vaccine-strain measles viral infection* is defined as a disease caused by poliovirus that is isolated from the affected tissue and should be determined to be the vaccine strain by oligonucleotide or polymerase chain reaction tests.

(9) *Vaccine-strain polio viral infection* is defined as a disease caused by poliovirus that is isolated from the affected tissue and should be determined to be the vaccine strain by oligonucleotide or polymerase chain reaction. Isolation of poliovirus from the stool is not sufficient to establish a tissue-specific infection or disease caused by vaccine-strain poliovirus.

······················

APPENDIX V.

State Immunization Requirements for School Attendance

The United States relies on child care and elementary and secondary school entry immunization requirements to achieve and sustain high levels of immunization coverage. This strategy has proven successful not only in dramatically decreasing communicable disease in settings where children gather and transmit infection but also in decreasing the opportunity for transmission of vaccine-preventable diseases to the unimmunized, the underimmunized, and the immunologically frail. All states require immunization of children at the time of entry into school, and most states require immunization for entry into licensed child care. In addition, many states require immunization of older children in upper grades as well as those entering college. The most up-to-date information about which vaccines are required in a specific state can be obtained from the immunization program manager of each state health department, from a number of local health departments, and from www.immunize.org/laws/.

The Centers for Disease Control and Prevention collects and publishes state-specific data on current school entry laws, child care and Head Start immunization regulations, and college immunization requirements. This survey of school laws usually is published annually. Copies of the latest state immunization requirements survey may be obtained by sending a request to the Centers for Disease Control and Prevention, National Immunization Program, 1600 Clifton Rd, Mailstop E-52, Atlanta, GA 30333, by calling 1-800-311-3435, or by using the online publications order form (https://www2.cdc.gov/nchstp_od/PIWeb/niporderform.asp). The National Immunization Program's home page is www.cdc.gov/nip/.

APPENDIX VI.

Clinical Syndromes Associated With Foodborne Diseases*

Foodborne disease is a major cause of morbidity and mortality in children and adults in developed countries. The epidemiology of foodborne disease is complex and changing because of the number of organisms associated with illness, changes in food production and distribution, rapid international distribution of food, changes in dietary habits, potential for extraintestinal manifestations of disease, and the susceptibility of certain immunocompromised people to infection and severe disease.

The diagnosis of foodborne disease should be considered when 2 or more people who have ingested the same food develop an acute illness characterized by nausea, vomiting, diarrhea, neurologic symptoms, or other extraintestinal manifestations. The diagnosis of the specific causative agent is suggested by the clinical syndrome, incubation period, and epidemiologic clues. To aid in the diagnosis, syndromes of foodborne diseases are categorized by incubation period, causative agent, and foods commonly associated with specific causes. The foods listed in the Table (p 811) are representative and not inclusive. The diagnosis can be confirmed by laboratory testing of stool, emesis, and/or blood, depending on the causative agent. If an outbreak is suspected, local or state public health officials should be notified immediately so they can work with local health care professionals, corroborate other reports, and arrange for special laboratory testing not available at the clinical laboratory.

---

* Centers for Disease Control and Prevention. Diagnosis and management of foodborne illnesses: a primer for physicians. *MMWR Recomm Rep.* 2001;50(RR-2):1-69. Additional information can be found at www.cdc.gov/foodsafety/ and www.nal.usda.gov/foodborne/.

Table. **Clinical Syndromes Associated With Foodborne Diseases**

Clinical Syndrome	Incubation Period	Causative Agents	Commonly Associated Vehicles
Nausea and vomiting	<1–6 h	*Staphylococcus aureus* (preformed toxins, A, B, C, D, E)	Ham, poultry, cream-filled pastries, potato and egg salads, mushrooms
		Bacillus cereus (emetic toxin)	Fried rice, meats
		Heavy metals (copper, tin, cadmium, iron, zinc)	Acidic beverages, metallic container
Flushing, dizziness, burning of mouth and throat, headache, gastrointestinal symptoms, urticaria	<1 h	Histamine (scombroid)	Fish (bluefish, bonito, mackerel, mahi-mahi, marlin, tuna)
Neurologic, including paresthesias and gastrointestinal symptoms	<1–6 h	Tetrodotoxin	Puffer fish
		Ciguatoxin	Fish (amberjack, barracuda, grouper, snapper)
		Paralytic shellfish poisoning	Shellfish (clams, mussels, oysters, scallops, other mollusks)
		Neurotoxic shellfish poisoning	Shellfish
		Domoic acid	Mussels
		Monosodium glutamate	Chinese food
Neurologic, including confusion, salivation, hallucinations, and gastrointestinal tract manifestations	0–2 h	Mushroom toxins (early onset)	Mushrooms
Moderate-to-severe abdominal cramps and watery diarrhea, vomiting	6–24 h	*B cereus* enterotoxin	Meats, stews, gravies, vanilla sauce
	16–72 h	*Clostridium perfringens* enterotoxin	Meats, poultry, gravy, dried or precooked foods
		Caliciviruses, including Norwalk	Shellfish, salads, ice, cookies, water, sandwiches, fruit
	1–3 days	Rotavirus	Fecally contaminated foods (salads, fruits)

Table. Clinical Syndromes Associated With Foodborne Diseases, continued

Clinical Syndrome	Incubation Period	Causative Agents	Commonly Associated Vehicles
Moderate-to-severe abdominal cramps and watery diarrhea, vomiting, continued	1–4 days	Enterotoxigenic *Escherichia coli*	Fruits, vegetables, water
	1–5 days	*Vibrio cholerae* O1 and O139	Shellfish (including crabs and shrimp), fish, water
		V cholerae non-O1	Shellfish
	1–14 days	*Cyclospora* species	Raspberries, vegetables, water
	2–14 days	*Cryptosporidium* species	Vegetables, fruits, milk, water
	1–4 wk	*Giardia lamblia*	Water, food sources
Diarrhea, fever, abdominal cramps, blood and mucus in stools	16–≥72 h	*Salmonella* species	Poultry; pork; beef; eggs; dairy products, including ice cream; vegetables; fruit; orange juice; alfalfa sprouts
		Shigella	Egg salad, vegetables, scallions
		Campylobacter jejuni	Poultry, raw milk, water
		Enteroinvasive *E coli*	Vegetables
		Yersinia enterocolitica	Pork chitterlings, tofu, raw milk
		Vibrio parahaemolyticus	Fish, shellfish
Bloody diarrhea, abdominal cramps	72–120 h	Enterohemorrhagic *E coli*	Beef (hamburger; raw milk; roast beef; salami; salad dressings; lettuce; unpasteurized juices, including apple cider; alfalfa and radish sprouts; water
Hepatorenal failure	6–24 h	Mushrooms (late onset)	Mushrooms (especially *Amanita* species)
Gastrointestinal tract manifestations, then blurred vision, dry mouth, dysarthria, diplopia, descending paralysis	12–48 h	*Clostridium botulinum*	Home-canned vegetables, fruits and fish, salted fish, meats, bottled garlic, potatoes baked in aluminum foil, cheese sauce, honey

Table. **Clinical Syndromes Associated With Foodborne Diseases, continued**

Clinical Syndrome	Incubation Period	Causative Agents	Commonly Associated Vehicles
Chronic, urgent diarrhea	Varied	Brainerd diarrhea	Unpasteurized milk, water
Extraintestinal manifestations	Varied	*Brucella* species	Goat cheese, queso fresco, raw milk, meats
		Group A streptococcus	Egg and potato salads
		Hepatitis A virus	Shellfish, raw produce (ie, strawberries, lettuce)
		Listeria monocytogenes	Cheese, raw milk, hot dogs, cole slaw, ready-to-eat delicatessen meats
		Trichinella spiralis	Pork, wild game, meat
		Vibrio vulnificus	Shellfish (especially oysters)
		Toxoplasma gondii	Beef, pork, lamb, venison

APPENDIX VII.

Prevention of Disease From Potentially Contaminated Food Products*

Foodborne diseases are associated with significant morbidity and mortality in people of all ages. The Centers for Disease Control and Prevention (CDC) estimates that there are more than 76 million cases of foodborne diseases in the United States each year, resulting in approximately 325 000 hospitalizations and 5000 deaths. Young children, the elderly, and especially immunocompromised people particularly are susceptible to illness and complications caused by many of the organisms associated with foodborne illness. The following preventive measures can be implemented to decrease the risk of infection and disease from potentially contaminated food.

Unpasteurized milk and cheese. The American Academy of Pediatrics (AAP) strongly endorses the use of pasteurized milk and recommends that parents and public health officials be fully informed of the important risks associated with consumption of unpasteurized milk. Interstate sale of raw milk is banned by the US Food and Drug Administration (FDA). Children should not consume unpasteurized milk or milk products, such as cheese and butter. Serious systemic infections attributable to *Salmonella* species, *Campylobacter* species, *Mycobacterium bovis,* and *Escherichia coli* O157:H7 have been attributed to consumption of unpasteurized milk, including certified raw milk. In particular, an increasing number of outbreaks of campylobacteriosis among children are associated with school field trips to farms and consumption of raw milk. Raw milk consumption should be prohibited during educational trips. Unpasteurized cheese has been associated with illness attributable to *Brucella* species and *Listeria monocytogenes.*

Eggs. Children should not eat raw or undercooked eggs, unpasteurized powdered eggs, or products containing raw eggs. The major vehicles of transmission of *Salmonella* species are foods of animal origin, including eggs. Ingestion of raw or improperly cooked eggs can produce severe salmonellosis. Examples of foods that may contain undercooked eggs include some homemade frostings and mayonnaise, ice cream from uncooked custard, eggs prepared "sunny-side up," fresh Caesar salad dressing, Hollandaise sauce, and cookie and cake batter.

Raw and undercooked meat. Children should not eat raw or undercooked meat or meat products, particularly hamburger. Various raw or undercooked meat products have been associated with disease, such as poultry with *Salmonella* or *Campylobacter* infection; ground beef with *E coli* O157:H7, enterohemorrhagic *E coli,* or *Salmonella* infection; hot dogs with *Listeria* infection; pork with trichinosis; and wild game with brucellosis, tularemia, or trichinosis. Knives, cutting boards, plates, and other utensils used for raw meats should not be used for preparation of fresh fruits or vegetables until the utensils have been cleaned properly.

---

* Centers for Disease Control and Prevention. Diagnosis and management of foodborne illnesses: a primer for physicians. *MMWR Recomm Rep.* 2001;50(RR-2):1–69. Additional information can be found at www.cdc.gov/foodsafety/ and www.nal.usda.gov/foodborne/.

Unpasteurized juices. Children should drink only pasteurized juice products unless the fruit is washed and freshly squeezed (ie, orange juice) immediately before consumption. Consumption of packaged fruit and vegetable juices that have not undergone pasteurization or a comparable treatment has been associated with food-borne illness attributable to *E coli* O157:H7 and *Salmonella* species. To identify a packaged juice that has not undergone pasteurization or a comparable treatment, consumers should look for a warning statement that the product has not been pasteurized and, therefore, may contain harmful bacteria that can cause serious illness in children, elderly people, or people with compromised immune systems.

Seed sprouts. The FDA and the CDC have reaffirmed health advisories that people who are at high risk of severe foodborne disease, including children, people with compromised immune systems, and elderly people, should avoid eating raw seed sprouts until intervention methods are implemented to improve the safety of these products.* Raw seed sprouts have been associated with outbreaks of illness due to *Salmonella* species and *E coli* O157:H7.

Fresh fruits and vegetables and nuts. Many fresh fruits and vegetables have been associated with disease attributable to *Cryptosporidium, Cyclospora,* calici-viruses, *Giardia, E coli* species, and *Shigella* species. All fruits and vegetables should be cleaned before ingestion. Knives, cutting boards, utensils, and plates used for raw meats should not be used for preparation of fresh fruits or vegetables until the utensils have been cleaned properly. Raw shelled nuts have been associated with outbreaks of salmonellosis.

Raw shellfish and fish. Many experts recommend that children should not eat raw fish or shellfish, especially raw oysters. *Vibrio* species contaminating raw shellfish may cause severe disease in people with liver disease. Some experts caution against children ingesting raw fish. Raw shellfish, including mussels, clams, oysters, scallops, and other mollusks, have been associated with many pathogens and toxins (see Appendix VI, p 810), and raw fish has been associated with transmission of parasites.

Honey. Children younger than 1 year of age should not be given honey. Honey has been shown to contain spores of *Clostridium botulinum.* Light and dark corn syrups are manufactured under sanitary conditions. However, the product is neither packaged under aseptic conditions nor terminally sterilized. Because spores of *C botulinum* are found in the environment and potentially can be found in corn syrup, the manufacturer cannot ensure that any product will be free of *C botulinum* spores.

Food Irradiation†. There is no process to eliminate all foodborne diseases; however, most food safety experts believe irradiation of food can be an effective tool in helping control foodborne pathogens. Irradiation involves exposing food briefly to radiant energy (such as gamma rays, x-rays, or high-voltage electrons) and often is referred to as "cold pasteurization." More than 40 countries worldwide have approved the use of irradiation for various types of foods. In addition, every governmental and professional organization that has reviewed the efficacy and safety of

---

* For additional information, contact the FDA Food Information Line at 1-800-FDA-4010 or the US Department of Agriculture at 1-800-535-4555 or 1-202-720-2791 or visit the following Web sites: www.usda.gov/ *and* www.foodsafety.gov/.

† American Academy of Pediatrics, Committee on Environmental Health. Technical report: irradiation of food. *Pediatrics.* 2000;106:1505–1510

food irradiation has endorsed its use. Irradiated meat and some produce items are available to US consumers. The availability of irradiated foods will increase in the near future. Children can significantly decrease their risk of foodborne illness with the routine consumption of irradiated meat, poultry, and produce.

Shiga Toxin-Producing E coli *Infections.* Because of the significant morbidity and mortality associated with shiga toxin-producing *E coli* (STEC) infections, the following points should be emphasized:

- All children infected with STEC should be reported to their state health department with subsequent implementation of public health measures to facilitate prompt recognition of outbreaks.
- Children should not drink unpasteurized milk or juices; eat unpasteurized cheeses or raw sprouts; or eat raw or undercooked eggs, seafood, poultry, or meat.
- Cross-contamination of foods should be avoided. Specifically, uncooked meats should not come in contact with other foods; hands, cutting boards, knives, and other cooking utensils should be washed after contact with uncooked meat.
- Education of parents and health care professionals about benefits of irradiation of meat, fruits, and vegetables to help minimize spread of any enteric pathogen, including STEC, needs to be increased.

APPENDIX VIII.

Diseases Transmitted by Animals

The transmission of diseases of animals to humans is of special interest in the care of children who interact with pets, unwanted rodents and other animals. Important zoonoses that may be encountered in North America are reviewed in the *Red Book* (see disease-specific chapters in Section 3 for further information) and listed in the table (p 818). Primary modes of transmission from animals to humans include direct contact, scratch, bite, inhalation, contact with urine or feces, and ingestion of contaminated food, water, or feces as well as contact with arthropod intermediate hosts. To minimize transmission of enteric disease at petting farms, the following infection control activities should be enforced: handwashing facilities should be readily available and configured for use by children; food-related activities should be separated from areas housing animals; and children should be supervised during contact with animals and during handwashing. Human-to-human transmission may occur for some zoonotic diseases. For a more complete listing of these diseases, standard textbooks in infectious diseases should be consulted.

Morbidity resulting from selected zoonotic diseases in the United States is reported annually by the Centers for Disease Control and Prevention (see "Summary of Notifiable Diseases" available at: www.cdc.gov/epo/dphsi/annsum/). Information also can be obtained at the following Web sites:

- National Center for Infectious Diseases, Bacterial Zoonoses Branch Web site. Available at: www.cdc.gov/ncidod/dvbid/misc/bzb.htm
- Rosenman K. *Zoonoses—Animals Can Make You Sick.* Lansing, MI: Michigan State University; 1992. Available at: www.cdc.gov/nasd/docs/d000701-d000800/d000752/d000752.html

Table. Diseases Transmitted by Animals

Disease and/or Organism	Common Animal Sources	Vector or Modes of Transmission
Bacterial Diseases		
Aeromonas species	Aquatic animals	Wound infection, ingestion of contaminated food
Bartonella henselae (cat-scratch disease)	Cats, infrequently other animals (<10%)	Scratches, bites, fleas, important in cat-to-cat transmission
Brucellosis (*Brucella* species)	Cattle, goats, sheep, swine, rarely dogs	Direct contact with birth products, ingestion of contaminated milk, inhalation of aerosols
Campylobacteriosis (*Campylobacter jejuni*)	Poultry, dogs (especially puppies), cats, ferrets, hamsters	Ingestion of contaminated food, direct contact (particularly with animals with diarrhea), person-to-person (fecal oral)
Capnocytophaga canimorsus	Dogs, rarely cats	Bites, contact
Erysipelothrix rhusiopathiae	Farm animals, fish, shellfish	Direct contact with animal or contaminated animal product
Hemolytic-uremic syndrome (enterohemorrhagic *Escherichia coli*)	Cattle	Ingestion of undercooked contaminated ground beef, or other contaminated foods or water, person-to-person (fecal oral), tick bite
Leptospirosis (*Leptospira* species)	Dogs, rats, livestock	Contact with urine, particularly in contaminated water
Lyme disease (*Borrelia burgdorferi*)	Wild rodents, birds	Tick bite
Mycobacteriosis (*Mycobacterium marinum*, others)	Fish (and cleaning aquaria)	Skin injury or contamination of existing wound
Pasteurella multocida	Cats, infrequently dogs	Bites, scratches, licks
Plague (*Yersinia pestis*)	Rodents, wild rabbits, cats	Bite of rodent fleas, direct contact with infected animals
Rat-bite fever (*Streptobacillus moniliformis, Spirillum minus*)	Rodents (particularly rats)	Bites
Relapsing fever (tickborne) (*Borrelia* species)	Wild rodents	Tick bite
Salmonellosis (*Salmonella* species)	Poultry, reptiles, dogs, cats, rodents, ferrets, turtles, other wild and domestic animals	Ingestion of contaminated food, direct contact, contact with fecally contaminated surfaces, person-to-person

Table. Diseases Transmitted by Animals, continued

Disease and/or Organism	Common Animal Sources	Vector or Modes of Transmission
Streptococcus iniae	Fish grown by aquaculture	Skin injury during handling of fish
Tetanus (*Clostridium tetani*)	Any animal, usually indirect via soil	Wound infection versus skin injury or soft tissue injury with inoculation of bacteria, contaminated bites
Tularemia (*Francisella tularensis*)	Wild rabbits, rodents, muskrats, moles, cats	Tick bites, occasionally deerfly or mosquito bite, direct contact with infected animal, ingestion of contaminated water, mechanical transmission from claws or teeth (cats), aerosolization of tissues or excreta
Vibrio species	Shellfish	Skin injury or contamination of existing wound, ingestion of contaminated food
Yersiniosis (*Yersinia enterocolitica*)	Swine; rarely dogs, cats, rodents	Ingestion of contaminated food or water, rarely direct contact, person-to-person (fecal oral)
Fungal Diseases		
Cryptococcosis (*Cryptococcus neoformans*)	Birds, particularly pigeons	Inhalation of aerosols from accumulations of pigeon feces
Histoplasmosis (*Histoplasma capsulatum*)	Bats, birds, particularly starlings	Inhalation of aerosols from accumulations of bat and bird feces
Ringworm (*Microsporum* and *Trichophyton* species)	Cats, dogs, rabbits, rodents	Direct contact
Sporotrichosis (*Sporothrix schenckii*)	Cats	Direct contact
Parasitic Diseases		
Anisakiasis (*Anisakis* species)	Saltwater and anadromous fish	Ingestion of undercooked or raw fish (eg, sushi)
Babesiosis (*Babesia* species)	Wild rodents	Tick bite
Balantidiasis (*Balantidium coli*)	Swine	Ingestion of contaminated food or water
Dwarf tapeworm (*Hymenolepis nana*)	Hamsters, rodents	Ingestion of eggs from feces (contaminated food, water)

Table. Diseases Transmitted by Animals, continued

Disease and/or Organism	Common Animal Sources	Vector or Modes of Transmission
Parasitic Diseases, continued		
Cryptosporidiosis (*Cryptosporidium* species)	Domestic animals, particularly cattle	Ingestion of contaminated water or foods, person-to-person
Cutaneous larva migrans (*Ancylostoma* species)	Dogs, cats	Penetration of skin by larvae, which develop in soil contaminated with eggs shed in animal feces
Cysticercosis (*Taenia solium*)	Swine (intermediate host)	Ingestion of eggs from fecal-oral contact or contaminated food, water, ingestion of cysts in raw or undercooked meat (adult tapeworm infection)
Dog tapeworm (*Dipylidium caninum*)	Dogs, cats	Ingestion of fleas infected with larvae
Echinococcosis, hydatid disease (*Echinococcus* species)	Dogs, foxes, possibly other carnivores	Ingestion of eggs shed in animal feces
Fish tapeworm (*Diphyllobothrium latum*)	Saltwater and freshwater fish	Ingestion of larvae in raw or undercooked fish
Giardiasis (*Giardia lamblia*)	Wild and domestic animals, including dogs, cats, beavers	Ingestion of cysts from fecal-oral contact or in contaminated food, water, person-to-person
Beef, pork tapeworm, taeniasis (*Taenia saginata* and *Taenia solium*)	Cattle, swine	Ingestion of larvae in undercooked beef or pork
Toxoplasmosis (*Toxoplasma gondii*)	Cats, livestock	Ingestion of oocysts from cat feces, consumption of cysts in undercooked meat, contact with birth products of cats
Trichinosis (*Trichinella spiralis*)	Swine, bears, possibly other wild carnivores	Ingestion of larvae in raw or undercooked meat
Visceral larva migrans (*Toxocara canis* and *Toxocara cati*)	Dogs, cats	Ingestion of eggs, usually from soil contaminated by animal feces
Chlamydial and Rickettsial Diseases		
Ehrlichiosis (*Ehrlichia* species)	Deer, dogs, ruminants, horses	Tick bites
Psittacosis (*Chlamydia psittaci*)	Psittacine and domestic birds, farm animals	Inhalation of aerosols from feces
Q fever (*Coxiella burnetii*)	Sheep, other livestock, wild rodents, rabbits	Direct contact and aerosols from birth products, ingestion of contaminated milk, occasionally tick bite

Table. Diseases Transmitted by Animals, continued

Disease and/or Organism	Common Animal Sources	Vector or Modes of Transmission
Rickettsialpox (Rickettsia akari)	House mouse	Mite bites
Rocky Mountain spotted fever (Rickettsia rickettsii)	Dogs, wild rodents, rabbits	Tick bites; rarely by direct contamination with infectious material from ticks
Typhus, flea-borne endemic typhus (Rickettsia typhi)	Rats, opossums, domestic cats	Flea feces scratched into abrasions
Typhus, louse-borne epidemic typhus (Rickettsia prowazekii)	Flying squirrels	Body louse, contact with squirrels, their nests, or ectoparasites, person-to-person via body louse
Viral Diseases		
Colorado tick fever	Wild rodents, particularly squirrels	Tick bites
Encephalitis		
California	Wild rodents	Mosquito bites
Eastern equine	Wild birds, poultry, horses	Mosquito bites
Western equine	Wild birds, poultry, horses	Mosquito bites
St Louis	Wild birds, poultry	Mosquito bites
Venezuelan equine	Horses	Mosquito bites
Powassan	Rodents, rabbits	Tick bites
West Nile	Birds	Mosquito bites
Hantaviruses	Wild rodents	Inhalation of aerosols of infected secreta and excreta
B virus (formerly herpesvirus simiae)	Macaque monkeys	Bite or exposure to secretions
Lymphocytic choriomeningitis	Rodents, particularly hamsters, mice	Direct contact, inhalation of aerosols, ingestion of contaminated food
Rabies	Bats, cats, ferrets, skunks, foxes, dogs	Bites, contact of open wounds with infected materials (eg, saliva)

....

APPENDIX IX.

Nationally Notifiable Infectious Diseases in the United States

Public health officials at state health departments and the Centers for Disease Control and Prevention (CDC) collaborate in determining which diseases should be nationally notifiable (see Table, p 823). The Council of State and Territorial Epidemiologists, with advice from the CDC, makes recommendations annually for additions and deletions to the list of nationally notifiable diseases. A disease may be added to the list as a new pathogen emerges, or a disease may be deleted as its incidence decreases. However, reporting of nationally notifiable diseases to the CDC by the states is voluntary. Reporting currently is mandated (ie, by state legislation or regulation) only by individual states. The list of diseases that are considered notifiable, therefore, varies slightly by state. Additional and specific requirements should be obtained from the appropriate state health department. All states generally report diseases that are quarantined internationally (ie, cholera, plague, and yellow fever) in compliance with the World Health Organization's International Health Regulations.

When health care professionals suspect or diagnose a case of a disease considered notifiable in the state, they should report the case by telephone or by mail to the local, county, or state health department. Clinical laboratories also report results consistent with reportable diseases. Staff members in the county or state health department implement disease control measures as needed. The written case report is forwarded to the state health department.

The CDC acts as a common agent for the states and territories for collecting information and reporting of nationally notifiable diseases. Reports of the occurrences of nationally notifiable diseases are transmitted to the CDC each week from the 50 states, 2 cities (Washington, DC, and New York, NY), and 5 territories (American Samoa, Commonwealth of Northern Mariana Islands, Guam, Puerto Rico, and the Virgin Islands). Provisional data are published weekly in the *Morbidity and Mortality Weekly Report;* final data are published each year by the CDC in the annual "Summary of Notifiable Diseases, United States." The timelines of the provisional weekly reports provide information that the CDC and state or local epidemiologists use to detect and more effectively interrupt outbreaks. Reporting also provides the timely information needed to measure and demonstrate the effect of changed immunization laws or a new therapeutic modality. The finalized annual data also provide information on reported disease incidence that is necessary for study of epidemiologic trends and development of disease prevention policies. The CDC is the sole repository for these data, which are used widely by schools of medicine and public health, communications media, and pharmaceutical or other companies producing health-related products as well as by local, state, and federal health agencies and other agencies or people concerned with the trends of reportable conditions in the United States.

Table. Infectious Diseases Designated as Notifiable at the National Level—United States, 2002

Acquired immunodeficiency syndrome
Anthrax
Botulism
Brucellosis
Chancroid
Chlamydia trachomatis, genital infections
Cholera
Coccidioidomycosis (regional)
Cryptosporidiosis
Cyclosporiasis
Diphtheria
Ehrlichiosis, human granulocytic
Ehrlichiosis, human monocytic
Encephalitis, California serogroup
Encephalitis, eastern equine
Encephalitis, Powassan
Encephalitis, St Louis
Encephalitis, western equine
Encephalitis, West Nile
Enterohemorrhagic *Escherichia coli* O157:H7
  Shiga toxin positive, serogroup non-0157

Giardiasis
Gonorrhea
Haemophilus influenzae (invasive disease)
Hansen disease (leprosy)
Hantavirus pulmonary syndrome
Hemolytic-uremic syndrome, postdiarrheal
Hepatitis A
Hepatitis B
Hepatitis C/non-A, non-B hepatitis
Human immunodeficiency virus infection
  Adult (≥13 years of age)
  Pediatric (<13 years of age)
Legionellosis
Listeriosis
Lyme disease
Malaria
Measles
Meningococcal disease
Mumps
Pertussis
Plague
Poliomyelitis, paralytic
Psittacosis

Q fever
Rabies, animal
Rabies, human
Rocky Mountain spotted fever
Rubella
Rubella, congenital syndrome
Salmonellosis
Shigellosis
Streptococcal disease, invasive, group A
Streptococcus pneumoniae, drug-resistant invasive disease
Streptococcus pneumoniae, invasive in children <5 years of age
Streptococcal toxic shock syndrome
Syphilis
Syphilis, congenital
Tetanus
Toxic shock syndrome
Trichinosis
Tuberculosis
Tularemia
Typhoid fever
Varicella deaths[1]
Yellow fever

---

[1] Although varicella is not a nationally notifiable disease, the Council of State and Territorial Epidemiologists recommends reporting of cases of this disease to the Centers for Disease Control and Prevention.

....

APPENDIX X.

Services of the Centers for Disease Control and Prevention (CDC)

The Centers for Disease Control and Prevention (CDC), US Public Health Service, Department of Health and Human Services (Atlanta, GA) is the federal agency charged with protecting the public health of the nation by preventing disease and other disabling conditions. The CDC administers national programs for prevention and control of the following: (1) infectious diseases; (2) vaccine-preventable diseases; (3) occupational diseases and injury; (4) chronic diseases; (5) environment-related injury and illness; and (6) birth defects and developmental disabilities. The CDC also provides consultation to other nations and participates with international agencies in the control of preventable diseases. In addition, the CDC directs and enforces foreign quarantine activities and regulations and provides consultation and assistance in upgrading the performance of clinical laboratories.

The CDC provides a number of services related to infectious disease management and control. Although the CDC principally is a resource for state and local health departments, it also offers direct and indirect services to hospitals and practicing health care professionals. The range of services includes reference laboratory diagnosis and epidemiologic consultation, both usually arranged through state health departments.

The CDC Drug Service supplies some specific prophylactic or therapeutic drugs and biologic agents. Specific immunobiologic products available include botulinal equine (trivalent, ABE) antitoxin, Vaccinia Immune Globulin (VIG), botulinus pentavalent toxoid, and vaccinia vaccine. In addition, several drugs for the treatment of parasitic disease, which currently are not licensed for use in the United States, are handled under an investigational new drug permit. These antiparasitic drugs include bithionol, dehydroemetine, diethylcarbamazine citrate, melarsoprol, nifurtimox, sodium stibogluconate, and suramin.

Requests for biologic products, antiparasitic drugs, and related information should be directed to the CDC Drug Service (see Appendix I, Directory of Resources, p 789).

Index

Page numbers followed by "t" indicate a table. Page numbers followed by "f" indicate a figure.

interchangeability of, 32
for internationally adopted children, 178
for low-birth weight infants, 66
NCVIA reporting and compensation table
    for, 803t
for premature infants, 66
scheduling of, 27t
storage of, 11t, 13t
Diphtheria toxoid. *See also* Diphtheria,
    tetanus, acellular pertussis
    (DTaP) vaccine; Diphtheria,
    tetanus, pertussis (DTP) vaccine
for carriers, 264
for exposed people, 265
storage of, 11t
universal immunization with, 265
Diphtheria vaccine. *See also* Diphtheria,
    tetanus, acellular pertussis
    (DTaP) vaccine; Diphtheria,
    tetanus, pertussis (DTP) vaccine
in pregnancy, 68
for school attendance, 138
Diphyllobothrium latum infections, 610–611,
    765t
Dipylidium caninum infections, 610–611, 765t
Dipyridamole, for Kawasaki syndrome, 395
Direct-contact transmission, 140–142, 149
Direct-direct transmission, 149
Direct fluorescent antibody (DFA) test
for *Burkholderia,* 225
for giardiasis, 284
for rickettsialpox, 532
for syphilis, 596
for tularemia, 667
for varicella-zoster virus, 675t
Direct immunofluorescence test
for *Bordetella pertussis,* 473
for *Legionella pneumophila,* 397
Directly observed therapy, for tuberculosis,
    642
Disinfection, for adenoviruses, 191
Disseminated infections, from adenoviruses,
    190
Disseminated intravascular coagulation
from African trypanosomiasis, 639
from bioterrorist agents, 100t
from *Ehrlichia* infections, 267
from meningococcal infections, 430
from plague, 487
from Rocky Mountain spotted fever, 532
from smallpox, 555

Dizziness
from foodborne diseases, 811t
from hantavirus pulmonary syndrome, 301
DNA probes
for adenoviruses, 191
for *Blastomyces dermatitidis,* 219
for *Chlamydia trachomatis,* 240
for *Escherichia coli,* 278
for *Histoplasma capsulatum,* 354
for *Salmonella,* 543
for streptococci group A, 576
for tuberculosis, 644
Dobrava virus, hemorrhagic fevers from,
    307–309
Dog bites, 182–186
chemoprophylaxis for, 182, 183t,
    185t, 186
epidemiology of, 182
Pasteurella multocida infections
    in, 462–463
rabies from, 514–515, 517t
treatment of, 182, 183t–185t, 186
Dogborne diseases
cutaneous larva migrans (dog hookworm),
    257
hydatid disease, 610–611
tapeworm *(Dipylidium caninum),* 610–611,
    765t
toxocariasis, 630–631
Domoic acid poisoning, 811t
Donovanosis (granuloma inguinale), 292–293
clinical manifestations of, 292
control measures for, 293
diagnosis of, 292
epidemiology of, 292
etiology of, 292
hospital isolation for, 293
treatment of, 292–293
Dopamine, for anaphylaxis, 64, 65t
Down syndrome, *Mycoplasma pneumoniae*
    infections in, 443
Doxycycline
for actinomycosis, 190
for anthrax, 102t, 198
for brucellosis, 103t, 223
for *Campylobacter* infections, 228
for cat-scratch disease, 233
for cervicitis, 713t
for *Chlamydia (Chlamydophila) pneumoniae*
    infections, 236
for *Chlamydia trachomatis* infections, 165t,
    166t, 241, 242
for cholera, 687
dosage of, beyond newborn period, 712t

Z